Handbook of Rehabilitation Psychology

THIRD EDITION

Handbook of Rehabilitation Psychology

THIRD EDITION

EDITED BY

Lisa A. Brenner, Stephanie A. Reid-Arndt, Timothy R. Elliott, Robert G. Frank, and Bruce Caplan

American Psychological Association
Washington, DC

Published by
American Psychological Association
750 First Street, NE
Washington, DC 20002
https://www.apa.org

Order Department
https://www.apa.org/pubs/books
order@apa.org

In the U.K., Europe, Africa, and the Middle East, copies may be ordered from Eurospan
https://www.eurospanbookstore.com/apa
info@eurospangroup.com

Typeset in Berkeley by Circle Graphics, Inc., Reisterstown, MD

Printer: Sheridan Books, Chelsea, MI
Cover Designer: Anne C. Kerns, Anne Likes Red, Inc., Silver Spring, MD

Library of Congress Cataloging-in-Publication Data

Names: Brenner, Lisa A., editor.
Title: Handbook of rehabilitation psychology / edited by Lisa A. Brenner, Stephanie A. Reid-Arndt, Timothy R. Elliott, Robert G. Frank, and Bruce Caplan.
Description: Third edition. | Washington, DC : American Psychological Association, [2019] | Includes bibliographical references and index.
Identifiers: LCCN 2018049833 (print) | LCCN 2018050435 (ebook) | ISBN 9781433829840 (eBook) | ISBN 1433829843 (eBook) | ISBN 9781433829857 (hardcover) | ISBN 1433829851 (hardcover)
Subjects: LCSH: Clinical health psychology—Handbooks, manuals, etc. | Medical rehabilitation—Psychological aspects—Handbooks, manuals, etc.
Classification: LCC R726.7 (ebook) | LCC R726.7 .H366 2019 (print) | DDC 616.001/9—dc23
LC record available at https://lccn.loc.gov/2018049833

http://dx.doi.org/10.1037/0000129-000

Printed in the United States of America

10 9 8 7 6 5 4 3 2 1

Contents

Contributors

Kevin N. Alschuler, PhD, Departments of Rehabilitation Medicine and Neurology, University of Washington, Seattle

Erin E. Andrews, PsyD, Central Texas Veterans Health Care System, Dell Medical School, University of Texas, Austin

Nazanin H. Bahraini, PhD, VHA Rocky Mountain Mental Illness Research Education Clinical Center, Rocky Mountain Regional VA Medical Center, Aurora, CO, and Departments of Psychiatry and Physical Medicine and Rehabilitation, University of Colorado Anschutz Medical Campus, Aurora

Kathleen T. Bechtold, PhD, Department of Physical Medicine and Rehabilitation, Johns Hopkins University, Baltimore, MD

Jacob Bentley, PhD, Department of Physical Medicine and Rehabilitation, Johns Hopkins University, Baltimore, MD, and Department of Clinical Psychology, Seattle Pacific University, Seattle, WA

Kimberly E. Bodner, PhD, Thompson Center for Autism and Neurodevelopmental Disorders, Department of Health Psychology, University of Missouri, Columbia

Charles H. Bombardier, PhD, ABPP, Clinical and Neuropsychology Departments and Department of Rehabilitation Medicine, University of Washington, Seattle

Lisa A. Brenner, PhD, ABPP, Departments of Physical Medicine and Rehabilitation, Psychiatry, and Neurology, University of Colorado Anschutz Medical Campus, Aurora, and VHA Rocky Mountain Mental Illness Research Education Clinical Center, Rocky Mountain Regional VA Medical Center, Aurora, CO

Kathleen S. Brown, PhD, independent consultant, Fort Myers, FL

Letitia Burridge, PhD, The Hopkins Centre, Division of Rehabilitation, Metro South Health & Menzies Health Institute Queensland, Griffith University, Queensland, Australia

Shane S. Bush, PhD, ABPP, Long Island Neuropsychology PC, Lake Ronkonkoma, NY, and Department of Psychology, University of Alabama, Tuscaloosa

Bruce Caplan, PhD, ABPP (CN, RP), independent practice, Wynnewood, PA

Michele Catena, PT, DPT, College of Public Health and Human Sciences, Oregon State University, Corvallis

Nancy D. Chiaravalloti, PhD, Neuropsychology & Neuroscience Research, and Traumatic Brain Injury Research, Kessler Foundation, East Hanover, NJ, and Department of Physical Medicine and Rehabilitation, Rutgers—New Jersey Medical School, Newark

Laura Coffey, PhD, Department of Psychology, Maynooth University, Maynooth, Ireland, and Dublin Psychoprosthetics Group, Dublin, Ireland

John D. Corrigan, PhD, Department of Physical Medicine and Rehabilitation, Ohio State University, Columbus

Molly K. Cox, MS, Department of Ophthalmology and Visual Sciences, University of Alabama at Birmingham

Patrick H. DeLeon, PhD, Uniformed Services University of the Health Sciences, Daniel K. Inouye Graduate School of Nursing and F. Edward Hebert School of Medicine, Bethesda, MD, and former APA President

Deirdre M. Desmond, PhD, Department of Psychology, Maynooth University, Maynooth, Ireland, and Dublin Psychoprosthetics Group, Dublin, Ireland

Alicia Dixon-Ibarra, PhD, MPH, College of Public Health and Human Sciences, Oregon State University, Corvallis

Laura E. Dreer, PhD, Department of Ophthalmology and Visual Sciences, University of Alabama at Birmingham

Dana S. Dunn, PhD, Department of Psychology, Moravian College, Bethlehem, PA

Rose A. Dunn, PhD, Rehabilitation Institute of Michigan, Wayne State University, Detroit

Dawn M. Ehde, PhD, Department of Rehabilitation Medicine, University of Washington, Seattle

Timothy R. Elliott, PhD, ABPP, Department of Educational Psychology, Texas A&M University, College Station, and Editor-in-Chief, *Journal of Clinical Psychology*

Michele Foster, PhD, The Hopkins Centre, Division of Rehabilitation, Metro South Health & Menzies Health Institute Queensland, Griffith University, Queensland, Australia

Robert G. Frank, PhD, Center for Innovation in Health and Education and Department of Family and Community Medicine, University of New Mexico, Albuquerque

Pamela Gallagher, PhD, School of Nursing and Human Sciences, Dublin City University Glasnevin Campus, Dublin, Ireland, and Dublin Psychoprosthetics Group, Dublin, Ireland

Priscille Geiser, MSc, independent advisor, Lyon, France

Lisa D. Goldberg, PhD, Department of Psychology, Virginia Commonwealth University, Richmond

Michelle M. Haddad, PhD, Department of Rehabilitation Medicine, Emory University, Atlanta, GA

Kristofer J. Hagglund, PhD, ABPP, School of Health Professions, University of Missouri, Columbia

Stephanie L. Hanson, PhD, College of Public Health and Health Professions, University of Florida, Gainesville

Ramzi Hasson, PhD, University Pediatricians Autism Center and Division of Neurology, Wayne State University, Detroit, MI

Philip Jefferies, PhD, Resilience Research Centre, Dalhousie University, Halifax, Nova Scotia, Canada, and Dublin Psychoprosthetics Group, Dublin, Ireland

Kelly Jones, PhD, Division of Neuropsychology, Dell Children's Medical Center, University of Texas, Austin

Stephen M. Kanne, PhD, Thompson Center for Autism and Neurodevelopmental Disorders, Department of Health Psychology, University of Missouri, Columbia

Elizabeth Kendall, PhD, The Hopkins Centre, Division of Rehabilitation, Metro South Health & Menzies Health Institute Queensland, Griffith University, Queensland, Australia

Thomas R. Kerkhoff, PhD, Department of Clinical and Health Psychology, University of Florida, Gainesville

Sebastian T. Koenig, PhD, Katana Simulations Pty Ltd, Adelaide, Australia

Gloria Krahn, PhD, MPH, College of Public Health and Human Sciences, Oregon State University, Corvallis

Anna L. Kratz, PhD, Department of Physical Medicine and Rehabilitation, University of Michigan, Ann Arbor

Denise Krch, PhD, Traumatic Brain Injury Research, Kessler Foundation, East Hanover, NJ, and Department of Physical Medicine and Rehabilitation, Rutgers—New Jersey Medical School, Newark

Pim Kuipers, PhD, The Hopkins Centre, Division of Rehabilitation, Metro South Health & Menzies Health Institute Queensland, Griffith University, Queensland, Australia

Belinda S. Lange, PhD, College of Nursing and Health Sciences, Flinders University, Adelaide, South Australia

Karen G. Langer, PhD, Department of Rehabilitation Medicine, NYU School of Medicine, New York

Richard Lombard-Vance, PhD, School of Nursing and Human Sciences, Dublin City University Glasnevin Campus, Dublin, Ireland, and Dublin Psychoprosthetics Group, Dublin, Ireland

David D. Luxton, PhD, Department of Psychiatry and Behavioral Sciences, University of Washington School of Medicine, Seattle

Malcolm MacLachlan, PhD, Assisted Living & Learning Institute and Department of Psychology, Maynooth University, Maynooth, Ireland

Hasheem Mannan, PhD, School of Nursing Midwifery and Health Systems, University College Dublin, Ireland

Victor W. Mark, MD, Department of Physical Medicine and Rehabilitation, University of Alabama at Birmingham

Hannah R. Martinez, Doctoral Candidate, Department of Medical and Clinical Psychology, Uniformed Services University of the Health Sciences, Bethesda, MD

Suzanne McGarity, PhD, Department of Physical Medicine and Rehabilitation, University of Colorado Anschutz Medical Campus, Aurora, and VHA Rocky Mountain Mental Illness Research Education Clinical Center, Rocky Mountain Regional VA Medical Center, Aurora, CO

Michael D. Mohrland, PsyD, Thompson Center for Autism and Neurodevelopmental Disorders, Department of Health Psychology, University of Missouri, Columbia

Kerri P. Nowell, PhD, Thompson Center for Autism and Neurodevelopmental Disorders, Department of Health Psychology, University of Missouri, Columbia

Jennifer H. Olson-Madden, PhD, VHA Rocky Mountain Mental Illness Research Education Clinical Center, Rocky Mountain Regional VA Medical Center, Aurora, CO, and Departments of Psychiatry and Physical Medicine and Rehabilitation, University of Colorado Anschutz Medical Campus, Aurora

Paul B. Perrin, PhD, Department of Psychology, Virginia Commonwealth University, Richmond

Bradford S. Pierce, Doctoral Candidate, Department of Psychology, Virginia Commonwealth University, Richmond

Joseph F. Rath, PhD, Postdoctoral Fellowship in Rehabilitation Research, Rusk Rehabilitation, New York University Langone Health, New York

Stephanie A. Reid-Arndt, PhD, ABPP, School of Health Professions, University of Missouri, Columbia

Laurel D. Riek, PhD, Department of Computer Science and Engineering, University of California, San Diego

Albert "Skip" Rizzo, PhD, Institute for Creative Technologies, University of Southern California, Playa Vista

Beth K. Rush, PhD, Department of Psychiatry and Psychology, Mayo Clinic, Jacksonville, FL

Beth S. Slomine, PhD, ABPP, Department of Neuropsychology, Kennedy Krieger Institute, Johns Hopkins University School of Medicine, Baltimore, MD

William Stiers, PhD, Department of Physical Medicine and Rehabilitation, Johns Hopkins University School of Medicine, Baltimore, MD

Kirk Stucky, PsyD, Hurley Medical Center, Department of Behavioral Health, Flint, MI

M. Jan Tackett, PhD, VA Puget Sound Healthcare System, Seattle, WA

Aaron P. Turner, PhD, ABPP, Rehabilitation Psychology, VA Puget Sound Health Care System, and Department of Rehabilitation Medicine, University of Washington, Seattle

Philip M. Ullrich, PhD, Department of Rehabilitation Medicine, University of Washington, Seattle

Gitendra Uswatte, PhD, Department of Psychology, University of Alabama at Birmingham

Marie Van Tubbergen, PhD, Department of Physical Medicine and Rehabilitation, University of Michigan, Ann Arbor

Seth Warschausky, PhD, Department of Physical Medicine and Rehabilitation, University of Michigan, Ann Arbor

Ann Marie Warren, PhD, Department of Trauma, Critical Care and Acute Care Surgery, Baylor University Medical Center, Baylor Scott & White, Dallas, TX

Erica Weber, PhD, Traumatic Brain Injury Research, Kessler Foundation, East Hanover, NJ, and Department of Physical Medicine and Rehabilitation, Rutgers—New Jersey Medical School, Newark

Stephen T. Wegener, PhD, Department of Physical Medicine and Rehabilitation, Johns Hopkins University, Baltimore, MD

Shelley Wiechman, PhD, ABPP, Department of Rehabilitation Medicine, University of Washington, Seattle

Haibin Zou, MA, independent consultant, Beijing, China

Preface

Robert G. Frank and Timothy R. Elliott

More than 20 years ago, we (Tim Elliott and Bob Frank) began to work on the first edition of the *Handbook of Rehabilitation Psychology*. For several years, we had chatted about the progress in our field and the need to consolidate knowledge in one comprehensive, contemporary text. We shared a common vision of opportunities for the field, including a need for greater theoretical development, the value of the scientist–practitioner as a metamodel encouraging adaptive thinking as a discipline, and the need for stronger recognition of the changing models of health care on psychologist practice. In 1995, we began to outline current knowledge and areas in which we hoped to inspire future growth. By 1997, we set to work in earnest to bring together leaders in the field to craft a compendium of knowledge defining the discipline and its potential for the future. It took 3 years to realize our vision: The first edition was published in 2000, at the dawn of a new century.

Rehabilitation psychology was in an exciting phase at that point as the discipline struggled to become a specialty and to integrate the momentous changes occurring in the larger health care environment. In our final chapter "Afterword: Drawing New Horizons" (Elliott & Frank, 2000), we considered the promise of the century in light of the status of the field of rehabilitation psychology. This "look forward" to consider issues the discipline needed to address in the near and distant future focused on professional identity, the importance of integrating rehabilitation psychology into the larger changes in health care and science, and the need to move away from "naïve empiricism" that dominated the literature at that point. Our thinking reflected a distinct bias toward the value of the "scientist–practitioner model" as the most critical element of growth for rehabilitation psychology. We recognized the importance of rehabilitation psychologists engaging in national experiments to create alternative health care delivery models focused on cost-effective, integrated care for all aspects of people's lives (physical, psychological, functional, environmental) and whatever challenges they faced. We noted the likely transformative power of new brain imaging models such as functional magnetic resonance imaging to change assessment and our understanding of brain–behavior relationships. We concluded that psychologists must be catalysts in changing the focus from acute care to integrated care addressing chronic health limitations and psychological health.

As the first compilation of expert perspectives on theory, research, and clinical practice in rehabilitation psychology, the first edition of this handbook quickly became the primary resource for the discipline. In 2004, Tim Elliott suggested the need for a second edition reflecting the progress of the field, though he would not be able to participate. Mitch Rosenthal had previously approached Bob Frank indicating his interest in being involved in future editions of the handbook, so he joined the team, replacing Tim. A few weeks later, Bruce Caplan joined us as third editor. By 2007 we had the project on track. However, in May of that year, we and our colleagues around the world in rehabilitation psychology were stunned by Mitch's untimely death. Given our close friendship and his significant role in managing the development of a number of chapters in the second edition, we lost a year recovering from his death and coming to terms with the need to push the project forward without his involvement. The second edition of the *Handbook of Rehabilitation Psychology* was published in 2010.

We asked one of the truly innovative thinkers in the field of rehabilitation psychology, John Corrigan, to write the last chapter of the second edition. In his chapter, "Afterword: Of Bins and Arrows" (Corrigan, 2010), he recognized the history of theoretical fragmentation that Elliott and Frank (2000) described as "naïve empiricism" disconnected from theoretical models. Corrigan described the phenomenon as "bins" of theory that "did not inform each other, but rather sat side-by-side as competing models" (Corrigan, 2010, p. 477). He noted that the development of the World Health Organization's *International Classification of Functioning, Disability and Health* (2000) was important for creating critical "bins" for rehabilitation psychology with the inclusion of health and function, and for creating an overarching model that highlighted influences between the bins. Pointing to the scientific advances that occur when research focuses on interactions of multiple influences on behavior, Corrigan (2010) provided the example of the increasing importance of understanding genotypic expression as a function of environmental influences. He noted that phenotypic plasticity, the differential expression of genotypic expression as a function of the environment, potentially interacts with the bins affecting behavior and may cause plasticity to be expressed within the lifetime of an organism (Corrigan, 2010). Corrigan further reflected on the value of research on interactions between bins as exemplified in the growing interest in applying "big data" (i.e., sifting through large databases to identify relationships) to understand how environmental factors in neighborhoods impact health and social well-being. For example, Corrigan and Bogner (2008) found that neighborhood characteristic improved predictions of subjective well-being among individuals with traumatic brain injury. Corrigan (2010) concluded, "It may be time to look beyond disability and chronic illness as complex conditions with multiple interactions and attend to ways these influences interact and influence with each other in their own right" (p. 480).

As the second edition aged, we began to consider the need for a third edition reflecting changes within the field. Tim Elliott returned as a coeditor, and we recognized a need to better reflect the dynamics of the Division of Rehabilitation Psychology. Lisa Brenner and Stephanie Reid-Arndt agreed to join our team, adding their experience and perspectives reflecting the best and brightest of the new demographic of the Division of Rehabilitation Psychology. The third edition of the *Handbook of Rehabilitation Psychology* addresses a more mature specialty, now recognized by the APA Council of Specialties. The number of individuals with Diplomates in rehabilitation psychology has rapidly moved to match the numbers of much more historic specialties.

As noted by John Corrigan (2010) in his conclusion to the second edition, rehabilitation psychology increasingly interfaces with the health of the population. Population health recognizes multiple determinants of health outcomes, "including medical care, public health interventions, aspects of the social environment (income, education, employment, social support, culture) and of the physical environment (urban design, clean air and water), genetics, and individual behavior" (Kindig & Stoddart, 2003, p. 381). Recognizing the changing emphasis on health outcomes and the need to understand multiple determinants of health, the third edition includes chapters on public health, global health, community rehabilitation, and the epidemiology of disability. Recognizing the many new technologies impacting rehabilitation, chapters on artificial intelligence and technology changes in rehab are included.

As with the previous edition of the handbook, approximately 30% of the material in the third edition is new to the volume, and the remainder is dedicated to updated content on foundational issues such as spinal cord injury, traumatic brain injury, acquired disability, amputation, burn injuries, chronic pain, and disability associated with aging. The third edition also provides current guidance regarding education and training, health policy, ethics, and various roles that rehabilitation psychologists face in assessment, intervention, critical care, and consultation.

References

Corrigan, J. D. (2010). Afterword: Of bins and arrows. In R. G. Frank, M. Rosenthal, & B. Caplan (Eds.), *Handbook of rehabilitation psychology* (2nd ed., pp. 477–482). Washington, DC: American Psychological Association.

Corrigan, J. D., & Bogner, J. A. (2008). Neighborhood characteristics and outcomes after traumatic brain injury. *Archives of Physical Medicine and Rehabilitation*, *89*, 912–921. http://dx.doi.org/10.1016/j.apmr.2007.12.027

Elliott, T. R., & Frank, R. G. (2000). Afterword: Drawing new horizons. In R. G. Frank & T. R. Elliott (Eds.), *Handbook of rehabilitation psychology* (pp. 645–653). Washington, DC: American Psychological Association.

Kindig, D., & Stoddart, G. (2003). What is population health? *American Journal of Public Health*, *93*, 380–383.

World Health Organization. (2000). *International classification of functioning, disability and health.* Retrieved from http://www.who.int/classifications/icf/icf_more/en/

HANDBOOK OF REHABILITATION PSYCHOLOGY

THIRD EDITION

INTRODUCTION

Stephanie A. Reid-Arndt and Lisa A. Brenner

We are in the midst of a decade of seismic changes in the United States health care system associated with the Patient Protection and Affordable Care Act (2010) and subsequent efforts to repeal the legislation. Looking forward, modifications to this health care legislation are likely, although the current partisan political divide renders hazardous any prediction of specific alterations. Nonetheless, changes may be substantial, again altering the landscape of health care services. Efforts surrounding polices have reignited discussion regarding access to health care as a basic human right, a topic of particular salience to those living with chronic health conditions and disability. As such, principles and practices that are the foundation of rehabilitation psychology (e.g., the person–environment interaction; Wright, 1983) and an emphasis on integrated, team-based care have affected approaches to health care and have the potential to have an enduring influence. Opportunities abound for expanding the impact of the principles, research, and practice of rehabilitation psychology.

Simultaneously, other national and global events have affected the U.S. health care system and the practice and science of rehabilitation psychology. In particular, the United States' involvement in two sustained wars—in Iraq (2003–2012) and Afghanistan (the longest war in its history, 2001–present)—has modified the health care landscape. Innovations in health care historically have occurred to meet the needs of military personnel following engagement in military action or war. Such innovations have had profound effects during Operation Enduring Freedom and Operation Iraqi Freedom, as "modern changes in medical management, coupled with improved protective gear and evacuation capabilities, have facilitated the highest survival rate in combat history" (Ling, Rhee, & Ecklund, 2010, p. 457). In many cases, survival has increased the need for rehabilitation services for symptoms associated with traumatic brain injuries, mental and behavioral health issues, and other chronic conditions and disabilities, as well as for growth in research and practice in all health care disciplines engaged in rehabilitation.

Although the relative youth of rehabilitation psychology contributes to its position as one of the best-kept secrets in a whole-person approach to interdisciplinary health care practice and research, it arguably renders rehabilitation psychology nimbler and therefore better able to respond to changes in the health care environment. To remain relevant, we must continually examine our research and clinical practices to refine the essential knowledge base and clinical skills required for the practice of rehabilitation psychology. This will also facilitate the best outcomes for patients, families, and providers. We also must demonstrate how principles rooted in care provided to persons with disability are relevant to experiences of persons with acute and chronic health conditions, previously less associated with rehabilitation psychology care (e.g., a patient receiving care in intensive settings).

http://dx.doi.org/10.1037/0000129-001
Handbook of Rehabilitation Psychology, Third Edition, L. A. Brenner, S. A. Reid-Arndt, T. R. Elliott, R. G. Frank, and B. Caplan (Editors-in-Chief)

FUNDAMENTALS OF REHABILITATION PSYCHOLOGY

Rehabilitation psychology is a specialty area within psychology that focuses on the study and application of psychological knowledge and skills on behalf of individuals with disabilities and chronic health conditions to maximize health and welfare, independence and choice, functional abilities, and social role participation (Scherer, 2010). Rehabilitation psychologists are uniquely trained in this specialty area of practice, which includes a broad range of activities: clinical practice; consultation; program development; service provisions; research; teaching and education; training; administration; development of public policy; and advocacy (American Psychological Association, 2018a).

The field of rehabilitation psychology is distinct from other psychological specialties and from rehabilitation medicine for its early adoption of principles later espoused in the International Classification of Functioning, Disability and Health (ICF; World Health Organization, 2001) regarding the role of the environment in the experiences of persons living with chronic health conditions and disability. In his seminal work published in 1948, Lee Meyerson suggested that adjustment to physical disability is promoted by creating favorable social psychological situations for individuals living with disabilities (i.e., positive person–environment relations). Adjustment to physical disability was recognized as not just an issue for people living with disabilities; rather, Meyerson proposed that society as a whole must also learn to adjust to the experiences and outlooks of those living with physical disabilities. More recently, these tenets have also been expanded to those living with psychological disabilities and chronic health conditions.

Foreshadowed by founders of the field of rehabilitation psychology, this evolution of concepts regarding health and disability are evidenced in the creation and implementation of the ICF. As depicted in Figure 1, "The ICF is based on an integration of the medical and social models of disability, addressing the biological, individual, and societal perspectives of health in a biopsychosocial approach," which is, in part, accomplished by a model in which "functioning and disability are conceptualized within the dynamic interaction between health conditions and contextual factors" (World Health Organization, 2001, p. 106). The ICF model is ideal for community and community-based work, encouraging a focus on environmental factors that can be levers for maximizing opportunities for all persons to engage in

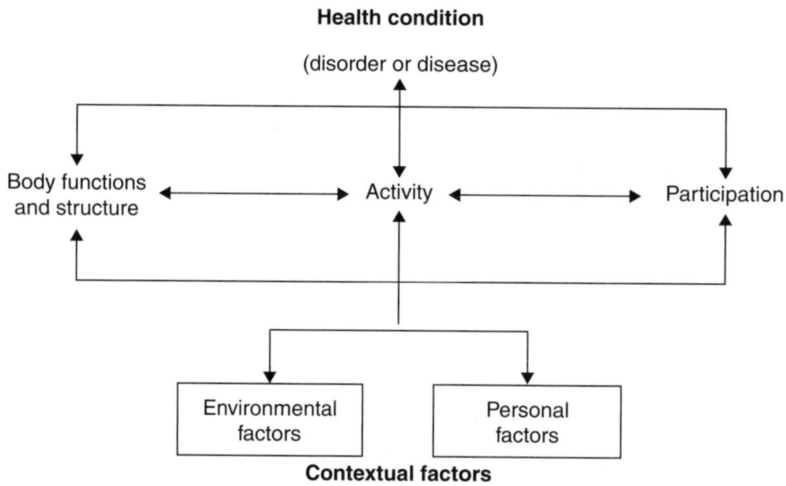

FIGURE 1. International Classification of Functioning, Disability and Health model. From *International Classification of Functioning, Disability and Health* (p. 18), by World Health Organization, 2001, Geneva, Switzerland: Author. Copyright 2001 by the World Health Organization. Reprinted with permission.

all aspects of community life (e.g., universal design principles).

The third edition of the *Handbook of Rehabilitation Psychology* was developed in the context of a changing health care environment, with reflections on both the foundations of rehabilitation psychology and the opportunities for expanding the field's influence. Relative to other psychological specialties, rehabilitation psychology is arguably still in its formative years. Though it has existed for more than 55 years (since World War II), the first training guidelines for rehabilitation psychology were published just over a decade ago (Patterson & Hanson, 1995), and rehabilitation psychology was recognized as a specialty by the American Board of Professional Psychology in 1997 (American Psychological Association, 2018a). More recently, in large measure due to the efforts of a dedicated team led by William Stiers, the American Psychological Association Education Directorate recognized rehabilitation psychology as a specialty in 2015. This designation confirms that rehabilitation psychology is "a defined area of psychological practice which requires advanced knowledge and skills acquired through an organized sequence of education and training" (American Psychological Association, 2018b, "About Specialties," para. 1; see also Stiers et al., 2012). For additional information, see the comprehensive examination of competencies unique to rehabilitation psychology by Cox, Cox, and Caplan (2013) and the discussion of competencies in this volume (see Chapter 1, this volume).

NEW FEATURES OF THE THIRD EDITION *HANDBOOK*

The first edition of the *Handbook of Rehabilitation Psychology* was published in 2000 and was recognized as an essential text in the field (Ryan & Tree, 2004). It was followed by an updated second edition in 2010. Both editions are intended to be source books for theory and practice in rehabilitation psychology and include state-of-the-science reviews of assessment and intervention strategies for core clinical conditions, as well as advances in the field and innovations on the horizon.

This third edition of the *Handbook* highlights the progress in theory application and research since 2010, and remains forward-thinking in identifying areas of opportunity for the growth of rehabilitation psychology in the context of an ever-changing health care environment. In this edition, chapters highlight the evidence base for assessment and intervention activities, integrating evidence-based care principles that have been explored with other clinical conditions and patient populations and noting where additional research is needed. Updated coverage of the foundations and core areas of expertise within rehabilitation psychology is provided, both in terms of clinical conditions that are often linked with rehabilitation psychology and the foundational psychological principles that inform practice and research in rehabilitation psychology. Toward this end, a chapter focused on rehabilitation psychology and competency-based training and practice has been added (Chapter 1, this volume). In addition, chapter authors have integrated references to clinical competencies throughout the handbook (American Board of Professional Psychology and American Board of Rehabilitation Psychology, 2018).

To reflect the changing health care environment and the need for rehabilitation psychologists to engage with expanding opportunities in health care, multiple new topics are covered in this third edition. The importance of viewing disability and chronic illness from a public health perspective is reflected in the inclusion of chapters reviewing the epidemiology of disability, public health models of care, and global health needs. Opportunities for expanding the influence of rehabilitation psychology to other settings and with other medical populations are highlighted in chapters on critical care, polytrauma, and community rehabilitation. Finally, reflecting technological advances since 2010, this edition includes chapters examining the application of technology in rehabilitation settings and with persons having chronic health conditions and disability.

ORGANIZATION OF THIS VOLUME

This third edition of the *Handbook* is divided into three parts. Part I, Core Areas and Professional Competencies, includes chapters on topics that are transdiagnostic, covering material that is germane to the study and implementation of rehabilitation psychology regardless of the scenario or clinical condition at hand. The first chapter is focused on rehabilitation psychology and competency-based training and practice. Additional chapters in this section reflect the latest advances in broad areas relevant to psychology education, practice, research, and policy. They include reviews of evidence-based, best-practice approaches to assessment, intervention, and consultation. Chapters in this section also explore issues related to disability across the lifespan, the social psychology of living with a disability, as well as implications for family members and the importance of multicultural awareness in rehabilitation psychology. Foundational principles of the field are explored, as are the applications of ethical principles in rehabilitation psychology. Within this section, readers will also find chapters on the epidemiology of disability with implications for research to inform care and health policy, as well as an examination of the state of the field's evidence base and research foundation, noting gains since the prior *Handbook* edition as well as areas of opportunity.

In Part II, Clinical Conditions, readers will find updated reviews of evidence-based practice in assessment, intervention, consultation, and advocacy with populations that have long been served by rehabilitation psychologists (e.g., persons with pediatric acquired conditions, amputations, spinal cord injuries, traumatic brain injuries, burns) as well as new areas of focus, including rehabilitation in the post–9/11 era. In the chapters, authors have highlighted links between the research and theory and the newly modified competencies for board certification in rehabilitation psychology (see Chapter 1, this volume).

In Part III, Topics in Practice and Public Health, chapters are offered that cover multiple issues not reviewed in previous editions of the *Handbook*. Specifically, topics are focused on those pertinent to the continued growth and expansion of rehabilitation psychology, including public health models of care, rehabilitation psychology in the global setting, rehabilitation psychology in public service settings, artificial intelligence and rehabilitation, and applications of virtual reality. These chapters point to evolving opportunities in new practice and research settings, as well as advances in rehabilitation science and technology that will shape the field of rehabilitation psychology.

This *Handbook* aims to serve as the essential sourcebook regarding the specialty practice of rehabilitation psychology for psychologists at all stages of their careers. For students exploring rehabilitation psychology and seeking to expand their knowledge of key concepts regarding health and disability, chapters discussing the foundations of rehabilitation psychology and those detailing the application of rehabilitation psychology principles to practice and research may be particularly informative. Early career psychologists seeking American Board of Professional Psychology board certification in rehabilitation psychology will find the integration of core competencies throughout the chapters, particularly in Parts I and II, a useful resource for expanding understanding, honing skills, and preparing for the examination process. It is our hope that all readers, and perhaps particularly those well-established in their careers, recognize the critical need to stay apprised of developments in the field and appreciate this edition's focus on advances in evidence-based practice. Furthermore, we propose that core principles of rehabilitation psychology (e.g., person–environment interaction) can positively influence practice and research in other health care disciplines as well as related psychological specialties. As such, we also see this volume as an important source of information for practitioners and researchers in a wide range of fields, including medicine, nursing, physical therapy, occupational therapy, speech-language pathology, and health care administration. We hope that this *Handbook* will serve as an informative collection of rehabilitation psychology's significant contributions to the care of persons with chronic health conditions and disabilities and as a source of inspiration—a compilation of advances and opportunities that will stimulate additional efforts to move the field of rehabilitation psychology forward.

References

American Board of Professional Psychology and American Board of Rehabilitation Psychology. (2018). *Certification guidelines and procedures: Candidates manual 2018*. Retrieved from https://abpp.org/BlankSite/

media/Rehabilitation-Psychology-Documents/Candidate-manual-september-10-2018.pdf

American Psychological Association. (2018a). *Recognized specialties and proficiencies in professional psychology*. Retrieved from https://www.apa.org/ed/graduate/specialize/recognized.aspx

American Psychological Association. (2018b). *Specialties and proficiencies*. Retrieved from http://www.apa.org/ed/graduate/specialize/index.aspx

Cox, D. R., Cox, R. H., & Caplan, B. (2013). *Specialty competencies in rehabilitation psychology*. New York, NY: Oxford University Press. http://dx.doi.org/10.1093/med:psych/9780195389241.001.0001

Ling, G. S., Rhee, P., & Ecklund, J. M. (2010). Surgical innovations arising from the Iraq and Afghanistan wars. *Annual Review of Medicine*, *61*, 457–468. http://dx.doi.org/10.1146/annurev.med.60.071207.140903

Meyerson, L. (1948). Physical disability as a social psychological problem. *Journal of Social Issues*, *4*, 2–10. http://dx.doi.org/10.1111/j.1540-4560.1948.tb01513.x

Patient Protection and Affordable Care Act, 42 U.S.C. § 18001 (2010).

Patterson, D. R., & Hanson, S. L. (1995). Joint Division 22 and ACRM guidelines for postdoctoral training in rehabilitation psychology. *Rehabilitation Psychology*, *40*, 299–310. http://dx.doi.org/10.1037/0090-5550.40.4.299

Ryan, J. J., & Tree, H. A. (2004). Essential readings in rehabilitation psychology. *Health Psychology*, 6, 15–27.

Scherer, M. J. (2010). Rehabilitation psychology. In I. B. Weiner & W. E. Craighead (Eds.), *The Corsini encyclopedia of psychology* (Vol. 4, pp. 1444–1447). New York, NY: Wiley.

Stiers, W., Hanson, S., Turner, A. P., Stucky, K., Barisa, M., Brownsberger, M., . . . Kuemmel, A. (2012). Guidelines for postdoctoral training in rehabilitation psychology. *Rehabilitation Psychology*, *57*, 267–279. http://dx.doi.org/10.1037/a0030774

World Health Organization. (2001). *International classification of functioning, disability and health*. Geneva, Switzerland: Author.

Wright, B. A. (1983). *Physical disability—A psychosocial approach* (2nd ed.). New York, NY: HarperCollins. http://dx.doi.org/10.1037/10589-000

Part I

CORE AREAS AND PROFESSIONAL COMPETENCIES

CHAPTER 1

REHABILITATION PSYCHOLOGY AND COMPETENCY-BASED TRAINING AND PRACTICE

Timothy R. Elliott and Stephanie A. Reid-Arndt

As a specialty within professional psychology, rehabilitation psychology has proposed competency-based training initiatives for internship programs and postdoctoral fellowships (e.g., Stiers et al., 2015). Less attention has been directed to current initiatives in doctoral training, as there are no accredited rehabilitation psychology doctoral training programs. Recent shifts in competencies now expected of accredited clinical, counseling, and school psychology doctoral programs are also relevant to rehabilitation but will not be discussed within this text (for more information, see Bell et al., 2017). Considerable work has occurred in developing guidelines for competencies required for board certification in rehabilitation psychology (American Board of Professional Psychology and American Board of Rehabilitation Psychology, 2017; Cox, Cox, & Caplan, 2013). A brief synopsis of the existing competencies for doctoral programs, internship, and postdoctoral training and specialty/board certification serve as a reference point for the subsequent chapters in this book.

Competency-based training in professional psychology doctoral programs became established as policymakers and regulators responded to an array of factors that called into question the traditional emphasis on standing curricular approaches, advocating instead for an emphasis on attainment of well-defined skills and competencies essential to the profession. The movement toward competency-based training stimulated an influential (and aspirational) "cube" conceptualization of functional and foundational competencies for every stage of professional development (see Figure 1.1; Rodolfa et al., 2005, p. 350). Foundational competencies are construed as "building blocks" for what all professional psychologists do, and mastery of skills in these domains provides a bedrock for acquisition of functional skills, knowledge, and values that are necessary to work as a psychologist.

This model had an immediate impact on accreditation policies and procedures for doctoral programs. The most recent iteration of expected competencies for doctoral training effectively institutes a model for health service psychology (Bell et al., 2017). This overarching term applies to all professional psychology training programs—clinical, counseling, and school—to emphasize the focus on the "application of the discipline of psychology to health-related service" and to communicate to the general public "that graduates of accredited programs have been trained in the competencies needed to promote psychological health" (Bell et al., 2017, p. 211).

As delineated in Section C of the *Implementation Regulations* from the Commission on Accreditation (n.d.), doctoral programs must provide training in and evidence of competency in four categories of discipline-specific knowledge and nine domains of professionwide competencies considered essential

http://dx.doi.org/10.1037/0000129-002
Handbook of Rehabilitation Psychology, Third Edition, L. A. Brenner, S. A. Reid-Arndt, T. R. Elliott, R. G. Frank, and B. Caplan (Editors-in-Chief)

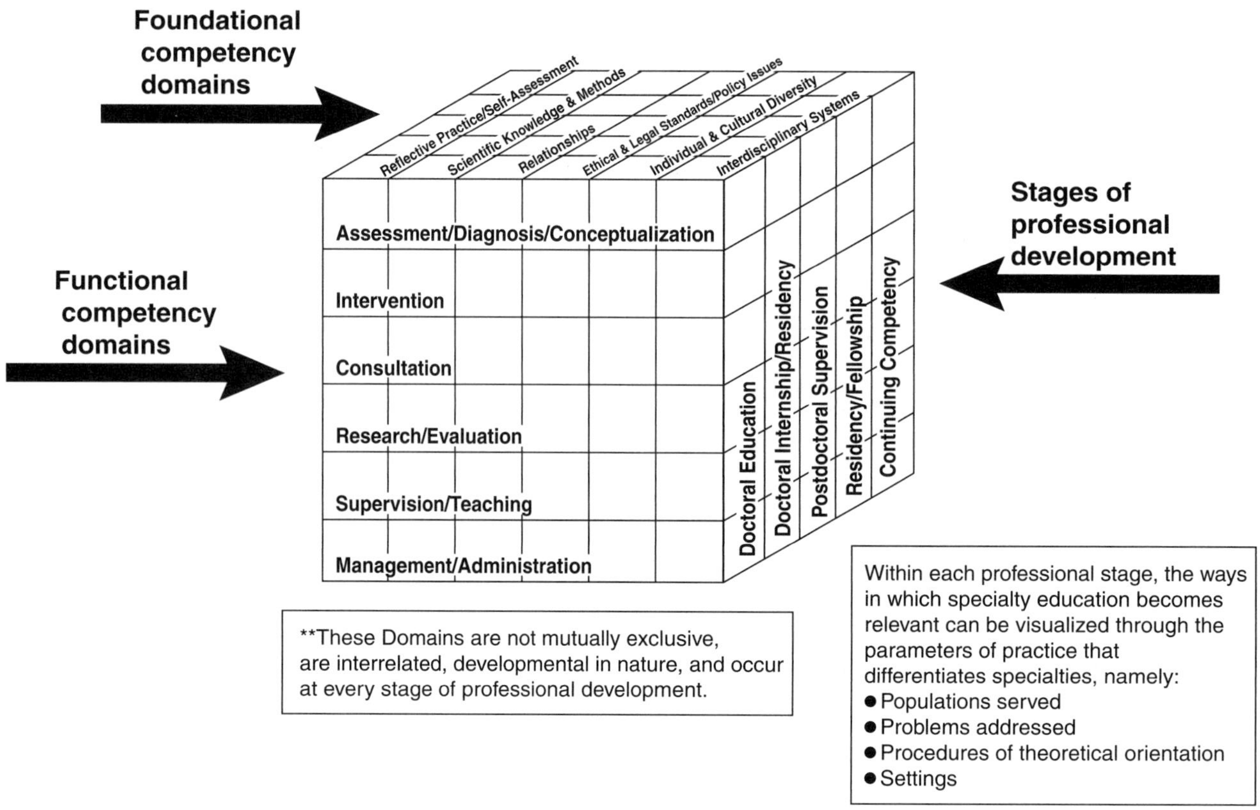

FIGURE 1.1. Competencies cube** for training in professional psychology. Reprinted from "A Cube Model for Competency Development: Implications for Psychology Educators and Regulators," by E. Rodolfa, R. Bent, E. Eisman, P. Nelson, L. Rehm, and P. Ritchie, 2005, *Professional Psychology: Research and Practice, 36*, p. 350. Copyright 2005 by the American Psychological Association.

for health service psychology (see Exhibit 1.1). The discipline-specific knowledge is essential for attaining the professionwide competencies. Programs can add to this list competencies that may reflect the unique aspects or emphasis areas of their particular program (e.g., forensic, clinical health), but all accredited doctoral programs must address these competencies and provide evidence of their implementation and student attainment. Of particular interest to rehabilitation psychology is the explicit emphasis on consultation and interdisciplinary–interprofessional interaction as a critical component of health service psychology. Interdisciplinary work is central to the rehabilitation enterprise. Furthermore, it is telling that disability is listed as an important aspect of cultural diversity that should be addressed throughout all accredited doctoral training programs.

POSTDOCTORAL TRAINING

The competencies highlighted in Exhibit 1.1 also apply to internship and postdoctoral residency programs. In many respects internship programs are an extension of doctoral training, but certain activities are expected of interns that may not be fairly expected of trainees in the doctoral program (e.g., supervising other trainees or other health professionals, direct consultation with other health care professionals). Examples of "level-appropriate" training and expectations are provided in Section C of the *Implementation Regulations* to guide internship and postdoctoral training programs. The degree to which these training competencies can be expanded in rehabilitation psychology postdoctoral programs is discussed later in this handbook (Chapter 2, this volume).

EXHIBIT 1.1

Standards of Accreditation Training and Practice Competencies for Doctoral Graduate, Internship, and Postdoctoral Residency Programs (Revised July 2017)

Discipline-specific knowledge

Category 1: *History and Systems*
Understanding and knowledge of the origins and development on major ideas in psychology

Category 2: *Basic Content Areas in Scientific Psychology*
Understanding and knowledge of the basic content areas in psychology including the five contents areas: affective aspects of behavior, biological aspects of behavior, cognitive aspects of behavior, developmental aspects of behavior, and social aspects of behavior

Category 3: *Advanced Integrative Knowledge in Scientific Psychology*
Understanding and demonstrating advanced integrative knowledge of multiple basic discipline-specific content areas (listed in Category 2)

Category 4: *Research Methods, Statistical Analysis & Psychometrics*
Understanding and demonstrating advanced integrative knowledge of research methods, statistical analyses, and psychometrics

Professionwide competencies

Understanding and demonstrating advanced integrative and independent ability to formulate and conduct research or other scholarly activity, and critically evaluate and disseminate research and scholarship that contributes to the knowledge base

Understanding of and competency in professional ethical and legal standards and laws, recognize ethical dilemmas that may occur and apply ethical decision-making processes to resolve these, and conduct self in an ethical manner in all professional activities

Understanding of and competency in individual and cultural diversity, relevant theories and the empirical knowledge base, ability to work effectively with others from diverse background and identities, and be able to integrate awareness of their own personal attitudes may affect how they understand and interact with others

Understanding and demonstrating professional values and attitudes (including integrity, deportment, professional identity, lifelong learning, self-reflection, responsiveness to feedback, and overall professional effectiveness) in complex situations and with appropriate degree of independence

Understanding and demonstrating professional communication and interpersonal skills (including maintenance of effective relationships, ability to produce and comprehend verbal, nonverbal, and written communication for various audiences) across academic, social and professional arenas, and an ability to manage difficult communications well

Understanding of and competency in diagnostic classification systems, client strengths and psychopathology, and psychological assessment practices grounded in the best available empirical literature, within appropriate contexts, accurately interpreting and effectively communicating assessment results orally and in writing to appropriate audiences

Understanding and demonstrating competency with psychological interventions and associated literature base, utilizing evidence-based approaches effectively, and modifying these approaches consistent with ongoing evaluation and as indicated

Understanding of and competency in supervision models and practices

Understanding and demonstrating competency with consultation models and practices, and demonstrating knowledge and respect for the roles and perspectives of other professions

Note. Professionwide competencies have been abbreviated from Commission on Accreditation (n.d.; see the 2019 Table 3 for Professionwide competencies under Standard II: Aims, Competencies, Curriculum and Outcomes; https://www.apa.org/ed/accreditation/about/policies/self-study-worksheets.aspx).

BOARD CERTIFICATION

All member boards of the American Board of Professional Psychology are required to articulate the specific competencies that characterize individuals with the expertise for certification with that board. Whereas all practicing psychologists are expected to be skilled in core functional and foundational areas considered professionwide competencies under the health service psychology model adopted by the American Psychological Association Commission on Accreditation, specialties reveal how practice parameters (e.g., client populations served, setting–context, theoretical framework) influence the implementation of these competencies. Reflecting this, the *Competencies of the Specialty of Rehabilitation Psychology* (American Board of Professional Psychology and American Board of Rehabilitation Psychology, 2017) highlight the distinct knowledge base and skill set of board-certified rehabilitation psychologists. They also provide guideposts for education in rehabilitation psychology and were integral to consensus guidelines on postdoctoral training that were developed following the Baltimore Conference on Rehabilitation Psychology Postdoctoral Training held in April 2011 in Baltimore, Maryland (Stiers et al., 2012, 2015).

The competencies adopted by the American Board of Rehabilitation Psychology on June 8, 2017, are presented in Table 1.1. These are referenced in chapters throughout this edition of the handbook. When viewed comprehensively, it is apparent that these competencies have retained the knowledge base and set of professional activities that as a whole are considered unique to rehabilitation psychology. Instead of two clusters of competencies that appeared in earlier iterations (Cox et al., 2013), the 2017 competencies have three—Foundations, Assessment/Evaluation, and Intervention. Yet this largely reflects a reorganization of competencies, shifting some to the cluster identified as Foundations (e.g., Consultation-related competencies/Interdisciplinary systems; Evidence-based practice) and sometimes renaming or regrouping them (e.g., Consumer Protection has been integrated into Ethical and Legal Principles).

TABLE 1.1

Competencies of the Specialty of Rehabilitation Psychology

Competency cluster	Competency name (no. of behavioral anchors)	Foci of behavioral anchors
Foundations	Specialty identification (2 of 2)	▪ Articulation of a working knowledge of the history of rehabilitation psychology; demonstration of an incorporation of the biopsychosocial foundations of rehabilitation psychology in practice as evidenced by a reference to the influence of any model, study, or leader in the rehabilitation psychology field ▪ Demonstration of clinical skills that are reflective of a rehabilitation psychologist as evidenced by a work history or experience congruent with this specialized field
	Professionalism (2 of 2)	▪ Comportment reflects integrity and demonstrates concern for the welfare of others as evidenced by a reference to standards of care, client well-being, or social justice ▪ Demonstration of knowledge and understanding of current issues in the field of rehabilitation psychology as evidenced by a reference to one or more of those issues in the exam process
	Reflective practice/ self-assessment/ self-care (3 of 4)	▪ Articulation of the ability to self-assess competencies relevant to practice and professional activities as evidenced by description of their own specific strengths and weaknesses ▪ Demonstration of an awareness of the responsibility to address limits in their knowledge base or skill set as evidenced by the articulation of steps to resolve these clinical weaknesses ▪ Description of a commitment to continued professional development as evidenced by ongoing and long-term plan to enhance competencies, either through education, specific training, and/or consultation ▪ Demonstration of active self-reflection as evidenced by the demonstration of regular self-monitoring through consultation and/or supervision, when required

TABLE 1.1

Competencies of the Specialty of Rehabilitation Psychology (*Continued*)

Competency cluster	Competency name (no. of behavioral anchors)	Foci of behavioral anchors
	Scientific knowledge and methods (2 of 4)	▪ Description of the impact of a recognized model, standard of care, or approach on the case formulation ▪ Reporting of the impact of a line of research, peer-reviewed articles, or expert consensus on the case formulation ▪ Reference to specific research methodologies, techniques of data collection, analysis, and interpretation, biological bases of behavior, cognitive-affective bases of behavior and development across the lifespan ▪ Description of the strengths and weaknesses of at least one scientific study
	Relationships (2 of 2)	▪ Description of the development and maintenance of adaptive working relationships with a wide range of clients/patients, colleagues, organizations, and communities ▪ Provision of informative, accurate, and well-integrated communication skills in written documentation and narrative presentation
	Ethical and legal principles/standards/ statutes and policy (2 of 2)	▪ Articulation of the American Psychological Association's (APA's) *Ethical Principles of Psychologists and Code of Conduct* (APA, 2017), relevant legal statutes, standards of care, and professional activities as they apply to rehabilitation populations and settings by describing actions consistent with the code, and referencing two or more elements of the code ▪ Description of effective integration of APA ethical principles in everyday practice as evidenced by the demonstration of ethical decision-making procedures to address at least three ethical dilemmas across the entire exam process
	Individual and cultural diversity (2 of 3)	▪ Articulation of an awareness of, sensitivity to, and mastery of skills related to working with diverse individuals, groups, populations and communities as evidenced by reference to the impact of those differences in culture, personal background, or other characteristic (e.g., culture of disability) ▪ Description of self-awareness as a cultural being in assessment, treatment, consultation, and advocacy/consumer protection as evidenced by a reference to the impact of the candidate's own cultural characteristics in a case or situation ▪ Demonstration of an awareness, interest, or knowledge of literature and resources available to enhance mastery of skills to work with diverse individuals, groups, populations, and communities
	Interdisciplinary systems (1 of 3)	▪ Articulation of fundamental concepts related to treatment team function within the context of rehabilitation team member identity and approach to care delivery as evidenced by referencing the impact of team treatment in a case or situation ▪ Demonstration of consultation or collaboration with team colleagues specifying how the consultation or collaboration was utilized to benefit both persons served and treatment team function ▪ Description of active leadership within an interdisciplinary team
	Evidence-based practice (4 of 5)	▪ Description of integration of a line of research, peer-reviewed articles, or expert consensus in support of the candidate's decision to use specific assessment tools and intervention strategies (includes literature citations) ▪ Description of ongoing changes in the evidence related to rehabilitation populations and its impact on case formulation and treatment decisions ▪ Articulation of the impact of a recognized model, standard of care, or approach on decision to use specific assessment tools and intervention strategies (includes literature citations) ▪ Description of a clinical approach derived from supervised practice or consultation with a specific colleague ▪ Description of the impact of knowledge gained from personal professional experience with similar cases

(*continues*)

TABLE 1.1

Competencies of the Specialty of Rehabilitation Psychology (*Continued*)

Competency cluster	Competency name (no. of behavioral anchors)	Foci of behavioral anchors
Assessment/ evaluation	General principles (4 of 6)	▪ Articulation of the rationale for assessment (e.g., who to assess, what to assess, why assess) in the context of the referral question ▪ Articulation of the impact of demographic (e.g., age, education, culture, race) data and reliability/validity/clinical utility data on assessment outcomes ▪ Articulation of recommendations for accommodations related to assessed conditions ▪ Discussion of the rationale for specific assessment measures (to include benefit of objective/subjective measures, limitations of the findings, and validity of the data) ▪ Discussion of the impact of assessment data on treatment intervention choices and implementation ▪ Reference to relevant current literature related to assessment in this specific population
	Sensory-perceptual, motor, language, cognitive functioning (2 of 2)	▪ Demonstration of knowledge of the impact of an injury or condition impact on anatomy, thinking, behavior, recovery, and outcomes ▪ Demonstration of test interpretation, reporting, and feedback relevant to the needs of the individual client/patient, family, or the treatment team
	Adjustment to disability: individual (2 of 2)	▪ Discussion of the patient's emotional adjustment and methods of evaluation (e.g., self-report vs. other report) ▪ Discussion of the factors considered in evaluating emotional adjustment
	Adjustment to disability: family (2 of 2)	▪ Discussion of client-specific variables (intrapersonal, family dynamics, environmental, etc.) included in evaluation ▪ Discussion of a theoretical and/or evidence-based approach to evaluating family response to changes in role and function, and discusses how findings/recommendations relate to the specific patient and family
	Sexuality (2 of 3)	▪ Discussion of how a person's sexual function could be impacted by the condition of interest or his or her status (to include physiology, emotional impact, medication impact) ▪ Reference to theory and/or scientific literature regarding sexual adjustment in varied disabling conditions ▪ Discussion of sexual health assessment and evaluative data in the context of individual client/patient needs and treatment planning
	Substance abuse (2 of 4)	▪ Inclusion of epidemiology data (e.g., incidence, prevalence, relapse risk) on substance abuse risk in the disability population of interest if/when appropriate ▪ Documentation of the impact and effects of substance abuse upon person and condition of interest using examples ▪ Demonstration of a specific rationale for selected method of assessing and evaluating substance use given the person and his/her condition of interest ▪ Discussion of at least one substance abuse screening tool and the limitations of these tools
	Pain (2 of 3)	▪ Discussion of the incidence/prevalence and functional effects of acute/chronic pain upon varied disabling health conditions, including reference to any germane literature ▪ Demonstration of knowledge of secondary factors that must be evaluated/assessed in the conceptualization of pain ▪ Demonstration of a specific rationale for selected method of assessing and evaluating pain given the person and his/her condition of interest
	Vocational/educational issues (1 of 2)	▪ Demonstration of the understanding of a vocational assessment model, approach, or tool ▪ Demonstration of an understanding of how the condition of interest will likely impact education and work future

TABLE 1.1

Competencies of the Specialty of Rehabilitation Psychology (*Continued*)

Competency cluster	Competency name (no. of behavioral anchors)	Foci of behavioral anchors
Intervention	General principles (3 of 4)	▪ Discussion of intervention in the context of the rehabilitation psychology consult referral question, patient/family goals, and assessment results ▪ Selection of appropriate intervention in the contexts of client/patient needs, the rehabilitation treatment milieu, treatment plan implementation, and discharge planning ▪ Discussion of varied evidence-based intervention strategies, their strengths/limitations, and their appropriateness to client/patient and the psychosocial environment ▪ Demonstration of psychotherapeutic interventions across multiple psychotherapy sessions and documentation of intervention effectiveness throughout the treatment course and outcome
	Behavior management (4 of 6)	▪ Discussion of target behavior(s) that improve or hinder behavioral health management or facilitate or serve as a barrier to patient engagement in the rehabilitation process/outcome ▪ Discussion of patient, family, team, and/or environmental or other factors, including probable antecedents, consequences, contingencies that impact behavior ▪ Discussion of a plan for managing reinforcers, contingencies, patient education, team teaching approach, or managing the physical, social, and contextual environment to support attainment of behavioral goal(s) ▪ Demonstration of communication with pertinent stakeholders regarding the behavior management plan and their willingness/objections to support it ▪ Discussion of a system to measure the effectiveness of the behavior management plan ▪ Citation of scientific literature pertinent to a specific behavioral problem or approach, and the integration of this literature into case conceptualization
	Adjustment to disability: individual (4 of 7)	▪ Articulation of a rational link between assessment findings and intervention plan specific to the rehabilitation process or adaptation to disability ▪ Discussion of client-specific variables (intrapersonal, support system, environmental, etc.) influencing the intervention approach ▪ Discussion of a theoretical and/or evidence-based approach to planning and implementing interventions ▪ A reference to at least one peer reviewed journal article relevant to the candidate's choice of intervention strategy, and discussion of how findings/recommendations relate to the specific patient ▪ Description the implementation of a theoretical/evidence-based approach to one of the client's problems ▪ Discussion of the limitations in the use of an intervention approach with this particular client ▪ Demonstration of suggestions for resources (e.g., educational material, support groups) that may support client's ongoing adjustment
	Adjustment to disability: family (4 of 7)	▪ Articulation of a rational link between assessment findings and intervention plan ▪ Discussion of client-specific variables (intrapersonal, family dynamics, environmental, etc.) influencing the intervention approach ▪ Discussion of a theoretical and/or evidence-based approach to planning and implementing interventions to enable family integration and support of the person with the disability ▪ Reference to at least one peer reviewed journal article relevant to the choice of intervention strategy, and discussion of how findings/recommendations relate to the specific patient and family ▪ Discussion of at least one example of an action implementing a theoretical/evidence-based approach to one of the family's problems ▪ Discussion of the limitations of the use of the intervention approach with this particular family ▪ Communication of suggestions for resources (e.g., educational material, support groups) that may support the family's ongoing adaptation to disability

(*continues*)

TABLE 1.1

Competencies of the Specialty of Rehabilitation Psychology (*Continued*)

Competency cluster	Competency name (no. of behavioral anchors)	Foci of behavioral anchors
	Sexuality (5 of 8)	▪ Discussion of medical variables affecting sexual desire and sexual response ▪ Assessment of patient's willingness to discuss sexual issues, and individualizes discussions according to patient's preferences ▪ Discussion of patient's emotional response to changes/limitations in sexual functioning ▪ Discussion of the impact of changes in sexual functioning on patient's identity ▪ Identification of sexual intercourse as one element of a person's sexual behavior, and articulation of multiple ways to support sexual activity and sexual identity ▪ Involvement of patient's partner in treatment, based on patient's consent and goals (as appropriate) ▪ Suggestion of resources that can be helpful in addressing patient's sexual concerns and in facilitating patient's access to those resources ▪ Citation of relevant professional literature and integration of that literature into case conceptualization
	Substance abuse (3 of 4)	▪ Discussion of intervention approaches appropriate to the needs of the specific population and the assessed substance use history ▪ Selection of appropriate evidence-based substance use intervention and prevention integrated into a team treatment approach ▪ Description of community resources and referrals related to substance use prevention and intervention ▪ Demonstration of serial evaluation and documentation of intervention effectiveness of substance use intervention
	Pain (2 of 3)	▪ Discussion of how findings from pain assessment impact patient intervention, course, and outcome ▪ Selection of evidence-based pain intervention strategies with attention to specific population-based needs integrated into the interprofessional team treatment context ▪ Description of a comprehensive approach to pain management including nonpharmacological interventions and focus on participation and quality of life
	Vocational/educational issues (2 of 3)	▪ Discussion of the client/patient's vocational and education history, and the influence of disability upon current vocational and education status, as well as future goals ▪ Demonstration of awareness and utilization of community vocational resources (e.g., state vocational rehabilitation services) and educational resources (e.g., school-based disability services) as warranted ▪ Demonstration of willingness to communicate with employers, school personnel, university office of disability services, or managers of volunteer organizations to assist with disability education and implementation of accommodations
Consultation	Peer (1 of 2)	▪ Demonstration of active consultation among treatment team and disciplinary peers to enhance treatment team function and client/patient treatment effectiveness ▪ Discussion of the challenges involved in shared treatment planning, cotreatment, and timely shared data related to treatment
	Community and organizational (1 of 3)	▪ Description of the delivery of active consultation with community and organizational resources to enhance client/patient treatment outcomes ▪ Articulation of expertise related to community resources (referral to patient advocacy organizations such as the Brain Injury Association of America, United Spinal Association, etc.) ▪ Description of participation in rehabilitation community organizations such as educational seminars and presentations to groups serving rehabilitation populations, serving on boards of directors and committees for relevant local community groups

TABLE 1.1

Competencies of the Specialty of Rehabilitation Psychology (*Continued*)

Competency cluster	Competency name (no. of behavioral anchors)	Foci of behavioral anchors
Advocacy	Client/patient (2 of 2)	▪ Demonstration of commitment to individual client/patient rights, equitable treatment, privacy/confidentiality, and autonomy in all aspects of health care within the treatment team, with family-support system members, and in the community in the context of discharge planning and community reintegration ▪ Discussion of at least one instance of participation in intervention, education. or outreach in the service of client/patient rights, equitable treatment, privacy/confidentiality, and/or autonomy (with the client/patient, other health care providers, family, social support system, employer, or health care facilities/systems)
	Disability issues (2 of 3)	▪ Demonstration of active promotion of disability rights, recognition, equitable social opportunities, accommodations, cultural identity at individual client/patient, facility, local, state and/or national levels via intervention, education, legislative testimony, political activism, etc. ▪ Demonstration of at least one instance of intervention, education, or political action (at any level including patient, family, treatment team, healthcare facility, local, regional, state, or national levels or professional organizations) that promotes disability rights, recognition, equitable social opportunities, accommodations, and/or cultural identity ▪ Demonstration of awareness of current issues in disability by citing relevant literature, which may include foundational works on disability as an identity variable (e.g., writings of Beatrice Wright, Dana Dunn, Rhoda Olkin, etc.), case law, or issues/cases in the public domain
Consumer protection	Federal legislative statutes (2 of 4)	▪ Demonstration of a working knowledge of disability-relevant federal laws (e.g., Americans With Disability Act of 1990, Americans With Disabilities Amendments Act, 2008, Patient Protection and Affordable Care Act, 2010) as they apply to the individuals described in the Practice Sample, as well as the population of individuals with disabilities ▪ Discussion of at least one federal statute or case law (e.g., Americans With Disabilities Amendments Act, 2008, Rehabilitation Act of 1973, Individuals With Disabilities Education Act, 1990, Tarasoff v. Regents of the University of California, 1976, etc.) and its application to the case or candidate's clinical practice ▪ Discussion of at least one federal standard in practice (e.g., Health Insurance Portability and Accountability Act, 1996, Uniting and Strengthening America by Providing Appropriate Tools Required to Intercept and Obstruct Terrorism Act of 2001, etc.) as they apply to candidate's clinical practice ▪ Demonstration of awareness of the potential of a violation of patient privacy/confidentiality
	State legislative statutes (2 of 3)	▪ Demonstration of a working knowledge of state statutes regarding the practice of psychology, definitions of disability, and standards of care ▪ Discussion of at least one state statute or case law and its application in the practice sample or chosen vignette case (e.g., duty to warn, mandatory reporting of abuse/neglect, competency standards) ▪ Discussion of the application of at least one state standard in practice (e.g., worker's compensation, motor vehicle license, consent for therapy)
	Community health and safety resources (3 of 3)	▪ Demonstration of a working knowledge of community resources supporting client/patient safety and security (e.g., fire and police services, suicide hotline services, public health clinics, mental health services, social services, abuse hotline) ▪ Discussion of at least one community program and its application to the case (e.g., vocational rehabilitation, adult protective services) ▪ Discussion of at least one aspect of client safety (e.g., consideration of abuse reporting)

Note. Data from American Board of Professional Psychology and American Board of Rehabilitation Psychology (2017).

Notably, however, this revised set of competencies is distinct from the prior version in a few key ways. First, with this reorganization and the addition of several competencies (e.g., Relationships, Interdisciplinary Systems), the cluster of Foundations competencies closely mirrors those recommended by Rodolfa et al. (2005). Second, while a majority of the broad categories of knowledge and skill were unchanged, behavioral anchors were added for each competency to provide criteria for evidencing mastery of that competency. Third, while demonstration of a competency always assumed that the work was evidence based, the requirement of demonstration of knowledge and application of research evidence in practice is now specifically articulated and integrated throughout the document. Finally, additional competencies were more clearly articulated in the areas of Research, Management/Administration, Supervision, and Teaching, as mandated by the American Board of Professional Psychology for all specialty boards. These competencies are listed as Supplemental, with the stipulation that they are to be examined in individuals who have responsibilities in those areas in their work as rehabilitation psychologists. Additional detailed information about specialty competencies is provided in American Board of Professional Psychology and American Board of Rehabilitation Psychology (2017).

References

American Board of Professional Psychology and American Board of Rehabilitation Psychology. (2017). *Certification guidelines and procedures, candidates manual 2018*. Retrieved from https://abpp.org/BlankSite/media/Rehabilitation-Psychology-Documents/Candidate-manual-september-10-2018.pdf

American Psychological Association. (2017). *Ethical principles of psychologists and code of conduct* (2002, Amended June 1, 2010 and January 1, 2017). Retrieved from http://www.apa.org/ethics/code/index.aspx

Americans With Disability Act of 1990, 42 U.S.C.A. § 12101 et seq. (West 1993).

Americans With Disabilities Amendments Act of 2008, 42 U.S.C. ch. 126 § 12101 et seq.

Bell, D. J., Bieschke, K. J., Zlotlow, S., Paternite, C. E., Illfelder-Kaye, J., McCutcheon, S., . . . Wall, J. (2017). New standards of accreditation in health service psychology: Rationale, opportunities, and challenges. *Training and Education in Professional Psychology*, *11*, 207–218. http://dx.doi.org/10.1037/tep0000163

Commission on Accreditation. (n.d.). *Implementing regulations. Section C: IRs related to the standards of accreditation*. Retrieved from https://www.apa.org/ed/accreditation/section-c-soa.pdf

Cox, D. R., Cox, R. H., & Caplan, B. (2013). *Specialty competencies in rehabilitation psychology*. New York, NY: Oxford University Press. http://dx.doi.org/10.1093/med:psych/9780195389241.001.0001

Health Insurance Portability and Accountability Act, 10 Stat. 1936 (1996).

Individuals With Disabilities Education Act, Pub. L. 101-476 (1990).

Patient Protection and Affordable Care Act, 124 Stat. 119 through 124 Stat. 1025 (2010).

Rehabilitation Act of 1973, 29 U.S.C. § 701 et seq.

Rodolfa, E., Bent, R., Eisman, E., Nelson, P., Rehm, L., & Ritchie, P. (2005). A cube model for competency development: Implications for psychology educators and regulators. *Professional Psychology: Research and Practice*, *36*, 347–354. http://dx.doi.org/10.1037/0735-7028.36.4.347

Stiers, W., Barisa, M., Stucky, K., Pawlowski, C., Van Tubbergen, M., Turner, A. P., . . . Caplan, B. (2015). Guidelines for competency development and measurement in rehabilitation psychology postdoctoral training. *Rehabilitation Psychology*, *60*, 111–122. http://dx.doi.org/10.1037/a0038353

Stiers, W., Hanson, S., Turner, A. P., Stucky, K., Barisa, M., Brownsberger, M., . . . Kuemmel, A. (2012). Guidelines for postdoctoral training in rehabilitation psychology. *Rehabilitation Psychology*, *57*, 267–279. http://dx.doi.org/10.1037/a0030774

Tarasoff v. Regents of the University of California, 17 Cal. 3d 425, 551 P.2d 334, 131 Cal. Rptr. 14 (Cal. 1976).

Uniting and Strengthening America by Providing Appropriate Tools Required to Intercept and Obstruct Terrorism Act of 2001, 115 Stat. 272 (2001).

Chapter 2

EDUCATION AND TRAINING

William Stiers

In the penultimate decade of the 19th century, psychological research and education found its place in graduate education. Wilhelm Wundt established the first psychological laboratory at the University of Leipzig, Germany, in 1879. A few years later, in 1883, the first American psychology laboratory was established by G. Stanley Hall at Johns Hopkins University. The first American doctorate in psychology was granted at Johns Hopkins in 1886. In 1888, the first academic title of "Professor of Psychology" was granted to James Cattell, who was a professor at the University of Pennsylvania and Columbia University (American Psychological Association [APA], n.d.-a).

Today, there are more than 400 doctoral programs, 600 internship programs, and 130 postdoctoral programs accredited by the APA Office of Program Consultation and Accreditation (n.d.). This chapter discusses the organizations and concepts that govern psychology education and training in general, the structures and processes that are specific to training and education in rehabilitation psychology, how psychology training programs are evaluated and funded, and the future of rehabilitation psychology training.

CURRENT ORGANIZATIONS GOVERNING PSYCHOLOGY EDUCATION AND TRAINING

Three organizations focus on the education and training of health service psychologists in the United States: APA, the Association of State and Provincial Psychology Boards (ASPPB), and the Association of Psychology Postdoctoral and Internship Centers (APPIC).

American Psychological Association

APA has created "directorates" that address critical issues for the profession. Each directorate has a board (sometimes more than one board) composed of psychologists to collaborate with the directorate. For example, the APA Education Directorate oversees psychology education in all settings, including high school, community college, undergraduate, graduate, and continuing education levels. Also under the Education Directorate is the Committee on Accreditation that oversees accreditation of APA educational programs for graduate education, internships, and postdoctoral program (APA, Education Directorate, n.d.-a). APA resources for precollege and undergraduate psychology education are shown in Table 2.1.

APA has consistently affirmed that a doctoral degree is required for independent practice and historically has not interacted with master's level psychology programs (APA, 2016). The decision to focus on doctorate education has allowed other agencies to assume oversight of master's level programs, sometimes to the detriment of doctoral psychologists. For example, the Behavior Analyst Certification Board has opined that master's trained behavioral analysts can conduct behavioral analysis but that doctoral psychologists who are board certified

http://dx.doi.org/10.1037/0000129-003
Handbook of Rehabilitation Psychology, Third Edition, L. A. Brenner, S. A. Reid-Arndt, T. R. Elliott, R. G. Frank, and B. Caplan (Editors-in-Chief)

TABLE 2.1

American Psychological Association Resources for Precollege and Undergraduate Psychology Education

Education level	Organization	Model curriculum	Resources
High school	Teachers of Psychology in Secondary Schools (APA, Education Directorate, n.d.-b)	National Standards for High School Psychology Curricula (APA, 2011a)	▪ online lesson plans for teachers ▪ online psychology laboratory for students
Community college	Psychology Teachers at Community Colleges (PT@CC; APA, Education Directorate, n.d.-c)	Principles for Quality Undergraduate Education in Psychology (APA, 2011b)	▪ online lesson plans ▪ online psychology laboratory for students to participate in studies and engage in data analysis ▪ resources for faculty development
Undergraduate university	Psychology Teacher Network (APA, Education Directorate, 2018)	Principles for Quality Undergraduate Education in Psychology (APA, 2011b)	▪ online lesson plans ▪ online psychology laboratory for students to participate in studies and engage in data analysis ▪ resources for faculty development

by the American Board of Professional Psychology (ABPP) in Behavioral and Cognitive Psychology with subspecialization in Applied Behavior Analysis cannot. Similarly, accreditation standards promulgated by the Council for the Accreditation of Counseling and Related Educational Programs (CACREP), and the Master's in Psychology Accreditation Council, have stipulated that only CACREP-graduated master's level counselors can teach in master's level counseling programs but that doctoral psychologists may not. The APA Education Directorate, through the Board of Educational Affairs, has recently begun to interact with master's level psychology programs regarding educational goal setting and measurement, and it is developing plans for improving relationships between master's level and doctoral-level training programs, practitioners, and educators. APA is developing guidelines for training and accreditation of master's programs in psychology (APA, Education Directorate, n.d.-d, n.d.-e).

APA accredits doctoral training programs in psychology through its Commission on Accreditation (APA, Education Directorate, n.d.-f). The commission is recognized as a national accrediting authority for professional education and training in psychology by the U.S. Department of Education and the Council for Higher Education Accreditation. The Commission on Accreditation is currently the only body recognized by the Department of Education and accreditation council to accredit psychology training programs. Accreditation requires that doctoral programs submit a self-study document that describes how the program is in compliance with Commission on Accreditation *Standards of Accreditation for Health Service Psychology* (APA, 2015a). If the self-study describes an accreditable program, a site visit is conducted, and then accreditation is granted if the program is in full compliance with the *Standards of Accreditation.*

The Commission on Accreditation also accredits psychology internship and postdoctoral residency programs through a process similar to that for doctoral programs. While *doctoral and internship training* is defined as "broad and general preparation for practice at the entry level," *postdoctoral training* is defined as "advanced preparation for practice . . . in a focus area and/or recognized specialty" that "builds upon the breadth of knowledge attained in earlier doctoral and internship education" (APA, 2015a, p. 4). Although postdoctoral residency training is not currently required for licensure, psychologists wishing to be credentialed in hospitals, patient care medical homes (see U.S. Department of Health and Human Services, n.d.), or specialized facilities (e.g., subacute rehabilitation hospitals, pain treatment programs, ventilator units) may encounter the expectation of board certification in a specialty, like their physician colleagues.

APA also supports continuing education for psychologists, including self-study, regional programs, and national programs, and it approves continuing education sponsors (see APA, Education Directorate, n.d.-g; see also https://www.apa.org/ed/ce/index.aspx). APA's Continuing Education Committee does not approve individual continuing education programs; rather, approval is granted to organizations that provide continuing education programs and focuses on the capacity of the organization to deliver continuing education consistent with APA standards and criteria (APA, 2015b). One of the primary requirements is that continuing education offerings must "have overall consistent and credible empirical support in the contemporary peer reviewed scientific literature beyond those publications and other types of communications devoted primarily to the promotion of the approach" (APA, 2015b, p. 9, Standard D: Curriculum Content). Continuing education programs may also provide information related to ethical, legal, statutory or regulatory policies, guidelines, and standards that impact psychology, or "topics related to psychological practice, education, or research . . . that are supported by contemporary scholarship grounded in established research procedures" (APA, 2015b, p. 9).

Association of State and Provincial Psychology Boards

ASPPB (n-d.-a) "represents the psychology regulatory bodies throughout North America. Its primary objective is protection of the public and promotion of excellence in the regulation of the profession of psychology." It has created a "bank" for credentials (externship and internship and postdoctoral training verification, letters of recommendation); manages the Examination for Professional Practice in Psychology; and provides the Psychology Licensure Universal System, a universal application system for state licensure as a psychologist.

The Association of Psychology Postdoctoral and Internship Centers

APPIC is a membership organization for internship and postdoctoral training programs; it is not an accrediting organization. The association manages the national match program between psychology internship centers and internship applicants, and it provides a centralized site for postdoctoral training programs and applicants. It has stipulated that in order to participate in the psychology internship match, students must be enrolled in doctoral programs accredited by APA/Commission on Accreditation. However, in 2016, the Psychological Clinical Science Accreditation System of the Academy of Psychological Clinical Science also began accrediting doctoral psychology training programs. This accreditation system is not recognized by the Department of Education, but it is recognized by the Council for Higher Education Accreditation. The Veterans Administration has determined that both APA and the academy's doctoral accreditations are acceptable for students to be eligible for training positions and employment within the Veterans Administration. Therefore, APPIC has now revised its policies to allow internship match participation of students from doctoral programs that are accredited by an organization that is "recognized by an approved government agency," which includes programs accredited by organizations recognized by the Department of Education (currently, APA is the only such organization) and programs accredited by organizations recognized by the U.S. Veterans Administration in its training and hiring criteria (APPIC, 2018). There are also policies that allow students to participate in the match who are from programs working toward accreditation that have had their APA/Commission on Accreditation self-study accepted and that have a site visit pending.

CURRENT CONCEPTS GOVERNING PSYCHOLOGY EDUCATION AND TRAINING

Focus on Competencies

Educators are responsible for developing health care professionals who can work in interdisciplinary teams to provide health care and improve health outcomes (Stiers et al., 2015; see also Chapter 1, this volume). For the last 2 decades, APA has advanced competency-based training and developed specific competency definitions and measurements in doctoral training (e.g., the Joint

Council on Professional Education in Psychology, the Task Force on the Assessment of Competence in Professional Psychology, the Assessment of Competency Benchmarks Workgroup, the Competency Assessment Toolkit for Professional Psychology). These efforts have led to a number of training guidelines (health service psychology, primary care, clinical supervision, multicultural practice) as well as guidelines for developing and evaluating guidelines (APA, 2004), and a number of competency development benchmarks and ratings forms (APA, Education Directorate, n.d.-h). Trainee competencies are the training program outcomes, and it is by comparing these actual outcomes in relation to the intended outcomes that program improvement can occur. However, in order to develop trainee competency assessment methodologies, it is first necessary to specify the key competency domains and then the key competency items within domains.

Rodolfa et al. (2005) proposed the "competency cube" as a model to conceptualize psychological competencies (see Figure 1.1, this volume). This model differentiates foundational competency domains such as scientific knowledge and methods, relationship skills, and ethical and legal standards from functional competency domains such as assessment, intervention, and consultation. Although there have been a number of different taxonomies published for psychology competencies, much of the variation in the literature is simply a matter of variance in terminology; the Rodolfa et al. model appears to be a useful taxonomy to clarify and unify the literature.

Stiers et al. (2015) described the major published models of psychology competency assessment, and they suggested that these could be grouped into six categories for assessing knowledge, skills–abilities, and attitude–values related to the Rodolfa et al. (2005) functional competencies. They proposed the Assessment Cube for Functional Competencies in Psychology, which included performance appraisal ratings by supervisors, peers, and colleagues; oral and written examinations and clinical vignettes; structured observations and structured item checklist ratings; record review ratings; self-ratings and student portfolios; patient clinical outcomes; and patient satisfaction reports.

The authors noted that performance appraisals are the most commonly used types of assessment and that structured observation to guide these appraisals has significant strengths in reliability, validity, and feasibility (Stiers et al., 2015). They noted that chart reviews, exams, essays, and self-reflection are useful for competency assessment of knowledge, but these methods do not adequately assess skills and attitudes. Although measures of patient satisfaction have the potential to adequately measure skills and attitudes, these also have not been well-developed in psychology.

Certification of Competency

ASPPB conducts the Examination for Professional Practice in Psychology (EPPP), the national examination of psychologists that is required for licensing. The EPPP is a knowledge-based computer examination taken after completion of doctoral and internship training. The association is now developing the EPPP Part 2 (ASPPB, n.d.-b), which is a skills-based computer examination taken after the completion of the EPPP Part 1. These skills include relational skills, intervention and assessment skills, ethics, systems thinking, and professionalism. The exam is expected to be available in 2020.

After accredited graduate and internship programs certify students' competence, and after students pass the EPPP, then regulatory bodies assess applicants' qualifications for licensure. The association has decided that it is also important to include periodic assessment of ongoing competence for licensure to assure the public of the currency of practitioners' knowledge and skills (ASPPB, 2014). The nature of this periodic assessment is under discussion, but it is proposed to involve self-assessment and the creation of a Professional Development Plan (using self-reflection, peer review, self-administered or externally administered tests), implementation of the plan (using formal continuing education, academic courses, scientific and clinical literature reviews, review of practice and treatment guidelines supervision or consultation, certifications), and demonstration of competent professional performance (using practice outcome monitoring, external practice audits, patient or client surveys, 360-degree evaluations). Although the current process of continuing education and licensure renewal is designed to address maintenance of competencies, this proposed process formalizes needs assessment, goal identification, and evaluation of outcomes.

Specialties in Psychology

Specialties in professional psychology are defined by having a body of specialized scientific knowledge and professional application that is distinct from other specialties, although there may be some overlap among specialties (APA, Education Directorate, n.d.-i). *Specialties* are defined as having distinct and essential parameters of practice, including specialized (a) populations; (b) psychological, biological, or social problems; and (c) procedures and techniques.

Specialties are recognized by three different processes. The APA Commission for the Recognition of Specialties and Proficiencies in Professional Psychology (2018) recognizes specialties through an evaluation of the distinctiveness of the specialty practice parameters, including the specialized populations, problems, and procedures (APA, Education Directorate, n.d.-i). The ABPP is a governing body that recognizes separately incorporated specialty examining boards. The board defines the areas of practice and the required competencies; the requirements for education, training, and experience; the research bases of the specialty; and specialty practice guidelines. ABPP (n.d.-a) certifies that specialists have successfully completed the educational, training, and experience requirements of the specialty and have passed an examination assess the competencies required in that specialty. The Council of Specialties in Professional Psychology (see https://www.cospp.org/) represents and supports the development and functioning of the recognized specialties in professional psychology. In order for a psychology specialty to be a member of the council, specialties must develop a specialty council consisting of the relevant professional and stakeholder groups to provide for the organized development of the specialty.

Specialization in Psychology

According to APA accreditation guidelines, psychology doctoral and internship training programs are required to emphasize "broad and general training in scientific psychology and in the foundations of practice in health service psychology," while postdoctoral training programs "provide education and training in preparation for health service psychology practice at an advanced level of competency" (APA, 2015b). Doctoral and internship programs have historically occurred in one of three developed practice areas: clinical, counseling, and school psychology (APA, Education Directorate, n.d.-i). However, doctoral and internship programs do not occur within a specialty practice area, such as rehabilitation psychology, health psychology, neuropsychology, or others (although they may have a focus involving a specialty practice area). Specialization in a specialty practice area is usually completed through a postdoctoral residency. Postdoctoral residencies can also be completed for advanced training in the developed practice areas of clinical, counseling, and school psychology. Most psychology specialties have a council of specialty training programs that works to integrate training in the specialty across sites.

In addition to the process developed by ASPPB for maintaining general competencies for licensing, ABPP has developed a method by which specialists periodically engage in self-review to assure maintenance of specialty competencies. The board's Maintenance of Certification requires that specialists certified after January 1, 2015, must undertake a review of their professional development every 10 years in order to maintain their board-certified status granted by ABPP (n.d.-b). This review considers participation in ongoing consultation with peers and ongoing professional education, teaching and training activities, professional leadership roles, and clinical or research program development, as well as the methods by which specialists evaluate their professional work.

EDUCATION AND TRAINING FOR THE SPECIALTY OF REHABILITATION PSYCHOLOGY

Definition of the Specialty

The specialized populations, problems, and procedures that define rehabilitation psychology are listed in Stiers et al. (2012; for a brief summary, see APA, Education Directorate, n.d.-j). The current core competencies of rehabilitation psychology as described by American Board of Rehabilitation Psychology are presented in Chapter 1, this volume. As discussed below in more detail, in July 2017 the Rehabilitation Psychology Specialty Council created a draft revision of the core competencies of rehabilitation psychology for use in APA accreditation procedures, and these are undergoing review.

Education and Training for the Specialty

Education and training in rehabilitation psychology has developed over the past 50 years. Wright (1959) and then others (Cox et al., 2013; Shontz & Wright, 1980) suggested that the preparation of psychologists for work in rehabilitation should involve rehabilitation-specific didactic and experiential training in assessment, treatment, and team consultation regarding persons experiencing chronic injury and illness and their families. Gold, Meltzer, and Sherr (1982) recommended didactic and experiential training in the physical and medical aspects of disability (specialized populations), the psychological and social issues of persons with disabilities (specialized problems), and the relevant diagnostic and intervention techniques for this population (specialized procedures).

Rehabilitation psychology specialty training occurs at the postdoctoral level (Cox et al., 2013, pp. 5, 7). The *Joint Division 22 and ACRM Guidelines for Postdoctoral Training in Rehabilitation Psychology* (Patterson & Hanson, 1995) were the first formal published guidelines for this specialty. These guidelines primarily focused on the structural and process elements of training programs, modeled after the APA requirements for accreditation of training programs as they existed at that time, rather than on any specialty-specific competencies acquired by residents.

Stiers and Stucky (2008) surveyed psychology residency programs in the United States and Canada. They found that compliance with the Patterson and Hanson (1995) *Guidelines* for rehabilitation psychology resident training sites ranged from 73% to 100%. Programs had more variance in meeting the American Board of Rehabilitation Psychology–required competencies, ranging from 7% to 100%. These wide variations reflect the diverse nature of the training programs' structures and processes.

Rehabilitation psychology training guidelines were further developed at the Baltimore Conference on Rehabilitation Psychology Postdoctoral Training. The resulting *Guidelines for Postdoctoral Training in Rehabilitation Psychology* (Stiers et al., 2012, p. 270) recommend that these specialty training programs take place as a formal, organized program in a nationally accredited institution that provides direct interdisciplinary services to individuals with rehabilitation needs; incorporate direct applied experience with persons with acquired disabling conditions; and involve residents working regularly and closely with other rehabilitation practitioners with appropriate didactic series and scheduled supervision. In addition, such training programs were recommended to "consist of an organized, cumulative, logically sequenced program of didactic and experiential education and training activities . . . which are directly linked to the competency goals" (Stiers et al., 2012, p. 272). It is not known how these recommendations have affected education and training in Rehabilitation Psychology.

Foundational Principles of Rehabilitation Psychology

Wright (1983) described 20 value-laden beliefs and principles (pp. x–xxvii) as the foundation of rehabilitation psychology. Stiers (2016) organized these into three areas—individual psychological processes, social psychological processes, and values related to social integration—and reviewed the existing literature relevant to these. They also reviewed the existing literature relevant to teaching methods for the foundational principles, including methods for reducing group prejudice and promoting values related to the foundational principles. A "core curriculum" was identified with key readings and suggestions for teaching in each of these three areas.

American Board of Rehabilitation Psychology

The American Board of Rehabilitation Psychology (a member of ABPP; see ABPP, n.d.-d) specifies the competencies that are required of psychologists and conducts a credential review, a written practice sample review, and an oral examination to certify psychologists as specialists in rehabilitation psychology

(ABPP, n.d.-a). These expected practitioner competencies provide important direction for defining rehabilitation psychology training program goals.

PSYCHOLOGY TRAINING EVALUATION MODELS

Program Evaluation

Structures, processes, and outcomes. Stiers and Stucky (2008) used a program evaluation model to study rehabilitation psychology postdoctoral training programs, differentiating three elements: (a) structural elements (e.g., program, setting, population, and resources; faculty number and characteristics; resident characteristics); (b) process elements (e.g., didactic activities, numbers and types of patients seen, hours of supervision provided); and (c) outcome elements (e.g., resident competencies and program performance). These three elements constitute a means of conducting program evaluation and improving outcomes. As discussed earlier, in regard to resident competency outcomes, the Stiers et al. (2015) proposed competency assessment cube provided specific structured observations for the competencies specific to rehabilitation psychology. Structured observation has significant strengths in reliability, validity, and feasibility, and other methods listed in the assessment cube have not been well developed in psychology.

Workforce needs analysis. An important component of evaluating rehabilitation psychology training programs is to determine whether these programs meet an existing need. There are approximately 106,000 doctoral-level licensed psychologists in the United States (Lin, Christidis, & Stamm, 2016a), with higher concentrations located in the Northeast, along the Pacific coast, and generally in urban areas, but broad portions of the Midwest have few or none. In 2013, approximately 16% of behavioral and social science providers were psychologists, with larger numbers of counselors and social workers (APA, 2014). The highest numbers of persons experiencing disability are located in the Appalachia region (Myers, Greiman, von Reichert, & Seekins, 2016), but this area has the lowest numbers of psychologists (Lin, Christidis, & Stamm, 2016b). Thus, the areas with the largest number of persons with disability have few psychologists in general, and few rehabilitation psychologists specifically. This indicates an ongoing need for rehabilitation psychology training programs and especially for training programs that emphasize care in rural areas. This mismatch between the location of practitioners and those in need of services is common to all health professions.

Accreditation

The APA Commission on Accreditation accredits doctoral, internship, and residency training programs (APA, 2015a). The commission does not mandate program content or methods, but rather assesses the clarity of the program aims and outcomes, the sufficiency of resources and the adequacy of processes, and the effectiveness of achieving its outcomes. However, the commission does mandate that doctoral students must demonstrate competence in the following areas: research; ethical and legal standards; individual and cultural diversity; professional values, attitudes, and behaviors; communication and interpersonal skills; assessment; intervention; supervision; and consultation and interprofessional–interdisciplinary skills.

For each competency, the program must specify how it evaluates student performance and provide outcome data that demonstrate that all students have reached the appropriate level of achievement. For program graduates, the program must provide evidence of program effectiveness by tracking graduates' career paths after they have left the program. Recent changes in APA Standards on Accreditation (APA, 2015a) state that postdoctoral training programs must ensure that residents attain advanced competencies in the professionwide areas of integration of science and practice, individual and cultural diversity, and ethical and legal issues, and then also in the specialty competencies as defined by the specialty's education and training guidelines. The Rehabilitation Psychology Specialty Council, with its member organizations (APA Division 22, American Board of Rehabilitation Psychology, Council of Rehabilitation Psychology Postdoctoral Training Programs, and the Academy for Rehabilitation Psychology), has defined the specialty-specific competencies that will be used by the APA/Commission on Accreditation in their accreditation reviews of rehabilitation psychology postdoctoral training programs. At present those specialty-specific competencies are undergoing review by APA and will then be put out for public comment and revised accordingly.

PSYCHOLOGY POSTDOCTORAL FUNDING MODELS

Training programs, of course, require funding. Stiers and Stucky (2008) surveyed rehabilitation psychology postdoctoral training programs and found that most residents were supported through general hospital budgets or service line budgets (64%), faculty billing or collections (28%), Veterans Administration federal funds (25%), and training grants (11%). Very few (6%) received funding from the Center for Medicare and Medicaid Studies. Hospital or service line budgets may pay for resident salaries and benefits, to the extent that the residents can demonstrate that they contribute positively to patient care and program outcomes. Some training programs support residents out of clinical billing by training supervisors, and in some environments the residents' contribution to increased billing can help support this. In some states, psychology residents can receive a limited or provisional license that allows billing (ASPPB, n.d.-a). Although Medicare does not allow graduate students to bill as technicians (see Puente, 2015, Slide 300), postdoctoral residents are employees and can provide testing services. Postdoctoral residents cannot bill "incident to" or technician services in a hospital inpatient setting (Centers for Medicare and Medicaid Services, 2016), but they can do so in an outpatient practice, conducting both testing and intervention billable services under appropriate supervision.

The Veterans Administration emphasizes that training is one of the core missions, and it funds internships and residencies. Its psychology training slots expanded during the period 2011–2016, but most have been for new Neuropsychology programs. No proposals occurred for new Rehabilitation Psychology programs, and there have been unfilled residency positions in Rehabilitation Psychology (Kenneth Jones, Director, Associated Health Education, Office of Academic Affiliations, Department of Veterans Affairs, personal communication, September 12, 2016). Developing Veterans Administration Rehabilitation Psychology postdoctoral training programs appears important.

The Centers for Medicaid and Medicare Studies provides financial support for faculty and residents in psychology training programs, as is provided for medical residency programs (see Stucky, Buterakos, Crystal, & Hanks, 2008, for a description of center-funded psychology postdoctoral training programs). However, the psychology residents must be employed by a hospital (like medical residents). Most postdoctoral psychology residents are employed by a university. Psychology's inability to navigate this requirement has largely excluded it from Graduate Medical Education, the single largest source of funding for education in the United States.

The Graduate Psychology Education program, through the Bureau of Health Professions of the Health Resources and Services Administration, provides grants to APA-accredited psychology doctoral, internship, and postdoctoral training programs to create new training positions focusing on vulnerable and underserved populations such as older adults, children, individuals with chronic illness, veterans, victims of abuse, unemployed persons, and victims of natural disasters, in both rural and urban communities. Psychology trainees must train with two or more other health professions (e.g., medicine, nursing, allied health, and pharmacy).

The Health Resources and Services Administration's Behavioral Health Workforce Education and Training program also provides funds for training (Health Resources & Services Administration, n.d.). Programs are required to provide interprofessional training for services to underserved populations.

RESOURCES FOR REHABILITATION PSYCHOLOGY POSTDOCTORAL TRAINING PROGRAMS

Resources for Competency Development and Assessment

Rehabilitation psychology postdoctoral training programs may benefit from the wealth of information provided through APA's competencies benchmarks initiatives regarding conceptualization and measurement of psychology competencies (see APA, Education Directorate, n.d.-k). APA has defined competencies, the essential components of those competencies, and categories of competencies, and it has described each competency in terms of level expected for readiness for practicum, readiness for internship, and readiness for practice, illustrated by a set of observable behaviors. APA has developed and made available specific rating forms related to psychology competencies (APA, n.d.-b, n.d.-c) that can provide valuable resources for training programs.

Clearly, training and education in rehabilitation psychology must focus on development of the specialty-specific competencies that define the field. However, the specialty-specific competencies of rehabilitation psychology have been defined in different ways by different sources. In the publications arising from the Baltimore Conference on Rehabilitation Psychology Postdoctoral Training (Stiers et al., 2012, 2015), similar but not identical competencies were defined. Cox et al. (2013) proposed similar, but not identical, competencies. Although competencies may be grouped under different categories or have different names, there is a clear consensus about the populations and problems with which rehabilitation psychologists work, the procedures they employ, and the types of competencies that are required.

The Council of Rehabilitation Psychology Postdoctoral Training Programs is a membership organization that functions to promote state-of-the-art education and training in rehabilitation psychology training programs. Council members benefit by being able to obtain help in developing and maintaining rehabilitation psychology residency training programs, assistance in implementing specialty-specific competency-based curricula, support in the professional development of rehabilitation psychology trainers, opportunities to network with others involved in specialty-specific postdoctoral training, and assistance in developing empirical quality improvement evaluation methods.

Resources for Training Problems and Conflicts

Trainees with competency problems. APA (n.d.-c) has developed a template for documenting and addressing trainee competency issues. This template distinguishes problems with foundational competencies (professionalism, reflective practice–self-assessment–self-care, scientific knowledge and methods, relationships, individual and cultural diversity, ethical and legal standards and policy, and interdisciplinary systems) from problems with functional competencies (assessment, intervention, consultation, research–evaluation, supervision, teaching, management-administration, and advocacy). The template provides a structure to document the problem behaviors, expectations for acceptable performance, trainee's and supervisors' responsibilities to improve the competency problems, how competencies will be reassessed, a time frame for reassessment, and the consequences for unsuccessful remediation.

Trainees reporting values conflicts. Occasionally, a trainee may object to working with certain types of patients. For example, some trainees have objected to providing services to transgender individuals or to same-sex couples because their values conflict with the goal of treatment. This has led a few state legislators to propose legislation that would prohibit "public institutions of higher education from disciplining or discriminating against a student in a counseling, social work, or psychology program" who "refuses to counsel or serve a client as to goals, outcomes, or behaviors that conflict with a sincerely held religious belief of the student" (APA, 2015c).

APA has worked to distinguish these "conscience clauses" from competency issues and has emphasized that psychology training programs are responsible for preparing a workforce trained to meet the needs of a diverse client population. Therefore, psychology trainees must be able to provide services to diverse individuals, whether or not they would choose to work with such individuals after completion of training. This doesn't just apply to students who may object to same-sex relationships, but it also applies to any students with beliefs that might conflict with providing competent care; for example, a student should not refuse to provide services to clients with racist beliefs (Clay, 2015; see also APA, Education Directorate, n.d.-l). Suggestions for training programs is this area can be found in *Preparing Professional Psychologists to Serve a Diverse Public: Addressing Conflicts between Professional Competence and Trainee Beliefs* (APA, 2013).

THE FUTURE OF EDUCATION AND TRAINING IN REHABILITATION PSYCHOLOGY

A number of factors affect the future practice of rehabilitation psychologists, and therefore the education and training of rehabilitation psychologists must keep pace with these changing practice requirements. First, health care provision and payment structures are becoming increasingly focused on maintaining health rather than treating illness and on managing chronic diseases to reduce illness episodes. Chronic diseases are responsible for seven in 10 deaths among Americans each year and account for 86% of the approximate $3 trillion U.S. annual health care costs (National Center for Chronic Disease Prevention and Health Promotion, n.d.). Health care systems and teams will become increasingly responsible for the health of defined populations. In the past, psychologists were primarily thought of as mental health providers. Today, psychologists are behavioral health providers and will go on to be simply health care providers, working in interprofessional teams focused on illness prevention and health management. Rehabilitation psychologists have specialized competencies in working with recovery from illness or injury, and self-management of chronic disease and disability, including work with patients, families, treatment teams, and institutions. Training in rehabilitation psychology has emphasized work with interdisciplinary teams for more than 60 years. It is important to communicate this expertise to other health care disciplines through interprofessional publications and presentations.

Second, rehabilitation specialists are recognized as specialists in function. Function cuts across levels of care (acute, subacute, and chronic), across demographics (age, gender, race), and across types of conditions (physical, cognitive, emotional); thus, it is an appropriate focus for all persons with acute or chronic health conditions. Rehabilitation psychologists have specialized competencies in assessing functional outcomes and using these data to improve clinical care. Rehabilitation psychology education and training needs to have an increasing focus on the collection and application of basic functional data regarding our patients and teams and the use of these data for program improvement.

Third, rehabilitation services in general are undergoing a transformation from traditional practice models to expanded practice models. Rehabilitation practitioners are applying their specialization in assessing and treating function in many settings beyond inpatient rehabilitation hospitals and outpatient rehabilitation clinics, including "pre-habilitation" for persons with pending health crises (e.g., approaching a major surgery), early mobilization in intensive care settings, and increasing functional activities in acute medical settings, subacute community rehabilitation centers, and long-term care centers. Thus, rehabilitation psychology education and training should also provide opportunities for exposure to these varieties of settings. Although such opportunities may be limited in some programs, it may be possible to arrange minor experiences, brief rotations to other institutions, or directed readings and discussions focused on these developing rehabilitation settings.

Fourth, the use of web-based resources to support disease and chronic-condition self-management, supported by e-mail and telephone consultation, has the demonstrated potential to improve health outcomes while increasing the efficiency of rehabilitation psychologist's work (Castillo et al., 2013; Dattalo et al., 2012; Skolasky, Maggard, Wegener, & Riley, 2018). Training programs should ensure that trainees are familiar with these existing resources.

Fifth, another consideration is whether psychology at large, and rehabilitation psychology specifically, might follow the models developed by physician, nursing, and rehabilitation therapy colleagues. Each of those rehabilitation specialties has fully qualified and licensed professionals and auxiliary or mid-level providers, such as physician assistants, nurses aids, and physical therapy aids. Rehabilitation psychologists could benefit from working with master's level providers to help carry out plans of care established by the psychologist. As has been discussed, there are tensions between doctoral psychologists and some master's level counselors because of the long history of APA focusing only on doctoral-level psychologists. However, there are a large number psychology master's programs, and a number of states allow persons with master's degrees to work as psychology associates under the supervision of a licensed psychologist. This is a natural model for rehabilitation psychologists and could facilitate the expanded practice models described above. This model has also been suggested as a valuable approach to providing rehabilitation psychology services in underserved international areas (Frank, 2017).

Finally, a significant challenge for rehabilitation psychologists is the workforce pipeline. This is a problem for psychology specialties in general. Neuropsychology has become widely known, but often doctoral students and interns are not familiar with rehabilitation psychology or other specialties. There are efforts to make information about psychology specialties more commonly available to doctoral students and interns, including efforts by the ABPP (n.d.-c) and the Council of Specialties in Professional Psychology (2016; see the entry specific to rehabilitation psychology). The APA Division 22-Rehabilitation Psychology Student Leadership Network (Rehabilitation Psychology, n.d.), involving 13 doctoral training programs, is an important means of helping doctoral students become familiar with this specialty.

CONCLUSION

Discussion about the best education and training in rehabilitation psychology has been an important topic for as long as the specialty has existed. Today, rehabilitation psychology has clearly established parameters in relation to other psychology specialties. Rehabilitation psychology is developing increasingly sophisticated and detailed approaches to defining, teaching, and measuring the specialty competencies. Rehabilitation psychology is creating expanded opportunities to use these skills outside of traditional rehabilitation settings, necessitating that training programs keep pace with these new developments. In regard to future research, new types of assessments of trainee competencies specific to rehabilitation psychology need to be developed, and their psychometric properties studied, so that accurate and effective data can be examined for training program improvement.

References

American Board of Professional Psychology. (n.d.-a). *The certification & examination process*. Retrieved from https://legacy.abpp.org/i4a/pages/index.cfm?pageid=3475

American Board of Professional Psychology. (n.d.-b). Maintenance of certification information. Retrieved from https://legacy.abpp.org/i4a/pages/index.cfm?pageid=3892

American Board of Professional Psychology. (n.d.-c). Information for educators & trainers. Retrieved from https://legacy.abpp.org/i4a/pages/index.cfm?pageid=3793

American Board of Professional Psychology. (n.d.-d). *Member specialty boards*. Retrieved from https://www.abpp.org/Applicant-Information/Specialty-Boards.aspx

American Psychological Association. (n.d.-a). *125th Anniversary APA timeline*. Retrieved from http://www.apa.org/about/apa/archives/timeline.aspx

American Psychological Association. (n.d.-b). *Competency benchmarks in professional psychology: Appendix*. Washington, DC: Author. Retrieved from http://www.apa.org/ed/graduate/rating-form-appendix.doc

American Psychological Association. (n.d.-c). *Competency remediation plan*. Washington, DC: Author. Retrieved from http://www.apa.org/ed/graduate/competency-remediation-template.doc

American Psychological Association. (2004). *Developing and evaluating standards and guidelines related to education and training in psychology: Context, procedures, criteria, and format*. Retrieved from https://www.apa.org/about/policy/bea-guidelines.pdf

American Psychological Association. (2011a). *National standards for high school psychology curricula*. Retrieved from http://www.apa.org/education/k12/psychology-curricula.pdf

American Psychological Association. (2011b). *Principles for quality undergraduate education in psychology*.

Retrieved from https://www.apa.org/education/undergrad/principles.aspx

American Psychological Association. (2013). *Preparing professional psychologists to serve a diverse public*. Retrieved from http://www.apa.org/ed/graduate/diversity-preparation.aspx

American Psychological Association. (2014). *What proportion of the nation's behavioral health providers are psychologists?* Retrieved from http://www.apa.org/monitor/2014/09/datapoint.aspx

American Psychological Association. (2015a). *Standards of accreditation for health service psychology*. Retrieved from http://www.apa.org/ed/accreditation/about/policies/standards-of-accreditation.pdf

American Psychological Association. (2015b). *Standards and criteria for approval of sponsors of continuing education for psychologists*. Washington, DC: Author. Retrieved from https://www.apa.org/about/policy/approval-standards.pdf

American Psychological Association. (2015c). *The "conscience clause" in professional training*. Retrieved from http://www.apa.org/ed/graduate/conscience-clause-brief.aspx

American Psychological Association. (2016). *Proceedings of the summit on master's training in psychological practice*. Retrieved from http://www.apa.org/pi/mfp/masters-summit/training-proceedings.pdf

American Psychological Association, Commission for the Recognition of Specialties and Proficiencies in Professional Psychology. (2018). *Mission*. Retrieved from https://www.apa.org/ed/graduate/specialize/crsppp.aspx

American Psychological Association, Education Directorate. (n.d.-a). *Programs and services*. Retrieved from https://www.apa.org/ed/index.aspx

American Psychological Association, Education Directorate. (n.d.-b). *APA teachers of psychology in secondary schools*. Retrieved from http://www.apa.org/ed/precollege/topss/index.aspx

American Psychological Association, Education Directorate. (n.d.-c). *About PT@CC*. Retrieved from http://www.apa.org/ed/precollege/undergrad/ptacc/about-ptacc.aspx

American Psychological Association, Education Directorate. (n.d.-d). *BEA Task force on Guidelines for Master's programs in psychology*. Retrieved from https://www.apa.org/ed/governance/bea/masters-guidelines.aspx

American Psychological Association, Education Directorate. (n.d.-e). *BEA Task Force to develop a blueprint for APA accreditation of master's programs in health service psychology*. Retrieved from https://www.apa.org/ed/governance/bea/masters-accreditation-blueprint.aspx

American Psychological Association, Education Directorate. (n.d.-f). *Office of Program consultation and accreditation*. Retrieved from https://www.apa.org/ed/accreditation/index.aspx

American Psychological Association, Education Directorate. (n.d.-g). *About the Office of CE Sponsor Approval*. Retrieved from https://www.apa.org/ed/sponsor/about.aspx

American Psychological Association, Education Directorate. (n.d.-h). *Benchmarks evaluation system*. Retrieved from https://www.apa.org/ed/graduate/benchmarks-evaluation-system.aspx

American Psychological Association, Education Directorate. (n.d.-i). *Principles for the recognition of specialties in professional psychology*. Retrieved from https://www.apa.org/about/policy/principles-recognition.pdf

American Psychological Association, Education Directorate. (n.d.-j). *Rehabilitation psychology*. Retrieved from https://www.apa.org/ed/graduate/specialize/rehabilitation.aspx

American Psychological Association, Education Directorate. (n.d.-k). *Competency initiatives in professional psychology*. Retrieved from https://www.apa.org/ed/graduate/competency.aspx

American Psychological Association, Education Directorate. (n.d.-l). *Serving a diverse public*. Retrieved from https://www.apa.org/ed/graduate/diversity-preparation.aspx

American Psychological Association, Education Directorate. (2018). *Psychology teacher network, 28*(3). Retrieved from http://www.apa.org/ed/precollege/ptn/index.aspx

American Psychological Association, Office of Program Consultation and Accreditation. (n.d.). *Search for accredited programs*. Retrieved from https://apps.apa.org/accredsearch/?_ga=2.15514358.155290998.1538972981-1039252151.1538972981

Association of Psychology Postdoctoral and Internship Centers. (2018). *APPIC policy on doctoral program associates*. Retrieved from https://www.appic.org/About-APPIC/APPIC-Policies/DPA-Policy

Association of State and Provincial Psychology Boards. (n.d.-a). *ASPPB PSY|book: Psychology licensing requirements*. Retrieved from http://psybook.asppb.org

Association of State and Provincial Psychology Boards. (n.d.-b). *Current ASPPB activities*. Retrieved from https://www.asppb.net/page/CurrentActivities

Association of State and Provincial Psychology Boards. (2014). *Maintenance of competence for licensure (MOCL) white paper*. Retrieved from https://c.ymcdn.com/

sites/www.asppb.net/resource/resmgr/Guidelines/Maintenance_of_Competence_fo.pdf

Castillo, R. C., Wegener, S. T., Newell, M. Z., Carlini, A. R., Bradford, A. N., Heins, S. E., . . . Mackenzie, E. J. (2013). Improving outcomes at Level I trauma centers: An early evaluation of the Trauma Survivors Network. *The Journal of Trauma and Acute Care Surgery*, *74*, 1534–1540. http://dx.doi.org/10.1097/TA.0b013e3182921606

Centers for Medicare and Medicaid Services. (2016). *Medicare Learning Network matters* (No. SE0441). Retrieved from https://www.cms.gov/Outreach-and-Education/Medicare-Learning-Network-MLN/MLNMattersArticles/downloads/se0441.pdf

Clay, R. A. (2015). *Competence vs. conscience*. Retrieved from http://www.apa.org/monitor/2015/04/competence.aspx

Council of Specialties in Professional Psychology. (2016). *Resources*. Retrieved from https://www.cospp.org/resources

Cox, D., Cox, R., & Caplan, B. (2013). *Specialty competencies in rehabilitation psychology*. New York, NY: Oxford University Press. http://dx.doi.org/10.1093/med:psych/9780195389241.001.0001

Dattalo, M., Giovannetti, E. R., Scharfstein, D., Boult, C., Wegener, S., Wolff, J. L., . . . Boyd, C. (2012). Who participates in chronic disease self-management (CDSM) programs? Differences between participants and nonparticipants in a population of multimorbid older adults. *Medical Care*, *50*, 1071–1075. http://dx.doi.org/10.1097/MLR.0b013e318268abe7

Frank, R. G. (2017). Hither and thither: How do we innovate? *Rehabilitation Psychology*, *62*, 1–6. http://dx.doi.org/10.1037/rep0000114

Gold, J., Meltzer, R., & Sherr, R. (1982). Professional transitions: Psychology internships in rehabilitation settings. *Professional Psychology*, *13*, 397–403. http://dx.doi.org/10.1037/0735-7028.13.3.397

Health Resources & Services Administration. (n.d.). Behavioral Health Workforce Education and Training (BHWET) program. Retrieved from https://bhw.hrsa.gov/fundingopportunities/?id=67ee4161-1b08-433d-8224-d1e009af2663

Lin, L., Christidis, P., & Stamm, L. (2016a). Datapoint: Where are the highest concentrations of licensed psychologists? *Monitor on Psychology*, *47*(3). Retrieved from http://www.apa.org/monitor/2016/03/datapoint.aspx

Lin, L., Christidis, P., & Stamm, L. (2016b). *2015 County-level analysis of U.S. licensed psychologists and health indicators*. Retrieved from https://www.apa.org/workforce/publications/15-county-analysis/index.aspx

Myers, A., Greiman, L., von Reichert, C., & Seekins, T. (2016). *Rural matters: The geography of disability in rural America*. Missoula: The University of Montana Rural Institute for Inclusive Communities. Retrieved from http://rtc.ruralinstitute.umt.edu/research-findings/geography/

National Center for Chronic Disease Prevention and Health Promotion. (n.d.). *At a glance 2016: National Center for Chronic Disease Prevention and Health Promotion*. Retrieved from https://www.cdc.gov/chronicdisease/resources/publications/aag/pdf/2016/nccdphp-aag.pdf

Patterson, D., & Hanson, S. (1995). Joint Division 22 and ACRM Guidelines for Postdoctoral Training in Rehabilitation Psychology. *Rehabilitation Psychology*, *40*, 299–310. http://dx.doi.org/10.1037/0090-5550.40.4.299

Puente, A. E. (2015). *Coding, billing & documenting professional psychological services*. Retrieved from http://psychologycoding.org/wp-content/uploads/2015/09/CPT-09.15.151.pdf

Rehabilitation Psychology. (n.d.). *Student leadership network*. Retrieved from http://www.div22.org/student-leadership-network

Rodolfa, E., Bent, R., Eisman, E., Nelson, P., Rehm, L., & Ritchie, P. (2005). A cube model for competency development: Implications for psychology educators and regulators. *Professional Psychology: Research and Practice*, *36*, 347–354. http://dx.doi.org/10.1037/0735-7028.36.4.347

Shontz, F., & Wright, B. (1980). The distinctiveness of rehabilitation psychology. *Professional Psychology*, *11*, 919–924. http://dx.doi.org/10.1037/0735-7028.11.6.919

Skolasky, R. L., Maggard, A. M., Wegener, S. T., & Riley, L. H., III. (2018). Telephone-based intervention to improve rehabilitation engagement after spinal stenosis surgery: A prospective lagged controlled trial. *The Journal of Bone and Joint Surgery*, *100*, 21–30. http://dx.doi.org/10.2106/JBJS.17.00418

Stiers, W. (2016). Teaching the foundational principles of rehabilitation psychology. *Rehabilitation Psychology*, *61*, 54–64. http://dx.doi.org/10.1037/rep0000078

Stiers, W., Barisa, M., Stucky, K., Pawlowski, C., Van Tubbergen, M., Turner, A. P., . . . Caplan, B. (2015). Guidelines for competency development and measurement in rehabilitation psychology postdoctoral training. *Rehabilitation Psychology*, *60*, 111–122. http://dx.doi.org/10.1037/a0038353

Stiers, W., Hanson, S., Turner, A. P., Stucky, K., Barisa, M., Brownsberger, M., . . . the Council of Rehabilitation

Psychology Postdoctoral Training Programs. (2012). Guidelines for postdoctoral training in rehabilitation psychology. *Rehabilitation Psychology*, *57*, 267–279. http://dx.doi.org/10.1037/a0030774

Stiers, W., & Stucky, K. (2008). A survey of training in rehabilitation psychology practice in the United States and Canada: 2007. *Rehabilitation Psychology*, *53*, 536–543. http://dx.doi.org/10.1037/a0013827

Stucky, K., Buterakos, J., Crystal, T., & Hanks, R. (2008). Acquiring CMS funding for an APA-accredited post-doctoral psychology fellowship program. *Training and Education in Professional Psychology*, *2*, 165–175. http://dx.doi.org/10.1037/1931-3918.2.3.165

U.S. Department of Health and Human Services. (n.d.). *Defining the PCMH*. Retrieved from https://pcmh.ahrq.gov/page/defining-pcmh

Wright, B. (1959). *Psychology and rehabilitation*. Washington, DC: American Psychological Association. http://dx.doi.org/10.1037/10539-000

Wright, B. A. (1983). *Physical disability—A psychosocial approach* (2nd ed.). New York, NY: HarperCollins. http://dx.doi.org/10.1037/10589-000

Chapter 3

REHABILITATION PSYCHOLOGY RESEARCH, SCIENCE, AND SCHOLARSHIP

Timothy R. Elliott and Lisa A. Brenner

In 2015, the American Psychological Association (APA) formally recognized rehabilitation psychology as a "specialty," "a defined area of psychological practice which requires advanced knowledge and skills acquired through an organized sequence of education and training" (APA, 2018, "About Specialties," para. 1). Guidance put forth by APA also suggests that all professional specialties share a "core" of psychological "scientific and professional knowledge, skills, and attitudes" (APA Council of Representatives, 2011, p. 1). Although "dimensions" of formal training in a specialty may vary,

> every defined specialty in professional psychology will contain: (a) core scientific foundations in psychology; (b) a basic professional foundation; (c) advanced scientific and theoretical knowledge germane to the specialty; and, (d) advanced professional application of this knowledge through procedures and techniques that are validated for use with the problems, populations and settings specific to the specialty. (APA Council of Representatives, 2011, p. 3)

These criteria emphasize the importance of establishing rehabilitation psychology research in foundational psychological scientific principles, while at the same time addressing means of implementing evidence-based strategies among those with disabilities and chronic health conditions to maximize health, function, and participation across the lifespan.

In this chapter, we provide a brief overview of the evolution of the rehabilitation psychology research agenda to highlight the instrumental role that psychological science and scholarship played in the development of rehabilitation psychology. This is followed by an overview of the challenges faced by rehabilitation psychologists, which in part are related to rehabilitation psychology practice traditionally occurring in medical schools and settings (vs. community-based settings and psychology departments). We discuss issues in current rehabilitation psychology scholarship—an overarching term that encompasses the published literature germane to the specialty (including "thought" and opinion pieces, policy statements, pedagogical works, scientific epistemology, and empirical studies)—followed by several recommendations that stem from classic scientist–practitioner training models in professional psychology to advance rehabilitation psychology scholarship.

HISTORICAL CONTEXT

At the 1959 Princeton Conference, participants discussing the role of psychologists in rehabilitation agreed that most problems in rehabilitation were essentially psychological (Wright, 1959, p. 83).

http://dx.doi.org/10.1037/0000129-004
Handbook of Rehabilitation Psychology, Third Edition, L. A. Brenner, S. A. Reid-Arndt, T. R. Elliott, R. G. Frank, and B. Caplan (Editors-in-Chief)

With some minor editing to update the terminology, the research agenda for rehabilitation identified during the conference essentially reflects current interest areas (see Table 7, p. 80, and Appendix IV in Wright, 1959). Although conference participants recognized the stress inherent in balancing the dual role of clinician and "researcher," the conference proceedings noted that the psychologist should maintain "identification with the basic science of psychology" and stay current with advances in the field (Wright, 1959, p. 79).

At the subsequent 1960 Miami Beach conference, attendees addressed the unique perspectives and expertise psychological research could bring to the rehabilitation enterprise. They empaneled psychologists with established scholarly records in subareas of psychology to discuss these issues (Lofquist, 1960, p. 1). Participants recognized the interdisciplinary nature of rehabilitation and the critical need for external funding to advance psychological science and scholarship in rehabilitation.

Steady and remarkable changes have occurred over the years in rehabilitation research, with rehabilitation psychologists playing prominent roles in this process. For example, rehabilitation psychologists actively participate in many of the largest, ongoing research projects funded by federal agencies germane to persons with catastrophic injuries (Traumatic Brain Injury Model Systems, http://www.msktc.org/tbi/model-system-centers; Spinal Cord Injury Model Systems, http://www.msktc.org/sci/model-system-centers). At present, rehabilitation psychologists serve as editors of leading peer-reviewed journals in rehabilitation (*Archives of Physical Medicine and Rehabilitation*, *The Journal of Head Trauma Rehabilitation*), interdisciplinary journals associated with rehabilitation (*Brain Injury*, *Sexuality and Disability*), and journals affiliated with psychology (*Rehabilitation Psychology*, *Journal of Clinical Psychology*) and counseling (*Rehabilitation Counseling Bulletin*).

For decades, rehabilitation psychologists have served on grant panels for federal and private funding agencies and participated in committees to identify funding priorities. Rehabilitation psychologists have worked with interdisciplinary committees evaluating and documenting the evidence base for rehabilitation treatments (e.g., Cicerone et al., 2011) to establish the state of the science, influence policies, and spearhead efforts to refine and advance specific methodologies (e.g., participatory action research; Ehde et al., 2013). In physical medicine and rehabilitation departments, it is common practice for a rehabilitation psychologist to teach basic and advanced research methods and statistical procedures for departmental colleagues, staff, and fellows. Indeed, rehabilitation psychologists may be considered among the pioneers of interdisciplinary collaborations that are idealized in current models of interprofessional health care services and research (Spring, Hall, Moller, & Falk-Krzesinski, 2012).

Consistent with the spirit of the Princeton and Miami Beach conferences, we, along with other rehabilitation psychology researchers, have long advocated that "psychologists with a strong identity and commitment to the science and practice of psychology" (Elliott & Gramling, 1990, p. 765) benefit the field of rehabilitation. This commitment includes an ongoing appreciation of theory and testable hypotheses in psychological and rehabilitation research (Dunn & Elliott, 2008) and receptivity to and facility with contemporary and advanced research methodologies and statistical procedures (Elliott, 2002).

Rehabilitation is an interdisciplinary endeavor, and rehabilitation psychology is often conceptualized as being embedded in these collaborations (Elliott & Rath, 2012). This may present unintended challenges for active scholars in rehabilitation psychology because it necessitates staying current with cutting-edge theoretical and methodological innovations in both the extant psychological and physical medicine and rehabilitative literatures. This is likely compounded by existing challenges to contemporary science including (a) declines in financial support—from state and federal sources—for both individual scholars and academic institutions, (b) limitations with current methodologies, (c) challenges associated with replication and reproducibility, and (d) inattentiveness to the importance of communicating science to a wide range of stakeholders (Brenner, 2017). Controversies that erode the public trust in psychological research—including allegations of "*p*-hacking" (to find significant results; Simmons, Nelson, & Simonsohn, 2011), "HARK-ing" (i.e., hypothesizing after results are known), and clinician inattention to evidence-based practices (Baker, McFall, & Shoham, 2008)—amplify the need for us to examine ongoing and emerging issues relevant to both our scholarly base and consumers of scholarship. This includes some reflection about the relative merits and trade-offs of rehabilitation psychology and its role in an interdisciplinary environment.

INTERDISCIPLINARY RESEARCH: BENEFITS AND NATURAL LIMITATIONS

Interdisciplinary research merges knowledge and expertise across traditional professional boundaries to generate and examine potential solutions to the complex problems facing our communities and our society (Leahey, 2016; National Academies, 2005). Federal funding agencies place a high premium on interdisciplinary research projects that address priorities identified by an array of stakeholders that may include researchers, service providers, consumers, and policymakers (e.g., elected officials). This process values applied, pragmatic solutions in a multidisciplinary context.

Many professions participate in the delivery of clinical rehabilitation services, the development of meaningful and reasonable policies that support and advance them, and the nurturing of its literature and knowledge base. Interdisciplinary research projects and services work best when collaborators share a common agenda and regard each other with mutual respect, sensitivity, and a sense of trust and reciprocity that ideally facilitates an open and equitable exchange of ideas to benefit each participating member (Boix Mansilla, Lamont, & Sato, 2016; Elliott, 2016; Maton, Perkins, & Saegert, 2006). This includes decisions about what research ideas may be potentially fundable, what grant proposals are to be developed, who will serve as key team members, where studies from the project will be presented and eventually published, and who will serve as first and "trailing" authors (Leahey, 2016). Decisions about publication outlets and authorship may be influenced by concerns about promoting the reputation of the home department and by the needs of individual collaborators for promotion and tenure in their respective academic departments. Junior colleagues, in particular, stand to lose much in interdisciplinary endeavors if they appear on a preponderance of papers as a "trailing author," raising doubts about the quality and status of their research program, specifically, and their capacity to conduct and report research as an independent scholar, generally (Maton et al., 2006). Such decisions require ongoing deliberations and time commitments, and misalignments between any of these goals can contribute to an array of tensions, conflicts, and role strain, and undermine communication essential to the success of collaborative research endeavors (Leahey, 2016; O'Rourke, 2017).

Sechrest and Smith (1994) observed that interdisciplinary collaborations succeed as long as they can reconcile and navigate real differences that exist between professions. Each profession has legitimate differences in terms of content areas, epistemology, skills, and their "own idiosyncratic means of discovering and justifying knowledge" that may, at times, be irreconcilable (Sechrest & Smith, 1994, p. 12). Successful and productive collaborations between professions depend on the degree to which the parties agree on (a) the research problems to be studied, (b) the measurement methodology and corresponding instrumentation and tools, (c) the use of experimental and intervention methodologies, and (d) the theoretical accounts of the issues to be studied (Sechrest & Smith, 1994).

Points of Congruence and Divergence

Consistent with Sechrest and Smith's (1994) observations, we see successful and productive collaborations between colleagues from other professions and rehabilitation psychologists who have a primary identity with rehabilitation medicine. This is apparent in the funded research conducted by the various Model Systems sites (notably in traumatic brain injury, spinal cord injury, and burn rehabilitation). Other examples include projects that address contemporary issues that appear in the clinic (e.g., changes in etiology, secondary complications, demographics) and topics associated with the acute and postacute evaluation of individuals who received rehabilitation services. Information from the Model Systems projects has been critical to developing, planning, and updating inpatient and postacute rehabilitation services.

There is also considerable congruence between rehabilitation psychology and other rehabilitation professions in using research to inform policy that best shapes practice. Rehabilitation psychologists work with stakeholders on grant panels (to identify priorities to be addressed in future grant announcements and to evaluate potentially fundable projects) and on various committees empaneled by professional associations to identify evidence-based practices in rehabilitation research and service (e.g., see Issue 8, Supplement 2 of the 2012 volume of the *Archives of Physical Medicine and Rehabilitation*).

Shared values are also apparent between rehabilitation psychologists and interdisciplinary collaborators in regard to measurement methodology, a critical element in the Sechrest and Smith (1994) essay. In fact, rehabilitation psychologists play an integral and essential role in developing, studying, and refining assessment tools to measure issues germane to rehabilitation, including functional abilities and impairment, psychological adjustment, neurobehavioral functioning, quality of life, and rehabilitation outcomes. For example, Allen Heinemann, an eminent rehabilitation psychologist who has studied instrumentation and measurement issues in functional impairment and outcomes and quality of life following disability, is the fourth most-published author in the history of the *Archives of Physical Medicine and Rehabilitation* (according to current data obtained from the online Web of Science search engine). Heinemann and other rehabilitation psychologists were among the leaders in developing the standardized patient-oriented outcome measures for use in research and clinical protocols in an ambitious project supported by the National Institutes of Health (Patient-Reported Outcomes Measurement Information System; http://www.nihpromis.org/). These scales are now available to clinicians, researchers, and administrators to facilitate a common bank of outcome measures for research and practice across broad domains of physical, mental, and social health.

Other work concerning measurement and evaluation in rehabilitation illustrates the ways in which rehabilitation psychologists share common research goals with the larger interdisciplinary agenda. Rehabilitation psychologists use their expertise in assessment, scale development, and statistical techniques to evaluate the psychometric properties of instruments that may be used in the rehabilitation setting. This work often concerns determining the validity of certain instruments for use with individuals with different disabling conditions and examining the underlying structures of these instruments. This is evident in the preponderance of factor analytic studies of various depression measures throughout the rehabilitation literature. This research is needed to determine the suitability and the validity of instruments for use with individuals with different disabling conditions (e.g., spinal cord injury, traumatic brain injury). Unfortunately, this kind of research becomes needlessly incremental when it fails to inform clinical practice beyond what we already know (e.g., beyond the typical "cognitive–somatic" factor structure), attends to obscure or outdated instruments, or relies on flimsy "straw man" arguments as a study rationale that, in turn, result in uninteresting, atheoretical, and/or trivial findings.

Rehabilitation psychologists also contribute to advancements in rehabilitation science as they learn and promote new methods that engage stakeholders in the research process (e.g., participatory action research methods, focus groups, qualitative studies) and examine issues and propose solutions to methodological conundrums that adversely affect studies critical to evidence-based practice (in conducting randomized clinical trials [RCTs]: Hart & Bagiella, 2012; Tate, Kalpakjian, & Kwon, 2008; designing control groups: Hart, Fann, & Novack, 2008). Rehabilitation psychologists also recommend guidelines for improved use and reporting of statistical information (e.g., see the special issue on research and methodological issues and advances in the 2008 volume of *Rehabilitation Psychology*) and examine, demonstrate, and advocate for the use of contemporary analytic techniques in rehabilitation research (structural equation modeling: Chan, Lee, Lee, Kubota, & Allen, 2007; hierarchical linear modeling: Kwok et al., 2008).

The Kwok et al. (2008) paper on multilevel modeling (MLM) illustrates an interesting point of divergence. As discussed in their introduction, multilevel and growth modeling techniques were used in educational and psychological research for 2 decades; their first appearance in the rehabilitation literature occurred in 1995 (Clay, Wood, Frank, Hagglund, & Johnson, 1995). Despite the acceptance and usage in these broader fields of inquiry, Kwok et al. observed that few studies using MLM could be found in the rehabilitation psychology literature, "implying that the field has yet to realize the potential and the possibilities of these approaches" (p. 371). MLM and other growth modeling techniques were ideally suited for use in studies of any of the large, longitudinal databases available in rehabilitation.

In the years following Kwok et al. (2008), MLM techniques now appear regularly in the rehabilitation literature. This may be due, in part, to the influence of this article (the Kwok et al., 2008, paper is now listed by the online Web of Science search engine as the sixth-most frequently cited paper in the history of the *Rehabilitation Psychology* journal, $n = 134$; the majority of these citations occurred in outlets associated with the research terms *psychology*, *rehabilitation*, and/or *neurosciences neurology*). A subsequent paper in the 2013 volume of the *Archives of Physical Medicine and Rehabilitation* provided a demonstration of growth curve modeling with data from the Traumatic Brain Injury Model Systems project for the larger rehabilitation audience, in effect "vetting" these techniques for future use by rehabilitation researchers (Kozlowski, Pretz, Dams-O'Connor, Kreider, & Whiteneck, 2013).

The question remains, Why would it take 20 years after accepted use in education and psychology before rehabilitation researchers would embrace these techniques? Several dynamics may account for this delay. Interdisciplinary research is a time-consuming effort, and it is difficult for collaborators to stay current with innovations in their "home" disciplines while simultaneously participating in activities that address the problems shared by the interdisciplinary team. This cognitive "cost" and accompanying role strain for collaborators is an understudied aspect of interdisciplinary work that contributes to a "jack-of-all-trades, master of none" characterization of individuals in team science (Leahey, Beckman, & Stanko, 2017).

There may also be some degree of intellectual marginalization that occurs for rehabilitation psychologists participating in these efforts. Each profession in rehabilitation has recognized strengths and assets, and statistical and analytic expertise is often accorded to colleagues who have specialized and advanced training in these areas. Quite often, a designated "statistician" or "methodologist" for a research team is expected by a funding agency, and this role is then assumed by a colleague with an advanced degree in a discipline other than psychology. However, the best psychological research analytic techniques are dictated by the theoretical models that inform the hypotheses to be tested, and in this, analytic techniques are chosen because they provide appropriate tests of the theory. Consequently, differences in theoretical orientation between the professions may account for the delay in applying certain analytic techniques in rehabilitation research, in a fashion anticipated by the Sechrest and Smith (1994) essay.

Advanced modeling techniques—like growth curve and structural equation models (SEMs)—require a conceptualization of predictor and outcome variables that differs from more traditional approaches. For example, an *outcome* in growth modeling would be the trajectory of adjustment over time, rather than a discrete, single indicator of depression (i.e., the average depression score) or the occurrence of a pressure sore assessed 12 months after discharge. Rather than examine the degree of variance a predictor variable may account for in the single outcome assessed later in time, growth models examine the degree to which predictor variables contribute to the trajectory observed on these variables over time. This distinction is much more compatible with our understanding of individual and environmental differences that contribute to therapeutic and development changes (and a lack of change) over time, anticipated by most theoretical perspectives of adjustment and psychotherapy. Similarly, SEM allows for the study of observed variables (i.e., manifest) and latent constructs for advanced tests of theorized relationships between them (Chan et al., 2007; Weston, Gore,

Chan, & Catalano, 2008). These, too, necessitate a greater understanding of and facility with theoretical models and hypothesized relationships to be tested above and beyond a straightforward focus on a single independent variable and a single dependent variable (typically assessed by one measure or indicator).

SEM can accommodate more than one measure of a construct (an important feature in light of the overlapping variance between usual measures of adjustment). These features are unique strengths of SEM and MLM because they can examine specific dynamics within a larger context that simultaneously take into consideration several co-occurring relationships that exist among an array of variables and constructs. As one example, advanced applications of these contextual models can take into consideration hypothesized relationships between dyads over time and thus permit sophisticated investigations of how the behavior of one individual affects the other over time (e.g., latent growth modeling of caregiver and care recipient responses to a psychological intervention for the caregiver: Berry, Elliott, Grant, Edwards, & Fine, 2012; actor-independence modeling of caregiver and care recipient ratings of patient impairment on their subsequent ratings of caregiver psychosocial dysfunction: Perrin et al., 2017).

Decisions about the best and appropriate use of these techniques from a psychological perspective, then, require a command of the theoretical properties and issues to be tested rather than the expertise of a statistician who may have little, if any, interest in the theoretical matters at stake. Several of the attractive features of SEM and MLM techniques may not seem so to colleagues from other professions who might prefer measures of discrete, "tangible" variables encountered in routine clinical practice (rather than "manifest" variables in SEM). To be fair, there are topical areas in rehabilitation research in which theoretical perspectives have been championed and widely embraced. This is most obvious in the use of item response theory in the development and refinement of measures and scales for various applications (Velozo, Seel, Magasi, Heinemann, & Romero, 2012). This remarkably productive and far-reaching marriage of theory, research, and practice reflects the shared investment all rehabilitation professions have in the need for valid, reliable, and clinically meaningful measures for rehabilitation services and research.

Differences in the appreciation and use of theory exist when epistemological and methodological conflicts occur in identifying what problems are to be studied, why they are to be studied (and why they are important), and how they are to be studied. These questions represent the sine qua non of interdisciplinary endeavors, generally, and the answers are usually determined by group consensus (rather than the agenda of a single scholar or profession). As it is often described by proponents (and critics; see Olkin & Pledger, 2003), contemporary rehabilitation research is often centered on the issues and needs identified by the medical rehabilitation community; as such, this literature reflects the vested interests of health care delivery systems, the doctoral-level providers who operate within them, the policymakers and administrators who work to maintain the system, and the consumers who access them. Although rehabilitation psychology has arguably made great strides to adopt a more "social" model of disability, Olkin (2017) correctly observed that "the settings in which rehabilitation psychologists work tend to be medically oriented . . . entrenched in the medical model" (p. 84).

Most research projects supported by external funds operate within this enterprise. Framed in this context, we can understand why rehabilitation psychology's contributions in instrumentation and measurement are valued in rehabilitation research. But the long-standing affiliation with the medical model has the potential to exert an influence on rehabilitation psychology research that can thwart the application of cutting-edge theoretical models and accompanying variables used by other colleagues in psychology.

For example, rehabilitation psychologists continue to rely on demographic variables of "White," "Black," "Latino/a," and "Asian American" when including race or ethnicity in their studies. Although this is compatible with terminology preferred by federal funding agencies for reporting purposes, these variables have little theoretical and practical use in modern multicultural research. Models of acculturation have yet to be systematically studied in the rehabilitation psychology literature. Health and social psychologists have contributed to the rich and meaningful study of perceived discrimination experienced by individuals from racial and ethnic minority groups (Pascoe & Smart Richman, 2009; Schmitt, Branscombe, Postmes, & Garcia, 2014), and the deleterious effects of perceived discrimination on individuals from these groups throughout health care systems and encounters are well documented (Abramson, Hashemi, & Sánchez-Jankowski, 2015). Despite a historical interest in issues of stigma, we have yet to see a systematic, sustained research program in the rehabilitation psychology literature that documents the effects of perceived discrimination on individuals from ethnic or minority groups in rehabilitation settings. The current level of attention to this rich literature and implications for training, service, and policy for the rehabilitation enterprise suggests a gap.

Rehabilitation psychologists have a long and illustrious history of developing and refining important rehabilitation treatments that consist of face-to-face sessions with nondoctoral-level providers from other professions. These include cognitive remediation to individuals with traumatic brain injury (Cicerone et al., 2011), constraint-induced movement therapies in stroke rehabilitation (Taub, Uswatte, & Pidikiti, 1999), and chronic pain rehabilitation programs (Fordyce, 1976). Although face-to-face services with a doctoral-level psychologist may be provided, these are not essential to the treatments. To some extent, these services have been informed by theoretical models of behavior, they addressed clinical needs and issues presented by patients, and their current operations are sustained by ongoing institutional, financial, and collegial support.

In contrast, psychotherapy and counseling services from a doctoral-level psychologist during the inpatient rehabilitation program are not routinely provided. They are conceptualized within a recent taxonomy of rehabilitation treatments (Hart et al., 2014), but in practice, these services are often seen as tangential to the inpatient rehabilitation program. This is likely due to multiple factors: Counseling and psychotherapy are contingent on the interest of the patient, therapists providing other scheduled (and reimbursable) therapies would likely need to make changes in their appointment to allow time for the patient to participate in counseling, and counseling and psychotherapy in the inpatient rehabilitation setting is usually not reimbursed by third-party payers. When it is provided, Olkin (2017) again correctly observed that it is usually restricted to the presenting issues associated with recent-onset disability that may be addressed in short-term, time-limited therapy imposed by the clinical and practical realities of the inpatient setting. Rehabilitation psychologists have worked within these constraints in medical rehabilitation settings for several decades.

These conditions have had a suppressing effect on the evidence base for psychological interventions for adjustment issues reported by persons with disabilities. For many years, funding agencies did not provide support for studies of psychological interventions in this area, indicating that this work was not considered a priority by stakeholders. Studies that did appear were often characterized by a small number of participants and convenience samples. For example, in 2004, an evidence-based review of intervention research for a problem recognized for several decades by clinicians—depression following spinal cord injury—found no RCTs of psychological interventions or antidepressant therapy for depression in the peer-reviewed literature (Elliott & Kennedy, 2004). Recent increases in funding to support studies of psychological and medical interventions for psychological issues experienced by persons with a variety of disabilities have occurred over the past few years, and the corresponding benefits to the knowledge base are readily apparent in the literature (see Chapter 5, this volume). Meta-analytic studies published in 2011 reported nine (Mehta et al., 2011) and 10 studies of cognitive behavioral interventions for persons with spinal cord injury (Dorstyn, Mathias, & Denson, 2011a) and eight studies of telephone-based counseling for adults with physical disabilities (Dorstyn, Mathias, & Denson, 2011b). These meta-analytic reviews found positive effects. Yet a careful reading of the recently published intervention research supported by external funding reveals that most of this work emanates from a few select sites across the United States.

Context Matters

Following Popper's (1959) classic conceptualization, the bulk of the interdisciplinary research in rehabilitation occurs within the *context of discovery*, encompassing the study of observed relationships that may be pragmatic, informative, useful, and directly relevant to the stated priorities identified by the funding agencies and to the problems recognized by the interdisciplinary collaborators. This is true of most clinically driven research (O'Rourke, 2017; Sechrest & Smith, 1994), and it is a fair characterization of much of the funded, policy-relevant, translational, and solution-focused research conducted in medical rehabilitation settings as it is typically described and conducted (Frontera et al., 2017). It is also a fair characterization of most of the research conducted by rehabilitation psychologists, who use an inductive approach to derive many of their research ideas from existing theories and models in the extant literature and consider how a particular theory or model may help us understand a particular research problem or clinical issue.

Popper's (1959) *context of justification* describes the classic—if not stereotypic—image of the single, solitary scientist entrenched in the laboratory, intent on developing a theoretical model that addresses gaps in our existing knowledge that can be demonstrated in tests of a priori, potentially falsifiable hypotheses. Although many studies conduct tests of hypotheses that may be described as a priori and potentially falsifiable (see Dunn & Elliott, 2008, for an overview of the different types of theories and models germane to rehabilitation psychology), the classic ideal in academic psychology emphasizes a deductive approach in which a novel, innovative perspective is developed to break new ground, resolve thorny theoretical issues or provide new insights about a clinical concern, and stimulate a programmatic series of studies that may have far-reaching implications across the various domains and specialties in psychology.

Put another way, research conducted within a context of discovery entails the "description of phenomena," and research conducted within a context of justification involves the "creation and testing of theories to explain the phenomena" (Rozin, 2009, p. 435). Studies of the factor structure of a depression measure, of the degree to which demographic (e.g., age, biological sex) or injury-specific (e.g., completeness of lesion, functional impairment) variables predict quality of life over a year, of the number of individuals with mild traumatic brain injury who meet criteria for post-traumatic stress disorder in a particular clinic, or of a focus group with family members to identify the problems they experience as a caregiver of a person with a spinal cord injury all describe "phenomena." So, too, do studies of simple associations between variables such as hope and depression and between resilience and anxiety. Although these are psychological variables and there are theoretical models for hope and resilience, correlational studies like these may (or may not) advance our existing understanding of these concepts, but they do not explain the relationships between these "independent variables" and the outcomes beyond what is already known. An a priori rationale for a study does not necessarily mean it is concerned with testing potentially falsifiable hypotheses about the theorized mechanisms that account for—or explain—associations between variables.

Popper (1962) was well aware of the gray areas between these two broad categorizations of research, observing that "all this classification and distinction is a comparatively unimportant and superficial affair. We are not students of some subject matter but students of problems. And problems may cut across the borders of any subject matter or discipline" (p. 88). With this in mind, then, incremental applications of contemporary psychological theories of relevance to rehabilitation psychology include theory-driven studies that weed out bad variables and faulty reasoning and that refine knowledge and advance our understanding of the mechanisms that explain relationships (e.g., Does resilience predict well-being through its presumed effects on positive emotions?). Identifying and clarifying the theorized mechanisms that influence important outcomes is critical to understanding the behaviors that should be targeted in interventions and the process of change in response to interventions, and it is an essential step in developing potentially replicable trials of interventions (Craig et al., 2008). Potentially useful theories for rehabilitation psychology will provide clear and testable explanations for why things work the way they do, how they work, and the conditions in which they work. An absence or awkward application of theoretical models in research results in a literature typified by descriptive, correlational designs in ex post facto studies that lack coherence and are unable to meaningfully predict, explain, or refine our understanding of behavior, resulting in no real implications for clinical services, practice, or policy.

Some theory-driven variables withstand systematic, empirical scrutiny and emerge as useful in clinical practice (e.g., social problem-solving abilities; Nezu, Nezu, & D'Zurilla, 2013). Other variables that appear promising in initial field work but fail to stimulate advances in clinical assessment or intervention practices should probably be shelved until substantial evidence for clinical use appears (e.g., we have known for over 25 years that hope is correlated with depression, but we have yet to see a sustained research program that provides systematic empirical evidence of a "hope intervention" that benefits individuals in rehabilitation settings). Developing, testing, refining, and advancing theoretical models in this manner is a difficult business, and it may appear incremental or derivative to colleagues more accustomed to the academic images of the solitary scientist. But it is essential to rehabilitation psychology science and practice.

REEVALUATE THE BOUNDARIES, EXPAND THE HORIZON

Rehabilitation psychology balances its strong interdisciplinary tradition and its professional identity in core psychological training, theory, and practice. Its long-standing affiliation with medical rehabilitation will and should undoubtedly continue. Yet it is essential that rehabilitation psychology research respect its core identity as a practice-oriented branch of psychology. Without neglecting or circumscribing successful interdisciplinary endeavors, it is instructive to evaluate several areas that present issues that may be addressed in a manner to benefit rehabilitation psychology research and scholarship.

Overidentification With the Medical Model

The traditional identity of rehabilitation psychology within medical settings, institutions, and activities has been a concern of disability advocates for some time. There are clear benefits to this long-standing relationship, and Malec (2013) saw a bright future for the next generation of psychologists who will participate in evaluating rehabilitation procedures and services, assist in ushering in a chronic disease model for rehabilitation services across the lifespan, and collaborate in advances in neuroscience research that will likely direct the next wave of rehabilitation services.

But there are at least two areas that may be better addressed from perspectives that are not traditionally aligned with the "medical model." First, whereas a chronic disease model of disability is sensible from a clinical service and health policy perspective, it is a concern of disability advocates, who chafe at the notion of being construed as "patients" first rather than citizens (or consumers; Olkin & Pledger, 2003). This opinion is consistent with Wright's (1991) fundamental negative bias; our health care systems focus first on chronic disease as a problem to manage, rather than appreciate the individuals who live lives and who also happen to have certain health conditions. To a great extent, rehabilitation psychologists are cognizant of these matters and have shown the value of participatory action methods to involve consumers in research and service delivery activities (Ehde et al., 2013) and in developing "patient-oriented" assessment methods.

But there are more subtle issues that require some recalibration of the lens in which we view, understand, and appreciate those who are occasionally described in our research articles as "community-residing" adults. For example, it is fair to ask, "Where else would they live?" With a vantage point firmly ensconced in a medical or hospital setting, rehabilitation researchers rely on their perspective (i.e., the medical setting) to define others in relation to that particular system. It is important to make some distinction about a sample that was not recruited from within the medical system, but the point of reference is salient to the researcher and most readers of the scientific report.

Our research "samples" are usually defined first and foremost in terms of their relationship to the medical rehabilitation setting. The degree to which we are aware of this problem varies. There are several studies over the years that compare the samples participating in the Model Systems projects with other available databases, and lately, we see studies comparing these samples with those now participating in large-scale projects conducted in Veterans Affairs medical centers. Most individuals who volunteer to participate in rehabilitation research usually have some degree of interface with the system, and they are motivated for a variety of reasons to participate. We do not always know what these motivations are, and these factors have to be considered in our field studies and our RCTs because we are unsure of the degree to which they affect our results and limit generalizability.

Many of our projects are problem focused for understandable reasons. Consequently, our projects typically recruit individuals who have some contact with the system hosting the project and who share some level of interest in the problem. This does not necessarily ensure a fair sample of individuals throughout our communities who may also have some level of familiarity with the problem but who are also not in contact with the system and, if so, are not motivated or able to participate. Recent research from a population-based, case-controlled, nationwide sample of family caregivers of individuals experiencing stroke illustrated some of the information that may be learned from projects that obtain more representative "community" samples. In contrast to prevailing notions of family caregiving as a long-term burden with accompanying problems in health and adjustment, family caregivers of stroke survivors did not differ from matched noncaregivers in physical health quality of life, and within 3 years observed differences between these groups on life satisfaction, depression, and mental health quality of life were no longer present (Haley, Roth, Hovater, & Clay, 2015). Studies like this provide a more sophisticated view of the issues facing those living with disabling conditions above and beyond projects that rely on samples that volunteer to participate in projects at specific medical settings.

A more sophisticated appreciation of adjustment, well-being, and health promotion essential to a chronic disease management model would necessitate a wider lens and greater familiarity with research methods and designs more common in public health than typically used in medical rehabilitation research. One of the intellectual pioneers of rehabilitation psychology, Lee Meyerson (1988), spoke to these issues and possibilities, observing "if clinical psychologists, like their medical counterparts, center their attention on defects, deformities, and disease whose origins and treatment are within the individual," the clinical focus will be on the individual, and less attention would be given to the environmental and social issues in which these issues occur. But a broader perspective could occur if "psychologists, like their counterparts in public health, orient themselves toward person–environment interactions, so central to the Lewinian tradition, a new and even more favorable Zeitgeist for people with disabilities may be in the offing" (pp. 186–187).

Defining Evidence for Science and Policy

Malec (2013) argued for greater diversity in research methods, particularly in determining effectiveness and evaluating rehabilitation interventions, noting the limitations and shortcomings of the RCT as the lodestar in this endeavor. Others have made similar requests for using diverse research methods (Elliott, 2002) and for expanding our understanding of "evidence" in rehabilitation psychology intervention research (Tucker & Reed, 2008). Dijkers's (2009) essay may be the most definitive statement concerning the shortcomings of the RCT as a gold standard in rehabilitation research, generally, arguing that a focus on its selection as the "strongest" design obscures clear thinking about the more appropriate, "What is the best design to answer this research question?"

Rather than restate the arguments and issues articulated in the Dijkers (2009) monograph, our discussion concerns the evidence base for psychotherapy and counseling approaches used by rehabilitation psychologists. RCTs are sometimes argued to be the best way to determine whether it is "good policy" to favor one treatment over another or a specific treatment to none at all. This position raises concerns among those of us who value theory-driven research, who want to establish empirical support for our interventions, and who work with underserved individuals who have low-incidence, high-impact conditions and who are underrepresented in the psychotherapy and counseling outcome literature (Olkin, 2017). For some groups—such as family caregivers—there is no "standard" of mental health care; an absence of mental health services is the "routine treatment of choice" (several papers by Hart and colleagues on the selection of control groups and RCTs are relevant here: Hart & Bagiella, 2012; Hart et al., 2008). The emphasis on policy belies a greater value on administrative and financial support for services rather than advancing theory, obtaining empirical support, and nurturing an evidence base essential for providing effective psychological interventions.

Reliance on RCTs as the source of the highest grade of evidence discourages novel and creative investigations of psychotherapy outcomes in rehabilitation psychology research. But psychotherapy and counseling with individuals with disabilities routinely occurs in the context of multiple and chronic health issues and pressing social and environmental constraints that limit a client's full inclusion in society. These factors dictate individually tailored interventions. It is rare that a single manualized treatment as presented in most evidence-based protocols could be applied from start to finish with any single individual in a real-life, rehabilitation psychology setting. Although we see great strides in currently funded RCTs of psychological interventions in rehabilitation, it is unlikely that most of these will be adapted into multisite RCTs with sufficient sample sizes of individuals with low-incidence conditions required to meet the "highest grade of evidence" that are presumably necessary to impress policymakers and third-party payers.

Furthermore, a routine, pro forma use of the RCT design typically assumes a linear response to treatment, unless the researcher has a strong and explicit theoretical reason to expect otherwise. Occasionally, tests of psychological treatments in RCTs implicitly assume a linear therapeutic response that is at odds with what is known about therapeutic change in response to psychotherapy and counseling. The assumption of a linear change, as represented by an average score on an outcome measure for a group that received a treatment and compared with an average score for a group that did not receive the treatment, is a conservative and rather straightforward indicator of a difference that may or may not reflect realities. We know from the relevant psychotherapy outcome literature that linear change is but one of several possible trajectories, and in chronic mental health disorders, it is highly unlikely (Hayes, Laurenceau, Feldman, Strauss, & Cardaciotto, 2007; Laurenceau, Hayes, & Feldman, 2007). Therapeutic change in response to therapy may be quadratic, discontinuous, or curvilinear. These trajectories would not be detected—and in fact, would be obscured—in a traditional application of the RCT template. For some psychotherapy researchers, the real questions concern under what conditions and circumstances linear change does occur. Others argue that the type of trajectory should be hypothesized, and appropriate modeling techniques should then be selected to test this assumption (Rodgers, 2010).

Modeling techniques—such as MLM and SEM-based procedures—are ideally suited for this purpose, and they are also preferred when analyzing treatment effects with samples that may have suspected (if not documented) differences at baseline that may affect their response (Kahn & Schneider, 2013). The ability to isolate individual-level trajectories has additional advantages in isolating individual responses to therapy and possible characteristics of those individuals. These techniques can be used in RCTs, and they can also be used in analyzing outcome data from an ongoing practice to evaluate effectiveness (Kahn & Schneider, 2013). These applications are found in the psychotherapy and counseling outcome literature.

Psychologists have demonstrated many ways to conduct meaningful, informative studies of psychological interventions across clinical and community settings. These are available to rehabilitation psychology researchers. It is safe to state that the empirical investigation of psychological interventions used by rehabilitation psychologists has not followed the linear path usually observed in the research supporting evidence-based therapies used in more traditional areas of psychological practice or other areas of medical and health psychology, and current intervention research appears dependent on external funding. This is a precarious situation for a practice-oriented psychological profession, and the specialty must consider ways to advance the study of psychotherapy and counseling with persons with disabilities, across treatment settings, and in community sites away from the traditional confines of inpatient medical rehabilitation to shore up the evidence base. This will require new streams of funding and, perhaps, a new generation of scholars who are committed to this work regardless of available funding and who are open to a variety of alternative designs routinely used in the larger psychotherapy and counseling literature.

Environmental Press, Institutional Realities

Psychologists conducting research in academic medical settings usually have a mandate to pursue external funding to support their work, and as a group, rehabilitation psychologists have excelled in this activity for many years. The relative benefits and pitfalls of grantsmanship—and its relationship to scholarship, generally—in rehabilitation psychology research have been discussed elsewhere (Dunn & Elliott, 2008). Current budgetary constraints imposed on state-supported universities has increased pressure on almost all academic psychologists, and these issues are often compounded for rehabilitation psychologists who face additional financial shortfalls in clinical reimbursements. Lilienfeld (2017) argued that to obtain external funding, the environmental press has increased to the extent that it stifles creativity and critical thinking and increases the risks of questionable research practices (QRPs; including *p*-hacking and "just publishable units") in the pursuit of continued funding and the rewards associated with it.

Rehabilitation psychologists are somewhat familiar with this scenario, but there is little in the extant literature about the ethical dilemmas colleagues encounter when facing administrative expectations to obtain external funding. Most rehabilitation psychologists work to meet the needs of their home department and serve as involved citizens, collaborating on research projects and publishing their work in outlets that reflect well on their departments. The degree to which the pressure to keep external funds adversely affects innovation and creativity and results in unethical research practices is unknown.

Differences in power and status can exert a negative effect on interdisciplinary collaborations (Klein, 2014). Most histories of rehabilitation psychology emphasize the positive aspects of its involvement in medical settings and avoid the unpleasant account of how rehabilitation therapy services were subsumed into the administration of a medical department (Gritzer & Arluke, 1985). It is likely that some colleagues in these departments feel compelled to develop proposals to study topics that may be tangential to their scholarly interests or at the expense of real needs in the rehabilitation psychology literature base (and, perhaps, of their own research program) to obtain financial support. These pressures can thwart potentially creative and innovative scholarly pursuits, and it may have a long-lasting detrimental effect on junior colleagues who may be primed to study new and emerging topics that are not yet fundable but might potentially become the next "hot topics" for future funding priorities.

RECOMMENDATIONS FOR THE NEXT DECADE

In the coming years, graduates of APA-accredited health service psychology doctoral programs—which includes clinical, school, and counseling psychology—should demonstrate competencies in conducting, evaluating, and applying research across all areas of professional identity and practice (as presented in Chapter 1, this volume). This includes expectations that a graduate possesses the abilities to develop, apply, modify, and evaluate evidence-based interventions. Ideally, then, the next wave of graduates entering rehabilitation psychology will possess a core set of competencies that will enable them to accommodate and integrate rehabilitation psychology-specific knowledge and skill that will result in new and innovative ideas and approaches. We suspect these colleagues may find it challenging to stay up to date with the ever-evolving professional psychology literature while simultaneously attending to the increasingly complex rehabilitation science literature.

To advance the existing body of knowledge, a potentially important, ground-breaking theoretical model must be tested and refined in a systematic series of studies that constitute a coherent, well-developed research program (for a discussion of research programs in rehabilitation psychology research, see Dunn & Elliott, 2008). And a research program reaches an admirable level of maturity when it provides clear implications for practice and policy. We hope the next generation of rehabilitation psychology scholars understands this process and will develop new research programs that command the attention of other scholars invested in the topical area. We also hope that home departments and institutions place a premium on theory-driven research programs and find ways to invest in and support promising scholars who propose compelling and potentially fundable work.

For a theory-driven research program to inform psychological interventions, it must establish the "empirically supported principles of change" (Tolin, McKay, Forman, Klonsky, & Thombs, 2015, p. 320). This is a critical element for developing psychological interventions that strategically target these mechanisms in a manner that effects predictable therapeutic responses. Although professional practice involves many activities in rehabilitation psychology (e.g., assessment, consultation, policy formation), our obvious concern here is with the current state of intervention research.

For over a decade some observers have argued that evidence-based practices for counseling and psychotherapy with persons with disabilities are lacking (Artman & Daniels, 2010; Olkin & Taliaferro, 2006). This neglect was presumably due, in part, to a perception that such intervention research was "relegated to the specialization of rehabilitation psychology" (Artman & Daniels, 2010, p. 443). This may be a fair characterization. Despite an early history of studying counseling issues among persons with disabilities, for example, an analysis of counseling psychology journals found only 1% to 2.7% of the articles published over a 20-year span (from 1990 to 2010) could be categorized as "disability research" (Foley-Nicpon & Lee, 2012).

As we discussed earlier, rehabilitation psychology outlets have recently published an impressive number of psychological intervention studies with persons living with disabilities (and we could easily argue that there has been an increase in the number of similar studies published in the clinical psychology literature, particularly with veterans who incurred traumatic brain injuries during war zone service). But much of the intervention research in the rehabilitation psychology literature was sponsored by external grant funds awarded to colleagues at a few medical rehabilitation facilities to conduct these trials. Without this funding, these studies would probably not have occurred. To expand our knowledge base, it is important that we encourage intervention research with other designs and in "nonacademic" and "nonresearch" settings. Rather than rely on a select few to obtain the kind of evidence we need to expand our knowledge base, other colleagues could conduct studies to demonstrate the effectiveness of interventions provided in community settings to individuals requesting and receiving psychological services. This kind of research, common in the psychotherapy outcome literature, is important in identifying empirically supported treatments, and it can be particularly informative in understanding useful approaches to working with complex cases (Tolin et al., 2015). It also addresses a serious gap in the psychotherapy literature, generally, that has concerned disability advocates for some time (Olkin & Pledger, 2003).

Contemporary rehabilitation psychology is far removed from an earlier time in which it often seemed "isolated from the mainstream of psychology" (Jansen & Eisenberg, 1982, p. 3). Issues experienced by our colleagues in clinical psychology science can affect us. We share the concerns expressed by some clinical psychologists that QRPs will require more constructive and preventive efforts to ensure the quality of our work and to uphold public trust (Tackett et al., 2017). Many journal editors already use software programs to check submissions for duplication and plagiarism and to ensure originality (and the *Archives of Physical Medicine and Rehabilitation* recently retracted an article for egregious duplication of a previously published article; Gu & Ran, 2016). Some scholars in nonmedical settings are uncomfortable with studies that rely on secondary data (Donnellan & Lucas, 2013), but this is a common practice in rehabilitation, and many rehabilitation psychologists are remarkably skilled in this kind of research. Unfortunately, some rehabilitation psychology researchers have encountered dismissive criticisms about ex post facto studies and piecemeal publications from some journal editors and manuscript reviewers who may be uncomfortable with these designs. Rather than endorse a registration process to ensure transparency to improve confidence and reduce the likelihood of QRPs in clinical psychology research (Tackett et al., 2017), rehabilitation psychologists could offer considerable expertise in these discussions should they gain traction.

This, too, requires ongoing attention to and involvement in initiatives that may occur in the larger arena of professional psychology that, at times, competes for the time and attention required to do cutting-edge work in the interdisciplinary world of rehabilitation research and practice. The special issue of *Rehabilitation Psychology* in 2008 dedicated to advances and issues in research methods and analyses provided an excellent forum for colleagues to report new perspectives from other areas of psychological research. Interestingly, the *Journal of Consulting and Clinical Psychology* and the *Journal of Counseling Psychology* occasionally devote special issues to advances and issues in research methods and analyses. Perhaps the *Rehabilitation Psychology* journal could follow suit, as part of its mission to maintain and perpetuate "an identity for rehabilitation psychologists, be they in academic or research settings, clinical practice, or administrative or policy settings" (Jansen & Eisenberg, 1982, p. 3).

CONCLUDING OBSERVATIONS

A science-based profession that does not nurture and maintain its scientific base loses control of its future. Toward this end, we encourage members of the rehabilitation psychology community to consider both the intended and unintended consequences of focusing our scholarly efforts on activities that are primarily construed from the medical context. We are not suggesting that such work is not valuable to both consumers and the field of rehabilitation psychology as a whole. We are highlighting the importance of both core psychological scientific foundations and research efforts and collaborations with those outside the traditional interdisciplinary medical team. In our view, prioritizing the latter will enhance our ability to work as members of interdisciplinary medical teams and promote innovative psychological scholarship that facilitates function and participation among those living with disabling health conditions.

References

Abramson, C. M., Hashemi, M., & Sánchez-Jankowski, M. (2015). Perceived discrimination in U.S. healthcare: Charting the effects of key social characteristics within and across racial groups. *Preventive Medicine Reports*, 2, 615–621. http://dx.doi.org/10.1016/j.pmedr.2015.07.006

American Psychological Association. (2018). *Specialties and proficiencies*. Retrieved from https://www.apa.org/ed/graduate/specialize/index.aspx

APA Council of Representatives. (2011). *Principles for the recognition of specialties in professional psychology*. Retrieved from https://www.apa.org/about/policy/principles-recognition.pdf

Artman, L. K., & Daniels, J. A. (2010). Disability and psychotherapy practice: Cultural competence and practical tips. *Professional Psychology: Research and Practice*, *41*, 442–448. http://dx.doi.org/10.1037/a0020864

Baker, T. B., McFall, R. M., & Shoham, V. (2008). Current status and future prospects of clinical psychology: Toward a scientifically principled approach to mental and behavioral health care. *Psychological Science in the Public Interest*, *9*, 67–103. http://dx.doi.org/10.1111/j.1539-6053.2009.01036.x

Berry, J. W., Elliott, T. R., Grant, J. S., Edwards, G., & Fine, P. R. (2012). Does problem-solving training for family caregivers benefit their care recipients with severe disabilities? A latent growth model of the Project CLUES randomized clinical trial. *Rehabilitation Psychology*, *57*, 98–112. http://dx.doi.org/10.1037/a0028229

Boix Mansilla, V., Lamont, M., & Sato, K. (2016). Shared cognitive–emotional–interactional platforms: Markers and conditions for successful interdisciplinary collaborations. *Science, Technology & Human Values*, *41*, 571–612. http://dx.doi.org/10.1177/0162243915614103

Brenner, L. A. (2017, February). *State of Division 22*. Paper presented at the meeting of the Division of Rehabilitation Psychology, Albuquerque, NM.

Chan, F., Lee, G. K., Lee, E. J., Kubota, C., & Allen, C. A. (2007). Structural equation modeling in rehabilitation counseling research. *Rehabilitation Counseling Bulletin*, *51*, 44–57. http://dx.doi.org/10.1177/00343552070510010701

Cicerone, K. D., Langenbahn, D. M., Braden, C., Malec, J. F., Kalmar, K., Fraas, M., . . . Ashman, T. (2011). Evidence-based cognitive rehabilitation: Updated review of the literature from 2003 through 2008. *Archives of Physical Medicine and Rehabilitation*, *92*, 519–530. http://dx.doi.org/10.1016/j.apmr.2010.11.015

Clay, D. L., Wood, P. K., Frank, R. G., Hagglund, K. J., & Johnson, J. C. (1995). Examining systematic differences in adaptation to chronic illness: A growth modeling approach. *Rehabilitation Psychology*, *40*, 61–70. http://dx.doi.org/10.1037/0090-5550.40.1.61

Craig, P., Dieppe, P., Macintyre, S., Michie, S., Nazareth, I., & Petticrew, M. (2008). Developing and evaluating complex interventions: The new Medical Research Council guidance. *British Medical Journal*, *337*, a1655. http://dx.doi.org/10.1136/bmj.a1655

Dijkers, M. P. J. M. (2009). *When the best is the enemy of the good: The nature of research evidence used in systematic reviews and guidelines*. Retrieved from http://ktdrr.org/ktlibrary/articles_pubs/ncddrwork/tfsr_best/

Donnellan, B., & Lucas, R. (2013). Secondary data analysis. In T. Little (Ed.), *The Oxford handbook of quantitative methods in psychology: Vol. 2. Statistical analyses* (pp. 665–677). New York, NY: Oxford University Press. http://dx.doi.org/10.1093/oxfordhb/9780199934898.013.0028

Dorstyn, D., Mathias, J., & Denson, L. (2011a). Efficacy of cognitive behavior therapy for the management of psychological outcomes following spinal cord injury: A meta-analysis. *Journal of Health Psychology*, *16*, 374–391. http://dx.doi.org/10.1177/1359105310379063

Dorstyn, D. S., Mathias, J. L., & Denson, L. A. (2011b). Psychosocial outcomes of telephone-based counseling for adults with an acquired physical disability: A meta-analysis. *Rehabilitation Psychology*, *56*, 1–14. http://dx.doi.org/10.1037/a0022249

Dunn, D. S., & Elliott, T. R. (2008). The place and promise of theory in rehabilitation psychology research. *Rehabilitation Psychology*, *53*, 254–267. http://dx.doi.org/10.1037/a0012962

Ehde, D. M., Wegener, S. T., Williams, R. M., Ephraim, P. L., Stevenson, J. E., Isenberg, P. J., & MacKenzie, E. J. (2013). Developing, testing, and sustaining rehabilitation interventions via participatory action research. *Archives of Physical Medicine and Rehabilitation*, *94*, S30–S42. http://dx.doi.org/10.1016/j.apmr.2012.10.025

Elliott, T. R. (2002). Defining our common ground to reach new horizons. *Rehabilitation Psychology*, *47*, 131–143. http://dx.doi.org/10.1037/0090-5550.47.2.131

Elliott, T. R. (2016). External funding and competing visions for academic counseling psychology. *The Counseling Psychologist*, *44*, 525–535. http://dx.doi.org/10.1177/0011000016634867

Elliott, T. R., & Gramling, S. E. (1990). Psychologists and rehabilitation: New roles and old training models. *American Psychologist*, *45*, 762–765. http://dx.doi.org/10.1037/0003-066X.45.6.762

Elliott, T. R., & Kennedy, P. (2004). Treatment of depression following spinal cord injury: An evidence-based review. *Rehabilitation Psychology*, *49*, 134–139. http://dx.doi.org/10.1037/0090-5550.49.2.134

Elliott, T. R., & Rath, J. F. (2012). Rehabilitation psychology. In E. M. Altmaier & J. I. C. Hansen (Eds.), *The Oxford handbook of counseling psychology* (pp. 679–702). New York, NY: Oxford University Press.

Foley-Nicpon, M., & Lee, S. (2012). Disability research in counseling psychology journals: A 20-year content analysis. *Journal of Counseling Psychology*, *59*, 392–398. http://dx.doi.org/10.1037/a0028743

Fordyce, W. E. (1976). *Behavioral methods for chronic pain and illness*. Saint Louis, MO: Mosby.

Frontera, W. R., Bean, J. F., Damiano, D., Ehrlich-Jones, L., Fried-Oken, M., Jette, A., . . . Thompson, A. (2017). Rehabilitation research at the National Institutes of Health moving the field forward (executive summary). *Rehabilitation Psychology*, *62*, 387–396. http://dx.doi.org/10.1037/rep0000164

Gritzer, G., & Arluke, A. (1985). *The making of rehabilitation: A political economy of medical specialization, 1890–1980*. Berkeley: University of California Press.

Gu, P., & Ran, J. J. (2016). Electrical stimulation for hemiplegic shoulder function: A systematic review and meta-analysis of 15 randomized controlled trials. *Archives of Physical Medicine and Rehabilitation*, *97*, 1588–1594. http://dx.doi.org/10.1016/j.apmr.2016.04.011

Haley, W. E., Roth, D. L., Hovater, M., & Clay, O. J. (2015). Long-term impact of stroke on family caregiver well-being: A population-based case-control study. *Neurology*, *84*, 1323–1329. http://dx.doi.org/10.1212/WNL.0000000000001418

Hart, T., & Bagiella, E. (2012). Design and implementation of clinical trials in rehabilitation research. *Archives of Physical Medicine and Rehabilitation*, *93*, S117–S126. http://dx.doi.org/10.1016/j.apmr.2011.11.039

Hart, T., Fann, J. R., & Novack, T. A. (2008). The dilemma of the control condition in experience-based cognitive and behavioural treatment research. *Neuropsychological Rehabilitation*, *18*, 1–21. http://dx.doi.org/10.1080/09602010601082359

Hart, T., Tsaousides, T., Zanca, J. M., Whyte, J., Packel, A., Ferraro, M., & Dijkers, M. P. (2014). Toward a theory-driven classification of rehabilitation treatments. *Archives of Physical Medicine and Rehabilitation*, *95*(Suppl.), S33–S44.e2. http://dx.doi.org/10.1016/j.apmr.2013.05.032

Hayes, A. M., Laurenceau, J. P., Feldman, G., Strauss, J. L., & Cardaciotto, L. (2007). Change is not always linear: The study of nonlinear and discontinuous patterns of change in psychotherapy. *Clinical Psychology Review*, *27*, 715–723. http://dx.doi.org/10.1016/j.cpr.2007.01.008

Jansen, M. A., & Eisenberg, M. G. (1982). Editorial. *Rehabilitation Psychology*, *27*, 3.

Kahn, J. H., & Schneider, W. J. (2013). It's the destination and it's the journey: Using multilevel modeling to assess patterns of change in psychotherapy. *Journal of Clinical Psychology*, *69*, 543–570. http://dx.doi.org/10.1002/jclp.21964

Klein, J. T. (2014). Communication and collaboration in interdisciplinary research. In M. O'Rourke, S. Crowley, S. D. Eigenbrode, & J. D. Wulfhorst (Eds.), *Enhancing communication & collaboration in interdisciplinary research* (pp. 11–30). Los Angeles, CA: Sage. http://dx.doi.org/10.4135/9781483352947.n2

Kozlowski, A. J., Pretz, C. R., Dams-O'Connor, K., Kreider, S., & Whiteneck, G. (2013). An introduction to applying individual growth curve models to evaluate change in rehabilitation: A National Institute on Disability and Rehabilitation Research Traumatic Brain Injury Model Systems report. *Archives of Physical Medicine and Rehabilitation*, *94*, 589–596. http://dx.doi.org/10.1016/j.apmr.2012.08.199

Kwok, O.-M., Underhill, A. T., Berry, J. W., Luo, W., Elliott, T. R., & Yoon, M. (2008). Analyzing longitudinal data with multilevel models: An example with individuals living with lower extremity intra-articular fractures. *Rehabilitation Psychology*, *53*, 370–386. http://dx.doi.org/10.1037/a0012765

Laurenceau, J. P., Hayes, A. M., & Feldman, G. C. (2007). Some methodological and statistical issues in the study of change processes in psychotherapy. *Clinical Psychology Review*, *27*, 682–695. http://dx.doi.org/10.1016/j.cpr.2007.01.007

Leahey, E. (2016). From sole investigator to team scientist: Trends in the practice and study of research collaboration. *Annual Review of Sociology*, *42*, 81–100. http://dx.doi.org/10.1146/annurev-soc-081715-074219

Leahey, E., Beckman, C. M., & Stanko, T. L. (2017). Prominent but less productive: The impact of interdisciplinarity on scientists' research. *Administrative Science Quarterly*, *62*, 105–139. http://dx.doi.org/10.1177/0001839216665364

Lilienfeld, S. O. (2017). Psychology's replication crisis and the grant culture: Righting the ship. *Perspectives on Psychological Science*, *12*, 660–664. http://dx.doi.org/10.1177/1745691616687745

Lofquist, L. H. (Ed.). (1960). *Psychological research and rehabilitation*. Washington, DC: American Psychological Association. http://dx.doi.org/10.1037/10041-000

Malec, J. F. (2013). Rehabilitation research: 30 years later; 30 years hence. *The Journal of Head Trauma Rehabilitation*, *28*, 227–231. http://dx.doi.org/10.1097/HTR.0b013e3182907c77

Maton, K. I., Perkins, D. D., & Saegert, S. (2006). Community psychology at the crossroads: Prospects for interdisciplinary research. *American Journal of Community Psychology*, *38*, 9–21. http://dx.doi.org/10.1007/s10464-006-9062-3

Mehta, S., Orenczuk, S., Hansen, K. T., Aubut, J. A. L., Hitzig, S. L., Legassic, M., & Teasell, R. W. (2011). An evidence-based review of the effectiveness of cognitive behavioral therapy for psychosocial issues post-spinal cord injury. *Rehabilitation Psychology*, *56*, 15–25. http://dx.doi.org/10.1037/a0022743

Meyerson, L. (1988). The social psychology of physical disability: 1948 and 1988. *Journal of Social Issues*, *44*, 173–188. http://dx.doi.org/10.1111/j.1540-4560.1988.tb02056.x

National Academies. (2005). *Facilitating interdisciplinary research*. Washington, DC: National Academics Press.

Nezu, A., Nezu, C., & D'Zurilla, T. (2013). *Problem-solving therapy*. New York, NY: Springer.

Olkin, R. (2017). *Disability-affirmative therapy*. New York, NY: Oxford University Press.

Olkin, R., & Pledger, C. (2003). Can disability studies and psychology join hands? *American Psychologist*, *58*, 296–304. http://dx.doi.org/10.1037/0003-066X.58.4.296

Olkin, R., & Taliaferro, G. (2006). Evidence-based practices have ignored people with disabilities. In J. C. Norcross, L. E. Beutler, & R. F. Levant (Eds.), *Evidence-based practices in mental health: Debate and dialogue on the fundamental questions* (pp. 353–359). Washington, DC: American Psychological Association.

O'Rourke, M. (2017). Comparing methods from cross-disciplinary research. In R. Frodeman, J. T. Klein, & R. C. S. Pacheco (Eds.), *The Oxford handbook of interdisciplinarity* (2nd ed., pp. 276–290). New York, NY: Oxford University Press.

Pascoe, E. A., & Smart Richman, L. (2009). Perceived discrimination and health: A meta-analytic review. *Psychological Bulletin*, *135*, 531–554. http://dx.doi.org/10.1037/a0016059

Perrin, P. B., Norup, A., Caracuel, A., Bateman, A., Tjørnlund, M., & Arango-Lasprilla, J. C. (2017). An actor–partner interdependence model of acquired brain injury patient impairments and caregiver psychosocial functioning: A dyadic-report, multinational study. *Journal of Clinical Psychology*, *73*, 279–293. http://dx.doi.org/10.1002/jclp.22324

Popper, K. (1959). *The logic of scientific discovery*. New York, NY: Basic Books.

Popper, K. (1962). *Conjectures and refutations: The growth of scientific knowledge*. New York, NY: Basic Books.

Rodgers, J. L. (2010). The epistemology of mathematical and statistical modeling: A quiet methodological revolution. *American Psychologist*, *65*, 1–12. http://dx.doi.org/10.1037/a0018326

Rozin, P. (2009). What kind of empirical research should we publish, fund, and reward? *Perspectives on Psychological Science*, *4*, 435–439. http://dx.doi.org/10.1111/j.1745-6924.2009.01151.x

Schmitt, M. T., Branscombe, N. R., Postmes, T., & Garcia, A. (2014). The consequences of perceived discrimination for psychological well-being: A meta-analytic review. *Psychological Bulletin*, *140*, 921–948. http://dx.doi.org/10.1037/a0035754

Sechrest, L., & Smith, B. (1994). Psychotherapy is the practice of psychology. *Journal of Psychotherapy Integration*, *4*, 1–29. http://dx.doi.org/10.1037/h0101150

Simmons, J. P., Nelson, L. D., & Simonsohn, U. (2011). False-positive psychology: Undisclosed flexibility in data collection and analysis allows presenting anything as significant. *Psychological Science*, *22*, 1359–1366. http://dx.doi.org/10.1177/0956797611417632

Spring, B., Hall, K. L., Moller, A. C., & Falk-Krzesinski, H. J. (2012). An emerging science and praxis for research and practice teams. *Translational Behavioral Medicine*, *2*, 411–414. http://dx.doi.org/10.1007/s13142-012-0180-1

Tackett, J. L., Lilienfeld, S. O., Patrick, C. J., Johnson, S. L., Krueger, R. F., Miller, J. D., . . . Shrout, P. E. (2017). It's time to broaden the replicability conversation: Thoughts for and from clinical psychological science. *Perspectives on Psychological Science*, *12*, 742–756. http://dx.doi.org/10.1177/1745691617690042

Tate, D., Kalpakjian, C., & Kwon, C. (2008). The use of randomized clinical trials in rehabilitation psychology. *Rehabilitation Psychology*, *53*, 268–278. http://dx.doi.org/10.1037/a0012974

Taub, E., Uswatte, G., & Pidikiti, R. (1999). Constraint-induced movement therapy: A new family of techniques with broad application to physical rehabilitation—a clinical review. *Journal of Rehabilitation Research and Development*, *36*, 237–251.

Tolin, D. F., McKay, D., Forman, E. M., Klonsky, E. D., & Thombs, B. D. (2015). Empirically supported treatment: Recommendations for a new model. *Clinical Psychology: Science and Practice*, *22*, 317–338. http://dx.doi.org/10.1111/cpsp.12122

Tucker, J. A., & Reed, G. M. (2008). Evidentiary pluralism as a strategy for research and evidence-based practice in rehabilitation psychology. *Rehabilitation Psychology*, *53*, 279–293. http://dx.doi.org/10.1037/a0012963

Velozo, C. A., Seel, R. T., Magasi, S., Heinemann, A. W., & Romero, S. (2012). Improving measurement methods in rehabilitation: Core concepts and recommendations for scale development. *Archives of Physical Medicine and Rehabilitation*, *93*, S154–S163. http://dx.doi.org/10.1016/j.apmr.2012.06.001

Weston, R., Gore, P. A., Jr., Chan, F., & Catalano, D. (2008). An introduction to using structural equation models in rehabilitation psychology. *Rehabilitation Psychology*, *53*, 340–356. http://dx.doi.org/10.1037/a0013039

Wright, B. A. (Ed.). (1959). *Psychology and rehabilitation*. Washington, DC: American Psychological Association. http://dx.doi.org/10.1037/10539-000

Wright, B. A. (1991). Labeling: The need for greater person–environment individuation. In C. R. Snyder & D. R. Forsyth (Eds.), *Handbook of social and clinical psychology* (pp. 469–487). New York, NY: Pergamon Press.

Chapter 4

ASSESSMENT

Shane S. Bush and Beth K. Rush

The provision of psychological treatment to persons receiving rehabilitative services is based on an assessment of psychological functioning, including deficits and assets. Assessment is the first step in the delivery of clinical services that allows clinicians to obtain a comprehensive understanding of a patient to promote rehabilitation and psychosocial functioning or identify targets for psychological intervention. Psychological assessment determines and clarifies the nature and severity of conditions (e.g., cognitive disorder, psychological adjustment, pain syndrome, relationship issues). When multiple clinical needs exist, assessment can provide empirical support for choosing specific interventions and methods. Assessment findings also can produce baseline data for outcome evaluations. Assessment is a core functional competency of rehabilitation psychologists. Rehabilitation psychologists should share a common knowledge base and skill set. These skills underlie psychological treatment in rehabilitation and serve as the foundation for more specialized, population-specific assessment and interventions.

TARGETS OF ASSESSMENT

Persons receiving rehabilitative services typically have needs that benefit from psychological intervention. Assessment needs vary within, or across, patients or clinical settings, but some commonalities exist. Frequent targets for assessment include cognition, behavior, emotional state, personality traits, daily functioning, insight/self-awareness, and coping skills. Additional issues, such as level of arousal or consciousness, pain, or community reintegration, typically are also assessed by rehabilitation psychologists.

Cognition

Formal assessment of cognition is essential to determine cognitive deficits and preserved abilities after a known or suspected neurological injury or illness. Assessment also fosters an understanding of the impact that many factors commonly experienced by rehabilitation patients have on cognitive functioning, including the acute effects of anesthesia, infections, medications, pain, emotional distress, and sleep disruption. Determining a patient's cognitive functioning is important to understanding deficits, preserved strengths, and decision-making capacity.

Premorbid functioning. The assessment competencies developed by the American Board of Rehabilitation Psychology (see Chapter 1, this handbook) do not include the estimation of premorbid abilities. This is an interesting omission, given that estimating optimal or premorbid intellectual/cognitive functioning is needed to determine whether current abilities reflect a decline from a previously higher level. Multiple performance-based and actuarial

http://dx.doi.org/10.1037/0000129-005
Handbook of Rehabilitation Psychology, Third Edition, L. A. Brenner, S. A. Reid-Arndt, T. R. Elliott, R. G. Frank, and B. Caplan (Editors-in-Chief)

methods allow for an estimation of optimal or premorbid functioning (Lezak, Howieson, Bigler, & Tranel, 2012). Common methods include (a) administration of "hold" tests, such as single-word reading; (b) consideration of best performances within a battery of tests; and (c) actuarial formulas based on demographic variables. Each method has limitations and can be more or less useful for a given patient. For example, reliance solely on a reading test as an indicator of premorbid functioning would be misleading for someone with a verbal learning disorder or with aphasia. A multimethod approach that includes all three methods with full awareness of their strengths and weaknesses is preferable.

Cognitive domains. Most cognitive evaluations cover a core set of abilities: intellectual functioning (or at least an estimate), attention and concentration (i.e., working memory), speed of information processing, language functions, visuospatial skills, memory, and executive functions, which include a variety of mental abilities (e.g., reasoning, planning, problem-solving; conceptual tracking and mental set shifting; initiation of behavior and inhibition of impulses; divided attention or multitasking; other higher level mental control functions).

Although not cognitive domains per se, sensory and motor functions also are commonly assessed. Awareness of sensory and motor deficits contributes to an understanding of cognitive limitations that guide rehabilitative and community reentry efforts. Because sensory or motor deficits can spuriously lower scores on measures assessing cognitive constructs, modification of standardized testing procedures may be needed to minimize the impact of sensory or motor deficits on cognitive test performance.

Following an injury or illness, it can be tempting to attribute cognitive changes to the proximate cause (i.e., the injury or illness). However, cognitive limitations may have existed before the most recent event either as a result of a prior injury or illness, or a developmental disorder. Depending on its nature, the presence of a developmental disorder can affect a patient's ability to process information. For example, some patients historically are better able to process visually based material compared with verbal information. The rehabilitation psychologist who identifies this style and understands the nature of a developmental disorder is well positioned to help other rehabilitation team members, school officials, and employers best communicate with the patient.

Behavior

A wide range of behavior problems can emerge during the course of rehabilitation from neurological injuries or illness, including acute confusion and/or frustration, or other psychological reactions. During rehabilitation, behavior problems can affect the recovery process and challenge family members, staff, and the patient. Behavioral symptoms can take the form of disruptive or harmful behaviors, or decreases in functioning, such as apathy or withdrawal. The specific type of behavioral problem can be diagnostic or anticipated with different types of injuries or psychological disorders; both types can be assessed and addressed.

Rehabilitation psychologists can determine if such behaviors are new or represent (perhaps exacerbated) developmental or otherwise long-standing difficulties. Often family members or prior health care or mental health professionals can provide answers to such questions. In the case of premorbid phenomena, they may be able to describe ways in which the behaviors were best managed or resolved in the past, as well as information about what makes the behaviors worse. A particularly important aspect of behavior to assess is the risk of self-harm or other harm, whether intentional or unintentional. The safety of the patient and others is an overarching priority.

Emotional State

The lives of people undergoing rehabilitation can change in fundamental and dramatic ways. Adjusting to these changes can be challenging for patients and their families. In addition, rehabilitation can be emotionally trying: It can create anxiety, frustration, and disappointment, as well as psychological denial with or without neurologically based diminished awareness of limitations. With ongoing assessment, all parties understand the patient's psychological functioning and work to maximize emotional adjustment.

The prognosis for patients who have strong social support is better than for those who lack such support (e.g., McKillop, Carroll, Jones, & Battié, 2017; Wade, Zhang, Yeates, Stancin, & Taylor, 2016). Rehabilitation psychologists are equipped to work with family members and friends to provide education and facilitate communication while ensuring that interpersonal resources are used to promote psychological adjustment. Assessment of social support also sets the foundation for individual, couples, or family therapy involving spouses or other family members. For these reasons, rehabilitation psychologists should inquire about current and past relationships, including supportive and more stressful ones.

Personality Traits and Behavioral Patterns

Patients' enduring emotional, behavioral, and interpersonal styles can make the rehabilitation process productive and rewarding, or can serve as obstacles. A person's beliefs or personality traits that previously were not problematic may be maladaptive during rehabilitation because of the nature of the injury or stress of the situation. For example, as a result of disinhibition caused by a neurological injury, a person with racist views who previously was able to inhibit the expression of those views may make hurtful racist comments to staff members from different ethnic groups. In contrast, a person with a history of hardiness or resilience in the face of challenging life situations may be able to cope with and adapt to significant limitations, and benefit more from rehabilitation than others who have been in similar situations (Alschuler, Kratz, & Ehde, 2016; Catalano, Chan, Wilson, Chiu, & Muller, 2011). For these reasons, the assessment of personality traits can be a valuable aspect of the psychological evaluation.

Functioning

Understanding a person's functional level—abilities and limitations—in the home and community before sustaining an injury or illness is valuable to establishing expectations and goals during rehabilitation. Assessing education level, vocational activities and achievements, daily domestic activities, leisure activities, and interpersonal functioning allows rehabilitation professionals to tailor treatment to the patient's specific needs.

Insight/Self-Awareness

A patient's understanding of his or her premorbid strengths and weakness is a key to maximizing rehabilitation outcome (Prigatano, 1999; Sherer et al., 1998). Comparing a patient's self-assessment of an ability, symptom, or trait with an assessment of those same factors by someone who knows the patient well (and has the patient's best interests in mind) helps establish the degree of insight or awareness possessed by the patient. Insight into one's assets and limitations is not an all-or-nothing concept; it commonly exists on a continuum and may differ across functional domains or over time. As a result, assessment of insight may need to occur periodically during rehabilitation. As insight improves, emotional adjustment may deteriorate.

As important as a patient's self-awareness is for establishing and achieving rehabilitation goals, understanding the level of insight of the patient's support system is equally critical. Rehabilitation psychologists are well suited to improve family members and others' awareness and understanding by providing evidence-based education about the condition in a supportive manner.

Coping Skills

Coping with the dramatic changes associated with illness or injury often is challenging and effortful, and challenges continue over time. Understanding the patient's premorbid methods of coping and current coping strategies allows the clinician to reinforce adaptive strategies and extinguish or revise maladaptive strategies. Of course, coping skills do not operate in a vacuum. Understanding a patient's ability to cope with challenges entails understanding surrounding factors that complicate or enhance coping skills.

FACTORS THAT INFLUENCE THE NATURE OF THE ASSESSMENT

Assessment needs vary, depending on such factors as the physical setting in which the assessment takes place, known or suspected disorder, patient's level of functioning, referral question, and assessment goals. For example, an assessment of an older adult on an inpatient brain injury rehabilitation unit will be different from the cognitive assessment of a young adult recently diagnosed with multiple sclerosis who is beginning to struggle with attentional focus and memory at work. To best meet patients' needs, rehabilitation psychologists commonly establish different assessment methods for different conditions and settings.

The Multimethod Assessment Process

A thorough psychological assessment is more than "testing"; it is a multimethod process. To obtain an accurate understanding of patients that promotes an individualized rehabilitation process, psychologists must consider multiple sources of information, perform multiple tasks, and integrate the information and results in the context of an empirical evidence base.

Record review. Patient records provide valuable information that informs diagnostic decision making. Key documents to review include medical records that describe the presenting condition and medical history, laboratory and imaging test results, and prior psychological assessment reports. When possible, it is advantageous to review education and/or employment records, relevant legal documents, and disability claims. Obtaining the necessary permissions before pursuing such records facilitates the process.

Interviews. Except for very low-functioning patients who are unable to engage in an interview, initial discussions with patients about their problems, strengths, and background are a critical component of assessment. For patients who are cognitively compromised, interviews with family members or others closely involved in their lives can provide a perspective that further illuminates aspects of psychological functioning across settings, situations, and time. Other health care professionals who work with the patient can offer information that contributes to a better understanding of the patient's cognitive, emotional, and interpersonal functioning.

Observations. Observation of the following nine factors is informative: (a) physical appearance, (b) level of alertness, (c) sensory and motor functions, (d) receptive and expressive language, (e) affect and mood, (f) cognitive limitations, (g) signs of psychosis, (h) presence or absence of behavioral problems, and (i) degree of insight into strengths and limitations.

Course of symptoms. Rehabilitation psychologists who understand the natural history of an injury or illness can help patients and their families with expectations and planning. Deviations from an expected course of recovery can result from many factors, including infection, medication issues, acute medical process, or a psychological adjustment or behavior problem. Close attention to a patient's recovery course compared with evidence-based expectations promotes good patient care.

Psychometric instruments. Screening measures exist for assessing level of arousal, various cognitive and sensorimotor domains, and emotional and behavioral functioning. When assessing cognitive abilities, attention to multiple sensory modalities is indicated. This approach allows psychologists to make specific recommendations according to the patient's strengths and weaknesses. The selection of specific measures is guided by (a) the patient's functional level, (b) context in which the assessment is performed, (c) referral questions, (d) psychometric properties of the instruments for the case, (e) suitability of available normative data, and (f) clinical utility and ecological validity of the measures. The degree to which standardized administration procedures can be followed or modified must be considered because modifications may affect the ability of the clinician to understand the constructs of interest. In the psychological report, the clinician should explain any deviations from standardized administration and the reasons for such deviations.

Interdisciplinary collaboration. Input from all team members facilitates assessment. Juxtaposition of different views of the patient provided by the rehabilitation team may reveal unforeseen areas for assessment, symptom monitoring, or intervention. The potential bias of any single assessment unintentionally introduced by a single evaluator can be counterbalanced by examining similarities and contrasts between raters of the same patient. Questionnaires and rating scales that are developed to evaluate the same constructs with varied raters can be particularly helpful. For example, the Functional Assessment Measure and the Functional Independence Measure (Hamilton, Granger, Sherwin, Zielzny, & Tashman, 1987) are the most well-known interdisciplinary evaluation instruments in brain injury rehabilitation. Patient summaries from team conferences may be particularly helpful. Interdisciplinary collaboration may assist with the assessment content and aid intervention design. Contrasts in approach with a patient may be revealed, allowing the team to acknowledge synergy when possible and to address conflicts in the patient's experience of rehabilitation.

Demographics and Culture in the Selection of Assessment Measures

The utility and value of an assessment depends on whether the construct being assessed is valid for the individual. Assessment (especially quantitative assessment) is a Western construct that is grounded in an individual rather than collectivist orientation. Even within individual-focused cultures, assessment "literacy" may not be uniform. Rather, assessment literacy may vary considerably, depending on education (i.e., level and quality). For example, in the cognitive assessment literature, several studies have demonstrated that educational privilege (i.e., better quality) influences both performance on assessment measures and interpretation of the results (e.g., Contador et al., 2017; Manly, Byrd, Touradji, & Stern, 2004; Spering et al., 2012). Those with higher educational privilege are more likely to have favorable assessment findings but may be at a greater risk of a false negative finding (i.e., conclusion of no impairment when impairment exists). Likewise, individuals with lower educational privilege are more likely to have unfavorable assessment findings. For patients with lower educational privilege, a clinician can be at a greater risk of obtaining a false positive finding (i.e., conclusion of impairment when no impairment exists).

When selecting measures for rehabilitation psychology evaluations, careful attention should be devoted to the patient's native language, reading literacy, estimated premorbid cognitive function, and culture. Demographic and cultural factors are commonly considered in the selection of cognitive assessment measures but less frequently in the selection and administration of measures of pain, adjustment to disability, sexual functioning, personality, and other constructs important to rehabilitation psychology. In an ideal world, an assessment measure would be developed and normed on a population of people comprising similar demographics, culture, and language. Validity and reliability studies should be conducted for each measure. When such assessment measures are available, it is more likely the assessment findings accurately reflect a person's status. Unfortunately, short of assessing cognition and some aspects of mood and personality, few rehabilitation psychology assessment measures have demonstrated validity and reliability for non-American English-speaking samples.

Many providers try to approach the challenge of demographics, language, and culture by pursuing assessment with a direct translation of an assessment measure (i.e., from one language to another) or with the assistance of an interpreter. In such attempts, it is important to caution the consumer of the evaluation about potential limitations in the application of the results. Translation of a measure from one language into another via direct translation or use of an interpreter may not be valid. This approach unintentionally may omit essential information due to a lack of one-to-one correlation between language, culture, and values. If and when interpretation services are used, it is important to explain the assessment process to the person being assessed and to the interpreter. The interpreter must be aware of standardization processes, verbatim translation, and maintaining the same valence, prosody, and tone when interpreting assessment items to the patient and interpreting the patient's responses. Even with these issues addressed and cautions provided, it is possible that assessment findings could contain "error" in reflection of the construct being assessed.

Casas et al. (2012) argued that interpreter use should be avoided "particularly for tests with high demands on interpreter abilities and skills, with tests that have not been appropriately adapted and translated into the patient's target language and with interpreters who are not trained professionals" (p. 88). These authors cited Standard 9.03(c) of the American Psychological Association's (2017) *Ethical Principles of Psychologists and Code of Conduct*, which states that "psychologists use assessment methods that are appropriate to an individual's language preference and competence." The *Guidelines for Providers of Psychological Services to Ethnic, Linguistic, and Culturally Diverse Populations* (Office of Ethnic Minority Affairs, 1993) advises psychologists to interact with patients in the language they prefer or to make an appropriate referral.

Clinicians should bear in mind that, in some instances, such as when the goal of the evaluation is to determine how well a patient with a neurological disorder whose primary language is not English can function in a treatment or rehabilitation environment in which English is spoken, the evaluation may be best conducted in English (Judd et al., 2009). Thus, depending on the purpose of the evaluation, efforts to administer tests in the patient's primary language—when it is other than English—may be misplaced.

Psychometric Properties

The rationale for selecting assessment measures and for relying on the data emerging from the evaluation must be informed by the psychometric properties of the selected measure. It is not enough simply to have experience or familiarity with a test. Also, test selection should not be based solely on the rationale that many other providers use the measure. Responsible rehabilitation psychologists consider the empirical justification for selecting assessment measures and design the evaluation according to the best fit between the construct(s) to be assessed, discrimination power of the measures available, person being assessed, and setting of the assessment. Selected assessment measures must be valid, reliable, and clinically useful in the current episode of care and in the specific care situation.

Validity. *Validity* is defined by how well a measure captures the construct that it is supposed to measure. Without using assessment measures that maximize validity, it is difficult to know whether an assessment data point is useful. When selecting assessment tools, it is important to determine whether studies have been performed that strongly correlate with the findings from measures of similar constructs. *Convergent validity* describes the degree to which an obtained finding on a measure "agrees with" or is similar to the obtained finding on an independent measure of the same construct. For example, an obtained score on a measure of pain should be similar in valence to an obtained score on a similar measure of pain. Evidence to the contrary may call into question the degree to which the measure accurately assesses the individual's pain experience. *Divergent validity* describes the degree to which an obtained finding on a measure "disagrees with" the obtained finding on a measure of a different construct. A valid assessment measure should be similar enough to measures tapping into the same construct but different enough to demonstrate little or no relation with constructs unrelated to what is being measured. This concept reflects the important value of double dissociation.

A key feature (and frequent criticism) of psychological assessment measures is the degree to which an obtained finding reflects practical abilities or daily functioning. The ecological validity of a measure is evaluated by determining the degree to which assessment findings generalize to real-life settings. For instance, an assessment may find that a person has significant cognitive impairment, but, in everyday routine, the person functions well and can compensate for the impairment identified by the test. In rehabilitation psychology, special attention must be paid to ecological validity. For instance, assessing gait or coping in an inpatient setting may yield different results than assessing gait in a person's unique living setting or assessing coping in a person's particular family system at home. Although studies of ecological validity of cognitive measures are more common, evaluations of ecological validity for measures of pain and other multifaceted constructs, such as adjustment to disability, are rare.

There are several potential limitations or confounds to the validity of an assessment. For example, the rater of the assessment measure or the respondent may be biased or have an implicit or explicit interest in the outcome. Alternatively, the language and culture of the person being assessed may be different than the language and culture for which the assessment measure was validated. Sensory, motor, or perceptual challenges also can affect the endorsement of items on a given assessment measure. In reports, rehabilitation psychologists should document their opinions about the degree to which the findings are valid or applicable. Potential limitations to validity should be identified so that assessment data are accurately interpreted.

Reliability. Assessment aims to detect the "signal" of a given symptom or phenomenon in the presence of "noise" related to the measured variable. *Reliability* refers to the precision of an assessment finding. Reliable measures provide confidence that what is detected (or not detected) is accurate. Different facets to reliability influence the interpretation of a finding, including internal consistency, test–retest reliability, and alternate forms of reliability.

Internal consistency evaluates the degree to which items on a given test reflect similar content of the same construct. A measure of depression may have better internal consistency if test items focus primarily on affective manifestations of depression rather than affective, physiological, *and* cognitive manifestations of depression. Examining the internal consistency of a measure can help a psychologist determine if an area of clinical interest is truly being measured.

Test–retest reliability is essential to monitoring outcomes and evaluating interventions. Rehabilitation psychologists should understand that an assessment instrument measures the same phenomenon in the same way over time. In rehabilitation settings, baseline evaluation often is compared with a 3- or 6-month reassessment of the same construct. Variability in the reliability of a measure over time may result in an inaccurate understanding of the course of recovery or the success of an intervention. The rehabilitation psychologist must select baseline assessment measures with good test–retest reliability so that longitudinal data on the same measure can be interpreted.

In rehabilitation psychology, alternate forms of an assessment measure often are used because of the importance of longitudinal evaluation and documentation of outcomes and intervention success. If alternate forms of an assessment measure are available, it is important to select those with adequate alternate forms reliability to ensure that what is measured by Form A of the measure is similar to the construct evaluated with Form B. Rehabilitation psychologists who attend to the reliability of the assessment methods can establish greater clinical confidence in their conclusions.

Clinical utility. Psychologists use data from their assessments to establish and justify diagnoses and interventions and to evaluate outcomes. Perhaps the most important property of a psychological assessment measure is its *clinical utility*, that is, the usefulness of any given finding. Rehabilitation psychologists should answer the following questions when designing an evaluation: What is the best measure to evaluate the presence or absence of symptom? What does a given score on this assessment measure mean for the person being assessed? Is the score associated with a certain course of symptoms or prognosis? Is the score associated with a greater probability of recovery versus long-term disability? Do the results suggest a specific rehabilitative, compensatory, or coping strategy?

The clinical utility of a given assessment measure is evaluated by calculating sensitivity, specificity, positive predictive value (PPV), and negative predictive value (NPV); PPV and NPV require an estimate of the base rate of the clinical phenomenon in the care setting. Because there is no certainty to any diagnosis or outcome, clinical utility is evaluated with respect to probability.

The first layer of clinical utility has to do with selecting the most appropriate measure to evaluate the presence or absence of a deficit or problematic state or trait in a person. The clinician is inundated with options for assessing pain, mood, cognitive function, personality, and other factors that affect adjustment to disability. Before assessment, a clinician needs to determine what tests to use and have a rationale for the test that is selected. *Sensitivity* is defined by the number of people with a given condition who test positive for the symptom or condition. *Specificity* is defined by the number of people without a given condition who test negative for the condition. Therefore, a highly specific test helps to rule in the presence of a condition. No single test will have near perfect sensitivity and specificity.

The relation between sensitivity and specificity often is documented by a *receiver operating characteristic (ROC) curve*. An ROC curve helps to evaluate the discriminability of a measure. The data point on the ROC curve that best balances sensitivity and specificity is an ideal cutoff point for a given measure. By comparing ROC curves of different measures, a clinician can select the best measure for evaluating a person with a specific condition.

The second layer of clinical utility has to do with evaluating the usefulness of a given score on an assessment measure. No clinician can forecast the future as it relates to an individual person's rehabilitation course, but it can be helpful to know the probability or "chance" of a given outcome based on obtained test results. Knowing the chance of a given outcome, depending on the test score achieved, ultimately can influence care decisions and allocations of health care resources. *Predictive value* is the probability of having the condition or outcome, given the results of the test. Predictive values also are referred to as *posttest probabilities*, which determine whether a person has a condition of interest, given a specific test score. *PPV* is the probability of having a condition or outcome, given a positive test finding. *NPV* is the probability of not having a condition or outcome, given a negative test finding. Tests with high specificity yield higher PPV. Tests with high sensitivity yield higher NPV. No matter how sensitive or specific a test, though, there still will be a proportion of people misclassified by the test.

Consider a tangible example of how predictive values vary with the psychometric properties of a test. Imagine a test that determines whether individuals with a history of mild traumatic brain injury (mTBI) return to work after injury. Let us say that a positive finding on the test suggests a successful postinjury return to work. A negative finding on the test suggests a failed postinjury return to work. If this particular test has high PPV, then the clinician can have greater confidence that patients with a positive finding will successfully return to work. This finding informs the clinician's care decisions and recommendations, suggesting that fewer clinical resources and support may be allocated to this specific patient, thus freeing those resources for better use with others. If this particular test has high NPV, then the clinician can have greater confidence that patients with a negative finding will struggle with return to work. This finding also informs the clinician's care decisions and recommendations, suggesting a need to bolster clinical resources and support in this specific case. Thus, rehabilitation psychologists can select tests based on what they need to know in a clinical setting.

It is important to understand that the predictive value of a test varies not just as a function of sensitivity and specificity but also as a function of the prevalence (or base rate) of a condition in a given setting. If the clinician is trying to evaluate the odds that a person will have a specific outcome on the return to work measure, the PPV and NPV may vary as a function of the sample of individuals given the test. Because the measure was developed for use with mTBI populations, diagnostic tests are going to be most helpful when the prevalence of mTBI is high, such as in a traumatic brain injury (TBI) clinic sample. However, the same diagnostic tests may be less useful when the prevalence of mTBI is low, such as in an outpatient primary care practice. It benefits the clinician to use specific assessment measures in specific assessment settings, such as where the prevalence of the condition is high. Thus, the intensity of the diagnostic evaluation needs to be adjusted, depending on whether the prevalence of the condition is high or low. Information about base rates can be derived from literature searches, epidemiological studies, and formal studies of outcome, such as those of the TBI or spinal cord injury model systems. The clinical utility of an evaluation can be manipulated in a favorable way by administering measures to a known referral group, a group of individuals with similar demographics, and a group with other similar educational or other factors that influence the validity of the evaluation. Thus, it is essential for the clinician to critically examine the psychometric properties of all measures selected for an evaluation. The psychometric properties of a test greatly affect the confidence a clinician can have in the evaluation findings. The rehabilitation psychologist should select different assessment approaches and measures, depending on the clinical questions and the clinical settings in which the questions are posed.

Considerations for Obtaining Valid Results

There are many potential threats to the validity of assessment results. A proactive approach to preventing or managing the threats can improve the likelihood that valid and useful results will be obtained.

Aids, modifications, and accommodations. Standardized test administration typically is essential to obtaining results that accurately reflect the constructs of interest. However, there are situations in which deviations from the standardized procedures are necessary in the service of obtaining valid results. Controllable sources of error, such as sensory-perceptual or motor limitations that might produce spuriously low scores, need to be eliminated or reduced to the extent possible to avoid clouding interpretation of the skill(s) that a test is believed to measure. Persons with visual limitations may benefit from written materials being printed in a larger font, and persons who are hard of hearing may benefit from having written, rather than verbal, instructions and questions or may benefit from the use of a sound amplifier. Persons with oral-motor limitations may need to write responses or point to response options, or may benefit from augmentative communication devices or speech production apps on smartphones. Persons with compromised dominant hand function may be allowed to provide verbal responses or use their nondominant hand (Bush, 2000; Bush & Martin, 2004). Of course, eyeglasses, hearing aids, or other devices that the patient typically uses should be used during the assessment.

If fatigue is a concern, testing sessions should be brief. The rehabilitation psychologist may need to prioritize and limit the number of tests administered, and, for the assessment, may need to select a certain time of day that corresponds to the patient's period of greatest arousal. In such cases, it is important to document whether stimulant medication was taken at the time of the assessment (clearly, testing should not be done if the patient has ingested medicine with sedative effects). Research has been conducted on some aspects of testing modifications. A relatively quick literature search often can reveal studies on a specific modification that is being considered and can inform the clinician about what to expect from a given modification. For example, research may indicate that use of the nondominant hand is comparable with the dominant hand on a visuospatial task. In the psychological report, the clinician should explain any changes in standardized assessment procedures that could affect the validity of the findings.

Potential environmental challenges to the validity of results. A variety of environmental factors can compromise the validity of the psychological assessment results. In outpatient contexts, cell phones can be a disruptive presence, distracting the patient from assessment tasks. In inpatient settings, the presence of others—including other patients, family members, or staff—can be distracting during testing and can invalidate the results. In any context, such factors as temperature, lighting, and extraneous noise should be controlled to the extent possible and in a manner that is conducive to the psychological assessment process.

Patient factors. The ability of the patient to feel comfortable and engage fully in the evaluation process is necessary for the results to be valid. Emotional issues (e.g., depression, test-taking anxiety) and situational factors (e.g., hunger, the need to use a restroom) can affect the patient's ability to focus on assessment questions, instructions, or tasks. It is advisable for clinicians to check with patients about these issues before beginning the assessment, with instructions to patients to inform the clinician if problems along these lines arise.

Normative Data

Psychologists are tasked to assess people from different backgrounds and with various conditions. On any given day in many rehabilitation psychology practice settings, the provider may be asked to evaluate a range of patients, such as an African American teenager, an elderly Caucasian man, a woman with an eighth-grade education, or a trilingual young adult who recently moved to the United States from Mexico; each patient has different presenting problems. Many factors influence how people endorse or respond to test items or perform tasks. Age, culture, educational privilege, language, social norms, and other factors introduce variability in scores or data points when the same measure is administered to different people. Without normative data on a reference population with characteristics similar to those of the person being assessed, it is difficult to judge whether a specific data point suggests normal versus abnormal function or symptomatology. Normative studies are conducted with assessment measures in specific populations defined by a common demographic characteristic (e.g., age, ethnicity, educational attainment, language) or condition of interest (e.g., TBI, spinal cord injury, sensory impairment).

Demographically representative normative data are more commonly available for instruments used in cognitive evaluations but much less so for evaluations of personality, pain, substance abuse, sexual function, and mood. Without appropriate normative data for comparison to the case at hand, the examiner risks making a false negative diagnosis (i.e., concluding no impairment or disorder is present when it is) or a false positive diagnosis (i.e., concluding impairment or disorder when no impairment or disorder exists). Normative data help to determine the credence of a raw test score. In the absence of appropriate normative data, it is impossible to know whether obtained assessment findings are diagnostically valid and clinically relevant to case conceptualization, intervention design, or outcomes.

Subjective and Objective Symptom Assessment

Obtaining both a subjective and objective understanding of the patient's presenting problems facilitates rehabilitation efforts. The degree to which there is correspondence between the subjective and objective may provide critical information about the patient's insight into the problems.

The assessment of a patient's subjective awareness and understanding of strengths, limitations, emotional adjustment, and behavior has diagnostic and functional value. In addition to providing the psychologist essential information that helps in the development of targets for objective assessment and intervention, subjective information allows the psychologist to determine whether a patient has an understanding of the clinical condition necessary to work to compensate for limitations and pursue needed treatments. Subjective assessment is based primarily on self-report, the observations and impressions of collateral sources, and the psychologist's observations of signs of function and impairment. Symptom checklists that are based on patients' impressions of their problems but do not involve quantitative ratings or allow for normative comparisons also provide subjective information.

One-Time Versus Longitudinal Assessment

A *one-time psychological assessment* often is performed for purposes of case conceptualization and development of interventions. Longitudinal or serial assessments over the course of a patient's rehabilitation allow for the tracking of progress and the fine-tuning or appropriate discontinuation of rehabilitative efforts. In the *longitudinal assessment* process, the first assessment generates the information needed for case conceptualization and treatment planning. Multiple factors in rehabilitation contexts can affect assessment results in positive or negative ways from one time period to another. Such factors include, but are not limited to, the following: recovery; acute medical changes, such as infections or pain; situational issues, such as distractions in the setting, hunger, and emotional reactions; medication/substance effects; fatigue; opposition to the assessment; and litigation. Because of both expected recovery courses and the possible negative impacts on assessment performance, the spacing of repeated assessments typically varies according to the diagnosis but also is individually tailored to each patient's needs. The availability of prior test data can be valuable from both diagnostic and treatment perspectives.

Prior assessments, although advantageous in many ways, produce problems. A primary challenge involves determining the impact of prior involvement in the assessment process on current test performance. Particularly from the first assessment to the second assessment, individuals typically generate improved scores based solely on increased familiarity with the assessment process and the measures used (Beglinger et al., 2005; McCaffrey, Duff, & Westervelt, 2000). Known as *practice effects*, the potential benefit of prior assessments on the current results must be considered. Both improved performance and a lack of improvement can be clinically meaningful.

The expected degree of change can be estimated statistically by calculating a reliable change index or similar method, although these are not without their drawbacks, including large confidence intervals. Alternative forms of tests can help avoid problems that emerge from patients' remembering specific test items, but the prior assessment experience alone can have an overall beneficial effect, despite the use of different test forms. Multiple baseline practice assessments can help overcome the problem of practice effects but may not be feasible in many clinical contexts. Rehabilitation psychologists should be aware of practice effects and, using the most appropriate method or combination of methods, strive to estimate the extent of effects of prior assessments on the current assessment results.

Response, Symptom, and Performance Validity

The assessment of symptom and performance validity is another interesting oversight in the American Board of Rehabilitation Psychology's list of assessment competencies. The results of psychological assessment are only meaningful if the psychologist has confidence that the patient responded honestly to questions and put forth good effort on cognitive and sensorimotor tests. Psychologists have long understood that psychometric assessment of symptom validity is preferable to clinician judgment alone. Inclusion of validity scales in the Minnesota Multiphasic Personality Inventory family of tests dates back decades, and psychologists learn early in their education and training that interpretation of those test results begins with interpretation of the validity scales. Although the profession's understanding of the importance of quantitative assessment of effort on cognitive and sensorimotor tests came later, the use of quantitative assessment of effort has been a standard of practice for more than a decade (Bush et al., 2005); multiple professional organizations (e.g., British Psychological Society, 2009; Bush, Heilbronner, & Ruff, 2014; Heilbronner et al., 2009) have provided position statements that reinforce and further clarify the psychometric assessment of symptom and performance validity. Formal validity assessment measures exist because, despite training in assessing human behavior and confidence in their ability to do so, psychologists are not particularly good at determining whether patients put forth valid effort without using a formal validity assessment approach (Guilmette, 2013). A structured, multimethod approach to validity assessment is preferred (Slick & Sherman, 2013).

Response validity. Case conceptualization depends on patients' providing accurate responses to interview questions about their background, including education level, work history, substance use history, history of a learning disability, or history of psychiatric disorder. Failure to provide accurate responses may be intentional (as with oppositional behavior) or unintentional (as in cases of significant cognitive impairment). Obtaining information from multiple sources or across multiple time points helps to ensure its accuracy.

Symptom validity. Understanding the onset, course, and nature of current symptoms is necessary for rehabilitation psychologists to make accurate diagnoses and develop appropriate care plans. Consistency is a key feature of valid symptom reporting. Psychologists should evaluate consistency in the type and intensity of symptoms across time, assessment measures, and clinical providers. Similarly, consistency between reported problems and observed functioning, particularly when patients do not know they are being observed, is informative, as is consistency between reported problems and known manifestations of the patient's injury or illness. Efforts should be made to understand discrepancies among reported, observed, and expected symptoms and functioning.

Most comprehensive measures of emotional state and personality traits have validity scales. The 338-item Minnesota Multiphasic Personality Inventory, Second Edition, Restructured Form (Ben-Porath, 2012) has multiple validity scales that inform clinicians about a patient's response style. The validity scales address two general classes of threats to the validity of a protocol: (a) noncontent-based invalid responding (i.e., nonresponding, random responding, and fixed responding) and (b) content-based invalid responding (i.e., underreporting or overreporting; Ben-Porath, 2012). Additional validity scales have been developed since the test was published (e.g., Henry-Heilbronner Index, representing a "pseudosomatic factor"; Henry, Heilbronner, Algina, & Kaya, 2013). Awareness of validity scales available both in the test manual and in the literature enhances the rehabilitation psychologist's ability to make sound clinical decisions. In contrast to such omnibus measures of personality and psychopathology, the briefer measures commonly used in many rehabilitation contexts typically lack robust validity scales, leaving the clinician to rely more on the consistency among the various sources of information and behavior.

Performance validity. Patients must put forth adequate effort on ability measures for the results to meaningfully reflect the constructs of interest (e.g., memory). As with assessment of symptom validity, patients performing in a valid manner tend to present (barring any situational factors) in a manner consistent with known patterns of performance for the disorder, observed behavior, and reported problems. Freestanding and embedded empirical measures of performance validity exist to help clinicians determine whether a patient's approach to the testing was valid. Description of the various performance validity tests is beyond the scope of this chapter, but readers should review other sources on this topic (e.g., Carone & Bush, 2018; Larrabee, 2007; Morgan & Sweet, 2009).

Interpretation. There is a misconception among some psychologists that validity assessment is needed only in forensic contexts and that invalid responding reflects malingering. Although it is true that invalid results are obtained more often in forensic contexts than clinical contexts and can reflect malingering, many factors can affect the accuracy or consistency of a patient's responses. Such factors include acute mental status changes and situational issues, such as distractions in the setting, hunger, significant emotional reactions, medication/substance effects, severe physical pain and fatigue, and opposition to the assessment. The clinician must consider the various possible reasons for a patient's invalid results, taking into account the base rates of invalid reporting or performance in the specific assessment context and the clinician's own biases, and render an evidence-based opinion about the validity assessment results and the cognitive and emotional test results.

Validity assessment measures typically are not indicated for persons with severe neurological disorders who require 24-hour care. Use and interpretation of validity assessment measures with a specific patient should correspond with known groups on whom the normative data are based. That is, the results of a person who has a pain disorder and is not involved in litigation or pursuing disability benefits should be compared with groups of similar persons rather than to persons with a history of mTBI involved in litigation. However, cross-group comparisons also are informative. For example, if that same patient with pain is able to live and function independently but performs below groups of patients who have severe TBIs or advanced dementia, there is strong evidence for suboptimal performance.

CHALLENGES AND GAPS IN THE LITERATURE

Rehabilitation psychology assessments can be challenging. There are gaps in the assessment literature for the specialty; for example, whereas the modern cognitive evaluation incorporates assessment of symptom and performance validity into the assessment approach, rehabilitation psychology has yet to make this a consistent component of the evaluation. Further research is needed to evaluate how variations in symptom and performance validity affect assessment data points and the conceptualization and evaluation of interventions and outcomes. By acknowledging these areas in which greater understanding and research are needed, the competent provider can meet challenges, acknowledge the gaps, and perform an empirically supported evaluation.

The rehabilitation psychologist should be equipped to evaluate the psychometric properties of measures administered to establish diagnoses and to monitor interventions and outcomes. More research is needed on the diagnostic validity and clinical utility of data points from new measures before such measures are put into use and/or published. Knowledge of the psychometric properties of various measures informs test selection, case conceptualization, and outcome prediction. The most recently published test or revision of a test is not always the preferred test for a given patient population, particularly for patients who differ from the healthy populations that tend to be most widely represented in initial normative data samples (Bush et al., 2018).

As the U.S. population becomes more culturally and linguistically heterogeneous, assessment methods will be increasingly required to provide more detailed information about the influence of demographic and cultural factors on the assessment results. There are many demographic and cultural groups (e.g., low educational privilege; non-American English-speaking; non-American, non-English-speaking) for which there are no normative reference populations. Therefore, in rehabilitation settings, there may be a risk of diagnostic false positive errors and false negative errors. Consequently, more research is needed on the assessment and evaluation of these constructs in various normative reference samples and groups. In the future, there likely will be an increased use of technology for test administration, scoring, interpretation, and reporting of results. While enjoying the many advantages of technology-based assessment, rehabilitation psychologists must strive to maintain the human element of the assessment process that resonates so well with many patients and their families.

References

Alschuler, K. N., Kratz, A. L., & Ehde, D. M. (2016). Resilience and vulnerability in individuals with chronic pain and physical disability. *Rehabilitation Psychology*, *61*, 7–18. http://dx.doi.org/10.1037/rep0000055

American Psychological Association. (2017). *Ethical principles of psychologists and code of conduct* (2002, Amended June 1, 2010 and January 1, 2017). Retrieved from http://www.apa.org/ethics/code/index.aspx

Beglinger, L. J., Gaydos, B., Tangphao-Daniels, O., Duff, K., Kareken, D. A., Crawford, J., . . . Siemers, E. R. (2005). Practice effects and the use of alternate forms in serial neuropsychological testing. *Archives of Clinical Neuropsychology*, *20*, 517–529. http://dx.doi.org/10.1016/j.acn.2004.12.003

Ben-Porath, Y. S. (2012). *Interpreting the MMPI-2-RF*. Minneapolis: University of Minnesota Press.

British Psychological Society. (2009). *Assessment of effort in clinical testing of cognitive functioning for adults*. Leicester, England: Author.

Bush, S. (2000). Intermanual differences in performing a visuoconstructional task. *Archives of Physical Medicine and Rehabilitation*, *81*, 1151–1152. http://dx.doi.org/10.1053/apmr.2000.7169

Bush, S., & Martin, T. (2004). Intermanual differences on the Rey Complex Figure Test. *Rehabilitation Psychology*, *49*, 76–78. http://dx.doi.org/10.1037/0090-5550.49.1.76

Bush, S. S., Heilbronner, R. L., & Ruff, R. M. (2014). Psychological assessment of symptom and performance validity, response bias, and malingering: Official position of the Association for Psychological Advancement in Psychological Injury and Law. *Psychological Injury and Law*, *7*, 197–205. http://dx.doi.org/10.1007/s12207-014-9198-7

Bush, S. S., Ruff, R. M., Tröster, A. I., Barth, J. T., Koffler, S. P., Pliskin, N. H., . . . Silver, C. H. (2005). Symptom validity assessment: Practice issues and medical necessity NAN Policy & Planning Committee. *Archives of Clinical Neuropsychology*, *20*, 419–426. http://dx.doi.org/10.1016/j.acn.2005.02.002

Bush, S. S., Sweet, J. J., Bianchini, K. J., Johnson-Greene, D., Dean, P. M., & Schoenberg, M. R. (2018). Deciding to adopt revisions and new psychological and neuropsychological tests: An inter-organizational position paper. *Clinical Neuropsychologist*, *32*, 319–325. http://dx.doi.org/10.1080/13854046.2017.1422277

Carone, D. A., & Bush, S. S. (2018). *Validity assessment in rehabilitation psychology and settings*. New York, NY: Oxford University Press.

Casas, R., Guzmán-Vélez, E., Cardona-Rodriguez, J., Rodriguez, N., Quiñones, G., Izaguirre, B., & Tranel, D. (2012). Interpreter-mediated neuropsychological testing of monolingual Spanish speakers. *Clinical Neuropsychologist*, *26*, 88–101. http://dx.doi.org/10.1080/13854046.2011.640641

Catalano, D., Chan, F., Wilson, L., Chiu, C. Y., & Muller, V. R. (2011). The buffering effect of resilience on depression among individuals with spinal cord injury: A structural equation model. *Rehabilitation Psychology*, *56*, 200–211. http://dx.doi.org/10.1037/a0024571

Contador, I., del Ser, T., Llamas, S., Villarejo, A., Benito-León, J., & Bermejo-Pareja, F. (2017). Impact of literacy and years of education on the diagnosis of dementia: A population-based study. *Journal of Clinical and Experimental Neuropsychology*, *39*, 112–119. http://dx.doi.org/10.1080/13803395.2016.1204992

Guilmette, T. J. (2013). The role of clinical judgment in symptom validity assessment. In D. A. Carone & S. S. Bush (Eds.), *Mild traumatic brain injury: Symptom validity assessment and malingering* (pp. 31–43). New York, NY: Springer.

Hamilton, B. B., Granger, C. V., Sherwin, F. S., Zielzny, M., & Tashman, J. S. (1987). A uniform national data system for medical rehabilitation. In M. J. Fuhrer (Ed.), *Rehabilitation outcomes: Analysis and measurement* (pp. 137–147). Baltimore, MD: Brookes.

Heilbronner, R. L., Sweet, J. J., Morgan, J. E., Larrabee, G. J., Millis, S. R., & Conference Participants. (2009). American Academy of Clinical Neuropsychology Consensus Conference statement on the neuropsychological assessment of effort, response bias, and malingering. *Clinical Neuropsychologist*, *23*, 1093–1129. http://dx.doi.org/10.1080/13854040903155063

Henry, G. K., Heilbronner, R. L., Algina, J., & Kaya, Y. (2013). Derivation of the MMPI-2-RF Henry-Heilbronner Index-r (HHI-r) scale. *Clinical Neuropsychologist*, *27*, 509–515. http://dx.doi.org/10.1080/13854046.2012.739644

Judd, T., Capetillo, D., Carrión-Baralt, J., Mármol, L. M., Miguel-Montes, L. S., Navarrete, M. G., . . . Valdés, J., & the NAN Policy and Planning Committee. (2009). Professional considerations for improving the neuropsychological evaluation of Hispanics: A National Academy of Neuropsychology education paper. *Archives of Clinical Neuropsychology*, *24*, 127–135. http://dx.doi.org/10.1093/arclin/acp016

Larrabee, G. J. (Ed.). (2007). *Assessment of malingered neurocognitive deficits*. New York, NY: Oxford University Press.

Lezak, M. D., Howieson, D. B., Bigler, E. D., & Tranel, D. (2012). *Neuropsychological assessment* (5th ed.). New York, NY: Oxford University Press.

Manly, J. J., Byrd, D. A., Touradji, P., & Stern, Y. (2004). Acculturation, reading level, and neuropsychological test performance among African American elders. *Applied Neuropsychology*, *11*, 37–46. http://dx.doi.org/10.1207/s15324826an1101_5

McCaffrey, R. J., Duff, K., & Westervelt, H. J. (Eds.). (2000). *Practitioner's guide to evaluating change with neuropsychological assessment instruments*. New York, NY: Springer Science & Business Media.

McKillop, A. B., Carroll, L. J., Jones, C. A., & Battié, M. C. (2017). The relation of social support and depression in patients with chronic low back pain. *Disability and Rehabilitation*, *39*, 1482–1488. http://dx.doi.org/10.1080/09638288.2016.1202335

Morgan, J. E., & Sweet, J. J. (Eds.). (2009). *Neuropsychology of malingering casebook*. New York, NY: Psychology Press.

Office of Ethnic Minority Affairs, American Psychological Association. (1993). Guidelines for providers of psychological services to ethnic, linguistic, and culturally diverse populations. *American Psychologist*, *48*, 45–48.

Prigatano, G. P. (1999). Impaired awareness, finger tapping, and rehabilitation outcome after brain injury. *Rehabilitation Psychology*, *44*, 145–159. http://dx.doi.org/10.1037/0090-5550.44.2.145

Sherer, M., Bergloff, P., Levin, E., High, W. M., Jr., Oden, K. E., & Nick, T. G. (1998). Impaired awareness and employment outcome after traumatic brain injury. *Journal of Head Trauma Rehabilitation*, *13*, 52–61. http://dx.doi.org/10.1097/00001199-199810000-00007

Slick, D. J., & Sherman, E. M. S. (2013). Differential diagnosis of malingering. In D. A. Carrone & S. S. Bush (Eds.), *Mild traumatic brain injury: Symptom validity assessment and malingering* (pp. 57–72). New York, NY: Springer.

Spering, C. C., Hobson, V., Lucas, J. A., Menon, C. V., Hall, J. R., & O'Bryant, S. E. (2012). Diagnostic accuracy of the MMSE in detecting probable and possible Alzheimer's disease in ethnically diverse highly educated individuals: An analysis of the NACC database. *Journals of Gerontology: Series A*, *67*, 890–896. http://dx.doi.org/10.1093/gerona/gls006

Wade, S. L., Zhang, N., Yeates, K. O., Stancin, T., & Taylor, H. G. (2016). Social environmental moderators of long-term functional outcomes of early childhood brain injury. *JAMA Pediatrics*, *170*, 343–349. http://dx.doi.org/10.1001/jamapediatrics.2015.4485

CHAPTER 5

INTERVENTION

Aaron P. Turner and Charles H. Bombardier

Rehabilitation psychology has been defined as the "application of psychological knowledge and skills on behalf of individuals with disabilities and chronic health conditions in order to maximize health and welfare, independence and choice, functional abilities, and social role participation across the lifespan" (American Psychological Association, Division 22—Rehabilitation Psychology, 2018). In this chapter, we discuss how rehabilitation psychologists use their knowledge to develop and apply interventions that improve the lives of those they serve. We first describe the roles of rehabilitation psychologists and the settings in which these psychologists frequently are found. We then address the scope of rehabilitation psychology specialty practice as defined by the American Board of Professional Psychology (ABPP) competencies that guide this handbook. The majority of this chapter introduces a new conceptual model of intervention in rehabilitation psychology called *PANEP* that forms an organizing framework for identifying and tailoring treatments. In reviewing the evidence for rehabilitation interventions—the *E* in the PANEP model—intervention topics are categorized according to ABPP content areas. We present suggestions for future directions to extend the reach, impact, and rigor of the field.

CONTEXT OF INTERVENTION

The range of interventions performed by rehabilitation psychologists is diverse in scope and broad in application. Rehabilitation psychologists may work with patients, their families, and their larger social networks, as well as the medical and rehabilitation teams with which they come into contact. Individual treatment may be focused specifically on a clearly defined mental disorder, such as major depressive disorder or generalized anxiety disorder. In other instances, rehabilitation psychologists frequently find themselves working with individuals whose psychological concerns may be either secondary to, or fundamentally intertwined with, physical injury and illness, or health behavior change (see Chapter 9 in Cox, Cox, & Caplan, 2013). Patients identified by family or other rehabilitation team members as having mental health needs may not initially expect to meet with a psychologist or, in some cases, may not even have an interest in mental health treatment.

SCOPE OF INTERVENTION

Rehabilitation psychologists provide interventions for individuals across the entire lifespan of an injury, chronic illness, and acquired disability, and, as a result, they are found in a broad range of settings that may include critical care, acute and subacute inpatient rehabilitation, outpatient rehabilitation, and specialized outpatient clinics (e.g., sports medicine, pain) and community transition programs. Context may have a significant impact on the time frame of intervention, which may range from a limited number of visits over several days of a brief inpatient admission to a

http://dx.doi.org/10.1037/0000129-006
Handbook of Rehabilitation Psychology, Third Edition, L. A. Brenner, S. A. Reid-Arndt, T. R. Elliott, R. G. Frank, and B. Caplan (Editors-in-Chief)

lifetime of care as part of ongoing outpatient chronic illness management.

Expectations for the practice of rehabilitation psychology are defined most clearly by the ABPP competencies for specialty certification that include both foundational and intervention-specific competencies (see Chapter 1, this volume). These later competencies also serve to define the traditional scope of services rehabilitation psychologists provide. With respect to foundational principles, rehabilitation psychologists are expected to demonstrate professionalism and an identification with their specialty. They engage in reflective practice by identifying professional strengths and weaknesses, working toward ongoing knowledge and skill development, and seeking consultation and training, when necessary. They appreciate individual and cultural diversity by promoting awareness of, and sensitivity toward, the differences in the communities in which they operate. They implement ethical and legal principles in their daily practice and maintain knowledge of the American Psychological Association's (2017) *Ethical Principles of Psychologists and Code of Conduct* and other relevant statutes and legal standards. Rehabilitation psychologists must be able to develop and maintain good working relationships with patients, coworkers, and other individuals they serve; this includes the ability to communicate clearly and concisely across settings (e.g., team meetings, family conferences) and modalities (e.g., written reports, verbal interactions). They must function effectively in interdisciplinary systems, including working closely with treatment professionals from a variety of disciplines in a variety of roles (e.g., consultation, collaboration, leadership, support), as necessary, for different patients, treatment goals, or teams. They maintain up-to-date scientific knowledge to inform evidence-based practice.

The intervention-specific competencies are built on, and informed by, this foundation. They include general principles (e.g., intervention context, referral question, milieu, documentation), adjustment to disability (individual), adjustment to disability (family), behavior management, sexuality, vocational issues, and pain and substance abuse (discussed individually later in the section Evidence Base for Intervention) Notably, interventions with children and interventions specifically targeted toward cognitive outcomes (e.g., cognitive rehabilitation) frequently are the focus of rehabilitation psychology but regrettably are beyond the scope of this chapter.

TOWARD A CONCEPTUAL MODEL OF INTERVENTION

Over time, the process of selecting and implementing rehabilitation psychology interventions has evolved to include several core domains that can be combined into a conceptual framework. Not surprisingly, they arise from the experience of working with individuals with disability across a variety of issues and settings. Together, these factors can be categorized in the conceptual model PANEP, which reflects an understanding of guiding principles of rehabilitation intervention, specifically the individual and social context of disability; the ongoing process of adapting to disability; the natural history of injury and illness, and responses to it; the evidence base of for specific interventions; and modifications to interventions based on clinical presentation (see Figure 5.1). Each of these ideas is described in more detail in the sections that follow.

Guiding Principles of Intervention

Rehabilitation psychology is grounded in series of foundational principles articulated and revisited over the past 50 years of the field's history. The most widely known is the "value-laden beliefs and principles" articulated by Beatrice Wright in the preface to the second edition of her classic text on the social psychology of disability (Wright, 1983, pp. x–xvii). In it, she identifies 20 principles to serve as inspiration and road map to guide the field of rehabilitation; recently, Stiers (2016) summarized those principles into three distinct categories: (a) individual psychological processes, (b) social psychological processes, and (c) values.

Individual psychological processes. Rehabilitation psychology explicitly recognizes that every person, regardless of disability, possesses psychosocial assets on which he or she can draw. These assets can come

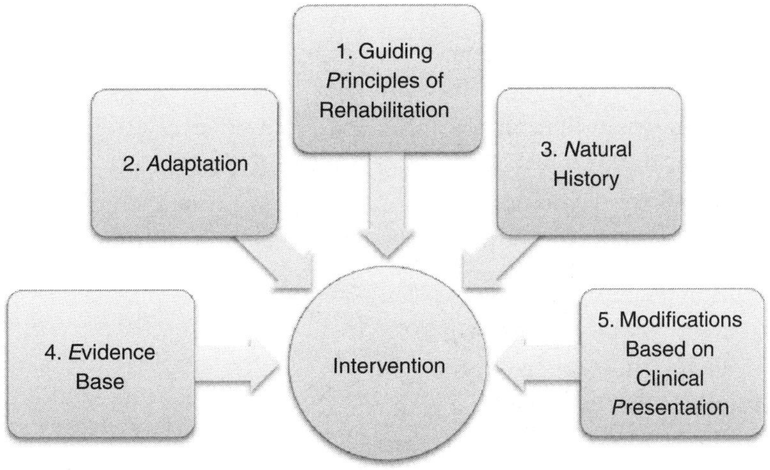

FIGURE 5.1. The PANEP (guiding *p*rinciples, *a*daptation, *n*atural history, *e*vidence base, clinical *p*resentation) model of rehabilitation psychology intervention.

in many forms, including those that are tangible (e.g., income, social network), personal qualities (e.g., sense of humor), previous attainments (e.g., education), and future goals and aspirations (Dunn, Ehde, & Wegener, 2016). Similarly, rehabilitation psychology focuses on, and emphasizes the development of, personal strengths, reminding people about their accomplishments even in the face of significant loss and encouraging the development of new skills even in the face of significant challenge (Dunn et al., 2016). With its affinity for identifying and fostering assets and strengths, rehabilitation psychology shares many commonalities with, and draws strongly from, the field of positive psychology. Several models of well-being and flourishing can provide conceptual targets for rehabilitation interventions. To provide one example, the PERMA model encourages the pursuit of five goals: *p*ositive emotions, *e*ngagement, *r*elationships, *m*eaning, and *a*chievement (Seligman, 2011).

Rehabilitation psychology recognizes the importance of self-perception in the context of illness and injury. It strives to promote a nondevaluating perspective on disability and promote personal appraisals that are realistic but do not unnecessarily and negatively impact self-worth and future outlook (Dunn et al., 2016; Wright, 1983).

Social psychological processes. Rehabilitation psychology acknowledges that the coping and adjustment of individuals with disability cannot be separated from the realities of the larger environment. Consequently, psychosocial functioning should be viewed in the context of families, support networks, social attitudes, structural environments, and economic, legal, and political factors that can increase or diminish the experience of disability.

Wright (1983) noted that individuals with disability "commonly share certain problems by virtue of their disadvantaged and devalued position" (p. xv). Several authors have argued that, as a result, individuals with disability share similarities with other minority groups in how they perceive themselves and how they are perceived by others, and that a minority model of disability provides important information about life challenges. Often, this perspective can be a source of strength by contributing to a sense of identity, opening opportunity for affiliation, and providing models for responding to discrimination (Olkin & Pledger, 2003). For additional discussion of social psychology and rehabilitation, see Chapter 9, this volume.

Values: Dignity and participation. Perhaps most centrally, rehabilitation psychology particularly emphasizes the promotion of human dignity. Wright (1987) asserted that a "core concept of human dignity is that a person is not an object, not a thing" (p. 12) and, as a result, "every individual needs respect and encouragement; the presence of a disability, no matter how severe, does not alter these fundamental rights" (p. xi). One outgrowth of this perspective is an emphasis on both independence and participation—that individuals with disability be active contributors to their rehabilitation programs, and that rehabilitation itself focus heavily on participation in the life of society, including independent living, meaningful work, and fulfilling social engagement.

Structural framework. Many of the guiding principles of rehabilitation psychology are codified in the World Health Organization's (2002) International Classification of Functioning, Disability and Health: ICF. The ICF establishes a framework that is not limited to the traditional medical conceptualization of disease and disability; instead, it recognizes that health conditions (e.g., injuries, diseases, disorders) interact with contextual factors that may be personal (e.g., age, gender) or environmental (e.g., built environment, social attitudes) to produce an overall level of health and function (World Health Organization, 2002). Further classification allows for the differentiation of limitations that may exist at the level of impairment of body structure or function (e.g., amputation), activity (e.g., ambulation), or participation (e.g., hiking with family), and the role of the environment in the experience of limitations (e.g., living near an accessible mall versus living in a community without sidewalks). The perspective extends to mental health, in which, for example, an anxiety disorder (i.e., impairment) may lead to significant difficulties communicating with friends and work colleagues (i.e., activity limitation), resulting in absences from work social gatherings (i.e., participation restriction). This system has considerable advantages: It shifts emphasis from cataloging discrete disease states to the identification of preserved abilities, allows for universal description of the functioning of all individuals regardless of underlying health conditions, and recognizes the role of the environment (World Health Organization, 2002).

Adaptation

A primary focus of work for rehabilitation psychologists is helping individuals come to terms with challenges posed by changes in sensory-perceptual, motor, language, and cognitive abilities. This immensely complex process frequently is described in the literature as adaptation to disability. Although individual responses to the onset of illness and injury vary considerably, the construct of adaptation provides a useful framework to help rehabilitation psychologists anticipate the potential needs of their patients and thus inform and guide their treatment.

Adaptation has been conceptualized dimensionally and pragmatically as consisting of nonadaptive responses to the onset of a disability (e.g., shock, anxiety, depression, anger) and adaptive responses (e.g., acknowledgment, adjustment; Livneh, Martz, & Bodner, 2006). More recent studies have indicated that denial and, alternatively, awareness of impairment represent a third dimension (Livneh et al., 2006).

A particularly rich description of adaptation has been proposed by Livneh and Antonak (2005), who posited that adjustment also consists of eight basic concepts: (a) *stress:* from the disruptions caused by disability; (b) *crisis:* the potentially sudden and traumatic nature of disability onset; (c) *loss and grief:* the mourning of a body part or function that may be repeatedly triggered by daily experiences; (d) *body image:* alterations in body schema, integrity, or self-concept, including impact on physical capabilities, pain, anxiety, depression, and fatigue; (e) *self-concept:* the sense of self that can be split into discordant private versus public ("disabled") selves based on mere appearance; (f) *stigma:* the impact of stereotypes and social restrictions on opportunities and self-esteem; (g) *uncertainty and unpredictability:* regarding prognosis, course, and outcomes that may pertain to some conditions (e.g., multiple sclerosis [MS]) more than others (e.g., complete spinal cord injury [SCI]); and (h) *quality of life:* including navigating intrapersonal, social, and role-functioning domains. Not every person will confront all the issues just described, but awareness of some of the common themes in the lived experience of individuals with disability is critical to understanding the challenges that make life both difficult and meaningful. These themes often form the therapeutic "grist for the mill" in treatment and the personal and social context through which traditional interventions are adapted and implemented. For example, behavioral activation for social engagement following limb loss might involve overcoming experiential avoidance of distress associated with body image and perceived stigma; cognitive behavior therapy (CBT) for depression following SCI might involve challenging pervasive negative thoughts about competence and worth following changes in physical function; and acceptance and commitment therapy for anxiety following a new diagnosis of MS or amyotrophic lateral sclerosis (ALS) might involve mindful acceptance of uncertainty surrounding disease course.

Natural History

Intervention is informed by an understanding of common trajectories of adaptation in the face of illness and injury, resulting in disability. In the early years of rehabilitation, the stages of grief model was used to describe normal longitudinal adaptation to acquired disability, especially in SCI but also in other disability groups (Vargo, 1978). This theoretical model was criticized for its lack of empirical grounding (Wortman & Silver, 1989). The stages of grief model gave way to a focus on a biopsychosocial model of adjustment (Elliott & Frank, 1996). Subsequent research focused more intently on measurable or diagnosable mental health conditions, such as depression, anxiety, and posttraumatic stress disorder (Craig, Hancock, & Dickson, 1994; Hibbard, Uysal, Kepler, Bogdany, & Silver, 1998). More recently, investigators have examined trajectories of symptoms, such as depression and anxiety, that might show the course of adjustment (Bonanno, Kennedy, Galatzer-Levy, Lude, & Elfström, 2012). This research has suggested four different adjustment trajectories after the onset of disability, most notably, the majority (66%) of individuals do well following a new injury, such as SCI. Approximately 13% will present with elevated distress that resolves over the course of the first year, 10% will report low initial distress that builds over the course of a year, and another 11% will display persistent distress. In addition, this research has shown that early appraisal and coping, the person's preinjury mental health and substance abuse history, and early pain, grief, and quality of life may impact depression trajectories 1 year to 2 years after disability onset.

Little is known about how adjustment trajectories may differ in various disability groups. Adjustment to traumatic disability in which some recovery is expected may differ from adjustment to diseases with uncertain or progressive courses, such as MS and ALS. Adjustment to traumatic injury may be different from other acquired disability (e.g., traumatic brain injury [TBI] versus stroke) because the person's age, socioeconomic background, and mental and physical health histories, as well as the circumstances surrounding disability onset, may differ between groups. Primary and secondary characteristics of the disabling condition (e.g., cognitive impairment, disfigurement, pain, immobility, fatigue) also should be considered when formulating expectations regarding adjustment trajectories.

Evidence Base for Intervention

In previous sections, we examined the first three components of our conceptual model of intervention that inform the contexts and targets of treatment. In this section, we review the knowledge base for the particular interventions highlighted in the ABPP competencies, beginning with the first and best developed: individual intervention. We then review additional areas by competency topic (e.g., pain, health behavior). As a review of the literature shows, the scientific underpinnings of our field remain in a nascent stage of development; however, emerging evidence is beginning to provide a base of knowledge to guide evidence-based practices in some areas. Because treatment outcome literature in rehabilitation psychology remains limited, we have included early evidence of promising practices.

Adjustment to disability: Individual. Selection of an appropriate intervention in rehabilitation psychology should be shaped by an understanding of current evidence in the field, specifically what works, for whom, and under what circumstances. In Table 5.1, we summarize current evidence on the treatment of two common mental health conditions (i.e., depression and anxiety) in three populations of individuals (i.e., TBI, SCI, and MS) seen in rehabilitation settings. The table is intended to provide a practical, 10,000-foot overview of the scientific literature for all rehabilitation psychologists. It is neither exhaustive (we do not mention every study) nor systematic (we do not grade every study using an

TABLE 5.1

Evidence for Psychosocial Interventions for Depression and Anxiety in Selected Rehabilitation Populations

Condition	Treatment	Outcome	Modality	Evidence	Comments	References
TBI	CBT vs. SUP	Dep Anx	I	b	Postacute comparative effectiveness RCT ($n = 77$) in which 16 sessions of CBT were equivalent to 16 sessions of SUP for people with MDD in the *Diagnostic and Statistical Manual of Mental Disorders* (4th ed.; *DSM–IV*; American Psychiatric Association, 1994); Anx also decreased significantly in both groups	Ashman, Cantor, Tsaousides, Spielman, & Gordon, 2014
TBI	PS and BA vs. UC	Dep	I, T	b	Secondary analysis of postrehabilitation RCT ($n = 126$) in which 7 scheduled T counseling sessions resulted in significantly lower Dep severity at 1 year	Bell et al., 2005; Bombardier et al., 2009
TBI	PA	Dep	I	b	RCT crossover study of 12-week home-based walking intervention vs. nutrition education; trend for Dep to decrease more with walking vs. nutrition class	Bellon et al., 2015
TBI	CBT	Dep	IN	a	Open trial of a 6-week IN-based CBT program postacute injury with Dep ($n = 21$); "completers" had significantly decreased Dep from baseline at 6 weeks and at 12 months	Topolovec-Vranic et al., 2010
TBI	MBCT vs. UC	Dep	G	a	Quasi-RCT of MBCT vs. UC ($n = 105$) in people with Dep; MBCT (15 hours over 10 weeks) resulted in a significantly greater reduction in Dep severity	Bédard et al., 2014
TBI	CST	Dep	G	a	Open trial of 6–8 weeks of group CST in veterans ($n = 21$) with mild cognitive disorder; completers demonstrated significant decline in Dep severity	Huckans et al., 2010
TBI	CBT vs. UC	Dep	I, T	b	Choice-stratified RCT of 12 sessions of in-person CBT or T CBT vs. UC in persons with MDD in *DSM–IV* ($n = 100$); post hoc analyses showed greater improvement on self-reported Dep severity in T CBT vs. UC	Fann et al., 2015
TBI	CBT + CR vs. WLC	Dep	I	a	RCT of 60 hours of CBT + CR vs. WLC over 11 weeks in patients with subjective cognitive dysfunction and emotional distress ($n = 29$); among completers ($n = 20$), Dep and Anx were significantly lower in the CBT + CR group	Tiersky et al., 2005
TBI	MI + CBT or NDC + CBT vs. WLC	Anx Dep	I	b	RCT of WLC vs. 3 weeks of MI or NDC, 9 weeks of CBT, and 3 CBT booster sessions postacute injury in people with Anx or Dep ($n = 75$); CBT groups had significantly greater reductions in Anx and Dep than WLC; no differences between MI vs. NDC subgroups	Ponsford et al., 2016

TABLE 5.1

Evidence for Psychosocial Interventions for Depression and Anxiety in Selected Rehabilitation Populations (*Continued*)

Condition	Treatment	Outcome	Modality	Evidence	Comments	References
TBI	EX	Anx Dep	G	a	RCT of 8 weeks (24 sessions) of aquatic aerobic plus strength training EX vs. vocational rehabilitation classes (*n* = 16); EX group had significantly better mood scores than control group	Driver & Ede, 2009
TBI	EX vs. WLC	Dep	G	b	RCT of 10 weekly aerobic EX sessions and home EX program vs. WLC in people with at least mild Dep; across both groups, those exercising 90 min/week or more were less depressed at follow-up	Hoffman et al., 2010
SCI	CBT	Anx, Dep	G	a	Trial of 10 weeks of group CBT for inpatients with SCI (*n* = 28) vs. historical and other controls (*n* = 41); among those depressed at baseline, CBT group was less depressed at 1 year compared with controls	Craig, Hancock, Dickson, & Chang, 1997
SCI	CET	Anx, Dep	G	a	Trial of 7 sessions of group CET among inpatients (*n* = 19) compared with matched historical controls; CET group had greater decreases in Dep and Anx than controls	C. King & Kennedy, 1999
SCI	CET	Anx, Dep	G	a	Trial of 7 sessions of group CET among inpatients (*n* = 45) compared with matched controls; Dep and Anx decreased significantly in CET group but not in control group at 6-week follow-up	Kennedy, Duff, Evans, & Beedie, 2003
SCI	CET vs. SGT	Anx Dep	G	a	RCT of 6 weekly sessions of CET vs. SGT among inpatients (*n* = 40); Dep and Anx decreased significantly in both groups from admission to discharge; CET used fewer sessions to obtain a similar effect	Duchnick, Letsch, & Curtiss, 2009
SCI, MS	AER	Dep	IVR	b	RCT of weekly IVR delivered AER calls over 6 months vs. UC in people who use a wheelchair for SCI (*n* = 106) or MS (*n* = 36); AER group reported significantly lower Dep severity than controls at 6 months	Houlihan et al., 2013
SCI	CBT	Dep	I	a	Open trial in community-residing persons with mostly chronic Dep comparing who accepted CBT (*n* = 28) and antidepressant treatment vs. declined treatment (*n* = 15); treated group had a 57% reduction in Dep severity	Kemp, Kahan, Krause, Adkins, & Nava, 2004

(*continues*)

TABLE 5.1

Evidence for Psychosocial Interventions for Depression and Anxiety in Selected Rehabilitation Populations (*Continued*)

Condition	Treatment	Outcome	Modality	Evidence	Comments	References
MS	CBT	Dep Anx	I	c	RCT of 6-session CBT with PMR vs. UC (*n* = 36); CBT group reported significantly lower Dep and Anx at 5-week posttreatment follow-up	Foley, Bedell, LaRocca, Scheinberg, & Reznikoff, 1987
MS	CBT	Dep	I	c	RCT of 16 weeks of weekly 50-minute CBT vs. 16 weeks of weekly 90-minute SEG vs. sertraline for individuals with MDD (*n* = 63); CBT group reported significantly greater improvement in Dep than SEG	Mohr, Boudewyn, Goodkin, Bostrom, & Epstein, 2001
MS	CBT	Dep	I, T	c	RCT of 16-weeks of weekly T CBT vs. 16 weeks supportive therapy for individuals with MDD (*n* = 127); CBT group reported greater improvement in Dep than supportive therapy; only 5.5% attrition	Mohr et al., 2005
MS	CBT	Dep	I, T	c	RCT of 8 weeks of T CBT vs. UC (*n* = 32) for individuals with elevated depressive symptoms; CBT group reported greater improvement in Dep at treatment completion	Mohr et al., 2000
MS	CBT	Dep	G	b	RCT of 6 week group-based CBT vs. UC (*n* = 20); CBT group reported greater improvement at 4-week follow-up	Larcombe & Wilson, 1984
MS	MI + PA	Dep	I, T	b	RCT of 9-session (7 T) of MI vs. UC (*n* = 92) to improve physical activity; MI condition reported greater physical activity and reduced Dep compared with controls at 12 weeks	Bombardier et al., 2013
MS	MI + PA	Dep	I, T	b	RCT of 6 weekly sessions of T MI + telehealth home monitoring vs. education and advice (*n* = 64) to improve physical activity; MI condition reported greater physical activity and reduced Dep compared with education at 6 months	Turner et al., 2016
MS	SM	Dep	I, T	b	RCT of 8 weekly sessions of T SM vs. 8 weekly sessions of T MS education (*n* = 163); there were significant reductions in Dep in the SM condition at posttreatment	Ehde et al., 2015
MS	SM	Dep	I, T, IN	a	RCT of SM consisting of 8 interactive IN modules combined with up to 3 T support sessions vs. UC (*n* = 40); SM condition reported greater improvement in Dep at 10-week follow-up	Moss-Morris et al., 2012

TABLE 5.1

Evidence for Psychosocial Interventions for Depression and Anxiety in Selected Rehabilitation Populations (*Continued*)

Condition	Treatment	Outcome	Modality	Evidence	Comments	References
MS	MBSR	Dep Anx	G	[b]	RCT of group-based MBSR vs. UC ($n = 150$); MBSR group reported greater improvements in Dep and Anx postintervention and 6-month follow-up among individuals with elevated symptom levels at baseline	Grossman et al., 2010
MS	MBCT	Dep Anx	G, IN	[b]	RCT of group-based teleconference-delivered MBCT vs. WLC ($n = 40$); MBCT reported greater improvements in Dep and Anx postintervention and 3-month follow-up.	Bogosian et al., 2015

Note. TBI = traumatic brain injury; CBT = cognitive behavior therapy; SUP = nondirective supportive counseling; Dep = depression; Anx = anxiety; I = individual; RCT = randomized controlled trial; MDD = major depressive disorder; PS = problem-solving; BA = behavior activation; UC = usual care; T = telephone; PA = physical activity; IN = Internet program; "completers" = individuals completing treatment; MBCT = mindfulness-based cognitive therapy; G = group; CST = cognitive strategy training; CR = cognitive remediation; WLC = wait-list control; MI = motivational interviewing; NDC = nondirective counseling; EX = exercise; SCI = spinal cord injury; CET = coping effectiveness training; SGT = supportive group therapy; MS = multiple sclerosis; AER = assessment, education, referral; IVR = telephone-based interactive voice response system; PMR = progressive muscle relaxation; SEG = supportive expressive group therapy; SM = self-management; MBSR = mindfulness-based stress reduction.
[a]Case study or series, pre–post improvement in a treatment arm, nonrandomized, historical, or other control group.
[b]RCT. [c]Multiple RCTs (study is supported by a separate study of same condition, treatment, outcome, and modality).

extensive list of criteria). Short descriptions are provided. Readers interested in additional specifics are encouraged to examine the studies that are listed.

Adjustment to disability: Family. Families are the principal source of social support for most individuals living with disability. They may be called on to provide practical, emotional, and financial assistance, and to advocate for medical and community services. Illness and injury often have a major impact on family members who may be asked to master complex medical information, develop new skill sets, alter their social and family roles, and, in many instances, assume responsibilities as a caregiver.

Numerous opportunities are available to rehabilitation psychologists to participate in intervention for families in several domains, such as education (e.g., providing information the course or symptoms of illness), skill training (e.g., behavior management) and treatment to promote caregiver emotional health (e.g., managing stress, guilt sadness), conflict management (e.g., couples therapy), social support (e.g., using social networks), and counseling for adjustment to new life circumstances (Chwalisz & Dollinger, 2010; Ramkumar & Elliott, 2010).

Caregivers represent one of the most immediate sources of support for persons living with disability; consequently, their health and well-being is a high priority and a primary focus of intervention. Many people report positive experiences serving in a caregiving role, including personal growth, strengthening of important relationships, and an increased appreciation of life (Pakenham, 2005; Wells, Dywan, & Dumas, 2005). At the same time, the demands of caregiving can represent a significant challenge because they impact physical, emotional, and social well-being. Available evidence has suggested that many caregivers report somatic symptoms and depression and anxiety, and report that the burden of caregiving results in relationship distress, increased social isolation, and reduced economic opportunity (Carlozzi et al., 2015; Kreutzer et al., 2009; Middleton et al., 2014).

Interestingly, far less is known about how the process of caregiving and the characteristics of caregivers impact those who are the actual recipients of care. Maladaptive caregiver coping styles characterized by impulsivity or passivity have been associated with greater functional deficits in individuals with TBI (Van Baalen et al., 2007) and greater likelihood of pressure ulcers in individuals with SCI (Elliott, Shewchuk, & Richards, 1999).

Growing evidence has suggested the efficacy of interventions aimed at improving caregiver satisfaction and well-being. In a large meta-analysis, Sorensen and colleagues reviewed 78 studies examining caregiver interventions and their impact on multiple caregiver outcomes (Sörensen, Pinquart, & Duberstein, 2002). On average, the interventions produced small but significant improvements across all outcomes; psychoeducational and psychotherapeutic interventions produced the biggest treatment effects Among caregiver interventions, the modality with the best empirical support is *problem-solving training*, which posits that the perceived burden and stress of caregiving demands is influenced by the cognitive and behavioral resources of the caregiver (Elliott, Shewchuk, & Richards, 2001). Individuals who perceive care provision as stressful and as exceeding personal coping resources, or who present with pessimism and low motivation for problem-solving, experience more distress over time in their caregiver roles (Chwalisz, 1996; Elliott et al., 2001; Grant et al., 2006). Based on the model developed by D'Zurilla and colleagues (e.g., D'Zurilla & Nezu, 2006), problem-solving training seeks to build problem-solving skills, including problem identification, goal setting, generating of solutions, decision making, and implementation (Pfeiffer et al., 2014).

Whether delivered in person or via a combination of face-to-face and telephone follow-ups, problem-solving training has been shown to produce reductions in depression and other distress for caregivers who provide support to individuals with stroke (Grant, Elliott, Weaver, Bartolucci, & Giger, 2002; Pfeiffer et al., 2014), TBI (Rivera, Elliott, Berry, & Grant, 2008), and SCI (Elliott, Brossart, Berry, & Fine, 2008), and mixed populations with disability (Elliott, Berry, & Grant, 2009).

Behavior management. The majority of individuals who participate in rehabilitation bring to the table a set of cognitive, personal, emotional, and social resources that differ in combination and degree but allow them to participate actively, collaboratively, and efficiently in the rehabilitation process. Sometimes however, individuals exhibit patterns of action that disrupt the provision of services or threaten the safety and welfare of themselves or others. Rehabilitation psychologists often are called on to assist teams in navigating these challenging behaviors (Kerkhoff & Butt, 2017).

Challenges include behavior that is disinhibited (e.g., lowered frustration tolerance, social and sexual language and behavior that is inappropriate for a particular context) or inhibited (e.g., lack of initiation, motivation, or engagement). Sources of behavior may include person-specific factors (e.g., premorbid coping style, anxious or depressed mood), characteristics of the injury (e.g., impairments in cognition, physical function, and emotional regulation), the environment (e.g., settings that expect a tolerance for stimulation, participation in treatment and social interaction that exceed the individual's coping resources), and the outcome (e.g., explicit or inadvertent reinforcement of the behavior; Sbordone, 1990).

Consistent with the guiding principles of rehabilitation, there is wide agreement that behavior management should be a collaborative process that strives to respect the autonomy of individuals to the greatest extent possible and operate in a context of mutual respect. This process can be challenging, particularly when patient behavior is distressing or unsafe. Often treatment teams turn to a psychologist to "fix" (meaning eliminate) unwanted actions quickly. Behavior management does not focus on establishing punitive contingencies to extinguish maladaptive target behaviors but, rather, seeks to promote adaptive behaviors that render disruptive behavior unnecessary.

The underpinning of behavior management is contextual analysis, and the widely recognized ABC model provides a useful framework for its implementation: Target behaviors can be understood in the context of their antecedents and consequences. The initial step is quantifying and clarifying the target behavior so that it is specific and explicit (e.g., "threw urinal at nurse at bedside at 9 a.m. medication administration" vs. "dysregulated outburst"). The second and third steps involve understanding the antecedent events that may have contributed to the behavior (e.g., time of day, location, task, persons involved, mental status, emotional state) and the consequences that might serve to reinforce the behavior (e.g., yelling that results in increased attention from nursing staff, skipping therapy that results in successful avoidance of painful or exhausting exercises).

With contextual analysis in mind, Sohlberg and Mateer (2001) proposed a continuum of intervention strategies to manage challenging behavior following neurologic injury that range from external (i.e., implemented by others on behalf of patients) to internal (i.e., implemented and sustained by patients themselves; see Chapter 11 in Sohlberg & Mateer, 2001). The selection of a particular strategy is guided by the insight and agency of particular participants, and matched to their current abilities and needs. Relevant considerations might include current cognitive status, time since an injury, and time since admission to a unit.

Farthest along the external end of the spectrum are *environmental management strategies*, which may include preventing visual, auditory, or social overstimulation and introducing calming influences like familiar objects or family members to reduce agitation. Paradoxically, understimulation and boredom also can serve as sources of agitation. Next are *communication strategies:* Caregivers and staff members can elect to strategically and consistently ignore some behaviors that may be reinforced by the responses they elicit or redirect attention when individuals have difficulty with perseveration or rumination. Sometimes, providing more choices and opportunities for meaningful input can counteract perceived loss of control and independence. Maintaining a calm demeanor and occasionally backing off a specific request, regrouping, and then trying again also may serve to defuse an escalating conflict or power struggle.

Moving along the continuum to more internally directed intervention, *behavioral strategies* seek to understand maladaptive behavior in the context of its antecedents and consequences, and gradually and sequentially build new patterns of behavior. As an example, an individual with quadriplegia and distressing respiratory secretions secondary to ALS who is admitted to inpatient rehabilitation develops an anxious pattern of pressing the nurse call light every 2 minutes. In collaborative discussion the patient, the physician and psychologist agree that there is no acute threat to safety and that the behavior is inconsistent with the shared goal of living with maximum independence after discharge. The patient and psychologist begin regular practice of anxiety coping strategies and develop a gradual and sequential plan for weaning use of the call light. Progress on the goal is tracked and presented as positive feedback to the patient.

Farthest along the internal end of the spectrum are *metacognitive and self-regulatory strategies* that involve self-monitoring and the deliberate use of problem-solving skills. In essence, they teach individuals to engage in their own process of identifying behaviors, increasing understanding of antecedents and consequences, and apply structured problem-solving rubrics, such as "stop, think, act." The scientific literature addressing the management of challenging behavior in rehabilitation is limited. Carnevale, Anselmi, Johnston, Busichio, and Walsh (2006) examined a natural setting behavior management program targeted at individuals with TBI and their caregivers. The intervention included 4 weeks of education followed by the development and implementation of an individualized behavior plan (based on the ABC model) over a subsequent 8 weeks. Target behaviors varied by individual but included disruptive vocalizations and perseverative and aggressive behaviors. At 30 weeks, individuals in the intervention condition experienced a significant reduction in target behaviors relative to controls.

Sexuality. Despite the effects of injury or illness, most individuals with disability maintain desires for closeness, affection, and sexual fulfillment (Torices Rodarte & Bonilla Muñoz, 2004). Even in the face of challenges that may impact satisfaction or interest, individuals frequently have reported a desire for greater sexual expression for themselves and for their partners (Sadoughi, Leshner, & Fine, 1971). Nonetheless, individuals with disability face considerable obstacles: They have reported more societal and personal barriers to dating, greater difficulty finding partners, and lower satisfaction with dating frequency than individuals without disabilities (Rintala et al., 1997). Limited evidence has suggested that they are more likely to divorce than the general population (DeVivo, Hawkins, Richards, & Go, 1995).

Most providers note that they do not consider themselves competent or are unsure of their role in delivering sexual health care (Esmail, Esmail, & Munro, 2001). It is perhaps unsurprising that many individuals with disability have reported that their sexual concerns were not addressed during rehabilitation (Esmail et al., 2001; McAlonan, 1996), and 50% have reported not having received any form of postdisability sexual education at all (McCabe, Cummins, & Deeks, 2000). Of those who did receive such education, half or less reported satisfaction with the quality (New, Seddon, Redpath, Currie, & Warren, 2016).

Considerable opportunity exists for rehabilitation psychologists to contribute to the promotion of sexual well-being among their patients across all treatment settings. The conceptual cornerstone of intervention has been the stepped care model known as PLISSIT: permission, limited information, specific suggestions, and intensive therapy. In this framework, individuals are provided with interventions of increasing intensity matched to their interests and needs. The first step, permission, involves raising the topic of sexuality as a health care issue. This important initial conversation both seeks permission from patients to ask about sex, reinforcing their role as the driver of their own sexual health, and provides permission to patients to discuss sexuality in the context of rehabilitation and identify sexual well-being as a target of treatment. The overall goal is to increase communication among patients, their partners, and the health care team, and challenge the notion that sexual expression is an unimportant or secondary consideration, or is only for typically abled individuals (Esmail et al., 2001).

The second step involves providing patients with limited information that is matched to their circumstances and interest. Educational content may range from specific to global. Examples of specific information might include a review of anatomy and the base rates, a presentation of physical impairments related to illness or injury, and a review of the prognosis for improvement and frequent complications, as well as reproductive issues, including fertility, contraception, and pregnancy (Esmail et al., 2001). Rehabilitation psychologists may have varying levels of expertise in these topics, and they frequently work in conjunction with other treatment team members (e.g., physicians, nurse specialists) to provide this information. Regardless of background, they are encouraged to familiarize themselves with these issues in the populations of individuals with whom they come into contact. Some evidence has suggested, for example, that greater knowledge about disability and its implications reduces the downstream impact of that disability on marital satisfaction (Williams, 1993).

Examples of global discussion might include conversations that move beyond a deficit model of impairment in individual sexual acts to a broader interpersonal perspective of sexuality that includes basic needs of being liked and accepted, displaying and receiving affection, feeling valued and attractive, and sharing thoughts and feelings (Esmail, Darry, Walter, & Knupp, 2010; Murphy & Elias, 2006). This expanded focus provides more opportunity to identify areas for intervention and to improve overall sexual health. Some evidence has showed that *intimacy*, more broadly defined as feelings of emotional closeness and willingness to participate in a range of sexual activities, may be at least as important for sexual fulfillment as the physiologic aspects of sex (Esmail et al., 2001).

The third and fourth steps of the PLISSIT model are most commonly implemented by individuals with specialized training. Specific suggestions may include practical education about positioning, devices and products, timing, and preparatory activities. At the level of intensive intervention, components of disability affirmative therapy, CBT, and acceptance and commitment therapy have been proposed to increase self-efficacy, self-esteem, and flexibility, and to reduce anxiety, unhelpful thought patterns, and avoidance (Carcieri & Mona, 2017).

Recently, Mona and colleagues proposed a disability and sexuality health care competency model (DASH-CM) for psychologists (Mona, Cameron, & Clemency Cordes, 2017). The DASH-CM model provides guidance to promote effective clinical assessment and, in turn, intervention in a number of specific arenas, including disability and sexuality awareness (e.g., social and political context of disability, personal perceptions of disability), knowledge (e.g., sexual anatomy, arousal, function, common presenting concerns, common sexual disorders), and skill development and application (e.g., use of affirming language; incorporation of patient perspective; routine assessment, including, as necessary, sexual history, activity, desire, preferred forms of expression, frequency, quality; satisfaction with intimate relationships).

Vocational issues. Work not only provides income and promotes financial independence, but it also contributes to identity and self-esteem, and creates opportunities to foster social networks and community engagement (Blessing, Golden, Pi, Bruyere, & Van Looy, 2012). Unfortunately, individuals with disability experience significant barriers to entering or reentering the workforce. In 2015, individuals with disability were less likely to be employed than their nondisabled counterparts (22.8% vs. 66.4%) and were more likely to live below the poverty line (33.6% vs. 19.5%; U.S. Census Bureau, 2017).

Rehabilitation psychologists can help to maximize vocational capacity directly through the use of individual intervention. Sleep and pain management, treatment of anxiety and depression, development of problem-solving strategies, and social skill building can be tailored to work settings and improved work performance (Ottomanelli, 2017). Rehabilitation psychologists also work with their treatment teams to promote employment as a goal and coordinate with in-house or community-based vocational rehabilitation counselors. Vocational rehabilitation services may include such things as an evaluation of interests, abilities, transferable skills; benefits counseling; job training; community-based situational assessment "tryouts"; individual job site consultation; job placement services; job site support services; transportation; and assistive technology (Fraser, 2010). Rehabilitation psychologists should strive to have an understanding of available services.

One potential avenue for collaborative intervention is *supported employment*, which consists of rapid engagement in job finding for competitive employment, ongoing job support, and a focus on individual participant preferences. Ideally, it is delivered by a vocational rehabilitation counselor who provides services in the community but also is closely integrated into a larger interprofessional rehabilitation team, thus providing an opportunity for consultation and coordinated intervention with other team members (including psychology). In a recent study, individuals with SCI who received supported employment were more likely to achieve competitive employment during their first year and retain it through 2-year follow-up (Ottomanelli, Barnett, & Goetz, 2014).

Pain. Chronic pain is thought to affect more than 116 million Americans and has an immense impact on the health and quality of life of those who experience it, as well as their families and support systems (Institute of Medicine, 2011). It is a particularly common concern among individuals with disability and chronic health conditions including (but not limited to) TBI, SCI, burns, amputation, MS, and stroke (Ullrich, 2017). Given its prevalence across health care settings, it is unsurprising that rehabilitation psychologists frequently are enlisted to participate in its management. Psychosocial interventions for pain are commonly guided by the realization that pain is a complex phenomenon resulting from the combination and interaction of multiple biopsychosocial factors. Jensen (2011) suggested an organizational structure of five factors that can be used to guide the development and implementation of specific pain treatments: (a) environment (e.g., reinforcement of pain behavior versus well behavior), (b) brain states (e.g., dissociation), (c) cognitive content (e.g., self-efficacy for functioning despite pain, belief one is disabled by pain), (d) cognitive coping (e.g., focusing on pain, rumination, acceptance), and (e) patient behavior (e.g., guarding, asking for assistance when in pain). Many of these factors form the targets for treatment intervention.

A growing body of outcome research has supported the use of several psychosocial treatments for pain. We review them briefly and refer readers to Chapter 14, this volume, for additional information. Hypnosis has been shown to reduce pain across a variety of pain conditions and rehabilitation populations, and mostly likely targets the experience of pain through brain states (Jensen, 2011). Relaxation training, including progressive muscle relaxation and biofeedback, is also linked to better pain outcomes and is thought to change both behavior and self-efficacy (Ostelo et al., 2005). The greatest body of evidence has supported the efficacy of CBT for pain, which frequently targets multiple factors, including behavior (e.g., pacing, activity scheduling), cognitive content and coping (e.g., restructuring maladaptive thought processes, such as rumination and catastrophizing), and environment (e.g., eliciting social support; Ehde, Dillworth, & Turner, 2014). More recently, acceptance-based therapies that emphasize pursuit of valued activities despite pain and mindfulness also have shown early promise (Pull, 2009). Treatment strategies that use graded exposure (to overcome pain-related avoidance), operant principles (i.e., social reinforcing well behaviors and ignoring pain behavior), and motivational interviewing have demonstrated potential in the treatment of chronic pain (Jensen, 2011).

Substance abuse and health behavior. The success or failure of rehabilitation efforts often hinge on whether patients make important health behavior changes. Rehabilitation psychologists often are called on to assist patients who are facing challenges adhering to medical regimens, participating fully therapy programs, adopting healthy lifestyle habits, or quitting harmful ones. For example, 30% to 50% of individuals with chronic conditions do not adhere to their medication regimen, and 37% have reported not completing their home physical therapy program (Forkan et al., 2006). Participation in inpatient rehabilitation varies significantly (Seel et al., 2015), influences outcomes, and can be responsive to psychosocial interventions (Pegg et al., 2005). Alcohol or other drug abuse can be disabling comorbid conditions in people with disabilities, such as SCI (Tétrault & Courtois, 2014) and TBI (Unsworth & Mathias, 2017).

Using different theoretical models and treatment approaches, rehabilitation psychologists can work individually with patients and with couples and families through rehabilitation teams or even on a broader systems level to promote health behavior change. Regardless of the treatment mechanism, interventions are more effective if they are theory based (Glanz & Bishop, 2010).

Health behavior interventions often begin with psychoeducation or persuasion. Rehabilitation psychologists use the health belief model (Rosenstock, 1982) when they review with patients the risk and protective behaviors associated with a particular health condition and factors, such as their perceived susceptibility to disease and the severity of the disease. For example, this model has been used to design self-management programs (Meade, 2009) and to frame assessment of skin care/wound prevention beliefs in SCI (R. B. King et al., 2012).

Motivational interviewing (Miller & Rollnick, 2012) is a counseling style that may be particularly useful when there is an important discrepancy between patient health behavior practices and health care provider recommendations. Motivational interviewing emphasizes specific strategies to build a strong therapeutic relationship (e.g., reflective listening), resolve ambivalence about initiating change (e.g., open questions to elicit desire, ability, reasons, or need to change), and negotiate action plans (e.g., open questions to elicit commitment and implementation intentions). This counseling style has a strong scientific evidence base and has been used to promote exercise and other healthy behaviors in populations of individuals with disability (Bombardier et al., 2008, 2013; Turner et al., 2016). However, it may not be more effective than other treatments or when participants are already motivated to participate in an intervention (Ponsford et al., 2016). Rather, motivational interviewing seems most appropriate for situations requiring a brief counseling intervention with people who express ambivalence regarding adoption of health behaviors and for therapists who can benefit from having a theoretically based structured approach to organize how to discuss the topic of change.

Rehabilitation psychologists use principles of social-cognitive theory (Bandura, 2004) when they focus on fostering self-efficacy, positive outcome expectations, and a sense of control. That theory has spawned disability-specific measures of self-efficacy (Amtmann et al., 2012) and influential correlational research (Robinson-Smith, Johnston, & Allen, 2000). Rehabilitation psychologists also use observational learning in peer support and group therapy programs (Forsythe & Horsewell, 2006), seeking to enhance self-efficacy through education, verbal persuasion, and incremental goal setting, and to ensure high rates of success toward rehabilitation goals (Jones & Riazi, 2011).

Newer and hybrid models of health behavior change include such concepts as intentions and subjective norms as determinants of behavior change (Martin Ginis, Papathomas, Perrier, Smith, & the SHAPE-SCI Research Group, 2017). Implementation intentions are thought to help bridge the gap between intentions and actions by helping people identify what they will do in specific circumstances to achieve their goals. Often operationalized as a series of if-then statements (e.g., "If it rains, then I will exercise on my treadmill instead"), this theory has been used in home-based rehabilitation programs (Kersten, McPherson, Kayes, Theadom, & McCambridge, 2015). The health action process model (HAPA; Schwarzer, Lippke, & Luszczynska, 2011) integrates the most salient social-cognitive factors with stage-based notions (e.g., identifying people as nonintenders, intenders, actors) and multiple types of self-efficacy and planning behaviors into a practical model. For example, beliefs about risks (e.g., "Can I get pressure ulcers?"), outcome expectancies (e.g., "Do routine pressure reliefs prevent pressure ulcers?"), and self-efficacy beliefs (e.g., "Can I remember to do routine pressure reliefs?") influence intentions to engage in those behaviors. Intentions then must be translated into *volition*, or action planning (e.g., "When, where, and how will I perform pressure reliefs?") and coping planning (e.g., "How will I deal with barriers and setbacks?"). The HAPA model was used to design a successful physical activity promotion pilot study for people with SCI (Brawley, Arbour-Nicitopoulos, & Martin Ginis, 2013).

Modifications Based on Clinical Presentation

Individuals seen in rehabilitation settings often face challenges associated with sensory-perceptual, motor, language, and cognitive limitations. These factors may not only impact mental health and well-being but also complicate the delivery of intervention services themselves. Effective treatment requires identification of, and accommodation for, individual limitations and strengths. Although it can be argued that this is true of all psychotherapy interventions, it is particularly salient in rehabilitation. Table 5.2 lists specific strategies used to adapt psychological interventions. It does not focus on specific patient populations (e.g., individuals with TBI, SCI, amputation) but, rather, presents concerns frequently found in rehabilitation and other medical settings.

THE FUTURE OF REHABILITATION PSYCHOLOGY INTERVENTION

Health care in the United States currently is undergoing a period of considerable transformation marked by widespread shifts in its political and economic underpinnings. Nonetheless, the past 2 decades have seen the emergence of several initiatives that have the potential to alter the day-to-day practice of rehabilitation psychology in the years to come and thus merit some consideration.

Two of the most prominent conceptual frameworks guiding discussion of health care transformation are the chronic disease model proposed by Wagner, Austin, and Von Korff (1996) and, later, the "Triple Aim" championed by the Institute for Healthcare Improvement (n.d.). Both share common themes directly relevant to rehabilitation psychology practice. At a global level, the chronic disease model attempts to reorient health care delivery away from a focus on the discrete treatment of acute illness to the management of chronic disease and promotion of wellness over the lifespan. The Triple Aim promotes the improvement of individual patient experience (i.e., quality and satisfaction) and population health, and reduction of per capita costs. Most important, both constructs share overlapping visions that encourage patient

TABLE 5.2

Adapting Interventions Based on Clinical Presentation

Area of impairment	Strategy
Motor function	▪ Coach individuals with impaired hand function to use voice-activated smartphone programs to access online tools such as relaxation apps. ▪ Consider telehealth delivery models when transportation is a barrier.
Attention	▪ Assess potential interference from auditory or visual stimuli and minimize distractions. ▪ When individuals have a short attention span, present information in smaller "chunks," break down complex tasks, stop and review, and ask patient to repeat back. ▪ Focus on one topic at a time and one task at a time (listen, then take notes). ▪ Provide written session outline/summary at beginning. ▪ Provide in-session breaks or conduct shorter sessions.
Memory	▪ Ask about preferred memory compensatory tools (e.g., notebook, digital recorder, photos, video recordings, voice-activated dictation) and encourage their use within sessions. ▪ When individuals do not complete homework, provide reminder calls or texts, or set up smartphone reminders to prompt completion of assignments. ▪ With permission, include family members in sessions to provide between-session support (e.g., cues, reminders to carry out homework). ▪ With problems encoding new information, provide more learning trials, encourage patients to focus on key words, and use visual imagery and semantic context (forming stories) to enhance learning. ▪ With problems retrieving learned information, use retrieval practice to aid recall. ▪ Encourage patient in session to summarize and highlight main points in materials, and make summary notes. ▪ Post instructional video demonstrating task.
Language	▪ For individuals with receptive language impairments, use simple concrete terms and minimize jargon. ▪ Use gestures, pictures, and graphics to reinforce verbal communication. ▪ Stop and confirm understanding frequently. ▪ Emphasize therapy options that are less language dependent (e.g., physical activity or behavioral activation for depression vs. cognitive restructuring). ▪ For individuals with expressive language impairments, make use of augmentative and alternative communication devices (e.g., alphabet, picture boards, dry erase board, computerized communication systems). ▪ Ask *yes* or *no* questions; determine the most reliable means of responding.
Processing speed	▪ Speak slowly and present information at slower rate, discuss with patient, and calibrate accordingly. ▪ Allow more time to formulate responses.
Executive function	▪ When individuals are tangential, agree on a signal to indicate conversation is off topic. ▪ When individuals are perseverative, negotiate strategies to interrupt process and explicitly practice turn-taking in conversations. ▪ For individuals who have difficulty sequencing and shifting cognitive sets, focus on one topic at a time; signal when switching topics. ▪ For individuals who think concretely, make interpretations and recommendations explicit and direct. ▪ When individuals have difficulty with generalization, model and role-play problem-solving behavior. ▪ Dedicate multiple sessions to generalization of tasks and relapse prevention.
Impulsivity	▪ Develop and practice metacognitive script (e.g., before action: stop, think, then act).
Initiation/motivation	▪ Include support person in treatment planning and implementation. ▪ Make greater use of scheduled activity and practice. ▪ Establish cues and reminders for sessions (e.g., reminder call), and activities (e.g., phone alarms, prompts). ▪ Focus on tasks that are intrinsically rewarding and aligned with goals.
Fatigue	▪ Schedule sessions at times when patient is most alert. ▪ Have shorter, more frequent sessions.
Emotion regulation	▪ Model calm composed behavior, problem solving, and interpersonal communication. ▪ Include explicit focus on distress tolerance skills.

Note. Data from Block and West (2013); Chiaravalloti, Sandry, Moore, and DeLuca (2016); Fann et al. (2015); Hibbard, Grober, Gordon, and Aletta (1990); and Sumowski, Coyne, Cohen, and DeLuca (2014).

participation in care, interprofessional collaboration, redesign of health care delivery to better align with patient needs, and routine monitoring of outcomes to foster ongoing quality improvement. There are opportunities for rehabilitation psychologists to participate in the development, implementation, and evaluation of these processes.

Patient Participation in Care: The Example of Self-Management

Self-management interventions seek to increase patients' skills and confidence in managing their chronic illness, including symptoms, treatments, psychosocial consequences, and lifestyle changes associated with health challenges (Barlow, Wright, Sheasby, Turner, & Hainsworth, 2002; Institute of Medicine, 2003). Many self-management programs provide disease specific information, but the emphasis is on building generalizable skills that include partnering with health care professionals, identifying problems, setting achievable health-related goals and acting on them, solving problems, engaging in ongoing monitoring, and enlisting support in a manner that promotes living well with illness (Bodenheimer, Lorig, Holman, & Grumbach, 2002; Lorig & Holman, 2003).

Outside of these general principles, the actual implementation of self-management interventions varies considerably. As noted by Barlow et al. (2002), programs may be based in health care or community settings, delivered in group or individual format (or a combination of the two) and may include information presented by a health care professional or peer, or both. They may use book or web-based content and group or individual exercises that are delivered face to face, over the telephone, via book or computer module, or via a combination of modalities (Barlow et al., 2002).

The content delivered in self-management interventions also varies substantially. Wegener and colleagues (Wegener, Mackenzie, Ephraim, Ehde, & Williams, 2009) examined the efficacy of a nine-session, group-based self-management intervention to improve functioning following amputation (i.e., the PALS [promoting amputee life skills] program). Topics included physical and emotional symptom management, communication and enlistment of support, the building of healthy habits, and maintenance of progress. Individuals receiving the intervention reported improved self-efficacy, physical functioning, and depression (Wegener et al., 2009).

Ehde and colleagues (Ehde et al., 2015) developed and tested a more targeted intervention for people with MS who had reported pain, fatigue, or depression. Participants received 8 weeks of telephone-delivered self-management. Topic areas included goal setting and problem-solving but focused less on disease-related education; instead, they heavily emphasized cognitive behavioral strategies, such as identifying and challenging thoughts; using relaxation strategies, mindfulness, gratitude, and guided imagery; and building resilience. More than half of individuals receiving self-management experienced a 50% or greater reduction in one or more of their target symptoms (Ehde et al., 2015). At their core, self-management interventions promote individual self-efficacy and the ongoing process of living well with illness, and thus are highly consistent with core values of rehabilitation.

Interprofessional Collaboration: The Example of Collaborative Care

Collaborative care does not have a singular definition but typically involves the management of one or more chronic conditions over time by a designated group of professionals who provide a structured intervention with close team communication and routine patient follow-up (Gunn, Diggens, Hegarty, & Blashki, 2006). The primary point of patient contact is a care manager who works with a medical/mental health team to execute an evidence-based treatment plan that may include education, health maintenance coaching, medication management, and counseling. Primarily serving in the role of care consultant, the rehabilitation psychologist contributes to the development, implementation, and ongoing monitoring of the intervention and target outcomes. Many chronic mental and physical health challenges typically addressed by rehabilitation psychologists (e.g., depression, pain, fatigue) are particularly well suited to this treatment model.

Evidence for the efficacy and utility of this approach is growing. In a landmark study, individuals in primary care clinics randomized to collaborative care demonstrated comparative improvements in a composite measure of blood sugar, LDL cholesterol, blood pressure, and depressive symptoms (Katon et al., 2010). Similarly, a meta-analysis of 79 randomized trials showed comparative benefits of collaborative care over care as usual for depression and anxiety at treatment completion and long-term (2-year) follow-up (Archer et al., 2012). In a follow-up analysis, trials that included psychological treatment improved depression more than those that did not (Coventry et al., 2014).

Health Care Redesign: The Example of Telehealth

Considerable attention in recent years has focused on the patient experience of health care, including the realignment of both medical infrastructure and services. Individuals with disabilities have long experienced barriers to care associated with geography, distance, and built environment. Telehealth represents an important opportunity to overcome some of these challenges and improve access and satisfaction with care (Hatzakis, Haselkorn, Williams, Turner, & Nichol, 2003). *Telehealth* has been defined as "the use of electronic information and telecommunications technologies to support and promote long-distance clinical health care, patient and professional health-related education, public health and health administration" (Health Resources & Services Administration, 2017). Typically, these technologies include videoconferencing, the Internet, store-and-forward imaging, streaming media, and terrestrial and wireless communications.

The telephone is the most widely available and most frequently studied communication platform. Telephone-based interventions have been used to treat depression and anxiety, and improve quality of life across multiple populations using a variety of intervention strategies, including structured CBT, self-management, and open-ended problem-solving (see Table 5.1). Increasingly, telephone intervention is blended with educational content and home monitoring (see, e.g., Moss-Morris et al., 2012; Turner et al., 2016). Mobile phone (i.e., mobile health or *mHealth*) interventions provide a degree of flexibility that is rapidly evolving and revolutionizing assessment and treatment by allowing continual and integrated assessment (e.g., structured assessment of mood via questionnaire, ecological momentary assessment of mood, information on physical activity via accelerometer, engagement in desired activity via geolocation) and treatment (e.g., telephone support, educational web- and text-based content, "just in time" intervention—"You are 5 minutes from home. Consider this walking route that will add an additional 10 minutes to your physical activity") in a single, portable, continuously available medium (Patrick et al., 2016).

Routine Monitoring of Outcomes

Standardized outcome assessment remains a significant challenge for rehabilitation psychologists in routine clinical practice. Nonetheless, medical systems increasingly are seeking individual- and organizational-level data for ongoing quality improvement, and external payers increasingly are intending to tie reimbursement to demonstrable improvements in treatment processes and outcomes. The result is a need to identify outcome instruments that not only are valid, reliable, broadly normed, and sensitive to change but also easy to administer and interpret (Heinemann & Mallinson, 2010). Furthermore, clinicians must navigate competing needs to use instruments that are specific to individual patients and presenting problems, and also be sufficiently global to be useful in comparing groups of patients across providers, clinics, or institutions. The National Institutes of Health–funded patient-reported outcomes measurement system, or PROMIS, and the National Institute for Neurological Disorders and Stroke-sponsored Neuro-QoL measurement system (normed for individuals with chronic health conditions and neurologic conditions respectively) represent two notable options (Northwestern University, n.d.). Instruments from these systems are freely available and can be administered in computer adaptive testing and paper-and-pencil short form (four–10 items) formats.

CONCLUSION

The professional life of a rehabilitation psychologist can be challenging and immensely rewarding. Successful intervention requires familiarity with an enormous array of physical, behavioral, cognitive, and emotional presenting problems, as well as an understanding of the ways in which they may unfold and interact over time. As reflected in the PANEP model introduced in this chapter, rehabilitation psychology brings a particular appreciation of the psychological and social experience of illness and disability, and emphasizes not only the amelioration of suffering but also recognition and support for strengths, growth, participation, and quality of life.

Few psychological disciplines work so closely and regularly with families, broader support networks, and large interprofessional teams. Rehabilitation psychologists have an underdeveloped yet growing base of empirical evidence that can be used to inform the selection and implementation of treatments that must be adapted both for the people they serve (e.g., particular impairments, activity restrictions) and the constraints of the settings in which they are found (e.g., short lengths of stay, limitations on reimbursement). Future interventions are increasingly likely to emphasize self-management and collaborative care, integrate developing technologies that increase the scope and reach treatment, and include routine outcome assessment to demonstrate efficacy.

References

American Psychiatric Association. (1994). *Diagnostic and statistical manual of mental disorders* (4th ed.). Washington, DC: Author.

American Psychological Association. (2017). *Ethical principles of psychologists and code of conduct* (2002, Amended June 1, 2010 and January 1, 2017). Retrieved from http://www.apa.org/ethics/code/index.aspx

American Psychological Association, Division 22—Rehabilitation Psychology. (2018). *Rehabilitation psychology: Life fully realized* [web site]. Retrieved from https://static1.squarespace.com/static/54fe580de4b0e762cd9f4d34/t/5a7341f5419202bff14db6b4/1517502967502/APA+Div+22+Leadership+Manual+2017.pdf

Amtmann, D., Bamer, A. M., Cook, K. F., Askew, R. L., Noonan, V. K., & Brockway, J. A. (2012). University of Washington self-efficacy scale: A new self-efficacy scale for people with disabilities. *Archives of Physical Medicine and Rehabilitation, 93,* 1757–1765. http://dx.doi.org/10.1016/j.apmr.2012.05.001

Archer, J., Bower, P., Gilbody, S., Lovell, K., Richards, D., Gask, L., . . . Coventry, P. (2012). Collaborative care for depression and anxiety problems. *Cochrane Database of Systematic Reviews, 2012*(10). http://dx.doi.org/10.1002/14651858.CD006525.pub2

Ashman, T., Cantor, J. B., Tsaousides, T., Spielman, L., & Gordon, W. (2014). Comparison of cognitive behavioral therapy and supportive psychotherapy for the treatment of depression following traumatic brain injury: A randomized controlled trial. *Journal of Head Trauma Rehabilitation, 29,* 467–478. http://dx.doi.org/10.1097/HTR.0000000000000098

Bandura, A. (2004). Health promotion by social cognitive means. *Health Education & Behavior, 31,* 143–164. http://dx.doi.org/10.1177/1090198104263660

Barlow, J., Wright, C., Sheasby, J., Turner, A., & Hainsworth, J. (2002). Self-management approaches for people with chronic conditions: A review. *Patient Education and Counseling, 48,* 177–187. http://dx.doi.org/10.1016/S0738-3991(02)00032-0

Bédard, M., Felteau, M., Marshall, S., Cullen, N., Gibbons, C., Dubois, S., . . . Moustgaard, A. (2014). Mindfulness-based cognitive therapy reduces symptoms of depression in people with a traumatic brain injury: Results from a randomized controlled trial. *Journal of Head Trauma Rehabilitation, 29,* E13–E22. http://dx.doi.org/10.1097/HTR.0b013e3182a615a0

Bell, K. R., Temkin, N. R., Esselman, P. C., Doctor, J. N., Bombardier, C. H., Fraser, R. T., . . . Dikmen, S. (2005). The effect of a scheduled telephone intervention on outcome after moderate to severe traumatic brain injury: A randomized trial. *Archives of Physical Medicine and Rehabilitation, 86,* 851–856. http://dx.doi.org/10.1016/j.apmr.2004.09.015

Bellon, K., Kolakowsky-Hayner, S., Wright, J., Huie, H., Toda, K., Bushnik, T., & Englander, J. (2015). A home-based walking study to ameliorate perceived stress and depressive symptoms in people with a traumatic brain injury. *Brain Injury, 29,* 313–319. http://dx.doi.org/10.3109/02699052.2014.974670

Blessing, C., Golden, T. P., Pi, S., Bruyere, S. M., & Van Looy, S. (2012). Vocational rehabilitation, inclusion, and social integration. In P. Kennedy (Ed.), *The Oxford handbook of rehabilitation psychology* (pp. 453–473). New York, NY: Oxford University Press.

Block, C. K., & West, S. E. (2013). Psychotherapeutic treatment of survivors of traumatic brain injury: Review of the literature and special considerations. *Brain Injury, 27,* 775–788. http://dx.doi.org/10.3109/02699052.2013.775487

Bodenheimer, T., Lorig, K., Holman, H., & Grumbach, K. (2002). Patient self-management of chronic disease in primary care. *JAMA, 288,* 2469–2475. http://dx.doi.org/10.1001/jama.288.19.2469

Bogosian, A., Chadwick, P., Windgassen, S., Norton, S., McCrone, P., Mosweu, I., . . . Moss-Morris, R. (2015). Distress improves after mindfulness training for progressive MS: A pilot randomised trial. *Multiple Sclerosis, 21,* 1184–1194. http://dx.doi.org/10.1177/1352458515576261

Bombardier, C. H., Bell, K. R., Temkin, N. R., Fann, J. R., Hoffman, J., & Dikmen, S. (2009). The efficacy of a scheduled telephone intervention for ameliorating depressive symptoms during the first year after traumatic brain injury. *Journal of Head Trauma Rehabilitation, 24,* 230–238. http://dx.doi.org/10.1097/HTR.0b013e3181ad65f0

Bombardier, C. H., Cunniffe, M., Wadhwani, R., Gibbons, L. E., Blake, K. D., & Kraft, G. H. (2008). The efficacy of telephone counseling for health promotion in people with multiple sclerosis: A randomized controlled trial. *Archives of Physical Medicine and Rehabilitation, 89,* 1849–1856. http://dx.doi.org/10.1016/j.apmr.2008.03.021

Bombardier, C. H., Ehde, D. M., Gibbons, L. E., Wadhwani, R., Sullivan, M. D., Rosenberg, D. E., & Kraft, G. H. (2013). Telephone-based physical activity counseling for major depression in people with multiple sclerosis. *Journal of Consulting and Clinical Psychology, 81,* 89–99. http://dx.doi.org/10.1037/a0031242

Bonanno, G. A., Kennedy, P., Galatzer-Levy, I. R., Lude, P., & Elfström, M. L. (2012). Trajectories of resilience, depression, and anxiety following spinal cord injury. *Rehabilitation Psychology, 57,* 236–247. http://dx.doi.org/10.1037/a0029256

Brawley, L. R., Arbour-Nicitopoulos, K. P., & Martin Ginis, K. A. (2013). Developing physical activity interventions for adults with spinal cord injury. Part 3: A pilot feasibility study of an intervention to increase self-managed physical activity. *Rehabilitation Psychology, 58,* 316–321. http://dx.doi.org/10.1037/a0032814

Carcieri, E. M., & Mona, L. R. (2017). Assessment and treatment of sexual health issues in rehabilitation: A patient-centered approach. In M. A. Budd, S. Hough, S. T. Wegener, & W. Stiers (Eds.), *Practical psychology in medical rehabilitation* (pp. 287–294). Cham, Switzerland: Springer. http://dx.doi.org/10.1007/978-3-319-34034-0_31

Carlozzi, N. E., Kratz, A. L., Sander, A. M., Chiaravalloti, N. D., Brickell, T. A., Lange, R. T., . . . Tulsky, D. S. (2015). Health-related quality of life in caregivers of individuals with traumatic brain injury: Development of a conceptual model. *Archives of Physical Medicine and Rehabilitation, 96,* 105–113. http://dx.doi.org/10.1016/j.apmr.2014.08.021

Carnevale, G. J., Anselmi, V., Johnston, M. V., Busichio, K., & Walsh, V. (2006). A natural setting behavior management program for persons with acquired brain injury: A randomized controlled trial. *Archives of Physical Medicine and Rehabilitation, 87,* 1289–1297. http://dx.doi.org/10.1016/j.apmr.2006.06.010

Chiaravalloti, N. D., Sandry, J., Moore, N. B., & DeLuca, J. (2016). An RCT to treat learning impairment in traumatic brain injury: The TBI-MEM trial. *Neurorehabilitation and Neural Repair, 30,* 539–550. http://dx.doi.org/10.1177/1545968315604395

Chwalisz, K. (1996). The perceived stress model of caregiver burden: Evidence from spouses of persons with brain injury. *Rehabilitation Psychology, 41,* 91–114. http://dx.doi.org/10.1037/0090-5550.41.2.91

Chwalisz, K., & Dollinger, S. C. (2010). Evidence-based practice with family caregivers: Decision-making strategies based on research and clinical data. In R. G. Frank, M. Rosenthall, & B. Caplan (Eds.), *Handbook of rehabilitation psychology* (2nd ed., pp. 301–311). Washington, DC: American Psychological Association. http://dx.doi.org/10.1037/15972-018

Coventry, P. A., Hudson, J. L., Kontopantelis, E., Archer, J., Richards, D. A., Gilbody, S., . . . Bower, P. (2014). Characteristics of effective collaborative care for treatment of depression: A systematic review and meta-regression of 74 randomised controlled trials. *PLoS One, 9,* e108114. http://dx.doi.org/10.1371/journal.pone.0108114

Cox, D. R., Cox, R. H., & Caplan, B. (2013). *Specialty competencies in rehabilitation psychology*. New York, NY: Oxford University Press.

Craig, A. R., Hancock, K. M., & Dickson, H. G. (1994). A longitudinal investigation into anxiety and depression in the first 2 years following a spinal cord injury. *Paraplegia, 32,* 675–679.

Craig, A. R., Hancock, K., Dickson, H., & Chang, E. (1997). Long-term psychological outcomes in spinal cord injured persons: Results of a controlled trial using cognitive behavior therapy. *Archives of Physical Medicine and Rehabilitation, 78,* 33–38. http://dx.doi.org/10.1016/S0003-9993(97)90006-X

DeVivo, M. J., Hawkins, L. N., Richards, J. S., & Go, B. K. (1995). Outcomes of post-spinal cord injury marriages. *Archives of Physical Medicine and Rehabilitation, 76,* 130–138. http://dx.doi.org/10.1016/S0003-9993(95)80022-0

Driver, S., & Ede, A. (2009). Impact of physical activity on mood after TBI. *Brain Injury, 23,* 203–212. http://dx.doi.org/10.1080/02699050802695574

Duchnick, J. J., Letsch, E. A., & Curtiss, G. (2009). Coping effectiveness training during acute rehabilitation of spinal cord injury/dysfunction: A randomized clinical trial. *Rehabilitation Psychology, 54,* 123–132. http://dx.doi.org/10.1037/a0015571

Dunn, D. S., Ehde, D. M., & Wegener, S. T. (2016). The foundational principles as psychological lodestars: Theoretical inspiration and empirical direction in rehabilitation psychology. *Rehabilitation Psychology, 61,* 1–6. http://dx.doi.org/10.1037/rep0000082

D'Zurilla, T. J., & Nezu, A. (2006). *Problem-solving therapy: A positive approach to clinical intervention* (3rd ed.). New York, NY: Springer.

Ehde, D. M., Dillworth, T. M., & Turner, J. A. (2014). Cognitive-behavioral therapy for individuals with chronic pain: Efficacy, innovations, and directions for research. *American Psychologist, 69,* 153–166. http://dx.doi.org/10.1037/a0035747

Ehde, D. M., Elzea, J. L., Verrall, A. M., Gibbons, L. E., Smith, A. E., & Amtmann, D. (2015). Efficacy of a telephone-delivered self-management intervention for persons with multiple sclerosis: A randomized controlled trial with a one-year follow-up. *Archives of Physical Medicine and Rehabilitation, 96,* 1945–1958 e1942. http://dx.doi.org/10.1016/j.apmr.2015.07.015

Elliott, T. R., Berry, J. W., & Grant, J. S. (2009). Problem-solving training for family caregivers of women with disabilities: A randomized clinical trial. *Behaviour Research and Therapy, 47,* 548–558. http://dx.doi.org/10.1016/j.brat.2009.03.006

Elliott, T. R., Brossart, D., Berry, J. W., & Fine, P. R. (2008). Problem-solving training via videoconferencing for family caregivers of persons with spinal cord injuries: A randomized controlled trial. *Behaviour Research and Therapy, 46,* 1220–1229. http://dx.doi.org/10.1016/j.brat.2008.08.004

Elliott, T. R., & Frank, R. G. (1996). Depression following spinal cord injury. *Archives of Physical Medicine and Rehabilitation, 77,* 816–823. http://dx.doi.org/10.1016/S0003-9993(96)90263-4

Elliott, T. R., Shewchuk, R. M., & Richards, J. S. (1999). Caregiver social problem-solving abilities and family member adjustment to recent-onset physical disability. *Rehabilitation Psychology, 44,* 104–123. http://dx.doi.org/10.1037/0090-5550.44.1.104

Elliott, T. R., Shewchuk, R. M., & Richards, J. S. (2001). Family caregiver social problem-solving abilities and adjustment during the initial year of the caregiving role. *Journal of Counseling Psychology, 48,* 223–232. http://dx.doi.org/10.1037/0022-0167.48.2.223

Esmail, S., Darry, K., Walter, A., & Knupp, H. (2010). Attitudes and perceptions towards disability and sexuality. *Disability and Rehabilitation, 32,* 1148–1155. http://dx.doi.org/10.3109/09638280903419277

Esmail, S., Esmail, Y., & Munro, B. (2001). Sexuality and disability: The role of health care professionals in providing options and alternatives for couples. *Sexuality and Disability, 19,* 267–282. http://dx.doi.org/10.1023/A:1017905425599

Fann, J. R., Bombardier, C. H., Vannoy, S., Dyer, J., Ludman, E., Dikmen, S., . . . Temkin, N. (2015). Telephone and in-person cognitive behavioral therapy for major depression after traumatic brain injury: A randomized controlled trial. *Journal of Neurotrauma, 32,* 45–57. http://dx.doi.org/10.1089/neu.2014.3423

Foley, F. W., Bedell, J. R., LaRocca, N. G., Scheinberg, L. C., & Reznikoff, M. (1987). Efficacy of stress-inoculation training in coping with multiple sclerosis. *Journal of Consulting and Clinical Psychology, 55,* 919–922. http://dx.doi.org/10.1037/0022-006X.55.6.919

Forkan, R., Pumper, B., Smyth, N., Wirkkala, H., Ciol, M. A., & Shumway-Cook, A. (2006). Exercise adherence following physical therapy intervention in older adults with impaired balance. *Physical Therapy, 86,* 401–410.

Forsythe, E., & Horsewell, J. E. (2006). Sexual rehabilitation of women with a spinal cord injury. *Spinal Cord, 44,* 234–241. http://dx.doi.org/10.1038/sj.sc.3101844

Fraser, R. T. (2010). Vocational rehabilitation. In R. G. Frank, M. Rosenthall, & B. Caplan (Eds.), *Handbook of rehabilitation psychology* (pp. 357–363). Washington, DC: American Psychological Association. http://dx.doi.org/10.1037/15972-023

Glanz, K., & Bishop, D. B. (2010). The role of behavioral science theory in development and implementation of public health interventions. *Annual Review of Public Health, 31,* 399–418. http://dx.doi.org/10.1146/annurev.publhealth.012809.103604

Grant, J. S., Elliott, T. R., Weaver, M., Bartolucci, A. A., & Giger, J. N. (2002). Telephone intervention with family caregivers of stroke survivors after rehabilitation. *Stroke, 33,* 2060–2065. http://dx.doi.org/10.1161/01.STR.0000020711.38824.E3

Grant, J. S., Elliott, T. R., Weaver, M., Glandon, G. L., Raper, J. L., & Giger, J. N. (2006). Social support, social problem-solving abilities, and adjustment of family caregivers of stroke survivors. *Archives of Physical Medicine and Rehabilitation, 87,* 343–350. http://dx.doi.org/10.1016/j.apmr.2005.09.019

Grossman, P., Kappos, L., Gensicke, H., D'Souza, M., Mohr, D. C., Penner, I. K., & Steiner, C. (2010). MS quality of life, depression, and fatigue improve after mindfulness training: A randomized trial. *Neurology, 75,* 1141–1149. http://dx.doi.org/10.1212/WNL.0b013e3181f4d80d

Gunn, J., Diggens, J., Hegarty, K., & Blashki, G. (2006). A systematic review of complex system interventions designed to increase recovery from depression in primary care. *BMC Health Services Research, 6,* 88. http://dx.doi.org/10.1186/1472-6963-6-88

Hatzakis, M., Jr., Haselkorn, J., Williams, R., Turner, A., & Nichol, P. (2003). Telemedicine and the delivery of health services to veterans with multiple sclerosis. *Journal of Rehabilitation Research and Development, 40,* 265–282.

Health Resources & Services Administration. (2017). *Telehealth programs.* Retrieved from https://www.hrsa.gov/rural-health/telehealth/index.html

Heinemann, A. W., & Mallinson, T. (2010). Functional status and quality of life measures. In R. G. Frank, M. Rosenthall, & B. Caplan (Eds.), *Handbook of rehabilitation psychology* (pp. 147–164). Washington, DC: American Psychological Association. http://dx.doi.org/10.1037/15972-009

Hibbard, M. R., Grober, S. E., Gordon, W., & Aletta, E. G. (1990). Modification of cognitive psychotherapy for the treatment of post-stroke depression. *Behavior Therapist, 13,* 15–17.

Hibbard, M. R., Uysal, S., Kepler, K., Bogdany, J., & Silver, J. (1998). Axis I psychopathology in individuals with traumatic brain injury. *Journal of Head Trauma Rehabilitation, 13,* 24–39. http://dx.doi.org/10.1097/00001199-199808000-00003

Hoffman, J. M., Bell, K. R., Powell, J. M., Behr, J., Dunn, E. C., Dikmen, S., & Bombardier, C. H. (2010). A randomized controlled trial of exercise to improve mood after traumatic brain injury. *Physical Medicine and Rehabilitation, 2,* 911–919. http://dx.doi.org/10.1016/j.pmrj.2010.06.008

Houlihan, B. V., Jette, A., Friedman, R. H., Paasche-Orlow, M., Ni, P., Wierbicky, J., . . . Williams, S. (2013). A pilot study of a telehealth intervention for persons with spinal cord dysfunction. *Spinal Cord, 51,* 715–720. http://dx.doi.org/10.1038/sc.2013.45

Huckans, M., Pavawalla, S., Demadura, T., Kolessar, M., Seelye, A., Roost, N., . . . Storzbach, D. (2010). A pilot study examining effects of group-based cognitive strategy training treatment on self-reported cognitive problems, psychiatric symptoms, functioning, and compensatory strategy use in OIF/OEF combat veterans with persistent mild cognitive disorder and history of traumatic brain injury. *Journal of Rehabilitation Research and Development, 47,* 43–60. http://dx.doi.org/10.1682/JRRD.2009.02.0019

Institute for Healthcare Improvement. (n.d.). *IHI Triple Aim initiative: Better care for individuals, better health for populations, lower per capita costs.* Retrieved from http://www.ihi.org/Engage/Initiatives/TripleAim/Pages/default.aspx

Institute of Medicine. (2003). *Priority areas for national action: Transforming health care quality.* Washington, DC: National Academies Press.

Institute of Medicine. (2011). *Relieving pain in America: A blueprint for transforming prevention, care, education, and research.* Washington, DC: National Academies Press.

Jensen, M. P. (2011). Psychosocial approaches to pain management: An organizational framework. *Pain, 152,* 717–725. http://dx.doi.org/10.1016/j.pain.2010.09.002

Jones, F., & Riazi, A. (2011). Self-efficacy and self-management after stroke: A systematic review. *Disability and Rehabilitation, 33,* 797–810. http://dx.doi.org/10.3109/09638288.2010.511415

Katon, W. J., Lin, E. H., Von Korff, M., Ciechanowski, P., Ludman, E. J., Young, B., . . . McCulloch, D. (2010). Collaborative care for patients with depression and chronic illnesses. *The New England Journal of Medicine, 363,* 2611–2620. http://dx.doi.org/10.1056/NEJMoa1003955

Kemp, B. J., Kahan, J. S., Krause, J. S., Adkins, R. H., & Nava, G. (2004). Treatment of major depression in individuals with spinal cord injury. *Journal of Spinal Cord Medicine, 27,* 22–28. http://dx.doi.org/10.1080/10790268.2004.11753726

Kennedy, P., Duff, J., Evans, M., & Beedie, A. (2003). Coping effectiveness training reduces depression and anxiety following traumatic spinal cord injuries. *British Journal of Clinical Psychology, 42,* 41–52. http://dx.doi.org/10.1348/014466503762842002

Kerkhoff, T. R., & Butt, L. (2017). Managing challenging behavior in an inpatient setting. In M. A. Budd, S. Hough, S. T. Wegener, & W. Stiers (Eds.), *Practical psychology in medical rehabilitation* (pp. 443–456). Cham, Switzerland: Springer. http://dx.doi.org/10.1007/978-3-319-34034-0_49

Kersten, P., McPherson, K. M., Kayes, N. M., Theadom, A., & McCambridge, A. (2015). Bridging the goal intention-action gap in rehabilitation: A study of if-then implementation intentions in neurorehabilitation. *Disability and Rehabilitation, 37,* 1073–1081. http://dx.doi.org/10.3109/09638288.2014.955137

King, C., & Kennedy, P. (1999). Coping effectiveness training for people with spinal cord injury: Preliminary results of a controlled trial. *British Journal of Clinical Psychology, 38,* 5–14. http://dx.doi.org/10.1348/014466599162629

King, R. B., Champion, V. L., Chen, D., Gittler, M. S., Heinemann, A. W., Bode, R. K., & Semik, P. (2012). Development of a measure of skin care belief scales for persons with spinal cord injury. *Archives of Physical Medicine and Rehabilitation, 93,* 1814–1821. http://dx.doi.org/10.1016/j.apmr.2012.03.030

Kreutzer, J. S., Rapport, L. J., Marwitz, J. H., Harrison-Felix, C., Hart, T., Glenn, M., & Hammond, F. (2009). Caregivers' well-being after traumatic brain injury: A multicenter prospective investigation. *Archives of Physical Medicine and Rehabilitation, 90,* 939–946. http://dx.doi.org/10.1016/j.apmr.2009.01.010

Larcombe, N. A., & Wilson, P. H. (1984). An evaluation of cognitive-behaviour therapy for depression in patients with multiple sclerosis. *British Journal of Psychiatry, 145,* 366–371. http://dx.doi.org/10.1192/bjp.145.4.366

Livneh, H., & Antonak, R. F. (2005). Psychosocial adaptation to chronic illness and disability: A primer for counselors. *Journal of Counseling & Development, 83,* 12–20. http://dx.doi.org/10.1002/j.1556-6678.2005.tb00575.x

Livneh, H., Martz, E., & Bodner, T. (2006). Psychosocial adaptation to chronic illness and disability: A preliminary study of its factorial structure. *Journal of Clinical Psychology in Medical Settings, 13,* 250–260. http://dx.doi.org/10.1007/s10880-006-9028-5

Lorig, K. R., & Holman, H. (2003). Self-management education: History, definition, outcomes, and mechanisms. *Annals of Behavioral Medicine, 26,* 1–7. http://dx.doi.org/10.1207/S15324796ABM2601_01

Martin Ginis, K. A., Papathomas, A., Perrier, M. J., Smith, B., & the SHAPE-SCI Research Group. (2017). Psychosocial factors associated with physical activity in ambulatory and manual wheelchair users with spinal cord injury: A mixed-methods study. *Disability and Rehabilitation, 39,* 187–192. http://dx.doi.org/10.3109/09638288.2015.1045991

McAlonan, S. (1996). Improving sexual rehabilitation services: The patient's perspective. *American Journal of Occupational Therapy, 50,* 826–834. http://dx.doi.org/10.5014/ajot.50.10.826

McCabe, M. P., Cummins, R. A., & Deeks, A. A. (2000). Sexuality and quality of life among people with physical disability. *Sexuality and Disability, 18,* 115–123. http://dx.doi.org/10.1023/A:1005562813603

Meade, M. A. (2009). *Facilitating Health Mechanics: A guide for care providers of individuals with spinal cord injury and disease.* Ann Arbor: The Regents of the University of Michigan.

Middleton, J. W., Simpson, G. K., De Wolf, A., Quirk, R., Descallar, J., & Cameron, I. D. (2014). Psychological distress, quality of life, and burden in caregivers during community reintegration after spinal cord injury. *Archives of Physical Medicine and Rehabilitation, 95,* 1312–1319. http://dx.doi.org/10.1016/j.apmr.2014.03.017

Miller, W. R., & Rollnick, S. (2012). *Motivational interviewing: Helping people change* (3rd ed.). New York, NY: Guilford Press.

Mohr, D. C., Boudewyn, A. C., Goodkin, D. E., Bostrom, A., & Epstein, L. (2001). Comparative outcomes for individual cognitive-behavior therapy, supportive-expressive group psychotherapy, and sertraline for the treatment of depression in multiple sclerosis. *Journal of Consulting and Clinical Psychology, 69,* 942–949. http://dx.doi.org/10.1037/0022-006X.69.6.942

Mohr, D. C., Hart, S. L., Julian, L., Catledge, C., Honos-Webb, L., Vella, L., & Tasch, E. T. (2005). Telephone-administered psychotherapy for depression. *Archives of General Psychiatry, 62,* 1007–1014. http://dx.doi.org/10.1001/archpsyc.62.9.1007

Mohr, D. C., Likosky, W., Bertagnolli, A., Goodkin, D. E., Van Der Wende, J., Dwyer, P., & Dick, L. P. (2000). Telephone-administered cognitive-behavioral therapy for the treatment of depressive symptoms in multiple sclerosis. *Journal of Consulting and Clinical Psychology, 68,* 356–361. http://dx.doi.org/10.1037/0022-006X.68.2.356

Mona, L. R., Cameron, R. P., & Clemency Cordes, C. (2017). Disability culturally competent sexual healthcare. *American Psychologist, 72,* 1000–1010. http://dx.doi.org/10.1037/amp0000283

Moss-Morris, R., McCrone, P., Yardley, L., van Kessel, K., Wills, G., & Dennison, L. (2012). A pilot randomised controlled trial of an Internet-based cognitive behavioural therapy self-management programme (MS Invigor8) for multiple sclerosis fatigue. *Behaviour Research and Therapy, 50,* 415–421. http://dx.doi.org/10.1016/j.brat.2012.03.001

Murphy, N. A., & Elias, E. R. (2006). Sexuality of children and adolescents with developmental disabilities. *Pediatrics, 118,* 398–403. http://dx.doi.org/10.1542/peds.2006-1115

National Institutes of Health. (n.d.). *Patient-reported outcomes measurement information system (PROMIS).* Retrieved from https://www.nia.nih.gov/research/resource/patient-reported-outcomes-measurement-information-system-promis

New, P. W., Seddon, M., Redpath, C., Currie, K. E., & Warren, N. (2016). Recommendations for spinal rehabilitation professionals regarding sexual education needs and preferences of people with spinal cord dysfunction: A mixed-methods study. *Spinal Cord, 54,* 1203–1209. http://dx.doi.org/10.1038/sc.2016.62

Northwestern University. (n.d.). *HealthMeasures: A national person-centered assessment resource.* Retrieved from http://www.healthmeasures.net/images/LearnMore/HealthMeasures_Brochure_-_for_emailing.pdf

Olkin, R., & Pledger, C. (2003). Can disability studies and psychology join hands? *American Psychologist, 58,* 296–304. http://dx.doi.org/10.1037/0003-066X.58.4.296

Ostelo, R. W., van Tulder, M. W., Vlaeyen, J. W., Linton, S. J., Morley, S. J., & Assendelft, W. J. (2005). Behavioural treatment for chronic low-back pain. *Cochrane Database of Systematic Reviews, 2005*(1). http://dx.doi.org/10.1002/14651858.CD002014.pub2

Ottomanelli, L. (2017). Vocational rehabilitation. In M. A. Budd, S. Hough, S. T. Wegener, & W. Stiers (Eds.), *Practical psychology in medical rehabilitation* (pp. 457–464). Cham, Switzerland: Springer. http://dx.doi.org/10.1007/978-3-319-34034-0_50

Ottomanelli, L., Barnett, S. D., & Goetz, L. L. (2014). Effectiveness of supported employment for veterans with spinal cord injury: 2-year results. *Archives of Physical Medicine and Rehabilitation, 95,* 784–790. http://dx.doi.org/10.1016/j.apmr.2013.11.012

Pakenham, K. I. (2005). The positive impact of multiple sclerosis (MS) on carers: Associations between carer benefit finding and positive and negative adjustment domains. *Disability and Rehabilitation, 27,* 985–997. http://dx.doi.org/10.1080/09638280500052583

Patrick, K., Hekler, E. B., Estrin, D., Mohr, D. C., Riper, H., Crane, D., . . . Riley, W. T. (2016). The pace of technologic change: Implications for digital health behavior intervention research. *American Journal of Preventive Medicine, 51,* 816–824. http://dx.doi.org/10.1016/j.amepre.2016.05.001

Pegg, Jr., P. O., Auerbach, S. M., Seel, R. T., Buenaver, L. F., Kiesler, D. J., & Plybon, L. E. (2005). The impact of patient-centered information on patients' treatment satisfaction and outcomes in traumatic brain injury rehabilitation. *Rehabilitation Psychology, 50,* 366–374. http://dx.doi.org/10.1037/0090-5550.50.4.366

Pfeiffer, K., Beische, D., Hautzinger, M., Berry, J. W., Wengert, J., Hoffrichter, R., . . . Elliott, T. R. (2014). Telephone-based problem-solving intervention for family caregivers of stroke survivors: A randomized controlled trial. *Journal of Consulting and Clinical Psychology, 82,* 628–643. http://dx.doi.org/10.1037/a0036987

Ponsford, J., Lee, N. K., Wong, D., McKay, A., Haines, K., Alway, Y., . . . O'Donnell, M. L. (2016). Efficacy of motivational interviewing and cognitive behavioral therapy for anxiety and depression symptoms following traumatic brain injury. *Psychological Medicine, 46,* 1079–1090. http://dx.doi.org/10.1017/S0033291715002640

Pull, C. B. (2009). Current empirical status of acceptance and commitment therapy. *Current Opinion in Psychiatry, 22,* 55–60. http://dx.doi.org/10.1097/YCO.0b013e32831a6e9d

Ramkumar, N. A., & Elliott, T. R. (2010). Family caregiving of persons following neurotrauma: Issues in research, service and policy. *NeuroRehabilitation, 27,* 105–112.

Rintala, D. H., Howland, C. A., Nosek, M. A., Bennett, J. L., Young, M. E., Foley, C. C., . . . Chanpong, G. (1997). Dating issues for women with physical disabilities. *Sexuality and Disability, 15,* 219–242. http://dx.doi.org/10.1023/A:1024717313923

Rivera, P. A., Elliott, T. R., Berry, J. W., & Grant, J. S. (2008). Problem-solving training for family caregivers of persons with traumatic brain injuries: A randomized controlled trial. *Archives of Physical Medicine and Rehabilitation, 89,* 931–941. http://dx.doi.org/10.1016/j.apmr.2007.12.032

Robinson-Smith, G., Johnston, M. V., & Allen, J. (2000). Self-care self-efficacy, quality of life, and depression after stroke. *Archives of Physical Medicine and Rehabilitation, 81,* 460–464. http://dx.doi.org/10.1053/mr.2000.3863

Rosenstock, I. M. (1982). The health belief model and nutrition education. *Journal of the Canadian Dietetic Association, 43,* 184–192.

Sadoughi, W., Leshner, M., & Fine, H. L. (1971). Sexual adjustment in a chronically ill and physically disabled population: A pilot study. *Archives of Physical Medicine and Rehabilitation, 52,* 311–317.

Sbordone, R. (1990). Psychotherapeutic treatment of the client with traumatic brain injury: A conceptual model. In J. S. Kreutzer & P. Wehman (Eds.), *Community integration following traumatic brain injury* (pp. 125–138). Baltimore, MD: Paul H. Brookes.

Schwarzer, R., Lippke, S., & Luszczynska, A. (2011). Mechanisms of health behavior change in persons with chronic illness or disability: The Health Action Process Approach (HAPA). *Rehabilitation Psychology, 56,* 161–170. http://dx.doi.org/10.1037/a0024509

Seel, R. T., Corrigan, J. D., Dijkers, M. P., Barrett, R. S., Bogner, J., Smout, R. J., . . . Horn, S. D. (2015). Patient effort in traumatic brain injury inpatient rehabilitation: Course and associations with age, brain injury severity, and time postinjury. *Archives of Physical Medicine and Rehabilitation, 96,* S235–S244. http://dx.doi.org/10.1016/j.apmr.2014.10.027

Seligman, M. E. (2011). *Flourish: A visionary new understanding of happiness and well-being.* New York, NY: Free Press.

Sohlberg, M. M., & Mateer, C. A. (2001). *Cognitive rehabilitation.* New York, NY: Guilford Press.

Sörensen, S., Pinquart, M., & Duberstein, P. (2002). How effective are interventions with caregivers? An updated meta-analysis. *Gerontologist, 42,* 356–372. http://dx.doi.org/10.1093/geront/42.3.356

Stiers, W. (2016). Teaching the foundational principles of rehabilitation psychology. *Rehabilitation Psychology, 61,* 54–64. http://dx.doi.org/10.1037/rep0000078

Sumowski, J. F., Coyne, J., Cohen, A., & DeLuca, J. (2014). Retrieval practice improves memory in survivors of severe traumatic brain injury. *Archives of Physical Medicine and Rehabilitation, 95,* 397–400. http://dx.doi.org/10.1016/j.apmr.2013.10.021

Tétrault, M., & Courtois, F. (2014). Use of psychoactive substances in persons with spinal cord injury: A literature review. *Annals of Physical and Rehabilitation Medicine, 57,* 684–695. http://dx.doi.org/10.1016/j.rehab.2014.10.002

Tiersky, L. A., Anselmi, V., Johnston, M. V., Kurtyka, J., Roosen, E., Schwartz, T., & DeLuca, J. (2005). A trial of neuropsychologic rehabilitation in mild-spectrum traumatic brain injury. *Archives of Physical Medicine and Rehabilitation, 86,* 1565–1574. http://dx.doi.org/10.1016/j.apmr.2005.03.013

Topolovec-Vranic, J., Cullen, N., Michalak, A., Ouchterlony, D., Bhalerao, S., Masanic, C., & Cusimano, M. D. (2010). Evaluation of an online cognitive behavioural therapy program by patients with traumatic brain injury and depression. *Brain Injury, 24,* 762–772. http://dx.doi.org/10.3109/02699051003709599

Torices Rodarte, I., & Bonilla Muñoz, M. P. (2004). Inventory of sexual experiences and response in disability (IEReSDi): Construction and validation of the scale of the sexual response in people with disabilities. *Sexuality and Disability, 22,* 181–195. http://dx.doi.org/10.1023/B:SEDI.0000039061.36054.b4

Turner, A. P., Hartoonian, N., Sloan, A. P., Benich, M., Kivlahan, D. R., Hughes, C., . . . Haselkorn, J. K. (2016). Improving fatigue and depression in individuals with multiple sclerosis using telephone-administered physical activity counseling. *Journal of Consulting and Clinical Psychology, 84,* 297–309. http://dx.doi.org/10.1037/ccp0000086

Ullrich, P. (2017). Pain. In M. A. Budd, S. Hough, S. T. Wegener, & W. Stiers (Eds.), *Practical psychology in medical rehabilitation* (pp. 397–404). Cham, Switzerland: Springer. http://dx.doi.org/10.1007/978-3-319-34034-0_44

Unsworth, D. J., & Mathias, J. L. (2017). Traumatic brain injury and alcohol/substance abuse: A Bayesian meta-analysis comparing the outcomes of people with and without a history of abuse. *Journal of Clinical and Experimental Neuropsychology, 39,* 547–562. http://dx.doi.org/10.1080/13803395.2016.1248812

U.S. Census Bureau. (2017). Selected economic characteristics for the civilian noninstitutionalized population by disability status: 2015 American Community Survey 1-year estimates. Retrieved from https://factfinder.census.gov/faces/tableservices/jsf/pages/productview.xhtml?src=bkmk

Van Baalen, B., Ribbers, G. M., Medema-Meulepas, D., Pas, M. S., Odding, E., & Stam, H. J. (2007). Being restricted in participation after a traumatic brain injury is negatively associated by passive coping style of the caregiver. *Brain Injury, 21,* 925–931. http://dx.doi.org/10.1080/02699050701553197

Vargo, J. W. (1978). Some psychological effects of physical disability. *American Journal of Occupational Therapy, 32,* 31–34.

Wagner, E. H., Austin, B. T., & Von Korff, M. (1996). Organizing care for patients with chronic illness. *Milbank Quarterly, 74,* 511–544. http://dx.doi.org/10.2307/3350391

Wegener, S. T., Mackenzie, E. J., Ephraim, P., Ehde, D., & Williams, R. (2009). Self-management improves outcomes in persons with limb loss. *Archives of Physical Medicine and Rehabilitation, 90,* 373–380. http://dx.doi.org/10.1016/j.apmr.2008.08.222

Wells, R., Dywan, J., & Dumas, J. (2005). Life satisfaction and distress in family caregivers as related to specific behavioural changes after traumatic brain injury. *Brain Injury, 19,* 1105–1115. http://dx.doi.org/10.1080/02699050500150062

Williams, S. E. (1993). The impact of aphasia on marital satisfaction. *Archives of Physical Medicine and Rehabilitation, 74,* 361–367.

Wortman, C. B., & Silver, R. C. (1989). The myths of coping with loss. *Journal of Consulting and Clinical Psychology, 57,* 349–357. http://dx.doi.org/10.1037/0022-006X.57.3.349

World Health Organization. (2002). *Toward a common language for functioning, disability and health.* Geneva, Switzerland: Author.

World Health Organization. (2008). *International classification of functioning, disability and health: ICF.* Geneva, Switzerland: Author.

Wright, B. A. (1983). *Physical disability: A psychosocial approach* (2nd ed.). New York, NY: Harper & Row. http://dx.doi.org/10.1037/10589-000

Wright, B. A. (1987). Human dignity and professional self-monitoring. *Journal of Applied Rehabilitation Counseling, 18,* 12–14.

CHAPTER 6

CONSULTATION

Joseph F. Rath and Karen G. Langer

Consultation is central to the rehabilitation psychologist's identity (Hibbard & Cox, 2010; Stiers et al., 2015). Along with assessment and intervention, consultation is one of three broad categories of services typically provided by rehabilitation psychologists (Cox, Hess, Hibbard, Layman, & Stewart, 2010; Elliott & Gramling, 1990; Rath, Bertisch, & Elliott, 2017). Although the role of rehabilitation psychologists as clinical consultants to the interdisciplinary team regarding patient behavior is well known (Butt & Caplan, 2010; Cox, Cox, & Caplan, 2013; Elliott & Rath, 2011), rehabilitation psychology consultation can be offered to a broader and more extensive network. Rehabilitation psychologists routinely provide consultations to attorneys and courts, government agencies, educational institutions and training programs, corporate facilities, insurance companies, case managers, and others. Broader still, consultation may include organizational and/or administrative bodies representing treatment facilities, fundraising/advocacy organizations, and regulatory systems (Cox et al., 2013), thereby allowing for systemic impact above and beyond individual patient-focused consultations.

CORE ATTITUDES AND VALUES

> Offered as possible guidelines with the intent that they be examined and improved, then kept in the foreground to remind and to prompt, to check and to challenge, lest they remain inactivated and submerged by the weight of social, political, and personal pressures of all sorts. (Wright, 1983, p. xi)

Regardless of clinical setting or professional scenario, identifiable core attitudes and values underlie the rehabilitation psychology consultant's perspective. High ethical standards, compassion, self-awareness, good relationships with others, multicultural sensitivity, conscientiousness, good stress management skills, and ability to establish boundaries are essential attributes for the rehabilitation psychology consultant (Cox et al., 2013; Hanson & Kerkhoff, 2011; Stiers et al., 2015). Consistent with the value-laden beliefs of rehabilitation psychology, postulated by Beatrice Wright (1972, 1983; for reviews, see Dunn, Ehde, & Wegener, 2016; Dunn & Elliott, 2005), key parameters of effective consultation include awareness of ethical guidelines, knowledge of applicable regulations and laws, willingness to consult with others who can assist with matters beyond the consultant's abilities or competencies, the valuing of diversity and the importance of differing views, awareness of local resources, and timeliness of response (Cox et al., 2013).

Comprehensive guidelines for consultation efficacy and competence have been developed (see Chapter 1, this volume). As is evident

http://dx.doi.org/10.1037/0000129-007
Handbook of Rehabilitation Psychology, Third Edition, L. A. Brenner, S. A. Reid-Arndt, T. R. Elliott, R. G. Frank, and B. Caplan (Editors-in-Chief)

in reviewing these guidelines, rehabilitation psychology consultation requires a broad spectrum of technical skills and abilities in assessment, behavioral management, family systems, and psychology of disability; however, going beyond these technical skills, rehabilitation psychologists play a crucial role as interdisciplinary team facilitators (Barry & O'Leary, 1989). Before addressing the specific skill sets that constitute the rehabilitation psychology perspective (Stiers et al., 2012), we first consider the role of the rehabilitation psychologist in working with the interdisciplinary team. Next, we address considerations relevant to consultation in specific settings and phases of rehabilitation (e.g., acute care hospitals, inpatient rehabilitation units, outpatient rehabilitation settings). The chapter concludes with a discussion of future directions and issues facing the field.

WORKING WITH THE INTERDISCIPLINARY TEAM

> The needs of individual clients are so diverse, encompassing all problems that one might expect to encounter in human affairs, that a variety of services is necessary. Comprehensive rehabilitation, therefore, requires the effort of many professions and close working relations among the various kinds of rehabilitation agencies. (Wright, 1983, p. xiv)

Rehabilitation psychologists are "expected to participate in inter-professional collaboration," involving the clinical team, program, and community to "provide comprehensive and effective care for persons with disability and to maximize rehabilitation team and program functioning" (Stiers et al., 2015, p. 116). Thus, in medical rehabilitation settings, rehabilitation psychologists typically operate as part of an interdisciplinary team. The consultant role is omnipresent when the psychologist works alongside professionals from other rehabilitation disciplines (i.e., physiatry, physical therapy, occupational therapy, speech and language pathology, vocational counseling, social work, rehabilitation nursing, horticulture and recreation therapy, neurology and primary care physician consultants).

Somewhat narrowly, *consultation* has been defined as "a deliberation between [health care providers] on a case or its treatment" (http://www.merriam-webster.com/dictionary/consultation), in which guidance or expertise is provided to another person, staff professional, patient, or member of the patient's support system. Extending this definition, Stiers et al. (2015) aptly noted that the consultation role typically involves team, interprofessional, or interpersonal dynamics; program evaluation and quality improvement plans; and issues of health, disability, and advocacy.

Addressing such diverse issues as adherence to treatment regimens, behavioral disturbances, vocational potential, motivational issues, and family concerns (Elliott & Gramling, 1990), rehabilitation psychology consultants provide guidance to the treatment team regarding the patient's specific learning style, needed accommodations, motivational needs, cognitive abilities, and emotional reactions. The consultant may be called on to optimize the patient's engagement in rehabilitation and identify factors that enhance or hinder such engagement to promote maximal rehabilitation effectiveness (Kortte, Falk, Castillo, Johnson-Greene, & Wegener, 2007; Kortte, Veiel, Batten, & Wegener, 2009). Perhaps more important, rehabilitation psychologists significantly contribute to the understanding of team dynamics, to the provision of feedback, and to the processes involved in the interdisciplinary team approach to patient care. By discussing, analyzing, and advising about management strategies for problematic behaviors displayed by patients (and family members), helping to resolve staff/patient conflicts, and teaching interdisciplinary team members psychologically informed ways of viewing and interpreting patient behaviors, the rehabilitation psychology consultant plays a crucial role (Caplan & Reidy, 1996; Caplan & Shechter, 1993; Stiers & the Rehabilitation Psychology Synarchy, 2015). Such multifaceted collaboration and facilitation help the interdisciplinary team establish realistic treatment goals (Diller, 1990; Elliott & Rath, 2011).

Consulting on interdisciplinary teams requires especially strong interpersonal skills, which are essential for effective communication and teamwork. As aptly noted by Cox et al. (2013), "Fostering effective communication among the referring source, team members, consultant, organization, patient, other disciplines outside the immediate rehabilitation team, and patient's family is a fundamental responsibility of the rehabilitation psychologist consultant" (p. 85). In particular, the consultant must be attuned to, and cognizant of, the reactions of consultees. Reactions such as disdain—and even hate (Gans, 1983)—are sometimes subtext of the consultation question, although they are masked by demands for the patient to change. Other reactions, such as overidentification leading to overinvolvement (or, conversely, avoidance) or extreme stress, may be common when staff is working with young patients, issues of mortality are salient (e.g., terminal illness), family or subcultural dynamics (e.g., age, background, vocation, life experience) are similar to those of the treating staff, or there are losses involving mutilation, profound cognitive changes, or significant behavioral issues in a previously high-functioning individual. Such reactions may manifest with the treating provider's stating that the patient is crying too often or not often enough (e.g., in denial), or is lacking in motivation or adherence to treatment recommendations and interventions. The rehabilitation psychologist must recognize, interpret, and decipher the complexity of the consultation question, and sensitively approach the interplay between the consultee's own needs—embedded within the question posed—and objective findings of the patient's performance.

Clearly defined boundaries and roles, needs, and relationships are useful in ensuring that the consultation is as effective, accurate, and unbiased as possible. In this vein, keen sensitivity as to when to refer to, or consult with, other specialists is key to effective consultation and displays sensitivity to administrative and organizational requirements as balanced with patient, support system, and interdisciplinary team needs. Overall, the complex interplay among consultant psychologist, patient, treatment team, and other organizational administrative or leadership staff must be considered when navigating the consultation role (Cox et al., 2013).

REHABILITATION PSYCHOLOGY CONSULTATION SKILL SETS

> Psychologists are able to describe principles and procedures that help to motivate a client, review mind–body relationships that are important to rehabilitation, assess client attributes, evaluate psychological and behavioral consequences of particular environmental situations . . . and sensitize personnel to social-emotional aspects of professional–client relations. (Wright, 1983, p. xiv)

Consistent with Wright's (1983) value-laden beliefs, specific skill sets in consultation related to personality and emotional factors, behavioral functioning improvement, cognitive functioning, substance abuse identification and management, vocational and/or educational considerations, and sexual functioning and disability have been identified as essential for rehabilitation psychologists (Hibbard & Cox, 2010; Stiers et al., 2015; see Exhibit 6.1). In providing expert consultation, the rehabilitation psychologist uses skills and knowledge drawn from a broad spectrum of psychological fields, including clinical, counseling, cognitive, educational, health, neuro-, developmental, and geropsychology.

Personality and Emotional Factors

One of the most common questions posed to the consulting psychologist in interdisciplinary rehabilitation settings concerns patients' emotional reactions and mood. Issues, such as adjustment and coping,

EXHIBIT 6.1

Six Consultation Skills in Rehabilitation Psychology

1. Personality and emotional factors
2. Behavioral functioning improvement
3. Cognitive functioning
4. Substance abuse identification and management
5. Vocational and/or education considerations
6. Sexual functioning and disability

depression and anxiety, denial and minimization, preexisting psychopathology, bereavement and grief, posttraumatic stress disorder, and suicidal ideation, are key aspects of psychological functioning that are especially relevant in rehabilitation settings. The rehabilitation psychology consultant's unique contribution to the interdisciplinary team includes highlighting positive personality and emotional factors, including strengths, coping skills, resilience, hopefulness, awareness, insight, and positive adaptation (Dunn & Dougherty, 2005; Kalpakjian et al., 2014; Kortte, Stevenson, Hosey, Castillo, & Wegener, 2012; Langer, 2017). In addition, the rehabilitation psychologist is uniquely qualified to consult regarding issues of significant distress, psychological disorders and diagnoses, psychopathological manifestations, and the special challenges posed thereby. These problems may be so extreme as to limit participation and active engagement in other therapies. Given insurer's requirements for active participation in rehabilitation efforts, patients no longer are permitted to stay on a rehabilitation unit when they are not actively engaged in treatment. Thus, the ability of the psychologist to intervene in such cases—consulting as a core member of the interdisciplinary team—facilitates timely and effective provision of necessary rehabilitation therapies for patients who otherwise may have been discharged (Stiers & the Rehabilitation Psychology Synarchy, 2015).

The value of psychological intervention for treatment of depression as an aspect of effective collaborative care is well established (Katon et al., 2010). In a meta-analysis, the success of collaborative care depended on provision of psychological treatment for depression by psychologists (as opposed to antidepressant pharmacotherapy; Coventry et al., 2014). Both accurate diagnosis and effective treatment for depression are considered critical for improved functional outcome in patients with traumatic brain injury (TBI; Bombardier et al., 2010), with similar research findings regarding poststroke depression (Gordon & Hibbard, 1997), spinal cord injury (SCI; Bombardier, 2014; Elliott & Frank, 1996), and multiple sclerosis (Siegert & Abernethy, 2005).

When working with patients who appear to deny or minimize aspects of disability (Caplan & Shechter, 1987; Langer, 1999a, 1999b; Langer & Padrone, 1992), the rehabilitation psychology consultant helps team members understand the context in which the disability is experienced and why denial/minimization is exhibited, as well as adaptive aspects of this emotional response (e.g., keeping overwhelming depression and anxiety at bay; titrating the path to "adjustment"). Furthermore, the consultant may assist in determining whether "denial" is a psychological response or neuropathologically based, or neuropsychologically and cognitively based anosognosia (Langer & Padrone, 1992). The consultant must handle the request in a diplomatic and sensitive manner, balancing the therapist's concerns with the needs and status of the patient.

Preexisting psychopathology can have a negative effect on the rehabilitation process and on interactions among patient, family, and staff. Thus, the rehabilitation psychologist may be consulted for staff education to help parcel out adjustment reactions from neurobehavioral features and call attention to preexisting psychiatric symptoms that can be exacerbated by the stress of illness, hospitalization, and loss. Anxiety regarding a myriad of aspects of the unknown in rehabilitation and recovery may affect the patients' response to suggested treatments, which can color staff perceptions of patient's cooperation; in this vein, consultation by the psychologist may clarify and enhance empathy.

Rehabilitation psychology consultants must be equipped to address bereavement and grief (Langer, 1995) as an additional complicating stressor in cases in which the patient has lost a significant other, possibly in the same traumatic accident in which the patient was injured. The relationship of the patient to the deceased loved one and their respective responsibilities for an accident that led to injury and death, need to be considered as the consultant weighs the emotional responses and advises the team regarding patient care. The effects of loss of limb, loss of home, loss of functional abilities, or loss of loved one (Parkes, 1972), and sometimes the co-occurrence of these events in rehabilitation settings, may have an impact on the expected emotional response and on the rehabilitation process. Staff may feel overwhelmed, along with the patient, and may benefit from expert consultation to assist with processing emotional responses and grief, as well as to modulate and assist with sensitive interactions. Furthermore, rehabilitation psychology consultants must be prepared to recognize signs of posttraumatic stress disorder, address its effects, and tailor interventions and staff recommendations in settings and circumstances in which traumatic injuries and loss occur (e.g., Veterans Administration and military settings; natural and manmade disasters, such as tornados, train collisions, terrorism; Bremner & Marmar, 1998).

Skill in assessing for suicidal ideation and risk assessment are core competencies for rehabilitation psychologists because devastating loss may precipitate or exacerbate thoughts of self-harm and undermine the will to live. In more rare circumstances, homicidal ideation may ensue (e.g., issues of anger after a loss caused by someone else's actions, whether intentional or due to carelessness or negligence). Legal aspects may be salient, and risk assessment is necessary if the patient possesses firearms or other means to carry out plans to cause harm (see, e.g., New York Secure Ammunition and Firearms Enforcement Act of 2013, also known as the NY SAFE Act).

Behavioral Functioning Improvement

Using strategies from learning theory, developmental psychology and the effectiveness of contingency rewards, and neuropsychology (Elliott & Rath, 2011; Rath & Elliott, 2012), the rehabilitation psychology consultant's role includes making recommendations for promoting positive adaptation, diminishing counterproductive or disruptive behaviors, minimizing avoidance or maladaptive attention-seeking behaviors, and educating about safety considerations for patients and staff alike. The consultant role involves, among other aspects, integrating feedback from interdisciplinary staff about patient behaviors or reactions that are less than adaptive, unsafe, or otherwise limit full participation in rehabilitation therapies. Depending on the nature of the problem, the consultation may include recommendations to staff members regarding optimal responses to patient behaviors, environmental modifications, and response modulation (i.e., reward and time-out reinforcement schedules).

It can be helpful to observe and/or cotreat the patient with therapists from other disciplines (e.g., physical therapy, occupational therapy) so that the psychologist's interactions with the patient can be observed and role-modeled while allowing the psychologist to better conceptualize the consultation request by observing the behavior in vivo. Observing cotreating patients with therapists from other disciplines also can form or reinforce an alliance between the consulting psychologist and the treating therapist while maintaining a focus on the patient's well-being.

For patients with neurobehavioral disorders, consultation typically involves development of behavior management plans with the interdisciplinary team. Effective behavior management plans use resources that are practical, relatively easy to implement, and relevant and useful to the consulting question. For example, for a sleep disturbance that affects behavior, the plan might include consideration of environmental factors (e.g., noise in the hospital hallways, television hours, roommates and visitors, lights), emotional features (e.g., seeing visiting friends and family members remove their belongings and leave the unit, which may induce anxiety and fear), and behavioral consistency (e.g., consistent bedtime and wake time with lights adjusted; limitations of daytime napping; the timing of fluids; encouragement of relaxation via tapes, music, exercise, breathing strategies at bedtime).

Patients may be administered rating scales (or staff may complete these scales) to measure disruptive behaviors, such as agitation (Corrigan, 1989; Corrigan & Bogner, 1994), with reductions in scores after implementation of behavioral plans being a sign of improvement. Given that the consultant often is expected to "fix" the problem, gentle reminders to staff to consider recency of onset, maintain reasonable expectations about the pace of improvement, weigh even small measurable or qualitative gains, and take into account other mediating variables that may affect the success of behavioral plans are vital in keeping the team motivated. The effectiveness of the consultation often is measured, even indirectly, by successful behavior change, so it is wise for the consultant to remind staff to consider even small gains as progress and to recognize that behavioral management is a process, not a "cure."

Cognitive Functioning

The rehabilitation psychology consultant can advise team members as to effective strategies for addressing cognitive difficulties that may limit a patient's ability to benefit from rehabilitation. Such consultation calls for expertise in the nuances of neurocognitive issues that affect functioning, behavior, and emotional presentation. For example, there are important distinctions to be made between apathy and aprosodia (Ross, 1981), abulia and adynamia, initiation and depressive psychomotor retardation, unawareness and denial (Caplan & Shechter, 1987; Langer, 1999a, 1999b), and attentional difficulties versus emotional withdrawal or avoidance because treatment implications will vary. On a systems level, empirically validated strategies developed by rehabilitation psychologists for remediating disorders of visual attention and visual neglect (Kortte & Hillis, 2011; Lisa, Jughters, & Kerckhofs, 2013; Weinberg et al., 1977) have long been integrated into many inpatient rehabilitation settings (e.g., bed placement on the side of the hemineglect to stimulate visual attention). The consultative applications of other cognitive remediation techniques and strategies are notable (see Haskins et al., 2012; Wilson, 2008).

Rehabilitation psychologists increasingly are called on to consult on complex issues in the area of cognitive loss and capacity assessment (see American Bar Association/American Psychological Association [APA] Assessment of Capacity in Older Adults Project Working Group, 2008). Capacity evaluations require not only the requisite assessment skills but also encompass reporting to, and consulting with, the referring team (whether the consultee is the physician, the treatment team, the care manager, a lawyer or other legal or judicial representative). Specific issues may include a patient's capacity to make decisions regarding discharge and disposition status (to what type of setting: home vs. facility vs. other), financial matters (e.g., testamentary, wills, health care directives), and other issues with significant short-term or longer term implications. The consulting psychologist must be sensitive to the possibility of competing or even conflicting needs, opinions, and perspectives that may influence the consultee's reaction to the findings.

Substance Abuse Identification and Management

The rehabilitation psychology consultant requires expertise in substance abuse identification and management, often a necessary component of treatment planning. For example, the psychologist working with a patient who sustained a TBI in an accident caused by alcohol use (see Heinemann, Corrigan, & Moore, 2004) may consult with the family and staff to secure discharge planning that includes a sobriety coach. Such consultation must be handled with sensitivity to environmental and interpersonal pressures within the patient's support system that might lead to recidivism and undermine abstinence. Psychoeducation regarding the deleterious effects of alcohol and substances post-TBI should be considered essential, as well.

Vocational and/or Educational Considerations

Consultations may involve evaluation of cognitive strengths and impairments with educational or vocational implications, as well as recommendations for reasonable accommodations on return to school or work. Effective consultation regarding educational and vocational interests, and options requires the rehabilitation psychologist to have specialized knowledge of the relevant legal frameworks in which vocational and educational activities take place, including the Improving Access to Assistive Technology for Individuals With Disabilities Act of 2004, Individuals With Disabilities Education Act of 1990, and Americans With Disabilities Act of 1990 (Stiers & the Rehabilitation Psychology Synarchy, 2015). The rehabilitation psychologist may collaborate with vocational counselors and consult with relevant personnel and significant others regarding the patient's readiness for vocational return. A patient, family member, or both may express eagerness to return to work prematurely (e.g., in the context of severe aphasic difficulties or cognitive dysfunction in the acute phase after stroke or brain injury, where the nature of the employment requires strong linguistic skills). In such cases, consultation serves a mediation role, helping to guide patients and families, as well as staff, to form realistic time frames with hopeful goals.

Sexual Functioning and Disability

Consultations regarding sexual functioning typically include educational and counseling strategies to encourage communication between partners, dispel erroneous inferences on the part of patients and partners, increase sexual satisfaction, and lessen the impact of disability (Cameron et al., 2011; Schover & Jensen, 1988). For example, the rehabilitation psychologist may be asked to consult with the spouse of a patient with SCI who has questions about sexual functioning (Elliott & Rath, 2011). Rehabilitation psychologists are mindful not to limit their consultations regarding sexual functioning to married couples or presume heterosexuality (Hanjorgiris, Rath, & O'Neill, 2004). Similarly, they are sensitive to the sexual concerns of individuals who are not in relationships and may be struggling with concerns about their attractiveness to potential partners and issues related to stigma and disability (Cox et al., 2013; Elliott & Rath, 2011; Hibbard & Cox, 2010; Stiers et al., 2015).

SETTING- AND PHASE-SPECIFIC CONSIDERATIONS

> Psychological factors are ever present and often crucial in all phases of rehabilitation. (Wright, 1983, p. xiv)

Rehabilitation psychologists consult across all settings and phases of rehabilitation, ranging from acute care hospitals to outpatient rehabilitation facilities to the community and beyond. The consultation may be focused on the individual clinical case or may target systemic change at the broadest possible levels. Setting-specific factors, such as size of the team (e.g., inpatient rehabilitation units in which there are large interdisciplinary teams) and degree of overlap of the psychologist's skills and/or training with those of other team members, may affect the nature and frequency of consultations (Karol & Sturm, 2017).

Acute Care Hospitals

In acute medical care settings, the psychologist may consult with staff from other disciplines (i.e., nurses, physicians, respiratory therapists, personal care technicians, medical students, medical residents, nutritionists, unit clerical staff, outpatient agencies.) who may not be as familiar with the skills and potential contributions of a rehabilitation psychologist as are staff members who work together on interdisciplinary rehabilitation teams. Nonetheless, there is ample evidence to support the crucial role of rehabilitation psychologists in acute medical settings because these psychologists contribute to medical education and teaching, patient care, consultation and recommendations regarding continuity of care, family intervention and guidance, solution-focused and biopsychosocial approaches, and staff support (Warren, Stucky, & Sherman, 2013).

Rehabilitation psychology consultants in acute medical settings typically work with patients and caregivers on an abbreviated time line (i.e., often measured in days as approved by insurance company guidelines) while providing valuable support, education (preparation for transfer to rehabilitation), and critical needs assessment (Warren et al., 2013). As in inpatient rehabilitation settings, timely response to consultation requests, usually within 24 hours of the request (Cox et al., 2013), often is vital because the referral question may be posed with varying degrees of urgency. Expectations inherent in the consulting question dictate the most appropriate means of communication (e.g., formal report, presentation at meeting, confidential discussion, other), which must consider and weigh respect for confidentiality and patient privacy against the need to communicate with multiple team members in a timely fashion.

The role played by the rehabilitation psychology consultant in acute care settings may be crucial for patients with acquired brain injury (e.g., TBI, stroke, encephalopathy, anoxic brain dysfunction) or other disorders with generalized behavioral or cognitive manifestations. For example, the rehabilitation psychologist may draw on specialized knowledge and skills to assess, define, and address sleep disorders after brain injury (Clinchot, Bogner, Mysiw, Fugate, & Corrigan, 1998; Lu, Krellman, & Dijkers, 2016). Consultation with nursing, medical, or other multidisciplinary staff may include recommendations for improving sleep hygiene and addressing environmental factors and mood symptoms. With the rehabilitation psychologist's evidence-based knowledge regarding the comparative effectiveness of psychopharmacology and behavioral strategies, staff training and education also may be part of the collaborative consultant role in acute care hospitals.

Inpatient Rehabilitation Unit

Recognizing the crucial role of rehabilitation psychologists on the interdisciplinary team, the Commission on Accreditation of Rehabilitation Facilities (CARF) has mandated that rehabilitation psychologists be on the staff of all inpatient rehabilitation facilities (Cox et al., 2010). On the inpatient rehabilitation unit, it is standard practice for the psychologist to evaluate and treat patients, report findings at interdisciplinary team meetings, document their findings in the electronic medical record, and use technological means to communicate findings (e.g., secure e-mail). To be effective and successful as a consultant on the interdisciplinary team, the psychologist must become accustomed to the constraints of competition for scheduling needs and environmental issues, including space and privacy concerns. In many inpatient rehabilitation settings, the psychologist formally communicates findings to team members during weekly meetings but is available for informal consultation with individual staff members between meetings. In addition to working directly with interdisciplinary teams, the rehabilitation psychologist plays a key role in providing consultations to authorized outside parties, such as family members, attorneys, courts, governmental and social services agencies, schools, employers, and insurance companies (Elliott & Rath, 2011), and also may develop larger scale psychoeducational training for staff.

The consulting psychologist typically evaluates and considers current emotional status; pre-onset psychological status; alcohol and substance use history; behavioral factors; positive coping skills and resilience; other personal preferences; life aspirations; creative pursuits, hobbies, and interests; and psychosocial issues and their impact on projections for rehabilitation planning. Furthermore, issues of psychosexual functioning, intimacy and loving, the existing social support system, additional and recent life stressors, and multiple or polytraumatic losses (e.g., lost loved ones in the accident in which the disabling condition occurred) may be salient. In addition, cognitive findings, neuropsychological status, history of abuse, and other risk factors can have a significant impact on rehabilitation prognosis and planning. The rehabilitation psychologist considers all of the aforementioned factors as aspects of what constitutes value and meaning, experience, goals, aspirations, and the fabric of life for the person who has become the focus of the clinical consultation (Langer, 2017).

The consulting psychologist must be familiar with the language and concepts of professional practice in other rehabilitation disciplines, including physiatry, rehabilitation nursing, physical therapy, occupational therapy, speech and language pathology, vocational counseling, and therapeutic recreation, as well as social work and care management. Understanding the languages, perspectives, and conceptualizations of the various disciplines is key to clarifying and implementing the team's ultimate consensus, thus allowing the rehabilitation psychology consultant to serve as an effective team leader.

Outpatient Rehabilitation Settings

In the outpatient setting, the rehabilitation psychologist typically provides consultation to the interdisciplinary staff, a member of a multidisciplinary team (for a discussion of distinctions between *multidisciplinary* and *interdisciplinary* teams, and the relative advantages of interdisciplinary teams, see Butt & Caplan, 2010; Cifu & Stewart, 1999), or a referring medical provider who wishes to have information about the referred patient's cognitive and emotional functioning. At times, outside agencies may consult the psychologist who, with the permission of the patient (or health care proxy) and the institution, may offer guidance regarding requested or needed services in the community, resources required for support, legal issues or forensic concerns, or agency referrals. The psychologist may be asked to consult with vocational counselors or representatives of vocational services agencies regarding functional status and vocational needs. If necessary, the consultant also may confer with other available experts for resources and guidance (e.g., APA's legal risk management program, professional LISTSERVs, other psychologists individually or in professional support networks, legal advisors affiliated with psychological organizations).

Home, Community, and Beyond

On the level of individual patient-focused consultations, the rehabilitation psychologist may address concerns of other professionals who serve the individual in the community (e.g., case managers, medical personnel, attorneys) or agencies that serve individuals with disabilities (e.g., certified home health agency, commissions for the blind and visually impaired, commissions for the deaf and hard of hearing, Social Security Administration).

On a systems level, rehabilitation psychologists consult with a variety of institutional/organizational entities seeking information regarding persons with disabilities and chronic health conditions. For example, a workplace may seek consultation about accommodations, adaptations, or disability cultural sensitivity training (Stiers & the Rehabilitation Psychology Synarchy, 2015). Broader still, consultation may include organizational and/or administrative bodies representing treatment facilities, advocacy organizations, and regulatory systems (Cox et al., 2013). For example, rehabilitation psychologists consult with key regulatory agencies that set and maintain standards of rehabilitative care, including the Joint Commission and CARF (Stiers & the Rehabilitation Psychology Synarchy, 2015).

Rehabilitation psychologists also consult with disability-based national organizations. For example, in consultation with the Consortium for Spinal Cord Medicine (formed by the Paralyzed Veterans of America), rehabilitation psychologists have played key roles in the preparation of consumer and provider guides to issues confronted by individuals with SCI (Stiers & the Rehabilitation Psychology Synarchy, 2015).

Another consideration in consultation is that of advocacy for disability rights, accessibility, and justice (Stiers & the Rehabilitation Psychology Synarchy, 2015). As aptly noted by Cox et al. (2013), "Becoming a contributor, advisor, or committee member or having other involvement in organizations that advocate for the challenged and/or disadvantaged in our society is considered by many to be an ethical responsibility of professionals in psychology" (p. 92). APA's Division of Rehabilitation Psychology espouses mission and vision statements that include "[to] champion disability as a human rights and social justice issue" (see http://www.div22.org/mission-and-vision-statements/). This aim reflects an important shift from the typical medical mind-set into an advocacy mode that is worthy of greater consideration by rehabilitation psychologists.

The advocacy potential of rehabilitation psychologists in consulting with colleagues, particularly with respect to training and accommodation issues, should not be underestimated. For years, rehabilitation psychologists have served on APA's Committee on Disability Issues in Psychology, frequently in the role of committee chair. In collaboration with rehabilitation psychologists serving on other APA committees, including the Committee on Women in Psychology and Committee on Early Career Psychologists, rehabilitation psychologists have provided expert consultation to APA's Board of Convention Affairs, convention/meeting services office, and Board for the Advancement of Psychology in the Public Interest regarding logistical considerations (e.g., architectural barriers, proximity to accessible restrooms, adequate time between scheduled events to allow those with mobility impairments to get from room to room) necessary to encourage full participation of psychologists with disabilities and chronic health conditions at APA's annual convention and consolidated meetings (see, e.g., Williams & Pilarski, 2014). In addition, through their work on the Committee on Disability Issues in Psychology, rehabilitation psychologists have played an important role consulting with other psychologists on such issues as providing necessary accommodations to doctoral students with disabilities who are learning to administer psychological tests (see, e.g., Carlos, 2014). Consultations such as these demonstrate the enormous potential of rehabilitation psychologists to impact psychology training programs through a consultative role.

Management of Competing Needs and Demands

Regardless of setting or phase of rehabilitation, a primary challenge in consultation revolves around establishing the identity of the consultee when multiple parties are involved, with each having differing needs or competing interests. For example, when consulting with insurance representatives and lawyers, psychologists often are in difficult positions, at times advocating on behalf of the patient while, at other times, defending treatment plans and staff decisions. Because these complex ethical issues tax the traditional ethics of psychological practice, the rehabilitation psychology consultant must remain cognizant of ethical issues and consult with experts regarding any questions concerning roles (Elliott & Gramling, 1990).

In the health care setting in which there are multiple roles for the rehabilitation psychologist (e.g., treatment provider for the patient, psychotherapist for the family, consultant to the rehabilitation team, staff person with administrative responsibilities), the challenges may be the most obvious. The consulting psychologist faces the multiple demands of the patient's needs and those of other treating staff, as well as family concerns and dynamics (Caplan & Reidy, 1996). For example, the psychologist may consider assuming the often requested task of helping to process and negotiate the circumstances of a patient whose discharge from the inpatient unit has stalled. This impasse, frustrating to all concerned and sometimes escalating to administrative levels, may involve caregivers' worries and fears, a desire to keep the patient on the unit longer for more intensive rehabilitation rather than discharge to a subacute facility, the feeling of being overwhelmed by the enormity of care needs that must be provided at home, concerns regarding availability of someone to provide such care in a home setting, or issues regarding the patient's capacity to understand discharge recommendations and implement them safely with an agreed on plan. On the one hand, the psychologist must consider the risks of losing the empathic neutrality needed to work with the patient and weakening the patient's experience of the therapeutic alliance; on the other hand, though, the psychologist is part of the rehabilitation team. Diplomatically negotiating this duality enhances respect for the psychologist's role and the sense of relevance of the psychologist on the interdisciplinary team.

FUTURE DIRECTIONS AND ISSUES FACING THE FIELD

The APA's Standards of Accreditation (Commission on Accreditation, 2017) recognizes consultation and interprofessional/interdisciplinary skills under professionwide competencies for purposes of accreditation review for doctoral training programs. Nonetheless, it seems that few such training programs—with the notable exception of some counseling psychology programs—routinely require consultation coursework. Although published data were not available to document the number of doctoral programs requiring such a course, an informal survey of 20 practicing rehabilitation psychologists found that 18 (90%) did not complete a consultation course during their training, whereas only two (10%) reported coursework in consultation that was offered in the context of broader "professional development" seminars. With the depth and breadth of foundational and functional competencies required for effective consultation in rehabilitation psychology, we are hopeful that the next generation of training programs will incorporate both formal coursework and practica in consultation.

Scope of practice is another salient issue facing the field because cross-disciplinary expertise may lead to role diffusion and conflict. Transdisciplinary education increasingly is valued in rehabilitation because all disciplines need to be aware of the special needs of patients with complex disorders, such as TBI and stroke; however, the particular expertise of each discipline, including that of the rehabilitation psychologist, must remain individualized and respected as such. Recognizing the particular expertise of each discipline is important for professional identity, the education of patients and families, and the optimization of service delivery and team communication and effectiveness. When clinicians have similar and perhaps overlapping skills and expertise, collaboration constitutes the core of professional standards of care. However, even in the psychosocial domain, the skill set is not interchangeable (Russell et al., 2016), and certainly this is the case when considering different disciplines that work together in the rehabilitation setting. For example, social work, rehabilitation psychology, psychiatry, and care management may deal with psychosocial aspects of patients' rehabilitation, and although the skill set may overlap, it is not identical. Thus, there may be some divergence of perspective when collaborating with professionals with similar but not identical scope of practice. Clear communication, clarification, and mutual respect are critical for optimal outcomes.

Assessment and diagnostic skills are highly valued in medical settings. Although these technical skills are well represented in rehabilitation psychology functional competencies, core beliefs and values also define the rehabilitation psychology perspective. As highlighted throughout this chapter, these value-laden beliefs underlie the rehabilitation psychology consultant's unique contributions to the team, including an appreciation of positive cognitive abilities (e.g., problem-solving skills; see Rath & Elliott, 2012), as well as personality and emotional factors, such as coping skills, resilience, hopefulness, and positive adaptation to disability (Bertisch, Rath, Long, Ashman, & Rashid, 2014). Although valued by the interdisciplinary team and accreditation, oversight, and regulatory agencies—particularly in the context of patient-centered care—more stringent length-of-stay requirements, along with decreasing support and reimbursement for psychological interventions, continue to limit therapeutic activities in the inpatient environment. With a steady growth of neuropsychology and other doctoral-level specialties that champion assessment, diagnosis, and medical interventions (Elliott & Rath, 2011), it is likely that these psychologists eventually will assume consultant positions in inpatient rehabilitation settings.

We anticipate that rehabilitation psychologists who are generalists in outlook and competence will be more likely to consult in public health programs to promote the health and well-being of community-residing individuals with disabling conditions, generally, regardless of specific medical diagnosis, in a manner congruent with the International Classification of Functioning, Disability and Health (World Health Organization, 2001) conceptualization of disability as "the outcome or result of a complex relationship between an individual's health condition and personal factors, and of the external factors that represent the circumstances in which the individual lives" (World Health Organization, 2001, p. 17). This perspective places a greater recognition on the disabling features of the environment and the person–environment interaction in a manner consistent with the long-standing value-laden beliefs and social psychological heritage of rehabilitation psychology (Wright, 1983; see also Elliott & Rath, 2011), and it is quite compatible with the views of most disability advocates (Pledger, 2003). Specific relevant areas of growth that can capitalize on the rehabilitation psychologist's unique perspective include consulting to "long-term care facilities, senior residences and communities, and medical equipment companies" (Cox et al., 2010, p. 84).

CONCLUSION

In addition to the six rehabilitation psychology consultation skill sets previously identified by others (see Exhibit 6.1), we concur with Cox et al. (2013) about the importance of additional skills related to ethical guidelines (e.g., boundaries, confidentiality) and local, state, and federal laws, and regulations relevant to people living with disabilities. In addition, we add familiarity with the language and concepts of other rehabilitation disciplines to the list of minimum requirements for effective consultation. These specific skill sets are necessary but insufficient for optimal functioning as a rehabilitation psychology consultant. Value-laden beliefs and core attitudes, first postulated by Wright (1972, 1983) and articulated throughout this chapter, also are crucial to consultation conducted from the rehabilitation psychologist's perspective.

In August 2016, the executive board of APA's Division of Rehabilitation Psychology voted to adopt new mission and vision statements that include "[to] set the standard of practice for culturally competent, evidence-based, wholistic, and personalized care" for people living with disability or chronic health conditions (see http://www.div22.org/mission-and-vision-statements/). To achieve this goal, it is incumbent on the division and its partners on the Rehabilitation Psychology Specialty Council to fully embrace and widely disseminate the unique and broad-based foundations of rehabilitation psychology that are valued for their far-reaching perspectives, which include, but extend beyond, technical skills.

References

American Bar Association/American Psychological Association Assessment of Capacity in Older Adults Project Working Group. (2008). *Assessment of older adults with diminished capacity: A handbook for psychologists.* Washington, DC: American Bar Association Commission on Law and Aging and American Psychological Association.

Americans With Disabilities Act[0] of 1990, 42 U.S.C.A. § 1201 et seq. (West 1993).

Barry, P., & O'Leary, J. (1989). Roles of the psychologist on a traumatic brain injury rehabilitation team. *Rehabilitation Psychology, 34,* 83–90.

Bertisch, H., Rath, J., Long, C., Ashman, T., & Rashid, T. (2014). Positive psychology in rehabilitation medicine: A brief report. *NeuroRehabilitation, 34,* 573–585. http://dx.doi.org/10.3233/NRE-141059

Bombardier, C. H. (2014). Depression and spinal cord injury. *Archives of Physical Medicine and Rehabilitation, 95,* 413–414. http://dx.doi.org/10.1016/j.apmr.2013.04.008

Bombardier, C. H., Fann, J. R., Temkin, N. R., Esselman, P. C., Barber, J., & Dikmen, S. S. (2010). Rates of major depressive disorder and clinical outcomes following traumatic brain injury. *JAMA, 303,* 1938–1945. http://dx.doi.org/10.1001/jama.2010.599

Bremner, J. D., & Marmar, C. R. (Eds.). (1998). *Trauma, memory, and dissociation* (Vol. 34). Washington, DC: American Psychiatric Press.

Butt, L., & Caplan, B. (2010). The rehabilitation team. In R. G. Frank, M. Rosenthal, & B. Caplan (Eds.), *Handbook of rehabilitation psychology* (2nd ed., pp. 451–457). Washington, DC: American Psychological Association. http://dx.doi.org/10.1037/15972-032

Cameron, R. P., Mona, L. R., Syme, M. L., Clemency Cordes, C., Fraley, S. S., Chen, S. S., . . . Lemos, L. (2011). Sexuality among wounded veterans of Operation Enduring Freedom (OEF), Operation Iraqi Freedom (OIF), and Operation New Dawn (OND): Implications for rehabilitation psychologists. *Rehabilitation Psychology, 56,* 289–301. http://dx.doi.org/10.1037/a0025513

Caplan, B., & Reidy, K. (1996). Staff-patient-family conflicts in rehabilitation: Sources and solutions. *Topics in Spinal Cord Injury Rehabilitation,* 2(2), 21–33.

Caplan, B., & Shechter, J. (1987). Denial and depression in disabling illness. In B. Caplan (Ed.), *Rehabilitation psychology desk reference* (pp. 133–170). Rockville, MD: Aspen.

Caplan, B., & Shechter, J. (1993). Reflections on the "depressed," "unrealistic," "inappropriate," "manipulative," "unmotivated," "noncompliant," "denying," "maladjusted," "regressed," etc patient. *Archives of Physical Medicine and Rehabilitation, 74,* 1123–1124. http://dx.doi.org/10.1016/0003-9993(93)90074-K

Carlos, M. (2014, July). Training clinical psychology students with disabilities in psychological testing assessment. *Spotlight on Disability Newsletter.* Retrieved from http://www.apa.org/pi/disability/resources/publications/newsletter/2014/07/clinical-psychology.aspx

Cifu, D. X., & Stewart, D. G. (1999). Factors affecting functional outcome after stroke: A critical review of rehabilitation interventions. *Archives of Physical Medicine and Rehabilitation, 80*(Suppl. 1), S35–S39. http://dx.doi.org/10.1016/S0003-9993(99)90101-6

Clinchot, D. M., Bogner, J., Mysiw, W. J., Fugate, L., & Corrigan, J. (1998). Defining sleep disturbance after brain injury. *American Journal of Physical Medicine & Rehabilitation, 77,* 291–295. http://dx.doi.org/10.1097/00002060-199807000-00006

Commission on Accreditation. (2017). *Implementing regulations. Section C: IRs related to the standards of accreditation.* Retrieved from https://www.apa.org/ed/accreditation/section-c-soa.pdf

Corrigan, J. D. (1989). Development of a scale for assessment of agitation following traumatic brain injury. *Journal of Clinical and Experimental Neuropsychology, 11,* 261–277. http://dx.doi.org/10.1080/01688638908400888

Corrigan, J. D., & Bogner, J. A. (1994). Factor structure of the Agitated Behavior Scale. *Journal of Clinical and Experimental Neuropsychology, 16,* 386–392. http://dx.doi.org/10.1080/01688639408402649

Coventry, P. A., Hudson, J. L., Kontopantelis, E., Archer, J., Richards, D. A., Gilbody, S., . . . Bower, P. (2014). Characteristics of effective collaborative care for treatment of depression: A systematic review and meta-regression of 74 randomised controlled trials. *PLoS One, 9,* e108114. http://dx.doi.org/10.1371/journal.pone.0108114

Cox, D. R., Cox, R. H., & Caplan, B. (2013). *Specialty competencies in rehabilitation psychology.* New York, NY: Oxford University Press. http://dx.doi.org/10.1093/med:psych/9780195389241.001.0001

Cox, D. R., Hess, D. W., Hibbard, M. R., Layman, D. E., & Stewart, R. K., Jr. (2010). Specialty practice in rehabilitation psychology. *Professional Psychology: Research and Practice, 41,* 82–88. http://dx.doi.org/10.1037/a0016411

Diller, L. (1990). Fostering the interdisciplinary team, fostering research in a society in transition. *Archives of Physical Medicine and Rehabilitation, 71,* 275–278.

Dunn, D. S., & Dougherty, S. B. (2005). Prospects for a positive psychology of rehabilitation. *Rehabilitation*

Psychology, 50, 305–311. http://dx.doi.org/10.1037/0090-5550.50.3.305

Dunn, D. S., Ehde, D. M., & Wegener, S. T. (2016). The foundational principles as psychological lodestars: Theoretical inspiration and empirical direction in rehabilitation psychology. *Rehabilitation Psychology, 61,* 1–6. http://dx.doi.org/10.1037/rep0000082

Dunn, D. S., & Elliott, T. R. (2005). Revisiting a constructive classic: Wright's physical disability: A psychosocial approach. *Rehabilitation Psychology, 50,* 183–189. http://dx.doi.org/10.1037/0090-5550.50.2.183

Elliott, T. R., & Frank, R. G. (1996). Depression following spinal cord injury. *Archives of Physical Medicine and Rehabilitation, 77,* 816–823. http://dx.doi.org/10.1016/S0003-9993(96)90263-4

Elliott, T. R., & Gramling, S. E. (1990). Psychologists and rehabilitation: New roles and old training models. *American Psychologist, 45,* 762–765. http://dx.doi.org/10.1037/0003-066X.45.6.762

Elliott, T. R., & Rath, J. F. (2011). Rehabilitation psychology. In E. M. Altmaier & J. C. Hansen (Eds.), *Oxford handbook of counseling psychology* (pp. 679–702). New York, NY: Oxford University Press.

Gans, J. S. (1983). Hate in the rehabilitation setting. *Archives of Physical Medicine and Rehabilitation, 64,* 176–179.

Gordon, W. A., & Hibbard, M. R. (1997). Poststroke depression: An examination of the literature. *Archives of Physical Medicine and Rehabilitation, 78,* 658–663. http://dx.doi.org/10.1016/S0003-9993(97)90433-0

Hanjorgiris, W. F., Rath, J. F., & O'Neill, J. H. (2004). Gay men living with chronic illness or disability: A sociocultural, minority group perspective on mental health. In B. Lipton (Ed.), *Gay men living with chronic illnesses and disabilities: From crisis to crossroads* (pp. 25–42). Binghamton, NY: Haworth Press.

Hanson, S. L., & Kerkhoff, T. R. (2011). The APA ethical principles as a foundational competency: Application to rehabilitation psychology. *Rehabilitation Psychology, 56,* 219–230. http://dx.doi.org/10.1037/a0024206

Haskins, E. C., Cicerone, K. D., Dams-O'Connor, K., Eberle, R., Langenbahn, D. M., Shapiro-Rosenbaum, A., & Trexler, L. E. (2012). *Cognitive rehabilitation manual: Translating evidence-based recommendations into practice.* Reston, VA: American Congress of Rehabilitation Medicine.

Heinemann, A. W., Corrigan, J. D., & Moore, D. (2004). Case management for traumatic brain injury survivors with alcohol problems. *Rehabilitation Psychology, 49,* 156–166. http://dx.doi.org/10.1037/0090-5550.49.2.156

Hibbard, M. R., & Cox, D. R. (2010). Competencies of a rehabilitation psychologist. In R. G. Frank, M. Rosenthal, & B. Caplan (Eds.), *Handbook of rehabilitation psychology* (2nd ed., pp. 467–475). Washington, DC: American Psychological Association. http://dx.doi.org/10.1037/15972-034

Improving Access to Assistive Technology for Individuals With Disabilities Act of 2004, Pub. L. No. 108-364, 118 Stat. 1707 (2004).

Individuals With Disabilities Education Act[0] of 1990, Pub. L. 101-476, 104 Stat. 1142 (1990).

Kalpakjian, C. Z., McCullumsmith, C. B., Fann, J. R., Richards, J. S., Stoelb, B. L., Heinemann, A. W., & Bombardier, C. H. (2014). Post-traumatic growth following spinal cord injury. *Journal of Spinal Cord Medicine, 37,* 218–225. http://dx.doi.org/10.1179/2045772313Y.0000000169

Karol, R. L., & Sturm, L. (2017). Models of consultation. In M. A. Budd, S. Hough, S. T. Wegener, & W. Stiers (Eds.), *Practical psychology in medical rehabilitation* (pp. 473–482). Cham, Switzerland: Springer. http://dx.doi.org/10.1007/978-3-319-34034-0_52

Katon, W. J., Lin, E. H. B., Von Korff, M., Ciechanowski, P., Ludman, E. J., Young, B., . . . McCulloch, D. (2010). Collaborative care for patients with depression and chronic illnesses. *The New England Journal of Medicine, 363,* 2611–2620. http://dx.doi.org/10.1056/NEJMoa1003955

Kortte, K. B., Falk, L. D., Castillo, R. C., Johnson-Greene, D., & Wegener, S. T. (2007). The Hopkins Rehabilitation Engagement Rating Scale: Development and psychometric properties. *Archives of Physical Medicine and Rehabilitation, 88,* 877–884. http://dx.doi.org/10.1016/j.apmr.2007.03.030

Kortte, K. B., & Hillis, A. E. (2011). Recent trends in rehabilitation interventions for visual neglect and anosognosia for hemiplegia following right hemisphere stroke. *Future Neurology, 6,* 33–43. http://dx.doi.org/10.2217/fnl.10.79

Kortte, K. B., Stevenson, J. E., Hosey, M. M., Castillo, R., & Wegener, S. T. (2012). Hope predicts positive functional role outcomes in acute rehabilitation populations. *Rehabilitation Psychology, 57,* 248–255. http://dx.doi.org/10.1037/a0029004

Kortte, K. B., Veiel, L., Batten, S. V., & Wegener, S. T. (2009). Measuring avoidance in medical rehabilitation. *Rehabilitation Psychology, 54,* 91–98. http://dx.doi.org/10.1037/a0014703

Langer, K. G. (1995). Depression and physical disability: Relationship of self-rated and observer-rated disability to depression. *Neuropsychiatry, Neuropsychology, & Behavioral Neurology, 8,* 271–276.

Langer, K. G. (1999a). Awareness and denial in psychotherapy. In K. G. Langer, L. Laatsch, & L. Lewis (Eds.), *Psychotherapeutic interventions for adults with brain injury or stroke: A clinician's treatment resource* (pp. 75–96). Madison, CT: Psychosocial Press.

Langer, K. G. (1999b). Depression and denial in psychotherapy of persons with disabilities. In R. Marinelli & A. Dell Orto (Eds.), *The psychological and social impact of disability* (pp. 316–328). New York, NY: Springer.

Langer, K. G. (2017). Psychological rehabilitation therapies. In *Reference module in neuroscience and biobehavioral psychology*. Elsevier. http://dx.doi.org/10.1016/B978-0-12-809324-5.05682-0

Langer, K. G., & Padrone, F. J. (1992). Psychotherapeutic treatment of awareness in acute rehabilitation of traumatic brain injury. *Neuropsychological Rehabilitation, 2,* 59–70. http://dx.doi.org/10.1080/09602019208401395

Lisa, L. P., Jughters, A., & Kerckhofs, E. (2013). The effectiveness of different treatment modalities for the rehabilitation of unilateral neglect in stroke patients: A systematic review. *NeuroRehabilitation*, *33*, 611–620.

Lu, W., Krellman, J. W., & Dijkers, M. P. (2016). Can cognitive behavioral therapy for insomnia also treat fatigue, pain, and mood symptoms in individuals with traumatic brain injury? A multiple case report. *NeuroRehabilitation, 38,* 59–69. http://dx.doi.org/10.3233/NRE-151296

New York Secure Ammunition and Firearms Enforcement Act, S. 2230, A. 2388, LBD12007-03-03 (January 15, 2013).

Parkes, C. M. (1972). Components of the reaction to loss of a limb, spouse or home. *Journal of Psychosomatic Research, 16,* 343–349. http://dx.doi.org/10.1016/0022-3999(72)90087-6

Pledger, C. (2003). Discourse on disability and rehabilitation issues. Opportunities for psychology. *American Psychologist*, *58*, 279–284. http://dx.doi.org/10.1037/0003-066X.58.4.279

Rath, J. F., Bertisch, H., & Elliott, T. R. (2017). Psychologists specializing in rehabilitation psychology. In R. Sternberg (Ed.), *Career paths in psychology: Where your degree can take you* (3rd ed., pp. 227–243). Washington, DC: American Psychological Association. http://dx.doi.org/10.1037/15960-015

Rath, J. F., & Elliott, T. R. (2012). Psychological models in rehabilitation psychology. In P. Kennedy (Ed.), *Oxford handbook of rehabilitation psychology* (pp. 32–46). New York, NY: Oxford University Press.

Ross, E. D. (1981). The aprosodias: Functional-anatomic organization of the affective components of language in the right hemisphere. *Archives of Neurology, 38,* 561–569. http://dx.doi.org/10.1001/archneur.1981.00510090055006

Russell, H. F., Richardson, E. J., Bombardier, C. H., Dixon, T. M., Huston, T. A., Rose, J., . . . Ullrich, P. M. (2016). Professional standards of practice for psychologists, social workers, and counselors in SCI rehabilitation. *Journal of Spinal Cord Medicine, 39,* 127–145. http://dx.doi.org/10.1080/10790268.2015.1119966

Schover, L. R., & Jensen, S. B. (1988). *Sexuality and chronic illness: A comprehensive approach.* New York, NY: Guilford Press.

Siegert, R. J., & Abernethy, D. A. (2005). Depression in multiple sclerosis: A review. *Journal of Neurology, Neurosurgery, & Psychiatry, 76,* 469–475. http://dx.doi.org/10.1136/jnnp.2004.054635

Stiers, W., Barisa, M., Stucky, K., Pawlowski, C., Van Tubbergen, M., Turner, A. P., . . . Caplan, B. (2015). Guidelines for competency development and measurement in rehabilitation psychology postdoctoral training. *Rehabilitation Psychology, 60,* 111–122. http://dx.doi.org/10.1037/a0038353

Stiers, W., Hanson, S., Turner, A. P., Stucky, K., Barisa, M., Brownsberger, M., . . . Kuemmel, A., & the Council of Rehabilitation Psychology Postdoctoral Training Programs. (2012). Guidelines for postdoctoral training in rehabilitation psychology. *Rehabilitation Psychology, 57,* 267–279. http://dx.doi.org/10.1037/a0030774

Stiers, W., & the Rehabilitation Psychology Synarchy. (2015). *Rehabilitation psychology petition for recognition of specialty in professional psychology.* Washington, DC: Commission for the Recognition of Specialties and Proficiencies in Professional Psychology (CRSPPP), American Psychological Association.

Warren, A. M., Stucky, K., & Sherman, J. J. (2013). Rehabilitation psychology's role in the Level I trauma center. *The Journal of Trauma and Acute Care Surgery*, *74*, 1357–1362.

Weinberg, J., Diller, L., Gordon, W. A., Gerstman, L. J., Lieberman, A., Lakin, P., . . . Ezrachi, O. (1977). Visual scanning training effect on reading-related tasks in acquired right brain damage. *Archives of Physical Medicine and Rehabilitation, 58,* 479–486.

Williams, J. L., & Pilarski, C. (2014, July). Disability-affirming considerations for professional meetings. *Spotlight on Disability Newsletter*. Office on Disability Issues in Psychology, American Psychological Association. Retrieved from http://www.apa.org/pi/disability/resources/publications/newsletter/2014/07/affirming-considerations.aspx

Wilson, B. A. (2008). Neuropsychological rehabilitation. *Annual Review of Clinical Psychology*, *4*, 141–162. http://dx.doi.org/10.1146/annurev.clinpsy.4.022007.141212

World Health Organization. (2001). *ICF: International classification of functioning, disability and health.* Geneva, Switzerland: Author.

Wright, B. A. (1972). Value-laden beliefs and principles for rehabilitation psychology. *Rehabilitation Psychology, 19,* 38–45. http://dx.doi.org/10.1037/h0090869

Wright, B. A. (1983). *Physical disability: A psychosocial approach.* New York, NY: Harper Collins. http://dx.doi.org/10.1037/10589-000

CHAPTER 7

APPLIED ETHICS

Thomas R. Kerkhoff and Stephanie L. Hanson

The fact that the American health care system is headed toward unsustainability at high cost that is nevertheless associated with variable quality and access has long been recognized (Centers for Disease Control and Prevention, 2013; Cheak-Zamora, Reid-Arndt, Hagglund, & Frank, 2012; Institute of Medicine [IOM], 2013; Keenan, 2014; Schoen et al., 2010). In addition, the health care system remains underprepared to serve people with disabilities (PWDs), among other underrepresented populations, as evidenced by a higher incidence of chronic health conditions and poorer health outcomes compared with people who do not have disabilities (Association of University Centers on Disabilities, 2016; Zack, 2013). The "future health system must reduce the burden of illness, injury, and disability, thereby enhancing the health status, functionality, and satisfaction of the U.S. population" (Fineberg, 2003, p. xi). This comment, made over a decade ago, is still relevant today.

Health care reform must improve on professionals' ability to deliver high-quality care to diverse groups of citizens, such as those served by rehabilitation psychologists, in a cost-effective manner. It also challenges the various health professions to consider how best to integrate their expertise into revised delivery systems and to prepare professionals in training for the changing health care landscape in a competent, ethical manner. As transformative change occurs in the structure and delivery of health care, so too do the challenges and opportunities for psychologists to guide and maintain competent, ethical practice.

In this chapter, we briefly describe health care reform under the Patient Protection and Affordable Care Act of 2010 to understand the backdrop of multiple ethics training and practice issues. We then present a summary of recent work in the psychology competency movement and the conceptualization of ethics within it. This is followed by a detailed presentation of ethics competency training and development in rehabilitation psychology. We also comment on current ethics issues delineated by the American Psychological Association (APA) and conclude the chapter with brief recommendations for training and practice.

HEALTH CARE REFORM

The IOM (2001) identified six aims for health care reform, all of which are intricately connected with the ethical principles embraced by APA's (2017) *Ethical Principles of Psychologists and Code of Conduct* (hereinafter APA Ethics Code), as shown in Table 7.1. All of these aims and knowledge about chronic care have been embodied in the activities leading to the adoption of the ACA, which was signed into law by then-President Obama in March 2010. The hope behind this legislation was that comprehensive health reform would help control the

http://dx.doi.org/10.1037/0000129-008
Handbook of Rehabilitation Psychology, *Third Edition*, L. A. Brenner, S. A. Reid-Arndt, T. R. Elliott, R. G. Frank, and B. Caplan (Editors-in-Chief)

TABLE 7.1

Alignment Between the Aims of Health Care Reform and the American Psychological Association (APA) *Ethical Principles of Psychologists and Code of Conduct*

Aim of an improved health care system	Definition	APA principles
Safe	▪ Avoid harm intended to help	▪ Beneficence and nonmaleficence
Effective	▪ Care based on science ▪ Avoid care that is unnecessary or overused	▪ Beneficence and nonmaleficence
Patient centered	▪ Care driven by the patient's values and preferences	▪ Respect for people's rights and dignity ▪ Fidelity and responsibility
Timely	▪ Minimize wait times and harmful delays for both provider and patient	▪ Beneficence and nonmaleficence
Efficient	▪ Avoid waste	▪ Justice ▪ Beneficence and nonmaleficence
Equitable	▪ Personal characteristics do not define quality received	▪ Justice

rate of growth in health care costs while improving access, efficiency, and quality, ultimately resulting in better health outcomes (for a review of the ACA, please see Kaiser Family Foundation, 2013, and Pozgar, 2014).

Several key provisions of the ACA directly affect behavioral health care and reflect stronger ethical mandates for access to services for America's citizens (i.e., social justice). The ACA provisions, as originally authorized, hold promise for populations served by rehabilitation psychologists (e.g., removal of both lifetime caps and denial of coverage based on preexisting conditions) and for general rehabilitation psychology practice, by devising incentives aimed toward team-based care. However, several areas that hold promise, such as coverage for persons with preexisting conditions, which can encompass acquired disabilities, are being challenged in the evolving health care reform debate. Although rehabilitation psychologists are well trained to lead in health care systems' emphasis on care in which patients and families are integrated into team-based decision making and treatment, like other providers, they must develop the integrated systems literacy necessary to advocate for appropriate leadership roles that influence policy and reimbursement (Nordal, 2012). They must also ensure that the training programs prepare students to become competent providers within the shifting sands of health care, as required by the APA Ethics Code. Health care reform clearly has the ability to shape the competencies all psychologists need in clinical practice.

COMPETENCE AND ETHICS

As overarching health care models have shifted, so too has the emphasis on the development of competence increased. This change in direction has occurred within and across health professions, influencing both individual (Hanson & Kerkhoff, 2012; IOM (US) Committee on the Health Professions Education Summit, 2003) and community- and population-focused training (Association of University Centers on Disabilities, 2016) based on the same underlying premise that competency training will improve service quality and ultimately influence health outcomes. For example, in 2003 the IOM identified five overlapping competencies all health practitioners should possess:

1. The ability to deliver patient-centered care, taking into account an increasingly diverse US population with varying cultural backgrounds, expectations, and values.

2. The ability to work in interdisciplinary teams and practice team-based skills, especially for patients with chronic conditions.
3. The training and ability to search and evaluate the scientific evidence base upon which health care decisions should be made in practice.
4. The knowledge and ability to analyze the root causes of medical errors and quality problems and fix them through system-wide approaches.
5. A solid foundation and skills in using cutting-edge information technology to deliver high-quality medical care, such as being able to search the medical literature online or being able to use computerized order entry systems that automatically flag pharmaceutical contraindications and errors. (Eastman, 2003, p. 75)

Similar to the aims of health care reform, these competencies generally align with the APA Ethical Principles shown in Table 7.2.

As part of its conceptualization of competence, IOM recognized that, although knowledge and application change as an individual moves from novice to expert, the fundamentals of competence do not shift significantly. IOM also recognized that assessment would be necessary if competency modeling were to be successfully incorporated into training. These themes would be echoed again as the psychology discipline began to grapple with how to more specifically define competence components and consider their implications for psychology training and practice.

FOUNDATIONAL AND FUNCTIONAL COMPETENCIES

Although different models incorporating ethics have been promulgated in the literature (see, e.g., Peterson, Peterson, Abrams, Stricker, & Ducheny, 2010), the three-dimensional model Rodolfa et al. (2005) proposed—the orthogonal cube model—remains the primary model underpinning psychology's efforts to operationalize professional competence (see Chapter 1, this volume). Because of the model's significance, we briefly review it here along with its ethics components

TABLE 7.2

Institute of Medicine Competencies and the American Psychological Association (APA) *Ethical Principles of Psychologists and Code of Conduct*

Institute of Medicine core competency	Component examples	Relevant APA principles
Provide patient-centered care	▪ Respect patients' preferences ▪ Share decision making ▪ Advocate prevention and wellness	▪ Respect for people's rights and dignity ▪ Beneficence and nonmaleficence
Work in interdisciplinary teams	▪ Communicate and integrate care in teams ▪ Ensure care is reliable	▪ Fidelity and responsibility ▪ Beneficence and nonmaleficence ▪ Integrity
Engage in evidence-based practice	▪ Use scientist–practitioner model to optimize care ▪ Participate in learning and research	▪ Beneficence and nonmaleficence ▪ Fidelity and responsibility
Apply quality improvement	▪ Identify errors and use safety design ▪ Measure quality of care at the individual and community levels ▪ Assess systems of care	▪ Beneficence and nonmaleficence
Use informatics	▪ Communicate and manage knowledge ▪ Mitigate error ▪ Support decision making	▪ Beneficence and nonmaleficence ▪ Integrity

and its influence on the development of competency benchmarks.

The orthogonal cube model is a continuation of work done at the 2002 Association of Psychology Postdoctoral and Internship Centers Competencies Conference, at which several themes about competence emerged (e.g., competencies include knowledge, skills, and attitudes; cross-cutting competencies exist across developmental levels; competencies should reflect evidence-based practice). The three dimensions of the cube reflect these themes and include foundational competencies, functional competencies, and developmental stages of professional development.

Foundational competencies are meant to represent the core knowledge, skills, and attitudes all psychologists need. They lay the groundwork (i.e., the foundation) for functional skill development. Ethical and legal precepts are included as a foundational competency, defined as the "application of ethical concepts and awareness of legal issues regarding professional activities with individuals, groups and organizations advocating for the profession" (Rodolfa et al., 2005, p. 351). As such, one can imagine this competency can be broadly applied in psychology practice. However, we argue later that conceptualizing ethics solely as a foundational competency falls short in our ability to prepare psychologists in training for competent everyday ethical practice.

The second dimension, *functional competencies*, focuses more on what psychologists do or how they engage their knowledge, skills, and attitudes in everyday activities (e.g., intervention, consultation).

The third dimension, *developmental stages of professional development*, represents a psychologist's progression in overall competence development from student and intern to postdoctoral fellow and practicing psychologist. Although Rodolfa et al. (2005) recognized different domains of practice—general practice relevant to all psychologists, domains of a specific practice area (e.g., clinical psychologist), and domains unique to specialty practice (e.g., rehabilitation psychology, neuropsychology)—the fundamental components of the cube remain unchanged across domains. That said, the cube components are interconnected and thus influence one other. Changes to scope of practice, for example, would be represented in the foundational competencies, which would then influence the functional competencies. New settings and populations would alter the contingencies of one's competence, such that an individual might require new skill development relevant to the maintenance of ethical practice in these novel circumstances. What Rodolfa et al. described as these parameters of practice—populations served, settings, problems addressed, and theoretical orientations—would define specialty competencies.

ETHICS AS A FOUNDATIONAL COMPETENCY

The orthogonal cube model became a driver for subsequent discussion regarding competency development and application in psychology. The APA Task Force on the Assessment of Competence in Professional Psychology (2006) extended Rodolfa et al.'s (2005) framework and delineated criteria (i.e., essential elements) and behavioral anchors characterizing the subcomponents of each competency across three levels of training: (a) readiness for practicum, (b) internship, and (c) entry-level practice. The 15 competencies originally identified by Rodolfa et al. were reorganized in 2012 by Hatcher et al. (2013) into six benchmark clusters, although the conceptualization of foundational and functional competencies across developmental levels remained in the overarching model. The Hatcher et al. (2013) work group developed assessment tools, including rating scales, to address concerns that the original benchmarking document was too cumbersome and difficult to include, creating a significant barrier to transforming to a culture of competence.

The Ethical, Legal Standards, and Policy competency is included as part of the Professionalism cluster. The other foundational clusters are Relational and Science, and the functional clusters are Application (e.g., evidence-based practice, consultation), Education, and Systems (Hatcher et al., 2013). The essential elements of the ethics competency are (a) knowledge of "ethical, legal, and professional standards and guidelines"; (b) "awareness and application of ethical decision making"; and (c) ethical conduct (Kaslow et al., 2009, p. S32). So, for example, displaying ethical attitudes and values demonstrates ethical conduct of a student ready to enter practicum, integrating moral principles and values into conduct demonstrates conduct of a student ready for internship, and independently integrating ethical and legal standards with all competencies demonstrates readiness for practice entry. We provide examples to further delineate the skills needed within each level to aid in rating a student's subcomponent performance. For example, readiness for practicum within the ethics component includes a desire to help others, showing honesty and integrity, and appropriate boundary management. This example seems to parse elements of the APA Ethics Code that already have an overall organizational structure within that code. We have argued for an alternative approach to ethics competence in which the APA Ethics Code itself is used to define and assess competency. This approach recognizes the fact that the code is field driven, incorporating the breadth of practice that is useful and adaptive over time, both of which are critical to creating a culture in which education and training are competency based (Hanson & Kerkhoff, 2011). Table 7.3 illustrates how the principles of the APA Ethics Code can be aligned with behavioral anchors from which to create a developmental framework and appropriate measurement tools for competency goal attainment. (See Hatcher et al., 2013; Kaslow et al., 2009; and Stiers et al., 2015, for examples of potential measurement tools.)

TABLE 7.3

American Psychological Association *Ethical Principles of Psychologists and Code of Conduct* and Behavioral Anchors for Foundational Competencies

Principles	Behavioral anchors
Beneficence and nonmaleficence: Benefit persons served and do no harm	▪ Safeguard welfare and rights ▪ Actively resolve conflicts ▪ Avoid misuse of professional and authoritative influence ▪ Demonstrate self-awareness of physical and mental health
Fidelity and responsibility: Establish relationships of trust with persons served and colleagues	▪ Fulfill professional and scientific societal responsibilities ▪ Uphold professional and social conduct ▪ Engage in frequent, active consultation ▪ Demonstrate proactive concern with ethical compliance of colleagues ▪ Provide pro bono services as circumstances warrant
Integrity: Promotion of accuracy, honesty, and trustworthiness in all professional activities	▪ Adhere to strict prohibitions against stealing, cheating, fraud, subterfuge, and intentional misrepresentation ▪ Keep professional promises ▪ Avoid unwise or unclear commitments ▪ Give careful consideration to potential consequences of scientifically justified deception ▪ Maintain familiarity with current literature
Justice: Provision of equal access to needed resources, while ensuring high quality in services, procedures, and processes delivered	▪ Demonstrate assurance that potential biases, boundaries of competence and expertise limitations do not condone unjust practices ▪ Demonstrate equitably distributed services, procedures and processes regarding individuals and organizations with which one may be affiliated ▪ Consistently develop and upgrade practice and scientific competencies to match the needs of the populations served
Respect for people's rights and dignity: Emphasis on individual rights to privacy, self-determination, and confidentiality	▪ Safeguard persons whose vulnerabilities may impair autonomous decision making and achievement and maintenance of satisfactory personal independence ▪ Demonstrate awareness of and respect for cultural, individual, and role differences while addressing personal biases or prejudices

REHABILITATION ETHICS AND SOCIETY

Both the health care reform and competency movements have had a substantial impact on the direction of leadership efforts in rehabilitation psychology. In the past decade, competencies have been promulgated for postdoctoral training (Stiers et al., 2015, 2012) and board certification (American Board of Professional Psychology/American Board of Rehabilitation Psychology, 2018; Cox, Cox, & Caplan, 2013; Hibbard & Cox, 2010), both based fundamentally upon foundational and functional competencies. We have also demonstrated in some detail the use of the APA Ethics Code as a foundational competency within a developmental framework for rehabilitation psychology (Hanson & Kerkhoff, 2011). These activities foster discussion around how we, as rehabilitation psychologists, define not only what we do or should do and the skills we need to do them, but also who we are as a specialty. As the Health Service Psychology Education Collaborative (2013) noted in its recommendations regarding education and training, "the competencies demonstrated by these graduates serve to identify them as health professionals whose distinctive contributions to health care are recognized and respected by other health professions, policymakers, and the public" (p. 411). The changing health care landscape forces rehabilitation psychologists to clarify our identity within the field of practice as reflected in how we define our core competencies as well as our professional expertise that uniquely contributes to the broader health care system. This represents an obligation fundamentally borne out of the APA Ethics Code, specifically the Principle of Fidelity and Responsibility, which, for rehabilitation psychologists, clearly includes professional responsibilities not only to our membership in APA and patients but also to society as a whole. We must grapple with how to appropriately advocate for both our patients and our profession in this new health care environment, consistent with our ethics framework.

Advocacy, one of the defining competencies of rehabilitation psychology (Cox et al., 2013), relates directly to ethical practice and requires that practitioners go beyond traditional individual evaluation and treatment paradigms (Dunn, 2015). Dunn (2015) asserted that advocacy on behalf of PWDs offers rehabilitation psychologists the opportunity to focus adaptive efforts toward reinforcing societal rights and responsibilities (respect for people's rights and dignity, justice, and beneficence), along with influencing social policy regarding disability (responsibility). Dunn reminded us that this approach in "adjustment to disability" extends beyond the individual PWD, arguing for "societal change at all levels (e.g., laws, culture, politics, accessibility)" (p. 134). Thus, the narrow vision of clinical practice, focusing predominantly on the PWD, minimizes the broader social–societal context in which the operational parameters of disability and the culture of disability are defined and play out (Kerkhoff & Hanson, 2015b). The ethical and professional responsibility incumbent on rehabilitation psychologists to meet their obligations as competent service providers is to broaden the scope of practice to include and value changing social–societal structures (e.g., physical barriers, policies, laws, regulations, health care agency procedures) that must adopt adaptive views of disability in order to offer equitable access to the goods of life that individuals without disabilities enjoy. Obviously, this requires a goal of reaching beyond the health care setting and into the community to effect change. Offering educational guidance, program and policy development consultancy, and expert testimony to the legislative process are some of the ways that we meet our ethical obligations in a larger societal context. These actions can also have the secondary effect of establishing the field's identity as a valued specialty within the broad system of psychological care.

From a practical perspective, in considering the normative moral responses to societal change, health care professionals are obligated to be aware of, adhere to, and be competent with regard to, ethical and legal prescriptions related to practice. The APA Ethics Code is a driver for ethical practice, and understanding and applying it is considered a core part of the ethical and legal competency issues in rehabilitation psychology advanced practice (Cox et al., 2013). Similarly, rehabilitation psychologists should have a "fundamental awareness of the significant laws that affect their practice and/or people whom they serve" as part of this ethical specialty core (Cox et al., 2013, p. 25). The American Board of Professional Psychology/American Board of Rehabilitation Psychology (2018) explicitly requires that rehabilitation psychologists have knowledge of and apply both the APA Ethics Code and relevant laws and standards of care in professional practice. Cox et al. (2013) provided a list of important federal legislative action directly relevant to rehabilitation psychology. Another important resource is the *Guide to Disability Rights Laws* (U.S. Department of Justice, 2009). Federal statutes and regulations detail obligations related to equitable allocation of health care resources as well as recognition of accommodations due PWDs (see U.S. Department of Justice, 2011).

Awareness of relevant state statutes is also essential. State statutes delimit the boundaries of practice for all health care disciplines. Classic ethics case scenarios reflect moral thinking about challenging social–ethical situations and recommend resolutions to those challenges that typically, but not always, square with legal mandates (Beauchamp & Childress, 2012). Independent of partisan political motivations underlying the statutory process, the variability of state statutes can then impact health care practice and cause confusion in this era of social hypermobility, with practitioners maintaining multiple practice residences and electronic practice at a distance. Consistent with the APA Ethics Code, these types of challenges require that health care providers be intricately knowledgeable about practice boundaries issues, such as geographic conundrums created by patients traveling long distances for inpatient rehabilitation who require subsequent follow-up (see APA, 2013, and Ragusea, 2012, for a discussion of ethical issues in telehealth). Fortunately, the Association of State and Provincial Psychology Boards (2018) made significant inroads into creating an E.Passport to allow telehealth across state lines. There has been even more progress within the Department of Veteran Affairs, which amended its rules in May 2018 (effective date June 11, 2018) to authorize telehealth across all states for its licensed health care providers. As noted in the *Federal Register*, this rule "ensures that all beneficiaries, specifically including beneficiaries in remote, rural, or medically underserved areas, have the greatest possible access to mental health care, specialty care, and general clinical care" ("Authority of Health Care," p. 3).

CHANGING THE TRAINING MODEL: ETHICS-GUIDED PRACTICE

Ethical–legal conflicts presented as high valence but often low incidence case examples have been a common focal point of applied ethics education in psychology as well as many other health care disciplines (e.g., Beauchamp & Childress, 2012; Hanson, Kerkhoff, & Bush, 2005; Kerkhoff & Hanson, 2013; Pozgar, 2016; Steinbock, Arras, & London, 2013; Vaughn, 2008). This level of case analysis has been introduced and episodically reinforced in the processes of critical philosophical discourse and ethical thinking. This traditional approach to ethics training has inestimable merit as a foundational basis for educating future health care professionals about ethical principles and standards, legal issues, critical thinking, and systematic decision-making schemata, as well as historical factors affecting the current ethical–legal professional health care practice interface. The traditional approach provides a structure on which to build adaptive moral professional behavior, in particular during graduate school. However, a notable limitation to this approach is that it continues to be a primary instructional model beyond graduate professional training, when the incidence of ethical–legal conflicts and dilemmas in independent professional practice is low. In addition, psychologists entering practice should already have acquired competence in understanding the ethical principles and standards these cases attempt to illustrate.

One result of the above instructional model is that health care providers use ethical–legal resources primarily for targeted events (e.g., licensure examination, specialty board examinations, legal testimony, professional presentations and publications, hot-button cases). In between those episodic performance events, the ethical resources are often relegated to office reference shelves. We contend that a transformation in ethics and medico–legal issues' education needs to occur at the very least by the time advanced applied clinical training begins in earnest. At that juncture (residency and continuing professional education), ethical principles should be intentionally and mindfully interleaved with every professional activity in which the psychology professional routinely engages. In this manner, ethics can be transferred to the desktop for daily use.

As we opined in a commentary (Kerkhoff & Hanson, 2015a, in response to Stiers et al., 2015), continuing to relegate ethics principles solely to foundational competencies, or considering them exclusively as having aspirational status, forfeits an opportunity to actively weave ethics into daily practice activities. They eventually become assumptions in the process of applying clinical skills to the real-life challenges of practice. Categorizing ethics principles solely as foundational competencies further distances these vital practice guidelines from functional ethical competency adoption.

Similar to other authors, for the past 15 years we and our colleagues have focused on refining a formal ethical decision-making model through classic case examples illustrating ethical conflicts and dilemmas (Hanson et al., 2005; Kerkhoff & Hanson, 2013). However, more recently (Hanson & Kerkhoff, 2011; Kerkhoff, 2015), we have begun to investigate the competency training process for applied ethics in everyday practice and moved away from dramatic low incidence ethics case conflicts and dilemmas, which the average rehabilitation psychologist may encounter only once or twice in her or his career. We have moved toward using more routine case examples that comprise daily practice as the environment in which to operationalize the ethical decision-making process. Until we, as a profession, routinely exercise the use of ethics principles and standards as part and parcel of everyday practice, we weaken the practical conceptual linkage between ethics and all other aspects of our professional services.

Developing the habit of intentionally incorporating ethics principles into active functional competency guidelines in the course of daily clinical decision making, active evaluation, case conceptualization and treatment planning, and intervention promotes a preventative perspective regarding applied ethics that has typically not been considered in traditional ethics training. We refer to this ethics educational approach as *ethics-guided practice* (Kerkhoff, 2015).

POSTDOCTORAL FOUNDATIONAL AND FUNCTIONAL COMPETENCIES

Tables 7.4 and 7.5 illustrate how this reconceptualization of ethics training can be framed with the competency model for rehabilitation psychology training. In Table 7.4, we offer a melding of ethics principles into the postgraduate rehabilitation psychology program training guidelines presented by Stiers et al. (2015). This is followed in Table 7.5 by an explication of ethical actions associated with case progression. Using these same foundational and functional ethics competencies, ingrained into the daily practice habits of the budding professional, helps licensed rehabilitation psychologists traverse the gulf between the supervised structure of training programs and establishing a career as an ethical independent practitioner and ultimately as a board-certified specialist in rehabilitation psychology. In essence, the conceptual model becomes grounded in routine practice and becomes part of the building blocks for the professional moral identity of the individual.

ETHICS DECISION MAKING

Although formal decision-making models lend themselves to structured ethics committee or rehabilitation team deliberations and ethical analysis, they are cumbersome for individual clinicians to use in the course of everyday practice. Individual practitioners typically move from identifying a critical ethical incident to searching for a resolution, bypassing the incremental investigative steps of the conceptual decision-making process. Instead of using this valuable but complex method of ethical analysis, and to complement our reconceptualization of ethics training, we have opted to incorporate ethical principles into every step of the clinical case analysis process (operationalized in standards of care/treatment) from the initial contact, interview and evaluation through assessment, treatment, and discharge planning. The clinician or trainee is tasked with intentionally and mindfully identifying the ethics

TABLE 7.4

American Psychological Association (APA) *Ethical Principles of Psychologists and Code of Conduct* Embedded in Rehabilitation Psychology Postdoctoral Training Competencies

Knowledge	Skills/abilities	Attitudes/values
1. Guidelines for Competencies and Structured Observation in Assessment and Intervention		
Demonstrate awareness and application of the APA Ethical Principles underlying all assessment and intervention modalities. Demonstrate understanding of implications of limited test validity and norms for populations served.	Operationalize the APA Ethical Principles and relevant standards in provision of varied assessment and intervention services. Weigh relative choices consistent with professional values and standards.	Actively acknowledge APA Ethical Principles as providing guidance in honoring the personal preferences of persons served, advocacy for personal choice in decision making, and self-awareness of strengths and limitations in practitioners.
2. Guidelines for Competencies and Structured Observation in Consultation		
Demonstrate knowledge of Ethical Principles underlying team functioning. Demonstrate an understanding of how to facilitate ethical decision making among team members.	Actively use Ethical Principles to guide strategic and tactical consultation efforts, anticipating potential conflicts of interest and focusing on facilitation of team decision making.	Advocate for recognition of Ethical Principles guiding team efforts in the following areas: owning personal responsibility, facilitating positive team function, respecting boundaries of competence, seeking feedback from colleagues, acknowledging and rectifying errors, maintaining composure during difficult interactions, and respecting diversity and differing perspectives.
3. Guidelines for Competencies and Structured Observation in Research and Evaluation		
Demonstrate knowledge of interpersonal relationships among ethical, legal, and regulatory standards for conducting research.	Achieve certification in and use research ethics standards established by the National Institutes of Health and other relevant oversight agencies in the design and implementation of research programs. Reconcile the above standards with the APA Ethics Code regarding research. Implement appropriate accommodations for persons with disabilities for research participation.	Demonstrate the importance of informed consent and ethical treatment of research participants; identify and describe values related to deception in research.

(*continues*)

TABLE 7.4

American Psychological Association (APA) *Ethical Principles of Psychologists and Code of Conduct* Embedded in Rehabilitation Psychology Postdoctoral Training Competencies (*Continued*)

Knowledge	Skills/abilities	Attitudes/values
4. Guidelines for Competencies and Structured Observation in Teaching and Supervision		
Demonstrate knowledge of ethics, guidelines, standards, and laws pertaining to teaching and supervisory relationships and methods. Demonstrate and explain Ethical Principles underpinning methods of teaching and supervision, evaluation of teaching and supervision effectiveness, and development of policies related to teaching and supervision.	Demonstrate and explain Ethical Principles underpinning methods of teaching and supervision, evaluation of teaching, and supervision effectiveness and development of policies related to teaching and supervision.	Advocate for incorporation of Ethical Principles in crafting teaching and supervision standards, methods, evaluation processes, and ongoing conduct of these professional activities.
5. Guidelines for Competencies and Structured Observation in Administration and Leadership		
Demonstrate knowledge of Ethical Principles, guidelines, standards, regulations and laws in rehabilitation, including informed consent and issues relating to patient confidentiality, privacy, and care access.	Demonstrate ethical guidance in decision making regarding matters of daily clinical operations; management team consultation; financial reimbursement processes; cost-effective service provision; resource allocation; quality assurance and improvement; treatment goal achievement parameters and treatment termination criteria; identifying, evaluating, and rectifying root causes of critical incidents; and in development and implementation of policies and procedures.	Advocate for utilization of health care organizational ethics in all matters of administration and management within the organization and in all interactions with the community in which the organization is nested.
6. Guidelines for Competencies and Structured Observation in Additional Areas		
Demonstrate knowledge of Ethical Principles and standards, including how they may be applied in everyday professional activities.	Demonstrate active use of ethics principles in professional comportment and behavior; seeking consultation in matters of ethical compliance and conflicts regarding regulatory and legal adherence; advocating for persons with disabilities; applying varied published APA practice standards and guidelines; applying federal statutes regarding disability; and seeking out and developing state and local resources for persons with disabilities, including caring for one's physical and mental health.	Demonstrate the ethics foundations of self-identification with the specialty of rehabilitation psychology, exemplified in emphasis on the worth of persons with disabilities and disability culture and respect for other aspects of diversity across individuals and populations.

Note. Adapted from "Guidelines for Competency Development and Measurement in Rehabilitation Psychology Postdoctoral Training," by W. Stiers, M. Barisa, K. Stucky, C. Pawlowski, M. Van Tubbergen, A. P. Turner, . . . B. Caplan, 2015, *Rehabilitation Psychology*, *60*, pp. 111–122; and "Applied Ethics: Have We Lost a Crucial Opportunity?," by T. R. Kerkhoff and S. L. Hanson, 2015, *Rehabilitation Psychology*, *60*, pp. 376–378. Copyright 2015 by American Psychological Association. See also Weber (2001) and Pozgar (2016, pp. 255–298).

TABLE 7.5

Clinical Evaluation and Treatment: Underlying Functional Competencies and Skills in the American Psychological Association *Ethical Principles of Psychologists and Code of Conduct*

Functional skills and stages	Functional competencies
Beneficence and Nonmaleficence	
Initial interview/ evaluation	Introduce the person with disability (PWD) to the rehabilitation process, and what to expect, in appropriate language. Ensure that the PWD's welfare is safeguarded and varied rights and responsibilities within the health care environment are explained and protected. Ensure that all rehabilitation psychology practices adhere to and comply with federal and state statutes and regulations, as well as health care organization policies and procedures.
Assessment	Be knowledgeable of and using current evidence-based assessment methodologies appropriate to the PWD's health condition. Identify benefits and limitations of tools selected and the resulting information and determining the PWD's understanding of these.
Treatment planning	Ensure that rehabilitation psychology and other team planned interventions are intentionally designed to benefit the PWD within her or his personal, health, family and social support system, and community environmental contexts. Ensure attention to risk reduction regarding the PWD's health, lifestyle, emotional, behavioral, cognitive, educational, vocational, and social contexts.
Intervention	Coordinate rehabilitation psychology services with other team treatment services to facilitate enhanced health, functional performance, welfare, and safety of the PWD. Ensure that risk reduction has been demonstrated as a treatment outcome metric.
Discharge planning	Demonstrate how treatment outcome goals are met. Understand whether functional status meets self- and/or assisted care capacity, consistent with a safe return to the community. Incorporate plans to minimize risk on return to the community.
Fidelity and Responsibility	
Initial interview/ evaluation	Establish the parameters of the working relationship between the rehabilitation psychologist and rehabilitation team and the PWD. Identify barriers to building rapport. Engage in consultative discussions with team members and other health care practitioners as required by the needs of the PWD. Ensure the PWD's understanding of the roles and responsibilities of a rehabilitation psychologist and other associated team members.
Assessment	Resolve potential conflicts among team members regarding who assesses what. Establish the PWD's understanding of the uses of resulting data for treatment planning in the team treatment milieu. Provide the PWD with feedback and ensure that he or she understands the personal and programmatic implications of test data, including a rationale for normative comparisons.
Treatment planning	Represent the PWD's goals regarding rehabilitation psychology services in the rehabilitation team treatment plan. Ensure the PWD's performance commitment regarding goal achievement within the treatment plan.
Intervention	Facilitate the consistent constructive participation of the PWD in the treatment process across all rehabilitation interventions. Determine reasonable performance progression toward goal achievement within or above the expected range for program continuation toward completion. Manage personal stresses affecting treatment effectiveness.

(*continues*)

TABLE 7.5

Clinical Evaluation and Treatment: Underlying Functional Competencies and Skills in the American Psychological Association *Ethical Principles of Psychologists and Code of Conduct* (Continued)

Functional skills and stages	Functional competencies
Discharge planning	Lay out a plan for continuity of care based on rate of recovery, ongoing care and treatment needs and availability of resources. Demonstrate adaptive relationships with the PWD and caregivers that foster ongoing rehabilitation services as required.
Integrity	
Initial interview and evaluation	Demonstrate open and accurate discussions of the workings of the rehabilitation team evaluation and treatment process. Establish the baseline of the PWD's understanding of his or her health condition and supporting realistic expectations regarding recovery trajectory and rehabilitation treatment outcome in the context of personal, familial, and social circumstances.
Assessment	Identify potential barriers to valid assessment, including engagement by the PWD. Demonstrate accurate test administration and interpretation within the context of the PWD's health status and individual needs. Ensure timely documentation of a written test interpretation summary.
Treatment planning	Demonstrate episodic treatment plan updates and responsiveness to the PWD's questions regarding treatment plan status and goal achievement progress. Ensure that the PWD has an accurate understanding of team performance metrics and implications for functional applications to the home and community environment.
Intervention	Demonstrate treatment adjustments on the basis of sufficient and accurate PWD awareness of performance status that influence decision making regarding the complexity of information disclosures and nature of activities to help the PWD maintain focus and effort on goal attainment.
Discharge planning	Ensure the PWD and caregivers (per the PWD's consent) have an accurate and thorough understanding of current health needs, along with an accurate prognosis of the continuing recovery course. Support use of a broad range of functional, cognitive, emotional, and behavioral outcome metrics to enhance the quality of rehabilitation program care.
Justice	
Initial interview/ evaluation	Determine fair distribution of time. Use current evidence-based practices and standards relevant to the PWD's presenting health issues.
Assessment	Recognize the impact of disability on assessment and implement appropriate accommodations in support of access to assessment tools. Ensure the PWD's understanding of the use of assessment across peers and diagnostic populations, if applicable, in the context of provision of rehabilitation services.
Treatment planning	Demonstrate advocacy for personal goals and methods of goal achievement regarding community integration by means of agency and resource access, including planning for continuity of care after discharge from rehabilitation services.
Intervention	Identify supplementary treatment resources and ensure that all PWDs served receive adequate material resources, information, recommendations, and assistance to optimize functional performance in the rehabilitation process.
Discharge planning	Anticipate postdischarge access issues and addressing barriers (e.g., emotional, cognitive) to maximize likelihood of following up on any needed ongoing treatment, care, or social assistance through community-based agencies. Advocating for equitable access should barriers to required treatment and care.

TABLE 7.5

Clinical Evaluation and Treatment: Underlying Functional Competencies and Skills in the American Psychological Association ***Ethical Principles of Psychologists and Code of Conduct*** **(Continued)**

Functional skills and stages	Functional competencies
Respect for People's Rights and Dignity	
Initial interview/ evaluation	Implement safeguards to protect the rights of individuals whose autonomous decision making is impaired. Determine the PWD's comprehension of information. Demonstrate awareness of biases affecting personal responses to the PWD; and respect for diversity represented in the disability culture; as well as diversity represented in ethnic, racial, cultural or other differentiating factors. Establish an advocacy role on behalf of the PWD when concerns or conflicts arise and regarding community reentry.
Assessment	Identify disability concerns related to garnering permission for assessment. Explain parameters of confidential records, release of information, and privacy rights. Ensure the PWD's understanding of these as well as normative data comparisons accounting for relevant diversity issues.
Treatment planning	Ensure that the PWD's self-identified health needs are addressed; integrate interview and evaluation and assessment data in the contexts of health history, expressed personal needs/preferences, and social environmental circumstances. Provide the PWD with sufficient information to make informed decisions regarding the treatment plan and community reintegration; alternatively, ensure that assistance and supervision regarding decision making is established for PWDs who have limited decisional capacity.
Intervention	Demonstrate understanding of a PWD's decision-making rights. Ensure the PWD understands his or her rights to participate in decisions regarding directing and modifying the treatment process, along with the right to refuse treatment. Incorporate sensitivity to and relevance of cultural, individual, and role differences in treatment processes. Set treatment outcome goals that reflect those characteristics.
Discharge planning	Support appropriate PWD control over use of health records by means of release-of-information procedures. Ensure optimal self-determination within an appropriate level of independent daily living as determined by the PWD's strengths, challenges, and support network.

Note. PWD = person with a disability.

principles and rationales underlying each step of the case analysis process as described in Table 7.5. In this manner, the ethics principles increase in relevance to the details of clinical service provision through habitually incorporating ethics concepts in case analysis and conceptualization. It also affords the opportunity to more directly and consistently explore personal biases and reactions that might be creating potential barriers to sound ethical judgment at different developmental phases. Traditional ethics training is commonly guided by specific applications of the APA Ethics Code without necessarily accounting for influential factors in moral reasoning, such as expectation of outcome, clarity of practice standards, and their alignment with professional judgment (Welfel, 2012). By infusing ethics-guided practice within the foundational and functional competencies as proposed, ideally one's developing moral identity will help mitigate poor decision making. The daily use of ethics principles to underpin all professional activities ingrains their applied perspective and reduces reactive negative affect related to enforcement fears borne of infrequent reference to ethics codes among health care professionals. If used to guide daily practice, ethics principles introduce safeguards into professional activities that can reduce the probability of occurrence of ill-conceived, distracted, or impulsive actions that may result in unintended errors (for which the health care professional is nonetheless morally culpable).

Ethics-guided practice does not obviate the necessity for further training in ethical standards and legal precedents and statutes given that these naturally evolve with changing societal moral norms. However, it is incumbent on educators to translate those advances in ethical and legal thinking into everyday clinical practice, actively relating standards of care and practice to their underlying ethics principles. Making this critical habitual linkage between ethics principles and routine professional behavior is key to preventing unintended ethical missteps. In the following list we summarize several arguments in support of adopting the tenets of ethics-guided practice.

1. *Utility*. The process of intentionally linking ethics principles to everyday professional practice provides repeated exposure to the five APA Ethical Principles throughout practicum, internship, and residency training, preparing clinicians for their routine incorporation into independent practice and creating linkages between moral judgment and practice standards.
2. *Ease of acquisition*. Learning the five APA Ethical Principles and their behavioral anchors, using the practice standards as reference material that further specify principles within challenging situations, is a relatively straightforward process provided their consistent use is a performance expectation in training, supervision, and in later independent practice (as evaluated via peer review).
3. *Emphasis on prevention*. Instead of relegating the APA Ethics Code to a status of situational reference, intentional and mindful incorporation of the ethics principles in the daily performance of one's professional activities serves to benefit and safeguard the persons served. Rehabilitation psychologists maintain a patient-centered focus in all clinical activities in addition to emphasizing this focal perspective in rehabilitation team interventions, reducing the risk of preventable errors.
4. *Valuing ethics standards*. The ethics-guided practice approach in no way diminishes the value of ethics standards. Their tripartite roles of specifying ethics principles, providing enforcement capability, and serving as mutable indices of societal evolution in succeeding iterations of the APA Ethics Code are preserved.

ETHICS TRAINING IMPLICATIONS

Consistent with the training outcomes explicated in the previous section, we can envision the training issues surrounding ethics-guided practice as falling into two phases or stages. The first is a graduate-level ethics course that introduces trainees to the tradition of moral–ethical analysis and decision making, along with focal training in ethical–legal precedents and classic case examples. In this initial educational process, foundational and functional ethics competencies and their behavioral anchors are introduced and exemplified by clinical and professional scenario analysis, the traditional approach to learning ethical conceptualization. A demonstrated, detailed, and historically grounded understanding of the APA Ethics Code principles and standards, the foundational and functional competencies tied to them, and the efficient reference to relevant legal precedents and state and federal statutes are the distal outcomes of this initial training phase.

The second phase involves an emphasis on incorporating the five APA General Principles, encompassing and justifying both foundational and functional competencies, into daily clinical and research skills training. Repeated exposure to this method of intentional incorporation of ethics principles into the details of everyday observed practice reinforces habit formation. The performance expectation in this phase of training is a trainee or clinician being able to detail ethics principles and rationales for different aspects of practice.

Practicum introduction to the proactive process of linking ethics principles to clinical work initially occurs during supervision and observation. The supervisor first determines the trainee's level of understanding of the APA Ethics Code through interviews and observations in the early stages of the supervisory relationship. (See Andrews et al., 2013; APA, 2014; and Kerkhoff & Hanson, 2015b). Supervisory querying as the trainee reports on data gathering, evaluation, assessment and intervention must be consistent across cases. Setting an expectation of trainee self-report of ethics principles and the underlying ethical rationale for each clinical case action should occur during initial supervisory meetings. Then, as the trainee becomes familiar with applying the principles, their linkage with all aspects of case analysis and conceptualization becomes adaptively habitual. Obviously, this approach requires supervisor orientation and training in order to ensure programmatic development of consistent trainee performance criteria. As junior trainees become comfortable with the process, group supervision involving more senior trainees will offer the experience of peer reinforcement in the learning process and exploration of values, beliefs, and biases.

The expectation for application of ethics principles during a broad and general internship will see ethics-guided practice habits applied to a wide array of cases in an applied experiential environment. This phase of training also introduces greater opportunities for culturally relevant discussion and reflection. The occasional ethics conflict or dilemma can be analyzed through further reference to APA Ethics Code, which specify details regarding the overarching principles and can effectively guide decision making and conflict resolution. However, the primary goal of ethics-guided practice is prevention through intentional linking of ethics principles and practice standards to daily practice activities.

Postdoctoral residency training in specialties further refines the application of ethics principles to specific evaluation and treatment modalities and populations (e.g., PWDs). At this level, training explores the particular individual characteristics of and social issues related to unique populations as ethics principles are applied to service provision. Specialty board certification then ensures, by means of a criterion-based peer review, advanced skill in application of ethics principles to clinical case scenarios. We consider it of equal importance that the written practice sample and oral examination processes related to board certification include both everyday application of ethics principles as well as mastery of a structured method of resolving ethics conflicts and dilemmas.

Both health care reform and the competency movement have shaped contemporary practice standards in rehabilitation psychology, including how we define our ethics competencies. In this chapter we have offered several practical examples reflective of both foundational and functional ethics competencies and have attempted to argue that as rehabilitation psychologists continue to shape the future of their specialty, trainees will benefit from an educational model incorporating ethics-guided practice in carrying out their daily professional responsibilities. This approach creates a culture of integrity in which ethics considerations are integrative rather than episodic.

Consistent with this ethics-guided approach, we offer the following recommendations regarding applied ethics in training and practice:

1. Graduate training programs, internship programs, and postdoctoral residency programs in rehabilitation psychology offer formal applied ethics study and training methodology with an additional focus on the development and maintenance of foundational and functional ethics competencies.
2. Specialty supervisors at the postdoctoral residency level are urged to adopt the ethics-guided practice model of training, incorporating the APA Ethics Code into everyday practice and developing behavioral evaluative indicators of trainee competence in applying this model to all professional activity. Enacting this recommendation depends on whether clinical and research supervisors have been trained to implement and are administratively supported in using this competency model.
3. Professionals using the specialist board certification process in rehabilitation psychology through the American Board of Professional Psychology/American Board of Rehabilitation Psychology (2018) is urged to create and incorporate a consistent set of behavioral anchors indicative of foundational and functional applied ethics competencies in both their initial and Maintenance of Certification examinations. In addition, this process are encouraged to reinforce their efforts by offering related continuing education experiences at professional conferences.

4. Rehabilitation psychologists are urged to advocate for professional ethics as the prioritized focus of the APA Ethics Code through membership on the APA Ethics committee, on state psychology ethics committees, participation in relevant APA and divisional discussions surrounding ethics and competency planning and implementation, and through opportunities to provide feedback, such as through calls for comments on the Ethics Code revisions.

CONCLUSION

Ethics practice reaches beyond student training, individual practice, and teamwork; it is a reflection of our values and identity as rehabilitation psychologists. The specialty of rehabilitation psychology has maintained a committed ethical focus on PWDs and underserved populations. Nonetheless, as society inexorably journeys toward an uncertain future, the APA Ethics Code will also episodically attempt to account for the moral implications of that journey in modifications to the standards. To the extent that we, as leaders, consider it our responsibility to create a culture of competence that embodies ethics as the moral groundwork on which we build our expertise that is applied in everyday practice (with attention paid to both technical skill and character development), we believe we will ultimately succeed in fulfilling our ethical obligations to both the persons we serve and society in general.

References

American Board of Professional Psychology/American Board of Rehabilitation Psychology. (2018). *Certification guidelines and procedures: Candidate's manual 2018.* Retrieved from https://abpp.org/BlankSite/media/Rehabilitation-Psychology-Documents/Candidate-manual-september-10-2018.pdf

American Psychological Association. (2006). *Final report of the APA Task Force on Assessment of Competence in Professional Psychology*. Retrieved from https://www.apa.org/ed/resources/competence-report.aspx

American Psychological Association. (2013). *Guidelines for the practice of telepsychology*. Retrieved from http://www.apa.org/practice/guidelines/telepsychology.aspx

American Psychological Association. (2014). *Guidelines for clinical supervision in health service psychology*. Retrieved from http://www.apa.org/about/policy/guidelines-supervision.pdf

American Psychological Association. (2017). *Ethical principles of psychologists and code of conduct* (2002, Amended June 1, 2010 and January 1, 2017). Retrieved from http://www.apa.org/ethics/code/index.aspx

Andrews, E. E., Kuemmel, A., Williams, J. L., Pilarski, C. R., Dunn, M., & Lund, E. M. (2013). Providing culturally competent supervision to trainees with disabilities in rehabilitation settings. *Rehabilitation Psychology*, *58*, 233–244. http://dx.doi.org/10.1037/a0033338

Association of State and Provincial Psychology Boards. (2018). *E.Passport program information*. Retrieved from https://www.asppb.net/page/EPassport?

Association of University Centers on Disabilities. (2016). *Including people with disabilities—Public health workforce competencies*. Retrieved from https://www.aucd.org/template/page.cfm?id=830

Authority of health care providers to practice telehealth. (2018, May 11). *Federal Register, 83*(92). Retrieved from https://www.gpo.gov/fdsys/pkg/FR-2018-05-11/pdf/2018-10114.pdf

Beauchamp, T. L., & Childress, J. F. (2012). *Principles of biomedical ethics* (7th ed.). New York, NY: Oxford University Press.

Centers for Disease Control and Prevention. (2013). CDC health disparities and inequalities report—United States, 2013. *Morbidity and Mortality Weekly Report*, *62*(Suppl. 3), 1–187. Retrieved from http://www.cdc.gov/mmwr/pdf/other/su6203.pdf

Cheak-Zamora, N., Reid-Arndt, S. A., Hagglund, K. J., & Frank, R. G. (2012). Health legislation and public policies. In P. Kennedy (Ed.), *The Oxford handbook of rehabilitation psychology* (pp. 511–524). Oxford, England: Oxford University Press.

Cox, D. R., Cox, R. H., & Caplan, B. (2013). *Specialty competencies in rehabilitation psychology*. Oxford, England: Oxford University Press. http://dx.doi.org/10.1093/med:psych/9780195389241.001.0001

Dunn, D. (2015). *The social psychology of disability*. New York, NY: Oxford University Press.

Eastman, P. (2003). IOM: Education of health professionals needs overhaul. Needed: More rigorous testing, better interdisciplinary teamwork. *Oncology Times*, *24*, 74–76. http://dx.doi.org/10.1097/01.COT.0000293348.41338.0a

Fineberg, H. (2003). Foreword. In A. C. Greiner & E. Knebel (Eds.), *Health professions education: A bridge to quality* (p. 1). Washington, DC: The National Academies Press.

Hanson, S. L., & Kerkhoff, T. R. (2010). Ethics. In R. Frank, M. Rosenthal, & B. Caplan (Eds.), *Handbook of rehabilitation psychology* (2nd ed., pp. 427–437). Washington, DC: American Psychological Association. http://dx.doi.org/10.1037/15972-030

Hanson, S. L., & Kerkhoff, T. R. (2011). The APA Ethical Principles as a foundational competency: Application to rehabilitation psychology. *Rehabilitation Psychology, 56*, 219–230. http://dx.doi.org/10.1037/a0024206

Hanson, S. L., & Kerkhoff, T. R. (2012). The health care setting: Implications for ethical psychology practice. In S. J. Knapp, M. C. Gottlieb, M. M. Handersman, & L. D. VanderCreek (Eds.), *APA handbook of ethics in psychology: Vol. 2. Practice, teaching, and research* (pp. 75–90). Washington, DC: American Psychological Association.

Hanson, S. L., Kerkhoff, T. R., & Bush, S. S. (2005). *Health care ethics for psychologists: A casebook*. Washington, DC: American Psychological Association. http://dx.doi.org/10.1037/10845-000

Hatcher, R. L., Fouad, N. A., Grus, C. L., Campbell, L. F., McCutcheon, S. R., & Leahy, K. L. (2013). Competency benchmarks: Practical steps toward a culture of competence. *Training and Education in Professional Psychology, 7*, 84–91. http://dx.doi.org/10.1037/a0029401

Health Service Psychology Education Collaborative. (2013). Professional psychology in health care services: A blueprint for education and training. *American Psychologist, 68*, 411–426. http://dx.doi.org/10.1037/a0033265

Hibbard, M. R., & Cox, D. R. (2010). Competencies in rehabilitation psychology. In R. Frank, M. Rosenthal, & B. Caplan (Eds.), *Handbook of rehabilitation psychology* (2nd ed., pp. 467–475). Washington, DC: American Psychological Association. http://dx.doi.org/10.1037/15972-034

Institute of Medicine. (2001). *Crossing the quality chasm: A new health system for the 21st century*. Washington, DC: The National Academies Press.

Institute of Medicine. (2013). *Delivering high-quality cancer care: Charting a new course for a system in crisis*. Washington, DC: The National Academies Press.

Institute of Medicine (US) Committee on the Health Professions Education Summit. (2003). The core competencies needed for health care professionals. In A. C. Greiner & E. Knebel (Eds.), *Health professions education: A bridge to quality* (pp. 45–74). Washington, DC: The National Academies Press.

Kaiser Family Foundation. (2013). *Summary of the Affordable Care Act*. Retrieved from http://kff.org/health-reform/fact-sheet/summary-of-the-affordable-care-act/

Kaslow, N. J., Grus, C. L., Campbell, L. F., Fouad, N. A., Hatcher, R. L., & Rodolfa, E. R. (2009). Competency assessment toolkit for professional psychology. *Training and Education in Professional Psychology, 3*(Suppl. 4), S27–S45. http://dx.doi.org/10.1037/a0015833

Keenan, P. S. (2014, November 24). *Issue Brief: What's driving health care costs?* Retrieved from http://www.commonwealthfund.org/~/media/files/publications/issue-brief/2004/nov/whats-driving-health-care-costs/keenan_whatsdrivingcosts_cong2004_707-pdf.pdf

Kerkhoff, T. R. (2015). Up close and personal: Ethics-guided practice. *Psychological Injury and Law, 8*, 300–310. http://dx.doi.org/10.1007/s12207-015-9233-3

Kerkhoff, T. R., & Hanson, S. L. (2013). *Ethics field guide: Applications in rehabilitation psychology*. Oxford, England: Oxford University Press.

Kerkhoff, T. R., & Hanson, S. L. (2015a). Applied ethics: Have we lost a crucial opportunity? *Rehabilitation Psychology, 60*, 376–378. http://dx.doi.org/10.1037/rep0000067

Kerkhoff, T. R., & Hanson, S. L. (2015b). Disability culture—Ethics perspectives. In J. Uomoto (Ed.), *Multicultural neurorehabilitation: Clinical principles for rehabilitation professionals* (pp. 169–202). New York, NY: Springer.

Nordal, K. C. (2012). Health care reform: Implications for independent practice. *Professional Psychology: Research and Practice, 43*, 535–544. http://dx.doi.org/10.1037/a0029603

Patient Protection and Affordable Care Act, Pub. L. 111-148, 42 U.S.C. §§ 18001—18121 (2010).

Peterson, R., Peterson, D. R., Abrams, J. C., Stricker, J., & Ducheny, K. (2010). The National Council of Schools and Programs of Professional Psychology: Educational model 2009. In M. B. Kenkel & R. L. Peterson (Eds.), *Competency-based education for professional psychology* (pp. 13–42). Washington, DC: American Psychological Association. http://dx.doi.org/10.1037/12068-001

Pozgar, G. D. (2014). *Legal and ethical essentials of health care administration*. Burlington, VT: Jones & Bartlett Learning.

Pozgar, G. D. (2016). *Legal and ethical issues for health professionals*. Burlington, VT: Jones & Bartlett Learning.

Ragusea, A. (2012). The more things change, the more they stay the same: Ethical issues in the provision of telehealth. In S. J. Knapp, M. C. Gottlieb, M. M. Handersman, & L. D. VanderCreek (Eds.), *APA handbook of ethics in psychology: Vol. 2. Practice, teaching, and research* (pp. 183–198). Washington, DC: American Psychological Association.

Rodolfa, E., Bent, R., Eisman, E., Nelson, P., Rehm, L., & Ritchie, P. (2005). A cube model for competency development: Implications for psychology educators and regulators. *Professional Psychology: Research and Practice, 36*, 347–354. http://dx.doi.org/10.1037/0735-7028.36.4.347

Schoen, C., Osborn, R., Squires, D., Doty, M. M., Pierson, R., & Applebaum, S. (2010). How health insurance design affects access to care and costs, by income, in eleven countries. *Health Affairs*, *29*, 2323–2334. http://dx.doi.org/10.1377/hlthaff.2010.0862

Steinbock, B., Arras, J. D., & London, A. J. (2013). *Ethical issues in modern medicine: Contemporary readings in bioethics* (8th ed.). New York, NY: McGraw-Hill.

Stiers, W., Barisa, M., Stucky, K., Pawlowski, C., Van Tubbergen, M., Turner, A. P., . . . Caplan, B. (2015). Guidelines for competency development and measurement in rehabilitation psychology post-doctoral training. *Rehabilitation Psychology*, *60*, 111–122. http://dx.doi.org/10.1037/a0038353

Stiers, W., Hanson, S., Turner, A. P., Stucky, K., Barisa, M., Brownsberger, M., . . . Council of Rehabilitation Psychology Postdoctoral Training Programs. (2012). Guidelines for postdoctoral training in rehabilitation psychology. *Rehabilitation Psychology*, *57*, 267–279. http://dx.doi.org/10.1037/a0030774

U.S. Department of Justice. (2009). *A guide to disability rights laws*. Retrieved from https://www.ada.gov/cguide.htm

U.S. Department of Justice. (2011). Information and technical assistance on the *Americans with Disabilities Act*. Retrieved from https://www.ada.gov/2010_regs.htm

U.S. House of Representatives, Office of the Legislative Council. (2010). *Compilation of Patient Protection and Affordable Care Act*. Retrieved from http://housedocs.house.gov/energycommerce/ppacacon.pdf

Vaughn, L. (2008). *Doing ethic: Moral reasoning and contemporary issues*. New York, NY: W. W. Norton.

Weber, L. J. (2001). *Business ethics in healthcare: Beyond compliance*. Bloomington: Indiana University Press.

Welfel, E. R. (2012). Teaching ethics: Models, methods, and challenges. In S. J. Knapp, M. C. Gottlieb, M. M. Handersman, & L. D. VanderCreek (Eds.), *APA handbook of ethics in psychology: Vol. 2. Practice, teaching, and research* (pp. 277–305). Washington, DC: American Psychological Association.

Zack, M. (2013). CDC health disparities and inequalities report: Health-related quality of life—United States, 2006 and 2010. *Morbidity and Mortality Weekly Report*, *62*(Suppl. 3), 105–111. Retrieved from https://www.cdc.gov/mmwr/preview/mmwrhtml/su6203a18.htm

CHAPTER 8

EPIDEMIOLOGY OF DISABILITY AND HEALTH

Alicia Dixon-Ibarra, Michele Catena, and Gloria Krahn

James is a 37-year-old man who lives with his wife, two children, and their dog in a mid-size U.S. city. He works as a mechanical engineer at a local design firm. James was a competitive runner in high school and college, married his college girlfriend, and embarked on his career. When he was 28, he was involved in a motor vehicle collision and sustained an incomplete C8 spinal cord injury (SCI), resulting in tetraplegia. He has intact sensation below the lesion but limited motor return. He uses an ultra-lightweight, custom manual wheelchair for mobility and drives his car independently with the use of hand controls. James participated in physical and occupational therapy for over a year after his injury and is currently seeing his physical therapist to manage shoulder pain related to use of his manual wheelchair. After the injury, James experienced significant depression and difficulty with all the changes in his life. His wife, their families, and the community are great supports, and he has not had a recurrence of clinical depression. He now peer-mentors others with recent SCIs. James tries to maintain physical activity but has a hard time working out regularly. He acknowledges that he eats too many fast foods and snacks, has gained 20 pounds since his injury, and has high cholesterol. James has worked with the same firm for more than 15 years and they added ramps and an accessible restroom to increase accessibility of his work environment. The firm is on two floors with no elevator access, so James can't access the management offices.

James is an example of one individual's experience of living with disability. In 2011, the *World Report on Disability* estimated that 1 billion people globally, or 15% of the world's population, live with some form of disability (World Health Organization [WHO], 2011). Disability has come to be recognized as a normal and universal human experience, affecting people in all countries, social strata, ages and genders. Rehabilitation professionals often serve the vital role of initiating a range of services at the person level to help people with disabilities maintain optimal health and functioning (WHO, 2011).

As a complement to person-level approaches, the field of public health represents a population-based approach to understanding and improving health. A public health approach relies on a portfolio of population-level methods for addressing health issues that includes epidemiology, public policy,

http://dx.doi.org/10.1037/0000129-009
Handbook of Rehabilitation Psychology, Third Edition, L. A. Brenner, S. A. Reid-Arndt, T. R. Elliott, R. G. Frank, and B. Caplan (Editors-in-Chief)

and broad-scale health communications campaigns, in addition to individually based interventions (Frieden, 2010). Public health efforts are credited historically with greatly reducing the incidence and prevalence of diseases and significantly increasing longevity and health status in much of the developed world (Salomon et al., 2012).

Population-based studies are valuable adjuncts to patient-based studies in many fields of health care, including disability and rehabilitation. For a clinician or a clinical researcher, a public health perspective can provide a context for understanding the larger circumstances of the individual's experience (Arah, 2009). Health is not solely controlled at the individual level; environmental factors, including social determinants of health, greatly influence the health and participation of persons with and without disabilities. The quote "Your zip code is a better predictor of your health than your genetic code" is attributed to Anthony Iton, former public health director of Alameda County in California, in communicating the determinants of the stark health disparities evident in his county (Hindery, 2009). The phrase aptly captures the strong influences of socioeconomic background, education, and available environmental supports in shaping health. When health is viewed within this rich contextual web of health determinants and environmental circumstances, the opportunities and barriers to improving health become more evident.

Epidemiology—the study of the distribution and determinants of health-related states or events (including disease), in specified populations, and the use of this knowledge to control health problems (Porta, 2014)—is a critical tool to discovering these relationships. Long recognized as a core discipline of public health science and practice (Institute of Medicine, 1988), it is included in the training of all schools and programs in public health. Core functions of epidemiology include public health surveillance, field investigation, analytic studies, evaluation, linking with health departments and health care providers, and policy development (Gordis, 2013). Rehabilitation professionals can use knowledge developed by epidemiologists to better understand the environmental influences on the current and future health outcomes of their patients with disabilities.

The purpose of this chapter is to provide an introduction to disability epidemiology for rehabilitation professionals and to describe how a population-level perspective can support individual care in the rehabilitation setting. In the final section of the chapter, we highlight ways to become an active voice in public policy and health promotion for people with disabilities.

DISABILITY UNDERSTOOD THROUGH THE *INTERNATIONAL CLASSIFICATION OF FUNCTIONING, DISABILITY AND HEALTH*

A number of frameworks are currently used to understand "disability." Within a clinical context, a medical model of disability is highly useful for determining diagnosis and implications for medical care. In our case example provided at the beginning of the chapter, the incomplete C8 SCI resulting in tetraplegia would be James's disability according to the medical model. *Functional models* of disability address the functional limitations of individuals and their participation in community, with less regard for etiology of the limitations. James's use of a manual wheelchair and hand controls for driving are examples of how he participates in the community given his functional limitations. A *social model* of disability emphasizes the social contexts in which people live. Street curb cuts and building ramps reflect policies and practices that facilitate a person's abilities to participate. For James, not having access to management offices on the upper floors would limit his participation in his company and illustrates disability from a social model. Summaries of these models have been provided elsewhere (e.g., Drum, 2009; Iezzoni & Freedman, 2008).

In 2001, WHO integrated many of these previous models of disability into the *International Classification of Functioning, Disability and Health* (ICF). The ICF regards *disability* as an umbrella term to refer to limitations due to health conditions that occur in the context of environmental and personal factors and that manifest in limitations of body function, activity, and participation.

The core of the ICF framework is a person's body functions and structures (physiological functions and anatomical parts), reciprocal influencing activities (functioning at the individual level and activity restrictions), and participation (involvement in all areas of life and participation restrictions). These elements reflect dynamic interaction with one's health condition (disorder or disease), environmental factors (facilitators or barriers), and personal factors (e.g., sex, age, educational background).

Numerous population surveys now incorporate an ICF perspective in their construction. For instance, the Multi-Country Survey Study on Health and Responsiveness (Üstün et al., 2001) and the World Health Survey (see https://www.who.int/healthinfo/survey/en/) use the ICF as a framework to measure the health status of populations in 71 countries. The ICF also served as the framework in the design of the National Paralysis Survey (NPS) to define paralysis and examine the health of a nationally representative sample of adults with paralysis across the United States (Fox, Krahn, Sinclair, & Cahill, 2015). In other surveys, the identification of persons with disabilities is shifting from questions based on a categorical identification ("Do you have [diagnosis]?") to questions based on functional limitation ("Because of a condition, do you experience difficulty with [function or activity]?").

Because of its use in both population-based public health and clinical practice, the ICF can serve as a bridge across these fields. For rehabilitation practice, it can serve as both a framework and a classification system to address the complex interaction between disability and functioning (Escorpizo et al., 2010). It is important to note that the ICF model explicitly incorporates environmental and personal factors that interact with functioning to influence a person's activities and participation. Furthermore, disability and disease are not static states; they often fluctuate over a lifetime. People can recover from their health condition (e.g., a broken bone), the condition may progress (e.g., Huntington's disease), or the condition may be intermittent (e.g., relapsing and remitting multiple sclerosis). The ways in which conditions manifest will influence the disability experience. For example, if James in our case example loses his wife or moves to another city, he will likely experience changes in social support and accessibility in his workplace. These changes would influence the dynamics of his disability experience, despite there being little to no change in his body functions and structures.

The ICF can be used by rehabilitation professionals to evaluate functional status, develop interventions and care, set goals, monitor treatment, and measure outcomes (Rauch, Cieza, & Stucki, 2008). A number of clinical tools have been developed using the ICF framework (e.g., Kisser et al., 2017; Steiner et al., 2002). The ICF supports a patient-centered approach and allows professionals working in multiple disciplines to speak a common language and use similar terms that can support more efficient, streamlined patient care (Steiner et al., 2002). Application of the ICF model to a person with an SCI, such as James, would include

- *body structure:* vertebrae, spinal cord, nerves and sensation, muscles, autonomic nervous system activation;
- *body function:* power of muscles in limbs and trunk, gait pattern functions, tone of muscles in lower extremities, bowel and bladder function, thermoregulation, pain in bilateral shoulders, mobility, posture;
- *activities:* standing, balance, walking short and long distances, transfers, toileting, fine-motor hand function, driving, health behaviors;
- *participation:* physical therapy, fitness center, life roles of family member (father, husband, son, dog owner), worker (engineer), neighbor and community member, peer mentor and advocate;
- *environmental factors:* use of technology for mobility and daily life, accessibility of home and work, support from family members, financial stability, health insurance; and
- *personal factors:* age, gender, college education, motivated for a "good life," belief in his own ability, ambitious career and family goals.

FUNDAMENTALS OF DISABILITY EPIDEMIOLOGY

Conventional epidemiologic methods are highly useful when applied to the study of disability, leading to the emergence of the subdiscipline of *disability epidemiology* (Adams, Krahn, Horner-Johnson, & Leman, 2009; Andresen, 2011; Gordis, 2013).

Disability epidemiology professionals describe the nature of disabilities while also examining outcomes and predictors of health that are important to improve the lives of persons with disabilities (Adams et al., 2009; Andresen, 2011). They typically use disability as a demographic variable in survey research to identify those with and without disability in order to describe health differences between them. Disability epidemiology addresses questions such as

- How many people with disabilities are there in a population?
- Who is counted, and why and how are they counted?
- What relates to improved health and quality of life for people with disabilities?
- What types of disabilities are associated with poorer health status?
- How can this information be used to improve health in these populations?

Answers to these questions can inform rehabilitation and public health professionals in intervening to improve the health of people with disabilities.

Goals of Disability Epidemiology

The goals are similar to those of epidemiology in general: to explain, predict, and control health problems (Gordis, 2013). Epidemiology helps explain the causal mechanisms of a health problem, such as the association between age at onset of disability and health status. A second goal is to predict or identify the likelihood of outcomes for a population. What are the likely outcomes given what we know about the population? As examples, persons with sedentary lifestyles are more likely to experience chronic disease, and persons with SCIs are more likely to have shoulder pain and injury compared with the general population. The third goal is to control health outcomes by promoting interventions that improve health and discourage disease, injury and other negative health outcomes. "Living Well with a Disability" is an example of an evidence-based wellness program that has shown reductions in secondary conditions, symptom days, and health care utilization among persons who have taken part in the intervention (Ravesloot et al., 2016; Ravesloot, Seekins, & White, 2005). Disability epidemiology can establish prevalence estimates of disability in given populations (explain), recognize predictors of decreased quality of life (predict), and identify interventions to address these factors (control; Adams et al., 2009).

Case Definition and Case Ascertainment

A *case definition* is a set of criteria to define a "case"; that is, who is included in the population under study and who is not included. *Case ascertainment* comprises the methods for finding cases in a population and may include direct observation, survey data, registry data, medical reports, education records, administrative data sets, and other sources (Porta, 2014). Because of the heterogeneity of populations, clear case definitions and case ascertainment are critical for understanding findings across different studies that may seem contradictory.

Determining common ways to define disability for surveillance has been an ongoing point of contention (Andresen, 2011). Without a consistent definition of *disability* across surveys, it is difficult to compare findings and impossible to combine data sets for increased statistical power. A major objective of Healthy People 2010 and 2020 was a standardized definition of disability for surveillance (U.S. Department of Health and Human Services [DHHS], 2001, 2011b). This requirement was included in the Patient Protection and Affordable Care Act of 2010 (ACA; Pub. L. 111-148), and standard identifiers were negotiated and published by the DHHS (2011b). These standard identifiers, although not perfect, provide common criteria with which to define disability. They are listed in Appendix 8.1 at the end of this chapter. It is important to note that this six-question set allows for differentiation by type of limitation. At present, 15 national surveys include the DHHS question set, including surveys of the U.S. Census Bureau and the U.S. Departments of Health and Human Services, Labor, Housing and Urban Development, and Justice (see https://www.cdc.gov/ncbddd/disabilityandhealth/datasets.html).

Incidence and Prevalence

Incidence is the number of new cases within a specified time frame and specified population (Porta,

2014)—for example, the number of new cases of SCI in a calendar year. Incidence is important for determining whether a disabling condition is increasing or decreasing across multiple years. Disabilities that appear at discrete times, such as birth-related disabilities or SCIs, are easier to identify and count. Determining incidence is more challenging for disabilities with slower onset or appearance, such as autism spectrum disorder, severe speech disorder, multiple sclerosis, or dementia. For disabling conditions with a longer latency for full expression, the time of diagnosis can be used as a proxy for calculating incidence, with the recognition that count is influenced by differential access to health care and diagnostic services.

Prevalence—the number of instances of disability at a certain time in a specific population (Porta, 2014)—is the most common tally of disability. It involves a basic count of everyone with the disability, new cases as well as those previously identified. In cross-sectional surveys whether the disability is a new case or long-standing one is often unknown. Data sources that include information about disability onset can allude to incidence, but these estimates may be inaccurate (Adams et al., 2009).

Incidence and prevalence of disability are highly dependent on case definition, as illustrated by the following study. The BRFSS is a population-based telephone survey that collects data on U.S. residents regarding their health-related risk behaviors, chronic health conditions, and use of preventive services. Until 2013, the BRFSS relied exclusively on the following two questions to determine disability: (a) "Are you limited in any way in any activities because of physical, mental, or emotional problems?" and (b) "Do you now have any health problem that requires you to use special equipment, such as a cane, a wheelchair, a special bed, or a special telephone?" Use of these questions grouped a heterogeneous population of people with diverse disabilities into one disability category. This cross-disability grouping facilitated self-report with a minimal number of questions but made it difficult to determine more finely grained associations among predictors and health outcomes; for example, a young, elite athlete with an SCI was grouped with an aging adult with visual impairment.

In 2013, the BRFSS added five of the six items from DHHS disability questions (the hearing question was not included), allowing a comparison of the two methods for case definition. Although the overall disability estimates were highly similar across the two measures (21.6% for the two-question set vs 22.7% for the five-question set), there were substantial differences in demographics and health among the people identified by the two-question versus the five-question set (Stevens, Courtney-Long, Okoro, & Carroll, 2016). Figure 8.1 depicts the overlap of prevalence estimates given these two criteria for defining disability.

Only about half (51.2%) of the disability respondents were identified as having disability on both the two-question and five-question set. The five-question set identified higher proportions of people aged 18 to 24 (8.5% vs 5.7%), females (58.2% vs. 47.2%), Hispanics (16.8% vs 11.4%), and persons with depression (30.2% vs. 22.7%); while the two-question set identified more people with arthritis (56.6% vs 51.8%; Stevens et al., 2016). Individuals identified by both question sets were those who reported more health conditions and poorer health status than those identified by only one of the question sets. Different disability identifiers identify different individuals, especially for people with less severe disability and better health, reflecting the importance of clearly operationalizing disability identification.

Prevalence of disability by type. With the introduction of the six HHS disability identifiers, which includes the five questions used in the BRFSS and a question about hearing difficulty (DHHS, 2011b), researchers can begin to disaggregate population data by type of disability. The prevalence of disability by disability type and sex is demonstrated in Figure 8.2, which is based on data from Courtney-Long et al. (2015).

Different types of functional limitations are associated with different profiles of health status and needed services. For example, data from the Medical Expenditure Panel Survey (MEPS) showed 47% of people with cognitive limitations required assistance for independent living, significantly more than any other disability types (Reichard, Stransky, Phillips, Drum, & McClain, 2015).

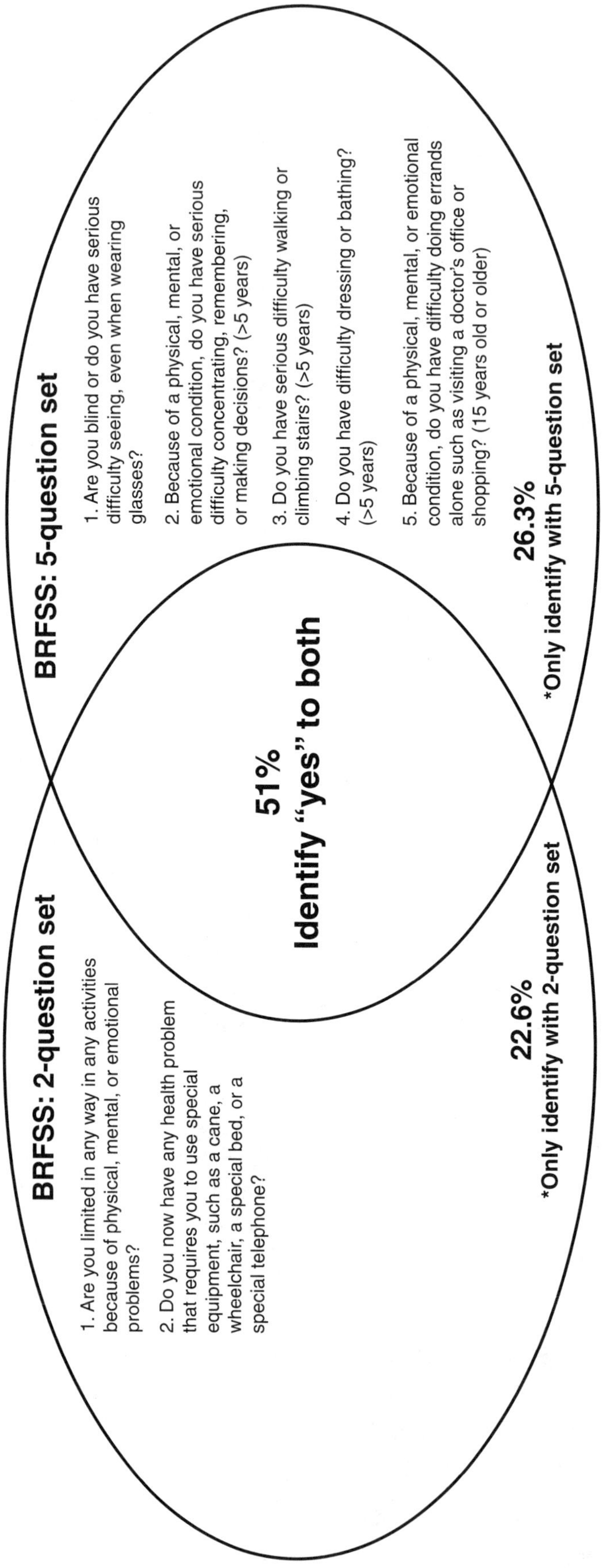
BRFSS: 2-question set
1. Are you limited in any way in any activities because of physical, mental, or emotional problems?
2. Do you now have any health problem that requires you to use special equipment, such as a cane, a wheelchair, a special bed, or a special telephone?
22.6%
*Only identify with 2-question set
51%
Identify "yes" to both
BRFSS: 5-question set
1. Are you blind or do you have serious difficulty seeing, even when wearing glasses?
2. Because of a physical, mental, or emotional condition, do you have serious difficulty concentrating, remembering, or making decisions? (>5 years)
3. Do you have serious difficulty walking or climbing stairs? (>5 years)
4. Do you have difficulty dressing or bathing? (>5 years)
5. Because of a physical, mental, or emotional condition, do you have difficulty doing errands alone such as visiting a doctor's office or shopping? (15 years old or older)
26.3%
*Only identify with 5-question set

FIGURE 8.1. Overlap of prevalence estimates across two disability criteria using the Behavioral Risk Factor Surveillance System (BRFSS).

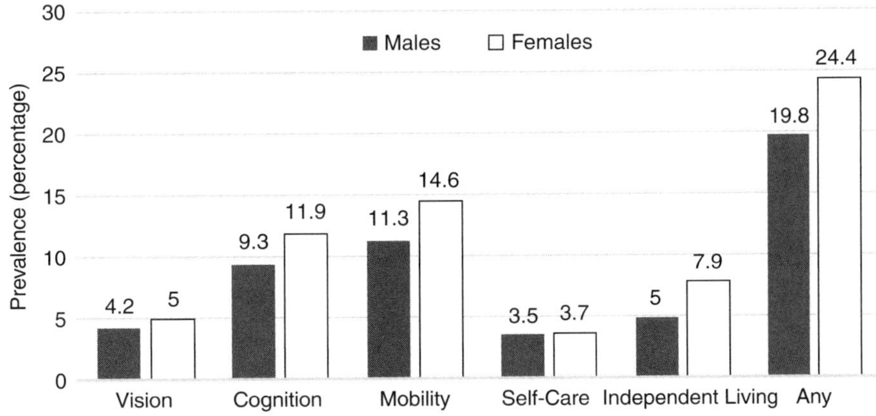

FIGURE 8.2. **Prevalence of disability by type, as identified by the Behavioral Risk Factor Surveillance System 2013.**

Descriptive and analytical studies. Epidemiologists conduct studies to inform population health, which is an approach that considers health outcomes and determinants within groups, including the distribution of these outcomes. Groups can be people in geographical areas (e.g., nations, communities) but can also include other groups, such as people with disabilities, employees, ethnic groups, prisoners, or any other defined group (Kindig, 2007).

Descriptive studies seek to describe disease or health status by person, place or time in population health (Porta, 2014), and are useful for generating hypotheses to test in analytic studies (Gordis, 2013). Descriptive studies do not attempt to look at cause and effect relationships, or to follow outcomes over time.

Analytical studies move beyond description to examine associations among exposures and their relationship to health outcomes. There are two types of analytical studies—observational and experimental studies. Study designs for observational research include cross sectional, case control, and cohort studies, which are described in detail elsewhere (Gordis, 2013; Porta, 2014). Intervention or experimental studies can also be analytic and deliberately modify an exposure to see if a change occurs in an outcome (e.g., randomized clinical trials and clinical lab-based research).

The fundamental elements of study design in epidemiology apply to disability populations. However, challenges in limited sample sizes to obtain a representative sample and adequate statistical power are a persistent problem (Andresen, 2011). For example, an analytic study (cross sectional) using the National Paralysis Survey examined associations between age at disability onset, current age, and health status. There were 94 individuals 65 years of age with disability onset less than 40 years compared with 318 older adults with disability onset after 40 years. While poorer health status was documented in adults aging into disability, more specific examination of relationship to variables such as sex and race was not possible, given limited power with wide confidence intervals and restricted covariates in the analysis models (Dixon-Ibarra, Krahn, Fredine, Cahill, & Jenkins, 2016).

Exposures and outcomes. Analytical studies examine the relationship between exposures and outcomes. These exposures can be harmful (e.g., toxins in the environment) or beneficial (e.g., access to treatment), with comparisons made on outcomes of interest (e.g., incidence of detected cancers) between the group exposed to the agent compared with those not exposed. In disability epidemiology, exposures can include social determinants (e.g., personal and environmental factors) or preventative measures (e.g., intervention), and outcomes typically include modifiable health outcomes (e.g., health-related quality of life).

Considered within a social determinants framework, exposures can be broad social experiences such as poverty, discrimination, or living in unsafe situations or neighborhoods. Social determinants of health are applicable to all populations and are those conditions in which people are born, grow, work, live and age, as well as the wider set of forces and systems that shape the conditions of their daily life (WHO, n.d.-b). Social determinants can include access to education, employment, health care, safe neighborhoods, and environments free of danger.

Confounders. Confounding factors can distort or inaccurately represent the true association between outcome and exposure. A classic study demonstrating confounders is that of Stark and Mantel (1966) who observed an association between birth order and Down syndrome, with higher birth order associated with increased likelihood of having a child with Down syndrome. However, when women were grouped by maternal age, the association between birth order and Down syndrome disappeared. Maternal age was confounding the relationship between birth order and having a child with Down syndrome (Stark & Mantel, 1966).

In disability epidemiology, a number of potential confounders are typically considered in interpretation: disability duration and onset, severity of the limitation, and supports for adaptation and accommodation (Adams et al., 2009). Persons with the same diagnosis may report much different experiences with their health in light of these and other disability specific covariates. Limiting bias in epidemiological studies requires knowing the population, developing good research questions, and utilizing study designs and statistical analyses to account for variables that distort true associations between exposures and outcomes.

Surveillance

Public health surveillance is the ongoing and systematic collection, analysis, and interpretation of health data followed by the dissemination of these data to those who need to know to stimulate public health action (Thacker, Qualters, Lee, & Centers for Disease Control and Prevention [CDC], 2012). Surveillance data are used to determine what health problems exist in the population; to describe trends in disease, exposures, and health behaviors; and to detect unexpected changes in disease and health outcomes. Public health surveillance can be used to examine the effects of policy changes (e.g., changes in health care), assess impacts of large health behavior campaigns, or generate hypotheses and confirm associations prior to initiating large scale studies (Gordis, 2013).

Surveillance methods include large-scale health surveys, registries, information systems environmental monitoring, clinical and public health research, and others (Thacker et al., 2012). In order for these methods to be considered surveillance, they need to include continuous collection, analysis, and interpretation of data with timely dissemination to the population (Porta, 2014). For noninfectious diseases, surveillance is often built on indicators from multiple data sources. Even when surveillance is not the primary aim of the data collection (e.g., medical records, administrative data sets), these methods can still be useful for monitoring trends and disease in populations (Hall, Correa, Yoon, Braden, & CDC, 2012).

Multiple federal and state surveillance systems provide data on periodic assessments of health of the U.S. population. Surveys of particular interest to rehabilitation professionals include the National Health Interview Survey (NHIS; CDC, 2017b), American Community Survey (U.S. Census Bureau, 2017), National Survey of Children's Health (CDC, 2015a), National Survey of Children with Special Health Care Needs (CDC, 2015b), Behavior Risk Factor Surveillance System (BRFSS; CDC, 2016), National Health and Nutrition Examination Survey (CDC, 2017a), the MEPS (Agency for Healthcare Research and Quality, 2016), among others—each with its unique constellation of data variables. These data sources are in the public domain, meaning there is free access to the data through online downloads. However, because of the complex sampling designs and sampling weight used to obtain these national data, researchers are often required to obtain additional statistical training in order to use them effectively (Kneipp & Yarandi, 2002; A. K. Smith et al., 2011).

Registries. Disease registries can serve an important role in surveillance-type activities. Because many high-impact disabling conditions occur at very low rates, collecting information on these diseases in population-based surveys often is not feasible. Although typically established for other purposes (e.g., participation in clinical trials, information dissemination, political advocacy), disease registries can provide information on large groups of people related to targeted health outcomes (Hall et al., 2012). However, they vary considerably in how well they represent the national population. Disability registries that provide valuable information include the model SCI systems (previously sponsored by the National Institute on Disability, Independent Living, and Rehabilitation Research; https://acl.gov/about-acl/about-national-institute-disability-independent-living-and-rehabilitation-research), the Healthy Athletes database of Special Olympics (https://resources.specialolympics.org/Taxonomy/Health/Healthy_Athletes_Software_INT.aspx), and the National Core Indicators™ data system for persons with intellectual and developmental disabilities (https://www.nationalcoreindicators.org/).

The value of disability surveillance. Although population-based surveillance is regarded as the gold standard for establishing prevalence rates of a condition or disorder, the low prevalence of many conditions makes surveillance seem unfeasible. However, population-based sampling can provide surprising and important findings. An example is SCI, for which researchers have historically relied on registries to count cases in the population. Those registry-based estimates suggest that approximately 270,000 people were living with SCI in the United States in 2012, representing roughly 0.086% of the overall U.S. population (National Spinal Cord Injury Statistical Center, 2012). In 2012–2013, the NPS, a national random–digit-dialed telephone survey, was conducted on the civilian, noninstitutionalized U.S. population. This survey used dual-frame sampling, which entailed the use of two sample frames (land lines and cell phones) to interview the population to reach a representative sample. The questions asked about anyone in the household having difficulty moving his or her arms or legs. Affirmative responses were followed with a question about the cause of the difficulty, with SCI as one response option. NPS researchers contacted 70,458 households, and 1,305 households that included a person with paralysis were identified. When weighted to account for selection and nonresponse and adjusted for known covariates, the estimated number of people living with SCI nationally was 1,462,220—more than 5 times the previous estimate (Armour, Courtney-Long, Fox, Fredine, & Cahill, 2016). Additional details regarding survey development, case definitions, and survey content can be found elsewhere (Armour et al., 2016; Dixon-Ibarra et al., 2016; Fox et al., 2015). Although not considered true surveillance because of the lack of ongoing data collection, the NPS is a unique and valuable data source.

EPIDEMIOLOGY TO INFORM HEALTH DISPARITIES

Across the multiple definitions of health inequities (Braveman, 2014; Institute of Medicine, 2002; WHO, n.d.-a), there is general agreement on three issues: (a) the term *health disparities* refers to differences in health outcomes at the population level; (b) these differences are linked to a history of social, economic, or environmental disadvantages; and (c) these differences are regarded as avoidable. The health status of a person with a disability is influenced by different types of health factors, with only some factors being preventable. One rubric for differentiating among types of conditions affecting health of persons with disabilities—associated conditions, comorbid conditions, and secondary conditions—was presented by Krahn, Hammond, and Turner (2006).

Associated conditions are those that result in the disability or limitation in functioning, such as an SCI, cerebral palsy, or Down syndrome. Associated conditions may have a number of health characteristics that are commonly part of that condition, such as paralysis for SCI, vision or motor impairment for cerebral palsy, or congenital heart defect or early-onset dementia for Down syndrome. These associated contributors to negative health are seen as unavoidable.

Comorbid conditions are concomitant or unrelated pathological or disease processes that have an adverse effect on health. Comorbid conditions for persons with SCI, for example, could be lung cancer or HIV/AIDS: negative health conditions that are largely unrelated to the primary disabling condition.

Secondary conditions are those for which people with preexisting disabilities are at a higher risk but are neither caused by nor are a direct result of the disability (Krahn et al., 2006). Examples of secondary conditions for persons with SCI include depression, decubitus ulcers, and obesity. As identified in the case study, James's high cholesterol would be considered a secondary condition if the condition is a result of his physical inactivity and poor nutrition and not a genetic factor. Secondary conditions are generally regarded as avoidable and are key targets of health promotion interventions for people with disabilities.

To identify health disparities, disability epidemiologists have called for including disability status as a demographic characteristic in many more surveillance systems (e.g., Andresen, 2011). Disability can then be used as an independent variable, such as a demographic characteristic, to identify health disparities, rather than used only as a dependent variable, such as a negative health outcome. This effort experienced important support through Title IV, Subtitle D, Section 4302 of the ACA, which now mandates the collection of data on disability status by "any federally conducted or supported health care or public health program, activity or survey" (ACA, 2010, pp. 478–479). Implementation of this mandate into other data sets will increase future knowledge about disability-related health disparities and how to reduce them.

The concept of health disparities stems from a social justice perspective and relies on epidemiologic methods to document population-level differences in health that are avoidable through changes in health care access, health promotion, or environmental changes that address broader social determinants. Determining whether chronic disease and other negative health outcomes are avoidable involves teasing apart associated, secondary, and comorbid health outcomes. Epidemiological studies have indicated clear disparities in health care access, health promotion, and health outcomes among people with disabilities compared with those without limitations. People with disabilities report 2.5 times the rate of unmet health care access (Altman & Bernstein, 2008; CDC, 2010; National Council on Disability, 2009). Despite passage of the Americans with Disabilities Act of 1990 (Pub. L. 101-336), the majority of health care facilities (Mudrick, Breslin, Liang, & Yee, 2012) and medical equipment were far from fully accessible in 2010. In general, persons with disabilities have poorer health status, less access to health care, and higher rates of chronic disease than the general population (Beatty et al., 2003; Drainoni et al., 2006; Krahn, Walker, & Correa-de-Araujo, 2015).

Carroll and colleagues (2014) published a seminal cross-sectional epidemiological study, using data from the National Health Interview Survey, to demonstrate that adults (ages 18–64 years) with disabilities were almost twice as likely as adults without disabilities to report inactive lifestyles (47.1% vs 26.1%). Compared with adults without a disability, 26% of whom reported no aerobic activity, those with mobility limitations had the highest percentage of no aerobic activity (57%) followed by those with cognitive (40%), vision (36%), and hearing limitations (33%). Inactivity corresponded with a greater likelihood for chronic disease. Among adults between ages 18 and 64 years, 46% of inactive individuals had one or more chronic conditions compared with 31% of active adults. Associations between inactivity and chronic disease were found across all disability types except for hearing (Carroll et al., 2014). Carroll et al.'s report highlights a key lifestyle disparity and highlights the role of health care providers in promoting physical activity and health. Rehabilitation professionals can use the recommendations and infographic in this seminal report to advocate for improved health of their patients.

Findings such as these beg the question of the temporal order between disability and poor health: Does having a disability put people at higher risk for developing chronic conditions, or do chronic conditions lead to disability? A study's research design helps address this question to some extent. For example, the annual number of new cases of diabetes is three times higher for people with disabilities compared with the general population, and the rate of cardiovascular disease is four times higher among young adults with disabilities, earlier than when cardiovascular disease might be expected to cause the disability (Krahn et al., 2015). Using data sources that provide information about disability onset are particularly useful in solving this conundrum. In a comparison of adults with lifelong disabilities (age of onset < 6 years of age) with the general adult population, adults with lifelong disabilities were more likely to have heart disease, cancer, diabetes, obesity, and hypertension, indicating that disability increases risk of developing future poor health (Dixon-Ibarra & Horner-Johnson, 2014).

An emerging approach in disability epidemiology is to consider disability within a life course perspective. Adults who acquired their disability later in life, typically as a consequence of multiple health conditions (i.e., aging *into* disability), account for the rising prevalence of disability with age. For this group, disability may reflect a more gradual decline in function (Molton & Jensen, 2010). For more information see Chapter 13, this volume. A second group includes adults who were born with or acquired their disability early in life and who have lived much of their lives with their disability (aging *with* disability; Monahan & Wolf, 2014). This group is more likely to have had lifelong experiences of poorer social determinants of health (less education, low income, difficulties with transportation). Age of disability onset appears to play a role in self-reported health, whereby older adults with early-onset paralysis (< 40 years of age) report significantly better health and fewer days of poor physical and mental health compared with older adults with paralysis and later onset disability (> 40 years of age; Dixon-Ibarra et al., 2016). The timing of disability onset presumably influences health trajectories when considered as to whether the disability (i.e., functional limitation) appears to be "off time" or "on time" in the life course (Elder, 1998). For example, James, in our case study, acquired his SCI at age 28; this would be considered off time. Someone 28 years old does not expect to be in a wheelchair for the rest of his or her life; in fact, James was likely expecting to run in college, obtain an education, and start a family without the complexity of having an SCI. James's depression subsequent to the accident demonstrates the cost of a debilitating injury at a young age. Conversely, if a 90-year-old man falls and has a hip fracture that results in him having to use a wheelchair this could be considered on time in the life course, given that disability is often considered as part of the natural process of aging. Although use of this perspective remains largely unexplored, the implications for the timing of disability onset and its intersection with age could provide key insights into the health of persons aging with disabilities (Dixon-Ibarra et al., 2016; Molton & Jensen, 2010; Putnam, Molton, Truitt, Smith, & Jensen, 2016).

Underlying many disparities for persons with disabilities are differences in broader social determinants of health, such as education, poverty, and community participation. Persons with disabilities are less likely to have a high school or college education, less likely to be employed, more likely to live in poverty as adults, and less likely to have access to reliable transportation and Internet connections (e.g., Krahn et al., 2015). These factors influence how they interact with their environment and health care and influence their awareness of health-promoting behaviors that could increase health-related quality of life and decrease negative health outcomes. The use of health disparity research in public health has utility in rehabilitation. The health of people with disabilities is multifaceted, involving multiple health conditions (avoidable and unavoidable), environmental factors, and personal factors such as the age at which their disability was acquired. Although individual-level information from patients provides insights into their disability experience and future health outcomes, population-level data can provide additional contextual knowledge about these populations.

IMPLICATIONS OF EPIDEMIOLOGY FOR DISABILITY AND REHABILITATION POLICY

For public policy in disability and rehabilitation to be relevant and effective, rehabilitation professionals need to be actively engaged in its development, as do those directly affected by the policies: persons with disabilities. Rehabilitation professionals can engage in public policy at multiple levels and in different ways. These include policy formation, advocacy for programs, or promoting increased support for research. Disability epidemiology can inform disability and rehabilitation policy on broad population concerns, such as improved access to health care to reduce health disparities; improved community accessibility, such as accessible public transportation; and individual concerns, such as reimbursement policies for specific therapy services and devices.

Stories and Data

Public policy is typically shaped by advocacy through stories and data. Individual stories are compelling and may be sufficient for some policy decisions on emotionally charged issues. However, data—in particular, population-based data—are often required by policymakers to identify the need for action ("Is there a problem?") or determine which among alternative policy decisions has the greatest likelihood for success ("What should be done?"; Birkland, 2014). Disability epidemiology can be an essential tool for policy decision making by documenting the prevalence and negative health outcomes in a population that might otherwise go unrecognized and unaddressed.

Disability epidemiology has played a critical role in the development of key research and policy-focused documents. The argument that "there's no substantiating data" can finally be put to rest with presentation of population-based data that document preventable differences in health determinants and health outcomes for persons with disabilities (e.g., Krahn et al., 2015). This designation is important for inclusion of persons with disabilities in health equity funding and policy development. As an example of a document pertinent to rehabilitation and health, Carroll et al. (2014) used population-level data to illustrate the importance of physical activity for persons with disabilities and its association with lower rates of chronic disease.

Knowing the policy context and potential implications of findings can help disability researchers improve the potential impact of their research findings. This policy awareness can inform decisions about types of participants, methods, variables, or analyses that may be of particular relevance for policymakers. A number of examples illustrate this. Public agencies at the state and federal levels have increasingly required evidence-based demonstration of a program's effectiveness before authorizing public funding for such services. Rehabilitation researchers have been responsive, and an increasing literature is amassing on the effectiveness of specific rehabilitation interventions (e.g., Kamper et al., 2015). However, a variable of particular interest to policymakers is cost, and comparative costs of interventions are frequently not reported in intervention studies. The advent of "big data analytics," especially analyses of administrative data sets, is anticipated to have major implications for disability and rehabilitation policy (e.g., Einav & Levin, 2013). Use of these methods were instrumental in identifying that the United States spends almost $400 billion annually on disability-related health expenditures (Anderson, Wiener, Finkelstein, & Armour, 2011), a finding that has garnered the attention of policymakers. Finally, national panels of disability and rehabilitation researchers have used epidemiological methods to develop a better understanding of the nature and size of populations of children with mental disorders (National Academies of Sciences, Engineering, and Medicine, 2015) and speech and language disorders (National Academies of Sciences, Engineering, and Medicine, 2016), as commissioned by the Social Security Administration.

The Practices and Politics of Counting

Although counting is a ubiquitous and seemingly simple practice, it is also highly political in nature (Martin & Lynch, 2009). What to count and whom to include or exclude in the counting process becomes highly contentious. The criteria for case definitions, and even whether to include case identifiers in surveillance systems, are political processes couched in scientific terminology. The classification of disability in surveillance systems has major implications for disability advocacy and policy. When "1 in 5" or "20% of the population" is considered to have a disability, this becomes one of the largest minority populations in the United States. People included in these broad definitions, however, may not view themselves or be viewed by others as having a disability (Andresen, 2011). When disability is defined more stringently, such as measuring "severe" limitation, the numbers and percentages are reduced substantially, from about

19% to 12% to 13% of adults, and when specific types of disability are counted separately, the numbers and percentages become quite low, such as 0.8% for severe vision difficulty or 0.5% for severe hearing impairment in all adults age 15 years and older (Brault, 2012). Disability subgroups can find advocacy value in aligning with the larger disability community on some policy issues and retaining distinct identity in others. This has been evident for the Deaf community or autism spectrum disorder advocates, with both groups eschewing a "disability" identity but allying with the disability community for issues such as discrimination protection under the Americans With Disabilities Act of 1990.

Multiple Levels of Policy Engagement

A systematic review of barriers and facilitators to the use of evidence by policymakers identified three important factors: (a) timely access to high-quality, relevant research evidence; (b) collaborations with policymakers; and (c) relationship building with policymakers (Oliver, Innvar, Lorenc, Woodman, & Thomas, 2014). For researchers and other professionals these findings mean ensuring that their knowledge is relevant and of good quality; connecting with organizations or advocates who have collaborative relationships with the policymaker; and learning how to develop relationships with policymakers and their staff.

Many researchers and professionals become involved in policy and advocacy secondarily on a specific issue and then may discontinue their engagement. Others enjoy the process of policy making and administrative rule setting and consider most issues from a policy perspective. Regardless, all need to know where responsibility resides for the policies of interest to them and how to engage with those policymakers. For example, Medicare is the federal U.S. program attached to Social Security that provides health care coverage for citizens 65 years and older and people with certain disabilities. Its regulations are generally federally determined and applicable across states. Medicaid, on the other hand, is a joint state and federal program for low-income individuals and families and provides coverage for health care and long-term care. Its regulations are more state determined, and eligibility and coverage are more state specific. As a result, Medicare policy advocacy is likely to occur at the federal level, and Medicaid advocacy at the state level.

State and local levels. Local and state policymakers are often your neighbors, and they usually are very interested in hearing the views and needs of people in their district or state. Strategies for engaging with state and local policymakers include volunteering on citizen committees or task forces; participating in the campaign process for candidates; and serving on organizations (both professional or as a citizen) to become more familiar with the people, the processes, and the ways of presenting information that are useful for policymakers. Universities and health care employers may have a government affairs office that serves as entry into the legislative process, including providing testimony to legislative committees. Some state professional associations have very active advocacy programs, with training to support their members in learning how to become more effective in their advocacy.

National level. At the national level, relationships with policymakers on rehabilitation issues often are managed through the policy arms of national organizations. These organizations disseminate information on current and emerging issues for their discipline and rehabilitation more broadly. The Healthy People framework creates a policy agenda. This "blueprint for the nation's health" provides science-based, 10-year, national objectives for improving the health of Americans (DHHS, 2018). The current version, Healthy People 2020 (DHHS, 2011a), contains 20 national objectives specific to the health of people with disabilities in four categories: (a) systems and policies to improve health, (b) barriers to health care, (c) environments for better health, and (d) activities and participation.

Improved data and targeted policy advocacy from multiple fronts are yielding policy changes at the national level. The Medicare and Medicaid programs account for about 70%of all disability-related health care expenditures. The Centers for Medicare and Medicaid (2015) recently expanded their health disparities populations to include people with disabilities and released their equity plan for improving quality in Medicare. The plan and subsequent initiatives include a specific priority to increase physical accessibility of health care facilities and to improve Medicaid-covered care for persons with limitations.

International level. Numerous international organizations that focus on disability and rehabilitation issues are engaged in policy advocacy internationally. The Convention on the Rights of Persons With Disabilities (CRPD; United Nations, 2006) may be the most visible global disability cause of the past 20 years. Led by the United Nations, CRPD is an international treaty that has strong advocacy support from many organizations and countries globally. It is grounded in general principles that recognize the inherent dignity and worth and the equal and inalienable rights of all humans, and it comprises 50 articles outlining specific actions in support of these principles. The United Nations General Assembly has repeatedly cited the lack of information on the circumstances of people with disabilities and the lack of comparable data across countries. Article 31 of CRPD specifically calls for statistics and data collection to enable the formulation and implementation of policies in support of the Convention (United Nations, 2006).

WHO is an agency of the United Nations concerned with international public health (WHO, n.d.-c). It is well known for its reports, guidelines, and actions to improve health. In conjunction with the World Bank, WHO sponsored the first *World Report on Disability* in 2011 (WHO & World Bank, 2011). This report of nine chapters, including a chapter on rehabilitation, provides a framework and set of specific recommendations for improving the health and well-being of persons with disabilities. They also note that "global data on the need for rehabilitation services, the type and quality of measures provided, and estimates of unmet need do not exist" (p. 102).

CONCLUSION

A public health perspective, as exemplified by disability epidemiology, offers important added value to an individual rehabilitation perspective by providing information about the social determinants of health for large populations of people with disabilities. The ICF model illustrates the merging of individual and population views, providing utility for both rehabilitation and public health practice. Its application to the case example of James ensures that attention is directed to his personal and environmental factors as well as his health condition, all to maximize his functioning; activities; and full participation in his family, work setting, and community. If these personal and environmental factors are not considered, key contributors to maximize his functional independence and quality of life may be ignored. Although some barriers, such as lack of elevator access to the second floor at his work site, are harder to overcome, others are more easily changed. Information from disability epidemiological studies can contribute to a deeper understanding of population-level health and environmental factors influencing long-term health outcomes for persons with disabilities.

Disability epidemiology is a new subdiscipline within the field of epidemiology. The methods and techniques of public health epidemiology are generally applicable to persons with disabilities, including measures of prevalence and incidence, study designs, and associations among health variables. Problems of small sample sizes and varied case definitions of disability require careful decisions by disability epidemiologists in choosing their study populations, research design, and analysis methods. With the inclusion and standardization of disability identifiers, the use of secondary surveillance data is an invaluable tool to describe the health of disability populations. Resources such as the NPS are useful in that they help highlight health needs among persons with disabilities, including health care access, secondary and chronic conditions, and overall health status. Disability epidemiology research findings have resulted in the identification of disability populations as a public health disparity group. The importance of this recognition is twofold: (a) the potential for additional public health funding to reduce differences in health and (b) political recognition that can result in improved services for persons with disabilities.

AREAS FOR FUTURE RESEARCH AND COLLABORATION

Disability epidemiology can be a useful tool for rehabilitation professionals to understand their role in reducing health disparities through patient care, clinical research, and policy advocacy. Practitioners can best serve patients, such as James, when they are aware of the potential health care disparities that persons with disabilities face. For instance, James's health care providers may consider patient and family education to emphasize the importance of physical activity to improve his current health status (e.g., weight gain, high cholesterol) and decrease his likelihood of developing secondary conditions (e.g., diabetes). Furthermore, clinicians and epidemiologists can work together, using stories and data, to advocate for strategies that close the gap in health care disparities for persons with disabilities. Each can use their expertise to bring these important issues to light in local, state, and national politics as well as support and inform their patients and families.

APPENDIX 8.1: U.S. DEPARTMENT OF HEALTH AND HUMAN SERVICES DATA COLLECTION STANDARDS FOR DISABILITY STATUS

The six item set of questions used on ACS and other major surveys to gauge disability is the data standard for survey questions on disability. Note the age thresholds for survey participants for the different disability questions.

<u>Data Standard for Disability Status</u>

1. Are you deaf or do you have serious difficulty hearing?
   a. ____ Yes b. ____ No

2. Are you blind or do you have serious difficulty seeing, even when wearing glasses?
   a. ____ Yes b. ____ No

3. Because of a physical, mental, or emotional condition, do you have serious difficulty concentrating, remembering, or making decisions? (5 years old or older)
   a. ____ Yes b. ____ No

4. Do you have serious difficulty walking or climbing stairs? (5 years old or older)
   a. ____ Yes b. ____ No

5. Do you have difficulty dressing or bathing? (5 years old or older)
   a. ____ Yes b. ____ No

6. Because of a physical, mental, or emotional condition, do you have difficulty doing errands alone such as visiting a doctor's office or shopping? (15 years old or older)
   a. ____ Yes b. ____ No

The six-item disability standard represents a minimum standard and the questions and answer categories cannot be changed. Additional questions on disability may be added to any survey as long as the minimum standard is included. If the ACS changes the disability questions in the future, HHS will revisit the standard and modify as necessary.

Note. ACS = American Community Survey; HHS = U.S. Department of Health and Human Services. From "Implementation Guidance on Data Collection Standards for Race, Ethnicity, Sex, Primary Language, and Disability Status," by U.S. Department of Health and Human Services, 2011, Washington, DC: Author. Retrieved from https://aspe.hhs.gov/basic-report/hhs-implementation-guidance-data-collection-standards-race-ethnicity-sex-primary-language-and-disability-status. In the public domain.

References

Adams, E., Krahn, G., Horner-Johnson, W., & Leman, R. (2009). Fundamentals of disability epidemiology. In C. E. Drum, G. L. Krahn, & Bersani, H., Jr. (Eds.), *Disability and public health* (pp. 105–124). Washington, DC: American Public Health Association.

Agency for Healthcare Research and Quality. (2016). *Medical Expenditure Panel Survey*. Retrieved from https://meps.ahrq.gov/mepsweb/

Altman, B., & Bernstein, A. (2008). *Disability and health in the United States, 2001–2005*. Hyattsville, MD: National Center for Health Statistics.

Americans With Disabilities Act of 1990, Pub. L. 101-336, 42 U.S.C. §§ 12101—12213 (2000).

Anderson, W. L., Wiener, J. M., Finkelstein, E. A., & Armour, B. S. (2011). Estimates of national health care expenditures associated with disability. *Journal of Disability Policy Studies*, *21*, 230–240. http://dx.doi.org/10.1177/1044207310391407

Andresen, E. M. (2011). Epidemiology and biostatistics. In D. J. Lollar & E. M. Andresen (Eds.), *Public health perspectives on disability* (pp. 15–54). New York, NY: Springer.

Arah, O. A. (2009). On the relationship between individual and population health. *Medicine, Health Care, and Philosophy*, *12*, 235–244. http://dx.doi.org/10.1007/s11019-008-9173-8

Armour, B. S., Courtney-Long, E. A., Fox, M. H., Fredine, H., & Cahill, A. (2016). Prevalence and causes of paralysis—United States, 2013. *American Journal of Public Health*, *106*, 1855–1857. http://dx.doi.org/10.2105/AJPH.2016.303270

Beatty, P. W., Hagglund, K. J., Neri, M. T., Dhont, K. R., Clark, M. J., & Hilton, S. A. (2003). Access to health care services among people with chronic or disabling conditions: Patterns and predictors. *Archives of Physical Medicine and Rehabilitation*, *84*, 1417–1425. http://dx.doi.org/10.1016/S0003-9993(03)00268-5

Birkland, T. A. (2014). *An introduction to the policy process: Theories, concepts and models of public policy-making* (3rd ed.). London, England: Routledge. http://dx.doi.org/10.4324/9781315706399

Brault, M. (2012). *Americans with disabilities: 2010 U.S. Census Bureau*. Washington, DC: U.S. Department of Commerce.

Braveman, P. (2014). What are health disparities and health equity? We need to be clear. *Public Health Reports*, *129*(Suppl. 2), 5–8. http://dx.doi.org/10.1177/00333549141291S203

Carroll, D. D., Courtney-Long, E. A., Stevens, A. C., Sloan, M. L., Lullo, C., Visser, S. N., . . . Centers for Disease Control & Prevention. (2014). Vital signs: Disability and physical activity—United States, 2009–2012. *Morbidity and Mortality Weekly Report*, *63*, 407–413.

Centers for Disease Control and Prevention. (2010, November 12). QuickStats: Delayed or foregone medical care because of cost concerns among adults aged 18–64 years, by disability and health insurance coverage status—National Health Interview Survey, United States, 2009. *Morbidity and Mortality Weekly Report*, *59*, 1456.

Centers for Disease Control and Prevention. (2012, July 27). CDC's vision for public health surveillance in the 21st century. *Morbidity and Mortality Weekly Report*, *61*(Suppl.).

Centers for Disease Control and Prevention. (2015a). *National Survey of Children's Health*. Retrieved from https://www.cdc.gov/nchs/slaits/nsch.htm

Centers for Disease Control and Prevention. (2015b). *National Survey of Children With Special Health Care Needs*. Retrieved from https://www.cdc.gov/nchs/slaits/cshcn.htm

Centers for Disease Control and Prevention. (2016). *Behavior Risk Factor Surveillance System*. Retrieved from https://www.cdc.gov/brfss/

Centers for Disease Control and Prevention. (2017a). *National Health and Nutrition Examination Survey*. Retrieved from https://www.cdc.gov/nchs/nhanes/

Centers for Disease Control and Prevention. (2017b). *National Health Interview Survey*. Retrieved from https://www.cdc.gov/nchs/nhis/

Centers for Medicare & Medicaid. (2015). *The CMS equity plan for improving quality in Medicare*. Retrieved from https://www.cms.gov/About-CMS/Agency-Information/OMH/OMH_Dwnld-CMS_EquityPlanforMedicare_090615.pdf

Courtney-Long, E. A., Carroll, D. D., Zhang, Q. C., Stevens, A. C., Griffin-Blake, S., Armour, B. S., & Campbell, V. A. (2015, July 31). Prevalence of disability and disability type among adults—United States, 2013. *Morbidity and Mortality Weekly Report*, *64*, 777–783. http://dx.doi.org/10.15585/mmwr.MM6429a2

Dixon-Ibarra, A., & Horner-Johnson, W. (2014). Disability status as an antecedent to chronic conditions: National Health Interview Survey, 2006–2012. *Preventing Chronic Disease*, *11*, 130251. http://dx.doi.org/10.5888/pcd11.130251

Dixon-Ibarra, A., Krahn, G., Fredine, H., Cahill, A., & Jenkins, S. (2016). Adults aging "with" and "into" paralysis: Epidemiological analyses of demography and health. *Disability and Health Journal*, *9*, 575–583. http://dx.doi.org/10.1016/j.dhjo.2016.06.003

Drainoni, M. L., Lee-Hood, E., Tobias, C., Bachman, S. S., Andrew, J., & Maisels, L. (2006). Cross-disability experiences of barriers to health-care access: Consumer perspectives. *Journal of Disability Policy Studies*, *17*, 101–115. http://dx.doi.org/10.1177/10442073060170020101

Drum, C. (2009). Models and approaches to disability. In C. Drum, G. Krahn, & H. Bersani (Eds.), *Disability and public health* (pp. 27–44). Washington, DC: American Public Health Association. http://dx.doi.org/10.2105/9780875531915ch03

Einav, L., & Levin, J. D. (2013). *The data revolution and economic analysis*. NBER Working Paper 19035. Cambridge, MA: National Bureau of Economic Research. http://dx.doi.org/10.3386/w19035

Elder, G. H., Jr. (1998). The life course as developmental theory. *Child Development*, *69*, 1–12. http://dx.doi.org/10.1111/j.1467-8624.1998.tb06128.x

Escorpizo, R., Stucki, G., Cieza, A., Davis, K., Stumbo, T., & Riddle, D. L. (2010). Creating an interface between the *International Classification of Functioning, Disability and Health* and physical therapist practice. *Physical*

Therapy, *90*, 1053–1063. http://dx.doi.org/10.2522/ptj.20090326

Fox, M. H., Krahn, G. L., Sinclair, L. B., & Cahill, A. (2015). Using the *International Classification of Functioning, Disability and Health* to expand understanding of paralysis in the United States through improved surveillance. *Disability and Health Journal*, *8*, 457–463. http://dx.doi.org/10.1016/j.dhjo.2015.03.002

Frieden, T. R. (2010). A framework for public health action: The Health Impact Pyramid. *American Journal of Public Health*, *100*, 590–595. http://dx.doi.org/10.2105/AJPH.2009.185652

Gordis, L. (2013). *Epidemiology* (5th ed.). Philadelphia, PA: Elsevier/W.H. Saunders.

Hall, H. I., Correa, A., Yoon, P. W., Braden, C. R., & the Centers for Disease Control and Prevention. (2012, July 27). Lexicon, definitions, and conceptual framework for public health surveillance. *Morbidity and Mortality Weekly Reports*, *61*(3), 10–14.

Hindery, A. I. (2009, January 30). Zip code, race, class trump genetics and health care as predictors of public health. *University of California San Francisco News Center*. Retrieved from https://www.ucsf.edu/news/2009/01/8246/zip-code-may-predict-health-expert-says

Iezzoni, L. I., & Freedman, V. A. (2008). Turning the disability tide: The importance of definitions. *Journal of the American Medical Association*, *299*, 332–334. http://dx.doi.org/10.1001/jama.299.3.332

Institute of Medicine. (1988). *The future of public health*. Washington, DC: The National Academies Press.

Institute of Medicine. (2002). *Unequal treatment: Confronting racial and ethnic disparities in health care*. Washington, DC: The National Academies Press.

Kamper, S. J., Apeldoorn, A. T., Chiarotto, A., Smeets, R. J. E. M., Ostelo, R. W. J. G., Guzman, J., & van Tulder, M. W. (2015). Multidisciplinary biopsychosocial rehabilitation for chronic low back pain: Cochrane Systematic Review and meta-analysis. *British Medical Journal*, *350*, h444. http://dx.doi.org/10.1136/bmj.h444

Kindig, D. A. (2007). Understanding population health terminology. *The Milbank Quarterly*, *85*, 139–161. http://dx.doi.org/10.1111/j.1468-0009.2007.00479.x

Kisser, U., Adderson-Kisser, C., Coenen, M., Stier-Jarmer, M., Becker, S., Sabariego, C., & Harréus, U. (2017). The development of an *ICF*-based clinical guideline and screening tool for the standardized assessment and evaluation of functioning after head and neck cancer treatment. *European Archives of Oto-Rhino-Laryngology*, *274*, 1035–1043. http://dx.doi.org/10.1007/s00405-016-4317-6

Kneipp, S. M., & Yarandi, H. N. (2002). Complex sampling designs and statistical issues in secondary analysis. *Western Journal of Nursing Research*, *24*, 552–566. http://dx.doi.org/10.1177/019394502400446414

Krahn, G. L., Hammond, L., & Turner, A. (2006). A cascade of disparities: Health and health care access for people with intellectual disabilities. *Mental Retardation and Developmental Disabilities Research Reviews*, *12*, 70–82. http://dx.doi.org/10.1002/mrdd.20098

Krahn, G. L., Walker, D. K., & Correa-de-Araujo, R. (2015). Persons with disabilities as an unrecognized health disparity population. *American Journal of Public Health*, *105*(Suppl. 2), S198–S206. http://dx.doi.org/10.2105/AJPH.2014.302182

Martin, A., & Lynch, M. (2009). Counting things and people: The practices and politics of counting. *Social Problems*, *56*, 243–266. http://dx.doi.org/10.1525/sp.2009.56.2.243

Molton, I. R., & Jensen, M. P. (2010). Aging and disability: Biopsychosocial perspectives. *Physical Medicine and Rehabilitation Clinics of North America*, *21*, 253–265. http://dx.doi.org/10.1016/j.pmr.2009.12.012

Monahan, D. J., & Wolf, D. A. (2014). The continuum of disability over the lifespan: The convergence of aging with disability and aging into disability. *Disability and Health Journal*, *7*(Suppl. 1), S1–S3. http://dx.doi.org/10.1016/j.dhjo.2013.10.002

Mudrick, N. R., Breslin, M. L., Liang, M., & Yee, S. (2012). Physical accessibility in primary health care settings: Results from California on-site reviews. *Disability and Health Journal*, *5*, 159–167. http://dx.doi.org/10.1016/j.dhjo.2012.02.002

National Academies of Sciences, Engineering, and Medicine. (2015). *Mental disorders and disabilities among low-income children*. Washington, DC: The National Academies Press.

National Academies of Sciences, Engineering, and Medicine. (2016). *Speech and language disorders in children: Implications for the Social Security Administration's Supplemental Security Income program*. Washington, DC: The National Academies Press.

National Council on Disability. (2009). *The current state of health care for people with disabilities*. Retrieved from http://www.ncd.gov/publications/2009/Sept302009

National Spinal Cord Injury Statistical Center. (2012). *Spinal cord injury facts and figures at a glance*. Retrieved from https://www.nscisc.uab.edu/PublicDocuments/fact_figures_docs/Facts%202012%20Feb%20Final.pdf

Oliver, K., Innvar, S., Lorenc, T., Woodman, J., & Thomas, J. (2014). A systematic review of barriers to and facilitators of the use of evidence by policymakers. *BMC Health Services Research*, *14*, 2. http://dx.doi.org/10.1186/1472-6963-14-2.

Patient Protection and Affordable Care Act, Pub. L. 111-148, 42 U.S.C. §§ 18001—18121 (2010).

Porta, M. S. (2014). *A dictionary of epidemiology* (6th ed.). New York, NY: Oxford University Press.

Putnam, M., Molton, I. R., Truitt, A. R., Smith, A. E., & Jensen, M. P. (2016). Measures of aging with disability in U.S. secondary data sets: Results of a scoping review. *Disability and Health Journal, 9*, 5–10. http://dx.doi.org/10.1016/j.dhjo.2015.07.002

Rauch, A., Cieza, A., & Stucki, G. (2008). How to apply the *International Classification of Functioning, Disability and Health (ICF)* for rehabilitation management in clinical practice. *European Journal of Physical and Rehabilitation Medicine, 44*, 329–342.

Ravesloot, C., Seekins, T., Traci, M., Boehm, T., White, G., Witten, M. H., . . . Monson, J. (2016, February 12). Living Well with a Disability, a self-management program. *Morbidity and Mortality Weekly Report, 65*, 61–67. http://dx.doi.org/10.15585/mmwr.su6501a10

Ravesloot, C., Seekins, T., & White, G. (2005). Living Well with a Disability health promotion intervention: Improved health status for consumers and lower costs for health care policymakers. *Rehabilitation Psychology, 50*, 239–245. http://dx.doi.org/10.1037/0090-5550.50.3.239

Reichard, A., Stransky, M., Phillips, K., Drum, C., & McClain, M. (2015). Does type of disability matter to public health policy and practice? *Californian Journal of Health Promotion, 13*, 25–36.

Salomon, J. A., Wang, H., Freeman, M. K., Vos, T., Flaxman, A. D., Lopez, A. D., & Murray, C. J. L. (2012). Healthy life expectancy for 187 countries, 1990–2010: A systematic analysis for the Global Burden Disease Study 2010. *The Lancet, 380*, 2144–2162. http://dx.doi.org/10.1016/S0140-6736(12)61690-0

Smith, A. K., Ayanian, J. Z., Covinsky, K. E., Landon, B. E., McCarthy, E. P., Wee, C. C., & Steinman, M. A. (2011). Conducting high-value secondary dataset analysis: An introductory guide and resources. *Journal of General Internal Medicine, 26*, 920–929. http://dx.doi.org/10.1007/s11606-010-1621-5

Stark, C. R., & Mantel, N. (1966). Effects of maternal age and birth order on the risk of mongolism and leukemia. *Journal of the National Cancer Institute, 37*, 687–698.

Steiner, W. A., Ryser, L., Huber, E., Uebelhart, D., Aeschlimann, A., & Stucki, G. (2002). Use of the *ICF* model as a clinical problem-solving tool in physical therapy and rehabilitation medicine. *Physical Therapy, 82*, 1098–1107.

Stevens, A. C., Courtney-Long, E. A., Okoro, C. A., & Carroll, D. D. (2016). Comparison of 2 disability measures, Behavioral Risk Factor Surveillance System, 2013. *Preventing Chronic Disease, 13*, 160080. http://dx.doi.org/10.5888/pcd13.160080

Thacker, S. B., Qualters, J. R., Lee, L. M., & Centers for Disease Control and Prevention. (2012, July 27). Public health surveillance in the United States: Evolution and challenges. *Morbidity and Mortality Weekly Report, 61*(Suppl.), 3–9.

United Nations. (2006). Convention on the Rights of Persons With Disabilities. Retrieved from https://www.un.org/development/desa/disabilities/convention-on-the-rights-of-persons-with-disabilities.html

U.S. Census Bureau. (2017). *American Community Survey (ACS)*. Retrieved from https://www.census.gov/programs-surveys/acs/

U.S. Department of Health and Human Services. (2001). *Healthy People 2010, Objective Report* (p. 20). Atlanta, GA: Disability and Secondary Conditions.

U.S. Department of Health and Human Services. (2011a). *Healthy People 2020*. Washington, DC: Author.

U.S. Department of Health and Human Services. (2011b). *Implementation guidance on data collection standards for race, ethnicity, sex, primary language, and disability status*. Retrieved from https://aspe.hhs.gov/basic-report/hhs-implementation-guidance-data-collection-standards-race-ethnicity-sex-primary-language-and-disability-status

U.S. Department of Health and Human Services. (2018). *About Healthy People*. Retrieved from https://www.healthypeople.gov/2020/About-Healthy-People

Üstün, T. B., Chatterji, S., Villanueva, M., Bendib, L., Çelik, C., Sadana, R., . . . Murray, C. J. L. (2001). *WHO Multi-Country Survey Study on Health and Responsiveness*. GPE Discussion Paper No. 37, World Health Organization. Geneva, Switzerland: World Health Organization. Retrieved from http://www.who.int/healthinfo/survey/whspaper37.pdf

World Health Organization. (n.d.-a). *Health Impact Assessment—Glossary of terms used*. Retrieved from http://www.who.int/hia/about/glos/en/index.html

World Health Organization. (n.d.-b). *About social determinants of health*. Retrieved from http://www.who.int/social_determinants/sdh_definition/en/

World Health Organization. (n.d.-c). Constitution of WHO: Principles. Retrieved from http://www.who.int/about/mission/en/

World Health Organization. (2001). *International classification of functioning, disability and health*. Geneva, Switzerland: Author.

World Health Organization & World Bank. (2011). *World report on disability*. Geneva, Switzerland: Author.

CHAPTER 9

ONLY CONNECT: THE SOCIAL PSYCHOLOGY OF DISABILITY

Dana S. Dunn

Only connect!
—*E. M. Forster* (1910/1989, p. 195)

> There is general agreement in the literature on physical disability that the problems of the handicapped are not physical, but social and psychological.
> —*Lee Meyerson* (1948, p. 2)

As I finished writing this chapter, a colleague told me a brief story. She took a friend to an oncology appointment at a doctor's office. They noticed a husband and wife in the waiting room. The husband, who used a wheelchair, looked somewhat frail. He and his wife sat next to each other, and he leaned into her, resting his head on her shoulder. She then rested her head on his. A little while later, they were called into an examination room. My colleague went to the restroom and passed the room where the couple was speaking with the doctor. She overheard the doctor ask, "How are you feeling?" and then heard the wife respond, "I'm doing okay." My colleague was surprised that the wife, not the disabled husband, was the patient. She sheepishly told me the story. Examples like this illustrate how easily our presumptions guide our social inferences. We often assume disability is associated with other pathology—that the person who needs medical help must be the one with an apparent disability rather than a nondisabled spouse.

As this anecdote illustrates, social life is inherently subjective. We believe we know ourselves well (although empirical evidence indicates otherwise; e.g., Helzer & Dunning, 2012; Wilson, 2002) and spend much of our psychological energies trying to understand other people, their feelings, beliefs, and intentions, as well as the rationale for their actions (e.g., Malle, 2011). Where disability is concerned, a particular social puzzle emerges: Nondisabled people often presume what the experience of disability must be like (i.e., primarily negative), whereas disabled persons know that disability is but one aspect of their lives and by no means necessarily the most important one. In effect, people with disabilities (PWDs) and nondisabled persons often fail to connect with one another in the course of social life. Understanding the dynamics of the social psychology of disability can enable rehabilitation and other professional psychologists, as well as interested laypersons, family members, and friends, to connect with PWDs in constructive, meaningful ways (and vice versa).

DEFINING THE SOCIAL PSYCHOLOGY OF DISABILITY

What does it mean to be disabled or to have a disability? Is disability a quality that is embodied, that is, something tied to a given person or persons? Or is disability something that is linked to the

http://dx.doi.org/10.1037/0000129-010
Handbook of Rehabilitation Psychology, Third Edition, L. A. Brenner, S. A. Reid-Arndt, T. R. Elliott, R. G. Frank, and B. Caplan (Editors-in-Chief)

nature of situations in which people find themselves? Answers to these and related questions are provided by the area of research known as the social psychology of disability (Dunn, 2015). Research on this topic examines the various psychological processes, including perception, emotion, cognition, judgment, and behavior, that influence the attitudes and actions of PWDs and those individuals they encounter in the course of daily life (Dunn, 2010).

The social psychology of disability is an important topic within rehabilitation psychology because it characterizes the quality and nature of social expectations of, as well as exchanges between, disabled and nondisabled persons. Nondisabled bystanders often erroneously infer the presence of certain personality or character traits when seeing a person with a disability (e.g., warmth; Fiske, 2011). At the same time, these bystanders may believe that feelings of pity or sympathy are appropriate, reactions that PWDs might not welcome. Disability, whether it's physical, intellectual, emotional, or cognitive, represents difference—or, more specifically, perceived difference—from nondisabled individuals' perspectives. Differences like disability elicit curiosity in some people; others respond with uncertainty, anxiety, fear, or even disgust. As a result, nondisabled people, including strangers, acquaintances, friends, even family members and health care professionals, often are unsure how best to engage PWDs. Should they ignore or comment on a disability, for example? Is it best to offer a disabled person assistance or to wait to be asked for help? Worse still, could an innocent offer of aid or a friendly overture be misconstrued as condescending or even infantilizing?

The social psychology of disability also is concerned with the experience of PWDs: How do they think about themselves? What role does disability play, if any, in their identities? To what degree does a disability affect daily life? Is disability something to be celebrated, tolerated, or ignored? How do PWDs relate to other PWDs versus nondisabled individuals? How do disabled persons navigate both their physical and social environments?

The remainder of this chapter examines the shared history of social psychology and rehabilitation psychology, highlighting the contributions of Kurt Lewin and two of his students who pursued the study of disability, Tamara Dembo, and Beatrice A. Wright. The focus then shifts to examining key social psychological constructs that promote understanding of the experience of disability. The chapter closes by considering an emerging topic—disability identity—and its potential importance for the social psychology of disability.

SOCIAL PSYCHOLOGY AND REHABILITATION PSYCHOLOGY: SHARED HISTORY, SHARED THEORY

Social psychology and rehabilitation psychology share a common ancestry due to the theoretical orientation of Kurt Lewin (1890–1947), the German American social psychologist who emigrated to the United States in 1933 (Marrow, 1977; see also Dunn, 2011). Contrary to everyday intuition, Lewin argued that people's behaviors are not due to themselves alone, that is, as a result of personality traits or particular self-motivations. Instead, Lewin suggested that behavior is a function of both people and the situations in which they find themselves. Neither those psychological forces routinely attributed to nature (e.g., intelligence, personality traits) nor nurture (e.g., physical settings, experiences in the social world) can completely explain why people act as they do. To be sure, personal and situational factors can affect behavior, but Lewin claimed that it is the interaction between these two forces that shapes the unique behavioral choices and outcomes of each individual.

Thus, Lewin (1935) proposed a field theory wherein behavior is a function of both the person and the psychological environment—or what he referred to as the person's *life space*. Indeed, he even developed a quasimathematical equation to explain his idea, where $B = f(P, E)$, or behavior is a function of the person and his or her perceived environment. Lewin was trained in the tradition of Gestalt psychology so that he viewed social perception as holistic, not elemental, and inherently subjective rather than objective. For this reason, an individual's own interpretation of the social world (via cognition) and the possession of strength to act (via motivation) also are important factors that influence behavioral outcomes.

Both social psychology and rehabilitation psychology embrace the idea that observers downplay the importance of situational influences (e.g., social norms, physical boundaries) by focusing on what they see as an actor's perceived qualities, such as a disposition, a disability, a cognitive impairment, or a combination of these things, that are presumed to drive his or her actions. As Lewin knew, other people's behaviors draw our attention so strongly that we neglect to attend to the influence of situational constraints on behavioral outcomes. Behavior is so salient that it "engulfs" a social perceiver's field of view—any situational factors generally are overlooked. As a result, we often make inferences about the causes of people's behavior in ways that emphasize their origins as being linked to underlying psychological characteristics or, in the case of some disabilities, as some embodied feature. In effect, Lewin's person–environment relation means that although our actions are due to what we bring to situations and the situations themselves, outside observers will see our behavior as governed largely by presumed internal qualities, such as traits (see Nisbett, 1980; Ross & Nisbett, 1991).

The social construal of the source or particular cause of behavior is the province of attribution theory (Heider, 1958). For their part, attribution theorists in social psychology explored—largely in research that was conducted in the 1970s and 1980s—how people overlook situational influences. One prominent line of inquiry examined what is known as the *actor-observer difference* in which actors—those behaving—explain their actions by identifying situational influences over personal ones (e.g., an individual knows his frustration at waiting in line is due to fatigue, not impatience). In contrast, following Lewin, observers see personality traits and other individuated qualities as being the drivers of behavior (e.g., an observer sees the person have words with an airline ticketing agent, attributing the behavior to an impatient disposition rather than fatigue; see Jones & Nisbett, 1971).

Social psychologist Lee Ross (1977) coined the term *fundamental attribution error* to characterize social observers' choices of personal attributions over situational ones to explain an actors' behaviors (see also, Gilbert & Malone, 1995). Pettigrew (2001) extended this construct by arguing that intergroup prejudice represents an *ultimate attribution error* when ingroup members believe that negative behaviors exhibited by outgroup members are dispositionally, and possibly even genetically, based. Naturally, both the fundamental attribution error and the ultimate attribution error can be called on to explain nondisabled individuals' reactions to disabled persons, whether the attributions in question are positively (e.g., "Disabled people are fighters!") or negatively (e.g., "People in wheelchairs expect special treatment") valenced. Such attributions tend to be negative; what some nondisabled observers believe is positive might not be received that way by a PWD.

Specific Attributional Strategies Tied to Disability

Two of Lewin's students, Tamara Dembo (1902–1993) and Beatrice A. Wright (1917–2018), identified two related attributional strategies that clarify the nature and often the reason for observers' conclusions regarding disability. Building on Lewin's person–environment relation, Dembo (1964, 1970, 1982) created a distinction between *insiders,* those who have a disability and truly know what that experience is like, and *outsiders,* those who are compelled to imagine what the experience of disability must be like (most outsiders are nondisabled, but Dembo's analysis also means that one PWD is effectively an outsider to the disability experience of another PWD). Conceptually related to the actor-observer effect, the insider-outsider distinction is important because it explains why outsiders presume that either congenital or acquired disabilities are negative or disruptive to daily life and must be defining for those affected. Unless prompted to do so, outsiders are unlikely to view disability as one quality among the many in a given person's life and instead are prone to think of disability as an ongoing and troublesome preoccupation.

Dembo (1964) pointed out that although outsiders project their presumptions onto PWDs, insiders are intimate with the experience of disability and know its presence does not necessarily predict quality of life or affect their well-being. Disability is one life quality that takes its place alongside many others, including physical and mental health, stress, career, recreational interests, and role as friend, spouse, parent, or volunteer (see Duggan & Dijkers, 2001). More to the point, disability only becomes a focus for insiders when outsiders or environmental constraints (e.g., lack of curb cuts, ramps, Braille signage) render it salient. Otherwise, as is discussed later in this chapter, disability may be an important aspect of insiders' identities, which means it is more of a positive than a negative quality (Dunn, 2015; Dunn & Burcaw, 2013). Indeed, there is some evidence that outsiders can be encouraged to adopt an insider perspective on their own perceived disabilities (broadly defined), thereby becoming more open-minded about disability as an aspect of other people's identities or their lives in general (Dunn, Fisher, & Beard, 2012).

Building on the insider-outside distinction, especially perceivers' neglect of environmental influences, led Wright (1988) to posit what she called the *fundamental negative bias*. Although individuals falling prey to the Ross's (1977) fundamental attribution error overlook situational factors in favor of perceived personal qualities, Wright noted that where disability is concerned, observers often bypass available positive information or qualities and instead focus exclusively on a person's presumed negative features.

Imagine the following scenario: A handsome young man using a wheelchair encounters an older woman on the street who smiles, shakes her head, and remarks to him, "Oh, you are much, much too young to be in a wheelchair." Such comments represent the fundamental negative bias because one personal characteristic stands out (the saliency of the wheelchair) and is coded for whatever reason as negative (value), and the setting in which it operates is vague, sparse, or otherwise poorly defined (context). Wright (1991) believed that context influences meaning, or, as she argued, "Context can refer to conditions external to the perceiver or to intrapsychic predispositions of various sorts" (p. 471). When the three criteria are satisfied, the negative value attached to the target person (here, the young man with the disability) will drive perceptions, thoughts, and feelings to match its negative character. The apparently innocent comment regarding being young and having to use a wheelchair actually contains a value judgment—young people don't use wheelchairs—and, beyond that, is the implication that they should not have disabilities either.

Thus, the fundamental negative bias intensifies the magnitude of whatever negative characteristics observers distinguish during social encounters. In the case of the current example, the observer seems to convey a belief that young people should navigate the physical environment only by walking upright. Other social psychological research supports the regrettably persuasive power of negative information: As Baumeister, Bratslavsky, Finkenauer, and Vohs (2001) demonstrated, "bad is stronger than good" (p. 323) in that perceived negative qualities routinely muffle the impact of any available positive information. In turn, the extensive literature concerning nondisabled individuals' attitudes towards disabled persons can be summarized readily: In the main, such attitudes are negative or, at best, ambivalent (Chan, Livneh, Pruett, Wang, & Zheng, 2009; Dunn, 2015; Vilchinsky, Findler, & Werner, 2010).

Countering Negative Views Using Foundational Principles of Rehabilitation

Besides developing attributional analyses applicable to disability, the work of Lewin, Dembo, Wright, and other rehabilitation psychologists has led to the recognition that a set of principles should guide empirical research, theory, and practice in rehabilitation psychology (e.g., the value-laden beliefs and principles for rehabilitation psychology; see Wright, 1972, 1983). More recently, such principles have been codified and referred to as the *foundational principles* (see Dunn, Ehde, & Wegener, 2016). Exhibit 9.1 lists the six core principles that clearly entail points of view hailing from rehabilitation psychology and social psychology. I refer back to some of these principles in the next section of this chapter, which reviews social psychological constructs that promote an understanding of disability and foster connections between disabled and nondisabled persons.

EXHIBIT 9.1

Foundational Principles of Rehabilitation Psychology

- *Person–environment relation:* Attributions about people with disabilities tend to focus on presumed dispositional rather than available situational characteristics. Environmental constraints usually matter more than personality factors to living with a disability.
- *Insider–outsider distinction:* People with disabilities (*insiders*) know what life with a chronic condition is like (e.g., sometimes challenging but usually manageable), whereas casual observers (*outsiders*) who lack relevant experience presume that disability is defining, all encompassing, and decidedly negative.
- *Adjustment to disability:* Coping with a disability or chronic illness is an ongoing dynamic process that is dependent on making constructive changes to the social and the physical environment.
- *Psychosocial assets:* People with disabilities possess or can acquire personal or psychological qualities that can ameliorate challenges posed by disability and also enrich daily living.
- *Self-perception of bodily states:* Experience of bodily states (e.g., pain, fatigue, distress) is based on people's perceptions of the phenomena, not exclusively the actual sensations. Changing attitudes, expectations, or environmental conditions can constructively alter perceptions.
- *Human dignity:* Regardless of the source or severity of a disability or chronic health condition, all people deserve respect, encouragement, and to be treated with dignity.

Note. Adapted from "The Foundational Principles as Psychological Lodestars: Theoretical Inspiration and Empirical Direction in Rehabilitation Psychology," by D. S. Dunn, D. M. Ehde, and S. T. Wegener, 2016, *Rehabilitation Psychology, 61,* p. 2. Copyright 2016 by the American Psychological Association.

SOCIAL PSYCHOLOGICAL CONSTRUCTS: UNDERSTANDING THE EXPERIENCE OF DISABILITY

In this section, I review social psychological constructs that augment the insider–outsider distinction and the fundamental negative bias and connect to the foundational principles. The discussion begins with the *somatopsychological relation,* which ties people's bodies to the social and psychological spaces they explore.

The Somatopsychological Relation

An important assumption within rehabilitation psychology is that people's physiques are inherently tied to their self-images, the execution of daily activities, and the character and quality of their social interactions with others. Rehabilitation psychologists encourage clients to carry out daily routines, navigate familiar and unfamiliar settings, and engage with others while managing outsider curiosity concerning their mental or physical disabilities, viable goals that should replace the need for their bodies to meet some set of expectations or standard of performance. According to the social psychology of disability (Barker, Wright, Meyerson, & Gonick, 1953; Wright, 1983), this somatopsychological relation influences people's psychology to a greater degree than any psychosomatic connection between other physical or organic disorders. As a result, any adjustment to disability, whether challenging or relatively easy, should not be attributed to the disability per se; instead, it should be seen as being influenced by the individuals and their physical, social, and psychological environments (see also Lewin, 1935). As noted in Exhibit 9.1, how PWDs experience their bodily states is largely a matter of perception, not necessarily actual sensations, which means that their expectations and beliefs as well as changes to their environments can be the means to alter their self-observations and conclusions.

Deindividuation, Individuation, and Labeling

One of social psychology's lessons is that people not only participate in groups but observers often see them as belonging to particular groups. Such social categorization can have its downsides when a person is perceived as part of a homogeneous group (e.g., "amputees") and not as an individual ("Irene, whose leg was amputated"). Considerable research has demonstrated that outgroup members (here, amputees or possibly any disabled person) are not only seen as all being similar to one another (i.e., "They're all alike") but are simultaneously perceived to be distinctly different from ad hoc ingroup members (here, nondisabled people), who, in turn, are characterized as heterogeneous. The results of this *deindividuation,* or the consolidation and distorting reduction of another's identity, includes showing favoritism to ingroup members while potentially derogating outgroup members (e.g., Hewstone, Rubin, & Willis, 2002).

Wright (1983, 1991) and other rehabilitation psychologists have advocated using person-first language constructions to promote individuation over a focus on group membership based on disability status. As a result, researchers and practitioners often write and speak of "persons with disabilities" rather than "the disabled" or "the handicapped" (indeed, the American Psychological Association, 2010, advocates person-first language for written and oral presentations; but see Dunn & Andrews, 2015). Similarly, people are not equated with or labeled by their disabilities, physical states, or medical diagnoses or prognoses; one is a "person who had a stroke" and never a "stroke patient" or, worse, a "stroke victim." As discussed earlier, negative information ("Zaha uses a prong cane") is more salient, memorable, and influential in subsequent social judgments than is positive information ("Zaha is a talented real estate broker"). For this reason, monolithic language and labels should be avoided in favor of descriptions or referents that promote dignity, worth, collaboration, and self-reliance in the rehabilitative process. Similarly, rehabilitation professionals routinely refer to PWDs using active terms, such as *clients* and *consumers* rather than with passive descriptions like *patients* (Dunn & Elliott, 2005).

Among members of disability culture and the disabilities studies communities (e.g., Brueggemann, 2013), however, arguments suggest that PWDs should claim disability—and, at times, even rely on pejorative labels and epithets (e.g., "crip") once used by outsiders to characterize disabled persons (e.g., Johnson, 2005)—by using *identity-first language* in place of person-first constructions (Dunn & Andrews, 2015). Identity-first language encourages use of phrases like "amputee," "diabetic," and "disabled person" in which disability identity comes first (labels like "victim" are still avoided). The supporting argument is straightforward: Using such honest, candid, and less euphemistic terms and phrases enables groups and the individuals within them to "claim" their disabilities with pride. As a social process, claiming can be about disability in general or in terms of highlighting a particular disability. By doing so, disabled individuals intentionally select an identity rather than allowing others—even well-meaning family, friends, and rehabilitation professionals—to do so for them.

Besides promoting autonomy, adopting an identity-first approach rather than a person-first approach can counter the criticism that the person-first linguistic approach sometimes can be seen as implying that there is something inherently negative about disability (Dunn & Andrews, 2015). Consider that the add-on phrase "with a disability," for example, effectively dissociates the disability from the person. Disabled people who choose identity-first language claim and celebrate, rather than distance themselves, from their disabilities. Furthermore, particular groups within the disability community have already established their language preferences. The National Federation of the Blind (1993) has long touted the use of identity-first language, preferring "blind person" in lieu of person-first constructions like "individual with blindness" or "person who is blind." Members of Deaf culture want their label to be capitalized with a *D*, which is a means for establishing unity and community (Solomon, 2012).

But what if you are not sure what to call PWDs or how to refer to them? How should nondisabled people refer to disabled persons? Dunn and Andrews (2015) recommended that all psychologists, not only rehabilitation professionals, develop cultural competence where disability language is concerned. Evolving language for disability can pose challenges because no one wants to offend or be insensitive to others. A reasonable accommodation is to use person-first and identity-first language interchangeably unless or until a given situation indicates one is clearly preferred. Following American Psychological Association (2010) guidance, too, calling people what they prefer to be called is a good solution. Discerning preference is not always easy; one individual with dwarfism might like to be referred to as a "dwarf," whereas another might prefer being called a "person with dwarfism." Asking people about their preference is always a good approach as is emphasizing possible qualities they possess or could (re)learn.

Existing or Potential Assets

Whether congenital or acquired, the presence and severity of any disability does not affect a person's opportunity to retain or develop psychosocial *assets*. Assets, which represent a foundational principle (see Exhibit 9.1), comprise the variety of real, perceived, or potential resources available to any person, including self-concept or identity; strengths or personal qualities; educational, professional, social, or even physical abilities; and work or career-linked talents. Some assets are apparent, such as social support from family, friends, and colleagues, as well as household income. Other assets are achieved or attained (e.g., degree, job title, honors, awards), imagined (e.g., goals), and psychological, for example, one's personality (e.g., optimistic, conscientious) or motivational qualities (e.g., self-discipline, tenacity). Even hobbies (e.g., collecting baseball cards, reading historical fiction), esoteric knowledge (e.g., Confederate Civil War generals), and more community-based activities (e.g., volunteering, blogging) can represent assets (for a broader discussion of assets, including more examples, see Dunn, 2015).

Emphasis should not be placed on the loss of assets or a lost asset (i.e., never being able to do *X* again in the future). Doing so is counterproductive and potentially dispiriting, not constructive. Instead, PWDs should be encouraged to reclaim interests or to develop new ones, which may entail a change in frames of reference and even values (e.g., Keany & Glueckauf, 1993). An asset points to something that has already been accomplished or as something that can be done by a PWD in the future. Thus, as a motivational resource, assets promote resilience (Craig, 2012) and encourage PWDs to thrive within their particularly situations. For this reason, rehabilitation professionals, health care providers, family, and friends should encourage the maintenance of interests or the cultivation of new ones. Character strengths and virtues, such as curiosity, forgiveness, and gratitude, which can be learned (Peterson & Seligman, 2004), also can serve as assets and promote well-being (Peterson & Park, 2011) and a meaningful life (Peterson & Park, 2012). Emphasizing assets can promote positive attitudes toward the self, but how should nondisabled people's attitudes toward PWDs be characterized?

Attitudinal Consequences of Disability

Attitudes represent people's likes and dislikes (Bem, 1970). In the main, nondisabled people's attitudes toward disabled individuals tend to be negative (e.g., Chan et al., 2009; Vilchinsky et al., 2010) or ambivalent, that is, a mix of positive and negative reactions (e.g., Barker et al., 1953). Based on research conducted with other diverse groups (e.g., Pettigrew & Tropp, 2008; Tropp & Mallett, 2011), positive attitudes are most likely to occur based on meaningful, constructive, and personal encounters between PWDs and nondisabled individuals (see also, Mason, Pratt, Patel, Greydanus, & Yahya, 2004). At present, however, there is no comprehensive review that has provided evidence for the effectiveness of the contact hypothesis where disability is concerned. Space constraints prohibit a review of the relevant but voluminous literature on attitudes. Instead, the focus here is on three consequences related to negative or ambivalent attitudes: stigma, the just world hypothesis, and the requirement of mourning.

Stigma. A *stigma* is any attribute or identity quality that others perceive to be negative within some context or culture (Corrigan, 2014; Goffman, 1963). Disability is recognized as a stigmatizing condition, a social marker indicating that PWDs are different and distinct from others in some usually apparent way. Although stigma is attributed to a myriad of causes, including low self-esteem and authoritarian tendencies (e.g., Adorno, Frenkel-Brunswik, Levinson, & Sanford, 1950; Fein & Spencer, 1997), contemporary accounts have suggested that stigmatizing reactions are due primarily to normative psychological processes (Dovidio, Pagotto, & Hebl, 2011). In effect, social perceivers categorize other people quickly and efficiently into groups (e.g., "like me" vs. "not like me," "foreign" vs. "familiar"; Macrae & Bodenhausen, 2001), enabling prejudiced attitudes, stereotypes, and the potential for indifferent or even discriminatory behavior to follow.

Social psychologist Gordon Allport (1954) advanced the idea that such categorization is a necessary part of social life and that the resulting ingroups and outgroups guide subsequent social interactions (see also, Fiske, 2005, on the normality of prejudgment due to categorization). The social challenge, of course, is that perceived similarities among outgroup members are amplified in the minds of the ingroup, often as negative, character-based traits or presumed faults (also referred to as the *outgroup homogeneity effect*; see, e.g., Boldry, Gaertner, & Quinn, 2007). At the same time, ingroup members see themselves and their peers as distinct, different from one another, and possessing positive character-based traits. Thus, the presence of a stigma like disability serves as an inferential, if oversimplified, trigger for thoughts, beliefs, expectations, and behaviors toward PWDs.

The just world hypothesis and the requirement of mourning. When a disability serves as a stigma trigger, one prominent social psychological theory that can explain negative reactions is the *just world hypothesis* (Lerner, 1980). If good things are anticipated to happen to good people, then when bad things befall some individuals, they must somehow be deserving of their fate. To maintain a consistent and placid view of the world (and, importantly, their place in it), nondisabled people must devalue, perhaps even derogate or blame, PWDs for being disabled ("That's what you get if you swim where you don't know how deep the water is," "It's his own fault he damaged his spinal cord"). In a recent examination of the influence of this and other injustice appraisals made by PWDs and their potential impact on rehabilitation outcomes, Monden, Trost, Scott, Bogart, and Driver (2016) suggested that just world beliefs generated by insiders, too, can have implications for psychosocial adjustment.

A conceptual relative of the just world hypothesis is the *requirement of mourning* (Dembo, Leviton, & Wright, 1956), a classic construct identified in the disability literature. In brief, when outsiders feel compelled to protect their cherished beliefs and values, they often behave as if those they deem to be unfortunate must necessarily be suffering—even when no signs of distress or upset are apparent on the part of the insider or insiders. When such suffering is missing, then a social script is being ignored; to "right" matters, outsiders must devalue or blame the target person because he or she should be anguished but, for whatever reason, is not. Thus, a nondisabled observer might presume that an individual with muscular dystrophy who appears to be happy and content must be dissembling ("Why is she pretending everything is fine when it can't possibly be? She can barely move!"). Considering an alternative possibility, for example, that disability does not represent ongoing loss is cognitively challenging because outsiders believe that all losses—whether physical, financial, mental, social (power, opportunity), or whatever—must be mourned (Vash & Crewe, 2004; for a more detailed discussion of the requirement of mourning, see Wright, 1983).

An additional reflection on attitudes toward disability: Not all are negative nor are they the result of stigma and stereotyping or other social psychology phenomena. Instead, some people attribute highly favorable and positive qualities to disabled persons because they assume that coping with a cognitive, physical, or even psychiatric disability must require great wherewithal or strength, and even may be indicative of outstanding personal success (e.g., Wright, 1983). The problem with such conclusions is that they represent mirror-image distortions that overemphasize disability compared with a person's other characteristics and abilities (Yuker, 1994). Coding disability as somehow ennobling is still simplifying a person's situation; PWDs may not wish to be characterized as either saints or victims (Fine & Asch, 1988; Wright, 1983). Instead of being put on a pedestal for "being brave"—however they came to terms with their situation—they likely would prefer to be treated like everyone else.

Adapting to, Adjusting to, and Accepting Disability

Rehabilitation psychologists are careful to draw distinctions among terms used to advance how and whether PWDs come to terms with disability (for a detailed review, see Smedana, Bakken-Gillen, & Dalton, 2009). Terms like *adapting to, adjusting to,* and *accepting* disability are applicable primarily to people with acquired disabilities, that is, following an accident, chronic illness, or some other acute event. In contrast, individuals with congenital disabilities do not know life without their disability; they do not have to adapt or adjust to their circumstance—they have not experienced any other state of being (Dunn, 2015).

Among people with acquired disabilities, disability onset leads the affected to start a process of psychosocial adaptation, that is, gradually understanding and integrating the disability into their sense of self, identity, body image, and daily life (recall the earlier discussion of somatopsychology). *Adaptation* is used to characterize the dynamic, ongoing somatopsychological process that PWDs experience as they move toward the idealized state of *adjustment* (Livneh & Antonak, 1997). Psychosocial adjustment to disability is reached once a person is satisfied with his or her own person–environment relation, whereby any loss or bodily changes are no longer preoccupations, and the person concentrates on his or her existing assets or potential abilities and what can be accomplished moving forward in time (Wright, 1983). Rehabilitation professionals argue that adjustment is indicated by an established connection between how a PWD sees his or her subjective experience and the actual external environment (Livneh & Antonak, 1997; Roessler & Bolton, 1978) based on criteria like those shown in Exhibit 9.2. Based on such criteria, some PWDs will adjust to their situations with greater ease than others, just as some will adapt more readily than others.

EXHIBIT 9.2

Qualities Demonstrating Psychosocial Adjustment to Disability

- Presence of positive self-concept and self-esteem
- Capability of navigating physical and social environments
- Belief in personal mastery
- Frequent engagement with vocational, social, and leisure activities
- Independent attitude
- Demonstrated active problem-solving skills relevant to daily living
- Demonstrated awareness of existing and potential assets, and any functional limitations

The *acceptance* of disability occurs when the disability or chronic illness becomes a part of the person's self-concept (Wright, 1983). In Wright's view, acceptance occurs when a PWD views the disability as a *nondevaluing outcome,* something that does not reduce self-worth, future opportunities or potential, or the general psychosocial performance of the person. Thus, acceptance is not resignation, hiding, or covering the disability in an attempt to "pass" as nondisabled, or trying to achieve a sense of normality. Rather, acceptance is marked by perspective: seeing things as they really are regarding disability and continuing to "improve the improvable" (Wright, 1983, p. 159).

FUTURE DIRECTIONS: EXPLORING DISABILITY IDENTITY

One way to characterize much of the social psychological literature pertaining to disability is by emphasizing the person–environment relation and related psychosocial constructs, highlighting the limited social connections that can occur between PWDs and nondisabled people. The challenge for researchers and practitioners is to recognize that much of the focus on the social experience of PWDs has emphasized negative issues. Research on the positive psychology of disability is an obvious and fruitful alternative (e.g., Dunn & Dougherty, 2005; Dunn, Uswatte, Elliott, Lastres, & Beard, 2013; Ehde, 2010; Wehmeyer, 2013). However, where the social psychology of disability is concerned, exploring the potential importance of disability identity is apt to be of great interest. After all, identities allow people to share their individuality, to make sense of themselves, and to connect with other individuals and even groups (Oyserman, Elmore, & Smith, 2012).

Disability identity entails those positive, beneficial self-beliefs that PWDs hold where their disabilities are concerned, as well as connections they may have to other members of the disability community (e.g., Dunn & Burcaw, 2013; Gill, 1997). Because adaptation, adjustment, and acceptance can vary among PWDs, the extent of development of a given person's disability identity will fall along a continuum (Dunn, 2015). People who feel close to the disability community and view their disability with some pride likely will possess a moderate to high level of identification, whereas people who are actively trying to advance disability rights by seeking economic, social, and political gains should have a high level of identity. Someone with a few friends who are disabled but who is not active in wider disability circles would have a moderate level of disability identity. In turn, people with low or no disability identity are those with little or no connection to the disability community or who see their own disability as a source of distraction or distress, or who want to "pass" as nondisabled.

Exhibit 9.3 contains six key themes related to disability identity. *Communal attachment* and *affirmation of disability* (see Exhibit 9.3) suggest that disability identity is rooted in connections with disability culture and affiliations with other PWDs. Moreover, self-affirmation has been identified as an effective coping strategy when it is freely chosen (Silverman, Logel, & Cohen, 2013). The next three aspects of disability identity—*self-worth, pride,* and *discrimination*—are based in research on disability politics and the ongoing struggle in the disability community for civil rights and equality. These three identity qualities also help PWDs in everyday life to deal with hassles, stigma, stereotyping, and the often negatively tainted interactions with nondisabled people. *Personal meaning,* the last entry in Exhibit 9.3, is linked to constructive thinking and coping with the onset and subsequent life with disability; it also can also entail a person's acceptance of his or her disability.

Bogart (2014) explored the role of *disability self-concept*—defined as consisting of disability identity and disability self-efficacy—in which adapting to congenital or acquired disability is concerned. Bogart hypothesized that disability self-concept would be developed to a greater extent among individuals with congenital disabilities so that they, in turn, would report higher levels of life satisfaction compared with those with acquired disabilities. More than 200 participants completed a cross-sectional survey that revealed that self-esteem, disability identity and self-efficacy, and income served as significant predictors of satisfaction with life. However, congenital onset of disability was associated with still higher levels of life satisfaction, and both disability identity and disability self-efficacy—but not self-esteem—partially mediated that relationship. The empirical upshot is that disability self-concept likely plays an important role in promoting and maintaining the well-being of PWDs. As Bogart (2014) suggested, health care professionals would be wise to avoid trying to "normalize" the experience of disability and instead foster disability self-concept through promoting disability pride and connection to the wider disability community (for further discussion of these issues, see Fernández, Branscombe, Gómez, & Morales, 2012; Olkin, 2008).

Subsequent research conducted by Bogart (2015) found that the affirmation of disability identity was associated with protective effects in a sample of PWDs. Specifically, Bogart anticipated that higher levels of disability identity would be associated with lower levels of anxiety and depression in a sample of persons with multiple sclerosis. Participants took part in a cross-sectional online survey that assessed disability identity, depression and anxiety, performance of activities of daily living, duration of multiple sclerosis, and impairment in walking.

EXHIBIT 9.3

Six Key Themes of Disability Identity

- *Communal attachment:* desiring to affiliate with other people with disabilities
- *Affirmation of disability:* holding thoughts, feelings, and beliefs of being part of society and sharing the same rights and responsibilities of other citizens
- *Self-worth:* valuing the self with disability and feeling equal to nondisabled individuals
- *Pride:* feeling proud of identity despite understanding that disability often is viewed by outsiders as being a devalued quality
- *Discrimination:* knowing that being a person with a disability means being a potential recipient of prejudicial thoughts and discriminatory behavior in the course of daily life
- *Personal meaning:* locating significance in, identifying benefits with, and making sense of the experience of disability

Note. Adapted from "Disability Identity: Exploring Narrative Accounts of Disability," by D. S. Dunn and S. Burcaw, 2013, *Rehabilitation Psychology, 58,* pp. 149–151. Copyright 2013 by the American Psychological Association.

Stronger disability identity predicted lower psychological distress linked to multiple sclerosis as did older age and performance of activities of daily living. Rehabilitation practitioners and researchers should consider ways to encourage participation in disability advocacy and support groups while also considering how best to develop interventions aimed at affirming disability identity.

CONCLUSION

Clearly, social psychology has much to contribute toward understanding the experience of disability and the development of successful rehabilitation interventions. Connections between PWDs and nondisabled persons probably can benefit both parties when uncertainty, discomfort, and even threat are reduced. Based on the lessons of social psychology, reduction of both prejudice and anxiety is likely to occur when meaningful, sustained contact is established. Such efforts will require greater attention to social environments and the contextual elements therein, possibly through the creation and development of positive social institutions (e.g., Dunlap, Kincaid, & Jackson, 2013).

At the same time, the promise of research on disability identity is that minimal or modest interventions may promote greater levels of constructive, self-affirmation of disability, which, in turn, may well translate into more relaxed connections between PWDs and nondisabled individuals. As Wright (1983) observed, "The extent of limitations is as much a function of physical and social environmental barriers, if not more so, than of personal disability" (p. 479).

References

Adorno, T. W., Frenkel-Brunswik, E., Levinson, D. J., & Sanford, R. N. (1950). *The authoritarian personality*. New York, NY: Harper.

Allport, G. W. (1954). *The nature of prejudice*. Reading, MA: Addison-Wesley.

American Psychological Association. (2010). *Publication manual of the American Psychological Association* (6th ed.). Washington, DC: Author.

Barker, R. G., Wright, B. A., Meyerson, L., & Gonick, M. R. (1953). *Adjustment to physical handicap and illness: A survey of the social psychology of physique and disability* (2nd ed.). New York, NY: Social Science Research Council.

Baumeister, R. F., Bratslavsky, E., Finkenauer, C., & Vohs, K. D. (2001). Bad is stronger than good. *Review of General Psychology*, *5*, 323–370. http://dx.doi.org/10.1037/1089-2680.5.4.323

Bem, D. J. (1970). *Beliefs, attitudes, and human affairs*. Belmont, CA: Brooks-Cole.

Bogart, K. R. (2014). The role of disability self-concept in adaptation to congenital or acquired disability. *Rehabilitation Psychology, 59,* 107–115. http://dx.doi.org/10.1037/a0035800

Bogart, K. R. (2015). Disability identity predicts lower anxiety and depression in multiple sclerosis. *Rehabilitation Psychology, 60,* 105–109. http://dx.doi.org/10.1037/rep0000029

Boldry, J. G., Gaertner, L., & Quinn, J. (2007). Measuring the measures: A meta-analytic investigation of outgroup homogeneity. *Group Processes & Intergroup Relations, 10,* 157–178. http://dx.doi.org/10.1177/1368430207075153

Brueggemann, B. J. (2013). Disability studies/disability culture. In M. L. Wehmeyer (Ed.), *The Oxford handbook of positive psychology and disability* (pp. 279–299). New York, NY: Oxford University Press.

Chan, F., Livneh, H., Pruett, S., Wang, C.-C., & Zheng, L. X. (2009). Societal attitudes toward disability: Concepts, measurements, and interventions. In F. Chan, E. da Silva Cordoso, & J. A. Chronister (Eds.), *Understanding psychosocial adjustment to chronic illness and disability: A handbook for evidence-based practitioners in rehabilitation* (pp. 333–367). New York, NY: Springer.

Corrigan, P. W. (Ed.). (2014). *The stigma of disease and disability: Understanding causes and overcoming injustices*. Washington, DC: American Psychological Association. http://dx.doi.org/10.1037/14297-000

Craig, A. (2012). Resilience in people with physical disabilities. In P. Kennedy (Ed.), *Oxford handbook of rehabilitation psychology* (pp. 474–491). New York, NY: Oxford University Press.

Dembo, T. (1964). Sensitivity of one person to another. *Rehabilitation Literature*, *25*, 231–235.

Dembo, T. (1970). The utilization of psychological knowledge in rehabilitation. *Welfare in Review*, *8*, 1–7.

Dembo, T. (1982). Some problems in rehabilitation as seen by a Lewinian. *Journal of Social Issues, 38,* 131–139. http://dx.doi.org/10.1111/j.1540-4560.1982.tb00848.x

Dembo, T., Leviton, G. L., & Wright, B. A. (1956). Adjustment to misfortune: A problem of social-psychological rehabilitation. *Artificial Limbs, 3,* 4–62.

Dovidio, J. F., Pagotto, L., & Hebl, M. R. (2011). Implicit attitudes and discrimination against people with physical disabilities. In R. L. Wiener & S. L. Willborn (Eds.), *Disability and age discrimination: Perspectives in law and psychology* (pp. 157–183). New York, NY: Springer. http://dx.doi.org/10.1007/978-1-4419-6293-5_9

Duggan, C. H., & Dijkers, M. (2001). Quality of life after spinal cord injury: A qualitative study. *Rehabilitation Psychology, 46,* 3–27. http://dx.doi.org/10.1037/0090-5550.46.1.3

Dunlap, G., Kincaid, D., & Jackson, D. (2013). Positive behavior support: Foundations, systems, and quality of life. In M. L. Wehmeyer (Ed.), *The Oxford handbook of positive psychology and disability* (pp. 303–316). New York, NY: Oxford University Press.

Dunn, D. S. (2010). The social psychology of disability. In R. G. Frank, B. Caplan, & M. Rosenthal (Eds.), *Handbook of rehabilitation psychology* (2nd ed., pp. 379–390). Washington, DC: American Psychological Association. http://dx.doi.org/10.1037/15972-026

Dunn, D. S. (2011). Situations matter: Teaching the Lewinian link between social psychology and rehabilitation psychology. *History of Psychology, 14,* 405–411. http://dx.doi.org/10.1037/a0023919

Dunn, D. S. (2015). *The social psychology of disability*. New York, NY: Oxford University Press.

Dunn, D. S., & Andrews, E. E. (2015). Person-first *and* identity-first language: Developing psychologists' cultural competence using disability language. *American Psychologist, 70,* 255–264. http://dx.doi.org/10.1037/a0038636

Dunn, D. S., & Burcaw, S. (2013). Disability identity: Exploring narrative accounts of disability. *Rehabilitation Psychology, 58,* 148–157. http://dx.doi.org/10.1037/a0031691

Dunn, D. S., & Dougherty, S. B. (2005). Prospects for a positive psychology of rehabilitation. *Rehabilitation Psychology, 50,* 305–311. http://dx.doi.org/10.1037/0090-5550.50.3.305

Dunn, D. S., Ehde, D. M., & Wegener, S. T. (2016). The foundational principles as psychological lodestars: Theoretical inspiration and empirical direction in rehabilitation psychology. *Rehabilitation Psychology, 61,* 1–6. http://dx.doi.org/10.1037/rep0000082

Dunn, D. S., & Elliott, T. R. (2005). Revisiting a constructive classic: Wright's *Physical disability: A psychosocial approach*. *Rehabilitation Psychology, 50,* 183–189. http://dx.doi.org/10.1037/0090-5550.50.2.183

Dunn, D. S., Fisher, D. J., & Beard, B. M. (2012). Revisiting the mine/thine problem: A sensitizing exercise for clinic, classroom, and attributional research. *Rehabilitation Psychology, 57,* 113–123. http://dx.doi.org/10.1037/a0027967

Dunn, D. S., Uswatte, G., Elliott, T. R., Lastres, A., & Beard, B. (2013). A positive psychology of physical disability: Principles and progress. In M. L. Wehmeyer (Ed.), *The Oxford handbook of positive psychology and disability* (pp. 427–441). New York, NY: Oxford University Press.

Ehde, D. M. (2010). Application of positive psychology to rehabilitation psychology. In R. G. Frank, M. Rosenthal, & B. Caplan (Eds.), *Handbook of rehabilitation psychology* (pp. 417–424). Washington, DC: American Psychological Association. http://dx.doi.org/10.1037/15972-029

Fein, S., & Spencer, S. J. (1997). Prejudice as self-image maintenance: Affirming the self through derogating others. *Journal of Personality and Social Psychology, 73,* 31–44. http://dx.doi.org/10.1037/0022-3514.73.1.31

Fernández, S., Branscombe, N. R., Gómez, A., & Morales, J. F. (2012). Influence of the social context on use of surgical-lengthening and group-empowering coping strategies among people with dwarfism. *Rehabilitation Psychology, 57,* 224–235. http://dx.doi.org/10.1037/a0029280

Fine, M., & Asch, A. (1988). Disability beyond stigma: Social interaction, discrimination, and activism. *Journal of Social Issues, 44,* 3–21. http://dx.doi.org/10.1111/j.1540-4560.1988.tb02045.x

Fiske, S. T. (2005). Social cognition and the normality of prejudgment. In J. F. Dovidio, P. Glick, & L. A. Rudman (Eds.), *On the nature of prejudice: Fifty years after Allport* (pp. 36–53). Malden, MA: Blackwell. http://dx.doi.org/10.1002/9780470773963.ch3

Fiske, S. T. (2011). *Envy up, scorn down: How status divides us*. New York, NY: Russell Sage Foundation.

Forster, E. M. (1989). *Howard's end*. New York, NY: Vintage Books. (Original work published 1910)

Gilbert, D. T., & Malone, P. S. (1995). The correspondence bias. *Psychological Bulletin, 117,* 21–38. http://dx.doi.org/10.1037/0033-2909.117.1.21

Gill, C. J. (1997). Four types of integration in disability identity development. *Journal of Vocational Rehabilitation, 9,* 39–46. http://dx.doi.org/10.1016/S1052-2263(97)00020-2

Goffman, E. (1963). *Stigma: Notes on the management of spoiled identity*. Englewood Cliffs, NJ: Prentice-Hall.

Heider, F. (1958). *The psychology of interpersonal relations*. New York, NY: Wiley. http://dx.doi.org/10.1037/10628-000

Helzer, E. G., & Dunning, D. (2012). On motivated reasoning and self-belief. In S. Vazire & T. D. Wilson (Eds.), *Handbook of self-knowledge* (pp. 379–396). New York, NY: Guilford Press.

Hewstone, M., Rubin, M., & Willis, H. (2002). Intergroup bias. *Annual Review of Psychology, 53,* 575–604. http://dx.doi.org/10.1146/annurev.psych.53.100901.135109

Johnson, H. M. (2005). *Too late to die young: Nearly true tales from a life*. New York, NY: Holt.

Jones, E. E., & Nisbett, R. E. (1971). The actor and the observer: Divergent perspectives of the causes of behavior. In E. E. Jones, D. E. Kanouse, H. H. Kelley, R. E. Nisbett, S. Valins, & B. Weiner (Eds.), *Attribution: Perceiving the causes of behavior* (pp. 79–94). Morristown, NJ: General Learning Press.

Keany, K. M. H., & Glueckauf, R. L. (1993). Disability and value change: An overview and reanalysis of acceptance of loss theory. *Rehabilitation Psychology, 38,* 199–210. http://dx.doi.org/10.1037/h0080297

Lerner, M. J. (1980). *The belief in a just world: A fundamental delusion*. New York, NY: Plenum Press. http://dx.doi.org/10.1007/978-1-4899-0448-5

Lewin, K. A. (1935). *A dynamic theory of personality*. New York, NY: McGraw-Hill.

Livneh, H., & Antonak, R. F. (1997). *Psychosocial adaptation to chronic illness and disability*. Gaithersburg, MD: Aspen.

Macrae, C. N., & Bodenhausen, G. V. (2001). Social cognition: Categorical person perception. *British Journal of Social Psychology, 92,* 239–255. http://dx.doi.org/10.1348/000712601162059

Malle, B. F. (2011). Attribution theories: How people make sense of behavior. In D. Chadee (Ed.), *Theories in social psychology* (pp. 72–95). Malden, MA: Wiley-Blackwell.

Marrow, A. J. (1977). *The practical theorist: The life and work of Kurt Lewin*. New York, NY: Teachers College Press.

Mason, A., Pratt, H. D., Patel, D. R., Greydanus, D. E., & Yahya, K. Z. (2004). Prejudice toward people with disabilities. In J. L. Chin (Ed.), *The psychology of prejudice and discrimination: Disability, religion, physique, and other traits* (Vol. 4, pp. 52–93). Westport, CT: Praeger.

Meyerson, L. (1948). Physical disability as a social psychological problem. *Journal of Social Issues, 4,* 2–10. http://dx.doi.org/10.1111/j.1540-4560.1948.tb01513.x

Monden, K. R., Trost, Z., Scott, W., Bogart, K. R., & Driver, S. (2016). The unfairness of it all: Exploring the role of injustice appraisals in rehabilitation outcomes. *Rehabilitation Psychology, 61,* 44–53. http://dx.doi.org/10.1037/rep0000075

National Federation of the Blind. (1993). Resolution 93–01. Retrieved from http://courses.csail.mit.edu/PPAT/fall2011/labs/01/NFB-resolution.pdf

Nisbett, R. E. (1980). The trait construct in lay and professional psychology. In L. Festinger (Ed.), *Retrospections on social psychology* (pp. 109–130). New York, NY: Oxford University Press.

Olkin, R. (2008). Disability-affirmative therapy and case formulation: A template for understanding disability in a clinical context. *Counseling and Human Development, 39,* 1–20.

Oyserman, D., Elmore, K., & Smith, G. (2012). Self, self-concept, and identity. In M. R. Leary & J. P. Tangney (Eds.), *Handbook of self and identity* (2nd ed., pp. 69–104). New York, NY: Guilford Press.

Peterson, C., & Park, N. (2011). Character strengths and virtues: Their role in well-being. In S. I. Donaldson, M. Csikszentmihalyi, & J. Nakamura (Eds.), *Applied positive psychology: Improving everyday life, health, schools, work, and society* (pp. 49–62). New York, NY: Routledge.

Peterson, C., & Park, N. (2012). Character strengths and the life of meaning. In P. P. Wong (Ed.), *The human quest for meaning: Theories, research, and applications* (2nd ed., pp. 277–295). New York, NY: Routledge.

Peterson, C., & Seligman, M. E. P. (2004). *Character strengths and virtues: A handbook and classification*. Washington, DC: American Psychological Association.

Pettigrew, T. F. (2001). The ultimate attribution error: Extending Allport's cognitive analysis of prejudice. In M. A. Hogg & D. Abrams (Eds.), *Intergroup relations: Essential readings* (pp. 162–173). New York, NY: Psychology Press.

Pettigrew, T. F., & Tropp, L. R. (2008). How does intergroup contact reduce prejudice? Meta-analytic tests of three mediators. *European Journal of Social Psychology, 38,* 922–934. http://dx.doi.org/10.1002/ejsp.504

Roessler, R., & Bolton, B. (1978). *Psychosocial adjustment to disability*. Baltimore, MD: University Park Press.

Ross, L. (1977). The intuitive psychologist and his shortcomings: Distortions in the attribution process. In L. Berkowitz (Ed.), *Advances in experimental social psychology* (Vol. 10, pp. 174–221). New York, NY: Academic Press. http://dx.doi.org/10.1016/S0065-2601(08)60357-3

Ross, L., & Nisbett, R. E. (1991). *The person in the situation*. New York, NY: McGraw-Hill.

Silverman, A., Logel, C., & Cohen, G. L. (2013). Self-affirmation as a deliberate coping strategy: The moderating role of choice. *Journal of Experimental Social Psychology, 49,* 93–98. http://dx.doi.org/10.1016/j.jesp.2012.08.005

Smedana, S., Bakken-Gillen, S. K., & Dalton, J. (2009). Psychosocial adaptation to chronic illness and disability: Models and measurement. In F. Chan, E. Da Silva Cordoso, & J. A. Chronister (Eds.), *Understanding psychosocial adjustment to chronic illness and disability: A handbook for evidence-based practitioners in rehabilitation* (pp. 51–73). New York, NY: Springer.

Solomon, A. (2012). *Far from the tree: Parents, children, and the search for identity*. New York, NY: Scribner.

Tropp, L. R., & Mallett, R. K. (Eds.). (2011). *Moving beyond prejudice reduction: Pathways to positive intergroup relations*. Washington, DC: American Psychological Association. http://dx.doi.org/10.1037/12319-000

Vash, C. L., & Crewe, N. M. (2004). *Psychology of disability* (2nd ed.). New York, NY: Springer.

Vilchinsky, N., Findler, L., & Werner, S. (2010). Attitudes toward people with disabilities: The perspective of attachment theory. *Rehabilitation Psychology, 55*, 298–306. http://dx.doi.org/10.1037/a0020491

Wehmeyer, M. L. (Ed.). (2013). *The Oxford handbook of positive psychology and disability*. New York, NY: Oxford University Press. http://dx.doi.org/10.1093/oxfordhb/9780195398786.001.0001

Wilson, T. D. (2002). *Strangers to ourselves: Discovering the adaptive unconscious*. Cambridge, MA: Harvard University Press.

Wright, B. A. (1972). Value-laden beliefs and principles for rehabilitation psychology. *Rehabilitation Psychology, 19*, 38–45. http://dx.doi.org/10.1037/h0090869

Wright, B. A. (1983). *Physical disability: A psychosocial approach*. New York, NY: Harper & Row. http://dx.doi.org/10.1037/10589-000

Wright, B. A. (1988). Attitudes and the fundamental negative bias. In H. E. Yuker (Ed.), *Attitudes towards persons with disabilities* (pp. 3–21). New York, NY: Springer.

Wright, B. A. (1991). Labeling: The need for greater person–environment individuation. In C. R. Snyder & D. R. Forsyth (Eds.), *Handbook of social and clinical psychology: The health perspective* (pp. 469–487). New York, NY: Pergamon Press.

Yuker, H. E. (1994). Variables that influence attitudes toward people with disabilities: Conclusions from the data. *Journal of Social Behavior and Personality, 9*, 3–22.

Chapter 10

MULTICULTURAL ISSUES AND INTERNATIONAL PERSPECTIVES ON DISABILITY

Paul B. Perrin, Lisa D. Goldberg, and Bradford S. Pierce

In 2002, the American Psychological Association (APA) published its *Guidelines on Multicultural Education, Training, Research, Practice, and Organizational Change for Psychologists*. There, *culture* is defined as a learned set of evolving beliefs and values "that influence customs, norms, practices, and social institutions" (p. 8). Multiculturalism appreciates that each individual's personal identity encompass characteristics such as race/ethnicity, language, gender, age, sexual orientation, disability, social class, religious/spiritual orientation, education, and other cultural components, and that these aspects of identity intersect and interact in nuanced ways (APA, 2002).

This chapter delves into how an individual's culture—and more specifically, race/ethnicity and nationality—affect the rehabilitation experience. We begin by describing some of the major research findings on rehabilitation disparities in the United States and internationally across several disability populations. We then address cultural bias in neuropsychological assessments, describes how cultural values and caregiving play a role in disability, and synthesizes the literature on cultural competencies necessary for rehabilitation psychologists. Finally, we identify a number of multicultural challenges facing rehabilitation psychologists and outline directions for future research.

REHABILITATION DISPARITIES IN THE UNITED STATES

Culture affects the prevalence, severity, and treatment of injuries; the outcome of treatments; and community attitudes concerning disabilities (Addo et al., 2012; Krause, Broderick, Saladin, & Broyles, 2006; Perrin et al., 2014; Stansbury, Jia, Williams, Vogel, & Duncan, 2005). Disparities among various cultural groups (e.g., race/ethnicity, gender, social class) are seen across a wide variety of injuries, such as traumatic brain injuries (TBIs; Perrin et al., 2014), spinal cord injury (SCI; Krause et al., 2006), stroke (Addo et al., 2012), and multiple sclerosis (MS; Naismith, Trinkaus, & Cross, 2006). Until more recently, multicultural rehabilitation research in the United States has focused primarily on identifying differences in prevalence rates and outcomes between Black and White Americans in various disability populations. This was an important first step toward recognizing and highlighting that rehabilitation disparities can exist in different populations. For example, some of the most consistent findings of disparities are that stroke incidence, recurrence rates, severity, and mortality are all higher for Black versus White Americans (Stansbury et al., 2005). Other research has found that, compared with White individuals with MS,

http://dx.doi.org/10.1037/0000129-011
Handbook of Rehabilitation Psychology, Third Edition, L. A. Brenner, S. A. Reid-Arndt, T. R. Elliott, R. G. Frank, and B. Caplan (Editors-in-Chief)

Black individuals have higher rates of primary progressive MS, develop gait difficulties faster and more frequently, and present more cerebellar dysfunction such as tremors and clumsy movements (Naismith et al., 2006). This study also found that Blacks were 30% more likely than Whites to score higher on Expanded Disability Status Scale at diagnosis (indicating higher levels of disability), and this trend continued at 4- and 6-year follow-ups.

Disparities have been found within TBI populations as well. Using data from the National Institute on Disability, Independent Living, and Rehabilitation Research's Traumatic Brain Injury Model Systems, Perrin and colleagues (2014) found that Black individuals with TBI have higher anxiety than Whites individuals over the first 2 years after injury. Black individuals also reported lower satisfaction with life than White individuals, and Black and Latino individuals with a TBI reported significantly higher depression compared with Whites. Another study found that even after controlling for etiology, age, gender, injury severity, and functional status at discharge from rehabilitation, Blacks and Latinos with TBI scored significantly lower than Whites on measures of community integration and employment status 1 year after injury (Rosenthal et al., 1996). Other research has found that satisfaction with life after TBI increased across 10 years after TBI for White individuals but actually decreased for Black individuals across the same time period (Williamson et al., 2016).

Research also suggests that Blacks have poorer outcomes after SCI compared with Whites. One study found that Black individuals with SCI reported a greater number of poor health days, along with more frequent and lengthier hospitalizations compared with White individuals (Krause, Broderick, Saladin, & Broyles, 2006). Another study of data collected over a 6-year period found that Black individuals with SCI scored lower than White individuals on subjective well-being and on measures of participation (e.g., physical independence, mobility, occupation, social integration, and economic self-sufficiency; Krause, Saladin, & Adkins, 2009). Krause and colleagues (2009) suggested that without intervention, the disparities would likely continue indefinitely because the trend differences between Black and White individuals did not change systematically during the 6-year period of the study.

Over the past few years, researchers have begun to expand from racial/ethnic comparisons to documenting disparities among populations based on language, socioeconomic status (SES), and other factors (Addo et al., 2012; Lequerica et al., 2015). For example, Lequerica and colleagues (2015) found that non-English speakers scored lower on functional communication outcomes relative to native English speakers following TBI. This is a critical finding because their study showed that emergency department and hospitals have a history of using English communication measures to assess functional impairment in individuals who are not completely fluent in English. One potential implication of this finding is that problems with measure selection may suggest a difference in outcomes when it is not clear that a difference actually exists. A meta-analysis by Addo and colleagues (2012) found that lower SES populations (measured by proxies such as area-level socioeconomic deprivation, social class, education, and annual income) within Western Europe, Australia, and the United States were 30% more likely to experience a stroke and suffer more cognitive and physical deficits and higher fatalities as a result of stroke. At the same time, individuals with lower SES were less likely to receive evidence-based stroke rehabilitation.

INTERNATIONAL DISPARITIES

Although much research has documented rehabilitation disparities in the United States, a body of research has found disparities internationally as well (e.g., Ackery, Tator, & Krassioukov, 2004; Paredes et al., 2016; Saltapidas & Ponsford, 2007). For example, in Colombia, gunshot and knife wounds account for a significant portion of SCIs as a result of violence in the region (Henao-Lema & Pérez-Parra, 2010). Although globally, SCI is 3 to 4 times more common for men than women, in lower income countries where men are more likely to encounter violence and face higher physical risks at work, men are up to 8 times more likely to experience SCI than women (Ackery, Tator, & Krassioukov, 2004).

In the context of stroke, Paredes and colleagues (2016) found that over the first year, individuals with stroke in Colombia had substantially lower scores on eight measures of health-related quality of life (physical functioning, role physical, pain, general heath, mental health, role emotional, social functioning, and vitality) compared with healthy control participants, and that the majority of these indices did not change at all over that time period, indicating no rehabilitation whatsoever. The authors attributed this to individuals with stroke in that region having few rehabilitation services available to them. Further, Colombians with stroke scored lower on health-related quality of life measures compared with those within countries with more nationalized health care systems and comprehensive stroke rehabilitation services (e.g., Spain, Netherlands; Paredes et al., 2016). These findings suggest that health disparity outcomes in various populations or global regions could be due in some instances to lack of access to rehabilitation care as opposed to solely multicultural factors such as discrimination or unique cultural values.

In the context of TBI, Australian individuals from culturally and linguistically diverse backgrounds with TBI have been found to be less likely than White individuals to return to work, tend to report more reliance on others for assistance with mobility and cognitive activities, and have less social interaction (Saltapidas & Ponsford, 2007). These differences between groups remained even when controlling for education, SES, employment status, and number of hours of rehabilitation therapy.

CULTURAL BIAS IN ASSESSMENTS

Although neuropsychological assessments are intended to provide reliable measurements of a person's current level of cognitive functioning in one or more domains, problems of validity arise when interpreting results without accounting for an individual's cultural background. This situation can diminish the accuracy of assessments and distort the interpretation of results in people from diverse backgrounds, often leading to under- or overdiagnosis of impairments (Pontón et al., 1996). It is important to keep these differences in mind when using norms created using homogeneous population samples (usually White Americans) to interpret results for individuals belonging to other racial/ethnic backgrounds or from diverse global regions. Culturally based norms are often needed to accurately interpret results for non-White samples and international populations.

Within the United States, these differences in scores among cultures have been found across a number of studies. Latinos' level of acculturation within the United States has been shown to affect scores on Halstead–Reitan Neuropsychological Test Battery subtests such as the Tactual Performance Test, Seashore Rhythm Test, and the Halstead Category Test (Arnold, Montgomery, Castañeda, & Longoria, 1994). Latinos also have been shown to perform worse on Digit Symbol-Coding and the Wisconsin Card Sorting Test relative to non-Latino Whites (Krch et al., 2015). Not surprisingly, those who learned English as a second language perform significantly lower on the Digit Span, Boston Naming Test, and Fatigue Assessment Scale compared with native English-speakers (Boone, Victor, Wen, Razani, & Pontón, 2007).

Disparities in testing exist in other countries outside of the United States, as well. For example, indigenous Mayans and Pame in Mexico have been found to have poorer performance on verbal memory tasks when given the NEUROPSI, a neuropsychological battery developed and standardized in Mexico, compared with nonindigenous Mexicans (Ostrosky-Solís, Ramirez, & Ardila, 2004). Yet they outperform nonindigenous Mexicans on visuospatial tasks, likely because economic survival within these indigenous cultures depends on similar skills for farming and basket-making (Ostrosky-Solís et al., 2004).

Because of these issues, culturally and linguistically appropriate norms are critical for neuropsychological assessment in rehabilitation psychology. Several recent studies have been conducted to overcome this barrier, with one of the strongest examples being a study that developed norms for 10 of the most common neuropsychological tests across more than 4,000 participants in 11 Latin American countries, with country-specific adjustments for gender, age, and education. These renormed tests include the

Boston Naming Test (Olabarrieta-Landa, Rivera, Morlett-Paredes, et al., 2015), the Stroop Color–Word Interference Test (Rivera et al., 2015), Verbal Fluency Tests (Olabarrieta-Landa, Rivera, Galarza-Del-Angel, et al., 2015), and the Modified Wisconsin Card Sorting Test (Arango-Lasprilla et al., 2015), among many others. When appropriate norms are unavailable for a specific population, it is critical that rehabilitation psychologists interpret the results of neuropsychological assessments with extreme caution and consider how clients' cultural background (e.g., language, race/ethnicity, SES, education) may have influenced their scores and whether those scores accurately reflect impairment level.

CULTURE AND FAMILY CAREGIVING

Willingness to provide care for a loved one with a disability, approaches to the assignment of caregiving roles, family communication, and regaining balance after injury within the context of the family system are linked to a family's larger culture (Sander et al., 2007). For example, Korean culture values dimensions of filial piety such as respect, responsibility, family harmony, and sacrifice (Sung, 1990), as well as the Confucian virtue of *Ren*, which can be translated as benevolence or altruism and can result in concern for the well-being of those within the family and community (Zhang & Ryden, 2002). Latino culture similarly places a high value on allocentrism, familialism, interdependence, and support for those in need (Zea, Quezada, & Belgrave, 1994). Black and Latino caregivers commonly identify faith and spirituality as an important source of support as they cope and find meaning with their role as a caregiver (Koerner, Shirai, & Pedroza, 2013). Additionally, caregivers within Black and Latino families are more likely to employ specific coping strategies such as emotional distancing, distraction, and acceptance as they attend to ongoing caregiving demands (Sander et al., 2007).

To gain insight into how family dynamics are associated with the mental health of family caregivers in Mexico, Perrin et al. (2013) studied TBI caregivers in Mexico City. Their results suggested that indices of family adaptability, cohesion, and communication predicted higher satisfaction with life and lower burden among caregivers (Perrin et al., 2013). A similar study in Mexico found that family functioning accounted for 47% and 36% of the variance in caregiver burden and depression, respectively, and that healthy family dynamics significantly buffered the effects of low patient social functioning on caregiver burden (Coy et al., 2013). These results suggest that rehabilitation psychology interventions designed to improve caregivers' mental health in Mexico, and perhaps in other similar countries in Latin America, could benefit from incorporating techniques to improve family dynamics (Coy et al., 2013; Perrin et al., 2013).

Family-systems therapy is an intervention that can be easily adapted for rehabilitation psychology and has shown strong promise for improving the mental health and family functioning of caregivers of individuals with SCI in Latin America. For example, Stevens, Lehan, Durán, Plaza, and Arango-Lasprilla (2016) designed and evaluated the effectiveness of an 8-week family intervention for caregivers of individuals with neurological conditions. This intervention integrates elements of cognitive behavior therapy, family therapy, narrative therapy, and solution-focused therapy to address issues such as managing emotions, meaning-making, effective communication, boundaries, self-care, and problem-solving. At posttreatment and 6 months, individuals with SCI in Colombia and their families demonstrated improved problem-solving and decreased depression, anxiety, and burden compared with the control group (Stevens et al., 2016). Although the study was conducted in Colombia, the findings suggest that family-systems therapy may also be useful for Latino families after traumatic injury in the United States or in other racial/ethnic groups with strong family values.

CULTURAL COMPETENCIES OF REHABILITATION PSYCHOLOGISTS

Cultural competence encompasses various aspects of clinical skill, including attempts to understand different experiences of people within a particular group, consideration of potential barriers to communication that exist as result of cultural differences, and possession of skills that increase cultural awareness and allow effective work with patients (Pope-Davis et al., 2001). APA (2002) has published guidelines for cultural competence based on the work of Sue, Arredondo, and McDavis (1992), and these have been incorporated into competency guidelines for rehabilitation psychology (see Exhibit 10.1). Clinicians should be aware of their own assumptions, values, and biases and have an understanding of the worldview and culture of the patient, including disability culture (Sue et al., 1992). Rehabilitation psychologists must be able to work with patients whose beliefs are different from their own (Lequerica & Krch, 2014) and develop appropriate and culturally sensitive strategies and techniques. Culturally competent clinicians have an awareness of how culture may influence every aspect of rehabilitation, including a patient's presentation of symptoms, use of services, adjustment to disability, and outcomes, as well as the clinician's interactions with the patient (Lee & Ditchman, 2016; Lequerica & Krch, 2014).

EXHIBIT 10.1

Multicultural Competency Guidelines for Rehabilitation Psychology

1. Rehabilitation psychologists demonstrate a working knowledge of rehabilitation psychology and an incorporation of the biopsychosocial model.
2. Rehabilitation psychologists are able to recognize that, as cultural beings, they may hold attitudes and beliefs that can detrimentally influence their assessment, treatment, and perceptions of and interactions with individuals who are culturally different from themselves (i.e., disability status, race/ethnicity).
3. Rehabilitation psychologists are encouraged to recognize the importance of multicultural sensitivity/responsiveness, knowledge, and understanding about culturally different individuals.
4. Rehabilitation psychologists demonstrate competency in assessment of emotional adjustment to disability as evidenced by articulation of a rational link between assessment findings and intervention plan specific to the rehabilitation process or adaptation to disability, discussion of client-specific variables influencing the intervention approach, discussion of theoretical or evidence-based approach to intervention, and resources that may support ongoing adjustment.
5. Rehabilitation psychologists demonstrate competency in addressing families' emotional adjustment to disability.
6. Rehabilitation psychologists strive to apply culturally appropriate skills in clinical and other applied psychological practices (i.e., selection of the appropriate intervention in the contexts of client needs, the rehabilitation treatment milieu, treatment plan implementation, and discharge planning).
7. Rehabilitation psychologists use organizational change processes to support culturally informed organizational (policy) development and practices.

Note. Data from American Psychological Association (2002) and American Board of Professional Psychology (2018).

Disability Competence

In rehabilitation settings, additional competence in awareness and understanding of disability is required beyond that outlined in the APA's (2002) guidelines, as a patient's individual and cultural beliefs about disability may greatly influence rehabilitation (Boston et al., 2015). According to Lee and Ditchman (2016), "the disability experience *is* a multicultural experience" (p. 27). Individuals with disabilities may have shared experiences and social identities, which can be positive, negative, or neutral. Like other minority statuses, individuals with disabilities may face stigma and discrimination as a function of that aspect of identity (Lee & Ditchman, 2016).

Previous literature has outlined three main models of disability that bear on one's attitudes, beliefs, and adjustment to disability (Olkin, 2002), and all have cultural underpinnings and assumptions. These are the moral, medical, and social models, and each model has unique perspectives about the meaning of disability, ethical implications, causes, and goals of intervention or rehabilitation. Whereas the moral and medical models view disability as a defect and connote stigma and shame, the social model suggests that disability is a social construct, thereby putting the onus on the environment that fails to accommodate the needs of those with disabilities (Olkin, 2002). An individual patient's beliefs about disability can be consistent with one model or can include aspects across two or all three of the models.

Although disability culture has been documented in the literature (Olkin, 2002), this is not to say that all persons with disabilities experience their disability in the same manner. Attitudes, beliefs, and understandings of disability may vary across cultures, and the experiences of persons with disabilities are determined by individual, familial, and societal structures (Boston et al., 2015). For example, research has documented a relationship between racial identity and multiple outcomes related to one's adjustment to disability (Lee & Ditchman, 2016). Furthermore, rehabilitation interventions for disabilities that are considered appropriate in one culture may be seen as discriminatory, oppressive, or harmful in another (Boston et al., 2015).

Different cultures may have their own perceptions of disability, rather than there being a universal cause, treatment, or understanding of disability (Boston et al., 2015; Olkin, 2002). For example, some Asian cultures view disability as a punishment for wrongdoing in one's past or a previous life (Miles, 2000), while the Ashanti in Ghana reject and abandon children with physical and intellectual disabilities and bar men with physical disabilities from becoming leaders (Munyi, 2012). Some cultures view disability as caused by medical and environmental factors, whereas others attribute it to spiritual causes. For example, while New Zealanders of European descent ascribe disability to biological factors, the Maori in New Zealand believe it to result from spiritual factors or happenstance (Sanders et al., 2011). Cultural beliefs about the cause of a disability may play a role in family and community attitudes toward the patient (Lee & Ditchman, 2016). In addition, because disability is a socially derived construct based on group norms and values of a given society, policies and procedures regarding disability are accordingly based on a culture's belief systems (Boston et al., 2015).

One's experience of disability as well as the rehabilitation process can also be influenced by one's family culture. It is important that providers be mindful of the cultural views not only of the individual with a disability but also those of the family (Boston et al., 2015; Lee & Ditchman, 2016; Middleton et al., 2000). Family members' attitudes about disability have the potential to either improve or impede the process of rehabilitation, and it therefore benefits clinicians to attend to how a patient's family perceives the individual's disability (Boston et al., 2015). At times, the services that an individual with a disability selects may be influenced by the perceptions and opinions of his or her family (Ravindran & Myers, 2012). As a result, treatment may benefit from directly discussing with patients their familial cultural beliefs and how rehabilitation interventions may be congruent with or dissonant from those beliefs. For example, a Latino individual with SCI may be encouraged by a health care team to participate in certain rehabilitation interventions at home (e.g., being challenged to tie one's own shoes, feed oneself, groom), yet Latino familial values of caring for sick or injured relatives may prevent family members or caregivers from allowing the individual with SCI to engage in these self-care activities, thereby limiting rehabilitation. In a case like this, a rehabilitation psychologist could engage in an open and nonjudgmental conversation with the family to help reframe their active involvement in the rehabilitation of their loved one with SCI as being consistent with their family values and discuss culturally relevant ways in which this can occur.

Models of Competence

Several primary models of cultural competence have been developed specifically for rehabilitation settings. Balcazar, Suarez-Balcazar, and Taylor-Ritzler (2009) proposed a four-component model to guide cultural competence in rehabilitation. They suggested that self-reflection and critical awareness of one's own personal biases and position in society are the first step in becoming culturally competent. Next, clinicians must familiarize themselves with the cultural characteristics, history, values, beliefs, and behaviors of their patients (Balcazar et al., 2009). Third, clinicians should work on the ability to effectively and empathically communicate with the patient, as well as integrate the patient's values and beliefs into treatment planning and execution. Finally, the clinician should understand how the knowledge and skills in the first three components are applied to the particular rehabilitation setting and population with which one works (e.g., Department of Veterans Affairs, academic medical center, private practice, or particular disability population such as TBI, SCI, burn).

A. N. Lewis (2006) presented a three-factor model of multicultural competence designed to guide rehabilitation clinicians to focus on a patient's adjustment to disability, stage of development, and cultural identity, as well as to help clinicians gain awareness of their own readiness to engage in multicultural interventions. According to the model, clinicians should explore a patient's stage of adjustment, meaning of adjustment, and commitment to the adjustment process; assess the developmental level of the patient; and gain an understanding of the patient's physical, mental, emotional, spiritual, social, and volitional functioning from the patient's cultural perspective. The model is flexible, and clinicians can put more focus on any one aspect (adjustment to disability, developmental stage, or cultural identity) depending on the goals of treatment at various stages of rehabilitation.

Most recently, the American Board of Professional Psychology (ABPP, 2018; see also Chapter 1, this volume) outlined several foundational competencies for rehabilitation psychologists with regard to working with diverse individuals, groups, populations, and communities. The ABPP states that rehabilitation psychologists should have an awareness of how differences in culture, background, and other characteristics affect assessment, treatment, consultation, and advocacy. The ABPP requires that those applying for board certification demonstrate awareness of their own individual and cultural diversity characteristics, as well as know how to seek out literature and resources to enhance one's own competency in working with diverse populations. Further, the ABPP includes disability as a central component of its cultural and social justice conceptualization, requiring that rehabilitation psychologists demonstrate active participation in the promotion of disability rights, equitable social opportunities, and cultural identity through their professional work.

Interventions to Enhance Competence

Research has suggested the need for improvement in multicultural competence among rehabilitation clinicians, including increased disability awareness and sensitivity, consideration of how culture impacts the ways in which the patient views and interacts with the world, and the need for clinicians to be mindful of the cultural views of the individual and family (Lee & Ditchman, 2016). Following a review of the literature, A. Lewis, Bethea, and Hurley (2009) suggested that there is a dearth of standards and guidelines for multicultural competencies across rehabilitation health professionals, which unfortunately can make training in rehabilitation cultural competence a moving target. Despite this challenge, a number of authors and researchers have outlined several interventions that have the potential to increase multicultural competence among rehabilitation clinicians.

Middleton and colleagues (2000) suggested several ways to improve multicultural competence in rehabilitation. First, they argued for "a clear commitment to multiculturalism in national rehabilitation policy and explicit objectives for its attainment" (p. 235), which would have the potential to begin overcoming the limitations outlined by A. Lewis and colleagues (2009). Furthermore, Middleton et al. advised rehabilitation professional organizations to adopt standards of practice that incorporate multicultural competencies and recommended that acceptable practice guidelines be specified for working with culturally and ethnically diverse patients. In addition, they suggested that the importance of multiculturalism in vocational and independent living rehabilitation be emphasized to providers. They urged leadership and governing bodies of various professional rehabilitation associations and organizations to endorse the spirit of the proposed competencies and recommended that national councils and boards identify effective educational strategies for ensuring culturally competent rehabilitation clinicians.

In addition to explicit standards from national organizations, one area in which multicultural competence can be improved is at the graduate level. Many graduate programs require only a single course on the topic, but many educators believe a more integrated curriculum in which stand-alone courses on multicultural competence are supplemented with an infusion of cultural competency throughout other courses and clinical work would be a superior form of training. A. Lewis and colleagues (2009) proposed a four-pronged approach to improving graduate training in multicultural competence: a stand-alone course on multicultural competence; integration of multicultural concepts into all courses; immersion, or an in-depth experiential exposure to multicultural content in one's clinical work; and a plan for continued professional development of cultural competence following the completion of coursework. The final aspect of this strategy would involve the development of a personal and proactive plan for continued engagement in cross-cultural exposure and would increase the likelihood of lifelong learning with regard to cultural competence. Other researchers have suggested that graduate training programs increase multicultural competence by not only changing the curriculum, but also by demonstrating a commitment to multicultural issues, recruiting minority faculty members, and providing minority role models (Pope-Davis, Liu, Toporek, & Brittan-Powell, 2001).

In addition to increasing cultural competence through graduate training, a second approach is on-the-job cultural competence training. Taylor-Ritzler et al. (2008) conducted an empirical study of the efficacy of an approach for improving cultural competence for working with individuals with disabilities, which can be applied in other rehabilitation settings as well. The training was designed to improve knowledge about cultural diversity as well as multicultural skills. It involved a review of various constructs related to multiculturalism (e.g., discrimination, oppression, White privilege), review of a cultural competence model, examination of factors that influence cultural diversity, and a discussion of effective outreach strategies for minority populations. The training, which lasted a full 8-hour workday, consisted of lectures, group discussions, group activities, and a goal-setting exercise to develop plans for improved effectiveness in serving multicultural patients. In total, 12 trainings were conducted across multiple cities in several states. Individuals who received the training indicated being moderately to highly satisfied with the content, presenters, exercises, and materials; demonstrated statistically significant improvements in multicultural knowledge; reported improvement over the following 2 months post-training in the physical environment and resources available at their agencies; and reported positive changes in values and attitudes regarding diversity. In addition, those who completed the training set goals related to organizational cultural competence, and the majority either achieved those goals or continued to pursue them at follow-up. The authors propose that goal-setting can be a useful tool to help clinicians receiving multicultural competency training to engage in organizational change (Taylor-Ritzler et al., 2008).

Finally, researchers have highlighted the need for incorporating patients' perspectives when evaluating multicultural competencies (Wiley, 2009). Pope-Davis et al. (2001) noted that although various measures have been developed to assess multicultural competence, most rely on self-report and fail to assess how patients view the clinician's competence or what preferences and expectations patients hold. They further contended that the research that has been conducted on multicultural competence has been biased by the worldviews and expectations of the researchers. For example, the paradigm for how cultural competence is measured has generally been based on definitions created by researchers rather than feedback from patients, raising the question of whether patients view cultural competence in the same way that researchers and clinicians have (Pope-Davis et al., 2001). The authors thus provided several recommendations for improving research on multicultural competence. They recommended assessing real patients in real clinical situations, rather than relying on potential patients who may have not experienced clinical intervention; using qualitative research methods to more accurately capture patients' experiences; exploring multiple roles a clinician may hold; and examining supervisors' multicultural competence and the impact on the trainee–supervisor relationship, as well as the clinician–patient relationship (Pope-Davis et al., 2001). Other researchers have highlighted the importance of participatory research and outcome evaluation to assess cultural competence and uncover needs that are not being addressed (Wiley, 2009).

MULTICULTURAL CHALLENGES FACING REHABILITATION PSYCHOLOGISTS

There have been strong movements in rehabilitation psychology, and particularly more so in recent years, to search for and document racial/ethnic or country-level differences in the prevalence and outcomes of various disabilities and health conditions. This has been an important and substantial first step in rehabilitation psychology coming to incorporate more of a multicultural and international perspective. In fact, most of our databases are ripe with demographic data to search for—and indeed, continue to identify—racial/ethnic disparities in important rehabilitation outcomes. However, we argue that to truly move the field forward and provide clinically applicable guidance for multicultural competence to practicing rehabilitation psychologists, researchers need to build in a cultural lens at the beginning of their studies, not simply analyze for racial/ethnic differences post hoc because the data are there.

As we look to the future, it will be increasingly important to move beyond traditional analytic approaches looking for Black versus White versus Latino versus Asian differences (at least in the United States) on variables that were included in a data collection for other purposes, relegating the racial/ethnic comparisons merely to an afterthought or perhaps at best to a secondary data analysis. Instead, culturally relevant variables should be selected a priori at the inception of a study to make the research truly multicultural or international in nature. Extremely ripe multicultural constructs for future rehabilitation psychology research include level of acculturation, fluency in English, immigration stressors, history of discrimination experiences or microaggressions, family dynamics and values, religiosity, level of cultural identity development, connectedness with others in one's cultural group, access to health care and rehabilitation services, perceived cultural competence of one's rehabilitation clinicians, and minority representation of students and professionals in the field of rehabilitation psychology, among many others. The incorporation into rehabilitation psychology research of multicultural variables such as these would provide substantial nuance beyond even our own research, which, for example, has found that Black and Latino individuals have worse mental health after TBI (Perrin et al., 2014). Obvious questions, such as "why?" emerge with only speculation for a response because these differences sometimes persist after accounting for all other theoretically relevant variables in the database; this will continue unless a more careful a priori variable selection and greater nuance is brought to multicultural rehabilitation psychology research.

Although research and theory have suggested that racial/ethnic disparities in health emerge from a confluence of societal, intrapersonal, and interpersonal factors (Penner et al., 2013; Williams & Mohammed, 2013), one of the most substantial influences is perceived discrimination. A large body of research culminating in meta-analyses (Schmitt, Branscombe, Postmes, & Garcia, 2014) has documented the connections between perceived discrimination and reduced health in diverse racial/ethnic minority populations. Despite this extremely robust and sophisticated area of research in social and health psychology, rehabilitation psychology has yet to examine in any serious way the influence of perceived discrimination on rehabilitation outcomes, health care satisfaction, mental health, or quality of life for individuals with disabilities in racial/ethnic minority communities. Experiencing perceived discrimination when adjusting to—or going through rehabilitation in the context of—an acquired disability may degrade interpersonal relationships in support groups, with important health care providers, and with friends, coworkers, and other associates who could otherwise provide strong social support that is critical for healthy adjustment to disability and engagement in rehabilitation, particularly for racial/ethnic minority populations (Zea, Quezada, & Belgrave, 1994).

Another growth area for the field in a multicultural sense is that rehabilitation psychology has only begun to incorporate intersectionality of disability and other various forms of identity. To an extent, the field has started to do this with race/ethnicity, as illustrated throughout this chapter, but intersectionality with other forms of cultural identity such as gender, sexual orientation, SES, religion, age, nationality, and education, among many others, is in its infancy (Warner & Brown, 2011). Gender comparisons, for example, have often been wrought with the same limitations as post hoc racial/ethnic comparisons, failing to incorporate important multicultural constructs that could account for observed differences such as gender-role conformity, history of sexist experiences, gender oppression, or endorsement of traditional gender-role belief systems. Future research can consider how masculinity or femininity plays a role in how one adapts to or copes with a disability. Again, these more nuanced variables would bring substantial meaning—and practical implications for clinical practice—beyond solely documenting gender disparities in traditional rehabilitation psychology outcomes. Similarly, little research has been conducted on the identity aspects of nonvisible disabilities (e.g., mild TBI, early stages of neurodegenerative disabilities), identity aspects of other nonvisible cultural identities (e.g., sexual orientation, religion), and on how those various forms of nonvisible identity might intersect with the more visible aspects of identity or disability specifically.

Future multicultural rehabilitation psychology research could benefit from continuing to focus on how disability may be defined and understood differently across cultures (Boston et al., 2015). It is critical that researchers and educators create better and more evidence-based programs for helping clinicians examine their own beliefs, come to understand that disability may be defined differently by various cultures, gain the ability to work with patients whose beliefs are salient to their attitudes about disability and learn to help patients overcome stigma attached to disability. A cross-cultural approach is also important in the context of the lack of culturally sensitive norms for many populations and the necessity of conducting more normative studies to overcome this significant problem.

Finally, to date, there is little consideration in the literature of the internalized stigma of disability, or "internalized ableism," which we define as the internalization by people with disabilities of ableist attitudes, behaviors, policies, and norms directed toward other individuals with disabilities and themselves, particularly including the belief in ableist stereotypes about their own disability status and identity. Future research should focus on developing a well-validated internalized ableism measure and eventually evidence-based interventions to reduce it in people with disabilities. This type of work would also spur research aimed at understanding how internalized ableism intersects with other aspects of internalized oppression including internalized racism, internalized ageism, internalized sexism, and internalized heterosexism, among others.

CONCLUSION

Rehabilitation psychology as a field has increasingly tried to incorporate multicultural and international perspectives into its core principles over the past several decades. Other authors and researchers have been quite loud advocates and pioneers in doing so. For example, many of the themes in this chapter are nicely underscored by Uomoto and Wong's (2015) encouragement that rehabilitation psychology consider the various ecosystems in which a patient lives and rehabilitates and that the field consider and use those ecosystems effectively in rehabilitation. Yet rehabilitation psychology has experienced challenges even defining cultural competence because historically cultural competence has been seen as focusing primarily on race/ethnicity, or only on disability competence in disability studies. But as the field moves into an era of stronger appreciation for intersectionality, it will be important to remain vigilant about maintaining an appropriate breadth for rehabilitation psychology's model of cultural competence and the diverse identities our patients bring into rehabilitation. Finally, there is a real need to move from a disparity-only lens to one that emphasizes the personal and collective strengths of people with disabilities. Doing so will help rehabilitation psychology continue to value and incorporate into clinical practice the unique strengths of people with disabilities from various cultural groups and diverse global regions.

References

Ackery, A., Tator, C., & Krassioukov, A. (2004). A global perspective on spinal cord injury epidemiology. *Journal of Neurotrauma*, *21*, 1355–1370. http://dx.doi.org/10.1089/neu.2004.21.1355

Addo, J., Ayerbe, L., Mohan, K. M., Crichton, S., Sheldenkar, A., Chen, R., . . . McKevitt, C. (2012). Socioeconomic status and stroke: An updated review. *Stroke*, *43*, 1186–1191. http://dx.doi.org/10.1161/STROKEAHA.111.639732

American Board of Professional Psychology. (2018). *American Board of Professional Psychology American*

Board of Rehabilitation Psychology: Certification Guidelines and Procedures, Candidates Manual 2018. Retrieved from https://abpp.org/BlankSite/media/Rehabilitation-Psychology-Documents/Candidate-manual-september-10-2018.pdf

American Psychological Association. (2002). *Guidelines on multicultural education, training, research, practice, and organizational change for psychologists*. Washington, DC: Author. Retrieved from https://www.apa.org/about/policy/multicultural-guidelines-archived.pdf

Arango-Lasprilla, J. C., Rivera, D., Longoni, M., Saracho, C. P., Garza, M. T., Aliaga, A., . . . Perrin, P. B. (2015). Modified Wisconsin Card Sorting Test (M–WCST): Normative data for the Latin American Spanish speaking adult population. *NeuroRehabilitation, 37*, 563–590. http://dx.doi.org/10.3233/NRE-151280

Arnold, B. R., Montgomery, G. T., Castañeda, I., & Longoria, R. (1994). Acculturation and performance of Hispanics on selected Halstead–Reitan neuropsychological tests. *Assessment, 1*, 239–248. http://dx.doi.org/10.1177/107319119400100303

Balcazar, F. E., Suarez-Balcazar, Y., & Taylor-Ritzler, T. (2009). Cultural competence: Development of a conceptual framework. *Disability and Rehabilitation, 31*, 1153–1160. http://dx.doi.org/10.1080/09638280902773752

Boone, K. B., Victor, T. L., Wen, J., Razani, J., & Pontón, M. (2007). The association between neuropsychological scores and ethnicity, language, and acculturation variables in a large patient population. *Archives of Clinical Neuropsychology, 22*, 355–365. http://dx.doi.org/10.1016/j.acn.2007.01.010

Boston, Q., Dunlap, P. N., Ethridge, G., Barnes, E., Dowden, A. R., & Euring, M. J. (2015). Cultural beliefs and disability: Implications for rehabilitation counsellors. *International Journal for the Advancement of Counselling, 37*, 367–374. http://dx.doi.org/10.1007/s10447-015-9250-7

Coy, A. E., Perrin, P. B., Stevens, L. F., Hubbard, R., Díaz Sosa, D. M., Espinosa Jove, I. G., & Arango-Lasprilla, J. C. (2013). Moderated mediation path analysis of Mexican traumatic brain injury patient social functioning, family functioning, and caregiver mental health. *Archives of Physical Medicine and Rehabilitation, 94*, 362–368. http://dx.doi.org/10.1016/j.apmr.2012.08.210

Henao-Lema, C. P., & Pérez-Parra, J. E. (2010). Lesiones medulares y discapacidad: Revisión bibliográfica [Spinal cord injuries and disabilities: A review]. *Aquichan, 10*, 157–172. http://dx.doi.org/10.5294/aqui.2010.10.2.5

Koerner, S. S., Shirai, Y., & Pedroza, R. (2013). Role of religious/spiritual beliefs and practices among Latino family caregivers of Mexican descent. *Journal of Latina/o Psychology, 1*, 95–111. http://dx.doi.org/10.1037/a0032438

Krause, J. S., Broderick, L. E., Saladin, L. K., & Broyles, J. (2006). Racial disparities in health outcomes after spinal cord injury: Mediating effects of education and income. *The Journal of Spinal Cord Medicine, 29*, 17–25. http://dx.doi.org/10.1080/10790268.2006.11753852

Krause, J. S., Saladin, L. K., & Adkins, R. H. (2009). Disparities in subjective well-being, participation, and health after spinal cord injury: A 6-year longitudinal study. *NeuroRehabilitation, 24*, 47–56.

Krch, D., Lequerica, A., Arango-Lasprilla, J. C., Rogers, H. L., DeLuca, J., & Chiaravalloti, N. D. (2015). The multidimensional influence of acculturation on Digit Symbol-Coding and Wisconsin Card Sorting Test in Hispanics. *The Clinical Neuropsychologist, 29*, 624–638.

Lee, E. J., & Ditchman, N. (2016). Working with people with disabilities within a multiculturalism framework. In J. M. Uomoto & T. M. Wong (Eds.), *Multicultural neurorehabilitation: Clinical principles for rehabilitation professionals* (pp. 25–46). New York, NY: Springer. http://dx.doi.org/10.1891/9780826115287.0002

Lequerica, A., & Krch, D. (2014). Issues of cultural diversity in acquired brain injury (ABI) rehabilitation. *NeuroRehabilitation, 34*, 645–653.

Lequerica, A., Krch, D., Lengenfelder, J., Chiaravalloti, N., Arango-Lasprilla, J. C., Hammond, F. M., . . . Sander, A. M. (2015). Comparison of FIM™ communication ratings for English versus non-English speakers in the traumatic brain injury model systems (TBIMS) national database. *Brain Injury, 29*, 1445–1451. http://dx.doi.org/10.3109/02699052.2015.1075144

Lewis, A., Bethea, J., & Hurley, J. (2009). Integrating cultural competency in rehabilitation curricula in the new millennium: Keeping it simple. *Disability and Rehabilitation, 31*, 1161–1169. http://dx.doi.org/10.1080/09638280902773760

Lewis, A. N. (2006). Three-factor model of multicultural counseling for consumers with disabilities. *Journal of Vocational Rehabilitation, 24*, 151–159.

Middleton, R. A., Rollins, C. W., Sanderson, P. L., Leung, P., Harley, D. A., Ebener, D., & Leal-Idrogo, A. (2000). Endorsement of professional multicultural rehabilitation competencies and standards: A call to action. *Rehabilitation Counseling Bulletin, 43*, 219–245. http://dx.doi.org/10.1177/003435520004300407

Miles, M. (2000). Disability on a different model: Glimpses of an Asian heritage. *Disability & Society, 15*, 603–618. http://dx.doi.org/10.1080/09687590050058206

Munyi, C. W. (2012). Past and present perceptions towards disability: A historical perspective. *Disability Studies Quarterly, 32*. Retrieved from http://dsq-sds.org/article/view/3197/3068

Naismith, R. T., Trinkaus, K., & Cross, A. H. (2006). Phenotype and prognosis in African-Americans with multiple sclerosis: A retrospective chart review. *Multiple Sclerosis*, *12*, 775–781. http://dx.doi.org/10.1177/1352458506070923

Olabarrieta-Landa, L., Rivera, D., Galarza-Del-Angel, J., Garza, M. T., Saracho, C. P., Rodríguez, W., . . . Arango-Lasprilla, J. C. (2015). Verbal fluency tests: Normative data for the Latin American Spanish speaking adult population. *NeuroRehabilitation*, *37*, 515–561. http://dx.doi.org/10.3233/NRE-151279

Olabarrieta-Landa, L., Rivera, D., Morlett-Paredes, A., Jaimes-Bautista, A., Garza, M. T., Galarza-del-Angel, J., . . . Arango-Lasprilla, J. C. (2015). Standard form of the Boston Naming Test: Normative data for the Latin American Spanish speaking adult population. *NeuroRehabilitation*, *37*, 501–513. http://dx.doi.org/10.3233/NRE-151278

Olkin, R. (2002). Could you hold the door for me? Including disability in diversity. *Cultural Diversity and Ethnic Minority Psychology*, *8*, 130–137. http://dx.doi.org/10.1037/1099-9809.8.2.130

Ostrosky-Solís, F., Ramirez, M., & Ardila, A. (2004). Effects of culture and education on neuropsychological testing: A preliminary study with indigenous and nonindigenous population. *Applied Neuropsychology*, *11*, 188–195. http://dx.doi.org/10.1207/s15324826an1104_3

Paredes, A. M., Landa, L. O., Chagualá, A. C., Peralta, H. C., Torres, G. V., Perrin, P. B., & Arango-Lasprilla, J. C. (2016). Health-related quality of life trajectories over the first year after stroke in Colombia, South America. *Topics in Stroke Rehabilitation*, *23*, 341–347. http://dx.doi.org/10.1080/10749357.2016.1143694

Penner, L. A., Hagiwara, N., Eggly, S., Gaertner, S. L., Albrecht, T. L., & Dovidio, J. F. (2013). Racial healthcare disparities: A social psychological analysis. *European Review of Social Psychology*, *24*, 70–122. http://dx.doi.org/10.1080/10463283.2013.840973

Perrin, P. B., Krch, D., Sutter, M., Snipes, D. J., Arango-Lasprilla, J. C., Kolakowsky-Hayner, S. A., . . . Lequerica, A. (2014). Racial/ethnic disparities in mental health over the first 2 years after traumatic brain injury: A model systems study. *Archives of Physical Medicine and Rehabilitation*, *95*, 2288–2295. http://dx.doi.org/10.1016/j.apmr.2014.07.409

Perrin, P. B., Stevens, L. F., Sutter, M., Hubbard, R., Díaz Sosa, D. M., Espinosa Jove, I. G., & Arango-Lasprilla, J. C. (2013). Exploring the connections between traumatic brain injury caregiver mental health and family dynamics in Mexico City, Mexico. *PM & R*, *5*, 839–849. http://dx.doi.org/10.1016/j.pmrj.2013.05.018

Pontón, M. O., Satz, P., Herrera, L., Ortiz, F., Urrutia, C. P., Young, R., . . . Namerow, N. (1996). Normative data stratified by age and education for the Neuropsychological Screening Battery for Hispanics (NeSBHIS): Initial report. *Journal of the International Neuropsychological Society*, 2, 96–104. http://dx.doi.org/10.1017/S1355617700000941

Pope-Davis, D. B., Liu, W. M., Toporek, R. L., & Brittan-Powell, C. S. (2001). What's missing from multicultural competency research: Review, introspection, and recommendations. *Cultural Diversity and Ethnic Minority Psychology*, *7*, 121–138. http://dx.doi.org/10.1037/1099-9809.7.2.121

Ravindran, N., & Myers, B. J. (2012). Cultural influences on perspectives of health, illness, and disability: A review and focus on autism. *Journal of Child and Family Studies*, *21*, 311–319. http://dx.doi.org/10.1007/s10826-011-9477-9

Rivera, D., Perrin, P. B., Stevens, L. F., Garza, M. T., Weil, C., Saracho, C. P., . . . Arango-Lasprilla, J. C. (2015). Stroop Color-Word Interference Test: Normative data for the Latin American Spanish speaking adult population. *NeuroRehabilitation*, *37*, 591–624. http://dx.doi.org/10.3233/NRE-151281

Rosenthal, M., Dljkers, M., Harrison-Felix, C., Nabors, N., Witol, A. D., Young, M. E., & Englander, J. S. (1996). Impact of minority status on functional outcome and community integration following traumatic brain injury. *The Journal of Head Trauma Rehabilitation*, *11*, 40–57. http://dx.doi.org/10.1097/00001199-199610000-00005

Saltapidas, H., & Ponsford, J. (2007). The influence of cultural background on motivation for and participation in rehabilitation and outcome following traumatic brain injury. *The Journal of Head Trauma Rehabilitation*, 22, 132–139. http://dx.doi.org/10.1097/01.HTR.0000265101.75177.8d

Sander, A. M., Davis, L. C., Struchen, M. A., Atchison, T., Sherer, M., Malec, J. F., & Nakase-Richardson, R. (2007). Relationship of race/ethnicity to caregivers' coping, appraisals, and distress after traumatic brain injury. *NeuroRehabilitation*, 22, 9–17.

Sanders, D., Kydd, R., Morunga, E., & Broadbent, E. (2011). Differences in patients' perceptions of Schizophrenia between Māori and New Zealand Europeans. *Australian and New Zealand Journal of Psychiatry*, *45*, 483–488. http://dx.doi.org/10.3109/00048674.2011.561479

Schmitt, M. T., Branscombe, N. R., Postmes, T., & Garcia, A. (2014). The consequences of perceived discrimination for psychological well-being: A meta-analytic review. *Psychological Bulletin*, *140*, 921–948. http://dx.doi.org/10.1037/a0035754

Stansbury, J. P., Jia, H., Williams, L. S., Vogel, W. B., & Duncan, P. W. (2005). Ethnic disparities in stroke: Epidemiology, acute care, and postacute outcomes. *Stroke*, *36*, 374–386. http://dx.doi.org/10.1161/01.STR.0000153065.39325.fd

Stevens, L. F., Lehan, T., Durán, M. A. S., Plaza, S. L. O., & Arango-Lasprilla, J. C. (2016). Pilot study of a newly developed intervention for families facing serious injury. *Topics in Spinal Cord Injury Rehabilitation*, *22*, 49–59. http://dx.doi.org/10.1310/sci2201-49

Sue, D. W., Arredondo, P., & McDavis, R. J. (1992). Multicultural counseling competencies and standards: A call to the profession. *Journal of Counseling & Development*, *70*, 477–486. http://dx.doi.org/10.1002/j.1556-6676.1992.tb01642.x

Sung, K. T. (1990). A new look at filial piety: Ideals and practices of family-centered parent care in Korea. *The Gerontologist*, *30*, 610–617. http://dx.doi.org/10.1093/geront/30.5.610

Taylor-Ritzler, T., Balcazar, F., Dimpfl, S., Suarez-Balcazar, Y., Willis, C., & Schiff, R. (2008). Cultural competence training with organization serving people with disabilities from diverse cultural backgrounds. *Journal of Vocational Rehabilitation*, *29*, 77–91.

Uomoto, J. M., & Wong, T. M. (2015). *Multicultural neurorehabilitation: Clinical principles for rehabilitation professionals*. New York, NY: Springer.

Warner, D. F., & Brown, T. H. (2011). Understanding how race/ethnicity and gender define age-trajectories of disability: An intersectionality approach. *Social Science & Medicine*, *72*, 1236–1248. http://dx.doi.org/10.1016/j.socscimed.2011.02.034

Wiley, A. (2009). At a cultural crossroads: Lessons on culture and policy from the New Zealand DISABILITY STRATEGY. *Disability and Rehabilitation*, *31*, 1205–1214. http://dx.doi.org/10.1080/09638280902773935

Williams, D. R., & Mohammed, S. A. (2013). Racism and health I: Pathways and scientific evidence. *American Behavioral Scientist*, *57*, 1152–1173. http://dx.doi.org/10.1177/0002764213487340

Williamson, M. L., Elliott, T. R., Bogner, J., Dreer, L. E., Arango-Lasprilla, J. C., Kolakowsky-Hayner, S. A., . . . Perrin, P. B. (2016). Trajectories of life satisfaction over the first 10 years after traumatic brain injury: Race, gender, and functional ability. *The Journal of Head Trauma Rehabilitation*, *31*, 167–179. http://dx.doi.org/10.1097/HTR.0000000000000111

Zea, M. C., Quezada, T., & Belgrave, F. Z. (1994). Latino cultural values: Their role in adjustment to disability. *Journal of Social Behavior & Personality*, *9*, 185–200.

Zhang, D., & Ryden, E. (2002). *Key concepts in Chinese philosophy*. New Haven, CT: Yale University Press.

Chapter 11

DEVELOPMENTAL PERSPECTIVES IN REHABILITATION PSYCHOLOGY

Seth Warschausky, Marie Van Tubbergen, and Ramzi Hasson

A lifespan developmental perspective on disability is essential for understanding and working effectively with persons with disabilities and their families. This chapter provides a brief overview of childhood disability, a review of important concepts and considerations from a developmental perspective, and a discussion of age-related psychosocial needs that are critical in achieving optimal levels of independence and happiness. The needs of children and adolescents with congenital or acquired conditions change through developmental phases, and age of onset has complex effects on functional outcomes. Although many childhood disabilities entail risks for poorer mental health and health-related quality of life, findings regarding life satisfaction are not clear cut, and there are differences in satisfaction among those with congenital versus acquired conditions. There are powerful moderators of developmental and recovery outcomes among children and adolescents with congenital and acquired conditions, many of which are potential targets for intervention.

To maximize developmental gains among children with disabilities, rehabilitation psychologists provide interventions both directly to patients and their families and indirectly through consultation with multidisciplinary teams and school systems. Core rehabilitation psychology competencies (see Chapter 1, this volume) are expanded to include additional skills and training specific to children and adolescents. From the foundational competencies, rehabilitation psychologists need broad expertise in relationships and interpersonal interactions, including the ability to interact with children and adolescents in a developmentally appropriate manner. Ethical and legal competencies are expanded to include child- and adolescent-specific guidelines regarding patient confidentiality and privacy and communication with parents, as well as knowledge of the Americans With Disabilities Act (ADA) and the Individuals With Disabilities Education Act (IDEA), which pertain to educational planning and services. Awareness of multicultural factors that affect family dynamics and parenting styles while raising a child with a disability is essential, as is an expanded notion of interdisciplinary systems to include various professionals in the educational system. Competencies in the assessment/evaluation cluster include familiarity with developmentally informed assessment tools, strategies, interpretations, and recommendations based on a knowledge of educational systems and special education rules and guidelines. Finally, in the domain of consumer protection, rehabilitation psychologists evaluate possible abuse and neglect and are familiar with associated reporting requirements.

http://dx.doi.org/10.1037/0000129-012
Handbook of Rehabilitation Psychology, Third Edition, L. A. Brenner, S. A. Reid-Arndt, T. R. Elliott, R. G. Frank, and B. Caplan (Editors-in-Chief)

CHILDHOOD DISABILITIES

In the last 100 years, there has been a significant decline in infant mortality in the United States from 10% to 0.6%, with a concomitant decline in childhood mortality (Centers for Disease Control and Prevention, 2002; Durkin, 2015; Hoyert & Xu, 2012; Murphy, Xu, & Kochanek, 2012). In recent years, however, evidence has suggested an increase in childhood disability associated with chronic conditions (Houtrow, Larson, Olson, Newacheck, & Halfon, 2014). Childhood disability prevalence is estimated at 4% of children with functional limitations and 8% of children with activity limitations. Although higher rates of disability are associated with low socioeconomic status, there has been an increase in prevalence among children and adolescents with high socioeconomic status. Furthermore, there has been a decrease in childhood disabilities classified as primarily physical (Houtrow et al., 2014). Several reasons have been cited for this increased prevalence: changes in data collection procedures (Halfon, Houtrow, Larson, & Newacheck, 2012), better access to health care, and advances in health care and diagnostic tools.

Special education enrollment has increased from 8% in the 1970s to the current level of 13% (Scull & Winkler, 2011). Most of the children and adolescents who receive services are eligible under Specific Learning Disability (39.5%) or Speech or Language Impairment (17.9%), and these levels have been stable for the past 35 years (Office of Special Education and Rehabilitative Services, 2015). The number of children and adolescents receiving services under Other Health Impairment (13.8%) or Autism (8.2%) have increased, whereas those receiving services under Intellectual Disability (7.1%) has slightly decreased. About 65% of children and adolescents receiving special education services spend at least 80% of their school day in a general education classroom, up from 33% 25 years ago. This trend toward mainstreaming has created a unique set of opportunities and challenges for children and adolescents with disabilities, their families, and rehabilitation psychologists.

DEVELOPMENTAL PERSPECTIVES

Several important concepts guide rehabilitation psychologists working with children and adolescents with disabilities and their families. Age effects on functioning are associated with age at onset, time since onset, and the age when assessed (Taylor & Alden, 1997). Regarding age at onset, neither the plasticity hypothesis (e.g., younger age of onset is associated with better outcomes) nor the vulnerability hypothesis (e.g., younger age of onset is associated with worse outcomes) is completely correct. Congenital neurodevelopmental conditions such as cerebral palsy (CP), spina bifida, and preterm birth entail risk for lower developmental trajectories, and there is evidence of poorer prognosis for acquired brain injuries sustained early in life. However, there is significant variability in outcomes within these populations and increasing evidence of factors that are associated with *developmental sparing*. Children's and adolescents' developing capabilities (e.g., social competencies, executive behaviors) are challenged by increased socioenvironmental demands. Competence in meeting those demands at younger ages is not a guarantee of being equipped to meet increased and changing demands later in childhood; there is the potential for emerging deficits and needs over time. These "latent deficits" can involve executive dysfunction that only becomes apparent in middle childhood when the need arises to complete more complex academic- and community-based tasks.

DEVELOPMENTAL TRAJECTORIES: PREDICTORS AND INTERVENING VARIABLES

Children and adolescents with disabilities frequently have atypical health care needs that require the development of more complex self-management skills (Tarazi, Mahone, & Zabel, 2007). In addition to accessibility issues associated with physical impairments, skill development can be affected by factors that include cognitive and emotional status, family and community support, and access to resources. At the person level, intellect has some effect on developmental trajectories. For example, among persons with CP, the ability to perform activities of daily living increases through childhood and adolescence. However, this happens at a lower level for those persons with CP who also have intellectual disabilities, which are a more important intervening variable than disabilities in gross motor function (Vos et al., 2013). Evidence suggests that executive functions are even stronger determinants of development of functional independence than IQ (Heffelfinger et al., 2008). Intriguingly, development of executive functions may be foreshadowed by early childhood mastery motivation, defined as an intrinsic desire to sustain goal-directed behavior in the face of challenge (Hauser-Cram, Woodman, & Heyman, 2014; Morgan, MacTurk, & Hrncir, 1991). Childhood disability has been associated with lower levels of mastery motivation (Majnemer, Shevell, Law, Poulin, & Rosenbaum, 2010), and levels of mastery motivation are associated with development of adaptive behaviors and response to intervention (Miller, Ziviani, Ware, & Boyd, 2015; Tuminello, Holmbeck, & Olson, 2012; Warschausky, Kaufman, Evitts, Schutt, & Hurvitz, 2017).

Social development and peer relations are critical determinants of quality of life for children and adolescents with disabilities. There has been limited longitudinal study of social participation in childhood and adolescence through the transition to early adulthood. Among children and adolescents with CP, developmental trajectories of social participation are affected by gross motor function, but this is typically only the case for those with the lowest levels of functional ability (Tan et al., 2014). Intellectual impairment attenuates the development of social participation to an even greater degree than physical functioning. Cross-sectional studies of differing aspects of social participation in childhood and adolescence have shown the importance of family and parenting factors including socioeconomic status, parent education level, and parent stress, as well as environmental factors like resources and accessibility (Chien et al., 2015; Smits et al., 2011; Voorman, Dallmeijer, Van Eck, Schuengel, & Becher, 2010). However, regarding parenting effects on social development, models that apply to families of typically developing children and adolescents may not apply to families of children and adolescents with disabilities. For example, whereas parenting factors are correlated with the quality of friendships in typically developing children and adolescents, the associations are less salient in children and adolescents with CP (Cunningham, Warschausky, & Dixon Thomas, 2009). There is evidence to suggest that direct parenting efforts to include children and adolescents with disabilities in social activities does not result in more successful development of friendships (Dixon Thomas, Warschausky, Golin, & Meiners, 2008). However, other factors like the availability of accessible activities and facilitated interactions may be particularly important.

Psychological well-being and family functioning are critical factors in development. Typically, children and adolescents with disabilities encounter stressors at rates above and beyond those of their peers, ranging from daily hassles associated with disability to significant vulnerabilities that can hamper educational/vocational success and social connectedness. Parents of children and adolescents with disabilities may strive to teach their children to manage stressors in a manner that will promote resilience. However, mothers of these children are at higher risk for depression and difficulties in family functioning (Rodenburg, Meijer, Deković, & Aldenkamp, 2007). Some evidence suggests that parental anxiety adversely affects use of optimal parenting strategies as well as adaptive functioning in children (Chapieski et al., 2005). In families of children and adolescents who sustain brain injury, siblings also are at risk for emotional and behavioral difficulties (Sambuco, Brookes, & Lah, 2008).

Children and adolescents with disabilities require greater assistance from parents than do their peers. It can be difficult to distinguish between appropriate helping and overprotection, which is often viewed as a pejorative term that may not adequately account for individual circumstances (Anderson & Coyne, 1991). There is an emerging emphasis on the role of larger social and economic circumstances in shaping outcomes. Regardless of parenting style, children from families with greater familial stressors (e.g., finances, health, employment) and fewer social supports (e.g., extended family, friends) exhibit more difficulties with executive functioning than do children from families with lesser stress levels

(Potter et al., 2011). Longitudinal studies of pediatric traumatic brain injury (TBI) indicate that parenting practices and quality of home environment are significant socioenvironmental moderators of general functional outcome (Wade, Zhang, Yeates, Stancin, & Taylor, 2016).

In the following sections, phase-specific developmental, educational, and psychosocial concepts and needs are examined.

INFANTS AND TODDLERS (0–3 YEARS)

The typically developing infant and toddler brain undergoes a rapid process of change and development that coincides with more complex cognitive and behavioral capacities (Volpe, 2008). Young children begin to survey and understand their environments and bodies as they gain greater motor control and cognitive capacities, including progressively expanding language and social functioning. There is a dynamic interplay among emerging abilities, developmental context, and child–caregiver interactions that ultimately shapes cognitive and psychological development.

Congenital Conditions and Cognitive Development

Congenital conditions that result in sensory, language, or motor impairments can have profound influence on the pace and trajectory of development. For instance, children with Down syndrome show a pattern of attaining early developmental milestones similar to that of typically developing children, but their trajectory is prolonged (Abbeduto, Warren, & Conners, 2007; Patterson, Rapsey, & Glue, 2013). Milestones achieved by typically developing children at 18 months (e.g., babbling, first words, and then short phrases) may take 3 years or more for children with Down syndrome (Abbeduto et al., 2007; Patterson et al., 2013).

The dynamic interplay among motor and cognitive systems that shape later development likely begins at this stage but is more reliably assessed in later developmental stages. For example, children with spina bifida myelomeningocele (SBM) have substantial motor deficits but also subtle cognitive, language, and visual-spatial deficits (Lomax-Bream, Barnes, Copeland, Taylor, & Landry, 2007). It has been speculated that early motor deficits may inhibit opportunities for exploration of the environment, which in turn may contribute to underdevelopment of visual-spatial processing experiences in later development (Wiedenbauer & Jansen-Osmann, 2008). Delays in language and motor functioning may also coincide with underdeveloped abilities to regulate emotions and behaviors. These difficulties with behavioral and emotional regulation may hinder greater exploration and positive child–caregiver interactions as well as other enriched opportunities, which can contribute to underdeveloped language development. These dynamic interactions highlight important foci for interventions that promote neurocognitive development.

Acquired Central Nervous System Insults and Cognitive Development

Central nervous system injuries can disrupt the connectivity and organization of brain networks that mediate the development of later skills (Jonsson, Horneman, & Emanuelson, 2004). Although very young children may possess greater neuroplasticity potential with some types of lesions, early brain insults also can inhibit plasticity and result in cascading detrimental effects on later development (Taylor & Alden, 1997). Early moderate to severe brain injuries are associated with less recovery than is noted in older children and adolescents (Jonsson et al., 2004; Taylor & Alden, 1997). Developing functions and abilities are the most likely to be disrupted by brain injuries, whereas previously acquired abilities are preserved (Taylor & Alden, 1997). Disruptions to language development may affect later development of verbal reasoning capacities and executive functions. Early language processing deficits involving phonology will likely affect further development of language capacity, vocabulary development, and preacademic and literacy skills. Overall, deficits in language, cognitive function, and executive function place very young children with TBI at significant risk for a global developmental delay, poor behavior regulation, and significant learning problems that require intensive rehabilitation interventions.

Special Education Services

Infants and toddlers up to 3 years old suspected of abnormal development of motor, cognitive, communicative, social/emotional, or adaptive functioning can obtain early intervention services under Part C of IDEA. Children can obtain services under the category of developmental delay, which provides access to speech and language, physical, and occupational therapy along with other required services (e.g., audiological assessment and treatment). An Individual Family Service Plan is developed to outline appropriate services and interventions.

Psychosocial Adjustment

The interaction of environmental factors, biological factors, attachment factors, and caregiver practices in early infancy has significant effects on behavioral and psychological adjustment (e.g., Easterbrooks, Bureau, & Lyons-Ruth, 2012; Greenberg, Speltz, & DeKlyen, 1993). Challenging temperament, child behavior, and parenting styles interact with developmental disruptions to predict internalizing and externalizing symptoms among older children (Easterbrooks et al., 2012). Temperament problems, in particular, are difficult to separate from poor regulatory mechanisms that may be secondary to developmental delay and poor emotional regulation capacity. Early childhood temperamental and attachment problems that persist into preschool will likely require clinical attention. During this developmental phase, rehabilitation psychologists typically focus direct services on child assessment and parent-focused intervention and advocacy.

Becoming a parent represents a dramatic shift in basic daily activities, overall priorities, and self-concept. The transition is well understood to be profound under typical circumstances; for parents of infants with disabilities, anxiety regarding their child's health, well-being, and prognosis can be overwhelming. Parents of typically developing children often find support and relief from comparing and contrasting experiences and problem-solving strategies among other parents in their extended family and community, deriving benefit from sharing common challenges and rewards. Parenting a child with a known disability can create an environment in which comparisons to typical norms and experiences feel discouraging or threatening rather than reassuring. Disability leads to a rapid immersion into an unfamiliar medical culture, and multidisciplinary health care providers can become primary touchstones regarding children's development. In addition to providing valuable education and intervention, focus on health providers may also inadvertently undermine parents' identity as the experts about their child.

Whether children have a congenital condition resulting in disability or an acquired disability through illness or injury, parents often experience grief (Fernandez-Alcántara et al., 2016; Whittingham, Wee, Sanders, & Boyd, 2013; Zinner, Ball, Stutts, & Philput, 1997). Parents of infants with congenital disabilities may grieve an unarticulated set of expectations for their child, and for the parents they imagined they would be. Parents of infants and toddlers who experience disability resulting from an injury or illness face similar issues on the heels of a traumatic experience. Rehabilitation psychologists working with families in this developmental phase recognize that parents are faced with significant daily practical challenges in the context of a grieving process. Families of children with disabilities show overall greater challenges in adaptation than those of typically developing children with unique patterns of waxing and waning concerns throughout development (Pedersen, Crnic, Baker, & Blacher, 2015).

PRESCHOOL-AGE CHILDREN (3–6 YEARS)

Preschool-age children show tremendous growth in cognitive, linguistic, social, and emotional development. There is greater integration of multisensory information at this age as well greater demand for self-regulation and self-organization, especially within structured school and daycare settings. Preschool-age children begin developing conceptual ideas of size and amounts and categorization-based reasoning skills (Piaget, 1964). These developing concrete abilities underlie future development of abstract reasoning and linguistic skills as well as complex executive functions. The later effects of congenital and acquired disabilities can include more specific and observable cognitive, academic, and behavioral deficits than are observed among younger children.

Congenital Conditions and Cognitive Development

Cognitive phenotypic variations begin to emerge across and within congenital conditions during this phase of development. For example, preschool-age children with a mild form of CP have been shown to develop relatively intact verbal abilities, but they can begin to exhibit significant lags within the nonverbal sphere (Gonzalez-Monge et al., 2009; Sigurdardottir & Vik, 2011). Children with physical impairments may have relatively intact higher-level cognitive functioning but show subtle deficits when compared with typically developing peers. For example, young children with muscular dystrophies can have substantial motor impairments but relatively intact global cognitive functioning. However, there is evidence of subtle deficits in verbal attention span and phonological processing as well as more notable deficits associated with adaptive functioning, memory, language, and fine motor dexterity (Cyrulnik et al., 2008).

Acquired Central Nervous System Insults and Cognitive Development

Like infants and toddlers who sustain moderate to severe TBIs, preschool-age children with TBI are at a tremendous risk for life-long neuropsychological impairments. Children with focal lesions may fare less well than toddlers because of reduced neuroplasticity; on the other hand, they may have more preserved abilities post-TBI. For example, infants and toddlers who sustain a focal injury to the language-motor dominant hemisphere may shift language representation to the nonaffected hemisphere (Bates et al., 1997); such plasticity is not typically observed among preschool-age and older children. In general, recovery of cognitive functions is more favorable when neurological insults are focal rather than diffuse, a pattern that is relatively consistent across development (Ewing-Cobbs et al., 2006). The impact of TBI on later functioning is difficult to determine at this age; small lesions may have small immediate effects but show greater effects later in development (Ewing-Cobbs et al., 2006). The most vulnerable areas of functioning at this age include motor, learning and memory, self-regulation, and expressive language functioning, which have important implications for academic and psychological functioning. Rehabilitation psychologists are instrumental in assisting families and other professionals with identifying and addressing emerging developmental needs. For example, children with a TBI may have significant difficulties with impulse control, emotion regulation, and attention while also having an average IQ and no physical impairments. Challenging behaviors in the absence of obvious disability may be misinterpreted by school personnel and result in disciplinary interventions. Rehabilitation psychologists can help families and school teams better understand behaviors, as well as provide recommendations to address behavioral concerns in the school setting. Behavior plans may include accommodations such as prearranged access to a "time out" space or use of a signal between student and staff to signal distress.

Academic Functioning

Preschool-age children demonstrate preacademic learning, general knowledge acquisition, and progressively sophisticated language functioning including improved phonological processing, syntax, and pragmatic skills. Observable functional deficits can be more pronounced at school than at home, secondary to interaction between learning demands and cognitive limitations. The level of academic difficulty varies across conditions and developmental phases and may be specific to an academic domain. For example, very preterm children with relatively intact language skills may initially develop basic alphabetics but are more likely to exhibit difficulties with more advanced skills such as word reading or mathematical concepts (Aarnoudse-Moens, Weisglas-Kuperus, van Goudoever, & Oosterlaan, 2009). Preschool-age children with neurodevelopmental disabilities, including children who were preterm and at a low birth weight, perform one half of a standard deviation below typically developing children across standardized measures of reading, mathematics, and spelling (Bhutta, Cleves, Casey, Cradock, & Anand, 2002).

Special Education Services

Infants and toddlers who received early intervention services under Part C of IDEA can transition to school-based services under Part B. This transition includes a shift from family-focused services to child-focused services. At this age, the school system assumes the primary educational responsibility and determination of appropriate services. Eligible children transition to an individualized education program (IEP) that outlines appropriate services, interventions, and progress goals. Rehabilitation psychologists facilitate communication between care providers and schools to inform development of targeted interventions and accommodations.

Psychosocial Adjustment

Preschool-age children show increasing motivation for interactive play with siblings and peers that underlies future development of social skills and overall social–emotional development. Impairments related to language and executive functions contribute to continued difficulties with communication and self-regulation (Lavigne, Nolan, & McLone, 1988). Preschool-age children with congenital or acquired neurological conditions are more likely to engage in disruptive, aggressive, and unsafe behaviors than their typically developing peers (Bhutta et al., 2002; Eisenhower, Baker, & Blacher, 2005; McDermott et al., 1996). Like their typically developing peers, boys with neurodevelopmental disabilities show greater externalizing and temperamental difficulties at this age (Bhutta et al., 2002; Lavigne et al., 1988). Although psychological adjustment difficulties may appear to be externalizing in nature, children's internalizing difficulties with mood may manifest as irritability, separation anxiety, or somatization. Difficulties with sleep onset and maintenance are also more prevalent among children with neuro-developmental conditions and may reflect an underlying mood disturbance (Lavigne & Faier-Routman, 1992). These challenges may result in neuro-developmental diagnoses such as attention-deficit/hyperactivity disorder (ADHD), which can have profound effects on social, emotional, and academic development (Spira, Bracken, & Fischel, 2005). Parental competence and socioeconomic status have important moderating effects on psychological adjustment, even when children are at significant risk for behavioral and emotional problems (Benn & McColl, 2004; Drotar, 1997; Lavigne et al., 1988).

Ideally, developmental processes involve increasing opportunities for positive social interactions that serve to build a sophisticated repertoire of positive social skills. As children experience positive social exchanges, they exhibit more behaviors showing cooperation, consideration, and reciprocity. These positive social behaviors generally lead to increased opportunity for more social interactions. Children with physical and/or cognitive disabilities are more vulnerable to disruptions in a positive cycle of social development because of barriers like diminished opportunity, less access to age-appropriate activities, or impairments in the cognitive skills that underpin social behaviors (Guralnick & Weinhouse, 1984).

During this developmental phase, physical impairments and needs tend to be the main focus for parents and caregivers, whereas cognitive and/or social deficits and needs may be underappreciated. Frequently, physical impairments require intensive management, intervention, or other treatment that can be onerous for children and parents. Poor behavior or social deficits can be underreported or minimized as a "natural" outcome of facing physical challenges; conversely, increased parental monitoring, control, and involvement in daily activities can render age-appropriate expressions of independence as unacceptable and labeled as noncompliance (Thomasgard, Metz, Edelbrock, & Shonkoff, 1995). Through direct, parent-focused psychotherapy and consultation with medical and school personnel, rehabilitation psychologists can play an important role in highlighting the social/emotional needs of children alongside the more obvious focus on physical impairments, while also assisting parents in managing challenging behaviors and developmental needs within the context of disability.

SCHOOL-AGE CHILDREN (6–12 YEARS)

During elementary school, children undergo a substantial increase in language, executive function, reasoning, memory, and learning abilities. Environmentally, there is greater demand at home, at school, and in social contexts. Consequently, cognitive deficits are more likely to be observed, and developmental gaps become more pronounced. In general, the assessment of distinct cognitive strengths and weaknesses is psychometrically more robust in school-age children compared with younger children, but assessments can be challenging when motor and/or language impairments preclude standardized assessment (Warschausky et al., 2012).

Congenital Conditions and Cognitive Development

There is significant variability in cognitive phenotypes within and among congenital neurodevelopmental conditions. For example, there is a significant risk for intellectual disability in children with CP, particularly in those with history of preterm birth and/or epilepsy. Yet, even among those with the greatest physical impairments, a subset exhibits intact level of intellect (Dalvand, Dehghan, Hadian, Feizy, & Hosseini, 2012). The cognitive profiles of children with SBM show a nuanced pattern of strengths and weaknesses within and across neuropsychological domains that have been described as distinctions between associative and assembled processing, with impairments in the latter (Dennis & Barnes, 2010). For example, for children with SBM, aspects of categorical perception (e.g., visual features, sequences) can be intact, but there are impairments in coordinated perception (e.g., spatial route finding, mental rotations).

Acquired Central Nervous System Insults and Cognitive Development

A moderate–severe TBI at a young age is associated with greater long-term neurobehavioral compromise. Like younger children, developmental outcomes for school-age children are associated with severity of injury, time since injury, and relative preservation of acquired skills. Deficits in speed of information processing, attention, memory inefficiency, executive dysfunction, impaired social pragmatics, and greater risks for mood disruptions are more common among children with moderate–severe TBI than are seen in typically developing children or children with orthopedic injuries (Dennis, Guger, Roncadin, Barnes, & Schachar, 2001; Yeates et al., 2002). Unlike infants and toddlers, school-age children who receive brain injuries show more negative effects on the development of visual-spatial skill and executive functions than on language functioning (Jonsson et al., 2004). For children who sustained an injury earlier in life, new deficits may emerge at this age because early brain damage may have disrupted the formation of new cognitive skills (Jonsson et al., 2004; Levin, 2003).

Academic Functioning

School-age children with neurodevelopmental disabilities are at risk for lower academic achievement, grade retention, and the need for special education services. Academic difficulties with math and reading are apparent as early as kindergarten and can persist throughout childhood and beyond. The severity of academic dysfunction is multidetermined, but extent of cognitive, language, and executive function impairments are important predictors. Academic deficits are among the most significant and pervasive areas of difficulty after pediatric TBI.

During the initial 6 months after TBI, core academic skills are commonly reduced (Prasad, Swank, & Ewing-Cobbs, 2017). These early deficits improve 6 months to 12 months postinjury, but long-term academic difficulties can persist well into late childhood and adolescence. Children with global developmental delay may later meet criteria for an intellectual disability and require specialized and alternative curricula. Even among children with largely intact global intellectual functioning, substantial academic delay may occur because of subtle cognitive, executive, and language deficits. For instance, deficits with visual-spatial working memory are predictive of lower mathematics achievement, even with intact intellectual functioning. Lower nonverbal abilities are also predictive of overall lower academic achievement, especially mathematics outcomes. Other executive function impairments affecting domains such as verbal working memory and cognitive flexibility/shifting adversely affect basic reading and writing skills (Jenks, van Lieshout, & de Moor, 2009).

Rehabilitation psychologists can be instrumental in communicating with school personnel about a school-age children's strengths and weaknesses. For example, many neurological conditions are linked with significant delays in cognitive processing speed. Rehabilitation psychologists can advocate for extra time in some situations (e.g., tests, quizzes) and avoid extended deadlines in other situations (e.g., daily classwork, homework), asking instead for reduced length and/or amount of work, preventing a back-pile of work, and facilitating a student's ability to maintain the pace of the classroom. These kinds of nuanced accommodations can address real-world challenges and support individualized interventions that may be different than the typical educational accommodations.

Special Education Services

Rehabilitation psychologists can play an important role in the updating of school-age children's IEP to reflect new developmental learning, social, behavioral, and emotional challenges. Typically, IEPs are annually updated, but parents can request a modification at any time. Completing a comprehensive psychological or neuropsychological evaluation can be a meaningful way of aiding communication between parents and school as well as developing targeted interventions. Another important role is to help parents monitor academic progress and work closely with the school-based evaluation team to develop goals that maximize academic and social development. Specific advocacy efforts may center on accommodations for accessibility. For instance, children with fine motor impairments may benefit from the aid of scribes, voice recognition, or keyboarding to improve writing efficiency. Physical accommodations to enhance mobility and transportation will be relevant for many children with motor limitations (e.g., wheel chair access, elevator access if there are multiple floors, eliminating or reducing need to carry materials/books). Additional common accommodations include augmentative communication assistance where there is a speech/language impairment and use of adaptive technology (e.g., personal frequency modulation systems, touch screens). It is common for parents and school personnel to have different views regarding children's cognitive abilities; in these instances, rehabilitation psychologists have an important role in developing appropriate expectations in the educational curriculum. This can be done by educating parents and teachers about children's strengths and weaknesses on the basis of comprehensive assessment and identifying resources that inform targeted educational accommodations and interventions.

Psychosocial Adjustment

School-age children with neurodevelopmental conditions face significant risk for psychological problems, including behavioral, emotional, self-esteem, and social maladjustment (Wallander, Thompson, & Alriksson-Schmidt, 2003). Type and severity of psychological dysfunction vary across condition and are moderated by comorbid health conditions, severity of disability, presence of pain, child temperament, parenting approaches, and coping style (Ramstad, Loge, Jahnsen, & Diseth, 2015; Wallander et al., 2003). A subset of children with neurodevelopmental conditions are 2 to 8 times more likely to meet behavioral criteria for ADHD, autism spectrum disorder, anxiety, and other mood symptoms (Fevang, Hysing, Markestad, & Sommerfelt, 2016). For instance, children with SBM are 2 to 3 times more likely to have behavior problems consistent with ADHD than are typically developing children (Bilenberg & Lie, 2001). In a population-based study, nearly half of children with CP screened positive for an emotional or behavioral problem and showed significantly higher rates of psychopathology when compared with typically developing peers (Rackauskaite, Bilenberg, Bech, Uldall, & Østergaard, 2016). Among children with CP, those with a comorbid intellectual disability are more likely to screen positive for a behavioral or emotional disorder (Parkes, White-Koning, McCullough, & Colver, 2009; Rackauskaite et al., 2016). It appears that low-average or very low IQ doubles the risk of having emotional and behavioral problems among children with CP (Rackauskaite et al., 2016). Generally, neurological abnormalities accompanied by impaired cognition place children at greater risk for behavioral and emotional problems that are likely to persist into adulthood.

Social opportunities and social skill development are important during this developmental phase, as school-age children's reference point shifts from family to peers. Among children with CP who were nonambulatory, social functioning decreased over the 2-year period of the study, and for those children who also had cognitive impairment, communication with peers also decreased (van Schie et al., 2013).

For children with disabilities, this developmental period marks an increasing self-awareness of disability, and specific physical, cognitive, or other impairments may take on new meaning as children compare themselves to peers. As such, rehabilitation psychologists may provide individual psychotherapy focused on developing a deeper understanding of diagnosis along with positive adaptive strategies. In addition, children may express or act out greater frustration with emerging awareness of their disability, requiring different parenting strategies.

Parenting styles are categorized as authoritative, authoritarian, and permissive, with consistent findings that authoritative parenting is associated with improved childhood outcomes (Baumrind, 1971; Ginsburg & Bronstein, 1993; Lamborn, Mounts, Steinberg, & Dornbusch, 1991). Authoritative parenting has also been linked with better behavioral outcomes among children who sustained TBI (Yeates, Taylor, Walz, Stancin, & Wade, 2010), whereas an authoritarian parenting style is related to more difficulties with executive functioning 12 and 18 months after TBI (Potter et al., 2011). Warm, responsive parenting, coupled with absent parental negativity, has been related to more positive behavioral outcomes in children who sustained TBI (Wade et al., 2011). Resources for parents and caregivers in health, education, and optimistic outlook ameliorate emotional and behavioral risks for children. However, caregiver anxiety is associated with suboptimal parenting styles and reduced adaptive functioning in school-age children (Chapieski et al., 2005; Ellingsen, Baker, Blacher, & Crnic, 2014). Parental use of emotion-focused coping behaviors predicts higher parenting stress (Rodenburg et al., 2007). Rehabilitation psychologists can continue to serve parents as they navigate these developmental transitions by providing guidance in parenting and behavioral strategies as well as supportive psychotherapy.

ADOLESCENTS (12–18 YEARS)

Adolescence is another period of rapid neurological development, as the brain undergoes major changes and reorganization. By middle adolescence many cognitive, memory, language, and executive function abilities approximate adult levels. There is greater capacity for analytical and abstract reasoning, improved executive functioning, highly developed memory capacity, and increasingly flexible self-regulation capabilities. Typically developing adolescents become functionally independent in the context of complex social and academic challenges.

Congenital Disabilities and Cognitive Development

There is a general trend of a widening gap between adolescents with congenital conditions and their typically developing peers, as deficits that were not evident at a younger age become more prominent. This may contribute to new social, psychological, academic, and functional challenges. For instance, higher-level executive abilities begin to mature in adolescence and are fundamental to successful execution of age-appropriate social, behavioral, and academic skills. Adolescents with congenital neurodevelopmental disabilities may find it more difficult to master age-appropriate grade-level content or successfully manage social situations compared with typically developing adolescents (Kuban et al., 2016). At this age, deficits in attention, working memory, and processing speed are significant predictors of academic attainment and activities of daily living (Aarnoudse-Moens et al., 2009; Mulder, Pitchford, & Marlow, 2010).

Acquired Central Nervous System Conditions and Cognitive Development

TBIs often have adverse effects on processing speed, attention, and executive functions. Adolescents with early-onset severe TBI are likely to present with mild to severe global intellectual functioning, whereas those with complicated mild TBI may display overall average intellectual functioning in the context of focal cognitive deficits. Processing speed is often affected, even when global cognitive functioning falls within average range or higher.

Academic Functioning

Deficits with higher level academic skills, such as reading comprehension, complex mathematics (e.g., prealgebra, geometry), and written expression, are more prevalent at this age. Difficulties with executive functioning can lead to learning inefficiencies despite intact cognitive and academic skills. Adolescents with congenital or acquired disabilities are less likely to earn a high school diploma, especially those with more pronounced cognitive impairments. Rehabilitation psychologists can help families to consider children's specific abilities, academic skills, and interests in developing realistic and desirable academic goals and postsecondary school plans. These considerations could inform specific vocational and adaptive skill development as prominent IEP objectives, leading to a certificate of completion rather than a diploma.

Special Education Services

Adolescents with disabilities are likely to continue to require special education services for previously identified learning difficulties in the context of new developmental challenges across social and academic domains. This developmental period presents some logistical challenges for updating and maintaining services as students transition from a structured elementary school setting to a less structured setting in middle school, junior high school, and high school. Schools are mandated to address transition goals in the IEP process starting at age 14, and students are to be included in the IEP process. For adolescents who do not have global cognitive impairment, the burden of requesting and using school accommodations may begin to shift to students, presenting a new layer of challenges for students with conditions that include deficits in executive functioning. Rehabilitation psychologists can advocate for students by identifying individual challenges and needs. For example, adolescents who "graduated" from speech services years ago may benefit from rehabilitation-based speech-language pathology services to address higher-level organization and memory challenges. As adolescents near the end of their secondary school experiences, they will require a focused collaboration between school staff, family, and community-based organizations to successfully implement a post–high school transition plan. Rehabilitation psychologists can provide guidance to the school team and the family as well as identify appropriate community resources to promote optimal levels of independence.

Psychosocial Adjustment

Adolescents with congenital and acquired disabilities may continue to face significant psychological challenges. Increased externalizing and internalizing symptoms are commonly identified among adolescents with a wide range of congenital disabilities (Fevang et al., 2016; Rackauskaite et al., 2016; Wallander et al., 2003). Stress related to greater independence, career, and educational goals may contribute to behavioral and emotional symptoms (Nassau & Drotar, 1995; Pinquart & Teubert, 2012). Poor self-image and low self-esteem are associated with increased anxiety and depressive symptoms, which can lead to further social problems and social isolation. Social difficulties may be affected by impairments in social information-processing secondary to cognitive processing deficits (Warschausky, Argento, Hurvitz, & Berg, 2003). Adolescents with TBI are likely to display less effective coping skills than those with congenital conditions and may present with increased apathy, irritability, anger, impulsivity, and emotional lability (Bogart, 2014; Hanks, Temkin, Machamer, & Dikmen, 1999). In young adults, use of task-oriented coping strategies and perceived social support in the 5 years after acquiring a TBI were independently and strongly predictive of measured resilience, more so than were injury severity, premorbid intelligence, or cognitive flexibility (Hanks, Rapport, Waldron Perrine, & Millis, 2016). Rehabilitation psychologists play an important role in education and development of adaptive strategies, while providing supportive psychotherapy to adolescents who are engaged in the critical work of identity formation.

Nonetheless, parenting and family factors continue to be key areas for rehabilitation psychologists to address in working with adolescents with disability. During this phase of development, as parents continue to set basic structures and limitations, adolescents pursue highly specialized motor skills, independent time management for daily and long-term projects/goals, vocational pursuits, unsupervised peer relationships, and use of trial-and-error strategies for many life skills. Adolescents with disabilities may have significant emotional reactions to physical limitations and may be acutely aware of cognitive and social difficulties. Social concerns are often significant, as typically developing peers make the transition to adult activities (e.g., driving, part-time jobs, dating) that may elude adolescents with disabilities.

Ideally, adolescents are provided with an increasing role in decisions as they transition to optimal independence, including decisions related to school participation, medical management, and social relationships. This presents a paradox for parents who know that opportunities to make poor decisions and encounter naturally occurring consequences are fundamental steps toward independence but are aware of their child's specific vulnerabilities (Holmbeck et al., 2002). Parents' fears of dramatic consequences from poor decisions in the realm of drugs/alcohol, driving/riding with peers, or sexual behaviors generate stress, which in turn can disrupt the development of independence. Rehabilitation psychologists can serve adolescents and parents in managing stress and adapting to disability in the context of greater independence for adolescents and reduced control for parents.

TRANSITION TO ADULTHOOD

Successful transition to adulthood can be examined in multiple domains including education, employment, independent living, and psychological and social well-being (Shogren, Shaw, & Little, 2016). It is important for the rehabilitation psychologist to be aware of significant transition needs and key predictors of achieving optimal outcomes. There is some evidence of a general decline in the percentage of typically developing young adults who achieve adult milestones in their 20s (Pinquart, 2014). Young adults with disabilities, however, are approximately 25% less successful than their peers in achieving adult milestones during their 20s and early 30s, though outcomes are highly variable. The risk for not becoming a parent in young adulthood is even higher than the risks involved in attaining education and employment milestones. Young adults with high incidence disabilities (e.g., learning disabilities) tend to have more positive outcomes than those with intellectual disabilities, conditions that affect cognition, sensory impairments, or TBI.

Competitive employment by the early to mid-20s is lower among young adults with disabilities, with evidence that employment is predicted by working in high school, computer skills, parental expectations of employment, no history of arrest, and the type of high school attended (Wehman et al., 2015). Employment in high school and computer skills are particularly strong predictors of employment outcomes. There is some evidence that income disparities between young adults with and without disabilities have been diminishing over time (Pinquart, 2014).

Young adults are expected to achieve health literacy, defined as the ability to obtain, process, and understand health information and services needed to make health-related decisions (Sansom-Daly et al., 2016). Greater health literacy has been associated with more positive health outcomes, except for substance abuse. The primary source of health information for adolescents and young adults is the Internet (Sansom-Daly et al., 2016). There is evidence that approximately one third of adolescents and young adults do not achieve health literacy with specific concerns about low levels of critical literacy defined as low understanding and application of information. Evidence suggests that although most young adults and their parents believe the young adult can self-manage his or her health, approximately one quarter report that they do not have a health care transition plan (Sawicki, Kelemen, & Weitzman, 2014).

There are few empirically validated interventions for health self-management for adolescents and young adults with physical disabilities, although there are a significant number of such interventions for those with chronic illnesses such as diabetes and asthma (Lindsay, 2016; Sattoe et al., 2015). In contrast with most health self-management intervention programs, interventions for young adults with physical disabilities tend to use a shared management model in which parents or caregivers are included in the intervention, and there is planned transfer of responsibility from the parents or caregivers to the young adult (Lindsay, Kingsnorth, Mcdougall, & Keating, 2014). Interventions tend to have positive effects in some domains, but exceptions include limited efficacy in youth responsibility for medication management.

CONCLUSION

At each stage of development, the capabilities of children and their families interact with changing social and environmental demands. Perspectives on disability change throughout childhood and adolescence. There are important social and environmental influences on children's ability to self-manage typical and atypical developmental demands. The rehabilitation psychologist maintains a developmental perspective, anticipating developmental needs and taking steps to prepare the child, family, and community to meet those needs in an optimal manner. Inevitably, the rehabilitation psychologist functions as an advocate for children and their families to support full integration into the community, drawing on a range of competencies that are specific to the needs of children with disabilities. Rehabilitation psychology competencies emerge from a value system of active collaboration with individuals and families to maximize independence, participation, emotional and physical health, and functional abilities.

References

Aarnoudse-Moens, C. S. H., Weisglas-Kuperus, N., van Goudoever, J. B., & Oosterlaan, J. (2009). Meta-analysis of neurobehavioral outcomes in very preterm and/or very low birth weight children. *Pediatrics*, *124*, 717–728. http://dx.doi.org/10.1542/peds.2008-2816

Abbeduto, L., Warren, S. F., & Conners, F. A. (2007). Language development in Down syndrome: From the prelinguistic period to the acquisition of literacy. *Mental Retardation and Developmental Disabilities Research Reviews*, *13*, 247–261. http://dx.doi.org/10.1002/mrdd.20158

Anderson, B. J., & Coyne, J. C. (1991). "Miscarried helping" in the families of children and adolescents with chronic diseases. In J. H. Johnson & S. B. Johnson (Eds.), *Advances in child health psychology* (pp. 167–177). Gainesville: University of Florida Press.

Bates, E., Thal, D., Trauner, D., Fenson, J., Aram, D., Eisele, J., & Nass, R. (1997). From first words to grammar in children with focal brain injury. *Developmental Neuropsychology*, *13*, 275–343. http://dx.doi.org/10.1080/87565649709540682

Baumrind, D. (1971). Current patterns of parental authority. *Developmental Psychology, 4*(1p2), 1–103. http://dx.doi.org/10.1037/h0030372

Benn, K. M., & McColl, M. A. (2004). Parental coping following childhood acquired brain injury. *Brain Injury*, *18*, 239–255. http://dx.doi.org/10.1080/02699050310001617343

Bhutta, A. T., Cleves, M. A., Casey, P. H., Cradock, M. M., & Anand, K. J. S. (2002). Cognitive and behavioral outcomes of school-aged children who were born preterm: A meta-analysis. *JAMA*, *288*, 728–737. http://dx.doi.org/10.1001/jama.288.6.728

Bilenberg, N., & Lie, H. R. (2001). Behavioral and emotional problems in children with myelomeningocele (MMC). *European Journal of Pediatric Surgery*, *11*(Suppl. 1), S44–S46.

Bogart, K. R. (2014). The role of disability self-concept in adaptation to congenital or acquired disability. *Rehabilitation Psychology*, *59*, 107–115. http://dx.doi.org/10.1037/a0035800

Centers for Disease Control and Prevention. (2002). United States life table, 2000. *National Vital Statistics Reports*, *51*(3), 1–42. Hyattsville, MD: US Department of Health and Human Services. Retrieved from https://www.cdc.gov/nchs/data/nvsr/nvsr51/nvsr51_03.pdf

Chapieski, L., Brewer, V., Evankovich, K., Culhane-Shelburne, K., Zelman, K., & Alexander, A. (2005). Adaptive functioning in children with seizures: Impact of maternal anxiety about epilepsy. *Epilepsy & Behavior*, *7*, 246–252. http://dx.doi.org/10.1016/j.yebeh.2005.05.002

Chien, A. T., Kuhlthau, K. A., Toomey, S. L., Quinn, J. A., Houtrow, A. J., Kuo, D. Z., . . . Schuster, M. A. (2015). Development of the children with disabilities algorithm. *Pediatrics*, *136*, e871–e878. http://dx.doi.org/10.1542/peds.2015-0228

Cunningham, S. D., Warschausky, S., & Dixon Thomas, P. (2009). Parenting and social functioning of children with and without cerebral palsy. *Rehabilitation Psychology*, *54*, 109–115. http://dx.doi.org/10.1037/a0014748

Cyrulnik, S. E., Fee, R. J., Batchelder, A., Kiefel, J., Goldstein, E., & Hinton, V. J. (2008). Cognitive and adaptive deficits in young children with Duchenne muscular dystrophy (DMD). *Journal of the International Neuropsychological Society*,

14, 853–861. http://dx.doi.org/10.1017/S135561770808106X

Dalvand, H., Dehghan, L., Hadian, M. R., Feizy, A., & Hosseini, S. A. (2012). Relationship between gross motor and intellectual function in children with cerebral palsy: A cross-sectional study. *Archives of Physical Medicine and Rehabilitation*, *93*, 480–484. http://dx.doi.org/10.1016/j.apmr.2011.10.019

Dennis, M., & Barnes, M. A. (2010). The cognitive phenotype of spina bifida meningomyelocele. *Developmental Disabilities Research Reviews*, *16*, 31–39. http://dx.doi.org/10.1002/ddrr.89

Dennis, M., Guger, S., Roncadin, C., Barnes, M., & Schachar, R. (2001). Attentional-inhibitory control and social–behavioral regulation after childhood closed head injury: Do biological, developmental, and recovery variables predict outcome? *Journal of the International Neuropsychological Society*, *7*, 683–692. http://dx.doi.org/10.1017/S1355617701766040

Dixon Thomas, P., Warschausky, S., Golin, R., & Meiners, K. (2008). Direct parenting methods to facilitate the social functioning of children with cerebral palsy. *Journal of Developmental and Physical Disabilities*, *20*, 167–174. http://dx.doi.org/10.1007/s10882-007-9087-z

Drotar, D. (1997). Intervention research: Pushing back the frontiers of pediatric psychology. *Journal of Pediatric Psychology*, *22*, 593–606. http://dx.doi.org/10.1093/jpepsy/22.5.593

Durkin, M. (2015). *Disability names and numbers: Challenges and opportunities in nosology, epidemiology, and equity/disparity*. Retrieved from http://sites.nationalacademies.org/cs/groups/dbassesite/documents/webpage/dbasse_170078.pdf

Easterbrooks, M. A., Bureau, J. F., & Lyons-Ruth, K. (2012). Developmental correlates and predictors of emotional availability in mother-child interaction: A longitudinal study from infancy to middle childhood. *Development and Psychopathology*, *24*, 65–78. http://dx.doi.org/10.1017/S0954579411000666

Eisenhower, A. S., Baker, B. L., & Blacher, J. (2005). Preschool children with intellectual disability: Syndrome specificity, behaviour problems, and maternal well-being. *Journal of Intellectual Disability Research*, *49*, 657–671. http://dx.doi.org/10.1111/j.1365-2788.2005.00699.x

Ellingsen, R., Baker, B. L., Blacher, J., & Crnic, K. (2014). Resilient parenting of children at developmental risk across middle childhood. *Research in Developmental Disabilities*, *35*, 1364–1374. http://dx.doi.org/10.1016/j.ridd.2014.03.016

Ewing-Cobbs, L., Prasad, M. R., Kramer, L., Cox, C. S., Jr., Baumgartner, J., Fletcher, S., . . . Swank, P. (2006). Late intellectual and academic outcomes following traumatic brain injury sustained during early childhood. *Journal of Neurosurgery*, *105*(4, Suppl.), 287–296.

Fernandez-Alcántara, M., García-Caro, M. P., Pérez-Marfil, M. N., Hueso-Montoro, C., Laynez-Rubio, C., & Cruz-Quintana, F. (2016). Feelings of loss and grief in parents of children diagnosed with autism spectrum disorder (ASD). *Research in Developmental Disabilities*, *55*, 312–321. http://dx.doi.org/10.1016/j.ridd.2016.05.007

Fevang, S. K. E., Hysing, M., Markestad, T., & Sommerfelt, K. (2016). Mental health in children born extremely preterm without severe neurodevelopmental disabilities. *Pediatrics*, *137*, 1–11. http://dx.doi.org/10.1542/peds.2015-3002

Ginsburg, G. S., & Bronstein, P. (1993). Family factors related to children's intrinsic/extrinsic motivational orientation and academic performance. *Child Development*, *64*, 1461–1474. http://dx.doi.org/10.2307/1131546

Gonzalez-Monge, S., Boudia, B., Ritz, A., Abbas-Chorfa, F., Rabilloud, M., Iwaz, J., & Bérard, C. (2009). A 7-year longitudinal follow-up of intellectual development in children with congenital hemiplegia. *Developmental Medicine & Child Neurology*, *51*, 959–967. http://dx.doi.org/10.1111/j.1469-8749.2009.03339.x

Greenberg, M. T., Speltz, M. L., & DeKlyen, M. (1993). The role of attachment in the early development of disruptive behavior problems. *Development and Psychopathology*, *5*, 191–213. http://dx.doi.org/10.1017/S095457940000434X

Guralnick, M. J., & Weinhouse, E. (1984). Peer-related social interactions of developmentally delayed young children—Development and characteristics. *Developmental Psychology*, *20*, 815–827. http://dx.doi.org/10.1037/0012-1649.20.5.815

Halfon, N., Houtrow, A., Larson, K., & Newacheck, P. W. (2012). The changing landscape of disability in childhood. *The Future of Children*, *22*, 13–42. http://dx.doi.org/10.1353/foc.2012.0004

Hanks, R. A., Rapport, L. J., Waldron Perrine, B., & Millis, S. R. (2016). Correlates of resilience in the first 5 years after traumatic brain injury. *Rehabilitation Psychology*, *61*, 269–276. http://dx.doi.org/10.1037/rep0000069

Hanks, R. A., Temkin, N., Machamer, J., & Dikmen, S. S. (1999). Emotional and behavioral adjustment after traumatic brain injury. *Archives of Physical Medicine and Rehabilitation*, *80*, 991–997. http://dx.doi.org/10.1016/S0003-9993(99)90049-7

Hauser-Cram, P., Woodman, A. C., & Heyman, M. (2014). Early mastery motivation as a predictor of executive function in young adults with developmental disabilities. *American Journal on Intellectual and Developmental Disabilities*, *119*, 536–551. http://dx.doi.org/10.1352/1944-7588-119.6.536

Heffelfinger, A. K., Koop, J. I., Fastenau, P. S., Brei, T. J., Conant, L., Katzenstein, J., . . . Sawin, K. J. (2008). The relationship of neuropsychological functioning to adaptation outcome in adolescents with spina bifida. *Journal of the International Neuropsychological Society*, *14*, 793–804. http://dx.doi.org/10.1017/S1355617708081022

Holmbeck, G. N., Johnson, S. Z., Wills, K. E., McKernon, W., Rose, B., Erklin, S., & Kemper, T. (2002). Observed and perceived parental overprotection in relation to psychosocial adjustment in preadolescents with a physical disability: The mediational role of behavioral autonomy. *Journal of Consulting and Clinical Psychology*, *70*, 96–110. http://dx.doi.org/10.1037/0022-006X.70.1.96

Houtrow, A. J., Larson, K., Olson, L. M., Newacheck, P. W., & Halfon, N. (2014). Changing trends of childhood disability, 2001–2011. *Pediatrics*, *134*, 530–538. http://dx.doi.org/10.1542/peds.2014-0594

Hoyert, D. L., & Xu, J. Q. (2012). *Deaths: Preliminary data for 2011* (Vol. 61). Hyattsville, MD: National Center for Health Statistics.

Jenks, K. M., van Lieshout, E. C. D. N., & de Moor, J. (2009). The relationship between medical impairments and arithmetic development in children with cerebral palsy. *Journal of Child Neurology*, *24*, 528–535. http://dx.doi.org/10.1177/0883073809335009

Jonsson, C. A., Horneman, G., & Emanuelson, I. (2004). Neuropsychological progress during 14 years after severe traumatic brain injury in childhood and adolescence. *Brain Injury*, *18*, 921–934. http://dx.doi.org/10.1080/02699050410001671900

Kuban, K. C., Joseph, R. M., O'Shea, T. M., Allred, E. N., Heeren, T., Douglass, L., . . . Leviton, A. (2016). Girls and boys born before 28 weeks gestation: Risks of cognitive, behavioral, and neurologic outcomes at age 10 years. *The Journal of Pediatrics*, *173*, 69–75. http://dx.doi.org/10.1016/j.jpeds.2016.02.048

Lamborn, S. D., Mounts, N. S., Steinberg, L., & Dornbusch, S. M. (1991). Patterns of competence and adjustment among adolescents from authoritative, authoritarian, indulgent, and neglectful families. *Child Development*, *62*, 1049–1065. http://dx.doi.org/10.2307/1131151

Lavigne, J. V., & Faier-Routman, J. (1992). Psychological adjustment to pediatric physical disorders: A meta-analytic review. *Journal of Pediatric Psychology*, *17*, 133–157. http://dx.doi.org/10.1093/jpepsy/17.2.133

Lavigne, J. V., Nolan, D., & McLone, D. G. (1988). Temperament, coping, and psychological adjustment in young children with myelomeningocele. *Journal of Pediatric Psychology*, *13*, 363–378. http://dx.doi.org/10.1093/jpepsy/13.3.363

Levin, H. S. (2003). Neuroplasticity following nonpenetrating traumatic brain injury. *Brain Injury*, *17*, 665–674. http://dx.doi.org/10.1080/0269905031000107151

Lindsay, S. (2016). Child and youth experiences and perspectives of cerebral palsy: A qualitative systematic review. *Child: Care, Health and Development*, *42*, 153–175. http://dx.doi.org/10.1111/cch.12309

Lindsay, S., Kingsnorth, S., Mcdougall, C., & Keating, H. (2014). A systematic review of self-management interventions for children and youth with physical disabilities. *Disability and Rehabilitation: An International Multidisciplinary Journal*, *36*, 276–288. http://dx.doi.org/10.3109/09638288.2013.785605

Lomax-Bream, L. E., Barnes, M., Copeland, K., Taylor, H. B., & Landry, S. H. (2007). The impact of spina bifida on development across the first 3 years. *Developmental Neuropsychology*, *31*, 1–20. http://dx.doi.org/10.1207/s15326942dn3101_1

Majnemer, A., Shevell, M., Law, M., Poulin, C., & Rosenbaum, P. (2010). Level of motivation in mastering challenging tasks in children with cerebral palsy. *Developmental Medicine & Child Neurology*, *52*, 1120–1126. http://dx.doi.org/10.1111/j.1469-8749.2010.03732.x

McDermott, S., Coker, A. L., Mani, S., Krishnaswami, S., Nagle, R. J., Barnett-Queen, L. L., & Wuori, D. F. (1996). A population-based analysis of behavior problems in children with cerebral palsy. *Journal of Pediatric Psychology*, *21*, 447–463. http://dx.doi.org/10.1093/jpepsy/21.3.447

Miller, L., Ziviani, J., Ware, R. S., & Boyd, R. N. (2015). Mastery motivation: A way of understanding therapy outcomes for children with unilateral cerebral palsy. *Disability and Rehabilitation: An International Multidisciplinary Journal*, *37*, 1439–1445. http://dx.doi.org/10.3109/09638288.2014.964375

Morgan, G. A., MacTurk, R. H., & Hrncir, E. J. (1991). Mastery motivation: Overview, definitions, and conceptual issues. In R. H. MacTurk & G. A. Morgan (Eds.), *Mastery motivation: Origins, conceptualizations, and applications* (pp. 1–18). Norwood, NJ: Ablex.

Mulder, H., Pitchford, N. J., & Marlow, N. (2010). Processing speed and working memory underlie academic attainment in very preterm children. *Archives of Disease in Childhood. Fetal and Neonatal Edition*, *95*(4), F267–F272. http://dx.doi.org/10.1136/adc.2009.167965

Murphy, S. L., Xu, J. Q., & Kochanek, K. D. (2012). *Deaths: Final data for 2010* (Vol. 61). Hyattsville, MD: National Center for Health Statistics.

Nassau, J. H., & Drotar, D. (1995). Social competence in children with IDDM and asthma: Child, teacher, and parent reports of children's social adjustment, social performance, and social skills. *Journal of Pediatric Psychology*, *20*, 187–204. http://dx.doi.org/10.1093/jpepsy/20.2.187

Office of Special Education and Rehabilitative Services. (2015). *37th Annual Report to Congress on the Implementation of the Individuals With Disabilities Education Act, 2015*. Retrieved from https://www2.ed.gov/about/reports/annual/osep/2015/parts-b-c/37th-arc-for-idea.pdf

Parkes, J., White-Koning, M., McCullough, N., & Colver, A. (2009). Psychological problems in children with hemiplegia: A European multicentre survey. *Archives of Disease in Childhood*, *94*, 429–433. http://dx.doi.org/10.1136/adc.2008.151688

Patterson, T., Rapsey, C. M., & Glue, P. (2013). Systematic review of cognitive development across childhood in Down syndrome: Implications for treatment interventions. *Journal of Intellectual Disability Research*, *57*, 306–318. http://dx.doi.org/10.1111/j.1365-2788.2012.01536.x

Pedersen, A. L., Crnic, K. A., Baker, B. L., & Blacher, J. (2015). Reconceptualizing family adaptation to developmental delay. *American Journal on Intellectual and Developmental Disabilities*, *120*, 346–370. http://dx.doi.org/10.1352/1944-7558-120.4.346

Piaget, J. (1964). Part I: Cognitive development in children: Piaget development and learning. *Journal of Research in Science Teaching*, *2*, 176–186. http://dx.doi.org/10.1002/tea.3660020306

Pinquart, M. (2014). Achievement of developmental milestones in emerging and young adults with and without pediatric chronic illness—A meta-analysis. *Journal of Pediatric Psychology*, *39*, 577–587. http://dx.doi.org/10.1093/jpepsy/jsu017

Pinquart, M., & Teubert, D. (2012). Academic, physical, and social functioning of children and adolescents with chronic physical illness: A meta-analysis. *Journal of Pediatric Psychology*, *37*, 376–389. http://dx.doi.org/10.1093/jpepsy/jsr106

Potter, J. L., Wade, S. L., Walz, N. C., Cassedy, A., Stevens, M. H., Yeates, K. O., & Taylor, H. G. (2011). Parenting style is related to executive dysfunction after brain injury in children. *Rehabilitation Psychology*, *56*, 351–358. http://dx.doi.org/10.1037/a0025445

Prasad, M. R., Swank, P. R., & Ewing-Cobbs, L. (2017). Long-term school outcomes of children and adolescents with traumatic brain injury. *The Journal of Head Trauma Rehabilitation*, *32*, E24–E32. http://dx.doi.org/10.1097/HTR.0000000000000218

Rackauskaite, G., Bilenberg, N., Bech, B. H., Uldall, P., & Østergaard, J. R. (2016). Screening for psychopathology in a national cohort of 8- to 15-year-old children with cerebral palsy. *Research in Developmental Disabilities*, *49–50*, 171–180. http://dx.doi.org/10.1016/j.ridd.2015.11.019

Ramstad, K., Loge, J. H., Jahnsen, R., & Diseth, T. H. (2015). Self-reported mental health in youth with cerebral palsy and associations to recurrent musculoskeletal pain. *Disability and Rehabilitation: An International Multidisciplinary Journal*, *37*, 144–150. http://dx.doi.org/10.3109/09638288.2014.913703

Rodenburg, R., Meijer, A. M., Deković, M., & Aldenkamp, A. P. (2007). Parents of children with enduring epilepsy: Predictors of parenting stress and parenting. *Epilepsy & Behavior*, *11*, 197–207. http://dx.doi.org/10.1016/j.yebeh.2007.05.001

Sambuco, M., Brookes, N., & Lah, S. (2008). Paediatric traumatic brain injury: A review of siblings' outcome. *Brain Injury*, *22*, 7–17. http://dx.doi.org/10.1080/02699050701822022

Sansom-Daly, U. M., Lin, M., Robertson, E. G., Wakefield, C. E., McGill, B. C., Girgis, A., & Cohn, R. J. (2016). Health literacy in adolescents and young adults: An updated review. *Journal of Adolescent and Young Adult Oncology*, *5*, 106–118. http://dx.doi.org/10.1089/jayao.2015.0059

Sattoe, J. N. T., Bal, M. I., Roelofs, P. D. D. M., Bal, R., Miedema, H. S., & van Staa, A. (2015). Self-management interventions for young people with chronic conditions: A systematic overview. *Patient Education and Counseling*, *98*, 704–715. http://dx.doi.org/10.1016/j.pec.2015.03.004

Sawicki, G. S., Kelemen, S., & Weitzman, E. R. (2014). Ready, set, stop: Mismatch between self-care beliefs, transition readiness skills, and transition planning among adolescents, young adults, and parents. *Clinical Pediatrics*, *53*, 1062–1068. http://dx.doi.org/10.1177/0009922814541169

Scull, J., & Winkler, A. M. (2011). *Shifting trends in special education*. Washington, DC: Thomas B. Fordham Institute. Retrieved from http://www.edexcellencemedia.net/publications/2011/20110525_ShiftingTrendsinSpecialEducation/ShiftingTrendsinSpecialEducation.pdf

Shogren, K. A., Shaw, L. A., & Little, T. D. (2016). Measuring the early adulthood outcomes of young adults with disabilities: Developing constructs using NLTS2 data. *Exceptionality*, *24*, 45–61. http://dx.doi.org/10.1080/09362835.2015.1064416

Sigurdardottir, S., & Vik, T. (2011). Speech, expressive language, and verbal cognition of preschool children with cerebral palsy in Iceland. *Developmental Medicine & Child Neurology*, *53*, 74–80. http://dx.doi.org/10.1111/j.1469-8749.2010.03790.x

Smits, D. W., Ketelaar, M., Gorter, J. W., van Schie, P., Dallmeijer, A., Jongmans, M., & Lindeman, E.

(2011). Development of daily activities in school-age children with cerebral palsy. *Research in Developmental Disabilities*, *32*, 222–234. http://dx.doi.org/10.1016/j.ridd.2010.09.025

Spira, E. G., Bracken, S. S., & Fischel, J. E. (2005). Predicting improvement after first-grade reading difficulties: The effects of oral language, emergent literacy, and behavior skills. *Developmental Psychology*, *41*, 225–234. http://dx.doi.org/10.1037/0012-1649.41.1.225

Tan, S. S., Wiegerink, D. J. H. G., Vos, R. C., Smits, D. W., Voorman, J. M., Twisk, J. W. R., . . . Roebroeck, M. E. (2014). Developmental trajectories of social participation in individuals with cerebral palsy: A multicentre longitudinal study. *Developmental Medicine & Child Neurology*, *56*, 370–377. http://dx.doi.org/10.1111/dmcn.12343

Tarazi, R. A., Mahone, E. M., & Zabel, T. A. (2007). Self-care independence in children with neurological disorders: An interactional model of adaptive demands and executive dysfunction. *Rehabilitation Psychology*, *52*, 196–205. http://dx.doi.org/10.1037/0090-5550.52.2.196

Taylor, H. G., & Alden, J. (1997). Age-related differences in outcomes following childhood brain insults: An introduction and overview. *Journal of the International Neuropsychological Society*, *3*, 555–567.

Thomasgard, M., Metz, W. P., Edelbrock, C., & Shonkoff, J. P. (1995). Parent–child relationship disorders. Part I. Parental overprotection and the development of the Parent Protection Scale. *Journal of Developmental and Behavioral Pediatrics*, *16*, 244–250.

Tuminello, E. R., Holmbeck, G. N., & Olson, R. (2012). Executive functions in adolescents with spina bifida: Relations with autonomy development and parental intrusiveness. *Child Neuropsychology*, *18*, 105–124. http://dx.doi.org/10.1080/09297049.2011.590470

van Schie, P. E. M., Siebes, R. C., Dallmeijer, A. J., Schuengel, C., Smits, D. W., Gorter, J. W., & Becher, J. G. (2013). Development of social functioning and communication in school-aged (5–9 years) children with cerebral palsy. *Research in Developmental Disabilities*, *34*, 4485–4494. http://dx.doi.org/10.1016/j.ridd.2013.09.033

Volpe, J. J. (2008). *Neurology of the newborn*. Amsterdam, the Netherlands: Elsevier Health Sciences.

Voorman, J. M., Dallmeijer, A. J., Van Eck, M., Schuengel, C., & Becher, J. G. (2010). Social functioning and communication in children with cerebral palsy: Association with disease characteristics and personal and environmental factors. *Developmental Medicine & Child Neurology*, *52*, 441–447. http://dx.doi.org/10.1111/j.1469-8749.2009.03399.x

Vos, R. C., Becher, J. G., Ketelaar, M., Smits, D. W., Voorman, J. M., Tan, S. S., . . . Dallmeijer, A. J. (2013). Developmental trajectories of daily activities in children and adolescents with cerebral palsy. *Pediatrics*, *132*, e915–e923. http://dx.doi.org/10.1542/peds.2013-0499

Wade, S. L., Cassedy, A., Walz, N. C., Taylor, H. G., Stancin, T., & Yeates, K. O. (2011). The relationship of parental warm responsiveness and negativity to emerging behavior problems following traumatic brain injury in young children. *Developmental Psychology*, *47*, 119–133. http://dx.doi.org/10.1037/a0021028

Wade, S. L., Zhang, N., Yeates, K. O., Stancin, T., & Taylor, H. G. (2016). Social environmental moderators of long-term functional outcomes of early childhood brain injury. *JAMA Pediatrics*, *170*, 343–349. http://dx.doi.org/10.1001/jamapediatrics.2015.4485

Wallander, J. L., Thompson, R. J., & Alriksson-Schmidt, A. (2003). Psychosocial adjustment of children with chronic physical conditions. In M. Robert (Ed.), *Handbook of pediatric psychology* (pp. 141–158). New York, NY: Guilford Press.

Warschausky, S., Argento, A. G., Hurvitz, E., & Berg, M. (2003). Neuropsychological status and social problem solving in children with congenital or acquired brain dysfunction. *Rehabilitation Psychology*, *48*, 250–254. http://dx.doi.org/10.1037/0090-5550.48.4.250

Warschausky, S., Kaufman, J. N., Evitts, M., Schutt, W., & Hurvitz, E. A. (2017). Mastery motivation and executive functions as predictors of adaptive behavior in adolescents and young adults with cerebral palsy or myelomeningocele. *Rehabilitation Psychology*, *62*, 258–267. http://dx.doi.org/10.1037/rep0000151

Warschausky, S., Van Tubbergen, M., Asbell, S., Kaufman, J., Ayyangar, R., & Donders, J. (2012). Modified test administration using assistive technology: Preliminary psychometric findings. *Assessment*, *19*, 472–479. http://dx.doi.org/10.1177/1073191111402458

Wehman, P., Sima, A. P., Ketchum, J., West, M. D., Chan, F., & Luecking, R. (2015). Predictors of successful transition from school to employment for youth with disabilities. *Journal of Occupational Rehabilitation*, *25*, 323–334. http://dx.doi.org/10.1007/s10926-014-9541-6

Whittingham, K., Wee, D., Sanders, M. R., & Boyd, R. (2013). Sorrow, coping and resiliency: Parents of children with cerebral palsy share their experiences. *Disability and Rehabilitation: An International Multidisciplinary Journal*, *35*, 1447–1452. http://dx.doi.org/10.3109/09638288.2012.737081

Wiedenbauer, G., & Jansen-Osmann, P. (2008). Manual training of mental rotation in children. *Learning and Instruction*, *18*, 30–41. http://dx.doi.org/10.1016/j.learninstruc.2006.09.009

Yeates, K. O., Taylor, H. G., Wade, S. L., Drotar, D., Stancin, T., & Minich, N. (2002). A prospective study of short- and long-term neuropsychological outcomes after traumatic brain injury in children. *Neuropsychology*, *16*, 514–523. http://dx.doi.org/10.1037/0894-4105.16.4.514

Yeates, K. O., Taylor, H. G., Walz, N. C., Stancin, T., & Wade, S. L. (2010). The family environment as a moderator of psychosocial outcomes following traumatic brain injury in young children. *Neuropsychology*, *24*, 345–356. http://dx.doi.org/10.1037/a0018387

Zinner, E. S., Ball, J. D., Stutts, M. L., & Philput, C. (1997). Grief reactions of mothers of adolescents and young adults with traumatic brain injury. *Archives of Clinical Neuropsychology*, *12*, 435–447. http://dx.doi.org/10.1093/arclin/12.5.435

Chapter 12

FAMILIES AND DISABILITY

Erin E. Andrews and Rose A. Dunn

> Life doesn't make any sense without interdependence. We need each other and the sooner we learn that the better for us all.
>
> —*Joan Erikson*

The above quote comes from a *New York Times* article published on June 14, 1988, and although widely attributed to her husband, Erik Erikson, Mrs. Erikson confirmed it was hers (Goleman, 1988). Erik Erikson—best known for his psychosocial identity stages theory of normal human development—and Joan had their fourth child in 1944. Their youngest son, Neil, was diagnosed with Down syndrome. He was institutionalized shortly after birth and remained so his entire life (Friedman, 1999). He was rarely visited by either of his parents, who kept his existence a secret for most of their lives. These autobiographical facts are congruent with societal norms of the times, but even today the existence of a disabled[1] family member is sometimes considered a source of shame.

Disability has historically been regarded as an individual phenomenon, but contemporary models of disability emphasize the importance of contextual factors (Watermeyer & Swartz, 2016). Some disability studies scholars argued that the individual is inseparable from the relational aspects of disability (Shakespeare, 2006). In this chapter, we make a case for disability as a family issue. Indeed, many disability and rehabilitation scholars have identified the importance of family support, and particularly the role of caregivers, in outcomes related to disability (Shewchuk & Elliott, 2000). Like nondisabled people, partnerships, family ties, and parenthood can have significant effects on the economic, social, and psychological well-being of people with disabilities (Clarke & McKay, 2014). Scant attention has been paid to the diverse roles that people with disabilities hold within their families, and the reciprocal and often interdependent relationships in which they engage. Disabled people are stereotypically portrayed as recipients of care from family members, and researchers have examined the supposed burden of such caregiving (Wates, 2004). As Banks (2003) pointed out, families tend to be completely unprepared for the birth of a disabled child or the acquired disability of a loved one. Family responses to disability are highly variable, and related to specific cultural, ethnic, generational, and gender norms held by families (Banks, 2003). Although several research studies using clinical-based samples have reported

[1]The term *disabled* is intentionally used throughout this chapter to honor identity-first language, preferred by many who identify proudly with disability identity and culture. Disability culture advocates have encouraged psychologists to adopt identity- and person-first language, which "ensures inclusion, addresses issues raised by disability studies and disability culture, respectively, and allows APA [American Psychological Association]-style writing to evolve along with contemporary trends" (Dunn & Andrews, 2015).

http://dx.doi.org/10.1037/0000129-013
Handbook of Rehabilitation Psychology, Third Edition, L. A. Brenner, S. A. Reid-Arndt, T. R. Elliott, R. G. Frank, and B. Caplan (Editors-in-Chief)

negative effects of disability on individuals and their families' well-being, more recent research using longitudinal designs and population-based samples have provided a more nuanced understanding. These findings demonstrated that many disabled individuals and their families experience psychological resiliency and life satisfaction (Elliott, Berry, Richards, & Shewchuk, 2014; Haley, Roth, Hovater, & Clay, 2015). The aim of this chapter is to present a perspective of disabled people and their families that acknowledges their inherent ability to pursue and maintain valued roles, relationships, and activities, while also underscoring the need for evidence-based services and public policies that promote resiliency and address existing systemic barriers.

DISABLED CHILDREN AND THEIR FAMILIES

A large body of literature describes the impact of childhood disability on families. The primary focus has been on the detrimental effects of disability on parents and siblings and the social and economic functioning of these families. Numerous studies confirmed that parents of disabled children experience additional stress and responsibility and have higher rates of physical and mental health problems compared with parents of nondisabled children (Brehaut et al., 2011). Economic strain and poverty can result from time spent away from work to care for disabled children and attend health care appointments and from having to pay for medical care and health insurance (Davidoff, 2004; Kuo, Cohen, Agrawal, Berry, & Casey, 2011). The likelihood of financial problems is commensurate with the severity of the child's disability (Kuhlthau, Hill, Yucel, & Perrin, 2005). Children with disabilities are less likely than their nondisabled peers to live in a home with two parents, and more likely to be raised by single mothers with lower household incomes (Cohen & Petrescu-Prahova, 2006).

Negative academic rhetoric around raising disabled children, called the "burden literature" by some disability studies scholars, has become the mainstream dialogue about the experience of families of disabled children (Davies & Watson, 2002). By focusing nearly exclusively on the stressors and negative aspects of parenting children with disabilities, opportunities to assess possible positive factors and identify strength-based approaches are greatly reduced (Scorgie, Wilgosh, & Sobsey, 2004). The traditional narrative of crisis initiated by a child's disability has overshadowed mediating factors and has failed to address the lack of appropriate support available to families of disabled children (Raina et al., 2005). In fact, emerging evidence indicates that some parents experience enrichment because of their child's disability, report value in facing adversity and learning to advocate as a family and appreciate their involvement in the disability community (Goodley & Cole, 2015). Scorgie and colleagues (2004) developed a model of resilience and transformational outcomes in which the lives of parents are initially disrupted and disoriented by a child's disability, as their worldview and beliefs are challenged. Their model suggests parents can release old assumptions and self-definitions that no longer work, while actively and intentionally creating new self-identities and perspectives following the onset of their child's disability. Indeed, disability studies scholars have postulated that resilience is a relational rather than individual concept (Runswick-Cole & Goodley, 2013). This social constructionist viewpoint places emphasis on the resilience not of the disabled person, but rather on available resources, including materials, relationships, identity, bodies and minds, power and control, community participation, community cohesion, and social justice (Runswick-Cole & Goodley, 2013).

Parents and families provide the primary environmental context in which children with disabilities engage (Rosenbaum & Gorter, 2012). Despite the central role of families, medical professionals have traditionally sidelined parents and other family members, missing crucial opportunities to intervene with families (Rosenbaum & Gorter, 2012). Ironically, it is these same parents who often make important medical decisions regarding their disabled children. Disability activists have been wary of attempts to undermine the self-determination of people with disabilities and have at times questioned the accuracy of "quality of life" assessments made by health care providers and family members (Asch, 2001). The interactions among disabled children, their parents, and health care providers exist in the context of a society where medical treatment can be withheld from infants with congenital disabilities, allowing them to die. Moreover, genetic testing and abortion are accepted as means to prevent the existence of disabled children, and the portrayal of disability is based on prejudicial and biased beliefs about the kind of lives that disabled children and their families lead (Asch, 2001). Scorgie and colleagues (2004) suggested that when health care providers present or reinforce a child's disability as a catastrophe, it is increasingly difficult for parents to effectively construct new narratives and meaning around this experience.

A major concern of children with disabilities and their families is reduced access to and participation in their communities. Families with low social integration in their communities have low expectations for disabled children to participate in family and recreational activities (Chiarello et al., 2016). Children with disabilities and their families are often excluded, implicitly or explicitly, from community and recreational opportunities because of physical, systemic, and attitudinal barriers.

The language used to describe disabled children also plays an important role with their families, in community and educational settings. One common phrase is "special needs" (Brehaut et al., 2011). McPherson et al. (1998) defined children with special health care needs as those who "have or are at increased risk for a chronic physical, developmental, or emotional condition, and who also require health and related services of a type or amount beyond that required by children generally" (p. 139). Children with disabilities are likely to be part of this group but may be referred to across settings as special needs. Like other terms that sound positive (e.g., "differently-able," "handi-capable"), special needs can be received as infantilizing (Dunn & Andrews, 2015). Although the disability community would agree that labeling children by their disabilities is detrimental, the supposition of special needs is that disabled children's needs are fundamentally different from those of nondisabled children, and that any related services are a special privilege, instead of fundamental to their right to education, respect, and human dignity.

Disability activists have taken offense to societal responses to publicized cases of child abuse and murder, where the perpetrator, usually a parent, is cast as a victim. This "overwhelmed guardian" defense for filicide stems from beliefs that disabled lives hold less worth and that the burden of caring for a disabled child is reasonable justification for murder. Autistic children are at an increased risk for filicide (Coorg & Tournay, 2013). In a review of cases, Sobsey (2007) revealed that parents who used feelings of stress or overwhelm as a defense were unlikely to be charged or prosecuted for criminal offenses. Few parents of disabled children are held criminally responsible for filicide; those who are convicted tend to face lesser charges and receive lighter sentences than parents who are convicted of killing nondisabled children (Sobsey, 2007).

PARTNERSHIPS

Almost by definition, relationships with disabled people tend to be interdependent. Like nondisabled peers, people with disabilities and their partners must navigate relationship formation and maintenance of personal and familial relations. Clarke and McKay (2014) argued that relational strain can result from difficulty negotiating and reciprocating care with respect to mutual dependence and autonomy.

Disabled people often encounter unique barriers affecting the creation and continuation of romantic and sexual partnerships. Adults with disabilities are more likely to be single than nondisabled adults and are less likely to raise children (Clarke & McKay, 2014). The medical model approach frames disability as a problem that creates difficulties within existing marriages and impedes the development of relationships (Shakespeare, 2006). This perspective has been reflected in the bulk of extant research, which has focused narrowly on caregiving and role changes following acquired disability. Unfortunately, there has been a dearth of attention paid to social and systemic factors affecting the formation and maintenance of intimate partnerships for disabled people.

Diverse barriers can hinder intimate relationship formation among disabled people. Negative social assumptions and stereotypes about disabled people that persist within the nondisabled community can interfere with disabled people's success in forming romantic and sexual relationships (Brodwin & Frederick, 2010). Although there have been several legislative, advocacy, and research efforts focused on the social integration of disabled people, social exclusion has continued to exist and even intensified in recent years (Tumin, 2016). Notably, Hergenrather and Rhodes (2007) concluded that attitudes toward disabled people were the most negative within the context of dating. For example, nondisabled people often perceive disabled people as being asexual, over-sexed, overly dependent, and/or disinterested in forming intimate relationships (Howland & Rintala, 2001; Louvet, 2007). These negative assumptions limit the inclusion of disabled people in social activities that could provide opportunities for initiating intimate relationships. Additionally, these misperceptions about disability can have a detrimental impact on disabled people's self-concept and self-expectations (Chance, 2002), leading them to expect rejection from potential nondisabled partners (Taleporos & McCabe, 2001). Developing platforms (e.g., media, public forums) for open dialogue and education about disability and sexuality would be a beneficial step in debunking these societal myths (Esmail, Darry, Walter, & Knupp, 2010).

In addition to the broader societal context, family, friends, and medical providers may also transmit negative messages to disabled people about their ability to engage in intimate relationships either through explicit statements or complete avoidance of the topic (Esmail et al., 2010; Nguyen, Liamputtong, & Monfries, 2016). For example, Clarke and McKay (2014) found that some young women with disabilities were discouraged by family members from cohabitation, dating, and marriage, and that many young disabled adults reported that their families did not consider their potential roles as romantic and sexual partners. Family members and health care providers may have apprehension about disabled adolescents and young adults exploring their sexuality, and as a result, a diffusion of responsibility for comprehensive sexual education can occur (East & Orchard, 2014). In addition to promoting safety and autonomy in sexuality, educational endeavors must also explicitly include discussions of consent, given that those with disabilities are at a higher risk of sexual abuse and assault, and that caregivers and family members are frequently the perpetrators (Williams & Colvin, 2016).

Although empirical data have demonstrated that disabled people experience more difficulty forming intimate partnerships, Clarke and McKay (2014) found that marriages with at least one a disabled partner experienced the same levels of stability as marriages with two nondisabled partners, although some factors (e.g., job loss after disability) may increase the likelihood of marriage dissolution (Charles & Stephens, 2004). Existing research has had a restricted focus on caregiver and care receiver roles, while neglecting the pre-existing dynamics and roles of the relationship that may be highly valued by the individuals (Clarke & McKay, 2014). There is a great need for empirical research and social policies aimed at helping disabled people maintain and develop valued partnership roles. As mentioned, job loss after disability was found to predict the likelihood of divorce (Charles & Stephens, 2004), suggesting that the forfeiture of this role of provider may be particularly harmful within the partnership. Access to appropriate workplace accommodations and independent income are important ways of ensuring that disabled people can maintain valued roles and exercise choice in maintaining or leaving partnerships.

PARENTS WITH DISABILITIES

The American Psychological Association's (APA; 2012) *Guidelines for Assessment of and Intervention With Persons With Disabilities* states that adults with various disabilities can and do effectively parent children. People with disabilities are believed to represent approximately 15% of parents in the United States, or anywhere from 6.9 million to 8.4 million people, and they are more likely to be single parents, African Americans, and/or Latinos (National Council on Disability, 2012). As the number of adults with disabilities grows, more disabled people are becoming parents (National

Council on Disability, 2012; Smeltzer, 2007). The limited evidence available indicates that disabled parents face substantial barriers to parenting, from restricted physical and attitudinal access, to a lack of knowledge, tools, and support for successful parenting (National Council on Disability, 2012; Olsen & Clarke, 2003; Wates, 2004).

The attitudinal prejudices against parents with disabilities include reduced societal expectation of partnership and parenthood, and stereotypes of disabled people as asexual, infertile, vulnerable, inadequate nurturers, and incapable of being caregivers for children (Andrews & Ayers, 2016; Kirshbaum & Olkin, 2002; Nario-Redmond, 2010). People with disabilities are often described as "selfish" for having children, are commonly presumed to be receiving governmental financial aid and, thus, disabled parents and their children are often judged to be a burden on society (National Council on Disability, 2012). In addition, disabled people are largely discouraged from reproduction through genetic testing, sterilization, and selective abortion because of the possibility of producing children with disabilities (Andrews & Ayers, 2016; Asch, 2001). Disabled parents are likely to face discrimination when pursuing assistive reproductive technology (ART), including fertility treatments, in vitro fertilization, artificial insemination, and embryo transfer and storage (Andrews & Ayers, 2016; National Council on Disability, 2012). ART can enable people with disabilities to produce children when they may otherwise be unable to do so (Collins, 1999). Despite protections under the Americans With Disabilities Act (ADA), discrimination can occur on the basis of direct risks (e.g., gestational concerns resulting in a child's inheritance of disability, the strong possibility of a harmful disability-related pregnancy outcome) and indirect risks (e.g., whether the parent's disability would limit the ability to safely and effectively care for a child; National Council on Disability, 2012). The risks are complicated by the fact that ART providers rarely receive culturally relevant and appropriate education and training to proficiently assess these disability factors (Pendo, 2008). Instead, providers may be susceptible to relying on bias and stereotypes, resulting in discrimination against disabled parents (Andrews & Ayers, 2016).

Similarly, people with disabilities face barriers when pursuing adoption as a means to parenthood. In domestic and international systems, the complex legal and administrative processes impede many disabled people from completing adoption (National Council on Disability, 2012). Many state adoption laws include exclusionary terminology, despite ADA protections that apply to agencies in the United States (Andrews & Ayers, 2016). Discrimination because of bias may occur at several stages of the process, particularly in the home study portion, during which agency evaluators primarily rely on their own discretion as to eligibility criteria and where reasonable accommodations are inconsistently provided (National Council on Disability, 2012). Birth parents, too, may express a preference for their child to be adopted by nondisabled parents, regardless of the fitness of potential adoptive parents with disabilities (Andrews & Ayers, 2016). International adoption holds unique challenges, including financial expenses and mandated travel to another country with variable accessibility. Although some countries will not consider any prospective parents with disabilities, others will make exceptions if parents intend to adopt children with disabilities, who are more difficult to place and expensive to care for (Saclier, 2000). Regardless of these challenges, some disabled parents indeed successfully adopt disabled and nondisabled children in the United States and internationally (Andrews & Ayers, 2016).

Parents with disabilities are disproportionately referred to the child welfare system and have their children removed from their custody at extremely high rates (National Council on Disability, 2012). The actions are often unjustified and destructive to families (Callow, Buckland, & Jones, 2011). Even today, multiple state statutes include the mere presence of disability as grounds for termination of parental rights. Custody determinations in U.S. courts are made on the basis of "the best interests of the child"; however, there is evidence that bias and speculation, in addition to lack of cultural competence and adequate training in disability issues, pollutes these decisions (Andrews & Ayers, 2016; National Council on Disability, 2012). Disabled parents are rarely provided reasonable and appropriate accommodations during family court proceedings (National Council on Disability, 2012). Despite evidence that suggested accommodations, adaptive parenting techniques, adequate social support, and parenting training interventions could facilitate more effective functioning, children are needlessly separated from their parents by courts and child welfare systems (Andrews & Ayers, 2016; National Council on Disability, 2012).

The United States has a shameful history of forcible sterilization of women with intellectual disabilities (Murphy & Feldman, 2002). Assumptions prevail that individuals with intellectual disabilities are incapable of making their own decisions related to sexuality and parenthood (National Council on Disability, 2012). Parenting is generally assumed contraindicated for people with intellectual disabilities (Mayes, Llewellyn, & McConnell, 2006). However, these beliefs are being challenged, by self-advocacy organizations and emerging research data, which suggests that with suitable early and ongoing support, many parents with intellectual disabilities can develop adequate childcare skills, or at least to have significant and meaningful involvement in child-rearing (Andrews & Ayers, 2016). Although children of intellectually disabled parents are at risk for developmental delay and behavioral problems (Feldman, 2002), there are few studies that investigate mediating factors such as social and environmental support, caregiving style, and training and education related to parenting; rather, these outcomes are attributed to cognitive impairments alone (Andrews & Ayers, 2016). Parent-training programs that provide skills and support to parents with intellectual disabilities are promising in demonstrating success but are rarely used and not readily available and accessible to parents (Murphy & Feldman, 2002; Olsen & Clarke, 2003).

Parents who have mental health issues have primarily been addressed in the literature from a deficits-based perspective. A body of research describes the various ways that children are adversely affected by mental illness among parents (Ackerson, 2003). Among the negative factors studied are anger, isolation, shame, fear, sadness, grief, frustration, confusion, identity problems, poor self-esteem and difficulties with trust and intimacy (Nicholson, Sweeney, & Geller, 1998). However, multiple co-occurring issues, including poverty, trauma, substance use, and homelessness, complicate the interpretation of these findings (Andrews & Ayers, 2016).

Assumptions persist that parental mental illness is universally detrimental to children, although the stigma of mental illness may contribute to poorer outcomes in families (Corrigan & Miller, 2004). For example, women with psychiatric disabilities often unnecessarily cease taking medications during pregnancy and worry about losing custody of children during periods of worsening mental health or hospitalization. Fear of separation by the legal system is legitimate; those with psychiatric disabilities have the highest rate of removal among all disability groups (National Council on Disability, 2012; Nicholson et al., 1998). Further research is needed to assess whether mitigating factors exist, like effective parenting strategies, parenting training programs, social support, and other social and interpersonal factors. The mere presence of mental illness must not be mistaken for parental incapability (Andrews & Ayers, 2016).

Evidence is clearer on the effects of parental physical disability; there is no adverse impact on children (National Council on Disability, 2012). Despite this research, physically disabled parents are subject to attitudinal, architectural, and environmental barriers (Bergerona, Vincenta, & Bouchera, 2012; Olsen & Clarke, 2003; Toms Barker & Maralani, 1997). Personal assistant services provided through public funding (i.e., Medicaid) cannot be used to assist with any parenting tasks (National Council on Disability, 2012). Concerns endure about children becoming caregivers for physically disabled parents, even though research has not supported this assertion (Kirshbaum & Olkin, 2002; National Council on Disability, 2012; Olsen & Clarke, 2003).

FAMILIES AND PERSONAL ASSISTANCE

Family caregiving for people with disabilities has been a prominent focus of research. Family caregivers are usually defined as unpaid relatives who routinely aid a disabled family member with activities of daily living (Shewchuk & Elliott, 2000). The well-being of family caregivers has received considerable attention, particularly related to detrimental caregiver outcomes, including burnout, increased depression and anxiety, and poorer health. Rehabilitation psychologists acknowledge that family caregiver relationships are complex and impacted by many individual and environmental factors, but that family caregivers do not inevitably have poor outcomes (Shewchuk & Elliott, 2000). For example, Elliott et al. (2014) found that a large percentage of family members providing care to individuals with traumatic spinal cord injury were resilient in the initial year following injury. Another study found that although individuals providing care to a family member after a stroke exhibited initial psychological distress, their levels of well-being were comparable to noncaregivers within 3 years after a stroke (Haley et al., 2015). Further, many family caregivers report that their role has positive aspects or has enriched their lives (Lloyd, Patterson, & Muers, 2016; Wells, Dywan, & Dumas, 2005).

From a disability studies perspective, the term *caregiver* is not preferred, as some disabled people believe the term is value laden (Parker & Clarke, 2002). Rather than conceptualizing the disabled person with agency, able to make choices and direct their own personal assistance, the term *caregiver* implies that disabled people must be taken care of in a way that can seem patronizing (Parker & Clarke, 2002). Similarly, family members who provide personal assistance may reject the label of caregiver, particularly if they think of their primary role in the relationship as wives, husbands, sisters, brothers, daughters, sons, mothers, or fathers. The term caregiver can overshadow these important identities and imply that the relationship is not reciprocal, or that the disabled person contributes no support or care to the family member (Parker & Clarke, 2002). Most people in the disability community use the term personal care attendant (PCA).

Disabled persons, especially those who rely on PCAs, often struggle to assert their autonomous adulthood. In Western cultures, the ideal of independent adulthood is based on participation in the labor market or responsibility for child-rearing (Priestley, 2003). Because disabled people stereotypically do not meet these criteria, they are often categorized as dependent, without either the responsibilities or rights of adulthood, and in need of supervision from nondisabled adults (Priestley, 2003). Family member are usually categorized as either requiring care or providing care, leaving little room for the complexities of interdependent family relationships (Banks, 2003).

Because professional PCA services are either unavailable or unaffordable to most families, the decision for a family member to act as a PCA may be based less on choice and more on necessity (Banks, 2003; Shewchuk & Elliott, 2000). In addition to concerns about caregiver distress, it is important to note that children and adults with disabilities are at heightened risk for sexual and physical abuse by those serving as caregivers and may feel trapped in relationships because of the limited resources available to them (Banks, 2003; Olkin, 2003). Ideally, people with disabilities would have access to PCA services that provide opportunity for maximum personal agency, with choices about how, when, and by whom the assistance is delivered.

PATIENT- AND FAMILY-CENTERED CARE

Patient- and family-centered care describes a health care delivery philosophy that is an "innovative approach to plan, deliver, and evaluate health care that is grounded in mutually beneficial partnerships among health care providers, patients, and families" (Joint Commission, 2010, p. 92). Family-centered care is integrative and collaborative health care aimed at improving communication and continuity of care (Rosenbaum & Gorter, 2012). Family-centered care is associated with lower stress levels, higher satisfaction, and improved mental health among parents of disabled children, and improved outcomes for children with disabilities (Rosenbaum & Gorter, 2012). Family-centered care is appropriate across the lifespan whenever disabled people identify the family unit as a central part of their life and as a source of strength or support (Bamm & Rosenbaum, 2008). By capitalizing on the family's strengths, family-centered care empowers people with disabilities to make informed choices and decisions with their families. Instead of focusing on the disabled member in the identified patient role, consideration is given to the family unit (Rosenbaum & Gorter, 2012). Because each family is unique and each relationship complex, family-centered care must be flexible to meet families' diverse needs (Dodd, Saggers, & Wildy, 2009). Patient- and family-centered care allows individuals with disabilities and their families to direct their care according to their own values, priorities, and needs (Rosenbaum & Gorter, 2012). The family-centered provider must be willing to relinquish power and share control of decision making by validating the expert role of those with the lived experience of disabilities and their families. Scorgie and colleagues (2004), however, pointed out that providers should be wary of a diffusion of responsibilities; clear communication in family-centered care can help providers gauge the extent to which families are able to self-advocate and the availability of resources to them. Similarly, Dodd and colleagues (2009) emphasized the gender disparities often observed in caregiving; providers should be careful not to place the onus on any one individual (usually a woman) to "coordinate the confusing array of services and manage the relationships of the diversity of professionals with whom they need to interact" (p. 17).

ROLE OF REHABILITATION PSYCHOLOGY

Rehabilitation psychologists and other health care professionals working with people with disabilities must consider the systems in which the individual exists. Rehabilitation psychologists are well positioned to model and coordinate patient- and family-centered care, explore the extent to which family involvement may be helpful or desirable, and intervene where there is a lack of resources and support. To maximize therapeutic impact, it is recommended that rehabilitation psychologists acquire specific competencies through specialized training and experience to adequately serve individuals with disabilities and their families (Cox, Cox, & Caplan, 2013). Table 12.1 is a summary of suggested competencies and specific skills relevant in rehabilitation psychology for working with families with disabilities (see also Chapter 1, this volume).

Self-Reflective Practice and Cultural Diversity

Delivering patient- and family-centered care requires rehabilitation psychologists to examine their own biases and emotional reactions, the meanings they associate with disability, and their own assumptions about the impact of disability on a client's life (Scorgie et al., 2004). Most individuals, including rehabilitation professionals, have deeply held beliefs, attitudes, and values regarding parenting, sexuality, and intimate relationships, and ongoing self-reflection is imperative to ensure that personal values are not being imposed on the individual and their family. It is important to be able to identify when a value-conflict or personal bias could impact treatment, and the rehabilitation psychologist must know when to seek consultation or supervision from a colleague or mentor who has experience in working with families and persons with disabilities.

Ethical and Legal Issues

Rehabilitation psychologists should be knowledgeable about the legal and ethical considerations relevant to people with disabilities and their families. For example, it is important for clinicians to be aware of the potential for harm and abuse within the disability population and understand that caregivers may perpetrate abuse (Hughes, Robinson-Whelen, Taylor, Swedlund, & Nosek, 2004; Williams & Colvin, 2016). Given this potential risk, there is a need to be well informed about effective methods of screening for abuse and/or neglect: psychologists should know the signs, symptoms, and dynamics of disability-related violence, including the unique areas of vulnerability, as well as state mandatory reporting requirements for violence against people with disabilities, including children, older adults, and dependent adults. Rehabilitation psychologists need to be able to engage in safety planning with patients, such as having a safe retreat, back-up PCA, and social supports. It is recommended that providers maintain current contact information for accessible local domestic violence/sexual assault programs and shelters and disability service providers (e.g., Centers for Independent Living).

TABLE 12.1

Suggested Competencies in Rehabilitation Psychology for Working With Families With Disabilities

Rehabilitation psychology competency	Specific skills relevant to families with disabilities
Individual and cultural diversity	Demonstrates willingness to examine own disability-related biases, assumptions, and emotional reactions Ensures that personal values are not being imposed on clients and their families Is able to identify when a value conflict or personal bias could impact treatment Knows when to seek consultation or supervision from a colleague or mentor who has experience in working with families and disability
Ethical and legal principles/standards/statutes and policy	Understands the legal and ethical considerations relevant to individuals with disabilities and their families Is educated on relevant disability laws (e.g., ADA) and has an understanding of how laws pertain to formation and maintenance of family relationships Knows the signs, symptoms, and dynamics of disability-related violence, including the areas of vulnerability Screens for abuse and neglect and intervenes appropriately Learns state mandatory reporting requirements for violence against people with disabilities
Assessment/evaluation	Involves family members in the process of assessment and intervention Considers the interaction between the individual with a disability and the environment, including family relationships Conducts thorough assessments to identify the family roles of disabled people and/or their desired family roles Explores families' personal values, strengths, resources, and challenges Includes assessment of strengths and adaptive coping skills Integrates direct observation, clinical interview, and objective measures to formulate a conceptualization of families' strengths and needs to guide future interventions
Intervention	Provides education about disabilities and how to navigate barriers within systems Offers disabled individuals and their families skill-based training toward the valued interpersonal roles Emphasizes resiliency models of family stress, adjustment, and adaptation, and uses a systems-based approach Obtains foundational knowledge in family systems theory and couples therapy approaches Has familiarity with local agencies and services to connect clients and their families with appropriate community resources Makes appropriate referrals to promote community integration for families
Consultation	Establishes rapport with disabled people and their families, medical providers, treatment teams, and advocacy organizations Facilitates system-level interventions Helps families and providers understand and respond to behavioral challenges Provides input about the effects of many disability- and psychology-related issues
Advocacy	Provides education about disability in public forums Conducts relevant research aimed at informing social policy issues Works to reduce systemic barriers and promote inclusive health care policies Promotes the importance of resources and access to adjunctive services Fosters accessible facilities and practice environments Offers a biopsychosocial and culturally competent perspective to systems issues Presents meaningful research findings that promote the well-being of families with disabilities Seeks out advocacy opportunities (e.g., active in local, regional, national, and international professional and consumer organizations)

Note. ADA = *Americans With Disabilities Act.*

Assessment

According to the *Guidelines for Assessment of and Intervention With Persons With Disabilities* (APA, 2012), clinicians should strive to involve family members in the process of assessment (see also Chapter 4, this volume) and intervention. Rehabilitation psychologists must consider the interaction between the individual with a disability and the environment, which includes the impact of relationships with family and/or caregivers. Rehabilitation psychologists need to be well versed in conducting a thorough assessment to identify the family roles in which disabled people find themselves or the family roles they desire. For many individuals, it is important to look beyond the "traditional" nuclear family unit and inquire about other relationships, such as those with close friends, step-relatives, and extended family that may be central to their lives. Ample time during the clinical interview should be devoted to exploring the family's values, strengths, resources, and challenges. In addition to being clinically informative, discussion of preinjury/illness strengths and coping skills can be therapeutic for individuals and their families as it can foster a sense of self-efficacy and cohesiveness. Rehabilitation psychologists should be able to effectively integrate direct observation, clinical interview, and objective measures to formulate a conceptualization of the family's strengths and needs to guide future interventions.

Intervention

Disabled individuals and their families have a right to education about disability and how to navigate systems barriers. Rehabilitation psychologists should be equipped to offer disabled individuals and their families' skill-based training (e.g., parenting skills, sexual education) to help them pursue valued roles. Approaches that emphasize resiliency models of family stress, adjustment and adaptation, and use a systems framework are particularly useful. Given that some families may require more intensive intervention services (see Chapter 5, this volume), providers are also encouraged to obtain foundational knowledge in family systems theory and couples therapy approaches. Rehabilitation psychologists also need to be familiar with agencies and services within their area to connect clients and their families with appropriate community resources (e.g., accessible facilities, support groups, respite services, options for child care, vocational counseling). Appropriate referrals are an important component of promoting community integration for these families.

Consultation

Cox and colleagues (2013) described consultation in rehabilitation psychology in broad terms; it is important to consider the role as a consultant (see also Chapter 6, this volume) to families, treatment teams, or even advocacy organizations. The ability to establish rapport with disabled people and their families and the ability to relate effectively to providers in the medical setting positions rehabilitation psychologists to facilitate system-level interventions, help families and providers understand and respond to behavioral challenges, and provide input about the effects of many disability- and psychology-related issues, including emotional, cognitive, and personality status, relevant laws and protections, vocational questions, and disability culture concerns.

Advocacy and Social Policy

There are important social policy implications for almost all the issues faced by families with disabilities, and to achieve optimal outcomes, rehabilitation psychologists must be aware of and address these systemic issues (e.g., access to affordable and accessible health care; McPherson et al., 1998). Contributing to caregiver stress is the difficulty that families face in coordinating complex systems of care, and a lack of resources to access adjunctive services such as paid PCA providers and respite care (Brehaut et al., 2011). Reforms that would provide universal health care would enable family members of disabled people to receive mental health services as warranted. Policies that govern the provision of public health care (i.e., Medicaid) could be expanded to include parenting tasks as essential activities of daily living, and coverage for adaptive parenting equipment as durable medical equipment. Health care providers could be required to offer accessible facilities and rewarded for demonstrating inclusive practices.

CONCLUSION

Without systemic change, implications for disabled people and their families are bleak, no matter how they are personally or relationally resilient. Rehabilitation psychology can inform many policy issues germane to disabled families and contribute to systemic changes as a profession. For example, there is a need for well-informed in-home assessments of family/child home-based and PCA services, incorporating a full biopsychosocial and culturally competent perspective on disability. Even terminology can influence the actions of policymakers, so it is crucial that providers advocate by presenting meaningful research findings on the ways that adequate social support services can improve the well-being and health of families with disabilities, and mitigate negative, and often costly, outcomes (Kuhlthau et al., 2005; Kuo et al., 2011; Raina et al., 2005). Professionals should seek out advocacy opportunities, within local, regional, national, and international professional organizations (e.g., Division 22 of the APA—Rehabilitation Psychology) and consumer organizations (e.g., National Multiple Sclerosis Society), providing education about disability in public forums, and conducting relevant research aimed at informing social policy issues. Perhaps more important, rehabilitation psychology must look to the future. By investing in training and quality preparation for psychology trainees, especially those with disabilities, who are interested in specializing in working with disabled families, the next generation will be prepared to assist with the expectation that these families can and should thrive.

References

Ackerson, B. J. (2003). Coping with the dual demands of severe mental illness and parenting: The parents' perspective. *Families in Society*, *84*, 109–118. http://dx.doi.org/10.1606/1044-3894.69

American Psychological Association. (2012). Guidelines for assessment of and intervention with persons with disabilities. *American Psychologist*, *67*, 43–62. http://dx.doi.org/10.1037/a0025892

Andrews, E. E., & Ayers, K. (2016). Parenting with disability: Experiences of disabled women. In S. Miles-Cohen & C. Signore (Eds.), *Eliminating inequities for women with disabilities: An agenda for health and wellness* (pp. 209–225). Washington, DC: American Psychological Association. http://dx.doi.org/10.1037/14943-011

Asch, A. (2001). Disability, bioethics, and human rights. In G. L. Albrecht, K. Seelman, & M. Bury (Eds.), *Handbook of disability studies* (pp. 297–326). Thousand Oaks, CA: Sage. http://dx.doi.org/10.4135/9781412976251.n12

Bamm, E. L., & Rosenbaum, P. (2008). Family-centered theory: Origins, development, barriers, and supports to implementation in rehabilitation medicine. *Archives of Physical Medicine and Rehabilitation*, *89*, 1618–1624. http://dx.doi.org/10.1016/j.apmr.2007.12.034

Banks, M. E. (2003). Disability in the family: A life span perspective. *Cultural Diversity and Ethnic Minority Psychology*, *9*, 367–384. http://dx.doi.org/10.1037/1099-9809.9.4.367

Bergerona, C., Vincenta, C., & Bouchera, N. (2012). Experience of parents in wheelchairs with children aged 6 to 12. *Technology and Disability*, *24*, 247–261.

Brehaut, J. C., Garner, R. E., Miller, A. R., Lach, L. M., Klassen, A. F., Rosenbaum, P. L., & Kohen, D. E. (2011). Changes over time in the health of caregivers of children with health problems: Growth-curve findings from a 10-year Canadian population-based study. *American Journal of Public Health*, *101*, 2308–2316. http://dx.doi.org/10.2105/AJPH.2011.300298

Brodwin, M. G., & Frederick, P. C. (2010). Sexuality and societal beliefs regarding persons living with disabilities. *Journal of Rehabilitation*, *76*, 37–41.

Callow, E., Buckland, K., & Jones, S. (2011). Parents with disabilities in the United States: Prevalence, perspectives, and a proposal for legislative change to protect the right to family in a disability community. *Texas Journal of Civil Liberties & Civil Rights*, *17*, 9–41.

Chance, R. S. (2002). To love and be loved: Sexuality and people with physical disabilities. *Journal of Psychology and Theology*, *30*, 195–208. http://dx.doi.org/10.1177/009164710203000303

Charles, K. K., & Stephens, M., Jr. (2004). Job displacement, disability, and divorce. *Journal of Labor Economics*, *22*, 489–522. http://dx.doi.org/10.1086/381258

Chiarello, L. A., Bartlett, D. J., Palisano, R. J., McCoy, S. W., Fiss, A. L., Jeffries, L., & Wilk, P. (2016). Determinants of participation in family and recreational activities of young children with cerebral palsy. *Disability and Rehabilitation: An International Multidisciplinary Journal*, *38*, 2455–2468. http://dx.doi.org/10.3109/09638288.2016.1138548

Clarke, H., & McKay, S. (2014). Disability, partnership and parenting. *Disability & Society*, *29*, 543–555. http://dx.doi.org/10.1080/09687599.2013.831745

Cohen, P. N., & Petrescu-Prahova, M. (2006). Gendered living arrangements among children with disabilities. *Journal of Marriage and Family*, *68*, 630–638. http://dx.doi.org/10.1111/j.1741-3737.2006.00279.x

Collins, C. (1999). Reproductive technologies for women with physical disabilities. *Sexuality and Disability*, *17*, 299–307. http://dx.doi.org/10.1023/A:1021325612563

Coorg, R., & Tournay, A. (2013). Filicide–suicide involving children with disabilities. *Journal of Child Neurology*, *28*, 745–751. http://dx.doi.org/10.1177/0883073812451777

Corrigan, P. W., & Miller, F. E. (2004). Shame, blame, and contamination: A review of the impact of mental illness stigma on family members. *Journal of Mental Health*, *13*, 537–548. http://dx.doi.org/10.1080/09638230400017004

Cox, D., Cox, R., & Caplan, B. (2013). *Specialty competencies in rehabilitation psychology*. New York, NY: Oxford University Press. http://dx.doi.org/10.1093/med:psych/9780195389241.001.0001

Davidoff, A. J. (2004). Insurance for children with special health care needs: Patterns of coverage and burden on families to provide adequate insurance. *Pediatrics*, *114*, 394–403. http://dx.doi.org/10.1542/peds.114.2.394

Davies, J., & Watson, N. (2002). Countering stereotypes of disability: Disabled children and resistance. In M. Corker & T. Shakespeare (Eds.), *Disability/postmodernity: Embodying disability theory* (pp. 159–174). London, England: Continuum.

Dodd, J., Saggers, S., & Wildy, H. (2009). Constructing the "ideal" family for family-centered practice: Challenges for delivery. *Disability & Society*, *24*, 173–186. http://dx.doi.org/10.1080/09687590802652447

Dunn, D. S., & Andrews, E. E. (2015). Person-first and identity-first language: Developing psychologists' cultural competence using disability language. *American Psychologist*, *70*, 255–264. http://dx.doi.org/10.1037/a0038636

East, L. J., & Orchard, T. R. (2014). Somebody else's job: Experiences of sex education among health professionals, parents, and adolescents with physical disabilities in Southwestern Ontario. *Sexuality and Disability*, *32*, 335–350. http://dx.doi.org/10.1007/s11195-013-9289-5

Elliott, T. R., Berry, J. W., Richards, J. S., & Shewchuk, R. M. (2014). Resilience in the initial year of caregiving for a family member with a traumatic spinal cord injury. *Journal of Consulting and Clinical Psychology*, *82*, 1072–1086. http://dx.doi.org/10.1037/a0037593

Esmail, S., Darry, K., Walter, A., & Knupp, H. (2010). Attitudes and perceptions towards disability and sexuality. *Disability and Rehabilitation: An International Multidisciplinary Journal*, *32*, 1148–1155. http://dx.doi.org/10.3109/09638280903419277

Feldman, M. A. (2002). Children of parents with intellectual disabilities. In R. J. McMahon & R. D. Peters (Eds.), *The effects of parental dysfunction on children* (pp. 205–223). Boston, MA: Springer. http://dx.doi.org/10.1007/978-1-4615-1739-9_10

Friedman, J. F. (1999). *Identity's architect: A biography of Erik H. Erikson*. New York, NY: Scribner.

Goleman, D. (1988, June 14). Erikson, in his own old age, expands his view of life. *The New York Times*. Retrieved from http://www.nytimes.com/1988/06/14/science/erikson-in-his-own-old-age-expands-his-view-of-life.html

Goodley, D., & Cole, K. R. (2015). Critical psychologies of disability: Boundaries, borders and bodies in the lives of disabled children. *Emotional & Behavioural Difficulties*, *20*, 51–63. http://dx.doi.org/10.1080/13632752.2014.947096

Haley, W. E., Roth, D. L., Hovater, M., & Clay, O. J. (2015). Long-term impact of stroke on family caregiver well-being: A population-based case-control study. *Neurology*, *84*, 1323–1329. http://dx.doi.org/10.1212/WNL.0000000000001418

Hergenrather, K., & Rhodes, S. (2007). Exploring undergraduate student attitudes toward persons with disabilities application of the disability social relationship scale. *Rehabilitation Counseling Bulletin*, *50*(2), 66–75. http://dx.doi.org/10.1177/00343552070500020501

Howland, C. A., & Rintala, D. H. (2001). Dating behaviors of women with physical disabilities. *Sexuality and Disability*, *19*, 41–70. http://dx.doi.org/10.1023/A:1010768804747

Hughes, R. B., Robinson-Whelen, S., Taylor, H. B., Swedlund, N., & Nosek, M. A. (2004). Enhancing self-esteem in women with physical disabilities. *Rehabilitation Psychology*, *49*, 295–302. http://dx.doi.org/10.1037/0090-5550.49.4.295

Joint Commission. (2010). *Advancing effective communication, cultural competence, and patient- and family-centered care: A roadmap for hospitals*. Oakbrook Terrace, IL: Author. Retrieved from https://www.jointcommission.org/assets/1/6/ARoadmapforHospitalsfinalversion727.pdf

Kirshbaum, M., & Olkin, R. (2002). Parents with physical, systemic, or visual disabilities. *Sexuality and Disability*, *20*, 65–80. http://dx.doi.org/10.1023/A:1015286421368

Kuhlthau, K., Hill, K. S., Yucel, R., & Perrin, J. M. (2005). Financial burden for families of children with special health care needs. *Maternal and Child Health Journal*, *9*, 207–218. http://dx.doi.org/10.1007/s10995-005-4870-x

Kuo, D. Z., Cohen, E., Agrawal, R., Berry, J. G., & Casey, P. H. (2011). A national profile of caregiver challenges among more medically complex children with special health care needs. *Archives of Pediatrics & Adolescent Medicine*, *165*, 1020–1026. http://dx.doi.org/10.1001/archpediatrics.2011.172

Lloyd, J., Patterson, T., & Muers, J. (2016). The positive aspects of caregiving in dementia: A critical review of the qualitative literature. *Dementia: The International Journal of Social Research and Practice*, *15*, 1534–1561. http://dx.doi.org/10.1177/1471301214564792

Louvet, E. (2007). Social judgments toward job applicants with disabilities' perception of personal qualities and competencies. *Rehabilitation Psychology*, *52*, 297–303. http://dx.doi.org/10.1037/0090-5550.52.3.297

Mayes, R., Llewellyn, G., & McConnell, D. (2006). Misconception: The experience of pregnancy for women with intellectual disabilities. *Scandinavian Journal of Disability Research*, *8*(2–3), 120–131. http://dx.doi.org/10.1080/15017410600774178

McPherson, M., Arango, P., Fox, H., Lauver, C., McManus, M., Newacheck, P. W., . . . Strickland, B. (1998). A new definition of children with special health care needs. *Pediatrics*, *102*, 137–149. http://dx.doi.org/10.1542/peds.102.1.137

Murphy, G., & Feldman, M. A. (2002). Parents with intellectual disabilities. *Journal of Applied Research in Intellectual Disabilities*, *15*, 281–284. http://dx.doi.org/10.1046/j.1468-3148.2002.00139.x

Nario-Redmond, M. R. (2010). Cultural stereotypes of disabled and non-disabled men and women: Consensus for global category representations and diagnostic domains. *British Journal of Social Psychology*, *49*, 471–488. http://dx.doi.org/10.1348/014466609X468411

National Council on Disability. (2012). *Rocking the cradle: Ensuring the rights of parents with disabilities*. Washington, DC: Author. Retrieved from http://www.ncd.gov/publications/2012/Sep272012/

Nguyen, T. T. A., Liamputtong, P., & Monfries, M. (2016). Reproductive and sexual health of people with physical disabilities: A metasynthesis. *Sexuality and Disability*, *34*, 3–26. http://dx.doi.org/10.1007/s11195-015-9425-5

Nicholson, J., Sweeney, E. M., & Geller, J. L. (1998). Mothers with mental illness: The competing demands of parenting and living with mental illness. *Psychiatric Services*, *49*, 635–642. http://dx.doi.org/10.1176/ps.49.5.635

Olkin, R. (2003). Women with physical disabilities who want to leave their partners: A feminist and disability-affirmative perspective. *Women & Therapy*, *26*, 237–246. http://dx.doi.org/10.1300/J015v26n03_05

Olsen, R., & Clarke, H. (2003). *Parenting and disability: Disabled parents experiences of raising children*. Bristol, England: Policy Press. http://dx.doi.org/10.2307/j.ctt1t89813

Parker, G., & Clarke, H. (2002). Making the ends meet: Do careers and disabled people have a common agenda? *Policy and Politics*, *30*, 347–359. http://dx.doi.org/10.1332/030557302760094711

Pendo, E. (2008). Disability, equipment barriers, and women's health: Using the ADA to provide meaningful access. *Saint Louis University Journal of Health Law & Policy*, *2*, 15–56.

Priestley, M. (2003). *Disability: A life course approach*. Oxford, England: Blackwell.

Raina, P., O'Donnell, M., Rosenbaum, P., Brehaut, J., Walter, S. D., Russell, D., . . . Wood, E. (2005). The health and well-being of caregivers of children with cerebral palsy. *Pediatrics*, *115*, e626–e636. http://dx.doi.org/10.1542/peds.2004-1689

Rosenbaum, P., & Gorter, J. W. (2012). The "F-words" in childhood disability: I swear this is how we should think! *Child: Care, Health and Development*, *38*, 457–463. http://dx.doi.org/10.1111/j.1365-2214.2011.01338.x

Runswick-Cole, K., & Goodley, D. (2013). Resilience: A disability studies and community psychology approach. *Social and Personality Psychology Compass*, *7*, 67–78. http://dx.doi.org/10.1111/spc3.12012

Saclier, C. (2000). In the best interest of the child? In P. Selman (Ed.), *Intercountry adoption developments, trends, and perspectives* (pp. 53–65). London, England: BAAF.

Scorgie, K., Wilgosh, L., & Sobsey, D. (2004). The experience of transformation in parents of children with disabilities: Theoretical considerations. *Developmental Disabilities Bulletin*, *32*(1), 84–110.

Shakespeare, T. (2006). The social model of disability. In L. J. Davis (Ed.), *The disability studies reader* (pp. 197–204). New York, NY: Routledge.

Shewchuk, R., & Elliott, T. R. (2000). Family caregiving in chronic disease and disability. In R. G. Frank & T. R. Elliott (Eds.), *Handbook of rehabilitation psychology* (pp. 553–563). Washington, DC: American Psychological Association. http://dx.doi.org/10.1037/10361-026

Smeltzer, S. C. (2007). Pregnancy in women with physical disabilities. *Journal of Obstetric, Gynecologic, & Neonatal Nursing*, *36*, 88–96. http://dx.doi.org/10.1111/j.1552-6909.2006.00121.x

Sobsey, R. (2007). Implementing the rights of children with disabilities. In K. Covell & R. B. Howe (Eds.), *A question of commitment: Children's rights in Canada* (pp. 373–394). Waterloo, Ontario, Canada: Wilfrid Laurier Press.

Taleporos, G., & McCabe, M. P. (2001). Physical disability and sexual esteem. *Sexuality and Disability*, *19*, 131–148. http://dx.doi.org/10.1023/A:1010677823338

Toms Barker, L., & Maralani, V. (1997). *Challenges and strategies of disabled parents: Findings from a national survey of parents with disabilities*. Oakland, CA: Berkeley Planning Associates.

Tumin, D. (2016). Marriage trends among Americans with childhood-onset disabilities, 1997–2013. *Disability and Health Journal*, *9*, 713–718. http://dx.doi.org/10.1016/j.dhjo.2016.05.004

Watermeyer, B., & Swartz, L. (2016). Disablism, identity, and self: Discrimination as a traumatic assault on subjectivity. *Journal of Community & Applied Social Psychology*, *26*, 268–276. http://dx.doi.org/10.1002/casp.2266

Wates, M. (2004). Righting the picture: Disability and family life. In J. Swain (Ed.), *Disabling barriers, enabling environments* (pp. 135–141). London, England: Sage.

Wells, R., Dywan, J., & Dumas, J. (2005). Life satisfaction and distress in family caregivers as related to specific behavioural changes after traumatic brain injury. *Brain Injury*, *19*, 1105–1115. http://dx.doi.org/10.1080/02699050500150062

Williams, J., & Colvin, L. (2016). Coming together to end violence against women and girls with disabilities. In S. Miles-Cohen & C. Signore (Eds.), *Eliminating inequities for women with disabilities: An agenda for health and wellness* (pp. 243–262). Washington, DC: American Psychological Association. http://dx.doi.org/10.1037/14943-013

Chapter 13

AGING AND DISABILITY

Laura E. Dreer and Molly K. Cox

As an unprecedented number of older adults (age 65 and older) are expected to be living with one or more chronic disabilities (Lin, Beck, Finch, Hummer, & Master, 2012; S. E. Rogers, Thrasher, Miao, Boscardin, & Smith, 2015), the landscape of medical rehabilitation and health care will substantially change over the next decade. According to the United States Census Bureau (2012), the number of older adults will exceed 70 million by 2030 and represent nearly 20% of the population. The fastest growing segment are those over age 80. Further complicating the health care landscape is the fact that the risk for disability increases with age and chronic illness (e.g., type 2 diabetes, stroke, hypertension, coronary heart disease, arthritis dementia, cancer), thereby contributing to the likelihood of a compromised quality of life. Also projected is a growing number of older adults who acquired a disability in early adulthood and who are now transitioning into late life and aging with that disability (Verbrugge & Yang, 2002). This trend will lead to increased medical expenditures and a significant economic toll on societal systems of care, families, and older adults over the next decade (Freedman, Stafford, Schwarz, Conrad, & Cornman, 2012; Jensen et al., 2012). As a result, rehabilitation and allied health institutions are on the cusp of confronting major challenges in health care training and delivery (Centers for Medicare and Medicaid Services, 2011; Freedman et al., 2014). Such challenges will be further complicated given (a) shorter lengths of stay in hospitals and rehabilitation facilities and (b) older adults are living longer because of advancements in medicine, despite potential decreases in their quality of life. As a result, aging and disability represents a major public health issue facing rehabilitation psychologists.

A key issue facing older adults with and without pre-existing disabilities is maintaining independence, health, and everyday functioning within their communities. Participating in meaningful and valued activities of daily living (ADL; e.g., personal care) and instrumental activities of daily living (IADL; e.g., driving, shopping, completing household tasks, managing finances and medical care) is reflective of independence (Bleijenberg, Zuithoff, Smith, de Wit, & Schuurmans, 2017; Connolly, Garvey, & McKee, 2017). These activities are also important for quality of life and social functioning. It has been well documented that with interventions, accommodations, support, and/or strategies to compensate for disabilities, older adults can successfully adapt in terms of maintaining active participation in valued activities (Freedman et al., 2014).

Rehabilitation psychologists play a critical role in assisting aging individuals with maintaining goals to remain independent while living with a disability. As such, rehabilitation psychologists in the workforce need to have a basic understanding of the aging process and issues confronting older

http://dx.doi.org/10.1037/0000129-014
Handbook of Rehabilitation Psychology, Third Edition, L. A. Brenner, S. A. Reid-Arndt, T. R. Elliott, R. G. Frank, and B. Caplan (Editors-in-Chief)

adults and their families, as well as competencies in conducting evidence-based practice with these individuals. Toward this end, the sections of this chapter will lay the foundation for working with older adults with an emphasis on the following: (a) aging into and with a disability, (b) risk factors related to aging and disability, (c) adjustment to disability in late life, (d) successful aging and disability, (e) unique issues related to working with older adults, (f) innovations in practice with older adults, and (g) recommended competencies for rehabilitation psychologists working with older adults.

AGING INTO AND WITH A DISABILITY

Along with changes related to the normal aging process (e.g., declines in intelligence, memory, vision, hearing, motor function, reaction time, etc.), older adults have a higher likelihood for being diagnosed with a chronic medical illness and/or experiencing an injury (e.g., falls) that can impact physical decline and result in disability (Puentes, Bradway, & Aselage, 2010; Stenholm et al., 2015). Additionally, given medical advancements and improved disease management, those who acquired a disability during early adulthood are now aging with that disability and/or may acquire new impairments or health conditions (Molton & Yorkston, 2017). The pathways of change and the adjustment process for individuals aging with a disability have only recently begun to be addressed (Molton & Yorkston, 2017; Yorkston, McMullan, Molton, & Jensen, 2010), and these differ from those individuals who are aging into disability. For instance, a more rapid decline in physical functioning because of a spinal cord injury may lead to the organ systems of an older adult aging at an increased rate (Frontera & Mollett, 2017). This process may also lead to the development of secondary health conditions (e.g., diabetes, cardiovascular complications). Aging with a disability may also result in long-term overuse of body parts necessary for mobility (e.g., problems with posture, shoulder deterioration, osteoporosis, arthritis) or the progression of decline in physical function related to the disease process (e.g., multiple sclerosis). Barriers to community participation is also greater for those adults with pre-existing disability. Despite having similar health care needs, older adults aging with and into disability are lacking the services, research, training, and policy networks prepared to address these issues.

RISK FACTORS RELATED TO AGING AND DISABILITY

Several risk factors for disability have been shown to increase with aging with or into a disability (Bleijenberg et al., 2017). For example, the number of comorbid, chronic medical illness increases as individuals age (Jensen et al., 2013; Lin, Beck, & Finch, 2014), particularly for those aging with a disability. Comorbid conditions can threaten independence, negatively impact emotional well-being, lead to institutionalization, or result in premature mortality (Chen, Chang, & Lan, 2015). Sociodemographic risk factors have also been related to poorer health and risk for disability as people age. Particularly at risk are those who live in rural areas and those who have lower household incomes and education, as well as those who have limited access to health-care services and/or no insurance (Fougère et al., 2016; C. Rogers, 2002). Like younger adults, there are well documented racial disparities across disabilities that extend into old age, with African Americans being at a disproportionally higher risk for unfavorable outcomes compared with Caucasians (Lin et al., 2014; Sun, Huang, Varadhan, & Agrawal, 2016). Health disparities in disability associated with race have been observed across a range of conditions. Secondary to socioeconomic challenges, similar patterns have been noted regarding limitations in ADLs, as well as IADLs. Much of the research has shown a persistent disadvantage for African Americans despite adjustment for socioeconomic differences, which have been suggested as a contributing factor for this disparity (Dreer, Girkin, & Mansberger, 2012; Dreer et al., 2013; Whitson et al., 2011). Studies suggest that sociocultural factors play a role in risk for disability, as research has found disadvantages in access to health care, treatment recommendations, and quality of care. Other contributing factors related to race and health disparities include a mistrust of health care providers, cultural differences, and a lack of understanding or appreciation for cultural diversity issues.

In addition to comorbidities and sociodemographic risk factors, the risk for falls also increases with age. Falls, the leading cause of disability among older adults, often result from slowed mobility or gait, problems with balance, loss of sensory functioning (e.g., vision), medication or polypharmacy effects, postural hypotension, health impairments/injuries (e.g., arthritis, joint diseases, hip fractures; Al-Momani, Al-Momani, Alghadir, Alharethy, & Gabr, 2016), living with other medical conditions (e.g., stroke, Parkinson's disease, multiple sclerosis), and/or depressive symptoms because of slow psychomotor functioning (Brodie et al., 2017). Fall risk is greater among those with existing disabilities and tends to increase among those age 80 years or older. Among older adults with or without a disability, falls can also result in serious injuries (e.g., traumatic brain injury [TBI]) or orthopedic injuries (e.g., hip fractures or broken bones; Cuthbert et al., 2015). Moreover, following injuries such as a TBI, older adults have slower recovery rates, higher mortality rates, and lower functional status at discharge compared with younger adults (Ramanathan, McWilliams, Schatz, & Hillary, 2012).

Another risk factor related to disability and aging that has received growing attention is obesity. Older adults are not immune to this epidemic. Obesity and problems with weight management among adults aging into or with a disability have been implicated in regards to early death, risk for other chronic medical conditions (e.g., stroke, diabetes, heart disease), and comorbidities. This growing epidemic is projected to place a substantial burden on health care systems over the next several decades (DeCaria, Sharp, & Petrella, 2012). On the positive side, several studies have found that obesity can be modified even in late life, and that doing so can help thwart the risk for chronic diseases, improve mood, health, and overall function (Rillamas-Sun et al., 2014). Adaptive sport and recreation programs based within communities can help maximize older adults' ability to remain independent. Lifestyle and exercise programs tailored to older adults can help influence their quality of life and social connectedness.

ADJUSTMENT TO DISABILITY IN LATE LIFE

Although most older adults learn to adapt to a disability over time (e.g., Kreutzer et al., 2016), research has consistently shown individual variability in the way in which older adults react and cope with aversive events (e.g., acquiring a chronic disability or a traumatic injury). Regarding an association between age, psychological functioning, and responses to disability, researchers have shown an inverse U-shaped curve across the lifespan, with depression more prevalent among middle-age adults relative to younger adults (Alschuler et al., 2013; Bombardier, Ehde, Stoelb, & Molton, 2010).

Disability has also been studied across the lifespan, with findings indicating differential effects on life satisfaction depending on age of disability onset. For instance, results suggest that compared with those in midlife (age 40 years–64 years), individuals who become disabled as younger adults or as older adults report greater declines in life satisfaction during the year within their disability onset and are less likely to adapt in the years after disability (Infurna & Wiest, 2016). Having a preexisting disposition for psychological problems has also been associated with health problems and behaviors that can be disabling or compromise health. Thus, it is critical that older adults receive appropriate treatment for mental health problems related to or comorbid with their disability.

Although the body of research studying emotional adjustment to disability has largely focused on understanding or identifying factors related to maladaptive adjustment (e.g., depression, poor quality of life), more recent work has focused on positive adaptive adjustment and even growth in response to aging with or into a disability. Key factors related to adaptive adjustment to disability have emerged and are highlighted in the sections that follow.

Resilience

Following a chronic illness or injury, many people undergo a process of posttraumatic growth, including enhanced personal relationships, a changed view of oneself, or change in life philosophy. Adults can reformulate a disability or reinterpret a life-long chronic disease diagnosis and the impact it has on physical or cognitive functioning, as well as develop a new and meaningful purpose in life (Dunn, Uswatte, & Elliott, 2009; T. R. Elliott, Uswatte, Lewis, & Palmatier, 2000). There is growing research on resilience and aging with a disability, in which several studies demonstrate resilience as a protective factor in supporting optimal functioning (Jeste et al., 2013; Silverman, Molton, Alschuler, Ehde, & Jensen, 2015). Out of this work, there are emerging trends in interventions that incorporate a focus on fostering resilience and aspects of positive psychology (e.g., gratitude, forgiveness). This type of framework may help older adults transition into old age and disability.

Social Support

Perceived satisfaction with social support has been repeatedly shown to influence well-being and adjustment for older adults and their caregivers (Grant et al., 2006; Jensen et al., 2014). Social support and meaningful social engagement in supportive relationships are critical factors that buffer the negative emotional effects associated with chronic health conditions (de Leon & Rajan, 2014). Thus, rehabilitation psychologists should emphasize social engagement therapies to cultivate successful adjustment and community integration (e.g., community-based behavioral health efforts).

Spirituality and Religious Beliefs

The role of spirituality and religious beliefs on health outcomes among older adults has also received attention in the scientific literature (Koenig, 2012). Several studies support the role of spirituality or religiosity as a positive predictor of life satisfaction, mental health, and perception of illness. It has also been shown that spirituality provides meaning and purpose related to adjustment to chronic disease or injury and is related to self-esteem, internal sense of control, well-being, marital stability, social support, and health behaviors. The benefits of religious involvement and spirituality have also been observed to help existential struggles among caregivers and their own process of adjustment (Koenig, Nelson, Shaw, Saxena, & Cohen, 2016). Traditionally, spirituality and religiosity have not been commonly addressed in health care settings. However, with the rise of integrative medicine approaches and evidence supporting the role of spirituality and mindfulness on mental and physical health, a greater focus is being placed on older adults' spiritual needs (Koenig, 2004).

Healthy Behaviors and Lifestyle

Research has repeatedly shown the therapeutic benefits of healthy lifestyle choices on health outcomes and successful aging into and with a disability (Chiuve, McCullough, Sacks, & Rimm, 2006; Gopinath, Russell, Kifley, Flood, & Mitchell, 2016; Hodge, English, Giles, & Flicker, 2013; Sabia et al., 2012). Unhealthy behaviors among the top 10 leading risk factors for death and disability are all preventable as well as modifiable, even in late life (Chiuve et al., 2008; Dreer & Linley, 2016). Eating a healthy diet, regularly exercising, and eliminating unhealthy behaviors (e.g., smoking, stress) are critical as adults age, and these can be achieved via nutritional counseling, adaptive sport/exercise therapies that range in intensity, and/or adherence to pharmacological therapies including lipid lowering and antihypertensive medications. Research has shown that the greatest influence on successful aging is from a combination of healthy behaviors rather than the individual behaviors alone (Sabia et al., 2012). However, prescriptions for lifestyle interventions that incorporate health promoting behaviors are often missing in traditional rehabilitation medicine, particularly for older adults (Dreer & Linley, 2016). Optimizing the benefits of exercise with adaptive instructions or equipment can have a positive effect on the physical functioning and health (e.g., lowering risk of falls, heart disease, and diabetes) of older adults who are disabled or at risk for a disability (Buford, Anton, Clark, Higgins, & Cooke, 2014). Some exercise programs (e.g., muscle strengthening) designed to target at-risk older adults, like those with cardiovascular disease or those who are aging with a disability (Evenson, Butler, & Rosamond, 2014), have shown benefits on maintaining independence and reducing late-life disability (Liu, Jones, Formyduval, & Clark, 2016). Several studies have demonstrated the positive benefits (e.g., improvement in emotional well-being) and feasibility of engaging older adults with and without disabilities in physical activity (Bauman, Merom, Bull, Buchner, & Fiatarone Singh, 2016; Loprinzi, 2016). This is critical given the magnitude of inactivity and obesity and the opportunity to maximize independence, health, and quality of life.

The Centers for Disease Control and Prevention (2017) recommend that, per week, older adults engage in at least 150 minutes of moderate intensity aerobic activity or 75 minutes of vigorous intensity aerobic activity and two or more days of muscle-strengthening activities that work major muscle groups (e.g., legs, hips, back, abdomen, chest, shoulders, and arms). The World Health Organization (2017) recommends similar guidelines for older adults and indicates that aerobic activity should be performed in bouts of at least 10 minutes. Older adults with poor mobility are advised to perform physical activity to enhance balance and prevent falls on three or more days per week. When older adults cannot do the recommended amounts of physical activity because of health conditions, the World Health Organization suggests that they should be as physically active as their abilities and conditions permit. There are specific guidelines for physical activities targeting balance, flexibility, strengthening, and aerobic exercise that can guide rehabilitation psychologists working with older adults with disabilities. Therefore, the integration of health promoting therapies into rehabilitation practice will help to reduce disability and/or enhance outcomes for older adults. Rehabilitation psychologists have not traditionally prescribed exercise, but they should prescribe it in conjunction with other rehabilitation team members (e.g., physicians), especially given the research demonstrating the benefits on physical and mental health, cognitive functioning, and obesity risk (Bauman et al., 2016; Bray, Smart, Jakobi, & Jones, 2016; Sink et al., 2015; Zaleski et al., 2016).

SUCCESSFUL AGING AND DISABILITY

Whereas the prior sections of this chapter have focused on the process of normal aging and common risk factors that increase the likelihood of living with a disability as adults age, a growing body of geriatric research has focused on understanding determinants related to "successful aging." It is important to study adults who adjust well to living with a disability in late life, as such information may be used to help foster adaptive adjustment (Molton & Yorkston, 2017). Definitions of successful aging have widely varied in the scientific literature. For example, some research has defined successful aging as being free of major chronic health conditions or the absence of disease while remaining cognitively robust and socially engaged (Depp & Jeste, 2006; Rowe & Kahn, 1998). However, more contemporary definitions propose that successful aging, chronic illness, and functional limitations can coexist if compensatory mechanisms are used (Woods et al., 2016; Young, Frick, & Phelan, 2009). This definition helps to account for the wide range of person–environment accommodations and adaptations that individuals with a disability can make to preserve function (Freedman, Kasper, & Spillman, 2017; Mejía, Ryan, Gonzalez, & Smith, 2017) and represents a newer perspective that accounts for adults aging with a disability.

Successful aging can also be conceptualized multidimensionally and include physiological, functional, social, spiritual, and psychological factors (Carver & Buchanan, 2016). It may also include gerotranscendence. A shift in perspective and the recognition that the task at hand is self-awareness and preparation for death in late life or being positive via retrospection with regards to end-of-life issues (Troutman-Jordan & Staples, 2014). Importantly, psychological or social compensations may offset physiological deficits and limitations. Examples of psychological compensations may include social problem-solving, resilience in response to adversity or risk, or spirituality, all of which positively influence successful aging with disability, as well as caregiving (Dreer et al., 2008; Dreer, Elliott, Fletcher, & Swanson, 2005; A. F. Elliott, Dreer, McGwin, Scilley, & Owsley, 2010; Grant, Elliott, Giger, & Bartolucci, 2001).

UNIQUE ISSUES RELATED TO WORKING WITH OLDER ADULTS

As part of working with older adults aging into or with a disability, there are unique issues that should be recognized among rehabilitation psychologists in the workforce. The following sections provide an overview of key issues relevant to working with older adults and their families including myths and stigma, long-term services, caregiving, abuse and neglect, end of life, medications, transportation, and health policies and initiatives.

Myths and Stigma

There are many misperceptions related to aging and disability (Lucchetti, Lucchetti, de Oliveira, Moreira-Almeida, & da Silva Ezequiel, 2017; Sarabia-Cobo & Castanedo Pfeiffer, 2015). Negative attitudes toward and stigmas around old age and disability persist even among professionals working in health care settings (King, Roberts, & Bowers, 2013). Old age is often considered a period of impending disability and/or death. However, many adults transition into late life just fine, with some adults even flourishing. Other misperceptions are related to stereotypes surrounding disability in late life, including adjustment (e.g., "older adults are depressed, lonely, unpleasant, and/or cannot participate in activities or learn new strategies"), sexual behavior (e.g., "older adults are not interested in sexual activity"), or technology use (e.g., "new technologies are too difficult for older adults to learn"; Benbow & Beeston, 2012; Wandke, Sengpiel, & Sönksen, 2012). Older adults can indeed learn and want to learn new strategies, reframe their circumstances, make changes in functioning (e.g., exercise), operate and learn new technologies, and engage in sexual activity. Stigma throughout the lifespan exists for people with disabilities as well (e.g., "people with disabilities cannot participate in sports; it is too dangerous or they will get hurt"). Many of these stereotypes can contribute to the problem of older adults not getting referred for necessary interventions or programs that could benefit their health, functioning, and well-being.

Long-Term Services and Supports

Most older adults who suffer from a medical condition or injury (e.g., stroke, heart attack) and undergo inpatient rehabilitation receive shorter stays in the hospital. This trend limits rehabilitation psychologists' ability to deliver effective treatments. Older adults, particularly the very old, are less likely to return to independent living, and transition instead to a residential or retirement community, a family member's home, an assisted living facility, or a skilled nursing home (Palmcrantz et al., 2012). Placement is often contingent upon whether the living situation is temporary or permanent, along with the availability of support systems and access to resources. The type of setting can also impact health outcomes (e.g., rehospitalization) and adjustment.

With the aging population rapidly changing, programs and policies that provide long-term support services are predicted to be overwhelmed. Existing programs and policies that provide long-term services and supports to adults in the United States have been traditionally segmented by age of consumer and the nature of the disability (e.g., developmental/intellectual, physical, psychiatric), which has created categorical service systems that divide aging and disability policies and programs at all levels of government (Putnam, 2014). The evolving landscape is changing with program initiatives to build structural bridges across aging and disability long-term services and support networks, particularly targeting Medicaid and Older Americans Act (OAA) programs. The emphasis for federal rebalancing is to reduce institutionalization and increase home and community-based services (Putnam, 2014). Changes and reforms are needed to support these infrastructures (e.g., professional training, organization structure, service delivery) to maximize independence for as long as possible (Putnam, 2014).

Caregiving

Older adults with chronic health conditions diagnosed in late life or those who are aging with a disability often need assistance (e.g., emotional or instrumental support). Family members typically take on the role of informal caregiver and serve as an extension of the health care system. Caregivers perform a variety of tasks and have been found to compromise their own health while performing caregiver duties. In most cases, caregivers do not receive payment for their services and are often strained as they reorganize their schedules, expectations, and roles. These circumstances can cause acute stress, psychological distress, loss of employment, and eventual burnout (T. R. Elliott, Shewchuk, & Richards, 2001). However, research has shown that proper training and education can reduce caregiver burden and risk for health problems, as well as improve their overall management of the stress of caregiving (T. R. Elliott, Berry, & Grant, 2009; Kurylo, Elliott, & Shewchuk, 2001; Rivera, Elliott, Berry, & Grant, 2008).

In 2016, the National Academies of Sciences, Engineering, and Medicine convened an expert Committee on Family Caregiving to examine what is known about family caregivers of older adults and to make recommendations regarding polices that will address their needs and minimize caregiver barriers. The report, "Families Caring for an Aging America" (Health and Medicine Division, 2016), suggested that family caregiving is an urgent public policy issue—at least 17.7 million individuals provide family caregiving for adults over age 65 with physical, mental, cognitive, or functional limitations. Given the growing aging population, this number is expected to grow.

Out of this effort, the committee challenged traditional practices that often assume the availability of family caregivers without adequate support services (Health and Medicine Division, 2016). Furthermore, the committee called for a transformation of policies and practices that focus on families in the care of older adults by evolving the focus from person-centered care to person-and-family-centered care (e.g., Medicare and Medicaid payment reform to motivate providers to involve family caregivers, evaluation and adoption of federal policies that provide economic support to working caregivers, and expansion of the national data collection infrastructure to develop a knowledge base about caregivers).

Abuse and Neglect

Given the physical or cognitive limitations associated with various chronic health conditions and need for assistance, older adults are at risk for abuse, violence, and/or neglect (e.g., physical, emotional, financial; Nerenberg, 1996). Self-neglect can occur as well. Unfortunately, research is lacking regarding those at greatest risk and caregivers who are at risk for being perpetrators of abuse. As such, it is important to assess abuse and neglect to prevent or intervene on behalf of those who are most vulnerable to becoming victims of violence. Assessment of caregiver burden and stress is important in this process. Related to abuse and neglect, older adults are also vulnerable to financial fraud and scams. Providing education to help older adults and their families avoid falling prey to such abuse is also important.

End-of-Life and Palliative Care

Given the risk for chronic disability among older adults, another unique issue is end-of-life care. These issues may surface during aging and ongoing medical appointments, medical procedures or surgeries, declines in health and functioning requiring hospitalization or institutionalization, or diagnosis and management of a terminal illness. Some of the changes (e.g., deterioration in health or appearance, perception of burden on others, need for greater assistance in ADLs) often emerge, particularly in more advanced stages of a disease or terminal illness. Older adults are often confronted with existential questions. Concerns and discussions may center around advance directives, code status, and pain management. Thus, health care plans that maximize patient medical decision-making and participation ahead of time, on the basis of discussions around the establishment of patient goals, values, and wishes, are critical with older adults and their families. These discussions can be particularly helpful for medical teams, families, and older adults when unexpected medical crises may arise.

Medications and Polypharmacy

Given the relationship between age and comorbid health conditions, older adults are often prescribed more medications than any other age group (Sirey, Greenfield, Weinberger, & Bruce, 2013). Medications are often prescribed for a variety of reasons (e.g., prevention or management of chronic health conditions, delay the progression of diseases). Although pharmacological management of chronic health conditions are important, medication nonadherence is high among older adults (Dreer et al., 2012; Marcum et al., 2013). Adherence to medications is critical for effective treatment or management of health conditions (Dreer & Linley, 2016). Reasons for nonadherence may vary and include problems with forgetfulness, attitudes and beliefs, cost, health literacy, and socioeconomic factors. On the positive side, several educational and psychoeducational health promotion programs have been found to improve medication adherence with many incorporating a motivational interviewing component (e.g., Dreer et al., 2016). However, continued improvement in such approaches are needed and should be tailored to disabilities.

Transportation

Given the impact of certain chronic health conditions on driving, greater research and resources are needed for alternative and accessible transportation for older adults (Curl, Stowe, Cooney, & Proulx, 2014). Driving is an important IADL that helps keep older adults active and engaged. When older adults are recommended to restrict or cease driving, they can benefit from public or alternative transportation options to buffer the transition (e.g., Uber, Lyft, churches, taxis, community or senior center bus transit service, friends/family/neighbors). Social engagement, mobility, and physical activity are important factors to help buffer against depression and other negative outcomes during such a transition in late life (Curl et al., 2014; Marottoli et al., 1997). However, those in rural communities or with low income are at a disadvantage in terms of access to such services. They are more likely to be at risk for social isolation, sedentary lifestyles, and depression and loneliness, and they may have trouble accessing medical care, all of which can further compromise their health and independence (Edwards, Lunsman, Perkins, Rebok, & Roth, 2009; Sanford et al., 2018).

Policies and Initiatives

Several federal, state, and local policies and initiatives support a wide range of social services, programs, and research focused on older adults. For example, the OAA, enacted in 1965, has been reauthorized and amended numerous times and is an important law that includes seven titles for policy efforts aimed at improving the lives of older adults, particularly by the availability and access to services at home and in the community. Most of these programs are administered under the Administration on Aging in the Administration for Community Living within the Department of Health and Human Services. Recently, the Consolidated Appropriations Act of 2018 provided discretionary appropriations for OAA programs and activities, with the largest proportion of OAA funding for Title III State and Community Programs on Aging (Colello & Napili, 2018). Although OAA funding increased from 2017–2018, with level funding for most core OAA programs, overall funding has declined over the last decade. More recent health policy initiatives have also been implemented that impact psychological practice. For example, section 4103 of the Patient Protection and Affordable Care Act (2010) mandates a health risk appraisal as part of the new Medicare annual wellness visits for older adults. The overall goal is for prevention and promotion of a healthy lifestyle and active living with greater quality of life (Hahn, Aronow, Rosario, & Guenther, 2013). The use among older adults with disabilities needs to be evaluated in terms of impact on health to continue to improve the identification of those at greatest risk and in need of treatment (Hahn et al., 2013). More recent initiatives, such as *Healthy People 2020* and the Surgeon General's wellness initiatives, acknowledge the importance of inclusion of all persons in health promotion efforts. Greater improvements are needed for policy strategy and evaluation of effectiveness that moves disease/disability management toward self-management and tailored systems of care. Although such programs have been developed for older adults, factors impacting funding initiatives, policies, and decisions include changes in administration priorities (e.g., partial repeal of the Affordable Care Act, repeal of Medicaid expansion, tighter spending on OAA programs), economic trends (e.g., sequestration, inflation), population estimates, health trends, legislation, and advocacy, which can affect aging services for those who provide as well as receive them.

INNOVATIONS IN PRACTICE WITH OLDER ADULTS

Innovations for all aspects of rehabilitation related to disability in late life have emerged in the literature on aging and disability. The following sections highlight some of the recent advancements.

Technology

Given advancements in health technologies and biomedical engineering, there is tremendous opportunity for tele-rehabilitation via assistive devices, software programs (e.g., mobile apps, gaming), and adaptive equipment (e.g., prosthetics, telemonitoring for caregivers) to improve health, maximize independence, and minimize consequences of disability (Egan & Pot, 2016; Putrino, 2014). With more and more baby boomers approaching older adulthood, user familiarity with technological devices may help lead to profound changes in health care practice, resulting in options that are more cost effective, easily accessible, and interactive compared with conventional rehabilitation efforts. Technological accommodations and devices are already being used by older adults with disabilities and appear to be well received with proper training (Skolarus, Burke, & Freedman, 2014). For example, the design and control of living environments can be accommodated to make houses more disability friendly and safer (e.g., smart homes, removing barriers to participating in outdoor mobility, allowing caregivers to work but monitor loved ones from afar; Smith, Chen, Clarke, & Gallagher, 2016). Other technologies in development and in testing could have a major impact on late-life adjustment (e.g., self-driving cars). Mobile or e-health apps for smartphones and tablets are being created daily to improve aspects of health care (e.g., monitor heart rate and physical activity) as well as quality of life (e.g., using Facetime or Skype to stay socially engaged). Advancements in technology also apply to innovation in medical treatments (e.g., surgical approaches, prosthetic legs), assessment devices, techniques, and procedures, which can lead to cutting edge breakthroughs and discoveries and virtual rehabilitation. With growing advancements and interest in technology, rehabilitation will most likely be revolutionized in the next decade. See Chapters 30 and 31, this volume, for additional discussion of innovations in technology for rehabilitation.

Community-Based Efforts

Several community-based efforts have emerged as extensions of medical rehabilitation for individuals aging with or into disabilities. Approaches that are preventative in nature and accessible in the community have received greater attention (Friedman et al., 2017). Educational and training-related health efforts are the focus of many community facilities and staff that interact with older adults. Examples of such efforts include online ordering and delivery for groceries, senior center health education classes, and interfaith organizations participating in medical screening campaigns. These "on-the-ground efforts" may help minimize the stigma and normalize the process of adjusting to disability in late life, within the context of peer support, thus providing a sense of social connectedness.

Integrative Medicine and Alternative Therapies

Attention has grown for integrative medicine approaches to supplement conventional rehabilitation. These types of programs are designed to help address physical, biological, lifestyle, emotional, and spiritual aspects of health and illness. This approach focuses on treating the whole person, as well as family caregivers, to optimize wellness and manage challenges throughout an older adult's chronic disease. Specialists in these complementary approaches to care include yoga instructors, pastoral counselors, nutritional and physical activity counselors, and mental health counselors. These efforts have been found beneficial as supplements to traditional approaches in treating disability and health.

RECOMMENDED COMPETENCIES FOR REHABILITATION PSYCHOLOGISTS WORKING WITH OLDER ADULTS

Given the rise of the aging population (20% of adults are over the age of 65), along with the shift in the demographic makeup of the United States and the estimated number of older adults living with comorbid health problems, older adults will undoubtedly represent a significant proportion of health care consumers over the next 15 years. It is imperative that rehabilitation psychologists working with this population have a fundamental understanding of disability, chronic health conditions, and behavioral health, and also meet basic competencies in geropsychology across aspects of traditional practice in psychology (e.g., evidence-based therapy for older adults, assessment, consultation, training). Unfortunately, most psychologists receive little or no training in these practice areas related to working with older adults (Hinrichsen, Emery-Tiburcio, Gooblar, & Molinari, 2018). This is particularly alarming as up to 8 million older adults experience mental health and/or substance use conditions each year (Bartels & Naslund, 2013), yet only an estimated 4% of psychologists specialize in geropsychology (Hoge, Karel, Zeiss, Alegria, & Moye, 2015). Therefore, the number of psychologists adequately trained to meet the behavioral health needs of older adults is disproportionally insufficient (Bartels & Naslund, 2013). Many psychologists provide services to a limited number of older adults and often do so without any specific or formal training in geriatrics. Furthermore, the geropsychology literature has focused on disability largely in terms of maximizing or compensating for ADLs and IADLs, whereas the traditional medical rehabilitation literature emphasizes more of a medical diagnostic focus (e.g., stroke, traumatic brain injury). The attention on the scope of behavioral health needs and role of rehabilitation psychology has not been as well articulated and continues to evolve. Therefore, it is critical that psychologists as a profession strengthen such requirements to meet developing practice guidelines and competencies as well as training in geriatric mental health and disability.

Pikes Peak Model for Training in Professional Geropsychology

One of the leading efforts to strengthen competencies in working with older adults is the "Pikes Peak Model for Training in Professional Geropsychology" (Knight, Karel, Hinrichsen, Qualls, & Duffy, 2009). The model represents an aspirational, competencies-based approach to training psychologists that allows for entry points at different levels of professional development. The model takes the stance that not all psychologists who work with older adults require specific training in the specialty of geropsychology; rather, they should meet the fundamental or basic competency requirements and recognize limits of competency that would require further consultation or a referral to a specialist in geropsychology. With increased frequency and complexity of interactions with older adults, there should be a greater need for meeting higher competencies related to geropsychology (e.g., American Board of Professional Psychology certification). In addition to roots in lifespan developmental psychology, geropsychology has certain elements distinctive as a specialty practice area including expertise in knowledge and skills relevant to late-life pathologies (e.g., dementia, late-life depression), presence of chronic medical conditions in older adults, age-specific environmental contexts (e.g., family, residential, community systems), and treatments designed specifically for older adults and their caregivers.

Although the Pikes Peak model provides guidance on a broad range of knowledge and competencies needed for psychologists who work with individuals in late life, the model does not identify which domains of knowledge would be most useful for those who practice with a small number of older adults or where to begin in the learning process postlicensure to gain specialty skills. To address this, Hinrichsen et al. (2018) conducted a survey among geropsychology experts that was based on the Pikes Peak model. The development of the survey was informed by a special Council of Professional Geropsychology Training Programs workgroup that was charged to review the issue of continuing education hours for training in geropsychology for psychologists with a minimal competency level ("exposure") to those with a more specialized level ("major area of study"). Hinrichsen et al. (2018) presented recommendations for foundational knowledge at the basic "exposure" level of training for psychologists serving older adults along with continuing education recommendations and time allocation (for more information, see http://copgtp.org). The workgroup also developed a Pikes Peak Geropsychology Knowledge and Skill Assessment Tool (https://gerocentral.org/competencies/competencies-tool-online/) for learners and supervisors to gauge their level of competence in psychological practice with older adults (Karel, Holley, et al., 2012).

American Psychological Association Guidelines for Psychological Practice With Older Adults

More recently, the Office on Aging and the Committee on Aging of the American Psychological Association (APA; 2014) expanded guidelines for psychological practice with older adults based off of the Pikes Peak model. The guidelines are organized into six groups and discussed in the following sections: competence and attitude; general knowledge about adult development, aging, and older adults; clinical issues; assessment; intervention, consultation, and other service provision; and professional issues and education. Rehabilitation psychologists working with older adults are advised to carefully review the guidelines in greater detail at https://www.apa.org/practice/guidelines/older-adults.

Competence and attitude. In terms of competence, psychologists are encouraged to work with older adults within the scope of their competence. For example, whereas some issues may present across the life span (e.g., depression, adjustment to a chronic medical condition or injury) that require psychologists to respond with basic skills and techniques, other problems may be more prevalent and unique among older adults (e.g., delirium, dementia) or manifest differently in this population (APA, 2014). These types of mental health related issues require competence in knowledge about normal and abnormal aging processes as well as different assessment and management techniques relevant for older adults (e.g., neuropsychological assessment, cognitive behavioral therapies tailored to late-life issues; Dreer, Copeland, & Cheavens, 2011). Thus, it is important for rehabilitation psychologists working with older adults be familiar of their scope of practice and have a basic understanding of the interplay between developmental issues unique to late life, generational perspectives and beliefs, comorbid medical conditions, potential effects of polypharmacy, cognitive and sensory impairments prevalent in late life, and history of medical/mental health problems that often influence aspects of practice.

In addition to competence, it is also important for rehabilitation psychologists to recognize how their attitudes and beliefs about older adults and aging may impact their work and to seek consultation and education about such issues. For example, ageism and stereotypes can lead to negative biases (e.g., "older adults will never change and are set in their ways" or "with age, comes dementia and decline") and unintentional discrimination that can result from lack of knowledge. For example, misattributing treatable symptoms of depression (e.g., lethargy) to aging can result in a lack of referral for needed treatment. Psychologists also need to be aware of the responses that are evoked when working with older adults, including their own issues with aging.

General knowledge about adult development, aging, and older adults. The second section of the APA guidelines focuses on general knowledge about adult development, aging, and older adults. APA-supported training in aspects of geropsychology related to aging with and into disability needs to be a priority across training programs in psychology as well as postlicensure. Many opportunities exist for rehabilitation psychologists and trainees to enhance their knowledge in working with older adults and caregivers (e.g., formal coursework, practicum/internship/fellowship clinical and/or research rotations, webinars, conference workshops, textbooks/journal articles). Training opportunities within a lifespan developmental perspective should include topics of age and aging, aging into and with a disability, longitudinal change and cross-sectional differences, and cohort effects. There are numerous professional organizations and committees, including the National Institute on Aging, Division 20 (Adult Development and Aging) or Division 12 (Society for Clinical Geropsychology) of APA, the Aging Special Interest Group of the Association for Cognitive and Behavioral Therapy, Council of Professional Geropsychology Training, and the Gerontological Society of America. More targeted efforts from doctoral training programs and internships should be spearheaded to attract trainees to focus on older adults and their caregivers (e.g., conducting greater outreach efforts to dispel myths about services; encouraging engagement in professional organizations, quality practicum sites, or community services involved in working with older adults; enhancing trainee knowledge about the range of opportunities for working with aging populations; providing extracurricular and career events to draw more into working with older adults; offering extra credit for volunteering in a setting with older adults; Moye et al., 2018). Suggestions have also been made for undergraduate and graduate programs to develop a gerontological competency curriculum that includes evaluation criteria (e.g., myths of aging checklist and expectations regarding aging survey; Galambos & Curl, 2013) to better prepare trainees to work with older adults following graduation. Other training programs for medical students to demystify myths related to aging have also been shown to improve attitudes and more favorable views about aging (Lucchetti et al., 2017). Finally, opportunities should exist for trainees to gain exposure to older adult populations (e.g., working with geropsychologists and multidisciplinary geriatric team members in clinical research activities; practicum placements).

Consistent with the APA's section on general knowledge about adult development, aging, and older adults, rehabilitation psychologists working at all levels of practice with older adults should strive to be aware of social/psychological dynamics of the aging process that challenges the aging person to make continued behavioral adaptations to normative later life transitions (Labouvie-Vief, Diehl, Jain, & Zhang, 2007), including retirement, residential relocations, changes in relationships, and bereavement as well as nonnormative events (e.g., stroke, social isolation). Furthermore, awareness of other psychosocial dynamics in late life is also important such as stability and change (Baltes, 1997); perspective of time and meaning in life as one ages; and changes in family, intimacy, friendships, and intergenerational relationships. Finally, psychologists should also strive to understand diversity in the aging process that influence expression of health and mental health problems later in life. For example, psychologists need to consider factors related to diversity, like the influence of cohort or generational issues that shape generational social and psychological perspectives throughout the lifespan, which may impact views on mental health issues, professionals, and treatment. Other factors that also affect aging dynamics include higher rates of women living into late life, gender and racial differences in the experience of aging and access to resources, chronic medical conditions and disability (e.g., vision or hearing impairments), and living environment (APA, 2014). Psychologists working with older adults also need to be familiar with biological and health-related aspects of aging, particularly in rehabilitation psychology as professionals work with those aging with and into a disability. For example, disease accelerates age-related decline in functioning in contrast to lifestyle and health promoting behaviors that can moderate aging effects to a certain extent. Having an understanding that the burden of biological and health aspects of aging can also be modified by factors such as psychological interventions, assistive devices, and technology is imperative to getting older adults' necessary resources. Rehabilitation psychologists also need to be familiar with and distinguish between normative patterns of change in terms of physical and cognitive functioning from nonnormative changes as well as medications that can impact functioning (APA, 2014).

Clinical issues. The third section of the APA guidelines for psychological practice with older adults focuses on clinical issues. For example, rehabilitation psychologists need be familiar with current knowledge about cognitive changes in older adults, including normative changes (e.g., subtle memory changes) versus nonnormative changes (e.g., Alzheimer's disease or other neurodegenerative diseases). Psychologists should also strive to understand the functional capacity of older adults in their social and physical environment. Functional ability and related factors (e.g., sociodemographic, culture) influence decisions older adults make about health care, rehabilitation, relationships, employment, living arrangements, and lifestyle. Participation in these types of ADLs can be challenging given the demands on time, transportation, and finances and limited access to resources and/or support. The balance between independence in everyday living and safety is often an issue for older adults as well as rehabilitation psychologists. These important decisions can have significant implications on older adults' social roles, quality of life, and autonomy and on their families. Aside from functional capacity, older adults are also living in a changing social world where family members' and/or friends' health declines and relationships change, and the emotional ramifications of these changes can affect their meaning of life.

Related to such changes, psychologists need to strive to be knowledgeable about psychopathology within late life, and aware of the prevalence and nature of psychopathology when practicing. For example, mental health disorders affect 20% to 22% of older adults, with higher rates among those adults in long-term care (Karel, Gatz, & Smyer, 2012). Compared with younger adults, unique issues affecting the mental health of older adults may include functional, physical/biological, and/or psychosocial changes (e.g., losses, relationships). Some mental health issues (e.g., late-life depression) may also coincide with other problems affecting cognition (e.g., stroke, mild cognitive impairment). Thus, it may be difficult to distinguish at the time of presentation unless rehabilitation psychologists have familiarity and knowledge about these issues. It is also important for psychologists to be familiar with the risk for specific mental health problems unique to late life. For example, studies have shown an elevated risk for suicide among older adults—Caucasian men over age 85 have the highest rate of suicide (Conwell, Van Orden, & Caine, 2011). Risk factors related to suicide among older adults include a history of psychiatric illness, a lack of or strained social connectedness, and an increase in physical illness and decline in functional capacity. Older age groups reported higher pain intensity scores, longer durations of pain, and higher percentages of chronic diseases. However, this group also reported better mood, better physical health, and more satisfaction with their social lives (Rustøen et al., 2005). Other research has found that older, married couples in which one individual has a disability tend to report worse subjective well-being, which may be influenced by pain symptoms and fatigue (Freedman et al., 2012). Finally, the risk for depression is higher with certain chronic health conditions (e.g., poststroke depression has been related to poorer recovery outcomes). Some mental health conditions (e.g., anxiety) are also more common in older adults, less prevalent in younger adults, different in content (e.g., comorbid health concerns), and not part of normal aging (Wolitzky-Taylor, Castriotta, Lenze, Stanley, & Craske, 2010). Other mental health issues unique to older adults may include problems with substance abuse (e.g., alcohol, opioids). This problem may be further complicated and dangerous among older adults given issues with polypharmacy and biological changes in late life (e.g., slowed metabolism). Familiarity with late-life mental health problems, along with other biopsychosocial contributions will help rehabilitation psychologists facilitate timely interdisciplinary assessment and interventions.

In terms of late-life psychological interventions, rehabilitation psychologists apply a range of evidence-based treatments tailored specifically for treating late-life mental health problems (Sorocco & Lauderdale, 2011; Zarit & Zarit, 2007). Many of these have been shown to be effective across settings (e.g., primary care, geriatric psychiatry, nursing homes; Jameson & Cully, 2011). Given the range of disciplines involved in geriatric health, consultation and delivery of such services will become even more important. Rehabilitation psychologists need to be knowledgeable of behavioral health issues relevant to disabilities, but also issues relevant to older adults and their caregivers in general (Dew et al., 2007). They also need to be flexible in adapting interventions for a disability (Dreer et al., 2011). For example, instead of monitoring thoughts, emotions, and feelings via written homework assignments, use of mobile apps or audio recorders might be more appropriate for monitoring symptoms among those who have a disability impacting their vision. Rehabilitation psychologists should also consult on behavioral health issues, like enhancing motivation for rehabilitation engagement, improving medication adherence, and promoting healthy lifestyles.

Assessment. The APA guidelines also suggest that psychologists should strive to be familiar with the theoretical and evidence-based methods of assessment that are culturally and psychometrically suitable for use with older adults (APA, 2014). Like rehabilitation approaches, working with older adults relies heavily on an interdisciplinary team approach. Given the changes related to normal aging and comorbid health conditions, many allied health professionals from various specialties play a unique role in the comprehensive and ongoing management and care of older adults (e.g., neurologists, urologists, cardiologists, social workers, physical/occupational therapists). Rehabilitation psychologists are an important part of the team as they provide evidence-based mental and behavioral health efforts in assessment, therapy and consultation, education, advocacy, and research. Their role is critical to conducting comprehensive assessments with older adults and their families in terms of evaluating mental health problems, decision-making capacity, management of difficult behaviors, sleep disturbances, suicide risk, pain management, and neuropsychological functioning. Familiarity with issues potentially impacting the presentation of symptoms and other contributing factors that can influence ADLs is important (e.g., depression, poor sleep, pain, medications, problems with hearing or vision, abuse, neurological problems; Lenze et al., 2005; Mantella et al., 2007). To appropriately evaluate older adults, it is critical that psychologists have a knowledge base of empirically supported psychological and neuropsychological assessment measures that are reliable, valid, and culturally appropriate, as well as a knowledge in test theory, test standardization, and factors that might impact performance (e.g., culture, gender, sleep, poor vision, hearing; Karp et al., 2009). Geriatric evaluations often consist of standardized measures that assess aspects of everyday living and function, support, emotional well-being, resources, compensatory strategies, neuropsychological functioning, and capacity to perform important activities (e.g., driving), among others. Recommendations for areas of concern outside of psychology also need to be used (e.g., ophthalmology, urology, endocrinology, oncology, neurology, cardiology). For example, understanding the difference in presentation of depression versus dementia, as well as the influence of medications, is essential to accurate diagnosis and selection of tests to evaluate functioning and quality of life, as well as scoring and interpretation of findings, prognosis, and treatment planning. Additionally, rehabilitation psychologists need to adapt or select psychological tests or interview strategies considering disabilities (e.g., limb weakness or loss, impaired hearing). Furthermore, depending on the degree of disability and/or the type of chronic health condition (e.g., dementia versus depression), it is important to collect collateral information from multiple sources (APA, 2014). Older adults may be misrepresenting, withholding or, lacking awareness of their behaviors, symptoms, and/or history for several reasons and/or motives (e.g., fear of losing their independence or being institutionalized, lack of insight into how much they can realistically do in terms of ADLs/IADLs). Family members or caregivers can provide critical pieces of information helpful in guiding difficult decisions (e.g., whether expired food is left in refrigerator, the number of crashes or citations incurred while driving). Behavioral assessments are particularly important when older adults are institutionalized temporarily or permanently. Thus, rehabilitation psychologists also play a critical role by conducting functional analysis of behaviors like wandering and aggression/agitation to identify and address potential contributing factors (e.g., change in medications; APA, 2014).

According to the APA guidelines, psychologists should also strive to develop skills in accommodating older adults' specific characteristics (e.g., hearing impairment, poor health literacy) and the assessment context (APA, 2014). Rehabilitation psychologists should try to maximize older adults' performance by modifying the presentation of test materials when necessary (e.g., oral versus vision-based administration). The same should apply for the context or setting where the evaluation is conducted (e.g., home versus office because of recent injury impacting mobility and pain). Dreer et al. (2011) provided specific strategies for adapting tests as well as cognitive–behavioral therapy strategies for older adults. The APA guidelines also recommend that psychologists strive to develop skill at administering and interpreting cognitive and functional ability evaluations. For example, some referral questions might center around determining changes in functioning or decline, assistance with diagnostic assessment, and differentiation (e.g., specific neurodegenerative disease processes, psychiatric issues, contribution of medications, poor sleep, and/or multiple factors). As mentioned earlier, an understanding of psychometrically validated measures ranging from cognitive or depression screening to full neuropsychological testing may be warranted with geriatric evaluations. Thus, an understanding of profile analysis, scoring with standardized and culturally appropriate norms, and knowledge of test interpretation as well as normative and nonnormative aging is critical to identifying problems and potentially reversible causes of impairment. Rehabilitation psychologists should be familiar with functional assessments to assess older adult capacity in everyday living.

Intervention consultation and other service provision. Psychologists strive to be familiar with the theory, research, and practice of various methods of intervention with older adults. The knowledge base of evidence-based approaches and theoretical frameworks for psychotherapy applied to older adults is imperative when practicing with this population. Current evidence supports that older adults respond well to a variety of forms of psychotherapy and can benefit from psychological treatments and behavioral medicine (Sorocco & Lauderdale, 2011). Psychotherapeutic approaches for older adults delivered as part of integrated care models have also been effective, particularly in primary care settings (Skultety & Zeiss, 2006). Examples of late-life interventions include reminiscence and life review, grief therapy, behavioral activation, expressive therapies for communication difficulties, psychoeducation, behavioral modification and strategies to compensate for physical limitations, and lifestyle approaches (Sorocco & Lauderdale, 2011). Psychotherapy can also provide support to caregivers and families (APA, 2011; Qualls, 2008). On a related note, selection of an appropriate intervention to use to treat late-life issues varies depending on the presenting problem, and it should to take into consideration cultural aspects. For example, given physical health problems and changes that increase with aging, selection of treatments might focus on helping older adults adapt and compensate for medical problems. In contrast, when problems are centered around terminal illness or life-threatening issues, older adults might benefit from processing such changes and end of life concerns and finding meaning in them. Psychologists should also strive to understand and address issues related to the provision of services depending on the specific setting where those services are available (e.g., nursing home, rehabilitation hospital, primary care facility; APA, 2014). For example, older adults in a hospice setting may be more likely to cope with end of life issues and pain management compared with older adults treated in outpatient rehabilitation settings.

In addition to late-life intervention approaches for treatment, rehabilitation psychologists should also strive to recognize issues related to provision of prevention and health promotion services with older adults (APA, 2014). Psychoeducation and wellness approaches are particularly important among rehabilitation psychologists given the greater prevalence of potential health complications following a disability and/or associated with aging (e.g., comorbid conditions). Rehabilitation psychologists should be familiar with community resources focused on older adult health and wellness preventative efforts. For example, local Area Agencies on Aging (see https://www.n4a.org) and other services for older adults might serve as an important supplement to traditional late-life psychotherapy or recovery from an injury (e.g., social support and prevention of loneliness and isolation). Along similar lines, psychologists working with older adults should also strive to understand issues related to consultation services and the importance of interfacing with other disciplines and sites. Psychologists are often called on to consult with different professionals, organizations, agencies, and families (e.g., training staff, program development). Therefore, familiarity of basic aging related issues (e.g., normative versus nonnormative aging, cultural and gender factors related to aging, processes and abnormalities, late-life psychotherapy approaches) and recognition of coordinated, comprehensive care (e.g., side effects or lack of response with antidepressant medication) is essential. Finally, psychologists should strive to understand the special ethical and/or legal issues in providing services with older adults (APA, 2014). For example, questions related to capacity in ADLs (e.g., medical decisions, financial management, driving, informed consent) are prominent dilemmas facing psychologists, health care providers, patients, and their families. These types of determinations require consideration of autonomy and safety, and psychologists should be familiar with an individual's rights to make his or her decisions to the extent possible (Marson & Dreer, 2007; Marson, Hebert, & Solomon, 2011). Being familiar with the unique issues related to capacity determinations is imperative. For example, a diagnosis of dementia is not equivalent to impairment or limitations in capacity, neither does a lack of capacity in one area of everyday living apply to other areas (APA, 2014). Rehabilitation psychologists working with older adults also need to be familiar with the process of having capacity to fully lacking capacity (e.g., neurodegeneration diseases) versus the process of temporary impairment of a capacity to full recovery (e.g., traumatic brain injury). Other ethical issues when providing services with older adults include confidentiality (e.g., living with a progressive dementia and concerns from family about safety), conflicts in working with or coordinating care, and/or suspected abuse or neglect of older adults. Consultation with professionals on such issues may be especially helpful when areas are not clear with regards to these important issues.

Rehabilitation psychologists may also function as advocates for the mental and behavioral health needs of older adults with disabilities. An example of advocacy in action came from a 2012 report by the Institute of Medicine Committee, which is part of the National Academy of Sciences and a nonprofit organization charged with providing unbiased information and recommendations to policymakers and the public with regards to health care (Hoge et al., 2015). The 2012 report highlighted the crisis regarding mental health and substance use among older adults and the need for training. The United States Congress commissioned this review in response to advocacy by the APA and other invested professions who interact with the health care workforce with older adults. This report represents one type of advocacy approaches rehabilitation psychologists are involved in across training and into postlicensure to keep this issue at the forefront of policy initiatives for practice, education/training, and research.

Professional issues and education. Psychologists need to strive to be knowledgeable about public policy and state and federal laws and regulations related to the provision and reimbursement of psychological services to older adults and the business of practice (APA, 2014). Related to this guideline and the growing aging population, rehabilitation psychologists need to stay updated on policy changes and laws affecting practice (e.g., the Affordable Care Act, changes in Medicare and Medicaid, Social Security payments and services). Psychologists need to increase their knowledge and skills in working with older adults through training, supervision, consultation, and continuing education (APA, 2014). Addressed earlier in this chapter, continual education and professional opportunities to develop, expand, and stay updated is critical. Being familiar with the organizations and affiliated divisions with a geropsychology emphasis on evidence-based training opportunities to ensure competency in practice is critical to arm psychologists with the knowledge base to provide empirically informed practice with this growing population. Being familiar with one's own scope of competence using the Pikes Peak Geropsychology Knowledge and Skill Assessment Tool will help professional psychologists working with older adults match the extent and types of their work with their competence and areas in need of further training to enhance knowledge and skills.

CONCLUSION

As the population of older adults aging into a disability increases along with people aging with a disability, our health care system will be challenged like no other time in history by unprecedented numbers of individuals living with one or more chronic health conditions. The urgency in strengthening our workforce to treat older adults represents a unique opportunity for rehabilitation psychologists. Bridging training between rehabilitation psychology and geropsychology and meeting basic competencies is warranted for training programs and continuing education efforts. With proper knowledge and continuing education of the issues surrounding late life, aging with a disability, and experience of disability in late life, rehabilitation psychologists will have much to offer in terms of behavioral health issues.

References

Al-Momani, M., Al-Momani, F., Alghadir, A. H., Alharethy, S., & Gabr, S. A. (2016). Factors related to gait and balance deficits in older adults. *Clinical Interventions in Aging, 11*, 1043–1049. http://dx.doi.org/10.2147/CIA.S112282

Alschuler, K. N., Jensen, M. P., Sullivan-Singh, S. J., Borson, S., Smith, A. E., & Molton, I. R. (2013). The association of age, pain, and fatigue with physical functioning and depressive symptoms in persons with spinal cord injury. *The Journal of Spinal Cord Medicine, 36*, 483–491. http://dx.doi.org/10.1179/2045772312Y.0000000072

American Psychological Association. (2011). *Resolution on family caregivers*. Retrieved from http://www.apa.org/pi/about/publications/caregivers/index.aspx

American Psychological Association. (2014). Guidelines for psychological practice with older adults. *American Psychologist, 69*, 34–65. http://dx.doi.org/10.1037/a0035063

Baltes, P. B. (1997). On the incomplete architecture of human ontogeny. Selection, optimization, and compensation as foundation of developmental theory. *American Psychologist, 52*, 366–380. http://dx.doi.org/10.1037/0003-066X.52.4.366

Bartels, S. J., & Naslund, J. A. (2013). The underside of the silver tsunami—Older adults and mental health care. *The New England Journal of Medicine, 368*, 493–496. http://dx.doi.org/10.1056/NEJMp1211456

Bauman, A., Merom, D., Bull, F. C., Buchner, D. M., & Fiatarone Singh, M. A. (2016). Updating the evidence for physical activity: Summative reviews of the epidemiological evidence, prevalence, and interventions to promote "active aging." *The Gerontologist, 56*(Suppl. 2), S268–S280. http://dx.doi.org/10.1093/geront/gnw031

Benbow, S. M., & Beeston, D. (2012). Sexuality, aging, and dementia. *International Psychogeriatrics, 24*, 1026–1033. http://dx.doi.org/10.1017/S1041610212000257

Bleijenberg, N., Zuithoff, N. P. A., Smith, A. K., de Wit, N. J., & Schuurmans, M. J. (2017). Disability in the individual ADL, IADL, and mobility among older adults: A prospective cohort study. *The Journal of Nutrition, Health & Aging, 21*, 897–903. http://dx.doi.org/10.1007/s12603-017-0891-6

Bombardier, C. H., Ehde, D. M., Stoelb, B., & Molton, I. R. (2010). The relationship of age-related factors to psychological functioning among people with disabilities. *Physical Medicine and Rehabilitation Clinics of North America, 21*, 281–297. http://dx.doi.org/10.1016/j.pmr.2009.12.005

Bray, N. W., Smart, R. R., Jakobi, J. M., & Jones, G. R. (2016). Exercise prescription to reverse frailty. *Applied Physiology, Nutrition, and Metabolism, 41*, 1112–1116. http://dx.doi.org/10.1139/apnm-2016-0226

Brodie, M. A., Coppens, M. J., Ejupi, A., Gschwind, Y. J., Annegarn, J., Schoene, D., . . . Delbaere, K. (2017). Comparison between clinical gait and daily-life gait assessments of fall risk in older people. *Geriatrics & Gerontology International, 17*, 2274–2282. http://dx.doi.org/10.1111/ggi.12979

Buford, T. W., Anton, S. D., Clark, D. J., Higgins, T. J., & Cooke, M. B. (2014). Optimizing the benefits of exercise on physical function in older adults. *PM & R: The Journal of Injury, Function, and Rehabilitation, 6*, 528–543. http://dx.doi.org/10.1016/j.pmrj.2013.11.009

Carver, L. F., & Buchanan, D. (2016). Successful aging: Considering nonbiomedical constructs. *Clinical Interventions in Aging, 11*, 1623–1630. http://dx.doi.org/10.2147/CIA.S117202

Centers for Disease Control and Prevention. (2017). *Nutrition, physical activity, and obesity: Data, trends, and maps*. Retrieved from https://www.cdc.gov/nccdphp/dnpao/data-trends-maps/index.html

Centers for Medicare and Medicaid Services. (2011). *Chronic conditions among Medicare beneficiaries. Chartbook: 2012 edition*. Baltimore, MD. Retrieved from https://www.cms.gov/research-statistics-data-and-systems/statistics-trends-and-reports/chronic-conditions/downloads/2012chartbook.pdf

Chen, C. M., Chang, W. C., & Lan, T. Y. (2015). Identifying factors associated with changes in physical functioning in an older population. *Geriatrics & Gerontology International, 15*, 156–164. http://dx.doi.org/10.1111/ggi.12243

Chiuve, S. E., McCullough, M. L., Sacks, F. M., & Rimm, E. B. (2006). Healthy lifestyle factors in the primary prevention of coronary heart disease among men: Benefits among users and nonusers of lipid-lowering and antihypertensive medications. *Circulation, 114*, 160–167. http://dx.doi.org/10.1161/CIRCULATIONAHA.106.621417

Chiuve, S. E., Rexrode, K. M., Spiegelman, D., Logroscino, G., Manson, J. E., & Rimm, E. B. (2008). Primary prevention of stroke by healthy lifestyle. *Circulation, 118*, 947–954. http://dx.doi.org/10.1161/CIRCULATIONAHA.108.781062

Colello, K. J., & Napili, A. (2018). *Older Americans act: Overview and funding*. Report prepared for Members and Committees of Congress. Retrieved August 1, 2018, from https://fas.org/sgp/crs/misc/R43414.pdf

Connolly, D., Garvey, J., & McKee, G. (2017). Factors associated with ADL/IADL disability in community dwelling older adults in the Irish longitudinal study on ageing (TILDA). *Disability and Rehabilitation, 39*, 809–816. http://dx.doi.org/10.3109/09638288.2016.1161848

Consolidated Appropriations Act of 2018, Pub. L. No. 115-141, 115 U.S.C. (2018).

Conwell, Y., Van Orden, K., & Caine, E. D. (2011). Suicide in older adults. *Psychiatric Clinics of North America, 34*, 451–468.

Curl, A. L., Stowe, J. D., Cooney, T. M., & Proulx, C. M. (2014). Giving up the keys: How driving cessation affects engagement in later life. *The Gerontologist, 54*, 423–433. http://dx.doi.org/10.1093/geront/gnt037

Cuthbert, J. P., Harrison-Felix, C., Corrigan, J. D., Kreider, S., Bell, J. M., Coronado, V. G., & Whiteneck, G. G. (2015). Epidemiology of adults receiving acute inpatient rehabilitation for a primary diagnosis of traumatic brain injury in the United States. *The Journal of Head Trauma Rehabilitation, 30*, 122–135. http://dx.doi.org/10.1097/HTR.0000000000000012

DeCaria, J. E., Sharp, C., & Petrella, R. J. (2012). Scoping review report: Obesity in older adults. *International Journal of Obesity, 36*, 1141–1150. http://dx.doi.org/10.1038/ijo.2012.29

de Leon, C. F. M., & Rajan, K. B. (2014). Psychosocial influences in onset and progression of late life disability. *The Journals of Gerontology. Series B, Psychological Sciences and Social Sciences, 69*, 287–302. http://dx.doi.org/10.1093/geronb/gbt130

Depp, C. A., & Jeste, D. V. (2006). Definitions and predictors of successful aging: A comprehensive review of larger quantitative studies. *The American Journal of Geriatric Psychiatry, 14*, 6–20. http://dx.doi.org/10.1097/01.JGP.0000192501.03069.bc

Dew, M. A., Whyte, E. M., Lenze, E. J., Houck, P. R., Mulsant, B. H., Pollock, B. G., . . . Reynolds, C. F., III. (2007). Recovery from major depression in older adults receiving augmentation of antidepressant pharmacotherapy. *The American Journal of Psychiatry, 164*, 892–899. http://dx.doi.org/10.1176/ajp.2007.164.6.892

Dreer, L., Copeland, J., & Cheavens, J. (2011). Integrating neuropsychological functioning into cognitive behavioral therapy: Implications for older adults. In K. H. Sorrocco & S. Lauderdale (Eds.), *Cognitive behavior therapy with older adults* (pp. 317–365). New York, NY: Springer.

Dreer, L., & Linley, A. (2016). Behavioral medicine: Nutrition, exercise, and medication management. In M. Budd, S. Hough, W. Steirs, & S. Wegener (Eds.), *Practical psychology in medical rehabilitation* (pp. 67–76). Basel, Switzerland: Springer International Publishing.

Dreer, L. E., Elliott, T. R., Berry, J., Fletcher, D. C., Swanson, M., & Christopher, J. M. N. (2008). Cognitive appraisals, distress and disability among persons in low vision rehabilitation. *British Journal of Health Psychology, 13*, 449–461. http://dx.doi.org/10.1348/135910707X209835

Dreer, L. E., Elliott, T. R., Fletcher, D. C., & Swanson, M. (2005). Social problem-solving abilities and psychological adjustment of persons in low vision rehabilitation. *Rehabilitation Psychology, 50*(3), 232–238. http://dx.doi.org/10.1037/0090-5550.50.3.232

Dreer, L. E., Girkin, C., & Mansberger, S. L. (2012). Determinants of medication adherence to topical glaucoma therapy. *Journal of Glaucoma, 21*, 234–240. http://dx.doi.org/10.1097/IJG.0b013e31821dac86

Dreer, L. E., Girkin, C. A., Campbell, L., Wood, A., Gao, L., & Owsley, C. (2013). Glaucoma medication adherence among African Americans. *Optometry and Vision Science, 90*, 883–897. http://dx.doi.org/10.1097/OPX.0000000000000009

Dreer, L. E., Owsley, C., Campbell, L., Gao, L., Wood, A., & Girkin, C. A. (2016). Feasibility, patient acceptability, and preliminary efficacy of a culturally informed, health promotion program to improve glaucoma medication adherence among African Americans: "Glaucoma management optimism for African Americans living with glaucoma" (GOAL). *Current Eye Research, 41*, 50–58. http://dx.doi.org/10.3109/02713683.2014.1002045

Dunn, D., Uswatte, G., & Elliott, T. (2009). Happiness, resilience, and positive growth following physical disability: Issues for understanding research, and therapeutic intervention. In S. Lopez & C. Snyder (Eds.), *Oxford handbook of positive psychology* (pp. 651–664). New York, NY: Oxford University Press.

Edwards, J. D., Lunsman, M., Perkins, M., Rebok, G. W., & Roth, D. L. (2009). Driving cessation and health trajectories in older adults. *The Journals of*

Gerontology. Series A, Biological Sciences and Medical Sciences, 64, 1290–1295. http://dx.doi.org/10.1093/gerona/glp114

Egan, K. J., & Pot, A. M. (2016). Encouraging innovation for assistive health technologies in dementia: Barriers, enablers and next steps to be taken. *Journal of the American Medical Directors Association, 17*, 357–363. http://dx.doi.org/10.1016/j.jamda.2016.01.010

Elliott, A. F., Dreer, L. E., McGwin, G., Jr., Scilley, K., & Owsley, C. (2010). The personal burden of decreased vision-targeted health-related quality of life in nursing home residents. *Journal of Aging and Health, 22*, 504–521. http://dx.doi.org/10.1177/0898264310361368

Elliott, T. R., Berry, J. W., & Grant, J. S. (2009). Problem-solving training for family caregivers of women with disabilities: A randomized clinical trial. *Behaviour Research and Therapy, 47*, 548–558. http://dx.doi.org/10.1016/j.brat.2009.03.006

Elliott, T. R., Shewchuk, R. M., & Richards, J. S. (2001). Family caregiver social problem-solving abilities and adjustment during the initial year of the caregiving role. *Journal of Counseling Psychology, 48*, 223–232. http://dx.doi.org/10.1037/0022-0167.48.2.223

Elliott, T. R., Uswatte, G., Lewis, L., & Palmatier, A. (2000). Goal instability and adjustment to physical disability. *Journal of Counseling Psychology, 47*, 251–265. http://dx.doi.org/10.1037/0022-0167.47.2.251

Evenson, K. R., Butler, E. N., & Rosamond, W. D. (2014). Prevalence of physical activity and sedentary behavior among adults with cardiovascular disease in the United States. *Journal of Cardiopulmonary Rehabilitation and Prevention, 34*, 406–419. http://dx.doi.org/10.1097/HCR.0000000000000064

Fougère, B., Aubertin-Leheudre, M., Vellas, B., Andrieu, S., Demougeot, L., Cluzan, C., & Cesari, M. (2016). Clinical research for older adults in rural areas: The MINDED study experience. *Age, 38*(2), 30. http://dx.doi.org/10.1007/s11357-016-9892-3

Freedman, V. A., Kasper, J. D., & Spillman, B. C. (2017). Successful aging through successful accommodations with assistive devices. *The Journals of Gerontology. Series B, Psychological Sciences and Social Sciences, 72*, 300–309.

Freedman, V. A., Kasper, J. D., Spillman, B. C., Agree, E. M., Mor, V., Wallace, R. B., & Wolf, D. A. (2014). Behavioral adaptation and late-life disability: A new spectrum for assessing public health impacts. *American Journal of Public Health, 104*, e88–e94. http://dx.doi.org/10.2105/AJPH.2013.301687

Freedman, V. A., Stafford, F., Schwarz, N., Conrad, F., & Cornman, J. C. (2012). Disability, participation, and subjective wellbeing among older couples. *Social Science & Medicine, 74*, 588–596. http://dx.doi.org/10.1016/j.socscimed.2011.10.018

Friedman, E. M., Ruini, C., Foy, R., Jaros, L., Sampson, H., & Ryff, C. D. (2017). Lighten UP! A community-based group intervention to promote psychological well-being in older adults. *Aging & Mental Health, 21*, 199–205. http://dx.doi.org/10.1080/13607863.2015.1093605

Frontera, J. E., & Mollett, P. (2017). Aging with a spinal cord injury: An update. *Physical Medicine and Rehabilitation Clinics of North America, 28*, 821–828. http://dx.doi.org/10.1016/j.pmr.2017.06.013

Galambos, C., & Curl, A. (2013). Developing gerontological competency: A curriculum approach. *Gerontological Geriatric Education, 34*, 309–321. http://dx.doi.org/10.1080/02701960.2013.782301

Gopinath, B., Russell, J., Kifley, A., Flood, V. M., & Mitchell, P. (2016). Adherence to dietary guidelines and successful aging over 10 years. *The Journals of Gerontology. Series A, Biological Sciences and Medical Sciences, 71*, 349–355. http://dx.doi.org/10.1093/gerona/glv189

Grant, J. S., Elliott, T. R., Giger, J. N., & Bartolucci, A. A. (2001). Social problem-solving abilities, social support, and adjustment among family caregivers of individuals with a stroke. *Rehabilitation Psychology, 46*, 44–57. http://dx.doi.org/10.1037/0090-5550.46.1.44

Grant, J. S., Elliott, T. R., Weaver, M., Glandon, G. L., Raper, J. L., & Giger, J. N. (2006). Social support, social problem-solving abilities, and adjustment of family caregivers of stroke survivors. *Archives of Physical Medicine and Rehabilitation, 87*, 343–350. http://dx.doi.org/10.1016/j.apmr.2005.09.019

Hahn, J. E., Aronow, H. U., Rosario, E. R., & Guenther, N. (2013). Multidimensional health risk appraisal among adults aging with acquired disabilities. *Disability and Health Journal, 6*, 195–203. http://dx.doi.org/10.1016/j.dhjo.2013.02.002

Health and Medicine Division. (2016). *Families caring for an aging America*. Washington, DC: National Academies of Sciences, Engineering, and Medicine. Retrieved from http://www.nationalacademies.org/hmd/~/media/Files/Report%20Files/2016/Caregiving-RiB.pdf

Hinrichsen, A. G., Emery-Tiburcio, E., Gooblar, J., & Molinari, V. (2018). Building foundational knowledge competencies in professional geropsychology: Council of Professional Geropsychology Training Programs (CoPGTP) recommendations. *Clinical Psychology: Science and Practice, 25*(2), 1–8.

Hodge, A. M., English, D. R., Giles, G. G., & Flicker, L. (2013). Social connectedness and predictors of successful ageing. *Maturitas, 75*, 361–366. http://dx.doi.org/10.1016/j.maturitas.2013.05.002

Hoge, M. A., Karel, M. J., Zeiss, A. M., Alegria, M., & Moye, J. (2015). Strengthening psychology's workforce for older adults: Implications of the Institute of

Medicine's report to Congress. *American Psychologist, 70*, 265–278. http://dx.doi.org/10.1037/a0038927

Infurna, F., & Wiest, M. (2016). The effect of disability onset across the adult life span. *The Journals of Gerontology. Series B, Psychological Sciences and Social Sciences, 72*, 1–12.

Institute of Medicine. (2012). *The mental health and substance use workforce for older adults: In whose hands?* Washington, DC: National Academies Press.

Jameson, J., & Cully, J. (2011). Cognitive behavioral therapy for older adults in the primary care setting. In K. H. S. Sorocco & S. Lauderdale (Eds.), *Cognitive behavior therapy with older adults* (pp. 291–316). New York, NY: Springer.

Jensen, M. P., Molton, I. R., Groah, S. L., Campbell, M. L., Charlifue, S., Chiodo, A., . . . Tate, D. (2012). Secondary health conditions in individuals aging with SCI: Terminology, concepts and analytic approaches. *Spinal Cord, 50*, 373–378. http://dx.doi.org/10.1038/sc.2011.150

Jensen, M. P., Smith, A. E., Bombardier, C. H., Yorkston, K. M., Miró, J., & Molton, I. R. (2014). Social support, depression, and physical disability: Age and diagnostic group effects. *Disability and Health Journal, 7*, 164–172. http://dx.doi.org/10.1016/j.dhjo.2013.11.001

Jensen, M. P., Truitt, A. R., Schomer, K. G., Yorkston, K. M., Baylor, C., & Molton, I. R. (2013). Frequency and age effects of secondary health conditions in individuals with spinal cord injury: A scoping review. *Spinal Cord, 51*, 882–892. http://dx.doi.org/10.1038/sc.2013.112

Jeste, D. V., Savla, G. N., Thompson, W. K., Vahia, I. V., Glorioso, D. K., Martin, A. S., . . . Depp, C. A. (2013). Association between older age and more successful aging: Critical role of resilience and depression. *The American Journal of Psychiatry, 170*, 188–196. http://dx.doi.org/10.1176/appi.ajp.2012.12030386

Karel, M. J., Gatz, M., & Smyer, M. A. (2012). Aging and mental health in the decade ahead: What psychologists need to know. *American Psychologist, 67*, 184–198. http://dx.doi.org/10.1037/a0025393

Karel, M. J., Holley, C. K., Whitbourne, S. K., Segal, D. L., Tazeau, Y. N., Emery, E. E., . . . Zweig, R. A. (2012). Preliminary validation of a tool to assess competencies for professional geropsychology practice. *Professional Psychology: Research and Practice, 43*, 110–117. http://dx.doi.org/10.1037/a0025788

Karp, J. F., Skidmore, E., Lotz, M., Lenze, E., Dew, M. A., & Reynolds, C. F., III. (2009). Use of the late-life function and disability instrument to assess disability in major depression. *Journal of the American Geriatrics Society, 57*, 1612–1619. http://dx.doi.org/10.1111/j.1532-5415.2009.02398.x

King, B. J., Roberts, T. J., & Bowers, B. J. (2013). Nursing student attitudes toward and preferences for working with older adults. *Gerontology & Geriatrics Education, 34*, 272–291. http://dx.doi.org/10.1080/02701960.2012.718012

Knight, B. G., Karel, M. J., Hinrichsen, G. A., Qualls, S. H., & Duffy, M. (2009). Pikes Peak model for training in professional geropsychology. *American Psychologist, 64*, 205–214. http://dx.doi.org/10.1037/a0015059

Koenig, H. G. (2004). Religion, spirituality, and medicine: Research findings and implications for clinical practice. *Southern Medical Journal, 97*, 1194–1200. http://dx.doi.org/10.1097/01.SMJ.0000146489.21837.CE

Koenig, H. G. (2012). Religion, spirituality, and health: The research and clinical implications. *International Scholarly Research Notices: Psychiatry, 2012*, 1–33. http://dx.doi.org/10.5402/2012/278730

Koenig, H. G., Nelson, B., Shaw, S. F., Saxena, S., & Cohen, H. J. (2016). Religious involvement and adaptation in female family caregivers. *Journal of the American Geriatrics Society, 64*, 578–583. http://dx.doi.org/10.1111/jgs.13929

Kreutzer, J. S., Marwitz, J. H., Sima, A. P., Bergquist, T. F., Johnson-Greene, D., Felix, E. R., . . . Dreer, L. E. (2016). Resilience following traumatic brain injury: A traumatic brain injury model systems study. *Archives of Physical Medicine and Rehabilitation, 97*, 708–713. http://dx.doi.org/10.1016/j.apmr.2015.12.003

Kurylo, M. F., Elliott, T. R., & Shewchuk, R. M. (2001). FOCUS on the family caregiver: A problem-solving training intervention. *Journal of Counseling & Development, 79*, 275–281. http://dx.doi.org/10.1002/j.1556-6676.2001.tb01972.x

Labouvie-Vief, G., Diehl, M., Jain, E., & Zhang, F. (2007). Six-year change in affect optimization and affect complexity across the adult life span: A further examination. *Psychology and Aging, 22*, 738–751. http://dx.doi.org/10.1037/0882-7974.22.4.738

Lenze, E. J., Mulsant, B. H., Mohlman, J., Shear, M. K., Dew, M. A., Schulz, R., . . . Reynolds, C. F., III. (2005). Generalized anxiety disorder in late life: Lifetime course and comorbidity with major depressive disorder. *The American Journal of Geriatric Psychiatry, 13*, 77–80. http://dx.doi.org/10.1097/00019442-200501000-00011

Lin, S. F., Beck, A. N., & Finch, B. K. (2014). Black-White disparity in disability among U.S. older adults: Age, period, and cohort trends. *The Journals of Gerontology. Series B, Psychological Sciences and Social Sciences, 69*, 784–797. http://dx.doi.org/10.1093/geronb/gbu010

Lin, S. F., Beck, A. N., Finch, B. K., Hummer, R. A., & Master, R. K. (2012). Trends in U.S. older adult disability: Exploring age, period, and cohort effects. *American Journal of Public Health, 102*, 2157–2163. http://dx.doi.org/10.2105/AJPH.2011.300602

Liu, C. J., Jones, L. Y., Formyduval, A. R. M., & Clark, D. O. (2016). Task-oriented exercise to reduce activities of daily living disability in vulnerable older adults: A feasibility study of the 3-step workout for life. *Journal of Aging and Physical Activity, 24*, 384–392. http://dx.doi.org/10.1123/japa.2015-0070

Loprinzi, P. D. (2016). Epidemiological investigation of muscle-strengthening activities and cognitive function among older adults. *Chronic Illness, 12*, 157–162. http://dx.doi.org/10.1177/1742395316641998

Lucchetti, A. L., Lucchetti, G., de Oliveira, I. N., Moreira-Almeida, A., & da Silva Ezequiel, O. (2017). Experiencing aging or demystifying myths? Impact of different "geriatrics and gerontology" teaching strategies in first year medical students. *BMC Medical Education, 17*, 35. http://dx.doi.org/10.1186/s12909-017-0872-9

Mantella, R. C., Butters, M. A., Dew, M. A., Mulsant, B. H., Begley, A. E., Tracey, B., . . . Lenze, E. J. (2007). Cognitive impairment in late-life generalized anxiety disorder. *The American Journal of Geriatric Psychiatry, 15*, 673–679. http://dx.doi.org/10.1097/JGP.0b013e31803111f2

Marcum, Z. A., Zheng, Y., Perera, S., Strotmeyer, E., Newman, A. B., Simonsick, E. M., . . . Hanlon, J. T. (2013). Prevalence and correlates of self-reported medication non-adherence among older adults with coronary heart disease, diabetes mellitus, and/or hypertension. *Research Social Administration Pharmacology, 9*, 817–827. http://dx.doi.org/10.1016/j.sapharm.2012.12.002

Marottoli, R. A., de Leon, C. F. M., Glass, T. A., Williams, C. S., Cooney, L. M., Jr., Berkman, L. F., & Tinetti, M. E. (1997). Driving cessation and increased depressive symptoms: Prospective evidence from the New Haven EPESE (established populations for epidemiologic studies of the elderly). *Journal of the American Geriatrics Society, 45*, 202–206. http://dx.doi.org/10.1111/j.1532-5415.1997.tb04508.x

Marson, D. C., & Dreer, L. E. (2007). Competence. In S. Gauthier (Ed.), *Clinical diagnosis and management of Alzheimer's Disease* (pp. 323–338). Abingdon, England: Informa.

Marson, D. C., Hebert, K., & Solomon, A. C. (2011). Assessing civil competencies in older adults with dementia: Consent capacity, financial capacity, and testamentary capacity. In G. J. Larrabee (Ed.), *Forensic neuropsychology. A scientific approach* (pp. 334–377). New York, NY: Oxford University Press.

Mejía, S. T., Ryan, L. H., Gonzalez, R., & Smith, J. (2017). Successful aging as the intersection of individual resources, age, environment, and experiences of well-being in daily activities. *The Journals of Gerontology. Series B, Psychological Sciences and Social Sciences, 72*, 279–289.

Molton, I. R., & Yorkston, K. M. (2017). Growing older with a physical disability: A special application of the successful aging paradigm. *The Journals of Gerontology. Series B, Psychological Sciences and Social Sciences, 72*, 290–299.

Moye, J., Molinari, V. A., Karel, M. J., Naik, A. D., Sakai, E., & Carpenter, B. D. (2018). Come, join, lead: Attracting students to careers in aging and promoting involvement in gerontological societies. *Gerontology & Geriatrics Education, 39*, 374–384.

Nerenberg, L. (1996). *Financial abuse of the elderly*. Washington, DC: National Center on Elder Abuse.

Palmcrantz, S., Holmqvist, L. W., Sommerfeld, D. K., Tistad, M., Ytterberg, C., & von Koch, L. (2012). Differences between younger and older individuals in their use of care and rehabilitation but not in self-perceived global recovery 1year after stroke. *Journal of the Neurological Sciences, 321*(1–2), 29–34. http://dx.doi.org/10.1016/j.jns.2012.07.024

Patient Protection and Affordable Care Act, 42 U.S.C. § 18001 et seq. (2010).

Puentes, W. J., Bradway, C. K., & Aselage, M. (2010). Older adult mental health: Teaching senior-level baccalaureate nursing students what they need to know. *Journal of Gerontological Nursing, 36*(7), 44–53. http://dx.doi.org/10.3928/00989134-20100528-99

Putnam, M. (2014). Bridging network divides: Building capacity to support aging with disability populations through research. *Disability and Health Journal, 7*(1, Suppl.), S51–S59. http://dx.doi.org/10.1016/j.dhjo.2013.08.002

Putrino, D. (2014). Telerehabilitation and emerging virtual reality approaches to stroke rehabilitation. *Current Opinion in Neurology, 27*, 631–636. http://dx.doi.org/10.1097/WCO.0000000000000152

Qualls, S. H. (2008). Caregiver family therapy. In B. Knight & K. Laidlaw (Eds.), *Handbook of emotional disorders in older adults* (pp. 183–210). Oxford, England: Oxford University Press. http://dx.doi.org/10.1093/med:psych/9780198569459.003.0008

Ramanathan, D. M., McWilliams, N., Schatz, P., & Hillary, F. G. (2012). Epidemiological shifts in elderly traumatic brain injury: 18-year trends in Pennsylvania. *Journal of Neurotrauma, 29*, 1371–1378. http://dx.doi.org/10.1089/neu.2011.2197

Rillamas-Sun, E., LaCroix, A. Z., Waring, M. E., Kroenke, C. H., LaMonte, M. J., Vitolins, M. Z., . . . Wallace, R. B. (2014). Obesity and late-age survival without major disease or disability in older women. *JAMA Internal Medicine, 174*, 98–106.

Rivera, P. A., Elliott, T. R., Berry, J. W., & Grant, J. S. (2008). Problem-solving training for family caregivers of persons with traumatic brain injuries: A randomized controlled trial. *Archives of Physical Medicine and Rehabilitation*, *89*, 931–941. http://dx.doi.org/10.1016/j.apmr.2007.12.032

Rogers, C. (2002). Rural health issues for the older population. *Rural America*, *3*, 1–6.

Rogers, S. E., Thrasher, A. D., Miao, Y., Boscardin, W. J., & Smith, A. K. (2015). Discrimination in healthcare settings is associated with disability in older adults: Health and retirement study, 2008–2012. *Journal of General Internal Medicine*, *30*, 1413–1420. http://dx.doi.org/10.1007/s11606-015-3233-6

Rowe, J. W., & Kahn, R. L. (1998). *Successful aging*. New York, NY: Pantheon/Random House.

Rustøen, T., Wahl, A. K., Hanestad, B. R., Lerdal, A., Paul, S., & Miaskowski, C. (2005). Age and the experience of chronic pain: Differences in health and quality of life among younger, middle-aged, and older adults. *The Clinical Journal of Pain*, *21*, 513–523. http://dx.doi.org/10.1097/01.ajp.0000146217.31780.ef

Sabia, S., Singh-Manoux, A., Hagger-Johnson, G., Cambois, E., Brunner, E. J., & Kivimaki, M. (2012). Influence of individual and combined healthy behaviours on successful aging. *Canadian Medical Association Journal*, *184*, 1985–1992. http://dx.doi.org/10.1503/cmaj.121080

Sanford, S., Rapoport, M. J., Tuokko, H., Crizzle, A., Hatzifilalithis, S., Laberge, S., & Naglie, G. (2018). Independence, loss, and social identity: Perspectives on driving cessation and dementia. *Dementia*. Advance online publication. http://dx.doi.org/10.1177/1471301218762838

Sarabia-Cobo, C. M., & Castanedo Pfeiffer, C. (2015). Changing negative stereotypes regarding aging in undergraduate nursing students. *Nurse Education Today*, *35*, e60–e64. http://dx.doi.org/10.1016/j.nedt.2015.06.006

Silverman, A. M., Molton, I. R., Alschuler, K. N., Ehde, D. M., & Jensen, M. P. (2015). Resilience predicts functional outcomes in people aging with disability: A longitudinal investigation. *Archives of Physical Medicine and Rehabilitation*, *96*, 1262–1268. http://dx.doi.org/10.1016/j.apmr.2015.02.023

Sink, K. M., Espeland, M. A., Castro, C. M., Church, T., Cohen, R., Dodson, J. A., . . . Williamson, J. D. (2015). Effect of a 24-month physical activity intervention vs. health education on cognitive outcomes in sedentary older adults: The LIFE randomized trial. *JAMA: Journal of the American Medical Association*, *314*, 781–790. http://dx.doi.org/10.1001/jama.2015.9617

Sirey, J. A., Greenfield, A., Weinberger, M. I., & Bruce, M. L. (2013). Medication beliefs and self-reported adherence among community-dwelling older adults. *Clinical Therapeutics*, *35*, 153–160. http://dx.doi.org/10.1016/j.clinthera.2013.01.001

Skolarus, L. E., Burke, J. F., & Freedman, V. A. (2014). The role of accommodations in poststroke disability management. *The Journals of Gerontology. Series B, Psychological Sciences and Social Sciences*, *69*(Suppl. 1), S26–S34. http://dx.doi.org/10.1093/geronb/gbu117

Skultety, K. M., & Zeiss, A. (2006). The treatment of depression in older adults in the primary care setting: An evidence-based review. *Health Psychology*, *25*, 665–674. http://dx.doi.org/10.1037/0278-6133.25.6.665

Smith, A. R., Chen, C., Clarke, P., & Gallagher, N. A. (2016). Trajectories of outdoor mobility in vulnerable community-dwelling elderly: The role of individual and environmental factors. *Journal of Aging and Health*, *28*, 796–811. http://dx.doi.org/10.1177/0898264315611665

Sorocco, K., & Lauderdale, S. (2011). *Cognitive behavior therapy with older adults*. New York, NY: Springer.

Stenholm, S., Westerlund, H., Head, J., Hyde, M., Kawachi, I., Pentti, J., . . . Vahtera, J. (2015). Comorbidity and functional trajectories from midlife to old age: The health and retirement study. *The Journals of Gerontology. Series A, Biological Sciences and Medical Sciences*, *70*, 332–338. http://dx.doi.org/10.1093/gerona/glu113

Sun, D. Q., Huang, J., Varadhan, R., & Agrawal, Y. (2016). Race and fall risk: Data from the national health and aging trends study (NHATS). *Age and Ageing*, *45*, 120–127. http://dx.doi.org/10.1093/ageing/afv173

Troutman-Jordan, M., & Staples, J. (2014). Successful aging from the viewpoint of older adults. *Research and Theory for Nursing Practice: An International Journal*, *28*, 87–104. http://dx.doi.org/10.1891/1541-6577.28.1.87

United States Census Bureau. (2012). *Projections of the population by selected age groups and sex for the United States: 2015 to 2060*. Retrieved from https://www.census.gov/data/tables/2012/demo/popproj/2012-summary-tables.html

Verbrugge, L., & Yang, L. (2002). Aging with disability and disability with aging. *Journal of Disability Policy Studies*, *12*, 253–267. http://dx.doi.org/10.1177/104420730201200405

Wandke, H., Sengpiel, M., & Sönksen, M. (2012). Myths about older people's use of information and communication technology. *Gerontology*, *58*, 564–570. http://dx.doi.org/10.1159/000339104

Whitson, H. E., Hastings, S. N., Landerman, L. R., Fillenbaum, G. G., Cohen, H. J., & Johnson, K. S. (2011). Black-White disparity in disability: The role of medical conditions. *Journal of the American*

Geriatrics Society, *59*, 844–850. http://dx.doi.org/10.1111/j.1532-5415.2011.03401.x

Wolitzky-Taylor, K. B., Castriotta, N., Lenze, E. J., Stanley, M. A., & Craske, M. G. (2010). Anxiety disorders in older adults: A comprehensive review. *Depression and Anxiety*, *27*, 190–211. http://dx.doi.org/10.1002/da.20653

Woods, N. F., Rillamas-Sun, E., Cochrane, B. B., La Croix, A. Z., Seeman, T. E., Tindle, H. A., . . . Wallace, R. B. (2016). Aging well: Observations from the women's health initiative study. *The Journals of Gerontology. Series A, Biological Sciences and Medical Sciences*, *71*(Suppl. 1), S3–S12. http://dx.doi.org/10.1093/gerona/glv054

World Health Organization. (2017). *Physical activity and older adults: Recommended levels of physical activity for adults aged 65 and above*. Retrieved from http://www.who.int/dietphysicalactivity/factsheet_olderadults/en/

Yorkston, K. M., McMullan, K. A., Molton, I., & Jensen, M. P. (2010). Pathways of change experienced by people aging with disability: A focus group study. *Disability and Rehabilitation*, *32*, 1697–1704.

Young, Y., Frick, K. D., & Phelan, E. A. (2009). Can successful aging and chronic illness coexist in the same individual? A multidimensional concept of successful aging. *Journal of the American Medical Directors Association*, *10*, 87–92. http://dx.doi.org/10.1016/j.jamda.2008.11.003

Zaleski, A. L., Taylor, B. A., Panza, G. A., Wu, Y., Pescatello, L. S., Thompson, P. D., & Fernandez, A. B. (2016). Coming of age: Considerations in the prescription of exercise for older adults. *Methodist Debakey Cardiovascular Journal*, *12*, 98–104. http://dx.doi.org/10.14797/mdcj-12-2-98

Zarit, S. H., & Zarit, J. M. (2007). *Mental disorders in older adults, second edition*. New York, NY: Guildford Press.

Part II

CLINICAL CONDITIONS

Chapter 14

CHRONIC PAIN

Dawn M. Ehde, Anna L. Kratz, and Kevin N. Alschuler

Rehabilitation psychologists have played a fundamental role in the assessment, treatment, and science of chronic pain since before 1968, the year Wilbert Fordyce published his seminal article on a behavioral approach to chronic pain (Fordyce, Fowler, & Delateur, 1968). This role has not diminished in the intervening years. Chronic pain remains a public health problem of alarming proportions, affecting more adults than diabetes, heart disease, and cancer combined (Jensen & Turk, 2014) and resulting in considerable costs to affected individuals, families, health care systems, and society (Institute of Medicine, 2011). No longer viewed from a disease model, chronic pain is regarded as a condition affected by biological, psychological, and social determinants, an understanding advanced by psychological theories and science (for a review of psychology's contributions to the field, see Jensen & Turk, 2014). Adoption of the biopsychosocial model of pain has led to the development and use of psychosocial interventions addressing chronic pain. The current opioid crisis, which intersects with inadequately or inappropriately treated chronic pain and opioid use disorders (National Academies of Sciences, Engineering, and Medicine, 2017), underscores the need for continued involvement of psychologists in advancing the understanding and treatment of chronic pain at the individual and public health level.

All rehabilitation psychologists working in health care will encounter individuals with chronic pain at some point in their clinical practice. This chapter provides an overview of essential assessment practices, evidence-based interventions, and practical considerations relevant to addressing chronic pain in rehabilitation psychology settings. Although one chapter cannot adequately summarize psychology's 50-plus-year history of contributions to the field, we highlight fundamental principles and provide key references for further erudition. This chapter focuses on chronic pain, that is, pain that persists or is recurrent for 6 months or more. Although psychologists practicing in rehabilitation settings may also treat acute pain, chronic pain is more commonly the focus of rehabilitation psychology services and, thus, the focus of this chapter. This chapter addresses several of the Rehabilitation Psychology Competencies, including those on the assessment, evaluation, and treatment of pain. Please see Chapter 1, this volume for further details.

BIOPSYCHOSOCIAL MODEL OF PAIN

The modern perspective of chronic pain uses a biopsychosocial model that considers the intersecting contributions of biological, psychological, and social factors to the experience of pain. Broadly,

http://dx.doi.org/10.1037/0000129-015
Handbook of Rehabilitation Psychology, Third Edition, L. A. Brenner, S. A. Reid-Arndt, T. R. Elliott, R. G. Frank, and B. Caplan (Editors-in-Chief)

the biopsychosocial model appreciates a biological basis for pain but suggests that psychological and social factors have a significant impact on how individuals experience and respond to that painful sensation. Although each domain is briefly reviewed separately in what follows, it is important to recognize that the biopsychosocial model is predicated on an interdependence between the domains, whereby they work together to account for the experience of chronic pain, as opposed to each functioning independently.

Biological Factors

Pain is understood to most commonly come from physical pathology (injury or damage to physical structure), although in chronic pain, such perspective is frequently insufficient. In chronic back pain, for example, efforts to use imaging to identify underlying pathology causing pain have revealed that many patients with chronic back pain have no identifiable structural source of their pain, whereas patients with no pain symptoms often have structural pathology that would be expected to cause pain (Geisser et al., 2007; Turk & Flor, 1999). Thus, although it is important to identify sources of pain, it is also the case that many have pain that persists beyond normal healing of an injury or illness or in the absence of any clear ongoing tissue damage or disease.

The neurobiology of pain is complex and multidimensional, with pain processing occurring in distinct regions of the brain including areas that process the sensory-discriminative and the affective emotional dimensions. In the presence of prolonged exposure to pain (such as in chronic pain), underlying changes to the central nervous system (CNS) alter subsequent brain processing of pain. Numerous theories have been offered to explain this phenomenon, including the concept of central sensitization, the reorganization of the CNS that results from the prolonged experience of neuropathic or musculoskeletal pain (Coderre, Katz, Vaccarino, & Melzack, 1993; Geisser et al., 2007), and the concept of the pain neuromatrix, such as that seen in phantom limb pain where the reorganization of the neural network results in peripheral stimulation in an adjacent area resulting in sensations in the nonexistent limb (R. Melzack, 2001). Thus, chronic pain may arise biologically from identifiable pain, CNS sensitization or reorganization, or a combination of sources. In addition, the pain system also shares common neurobiological pathways with regions in the brain associated with the processing of psychological distress, including both anxious and depressed mood (Goesling, Clauw, & Hassett, 2013), suggesting that pain is linked to other common targets of psychological treatment.

Psychological Factors

A vast body of research has focused specifically on the role of psychological factors in chronic pain, paying particular attention to the thoughts, beliefs, and behaviors individuals engage in when responding to pain. Numerous studies have established that maladaptive pain-related beliefs and coping responses are highly associated with increased pain intensity, psychological distress, and disability (Jensen, Turner, Romano, & Lawler, 1994; Robinson et al., 1997). *Pain catastrophizing*, defined as excessively negative thoughts and ruminative responses to pain and one's ability to cope with it (Sullivan, Bishop, & Pivik, 1995; Sullivan & D'Eon, 1990; Sullivan et al., 2001), has been repeatedly associated with poorer physical and psychosocial functioning, even after controlling for pain intensity and depressive symptoms (Quartana, Campbell, & Edwards, 2009). Other pain beliefs important to pain severity, physical functioning, and psychosocial adaptation include perceived control over pain, the belief that pain is a signal of physical harm, and self-efficacy for managing pain and related challenges (Jensen, 2011b). Adaptive beliefs that reflect the ideas that an individual can manage their pain or live well despite pain may increase activity and decrease disability (Jensen et al., 1994; Robinson et al., 1997). For example, pain acceptance has been associated with lower pain intensity, fewer anxiety and depressive symptoms, and higher levels of functioning (Kratz, Davis, & Zautra, 2007; Viane, Crombez, Eccleston, Devulder, & De Corte, 2004; Viane et al., 2003).

In parallel to pain catastrophizing and beliefs, behaviors can also be broadly dichotomized as adaptive or maladaptive. A common maladaptive behavior is avoidance, such that an individual avoids activities that they fear may increase their pain. Other common maladaptive behaviors include physically guarding the area where pain is experienced (e.g., through limping or not relaxing the back muscles when bending; Alschuler, Neblett, Wiggert, Haig, & Geisser, 2009) and communicating pain through behaviors such as grimacing. In fact, one of the most frequently cited theoretical models of pain psychology is a fear-avoidance model that emphasizes how an individual may fear the discomfort of pain and subsequently modify activity in an effort to avoid experiencing that pain, inadvertently decreasing activity and withdrawing from participation along the way (Vlaeyen & Linton, 2000). In contrast to the avoidant class of maladaptive behaviors, adaptive behaviors are generally considered to be those that emphasize engagement in appropriate levels of activity and engagement in valued activities despite the presence of pain (Tan, Teo, Anderson, & Jensen, 2011).

Although psychological research in pain has focused most significantly on the aforementioned domains, psychiatric conditions are also associated with greater pain severity and interference. For example, longitudinal research has shown the bidirectional influences of depression and pain, specifically demonstrating that depression is both a contributor to and effect of increased pain severity (Kroenke et al., 2011). Psychiatric conditions are associated with greater use of maladaptive coping strategies, such as we identified when comparing individuals with pain and PTSD to individuals with pain without PTSD (Alschuler & Otis, 2012). Finally, psychiatric conditions are associated with greater utilization of pain-related health services (Alschuler, Jensen, & Ehde, 2012). These relationships imply that pain treatment may be optimized if comorbid psychological conditions, such as depressive disorders, are concurrently treated in addition to pain.

Social and Environmental Factors

Important research has also revealed that the way individuals interact with persons in pain can have a significant impact on the way that individual experiences or responds to pain. The most studied social factor has examined how significant others' responses to pain impact self-reports of pain, mood, and disability through the reinforcement and punishment of pain behaviors (Fordyce, 1976, 1984; Turk & Flor, 1999). Responses may be punishing (a negative reaction to the individual's pain), solicitous (overly helpful to the individual in pain), or distracting (aiding the person in pain with being active or engaged despite pain; Kerns, Turk, & Rudy, 1985; Romano et al., 1995). It is generally believed that distracting responses are most effective for minimizing both disability and depressed mood (McCracken, 2005), whereas solicitous responses covertly reinforce pain and pain behaviors and thus increase the presence of these behaviors (Alschuler, Hoodin, Murphy, Rice, & Geisser, 2011; Leonard, Cano, & Johansen, 2006), and punishing responses may make the individual in pain feel an unintentional need to prove he or she truly is suffering (McCracken, 2005) and may be associated with greater depressive symptoms but not greater disability or pain severity (Kerns, Haythornthwaite, Southwick, & Giller, 1990; Kerns et al., 1985).

The impact of environmental factors on how individuals experience pain also extends beyond relationships to situational factors. For example, some have suggested that being involved in pain-related litigation is associated with greater pain-related disability (Blyth, March, Nicholas, & Cousins, 2003); similarly, others have noted an association of worker's compensation claims and other litigation with negative rehabilitation outcomes (Fredrickson, Trief, VanBeveren, Yuan, & Baum, 1988). Others have suggested that return to work after a painful injury may be impacted by factors within the workplace that may affect outcomes, such as differences in workplace accommodations, job satisfaction, or socioeconomic status of the employee in pain (Teasell & Bombardier, 2001). Some have suggested that a fear of not appearing disabled "enough" to be on disability may undermine efforts to rehabilitate individuals in pain, due to an implicit fear of the consequences of failing to qualify for disability. Although a small proportion of such individuals may be malingering, the more common context is simply related to principles of reinforcement, such that an ongoing legal matter may inadvertently reinforce sustained disability (Greve, Ord, Bianchini, & Curtis, 2009). Other environmental factors, such as the built environment (Schild, Reed, Hingston, Dennis, & Wilson, 2016) and racial and ethnic disparities (Tait & Chibnall, 2014), also play a role in the experience and treatment of pain, although they have received less attention in the literature.

PAIN ASSESSMENT

Pain is a complex and inherently subjective experience; physical, social–societal, affective, and environmental factors interact to produce the pain experience. These numerous inputs ensure that each person's experience of pain is as unique as they are. Despite ongoing efforts to quantify pain in an "objective" manner, such as with neuroimaging (Wager et al., 2013) or skin conductance (Ledowski et al., 2006), the dominant perspective of psychologists is that the best means of assessing pain is to ask the person about his or her pain, with empirically validated self-report measures, through clinical interview, or both. Some of the key aspects of the pain experience that can be assessed with existing self-report measures are described in Table 14.1.

TABLE 14.1

Commonly Assessed Pain Dimensions

Dimension	Definition
Intensity	Magnitude of the pain sensation
Interference	Impact of pain on multiple functional and quality-of-life domains
Quality	How the pain feels (e.g., achy, sharp, tingling)
Distribution	Spatial characteristics of pain; pain can be felt in different areas of the body as well as to different depths
Temporality	Experience of pain over time, including the frequency, duration, and variability of pain
Affect	General bothersomeness or unpleasantness of pain and the emotional responses that can go along with pain, such as fear or anger
Behavior	Verbal and nonverbal (posture, movement, facial) expressions of pain; can by either intentional or involuntary

Pain intensity is often the primary focus of pain interventions and commonly the only aspect of pain that is assessed in medical care. As such, many measures of pain intensity exist. Although less commonly assessed, pain interference is crucial to understanding a person's pain problem (Ballantyne & Sullivan, 2015) and is often an important target of psychological and rehabilitation interventions. Psychological interventions also commonly target pain affect and behavior. Assessing multiple dimensions of pain provides useful information to guide care and is thus recommended. For example, pain quality can be used both to characterize a person's experience of pain as well as to discriminate neuropathic pain (related to nerve damage or dysfunction) from nonneuropathic pain (nociceptive pain; Jensen, 2006, 2010).

Self-Report Measures

A growing number of empirically supported self-report measures, also known as *patient-reported outcomes* or *patient-reported outcome measures*, assess many facets of the pain experience. As outlined in what follows and summarized in Table 14.2, some measures assess a single facet, whereas others assess multiple aspects of the pain experience. Resources from the Initiative on Methods, Measurement, and Pain Assessment in Clinical Trials provide further guidance on selection of pain domains (Turk et al., 2003) and measures (Dworkin et al., 2005) in chronic pain research.

Two simple measures, the Visual Analogue Scale (VAS) and the Numerical Rating Scale (NRS), are most commonly used to assess pain intensity, particularly in clinical settings due to their brevity. The VAS is a single straight line, usually 100 mm long, where the left end point represents *no pain* and the right end point indicates *extreme pain*. The respondent places a mark on the line to indicate the severity of his or her pain. For the NRS, a series of numbers (usually 0–10 or 0–100) are presented with intensity end-point descriptors such as 0 = *no pain* and 10 = *pain as bad as you can imagine*; respondents indicate the number that best represents their pain intensity. The reliability and validity of the VAS and NRS have been supported across a wide spectrum of clinical populations (Jensen, 2011a).

TABLE 14.2

Empirically Supported Pain Measures

Measure	Pain domain(s)
Visual Analog Scale and Numerical Rating Scale (Jensen, 2011a)	Intensity
McGill Pain Questionnaire (MPQ; Melzack, 1975); Short-Form MPQ (SF–MPQ–2; Dworkin et al., 2009)	Intensity, quality, temporality, affect
Brief Pain Inventory (BPI; Cleeland, 2009); Modified Brief Pain Inventory (BPI; Osborne et al., 2006; Raichle et al., 2006; Tyler et al., 2002; for use with persons with disability)	Intensity, distribution, interference
PROMIS Pain Intensity Short Form	Intensity
PROMIS Pain Interference CAT and Short Forms (Amtmann et al., 2010)	Interference
PROMIS Pain Behavior CAT and Short Forms (Revicki et al., 2009)	Behavior
PROMIS Pain Quality—Neuropathic Pain Short Form (Askew et al., 2016)	Quality
PROMIS Pain Quality—Nociceptive Pain Short Form (Revicki et al., 2014)	Quality

Note. PROMIS = Patient Reported Outcome Measurement Information System; CAT = computer adaptive tests.

Because it offers a relatively large number of response options, allows for comparison with many data sets, and is less confusing than the VAS, the 0 to 10 NRS is generally recommended over the VAS (Dworkin et al., 2005).

The Brief Pain Inventory (BPI; Cleeland, 2009) is a self-report measure that assesses pain intensity, pain interference, and pain distribution. Worst, least, average pain, and current pain intensity and the degree to which pain interferes with seven life domains, such as sleep, mood, and relationships, are assessed on a 0 to 10 NRS. Distribution of pain is assessed with a body map where respondents indicate all body regions where pain is felt and mark the area of worst pain. Modifications to the BPI have been made for use with persons with disability, including changes in the wording of an item that asks about how much pain interferes with "walking ability" to "mobility (ability to get around)" as well as the addition of items that assess how pain interferes with a broader range of activities that are relevant to persons with disability, including self-care and recreational activities. The original BPI and the modified version have been extensively used in rehabilitation populations, and psychometric data provide support for their use (Osborne, Raichle, Jensen, Ehde, & Kraft, 2006; Raichle, Osborne, Jensen, & Cardenas, 2006; Tyler, Jensen, Engel, & Schwartz, 2002).

The McGill Pain Questionnaire (MPQ; R. Melzack, 1975) and short-form versions of the measure (Dworkin et al., 2009; Ronald Melzack, 1987) assess multiple pain domains, including pain quality, temporality, intensity, and the affect aspects of pain. The various versions of the MPQ have demonstrated reliability and validity for assessing the affective and qualitative domains of pain and this measure is useful for identifying neuropathic pain (Dworkin et al., 2009; Jensen, 2011a). The MPQ has been translated to and validated in multiple languages.

The National Institutes of Health funded the Patient-Reported Outcomes Measurement Information System (PROMIS; Cella et al., 2007, 2010) to develop and validate a broad range of measures of health-related quality of life for use in the general population and across chronic conditions. Among a wide range of measures of physical, emotional, and social health, PROMIS contains measures of five unidimensional pain domains: pain intensity, pain interference, pain behaviors, pain quality neuropathic, and pain quality nociceptive. The pain intensity and both pain quality measures are available only as short forms (a static set of items). The pain interference and pain behaviors measures are available as either short forms or computerized adaptive tests (CATs), which use an algorithm to administer a limited number (usually five–12) of items from a large item bank to provide a precise estimate of the target construct. CATs, or "smart tests," require a computer (e.g., tablet, smartphone) to administer. All PROMIS measures are freely available online (http://www.healthmeasures.net). Of interest to those in rehabilitation, PROMIS has been expanded to include condition-specific measurement systems for spinal cord injury (SCI–QOL; Slavin, Kisala, Jette, & Tulsky, 2010; D. Tulsky et al., 2011; D. S. Tulsky & Kisala, 2015; D. S. Tulsky et al., 2015),

Huntington's disease (HDQLife; Carlozzi et al., 2016), and traumatic brain injury (TBI–QOL; D. S. Tulsky et al., 2016).

Clinical Assessment of Pain

Given that pain is complex, ideally multiple rehabilitation professionals will play a role in assessing pain, with each discipline providing a different focus and perspective on the patient's pain problem. In addition to assessing the relevant aspects of the pain experience (e.g., intensity, quality, distribution, temporality) and the impact of pain (e.g., pain interference), a thorough clinical assessment of pain includes a broad-based evaluation of comorbid symptoms and conditions and consideration of the patient's treatment goals and expectations, current pain management strategies, and personal strengths and vulnerabilities. Clinical pain assessment typically requires some combination of the following:

1. Assessment of the pain experience (i.e., intensity, quality, distribution, temporality of the individual's pain) via interview, validated surveys, or both.
2. Conducting a thorough medical history via interview, medical records review, or both.
3. Assessment of other symptoms and problems that are commonly comorbid with pain, such as depressive disorders, anxiety, and fatigue. For example, the Patient Health Questionnaire—Depression Scale (Spitzer, Kroenke, & Williams, 1999), is validated in many populations and is one of the most widely used measures of depressive symptom severity due to its brevity and ability to indicate likelihood of a depressive disorder. Assessment of comorbid substance use and abuse is also recommended, including the use of opioid and nonopioid medications for pain.
4. Assessment of current pain coping strategies (e.g., cognitive and behavioral pain management strategies) and beliefs about pain. This assessment can be achieved through administration of surveys or interview. The clinician might ask: Besides medications, what sorts of things do you do to manage your pain? Does anything you do make the pain better or worse? Is there anything you do to help yourself feel better about the pain? The Chronic Pain Coping Inventory (Jensen, Turner, Romano, & Strom, 1995; Romano, Jensen, & Turner, 2003; Tan, Nguyen, Anderson, Jensen, & Thornby, 2005) and Coping Strategies Questionnaire (Rosenstiel & Keefe, 1983) both contain subscales that assess multiple types of adaptive and maladaptive types of coping. The Chronic Pain Acceptance Questionnaire (McCracken, Vowles, & Eccleston, 2004; Vowles, McCracken, McLeod, & Eccleston, 2008) is a measure of how willing one is to experience pain and how engaged in life activities despite pain. The Survey of Pain Attitudes (SOPA; Jensen, Turner, & Romano, 2000) and Pain Beliefs and Perceptions Inventory (Williams, Robinson, & Geisser, 1994) are two measures that assess the beliefs and attitudes one has about his or her pain. Notably, the SOPA assesses both adaptive and maladaptive beliefs about pain, allowing the clinician to identify potential vulnerabilities and resources in a person's thinking. Although originally developed for use specifically in arthritis, the Arthritis Self-Efficacy Scale (Lorig, Chastain, Ung, Shoor, & Holman, 1989; Lorig & Holman, 1998), has been widely used outside of rheumatological conditions to assess people's beliefs about their ability to manage pain. The PROMIS has a suite of five self-efficacy measures that assess perceived ability to manage daily activities, symptoms, medications and treatments, emotions, and social interactions, that was recently validated in a sample of individuals with chronic conditions, including neurological conditions (Gruber-Baldini, Velozo, Romero, & Shulman, 2017). The self-efficacy for managing symptoms measure is nonspecific to symptom type and could feasibly be used to assess self-efficacy for managing pain.
5. Evaluation of what the patient hopes to learn or gain from treatment and what his or her personal treatment goals are. Example questions for the clinician are: What sorts of things would you like to learn or try to manage your pain better? What are your hopes for this pain rehabilitation program or treatment? What is one thing you

would like to be able to do when you are done with treatment that you cannot do now?

6. Evaluation of personality, personal resources, strengths, social context, and literacy level are also helpful in planning treatment and advising other rehabilitation providers working with the patient.

Challenges to Assessing Pain in Rehabilitation Populations

Although pain may seem a relatively straightforward symptom to assess, there are a few challenges to its assessment in both clinical and research settings that warrant commentary. One challenge is the word *pain* itself. Many individuals who experience unpleasant physical sensations would not label these sensations pain per se. In such cases, a query about pain intensity on a 0 to 10 NRS, might result in the following response: "Zero. I don't have any pain; my legs do *ache* when the spasms are bad." Another challenge that might be especially common in rehabilitation populations is that pain is simply viewed as a part of "normal" life for many people, and as such, it is difficult to assess and rate. This may be particularly true for individuals who have had pain since they were very young and cannot recall a time when they did not have it or for older adults who incorrectly view pain as a necessary condition of aging. In such cases, a query about pain intensity in the past week on a 0 to 10 NRS might result in the following response: "Zero. I haven't had any pain flares recently. No headaches or anything—just my 'normal' pain." These challenges might be addressed by qualifying what one means by *pain* when conducting the pain assessment, such as specifying, as appropriate, that pain means any unpleasant physical sensation, including one's normal or usual discomfort. Providing education about pain, including its prevalence in the relevant disability or age group, and the potential for pain management strategies to decrease the associated suffering or limitations resulting from pain, may also facilitate assessment. Pain assessment can also be challenging when a person presents with cognitive impairment or a communication disorder, as well as in children and older adults; further information on assessment in these populations can be found, and fortunately guidelines for assessment in these populations are available (Hadjistavropoulos et al., 2007; Turk & Melzack, 2011).

Those interested in more information on assessment of pain are directed to the comprehensive *Handbook of Pain Assessment* (Turk & Melzack, 2011).

TREATMENT OF CHRONIC PAIN

Despite widespread acceptance of the biopsychosocial model of pain, biomedical interventions remain the dominant treatment approach to chronic pain. Opioid analgesics are commonly used across a range of noncancer chronic pain conditions, despite evidence that, over time, their benefits decrease while the risks of misuse and adverse effects increase (Chou et al., 2015; Krashin, Sullivan, & Ballantyne, 2013). Other biomedical interventions, including nonopioid analgesic medications (e.g., anticonvulsants, nonsteroidal anti-inflammatory drugs), antidepressants, surgery, and interventional therapies (e.g., epidural steroid injections, spinal cord stimulators) are also commonly used and can be beneficial in treating chronic pain, depending on the condition but also have potential adverse effects (National Academies of Sciences, Engineering, and Medicine, 2017). When prescribed or encouraged, physical therapy and exercise are effective in decreasing pain, particularly musculoskeletal pain, and improving function. However, numerous barriers, including nonadherence, fear of worsening pain, and excessive deconditioning, interfere with their widespread use (National Academies of Sciences, Engineering, and Medicine, 2017).

Since the early 1970s, interdisciplinary chronic pain rehabilitation programs, which incorporate medical, physical, psychological, and social principles and treatments, have documented efficacy for reducing pain and improving functioning as well as evidence for their cost-effectiveness (Gatchel, McGeary, McGeary, & Lippe, 2014). Psychologists are often integrated into these interdisciplinary teams, providing direct service to the patient in addition to consulting to and participating in the team care. Financial and system barriers have increasingly limited the availability of such interdisciplinary programs for most individuals affected by chronic pain (for a review, see Gatchel et al., 2014).

Outside of interdisciplinary rehabilitation programs, psychological interventions for pain, and the self-management strategies that stem from them, have been underutilized and too often viewed as an afterthought or the treatment of last resort after biomedical interventions have failed (National Academies of Sciences, Engineering, and Medicine, 2017). In its 2011 report, *Relieving Pain in America*, the Institute of Medicine (2011) recommended greater use of self-management interventions, including cognitive behavior therapy (CBT), in addressing the epidemic of inadequately treated chronic pain. More recently, the National Academies of Sciences, Engineering, and Medicine (2017) produced a scientific report on the opioid epidemic in which they emphasized the importance of nonpharmacological strategies, including physical activity, CBT, and mindfulness meditation, as "powerful tools in the management of chronic pain . . . they may provide effective pain relief for many patients in place of or in combination with pharmacologic approaches" (p. 91). Although challenges exist to implementation of these recommendations, this context also provides a number of opportunities for the integration of psychological interventions into the routine care of individuals affected by chronic pain. This section reviews several of the evidence-based psychological interventions for pain, followed by a discussion of practical considerations for their implementation in the practice of rehabilitation psychology.

Cognitive Behavior Therapy

CBT is the most researched and applied behavioral approach to addressing chronic pain across a wide range of conditions such as headaches, back pain, arthritis, cancer, and fibromyalgia (Ehde, Dillworth, & Turner, 2014). CBT has also been applied to pain associated with conditions commonly treated by rehabilitation psychologists, including spinal cord injury, brain injury, multiple sclerosis, and limb loss (Ehde & Hanley, 2006; Jensen et al., 2011). When used for pain, CBT aims to not only diminish pain intensity but also, if not more importantly, improve physical, psychological, and social functioning via cognitive behavioral principles. Common treatment targets include decreasing maladaptive pain coping, increasing adaptive coping, identifying and restructuring maladaptive or unhelpful pain thoughts and beliefs, and increasing self-efficacy for pain management (Ehde et al., 2014). CBT for pain varies in its content and delivery across different treatment manuals as well as treatment studies of its effects. Common techniques include relaxation training, behavioral activation, goal-setting (often focused on systematic increases in physical activity), instruction in activity pacing (to avoid a common cycle of over- and underactivity that can exacerbate pain), and problem-solving training. Cognitive therapy focused on helping individuals learn to identify and correct unhelpful pain catastrophizing cognitions is typically a central component of CBT for pain, given the salient role of pain catastrophizing in pain outcomes (Jensen, 2011b). Similar to most behavioral interventions, CBT often includes between-session home practice of new pain coping skills (e.g., relaxation practice, activity self-monitoring, completion of thought records). No single CBT treatment protocol exists; rather, several treatment manuals are available for guiding clinicians in delivering CBT and its components (Otis, 2007; Thorn, 2017).

Multiple systematic and meta-analytic reviews support the efficacy of CBT for reducing pain intensity, activity interference, distress, and disability across a range of chronic pain populations (Ehde et al., 2014). CBT has also been shown to be beneficial in the treatment of both youth (Palermo, Eccleston, Lewandowski, Williams, & Morley, 2010) and older adults (Molton & Terrill, 2014) with chronic pain, two age groups in which chronic pain is highly prevalent.

Mindfulness-Based Interventions

Although the practice of mindfulness dates back centuries, mindfulness-based interventions (MBIs), such as mindfulness-based stress reduction and mindfulness-based cognitive therapy (MBCT), have only recently become popular for addressing chronic pain and its associated suffering. Similar to other behavioral therapies, MBIs typically incorporate a variety of therapeutic techniques but have mindfulness meditation at their core. Mindfulness meditation encourages individuals to disengage from automatic thinking and to focus attention mindfully on an object of awareness (often the breath) with a sense of nonjudgmental awareness and acceptance of any sensory, emotional, or cognitive events (Day, Jensen, Ehde, & Thorn, 2014). Whereas most CBT interventions are rooted heavily in correcting deficits in thinking and behaving, MBIs builds on individual's strengths and innate ability to focus their attention at will, and to use these to work *for them* (as a way to mindfully perceive experience in a nonjudgmental, accepting way) rather than *against them* (as is often the case, with attention becoming "stuck" on pain, leading to hypervigilance and associated disability; Day et al., 2014).

MBIs are efficacious for treating chronic pain. A recent meta-analysis reported that MBIs reduced pain and depressive symptoms while also improving quality of life (Hilton et al., 2017). In addition to the most studied MBI, mindfulness-based stress reduction, another promising MBI for pain is MBCT (Day, 2017). MBCT integrates cognitive therapy techniques into mindfulness-based interventional strategies to form a streamlined approach to training the mind to respond adaptively to pain. MBCT focuses on enhancing awareness of how one is attending and responding to pain. This emphasis differs from traditional CBT, as the goal in MBCT is not to change thoughts, emotions, or behavior per se, but simply to notice moment-to-moment experience. With this awareness comes the opportunity to then mindfully choose how to respond wisely to the pain in a way that reduces stress and is most helpful or adaptive, rather than automatically react with habitual, unhelpful ways of thinking, feeling, and behaving that may exacerbate pain, distress, and dysfunction. Therapist manuals and patient workbooks are available to guide the application of mindfulness-based interventions to chronic pain (Day, 2017; Gardner-Nix & Costin-Hall, 2009).

Acceptance and Commitment Therapy

An alternative approach for managing pain-related cognitions and behaviors comes from acceptance and commitment therapy (ACT; Hayes, Luoma, Bond, Masuda, & Lillis, 2006; Hayes, Strosahl, & Wilson, 1999). Like CBT, ACT was originally developed to treat a range of psychological disorders. It shares commonalities with CBT, including an emphasis on cognitive processes and emotional experiences (McCracken & Vowles, 2014). The primary principles of ACT include being accepting of the presence of any of life's experiences (good, bad, or otherwise) and focusing behavior on living consistently with one's values. Whereas CBT places importance on overcoming problematic thought patterns, ACT focuses more on living well despite unpleasant thoughts or emotions. It uses mindfulness and acceptance strategies in addition to behavioral activation strategies.

When applied to pain, ACT promotes concepts such as being able to have pain (including its discomfort or unpleasantness) without having to suffer from pain, and focuses the individual on engaging in activities that are consistent with their values, rather than behaviors that are dictated by their pain (McCracken, Vowles, & Eccleston, 2005). Central to ACT's application to pain management is its emphasis on the concept of pain acceptance, which suggests that increases in both a willingness to experience pain and engagement in valued activities promotes better pain-related outcomes (McCracken, 1998; McCracken et al., 2004, 2005). ACT is considered an empirically supported treatment for chronic pain and has similar efficacy as CBT in one systematic review (McCracken & Vowles, 2014; Veehof, Oskam, Schreurs, & Bohlmeijer, 2011).

Self-Hypnosis Training

Similar to MBIs, hypnosis has long been used as a treatment for pain, both acute and chronic (Jensen & Patterson, 2014). Hypnosis essentially involves two phases: (a) an *induction phase* that is designed to increase the individual's receptiveness to clinical suggestions, followed by (b) a suggestion phase that focuses on changes in thoughts, physical sensations, emotions, or behavior (Jensen, 2011a). *Self-hypnosis* simply involves teaching individuals to increase their readiness to respond to their own suggestions, followed by purposefully thinking about the change they would like to experience. An example self-hypnosis training session may include an approximately

10-minute standard hypnotic induction followed by 10 minutes of suggestions for improvements in comfort, well-being, and function. Although self-hypnosis training typically involves an initial induction or series of inductions by a trained clinician, individuals may be taught how to engage in hypnosis outside of the therapy office on their own. This practice may be facilitated by audio-recordings or scripts, as well as instructions on building relevant suggestions. Thus, similar to other behavioral approaches to pain, self-hypnosis training is empowering: It teaches skills that people can implement to effectively self-manage their pain on their own outside of treatment. At least two treatment manuals provide guidance on the use of hypnosis in chronic pain (Jensen, 2011a; Patterson, 2010).

Research conducted over the past 2 decades provides evidence for the efficacy of hypnosis in the treatment of both acute (including procedural) pain and chronic pain (Jensen & Patterson, 2014). Its benefits include but are not limited to pain relief; they may also include improved energy, mood, and sleep, as well as increased positive affect and well-being, independent of whether pain relief was obtained (Jensen & Patterson, 2014). Similar to other pain treatments, individuals vary in their responsiveness to hypnosis, and research is now being conducted examining ways to enhance the effects of hypnosis by combining it with other treatments such as CBT or mindfulness meditation (Jensen & Patterson, 2014).

Guidelines for Treating Chronic Pain

A range of psychological interventions are available for treating chronic pain, with interventions benefiting many, but not all, individuals who receive them. Although comparisons between active psychological pain interventions often yield equivalent findings on average (Ehde et al., 2014), some studies have found that different interventions work for different individuals, suggesting a need for research informing how best to tailor treatments to individuals. Current scientific efforts are underway to better understand how to match patients with chronic pain to the treatments most likely to benefit them, increase the effectiveness of existing treatments, and combine different treatment approaches to maximize their efficacy. In the meantime, the following guidelines are offered to aid the rehabilitation psychologist in delivering psychological interventions for chronic pain.

1. *Educate the patient on the biopsychosocial model, linking it to the neurophysiology of pain.* Most effective psychological interventions for pain are built on the foundation of the biopsychosocial model of chronic pain. Pain education aims to arm the individual with a biopsychosocial framework for understanding pain, including modifiable factors (e.g., thoughts, physical activity, relaxation response, sleep) that are commonly the target of psychological interventions. Eliciting patients' understanding of their pain problem and the role of biopsychosocial factors will assist the clinician in tailoring education to that individual. Education-only interventions that educate patients on the biopsychosocial model, including the neurobiological processes linked to pain-related thoughts, emotions, and behaviors, have been shown to improve pain outcomes (Moseley & Butler, 2015; Thorn et al., 2011). They are likely most powerful when combined with other behavioral techniques. One educational approach in particular, "Explain Pain," may be particularly helpful in educating individuals about pain and its biopsychosocial underpinnings (D. S. Butler & Moseley, 2013).
2. *Cultivate a self-management mind-set.* The vast majority of pain management is done by the individual living with pain, not health care providers. As such, it is important to frame pain management as *self-management*; that is, that the individual living with pain is the primary manager, and the role of the psychologist and health care team is to provide self-management support. This mindset will readily resonate with some individuals with pain, whereas others may take a more passive approach or have difficulties viewing their role in this way. Thus, an assessment of the individual's readiness to engage in self-management is important. Motivational interviewing strategies (Jensen, 2018)

may facilitate a self-management mindset. These include using a nonjudgmental style, providing a menu of self-management options, encouraging an experimental attitude towards pain self-management, asking permission to suggest specific pain self-management strategies, and assessing existing self-management strengths and strategies to build on.

3. *Encourage self-management and participation goals rather than pain relief.* Effective behavioral interventions shift the focus of pain treatment from "how do I get rid of pain?" to "how do I manage pain so that I can live the life I value?" Thus, early in treatment, it is important to elicit the individual's goals and values for treatment beyond pain relief. It may be helpful to point out that although self-management strategies often focus on goals that do not specifically target alleviating pain, a decrease in pain intensity may be a side effect of improved coping, functioning, and participation.
4. *Promote success early in treatment.* Individuals who are highly disabled or distressed by chronic pain often have low self-efficacy for managing pain and its consequences. Thus, building self-efficacy is important and is facilitated by setting realistic, achievable goals that promote successful pain management gains early in treatment. Most empirically based treatments for pain start with strategies that are naturally reinforcing or comforting and build self-efficacy. For example, relaxation or mindfulness meditation practice is often an early strategy in therapy. Such treatments may be easier to implement than other strategies (e.g., cognitive restructuring) and may provide some immediate pain relief, stress reduction, comfort, positive experience, and success.
5. *Identify treatment strategies with potential benefits across different targets.* A potentially overwhelming number of psychosocial factors may be present in individuals with pain and thus the targets of treatment, may include but are not limited to physical inactivity, pain catastrophizing, self-efficacy, stress, depression, anxiety (e.g., fear of movement, pain anxiety), core beliefs (e.g., perceived injustice), insomnia, poor treatment adherence (e.g., to physical therapy), vocational dysfunction, relationship distress, substance use disorders, and pain flare-ups. When deciding which factor to target and therapeutic approach to use, it is essential to build on the patient's goals and preferences in addition to the approach indicated by the clinical assessment. It may also be helpful to start with strategies that address several symptoms at once, such as relaxation or hypnosis, which may be used for not only pain flare-ups but also sleep, fatigue, and anxiety. Often a combination approach (e.g., incorporating hypnosis with cognitive therapy or behavioral activation) may be indicated. Combination approaches are not only common in real-world practice, they are also increasingly recognized as potentially more effective than individual approaches alone (National Academies of Sciences, Engineering, and Medicine, 2017).
6. *Prescribe regular practice of pain self-management tools outside of treatment and regardless of pain levels.* As the primary pain manager, patients need to practice and use pain management strategies outside of the therapy session. Psychologists should encourage regular practice of preferred self-management skills, experimentation with new strategies, and routine "pain management habits" that promote the acquisition and maintenance of gains in pain, functioning, and well-being. Educating patients on the importance of practicing strategies when pain is minimal or manageable, and not only when it is severe, may build success and beneficial pain management routines. A variety of technological aids are also available to facilitate regular practice of skills, including apps (e.g., mindfulness apps, relaxation instruction), digital recordings, wearable devices (e.g., activity trackers), and web-based strategies. Electronic devices can also be used to cue individuals to engage in their self-management practices, such as alarms signaling a daily meditation practice.
7. *Facilitate behavioral activation goals that are "antipain."* As noted by Wilbert Fordyce (1976), "those with something better to do, don't hurt so much" (see also S. Butler, 2017). Behavioral

activation has thus long occupied a central role in behavioral approaches to pain (for a review of the benefits of activity in pain, see Fordyce, 1976, or Main et al., 2015). In pain treatment, behavioral activation often focuses not only on increasing physical activity but also on increasing activities that are enjoyable, meaningful, functional, and consistent with the values and goals of the individual. Behavioral goals should be "antidepressant" and "antipain," that is, reinforcing, valued, and "something better to do." Similar to behavioral activation strategies applied to other conditions such as depressive disorders, in pain, activities should be scheduled (vs. waiting until the person feels like engaging in them), time-contingent (vs. pain contingent), and increased gradually and systematically. Fordyce championed the use of quota-based reactivation, based on operant principles, designed to facilitate the gradual acquisition of activity and other wellness behaviors; see Fordyce (1976) and Main et al. (2015) for specific guidelines in these procedures.

8. *Use telehealth and other delivery models to increase the reach of psychological interventions for pain.* Psychological interventions for pain are typically delivered in person, limiting access to only a subset of individuals in pain clinical settings. However, remote technologies such as the telephone and the Internet are increasingly being used to deliver behavioral interventions. Remote technologies may improve the reach of our interventions, transcending geographic barriers and targeting larger populations. Remote delivery may also reduce stigma and lower the threshold for initiation of treatment, given that such technologies can be used in the privacy of one's home and outside the mental health system. They tend to be less expensive than traditional psychotherapies and are increasingly covered by payers and permitted by licensing boards. The evidence to date supports the efficacy of such interventions for treating pain (Ehde et al., 2014; Macea, Gajos, Daglia Calil, & Fregni, 2010), although web-based interventions have tended to have poorer uptake and higher dropout rates than other telehealth and in-person treatments. Thus, rehabilitation psychologists are encouraged to consider the use of telehealth technologies to improve access to pain interventions, particularly given the many barriers individuals with physical disabilities face in accessing in person care.
9. *Recognize potential opioid and other substance misuse and risks and address as indicated.* Given the risks associated with opioid misuse and other substance use disorders, psychologists treating individuals with pain should screen for and address such problems as indicated.
10. *Deploy evidence-based pain assessment and treatment strategies in integrated care settings.* Because rehabilitation psychologists are often integrated into rehabilitation and other health care settings, they play an important role in deploying evidence-based pain assessment and treatment strategies in integrated care. Assisting health care teams to recognize pain needs, develop assessment protocols, provide interdisciplinary care, promote physical activity adherence, and integrate self-management support and interventions into such settings are just some of the roles for psychologists in these settings beyond direct service to patients. Providers are likely to need education on the efficacy of psychological interventions, as well as how to discuss self-management interventions and referrals with patients.

CONCLUSION

For nearly 50 years, rehabilitation psychologists have advanced the science and practice of psychosocial assessment and treatment of chronic pain. Psychological research will continue to be central to the future of pain research and care. For example, as pain does not occur in a vacuum, future observational and experimental research should focus on elucidating relationships between pain and other commonly co-occurring problems such as sleep disturbance and cognitive dysfunction. Future intervention research should tackle issues central to improving the care of individuals with chronic pain, including identification of treatment mechanisms (moderators and mediators) for improving treatments and treatment matching, expanding the reach of psychological pain treatments to populations with poor access, and translating scientific evidence to community practice, Finally, in the context of emerging interest in positive psychology, research evaluating positive psychological constructs, as applied to pain, as well as the potential effects of positive psychology interventions (such as resilience) on chronic pain may be intriguing.

Although chronic pain is complex and multidimensional, numerous assessment tools and intervention options are available for effectively addressing this pervasive public health problem. Psychological interventions hold much appeal given their favorable safety profile (minimal risk, especially compared with the well-established risks of opioid therapies) and emphasis on self-management skills. Given their expertise in the biopsychosocial model, psychological assessment, interdisciplinary care, and psychological science, rehabilitation psychologists have much to contribute to the goal articulated by the Institute of Medicine of "relieving pain" and, we'd add, the impairment and suffering associated with it.

References

Alschuler, K. N., Hoodin, F., Murphy, S. L., Rice, J., & Geisser, M. E. (2011). Factors contributing to physical activity in a chronic low back pain clinical sample: A comprehensive analysis using continuous ambulatory monitoring. *Pain, 152,* 2521–2527. http://dx.doi.org/10.1016/j.pain.2011.07.017

Alschuler, K. N., Jensen, M. P., & Ehde, D. M. (2012). The association of depression with pain-related treatment utilization in patients with multiple sclerosis. *Pain Medicine, 13,* 1648–1657. http://dx.doi.org/10.1111/j.1526-4637.2012.01513.x

Alschuler, K. N., Neblett, R., Wiggert, E., Haig, A. J., & Geisser, M. E. (2009). Flexion-relaxation and clinical features associated with chronic low back pain: A comparison of different methods of quantifying flexion-relaxation. *Clinical Journal of Pain, 25,* 760–766. http://dx.doi.org/10.1097/AJP.0b013e3181b56db6

Alschuler, K. N., & Otis, J. D. (2012). Coping strategies and beliefs about pain in veterans with comorbid chronic pain and significant levels of posttraumatic stress disorder symptoms. *European Journal of Pain, 16,* 312–319. http://dx.doi.org/10.1016/j.ejpain.2011.06.010

Amtmann, D., Cook, K. F., Jensen, M. P., Chen, W. H., Choi, S., Revicki, D., . . . Lai, J. S. (2010). Development of a PROMIS item bank to measure pain interference. *Pain, 150,* 173–182. http://dx.doi.org/10.1016/j.pain.2010.04.025

Askew, R. L., Cook, K. F., Keefe, F. J., Nowinski, C. J., Cella, D., Revicki, D. A., . . . Amtmann, D. (2016). A PROMIS Measure of Neuropathic Pain Quality. *Value in Health, 19,* 623–630. http://dx.doi.org/10.1016/j.jval.2016.02.009

Ballantyne, J. C., & Sullivan, M. D. (2015). Intensity of chronic pain—The wrong metric? *The New England Journal of Medicine, 373,* 2098–2099. http://dx.doi.org/10.1056/NEJMp1507136

Blyth, F. M., March, L. M., Nicholas, M. K., & Cousins, M. J. (2003). Chronic pain, work performance and litigation. *Pain, 103,* 41–47. http://dx.doi.org/10.1016/S0304-3959(02)00380-9

Butler, D. S., & Moseley, G. L. (2013). *Explain pain* (2nd ed.). Adelaide, Australia: Noigroup Publications.

Butler, S. (2017). The wit and wisdom of Wilbert (Bill) Fordyce (1923–2009). *Scandinavian Journal of Pain, 16,* 160–163. http://dx.doi.org/10.1016/j.sjpain.2017.06.006

Carlozzi, N. E., Schilling, S. G., Lai, J. S., Paulsen, J. S., Hahn, E. A., Perlmutter, J. S., . . . Cella, D. (2016). HDQLIFE: Development and assessment of health-related quality of life in Huntington disease (HD). *Quality of Life Research: An International Journal of Quality of Life Aspects of Treatment, Care & Rehabilitation, 25,* 2441–2455. http://dx.doi.org/10.1007/s11136-016-1386-3

Cella, D., Riley, W., Stone, A., Rothrock, N., Reeve, B., Yount, S., . . . Hays, R., & the PROMIS Cooperative Group. (2010). The Patient-Reported Outcomes Measurement Information System (PROMIS) developed and tested its first wave of adult self-reported health outcome item banks: 2005–2008. *Journal of Clinical Epidemiology, 63,* 1179–1194. http://dx.doi.org/10.1016/j.jclinepi.2010.04.011

Cella, D., Yount, S., Rothrock, N., Gershon, R., Cook, K., Reeve, B., . . . Rose, M., & the PROMIS Cooperative Group. (2007). The Patient-Reported Outcomes Measurement Information System (PROMIS): Progress of an NIH Roadmap cooperative group during its first two years. *Medical Care, 45*(Suppl. 1), S3–S11. http://dx.doi.org/10.1097/01.mlr.0000258615.42478.55

Chou, R., Turner, J. A., Devine, E. B., Hansen, R. N., Sullivan, S. D., Blazina, I., . . . Deyo, R. A. (2015). The effectiveness and risks of long-term opioid therapy for chronic pain: A systematic review for a National Institutes of Health Pathways to Prevention Workshop. *Annals of Internal Medicine, 162,* 276–286. http://dx.doi.org/10.7326/M14-2559

Cleeland, C. (2009). *The Brief Pain Inventory: User guide*. Houston, TX: MD Anderson Cancer Center.

Coderre, T. J., Katz, J., Vaccarino, A. L., & Melzack, R. (1993). Contribution of central neuroplasticity to pathological pain: Review of clinical and experimental evidence. *Pain, 52*, 259–285. http://dx.doi.org/10.1016/0304-3959(93)90161-H

Day, M. A. (2017). *Mindfulness-based cognitive therapy for chronic pain: A clinical manual and guide*. Chichester, England: Wiley. http://dx.doi.org/10.1002/9781119257875

Day, M. A., Jensen, M. P., Ehde, D. M., & Thorn, B. E. (2014). Toward a theoretical model for mindfulness-based pain management. *The Journal of Pain, 15*, 691–703. http://dx.doi.org/10.1016/j.jpain.2014.03.003

Dworkin, R. H., Turk, D. C., Farrar, J. T., Haythornthwaite, J. A., Jensen, M. P., Katz, N. P., . . . Witter, J., & the IMMPACT. (2005). Core outcome measures for chronic pain clinical trials: IMMPACT recommendations. *Pain, 113*, 9–19. http://dx.doi.org/10.1016/j.pain.2004.09.012

Dworkin, R. H., Turk, D. C., Revicki, D. A., Harding, G., Coyne, K. S., Peirce-Sandner, S., . . . Melzack, R. (2009). Development and initial validation of an expanded and revised version of the Short-Form McGill Pain Questionnaire (SF–MPQ–2). *Pain, 144*, 35–42. http://dx.doi.org/10.1016/j.pain.2009.02.007

Ehde, D. M., Dillworth, T. M., & Turner, J. A. (2014). Cognitive-behavioral therapy for individuals with chronic pain: Efficacy, innovations, and directions for research. *American Psychologist, 69*, 153–166. http://dx.doi.org/10.1037/a0035747

Ehde, D. M., & Hanley, M. A. (2006). Pain in patient groups frequently treated by physiatrists. *Physical Medicine and Rehabilitation Clinics of North America, 17*, 275–285. http://dx.doi.org/10.1016/j.pmr.2005.12.009

Fordyce, W. E. (1976). *Behavioral methods for chronic pain and illness*. St. Louis, MO: Mosby.

Fordyce, W. E. (1984). Behavioural science and chronic pain. *Postgraduate Medical Journal, 60*, 865–868. http://dx.doi.org/10.1136/pgmj.60.710.865

Fordyce, W. E., Fowler, R. S., & Delateur, B. (1968). An application of behavior modification technique to a problem of chronic pain. *Behaviour Research and Therapy, 6*, 105–107. http://dx.doi.org/10.1016/0005-7967(68)90048-X

Fredrickson, B. E., Trief, P. M., VanBeveren, P., Yuan, H. A., & Baum, G. (1988). Rehabilitation of the patient with chronic back pain. A search for outcome predictors. *Spine, 13*, 351–353. http://dx.doi.org/10.1097/00007632-198803000-00022

Gardner-Nix, J., & Costin-Hall, L. (2009). *The mindfulness solution to pain: Step-by-step techniques for chronic pain management*. Oakland, CA: New Harbinger.

Gatchel, R. J., McGeary, D. D., McGeary, C. A., & Lippe, B. (2014). Interdisciplinary chronic pain management: Past, present, and future. *American Psychologist, 69*, 119–130. http://dx.doi.org/10.1037/a0035514

Geisser, M. E., Haig, A. J., Tong, H. C., Yamakawa, K. S., Quint, D. J., Hoff, J. T., . . . Phalke, V. V. (2007). Spinal canal size and clinical symptoms among persons diagnosed with lumbar spinal stenosis. *The Clinical Journal of Pain, 23*, 780–785. http://dx.doi.org/10.1097/AJP.0b013e31815349bf

Goesling, J., Clauw, D. J., & Hassett, A. L. (2013). Pain and depression: An integrative review of neurobiological and psychological factors. *Current Psychiatry Reports, 15*, 421. http://dx.doi.org/10.1007/s11920-013-0421-0

Greve, K. W., Ord, J. S., Bianchini, K. J., & Curtis, K. L. (2009). Prevalence of malingering in patients with chronic pain referred for psychologic evaluation in a medico-legal context. *Archives of Physical Medicine and Rehabilitation, 90*, 1117–1126. http://dx.doi.org/10.1016/j.apmr.2009.01.018

Gruber-Baldini, A. L., Velozo, C., Romero, S., & Shulman, L. M. (2017). Validation of the PROMIS® measures of self-efficacy for managing chronic conditions. *Quality of Life Research: An International Journal of Quality of Life Aspects of Treatment, Care & Rehabilitation, 26*, 1915–1924. http://dx.doi.org/10.1007/s11136-017-1527-3

Hadjistavropoulos, T., Herr, K., Turk, D. C., Fine, P. G., Dworkin, R. H., Helme, R., . . . Williams, J. (2007). An interdisciplinary expert consensus statement on assessment of pain in older persons. *The Clinical Journal of Pain, 23*(Suppl. 1), S1–S43. http://dx.doi.org/10.1097/AJP.0b013e31802be869

Hayes, S. C., Luoma, J. B., Bond, F. W., Masuda, A., & Lillis, J. (2006). Acceptance and commitment therapy: Model, processes and outcomes. *Behaviour Research and Therapy, 44*, 1–25. http://dx.doi.org/10.1016/j.brat.2005.06.006

Hayes, S. C., Strosahl, K., & Wilson, K. G. (1999). *Acceptance and commitment therapy: An experiential approach to behavior change*. New York, NY: Guilford Press.

Hilton, L., Hempel, S., Ewing, B. A., Apaydin, E., Xenakis, L., Newberry, S., . . . Maglione, M. A. (2017). Mindfulness meditation for chronic pain: Systematic review and meta-analysis. *Annals of Behavioral Medicine, 51*, 199–213. http://dx.doi.org/10.1007/s12160-016-9844-2

Institute of Medicine. (2011). *Relieving pain in America: A blueprint for transforming prevention, care, education, and research*. Retrieved from https://www.ncbi.nlm.nih.gov/pubmed/22553896

Jensen, M. (2006). Using pain quality assessment measures for selecting analgesic agents. *The Clinical Journal of Pain, 22*(Suppl.), S9–S13.

Jensen, M. (2010). Measurement of pain. In S. M. Fishman, J. C. Ballantyne, & J. P. Rathmell (Eds.), *Bonica's management of pain* (4th ed., pp. 251–270). Philadelphia, PA: Lippincott, Williams & Wilkins.

Jensen, M. P. (2011a). *Hypnosis for chronic pain management: Therapist guide* (Treatments That Work). New York, NY: Oxford University Press. http://dx.doi.org/10.1093/med:psych/9780199772384.001.0001

Jensen, M. P. (2011b). Psychosocial approaches to pain management: An organizational framework. *Pain, 152*, 717–725. http://dx.doi.org/10.1016/j.pain.2010.09.002

Jensen, M. P. (2018). Motivational interviewing and pain management. In P. Karoly & G. Crombez (Eds.), *Motivational perspectives on chronic pain: Theory, research, and practice*. New York, NY: Oxford University Press. http://dx.doi.org/10.1093/oso/9780190627898.003.0011

Jensen, M. P., Ehde, D. M., Gertz, K. J., Stoelb, B. L., Dillworth, T. M., Hirsh, A. T., . . . Kraft, G. H. (2011). Effects of self-hypnosis training and cognitive restructuring on daily pain intensity and catastrophizing in individuals with multiple sclerosis and chronic pain. *International Journal of Clinical and Experimental Hypnosis, 59*, 45–63. http://dx.doi.org/10.1080/00207144.2011.522892

Jensen, M. P., & Patterson, D. R. (2014). Hypnotic approaches for chronic pain management: Clinical implications of recent research findings. *American Psychologist, 69*, 167–177. http://dx.doi.org/10.1037/a0035644

Jensen, M. P., & Turk, D. C. (2014). Contributions of psychology to the understanding and treatment of people with chronic pain: Why it matters to ALL psychologists. *American Psychologist, 69*, 105–118. http://dx.doi.org/10.1037/a0035641

Jensen, M. P., Turner, J. A., & Romano, J. M. (2000). Pain beliefs assessment: A comparison of the short and long versions of the Survey of Pain Attitudes. *The Journal of Pain, 1*, 138–150. http://dx.doi.org/10.1016/S1526-5900(00)90099-3

Jensen, M. P., Turner, J. A., Romano, J. M., & Lawler, B. K. (1994). Relationship of pain-specific beliefs to chronic pain adjustment. *Pain, 57*, 301–309. http://dx.doi.org/10.1016/0304-3959(94)90005-1

Jensen, M. P., Turner, J. A., Romano, J. M., & Strom, S. E. (1995). The Chronic Pain Coping Inventory: Development and preliminary validation. *Pain, 60*, 203–216. http://dx.doi.org/10.1016/0304-3959(94)00118-X

Kerns, R. D., Haythornthwaite, J., Southwick, S., & Giller, E. L. (1990). The role of marital interaction in chronic pain and depressive symptom severity. *Journal of Psychosomatic Research, 34*, 401–408.

Kerns, R. D., Turk, D. C., & Rudy, T. E. (1985). The West Haven–Yale Multidimensional Pain Inventory (WHYMPI). *Pain, 23*, 345–356. http://dx.doi.org/10.1016/0304-3959(85)90004-1

Krashin, D., Sullivan, M., & Ballantyne, J. (2013). What are we treating with chronic opioid therapy? *Current Rheumatology Reports, 15*, 311. http://dx.doi.org/10.1007/s11926-012-0311-1

Kratz, A. L., Davis, M. C., & Zautra, A. J. (2007). Pain acceptance moderates the relation between pain and negative affect in female osteoarthritis and fibromyalgia patients. *Annals of Behavioral Medicine, 33*, 291–301. http://dx.doi.org/10.1007/BF02879911

Kroenke, K., Wu, J., Bair, M. J., Krebs, E. E., Damush, T. M., & Tu, W. (2011). Reciprocal relationship between pain and depression: A 12-month longitudinal analysis in primary care. *Journal of Pain, 12*, 964–973. http://dx.doi.org/10.1016/j.jpain.2011.03.003

Ledowski, T., Bromilow, J., Paech, M. J., Storm, H., Hacking, R., & Schug, S. A. (2006). Monitoring of skin conductance to assess postoperative pain intensity. *British Journal of Anaesthesia, 97*, 862–865. http://dx.doi.org/10.1093/bja/ael280

Leonard, M. T., Cano, A., & Johansen, A. B. (2006). Chronic pain in a couples context: A review and integration of theoretical models and empirical evidence. *Journal of Pain, 7*, 377–390. http://dx.doi.org/10.1016/j.jpain.2006.01.442

Lorig, K., Chastain, R. L., Ung, E., Shoor, S., & Holman, H. R. (1989). Development and evaluation of a scale to measure perceived self-efficacy in people with arthritis. *Arthritis & Rheumatism, 32*, 37–44. http://dx.doi.org/10.1002/anr.1780320107

Lorig, K., & Holman, H. (1998). Arthritis Self-Efficacy Scales measure self-efficacy. *Arthritis Care & Research, 11*, 155–157. http://dx.doi.org/10.1002/art.1790110302

Macea, D. D., Gajos, K., Daglia Calil, Y. A., & Fregni, F. (2010). The efficacy of Web-based cognitive behavioral interventions for chronic pain: A systematic review and meta-analysis. *The Journal of Pain, 11*, 917–929. http://dx.doi.org/10.1016/j.jpain.2010.06.005

Main, C. J., Keefe, F. J., Jensen, M. P., Vlaeyen, J. W. S., Vowles, K. E., Fordyce, W. E., & International Association for the Study of Pain. (2015). *Fordyce's behavioral methods for chronic pain and illness: Republished with invited commentaries*. Philadelphia, PA: Wolters Kluwer Health.

McCracken, L. M. (1998). Learning to live with the pain: Acceptance of pain predicts adjustment in persons with chronic pain. *Pain, 74*, 21–27. http://dx.doi.org/10.1016/S0304-3959(97)00146-2

McCracken, L. M. (2005). Social context and acceptance of chronic pain: The role of solicitous and punishing responses. *Pain, 113*, 155–159. http://dx.doi.org/10.1016/j.pain.2004.10.004

McCracken, L. M., & Vowles, K. E. (2014). Acceptance and commitment therapy and mindfulness for chronic pain: Model, process, and progress. *American Psychologist, 69*, 178–187. http://dx.doi.org/10.1037/a0035623

McCracken, L. M., Vowles, K. E., & Eccleston, C. (2004). Acceptance of chronic pain: Component analysis and a revised assessment method. *Pain, 107*, 159–166. http://dx.doi.org/10.1016/j.pain.2003.10.012

McCracken, L. M., Vowles, K. E., & Eccleston, C. (2005). Acceptance-based treatment for persons with complex, long standing chronic pain: A preliminary analysis of treatment outcome in comparison to a waiting phase. *Behaviour Research and Therapy, 43*, 1335–1346. http://dx.doi.org/10.1016/j.brat.2004.10.003

Melzack, R. (1975). The McGill Pain Questionnaire: Major properties and scoring methods. *Pain, 1*, 277–299. http://dx.doi.org/10.1016/0304-3959(75)90044-5

Melzack, R. (1987). The short-form McGill Pain Questionnaire. *Pain, 30*, 191–197. http://dx.doi.org/10.1016/0304-3959(87)91074-8

Melzack, R. (2001). Pain and the neuromatrix in the brain. *Journal of Dental Education, 65*, 1378–1382.

Molton, I. R., & Terrill, A. L. (2014). Overview of persistent pain in older adults. *American Psychologist, 69*, 197–207. http://dx.doi.org/10.1037/a0035794

Moseley, G. L., & Butler, D. S. (2015). Fifteen years of explaining pain: The past, present, and future. *The Journal of Pain, 16*, 807–813. http://dx.doi.org/10.1016/j.jpain.2015.05.005

National Academies of Sciences, Engineering, and Medicine. (2017). *Pain management and the opioid epidemic: Balancing societal and individual benefits and risks of prescription opioid use*. Washington, DC: The National Academies Press.

Osborne, T. L., Raichle, K. A., Jensen, M. P., Ehde, D. M., & Kraft, G. (2006). The reliability and validity of pain interference measures in persons with multiple sclerosis. *Journal of Pain and Symptom Management, 32*, 217–229. http://dx.doi.org/10.1016/j.jpainsymman.2006.03.008

Otis, J. D. (2007). *Managing chronic pain: A cognitive-behavioral therapy approach. Therapist guide*. Oxford, New York, NY: Oxford University Press. http://dx.doi.org/10.1093/med:psych/9780195329162.001.0001

Palermo, T. M., Eccleston, C., Lewandowski, A. S., Williams, A. C., & Morley, S. (2010). Randomized controlled trials of psychological therapies for management of chronic pain in children and adolescents: An updated meta-analytic review. *Pain, 148*, 387–397. http://dx.doi.org/10.1016/j.pain.2009.10.004

Patterson, D. R. (2010). *Clinical hypnosis for pain control*. Washington, DC: American Psychological Association. http://dx.doi.org/10.1037/12128-000

Quartana, P. J., Campbell, C. M., & Edwards, R. R. (2009). Pain catastrophizing: A critical review. *Expert Review of Neurotherapeutics, 9*, 745–758. http://dx.doi.org/10.1586/ern.09.34

Raichle, K. A., Osborne, T. L., Jensen, M. P., & Cardenas, D. (2006). The reliability and validity of pain interference measures in persons with spinal cord injury. *The Journal of Pain, 7*, 179–186. http://dx.doi.org/10.1016/j.jpain.2005.10.007

Revicki, D. A., Chen, W. H., Harnam, N., Cook, K. F., Amtmann, D., Callahan, L. F., . . . Keefe, F. J. (2009). Development and psychometric analysis of the PROMIS pain behavior item bank. *Pain, 146*, 158–169. http://dx.doi.org/10.1016/j.pain.2009.07.029

Revicki, D. A., Cook, K. F., Amtmann, D., Harnam, N., Chen, W. H., & Keefe, F. J. (2014). Exploratory and confirmatory factor analysis of the PROMIS pain quality item bank. *Quality of Life Research: An International Journal of Quality of Life Aspects of Treatment, Care & Rehabilitation, 23*, 245–255. http://dx.doi.org/10.1007/s11136-013-0467-9

Robinson, M. E., Riley, J. L., III, Myers, C. D., Sadler, I. J., Kvaal, S. A., Geisser, M. E., & Keefe, F. J. (1997). The Coping Strategies Questionnaire: A large sample, item level factor analysis. *The Clinical Journal of Pain, 13*, 43–49. http://dx.doi.org/10.1097/00002508-199703000-00007

Romano, J. M., Jensen, M. P., & Turner, J. A. (2003). The Chronic Pain Coping Inventory—42: Reliability and validity. *Pain, 104*, 65–73. http://dx.doi.org/10.1016/S0304-3959(02)00466-9

Romano, J. M., Turner, J. A., Jensen, M. P., Friedman, L. S., Bulcroft, R. A., Hops, H., & Wright, S. F. (1995). Chronic pain patient-spouse behavioral interactions predict patient disability. *Pain, 63*, 353–360.

Rosenstiel, A. K., & Keefe, F. J. (1983). The use of coping strategies in chronic low back pain patients: Relationship to patient characteristics and current adjustment. *Pain, 17*, 33–44. http://dx.doi.org/10.1016/0304-3959(83)90125-2

Schild, C., Reed, E. A., Hingston, T., Dennis, C. H., & Wilson, A. C. (2016). Neighborhood characteristics: Influences on pain and physical function in youth at risk for chronic pain. *Children (Basel, Switzerland), 3*, 35. http://dx.doi.org/10.3390/children3040035

Slavin, M. D., Kisala, P. A., Jette, A. M., & Tulsky, D. S. (2010). Developing a contemporary functional outcome measure for spinal cord injury research.

Spinal Cord, *48*, 262–267. http://dx.doi.org/10.1038/sc.2009.131

Spitzer, R. L., Kroenke, K., & Williams, J. B. (1999). Validation and utility of a self-report version of PRIME-MD: The PHQ primary care study. Primary Care Evaluation of Mental Disorders. Patient Health Questionnaire. *Journal of the American Medical Association*, *282*(18), 1737–1744. http://dx.doi.org/10.1001/jama.282.18.1737

Sullivan, M. J., & D'Eon, J. L. (1990). Relation between catastrophizing and depression in chronic pain patients. *Journal of Abnormal Psychology*, *99*, 260–263. http://dx.doi.org/10.1037/0021-843X.99.3.260

Sullivan, M. J., Thorn, B., Haythornthwaite, J. A., Keefe, F., Martin, M., Bradley, L. A., & Lefebvre, J. C. (2001). Theoretical perspectives on the relation between catastrophizing and pain. *The Clinical Journal of Pain*, *17*, 52–64. http://dx.doi.org/10.1097/00002508-200103000-00008

Sullivan, M. J. L., Bishop, S. R., & Pivik, J. (1995). The Pain Catastrophizing Scale: Development and validation. *Psychological Assessment*, *7*, 524–532. http://dx.doi.org/10.1037/1040-3590.7.4.524

Tait, R. C., & Chibnall, J. T. (2014). Racial/ethnic disparities in the assessment and treatment of pain: Psychosocial perspectives. *American Psychologist*, *69*, 131–141. http://dx.doi.org/10.1037/a0035204

Tan, G., Nguyen, Q., Anderson, K. O., Jensen, M., & Thornby, J. (2005). Further validation of the chronic pain coping inventory. *The Journal of Pain*, *6*, 29–40. http://dx.doi.org/10.1016/j.jpain.2004.09.006

Tan, G., Teo, I., Anderson, K. O., & Jensen, M. P. (2011). Adaptive versus maladaptive coping and beliefs and their relation to chronic pain adjustment. *The Clinical Journal of Pain*, *27*, 769–774. http://dx.doi.org/10.1097/AJP.0b013e31821d8f5a

Teasell, R. W., & Bombardier, C. (2001). Employment-related factors in chronic pain and chronic pain disability. *The Clinical Journal of Pain*, *17*(4, Suppl.), S39–S45. http://dx.doi.org/10.1097/00002508-200112001-00010

Thorn, B. E. (2017). *Cognitive therapy for chronic pain: A step-by-step guide* (2nd ed.). New York, NY: Guilford Press.

Thorn, B. E., Day, M. A., Burns, J., Kuhajda, M. C., Gaskins, S. W., Sweeney, K., . . . Cabbil, C. (2011). Randomized trial of group cognitive behavioral therapy compared with a pain education control for low-literacy rural people with chronic pain. *Pain*, *152*, 2710–2720. http://dx.doi.org/10.1016/j.pain.2011.07.007

Tulsky, D. S., Kisala, P. A., Victorson, D., Tate, D., Heinemann, A. W., Amtmann, D., & Cella, D. (2011). Developing a contemporary patient-reported outcomes measure for spinal cord injury. *Archives of Physical Medicine and Rehabilitation*, *92*(Suppl.), S44–S51. http://dx.doi.org/10.1016/j.apmr.2011.04.024

Tulsky, D. S., & Kisala, P. A. (2015). The Spinal Cord Injury—Quality of Life (SCI-QOL) measurement system: Development, psychometrics, and item bank calibration. *The Journal of Spinal Cord Medicine*, *38*, 251–256. http://dx.doi.org/10.1179/2045772315Y.0000000035

Tulsky, D. S., Kisala, P. A., Victorson, D., Carlozzi, N., Bushnik, T., Sherer, M., . . . Cella, D. (2016). TBI–QOL: Development and calibration of item banks to measure patient reported outcomes following traumatic brain injury. *The Journal of Head Trauma Rehabilitation*, *31*, 40–51. http://dx.doi.org/10.1097/HTR.0000000000000131

Tulsky, D. S., Kisala, P. A., Victorson, D., Tate, D. G., Heinemann, A. W., Charlifue, S., . . . Cella, D. (2015). Overview of the Spinal Cord Injury—Quality of Life (SCI–QOL) measurement system. *The Journal of Spinal Cord Medicine*, *38*, 257–269. http://dx.doi.org/10.1179/2045772315Y.0000000023

Turk, D. C., Dworkin, R. H., Allen, R. R., Bellamy, N., Brandenburg, N., Carr, D. B., . . . Witter, J. (2003). Core outcome domains for chronic pain clinical trials: IMMPACT recommendations. *Pain*, *106*, 337–345. http://dx.doi.org/10.1016/j.pain.2003.08.001

Turk, D. C., & Flor, H. (1999). Chronic pain: A biobehavioral perspective. In R. J. Gatchel & D. C. Turk (Eds.), *Psychosocial factors in pain: Critical perspectives* (pp. 18–34). New York, NY: Guilford Press.

Turk, D. C., & Melzack, R. (2011). *Handbook of pain assessment* (3rd ed.). New York, NY: Guilford Press.

Tyler, E. J., Jensen, M. P., Engel, J. M., & Schwartz, L. (2002). The reliability and validity of pain interference measures in persons with cerebral palsy. *Archives of Physical Medicine and Rehabilitation*, *83*, 236–239. http://dx.doi.org/10.1053/apmr.2002.27466

Veehof, M. M., Oskam, M. J., Schreurs, K. M., & Bohlmeijer, E. T. (2011). Acceptance-based interventions for the treatment of chronic pain: A systematic review and meta-analysis. *Pain*, *152*, 533–542. http://dx.doi.org/10.1016/j.pain.2010.11.002

Viane, I., Crombez, G., Eccleston, C., Devulder, J., & De Corte, W. (2004). Acceptance of the unpleasant reality of chronic pain: Effects upon attention to pain and engagement with daily activities. *Pain*, *112*, 282–288. http://dx.doi.org/10.1016/j.pain.2004.09.008

Viane, I., Crombez, G., Eccleston, C., Poppe, C., Devulder, J., Van Houdenhove, B., & De Corte, W. (2003). Acceptance of pain is an independent predictor of mental well-being in patients with chronic pain: Empirical evidence and reappraisal. *Pain*, *106*, 65–72. http://dx.doi.org/10.1016/S0304-3959(03)00291-4

Vlaeyen, J. W., & Linton, S. J. (2000). Fear-avoidance and its consequences in chronic musculoskeletal pain: A state of the art. *Pain, 85*, 317–332.

Vowles, K. E., McCracken, L. M., McLeod, C., & Eccleston, C. (2008). The Chronic Pain Acceptance Questionnaire: Confirmatory factor analysis and identification of patient subgroups. *Pain, 140*, 284–291. http://dx.doi.org/10.1016/j.pain.2008.08.012

Wager, T. D., Atlas, L. Y., Lindquist, M. A., Roy, M., Woo, C. W., & Kross, E. (2013). An fMRI-based neurologic signature of physical pain. *The New England Journal of Medicine, 368*, 1388–1397. http://dx.doi.org/10.1056/NEJMoa1204471

Williams, D. A., Robinson, M. E., & Geisser, M. E. (1994). Pain beliefs: Assessment and utility. *Pain, 59*, 71–78. http://dx.doi.org/10.1016/0304-3959(94)90049-3

CHAPTER 15

BURN INJURIES

Shelley Wiechman

Improvements in burn care, such as the development of comprehensive burn centers, advances in resuscitation, and surgical management of patients with large burns, have resulted in improved survival rates. According to the American Burn Association (2017) National Burn Repository Report, the survival rate for those sustaining burn injuries of any size was between 95% and 97%. Patients with burn injuries are surviving after increasingly large and severe injuries and are consequently posing unique physical and psychological rehabilitation challenges. Major burns (> 20% total body surface area) can have prolonged adverse effects on body functions and structures (pulmonary, cardiac, skeletal, hepatic organ systems; Porter, Hardee, Herndon, & Suman, 2015). These effects, including compromised lung function, decreased aerobic capacity, scarring, contractures, amputations, and pain, can exist even up to 5 years postinjury and beyond. Regardless of burn size, burn survivors also report high rates of secondary conditions, such as pain and itch, sleep disturbance, depression, anxiety, and body image dissatisfaction (Falder et al., 2009). These conditions can become chronic and disabling, and can adversely affect health and function and overall quality of life.

Patients with burns may require the aggressive range of motion, strengthening, and conditioning typically needed by those with an acquired disability, in addition to ongoing mental health treatment to cope with this chronic condition. Therefore, rehabilitation team members such as physical, occupational, and speech therapists and rehabilitation psychologists are ideally incorporated into the multidisciplinary burn team (Competency: Interdisciplinary Systems American Board of Rehabilitation Psychology [ABRP], n.d.). After the acute phase of burn care, many patients will require a more intensive, inpatient rehabilitation program and will continue to be followed in rehabilitation medicine as well as surgery clinics. Treatment to prevent these complications includes aggressive range-of-motion exercises, pressure garments, and splints, and these can be painful or uncomfortable for patients, making treatment adherence a challenge.

Burn recovery is a complex and dynamic process, and knowledge of the patient's history, support systems, coping style, secondary complications, and the nature of burn care will be necessary to appreciate and facilitate a full recovery (ABRP Competency: Specialty Identification). Rehabilitation psychologists have a unique understanding of the biopsychosocial model of recovery from injury and are a crucial member of the multidisciplinary burn team. However, given the relative infancy of the field of burn recovery and low incidence of burns compared with other disability groups, clinical trials of psychological interventions and assessment measures specific to burns are rare. Many of the assessment and intervention recommendations are not based

http://dx.doi.org/10.1037/0000129-016
Handbook of Rehabilitation Psychology, Third Edition, L. A. Brenner, S. A. Reid-Arndt, T. R. Elliott, R. G. Frank, and B. Caplan (Editors-in-Chief)

on empirical evidence but rather derive from clinical experience.

This chapter begins by addressing the demographics of people with burn injuries and moves on to a brief description of the recovery process and long-term outcomes of burn survivors. The chapter concludes with a discussion of specific topics relevant to burn care. The American Board of Professional Psychology has developed standard competencies required for board certification in rehabilitation psychology. (See Chapter 1, this volume for additional information.) Burn recovery addresses many of these competencies, and the corresponding ABRP competency is noted in parentheses in the chapter.

DEMOGRAPHICS AND TRENDS

According to the American Burn Association (2017), each year more than 486,000 people receive medical treatment and 40,000 are hospitalized for burn injury in the United States. With a 96% survival rate, more people are living with larger burns, and the focus has shifted from resuscitation and acute medical/surgical management to improving long-term quality of life. The American Burn Association verifies hospitals that meet their criteria as a regional burn center, and 30,000 patients each year are treated at verified burn centers. The etiology of a burn injury is related to age. The most common cause of burns is hot water scalds, with children, the elderly, and people with disabilities being most prone to this type of injury. Male adolescents typically suffer burn injuries resulting from risk-taking behavior, such as playing with fireworks or gasoline. People in certain occupations are at more risk for burn injuries, including electricians and workers in the food service, chemical, or fuel industries. The overwhelming majority of people who sustain burn injuries are men between the ages of 20 and 40 years.

The severity of this type of trauma is determined by the total body surface area (TBSA) of the burn and the depth of the burn. First degree or superficial burn injuries extend only into the epidermis. These burns rarely blister, are painful, and heal quickly without scarring. Partial-thickness burns extend through the epidermis and into the dermis. Burns in this category are harder to classify initially, they may or may not require grafting, and, if left to heal on their own, will likely cause scarring. These burns are typically quite painful. Full-thickness burns extend all the way through the dermis and into the subcutaneous fat. These burns will need to be excised and require a skin graft to promote healing. The practice of many burn centers is to debride burned skin on a daily basis to avoid infection and promote healing. This process involves scraping off the dead skin and washing the area. Such wound cleaning and grafting procedures are frequently painful for a period of weeks. Resulting pain can be worse than that experienced in the initial burn injury.

PHASES OF REHABILITATION

Hospitalization for burn injuries may vary in length from less than 1 week to several months, depending on the severity of the burn and the presence of other medical complications. Although not to be taken literally as a "stage theory," the physical and emotional recovery of patients often differs according to their phase of care. The recovery period can usually be broken down into three phases: the resuscitative or critical phase, typically spent in the intensive care unit (ICU); the acute phase, when patients are medically stable and able to begin rehabilitation; and the outpatient phase, after a patient has been discharged from the hospital, but continues in outpatient rehabilitation therapies. Although each phase represents accomplishment of a major milestone of recovery, it comes with an expectation of an increase in independence, which can increase anxiety for the patient. The transition to each phase can be challenging initially, and patients should be prepared for the transition by warning them of the initial distress that can occur with this increase in independence and decreased level of care. Each phase and the recommended corresponding treatments are described in the following subsections.

Resuscitative or Critical Phase: Assessment

Patients are usually treated in the ICU during the resuscitative or critical phase and may stay there for weeks. Characteristics of the resuscitative phase include uncertainty regarding outcome and a struggle for survival, particularly if the burn is severe. During this phase, patients typically undergo repeated medical procedures and must contend with severe physiological stressors, including electrolyte imbalance, infections, anoxia, and edema. The environment of the ICU can be both overstimulating, with its bright lights, machines, and multiple health care providers, yet also extremely monotonous, as patients are forced to lie in a hospital bed, often immobile for weeks at a time. Coping with this environment is affected by a patient's cognitive changes, such as extreme drowsiness, confusion, disorientation, and delirium (Mehta et al., 2015). These cognitive changes may be symptoms of infections, alcohol withdrawal, metabolic complications, or effects of high doses of medications. Recent attention has been paid to delirium and its negative consequences, including increased length of hospitalization, increased risk of contractures, and respiratory complications (Mehta et al., 2015). Screening for delirium, anxiety, and acute stress disorder should be conducted as soon as the patient is alert enough to participate in an assessment (Gibran et al., 2013).

Resuscitative or Critical Phase: Intervention

The primary role of psychologists during this phase is to help the patient feel safe and comfortable. If patients do become more alert, focusing on past or future concerns may be counterproductive. The patient's primary task now is physical recovery, if not survival. Patients should be encouraged to cope with the frighteningly unusual circumstances of the ICU through whatever defenses are available to them, such as denial and repression. Supportive psychological interventions should focus on immediate concerns, such as sleep, pain control, and protecting the coping strategies the patient uses. Nonpharmacological approaches to delirium, such as early mobilization and environmental interventions to enhance orientation, are important during this phase. In addition, nonpharmacological pain control strategies, such as hypnosis, meditation, and relaxation can be effective.

Rehabilitation psychologists can also help the medical staff to effectively intervene with the patient's family members (ABRP Competency: Adjustment to Disability: Family). Understandably, family members may be anxious and distressed while observing the patient undergo painful treatment. The patient may detect cues of anxiety and stress from the family and behave accordingly. It is important to help family members understand this process and encourage them to convey a sense of hope and calm to the patient. Frequent communication with the medical team on relevant medical information can reduce anxiety. It may also be important to introduce the family to peer support volunteers—burn survivors trained to provide support to current patients with burn injuries and their families. The Phoenix Society, a national advocacy group for the burn community, offers a peer support program called SOAR (Survivors Offering Assistance in Recovery; Phoenix Society, n.d.) that can be introduced at this time; visits should be offered throughout the hospitalization.

Acute Phase: Assessment

The acute phase of recovery focuses on restorative care such as nutritional support, excision and grafting, and topical wound care. Although patients are moved off the ICU to an environment that is more consistent and less intrusive, they must still undergo painful treatments. As cognition improves and patients become more alert during this phase, they face these painful procedures and physical therapy with less sedation. Consequently, symptoms of anxiety, posttraumatic stress disorder (PTSD), depression, and grief may become more apparent, and pain and sleep disturbance will need to be addressed. Screening for these issues is important during this phase. Additional information regarding rehabilitation psychology in critical care settings can be found in Chapter 28, this volume.

Acute Phase: Intervention

During this phase, when patients usually have the cognitive clarity to understand the impact of their trauma, medication management for anxiety, sleep, and depression should be considered. Brief counseling and psychoeducation may also be an option. Nonpharmacological approaches to pain management such as distraction, relaxation, imagery, and hypnosis become effective at this phase of recovery. (More on pain interventions can be found later in this chapter, as well in Chapter 14, this volume.) It can also be useful to provide brief interventions for alcohol and drug abuse, as indicated. Hospitalization often presents a window in which patients are receptive to behavior change.

Outpatient Phase: Assessment

The long-term phase of recovery typically begins when patients move from the acute floor to either an inpatient or outpatient rehabilitation setting and are challenged to reintegrate into society. For patients with severe burns injuries, this phase likely involves continued physical rehabilitation on an outpatient basis, along with possible continuation of procedures such as dressing changes and cosmetic surgery. Patients may encounter daily pain during rehabilitation, and they may also be forced to confront cosmetic or other existential changes that have occurred because of their injury. This is a period when patients slowly regain a sense of competence while simultaneously adjusting to the practical limitations of a burn injury. Studies have shown that the first year after hospitalization is a psychologically unique period of high distress (Patterson et al., 1993). Screening for difficulties during this phase is critical. Depression PTSD, sleep issues, pain, body image satisfaction, community integration, and overall quality of life should be assessed at the first outpatient clinic visit. Much attention has been paid recently to the best way to screen for these issues. Mental health providers can choose either general screening measures for these disorders or the few available burn-specific measures. Measures using computer-assisted technology that can be used to quickly assess outcomes for various domains of emotional adjustment are useful in the outpatient clinic.

Outpatient Phase: Intervention

Focus groups of burn survivors have repeatedly found that they feel isolated and alone when discharging from the burn unit to their community. They have requested more frequent and ongoing follow-up visits and more telehealth services from regional burn centers or training of rural providers unfamiliar with burn injuries (Wiechman & Holavanahalli, 2017). This is an ideal time to work with patients on their emotional recovery. It is likely that patients who have symptoms of distress in the months or years following discharge will need an evidence-based treatment by a mental health provider experienced with issues related to burn recovery. There have been few randomized controlled clinical trials specific to patients with burn injuries, so treatments should be used that have been effective for non–burn patients with these psychological problems. For example, depressed burn survivors may benefit from a combination of medication, cognitive behavior therapy (CBT), and exercise to treat depression. Exposure-based therapies may be effective for burn survivors with PTSD (Powers, Halpern, Ferenschak, Gillihan, & Foa, 2010). A multidisciplinary team approach should also be used because patients can benefit from support from a vocational or rehabilitation counselor to address issues related to return to work (Van Loey, Faber, & Taal, 2001). Social workers will also be needed to assist with a variety of matters, including financial resources. Support groups and peer counseling visitation may also be useful if carefully monitored by trained professionals (Williams et al., 2002). The Phoenix Society, mentioned earlier, provides a wide range of services for burn survivors and their families, including online support groups, peer visitors, a national conference, and valuable information on their website (http://www.phoenix-society.org). Ideally, patients should be introduced to their services early in their hospitalization and reminded of them after discharge.

Long-Term Outcomes After Burn Injury

Similar to people with other forms of disabilities, such as spinal cord injury and amputations, the biopsychosocial model is a helpful heuristic in understanding that the adjustment of burn survivors is a complex interplay of preinjury risk factors, burn-specific factors (e.g., TBSA, inhalation injury, sepsis), and coping style. With the support of more federal funding, research by rehabilitation psychologists has proven to be useful in understanding long-term burn recovery in the context of this model. For example, research support from the National Institute on Disability Independent

Living and Rehabilitation Research establishes model systems of care for burn survivors for both the acute phases of the burn and long-term management. These large databases allow researchers to track incidence rates for various mental health disorders and identify risk and protective factors to better predict who might need more intensive intervention. An important research finding is that large burns do not always lead to bad psychological outcomes, and conversely some patients with small burns struggle with emotional recovery. According to this model, preinjury factors, injury-related variables, and interpersonal factors all impact long-term outcomes. Specifically, risk factors for poorer mental and physical outcomes include uncontrolled or high acute pain levels (Edwards et al., 2007), prior mental health history (alcohol/drug use, anxiety, PTSD, depression; Patterson et al., 2003), personality characteristics (neuroticism; Fauerbach et al., 1997; Giannoni-Pastor, Eiroa-Orosa, Fidel Kinori, Arguello, & Casas, 2015), and poor social support. Although actual rates of major depressive disorder, anxiety disorders and PTSD are hard to pinpoint due to the differing methodologies and assessment tools used, the majority of studies show rates higher than the general population (Giannoni-Pastor et al., 2016). More important, even lower levels of distress can impact quality of life and should be treated (Wiechman et al., 2018). The variability in distress indicates how complicated the nature of burn recovery is and the importance of universal and routine screening for distress.

Although the field agrees that early screening is optimal, there is disagreement in the field as to whether burn-specific measures are needed or if it is preferable to use standardized general measures of outcome. For common issues such as depression, PTSD, and generalized anxiety, the use of well-validated, standardized measures, such as the Beck Depression Inventory—II, the Patient Health Questionnaire—9, the PTSD Checklist—Civilian Version, and the Seven-Item Generalized Anxiety Disorder Screener (Beck, Steer, & Brown, 1996; Kroenke, Spitzer, & Williams, 2001; Löwe et al., 2008; Miles, Marshall, & Schell, 2008) have been adequate and can be used to compare outcome trajectories across disability groups and the general population. A recent systematic review of depression measures in the burn population found that few of these general measures have been validated in the burn population. However, before taking on the monumental task of creating and validating a burn-specific measure for depression, researchers should validate the existing general measures for the burn population (Wiechman et al., 2016). This process entails the inclusion of psychometric statistics in published articles. Further, arguments have been made on both sides as to the value of disease-specific patient-reported quality-of-life outcome measures. The National Institutes of Health Patient-Reported Outcomes Measurement Information System (PROMIS) measures have been established based on item response theory to quickly assess a patient's outcomes on various domains and can be compared to standardized norms. The 12-Item Short-Form Health Survey (Ware, Kosinski, & Keller, 1996) is also widely used and has standardized norms. However, some argue that these measures are not sensitive or specific enough to capture the distress across the wide domains of function that are affected by a large burn injury (Blakeney et al., 1998).

To address the preceding issues, there has been a recent rise in multidimensional burn outcome measures both to screen for potential problem areas and to measure patient-reported outcomes. The Burn Outcomes Questionnaires for ages 0 to 5, 6 to 17, and 18 to 30 is one such project. Data were collected on burn survivors with a wide range of TBSA for 10 years. Norms were established, and recovery curves can be used to identify those outside the expected course of recovery. These measures can be administered in the waiting room before the outpatient visit, recovery curves can be established, and providers are then given this report to better tailor care to the patient's needs (Kazis et al., 2016). A similar approach was taken for adult burn survivors in establishing the Life Impact Burn Recovery Evaluation Profile. This is a self-reported outcome measure that uses computerized-assessment technology and measures seven domains related to the social impact of burn injuries. Norms are currently being established, and it is anticipated that the measure will be widely available soon (Marino et al., 2017). Given the current lack of norms for the various instruments mentioned here, a strong, thorough clinical interview is a crucial part of the assessment.

ADDITIONAL CONSIDERATIONS RELEVANT TO BURN CARE

Acute and chronic pain, body image, and physical activity are common issues for many people with various disabilities. Each topic has special considerations for those with burn injuries and is described in the following subsections.

Pain

A burn injury is one of the most painful injuries a person can experience, and persons hospitalized for acute burn injuries are often given high doses of opiates to cope with painful wound care and therapy procedures. This acute pain can continue for months after discharge as patients are now being discharged sooner with open wounds and extensive wound care to be done at home. It is not humane to completely wean a patient off of opiates before discharge, but continuing opiate use in the outpatient setting is fraught with potential dangers and complications with no clear guidelines on a reasonable time frame to continue prescribing these medications. When examining opioid prescription practices in the trauma population, it is clear that the transition from acute hospitalization to discharge is a critical time. One recent study examined prescribing practices at a verified regional burn center and found that more than 85% of patients with acute burn injuries are discharged with an opioid prescription with a morphine milligram equivalent (MME) of 114 (Wibbenmeyer, Oltrogge, Kluesner, Zimmerman, & Kealey, 2015). Adverse events and overdose deaths have been linked to the quantity of opioids prescribed ranging from 40 to 200 MMEs per day. Age, male sex, and total MME before discharge were associated with the amount of opiates prescribed at discharge. The number of refills was significantly associated with the average pain within 48 hours of discharge (Wibbenmeyer et al., 2015).

Burn pain can also go beyond the acute phase, with prevalence rates of chronic pain 10 years after burn injury ranging from 35% to 50%. Of those reporting chronic pain, 66% said that pain interfered with their ongoing rehabilitation, and 55% said it interfered with quality of life (Browne, Andrews, Schug, & Wood, 2011). Risk factors for chronic pain include high inpatient pain levels, depression, and PTSD. Furthermore, burn survivors can experience intense pruritus (itching), often classified as neuropathic pain. Pruritus can be a terrible problem for burn patients and is a common occurrence in the weeks when wounds begin to heal and hypertrophic scars form (Schneider et al., 2015).

Managing acute pain by clarifying pain treatment expectations increases patient satisfaction and may prevent long-term pain problems (Browne et al., 2011). In addition, both pharmacological and nonpharmacological (e.g., relaxation, distraction, imagery, mindfulness, hypnosis) treatments are necessary to control pain in the burn patient (ABRP Competency: Pain). There is considerable empirical evidence for the efficacy of nonpharmacological treatments, particularly when used as an adjunct to opioid medications (Wiechman & Sharar, 2017). These same techniques should be applied to postburn pruritus.

The impact of anxiety on pain is often underestimated, and its treatment is overlooked. Because anxiety greatly exacerbates pain, it is important to begin nonpharmacological treatments as early as possible in the patient's stay to help mitigate anticipatory anxiety and the subsequent anxiety–pain cycle (Patterson, Ptacek, Carrougher, & Sharar, 1997). Technological interventions, such as virtual reality, augmented reality, and gaming have received considerable attention in promoting pain control, reducing anxiety, and enhancing range of motion during burn recovery. Virtual reality and augmented reality can be used to provide distraction or induce hypnosis (Wiechman Askay, Patterson, & Sharar, 2009). Other computer games and tablet apps can be used to promote mobility by distracting a patient from the pain. Rehabilitation psychologists with unique expertise in the nonpharmacological approaches to pain management can implement the intervention themselves or teach other staff to use some of these techniques. For further discussion of pain assessment and management, see Chapter 14, this volume.

Body Image Issues

Burn injuries can cause significant changes in appearance, whether from scarring, contractures, changes in skin pigmentation, or amputations. The impact that these physical changes have on self-esteem and body image has received relatively limited attention to date. The majority of research on body image has focused on eating disorders or congenital differences (e.g., cleft palate), and there has been little study on acquired changes in appearance (e.g., trauma, burns). Across disability groups (craniofacial abnormalities, amputations, burns, spinal cord injuries), there is a wide range of individual differences in terms of coping with visible changes in appearance. Specifically, Egan, Harcourt, Rumsey, and the Appearance Research Collaboration (2011) estimated that 30% to 50% of individuals with visible differences may experience psychological difficulty at some time. Several studies of risk factors for the development of poor body image found that burn characteristics, such as the visibility of the scar and objective severity of a disfigurement, do not predict the extent of distress or negative body image (Egan et al., 2011). Instead, personal characteristics, such as depression, female gender, and coping style, best predicted body image dissatisfaction (Lawrence, Fauerbach, Heinberg, & Doctor, 2004).

An additional predictor of body image dissatisfaction is the importance that a patient placed on his or her appearance before the burn injury. Specifically, those who did not place much importance on their appearance before the burn tend to be much less distressed by scarring (Fauerbach et al., 2002). As such, viewing the visible difference as only a small part of their lives seems to be critical in developing body appreciation. Family and unconditional acceptance play a large role in this process. Parents can help children learn to talk about their scars in a casual way and model positive social responses toward teasing or other stigmatization. Developing hobbies, talents and exploring other aspects of identity (not just physical appearance) will help individuals to put their appearance in perspective (Quayle, 2015).

There has been recent attention on the concept of body appreciation, defined broadly as love and acceptance of one's body and appreciation of its uniqueness and the function it performs (Tylka & Wood-Barcalow, 2015). The concept of body appreciation is distinctly different from that of body dissatisfaction; interventions to promote body image appreciation may vary slightly from CBT approaches for body dissatisfaction. More research needs to be conducted in this area with the burn population. We do a disservice to our patients if we exclusively focus on alleviating symptoms of body image disturbance without recognizing opportunities to promote body image appreciation.

Most treatments to address body image concerns have focused on cognitive-behavioral strategies to address a person's appraisal of their appearance, teach adaptive coping strategies, and introduce social skills that enhance self-esteem and improve social competence. Programs such as these can be found through the Phoenix Society and the Changing Faces (n.d.) program in Great Britain.

Physical Activity

There is a tremendous focus on range-of-motion exercises for the burned areas over a joint. These exercises need to occur many times a day and can continue for several months after discharge. However, little attention has been paid to overall physical activity after a burn injury. A recent survey showed that burn survivors are exercising at rates significantly below the recommended guidelines of 30 minutes, five times per week. Even survivors who had previously been active have difficulty returning to previous levels of physical activity (Baldwin & Li, 2013). Barriers to physical activity after a burn injury include poor physical condition and lack of motivation.

Practice guidelines for prescribed exercise programs were established by an international group of burn care professionals and burn survivors (Nedelec et al., 2016). They call for assessment of strength and cardiovascular endurance for any burn survivor over age 7 years, and prescribed resistance and aerobic exercise programs for anyone below "normal" levels. These programs should begin as early as discharge from acute care and as late as 14 years postburn, but programs that are initiated as soon after discharge as feasible are desired. The guidelines specify that exercise programs should last from 6 to 12 weeks. This group of experts also identified barriers that included lack of resources for testing and training equipment, lack of rehabilitation personnel and lack of patient resources. Experts in this area recommend more structured and supervised outpatient exercise programs that focus on general physical activity in addition to range-of-motion exercises. Exercise has been shown to improve health-related quality of life, depression, anxiety, sleep, and body image across disability groups, including multiple sclerosis, spinal cord injury, and burns and in the general population (Motl, 2014; Rosenberg, Bombardier, Hoffman, & Belza, 2011). Given the secondary benefits that exercise can have on the issues of distress common to burn survivors, increasing physical activity is one of the most effective interventions for burn survivors, and the rehabilitation psychologist plays a crucial role in enhancing motivation for exercise.

CONCLUSION AND FUTURE DIRECTIONS

Rehabilitation psychologists are a critical part of the multidisciplinary burn treatment team across both the inpatient and outpatient settings. Issues relevant to burn survivors can impair quality of life for decades after the injury. In addition to having a unique understanding of the biopsychosocial model of burn recovery and the ability to treat various mental health conditions (depression, PTSD, anxiety), rehabilitation psychologists lead the way in research to improve the quality of life of burn survivors. Gaps in the literature remain that include nonpharmacological interventions for delirium and pruritus, body image interventions specific to those with acquired physical differences, and a better understanding of trajectories of burn recovery to aid in earlier identification of patients who may need more intense intervention. Further, larger randomized controlled trials of treatments unique to burn survivors that improve quality of life would make a tremendous contribution to the field. These treatments should be able to be delivered via telehealth to reach those in rural areas who feel isolated from services of regional burn centers.

References

American Board of Rehabilitation Psychology. (n.d.). *Competency requirements: Foundational & functional*. Retrieved from https://abpp.org/Applicant-Information/Foundational-Functional-Competencies.aspx

American Burn Association. (2017). *National burn repository report*. Chicago, IL: Author.

Baldwin, J., & Li, F. (2013). Exercise behaviors after burn injury. *Journal of Burn Care & Research, 34*, 529–536. http://dx.doi.org/10.1097/BCR.0b013e31827a2bcd

Beck, A. T., Steer, R. A., & Brown, G. K. (1996). *Manual for the Beck Depression Inventory—II*. San Antonio, TX: Psychological Corporation.

Blakeney, P., Meyer, W., III, Robert, R., Desai, M., Wolf, S., & Herndon, D. (1998). Long-term psychosocial adaptation of children who survive burns involving 80% or greater total body surface area. *The Journal of Trauma, 44*, 625–634. http://dx.doi.org/10.1097/00005373-199804000-00011

Browne, A. L., Andrews, R., Schug, S. A., & Wood, F. (2011). Persistent pain outcomes and patient satisfaction with pain management after burn injury. *Clinical Journal of Pain, 27*, 136–145.

Changing Faces. (n.d.). *Self-help guides*. Retrieved from https://www.changingfaces.org.uk/adviceandsupport/self-help-guides

Edwards, R. R., Magyar-Russell, G., Thombs, B., Smith, M. T., Holavanahalli, R. K., Patterson, D. R., . . . Fauerbach, J. A. (2007). Acute pain at discharge from hospitalization is a prospective predictor of long-term suicidal ideation after burn injury. *Archives of Physical Medicine and Rehabilitation, 88*(12, Suppl. 2), S36–S42. http://dx.doi.org/10.1016/j.apmr.2007.05.031

Egan, K., Harcourt, D., Rumsey, N., & the Appearance Research Collaboration. (2011). A qualitative study of the experiences of people who identify themselves as having adjusted positively to a visible difference. *Journal of Health Psychology, 16*, 739–749. http://dx.doi.org/10.1177/1359105310390246

Falder, S., Browne, A., Edgar, D., Staples, E., Fong, J., Rea, S., & Wood, F. (2009). Core outcomes for adult burn survivors: A clinical overview. *Burns, 35*, 618–641.

Fauerbach, J. A., Heinberg, L. J., Lawrence, J. W., Bryant, A. G., Richter, L., & Spence, R. J. (2002). Coping with body image changes following a disfiguring burn injury. *Health Psychology, 21*, 115–121. http://dx.doi.org/10.1037/0278-6133.21.2.115

Fauerbach, J. A., Lawrence, J., Haythornthwaite, J., Richter, D., McGuire, M., Schmidt, C., & Munster, A. (1997). Psychiatric history affects posttrauma morbidity. *Psychosomatics: Journal of Consultation and Liaison Psychiatry*, *38*, 374–385. http://dx.doi.org/10.1016/S0033-3182(97)71445-2

Giannoni-Pastor, A., Eiroa-Orosa, F. J., Fidel Kinori, S. G., Arguello, J. M., & Casas, M. (2016). Prevalence and predictors of posttraumatic stress symptomatology among burn survivors: A systematic review and meta-analysis. *Journal of Burn Care Research*, *37*, e79–e89. http://dx.doi.org/10.1097/BCR.0000000000000226

Giannoni-Pastor, A., Gomà-i-Freixanet, M., Valero, S., Fidel Kinori, S. G., Tasqué-Cebrián, R., Arguello, J. M., & Casas, M. (2015). Personality as a predictor of depression symptoms in burn patients: A follow-up study. *Burns*, *41*, 25–32. http://dx.doi.org/10.1016/j.burns.2014.07.028

Gibran, N. S., Wiechman, S. A., Meyer, W. M., Gamelli, R. L., Palmieri, T. L., Horton, J. W., . . . Latenser, B. A., & the American Burn Association Consensus Conference on Burn Sepsis and Infection Group. (2013). American Burn Association consensus statement. *Journal of Burn Care Research*, *34*, 361–385.

Kazis, L. E., Lee, A. F., Rose, M., Liang, M. H., Li, N. C., Ren, X. S., . . . Tompkins, R. G. (2016). Recovery curves for pediatric burn survivors: Advances in patient-oriented outcomes. *JAMA Pediatrics*, *170*, 534–542. http://dx.doi.org/10.1001/jamapediatrics.2015.4722

Kroenke, K., Spitzer, R. L., & Williams, J. B. W. (2001). The PHQ–9: Validity of a brief depression severity measure. *Journal of General Internal Medicine*, *16*, 606–613. http://dx.doi.org/10.1046/j.1525-1497.2001.016009606.x

Lawrence, J. W., Fauerbach, J. A., Heinberg, L., & Doctor, M. (2004). The 2003 clinical research award: Visible vs hidden scars and their relation to body esteem. *Journal of Burn Care & Research*, *25*, 25–32.

Löwe, B., Decker, O., Müller, S., Brähler, E., Schellberg, D., Herzog, W., & Herzberg, P. Y. (2008). Validation and standardization of the Generalized Anxiety Disorder Screener (GAD–7) in the general population. *Medical Care*, *46*, 266–274. http://dx.doi.org/10.1097/MLR.0b013e318160d093

Marino, M., Soley-Bori, M., Jette, A. M., Slavin, M. D., Ryan, C. M., Schneider, J. C., . . . Kazis, L. E. (2017). Measuring the social impact of burns on survivors. *Journal of Burn Care & Research*, *38*, e377–e383. http://dx.doi.org/10.1097/BCR.0000000000000398

Mehta, S. L., Cook, D., Devlin, J. W., Skrobik, Y., Meade, M., Fergusson, D., . . . Burry, L., SLEAP Investigators, and the Canadian Critical Care Trials Group. (2015). Prevalence, risk factors, and outcomes of delirium in mechanically ventilated adults. *Critical Care Medicine*, *43*, 557–66. PMID: 25493968.

Miles, J. N., Marshall, G. N., & Schell, T. L. (2008). Spanish and English versions of the PTSD Checklist-Civilian version (PCL–C): Testing for differential item functioning. *Journal of Traumatic Stress*, *21*, 369–376. http://dx.doi.org/10.1002/jts.20349

Motl, R. W. (2014). Benefits, safety, and prescription of exercise in persons with multiple sclerosis. *Expert Review of Neurotherapeutics*, *14*, 1429–1436. http://dx.doi.org/10.1586/14737175.2014.983904

Nedelec, B., Parry, I., Acharya, H., Benavides, L., Bills, S., Bucher, J. L., . . . Kloda, L. A. (2016). Practice guidelines for cardiovascular fitness and strengthening exercise prescription after burn injury. *Journal of Burn Care & Research*, *37*, e539–e558. http://dx.doi.org/10.1097/BCR.0000000000000282

Patterson, D. R., Everett, J. J., Bombardier, C. H., Questad, K. A., Lee, V. K., & Marvin, J. A. (1993). Psychological effects of severe burn injuries. *Psychological Bulletin*, *113*, 362–378. http://dx.doi.org/10.1037/0033-2909.113.2.362

Patterson, D. R., Finch, C. P., Wiechman, S. A., Bonsack, R., Gibran, N., & Heimbach, D. (2003). Premorbid mental health status of adult burn patients: Comparison with a normative sample. *The Journal of Burn Care & Research*, *24*, 347–350. http://dx.doi.org/10.1097/01.BCR.0000086070.91033.7F

Patterson, D. R., Ptacek, J. T., Carrougher, G. J., & Sharar, S. R. (1997). Lorazepam as an adjunct to opioid analgesics in the treatment of burn pain. *Pain*, *72*, 367–374. http://dx.doi.org/10.1016/S0304-3959(97)00064-X

Phoenix Society. (n.d.). Phoenix SOAR. Survivors Offering Assistance in Recovery. Retrieved from https://www.phoenix-society.org/our-programs/soar

Porter, C., Hardee, J. P., Herndon, D. N., & Suman, O. E. (2015). The role of exercise in the rehabilitation of patients with severe burns. *Exercise and Sport Sciences Reviews*, *43*, 34–40. http://dx.doi.org/10.1249/JES.0000000000000029

Powers, M. B., Halpern, J. M., Ferenschak, M. P., Gillihan, S. J., & Foa, E. B. (2010). A meta-analytic review of prolonged exposure for posttraumatic stress disorder. *Clinical Psychology Review*, *30*, 635–641.

Quayle, B. K. (2015). *Program that helped thousands began with one survivor*. Retrieved from https://www.phoenix-society.org/resources/entry/program-that-helped-thousands-began-with-one-survivor

Rosenberg, D. E., Bombardier, C. H., Hoffman, J. M., & Belza, B. (2011). Physical activity among persons aging with mobility disabilities: Shaping a research agenda. *Journal of Aging Research, 2011*, 708510. http://dx.doi.org/10.4061/2011/708510

Schneider, J. C., Nadler, D. L., Herndon, D. N., Kowalske, K., Matthews, K., Wiechman, S. A., . . . Ryan, C. M. (2015). Pruritus in pediatric burn survivors: Defining the clinical course. *Journal of Burn Care & Research*, *36*, 151–158. http://dx.doi.org/10.1097/BCR.0000000000000145

Tylka, T. L., & Wood-Barcalow, N. L. (2015). What is and what is not positive body image? Conceptual foundations and construct definition. *Body Image*, *14*, 118–129. http://dx.doi.org/10.1016/j.bodyim.2015.04.001

Van Loey, N. E., Faber, A. W., & Taal, L. A. (2001). Do burn patients need burn specific multidisciplinary outpatient aftercare: Research results. *Burns*, *27*, 103–110.

Ware, J., Jr., Kosinski, M., & Keller, S. D. (1996). A 12-Item Short-Form Health Survey: Construction of scales and preliminary tests of reliability and validity. *Medical Care*, *34*, 220–233. http://dx.doi.org/10.1097/00005650-199603000-00003

Wibbenmeyer, L., Oltrogge, K., Kluesner, K., Zimmerman, M. B., & Kealey, P. G. (2015). An evaluation of discharge opioid prescribing practices in a burn population. *Journal of Burn Care & Research*, *36*, 329–335. http://dx.doi.org/10.1097/BCR.0000000000000110

Wiechman, S., Kalpakjian, C. Z., & Johnson, K. L. (2016). Measuring depression in adults with burn injury: A systematic review. *Journal of Burn Care & Research*, *37*, e415–e426. http://dx.doi.org/10.1097/BCR.0000000000000384

Wiechman, S. A., & Holavanahalli, R. (2017). Burn survivor focus group. *Journal of Burn Care & Research*, *38*, e593–595.

Wiechman, S. A., McMullen, K., Carrougher, G. J., Fauerbach, J. A., Ryan, C. M., Herndon, D. N., . . . Roaten, K. (2018). Reasons for distress among burn survivors at 6, 12, and 24 months postdischarge: A burn injury model system investigation. *Archives of Physical Medicine and Rehabilitation*, *99*, 1311–1317. http://dx.doi.org/10.1016/j.apmr.2017.11.007

Wiechman, S. A., & Sharar, S. (2017). Burn pain: Principles of pharmacologic and nonpharmacologic management. *UptoDate*. Retrieved from https://www.uptodate.com/contents/management-of-burn-wound-pain-and-itching

Wiechman Askay, S. W., Patterson, D. R., & Sharar, S. R. (2009). Virtual reality hypnosis. *Contemporary Hypnosis*, *26*, 40–47. http://dx.doi.org/10.1002/ch.371

Williams, R. M., Patterson, D. R., Schwenn, C., Day, J., Bartman, M., & Engrav, L. H. (2002). Evaluation of a peer consultation program for burn inpatients. 2000 ABA paper. *The Journal of Burn Care & Rehabilitation*, *23*, 449–453. http://dx.doi.org/10.1097/00004630-200211000-00012

CHAPTER 16

LIMB LOSS

Pamela Gallagher, Laura Coffey, Deirdre M. Desmond, Richard Lombard-Vance, Philip Jefferies, and Stephen T. Wegener

Amputation involves the surgical or traumatic removal of a limb, and may involve one limb only (unilateral), both of the upper or lower limbs (bilateral), or a combination of upper and lower limbs (multiple amputations). Amputation can be performed at different anatomical levels: removal of one or more toes (transmetatarsal) or fingers (transmetacarpal), or part of the foot or hand; ankle or wrist disarticulation (i.e., amputation through the joint); amputation below the knee (transtibial) or elbow (transradial); knee or elbow disarticulation; amputation above the knee (transfemoral) or elbow (transhumeral); hip or shoulder disarticulation; and hemipelvectomy (removal of half of the pelvis) or forequarter amputation (amputation of the arm, clavicle, and scapula). Lower limb amputation (LLA) is significantly more common than amputation of the upper limb, accounting for 65% of all existing cases of amputation in the United States (Ziegler-Graham, MacKenzie, Ephraim, Travison, & Brookmeyer, 2008).

Upper and lower limb amputations are distinctly different in terms of their precipitating etiologies. Within economically developed countries the leading causes of upper limb amputation (ULA) are traumatic (e.g., because of workplace injury, motor vehicle accident, natural disaster, war), whereas peripheral vascular disease (PVD) and diabetes are the leading causes of LLA (Ziegler-Graham et al., 2008; National Amputee Statistical Database, 2009). In the United States, 54% of all existing cases of limb loss are secondary to PVD, two-thirds of which involve a comorbid diagnosis of diabetes (Ziegler-Graham et al., 2008). Amputation rates for trauma and cancer are falling (Varma, Stineman, & Dillingham, 2014). The incidence of amputation in people with PVD and diabetes has also decreased because of improvements in disease management and revascularization procedures, but remains high (Gregg et al., 2014; Jones et al., 2012; Varma et al., 2014), and the incidence of both PVD and diabetes is projected to continue rising (Alzamora et al., 2016; Boyle, Thompson, Gregg, Barker, & Williamson, 2010).

Although trauma is at present the most common cause of all-level amputations in countries with developing economies (Ephraim, Dillingham, Sector, Pezzin, & MacKenzie, 2003), the incidence of cardiovascular disease, diabetes, and PVD is also increasing rapidly (e.g., Hall, Thomsen, Henriksen, & Lohse, 2011; Mbanya, Motala, Sobngwi, Assah, & Enoru, 2010), which is likely to impact dysvascular amputation rates. Amputation as a result of military conflict or violence against civilians continues to constitute a serious public health problem in certain war-torn regions (Edwards et al., 2016; Salamon et al., 2016).

An individual's age and overall health status complicate the challenge of rehabilitation post-amputation. Patients with amputations secondary

http://dx.doi.org/10.1037/0000129-017
Handbook of Rehabilitation Psychology, Third Edition, L. A. Brenner, S. A. Reid-Arndt, T. R. Elliott, R. G. Frank, and B. Caplan (Editors-in-Chief)

to PVD or diabetes tend to be older, experience more comorbid health conditions, and are at increased risk of postoperative morbidity, mortality, and contralateral amputation, whereas traumatic limb loss is more prevalent among younger adults of working age who are otherwise healthy (Dillingham, Pezzin, & Shore, 2005; Dillingham & Pezzin, 2008; National Amputee Statistical Database, 2009). The age at which amputation is performed appears to be rising likely because of improved disease management and revascularization prior to critical limb ischemia (Carmona et al., 2005). Increasing age carries heightened risk of cognitive impairment and dementia, which present difficulties in terms of rehabilitation and recovery of mobility postamputation (Coffey, O'Keeffe, Gallagher, Desmond, & Lombard-Vance, 2012; Frengopoulos, Burley, Viana, Payne, & Hunter, 2017; Williams et al., 2014, 2015).

Regaining mobility and functioning is a primary function of rehabilitation after limb loss. A key component of this is the fitting of and learning to use a prosthetic limb. It is important to note, however, that some people are never fitted with a prosthesis, whereas others may be fitted but either abandon the prosthesis or do not maximize its use; this is particularly common among older individuals (Fletcher et al., 2001; Schoppen et al., 2003). There are many possible reasons for nonprescription or nonuse of a prosthetic limb including age, mortality, comorbidities, cognitive impairment, type and level of amputation, condition of the residual limb, dissatisfaction with the prosthesis, and individual choice or preference (Biddiss & Chau, 2007; Coffey et al., 2012; Desmond et al., 2012; Robinson, Sansam, Hirst, & Neumann, 2010).

In addition to the physical challenges associated with rehabilitation efforts and life following limb loss, there are numerous psychological and social consequences that individuals may encounter. Emotional responses including negative mood, depression, anxiety, and symptoms of posttraumatic stress, as well as changes in body image, self-concept, family and social relationships, occupational status, and personally meaningful life activities, can prove challenging. These varied and complex needs indicate the importance of including a psychologist in the multidisciplinary team (MDT). This chapter provides a detailed overview of psychosocial outcomes following limb loss and key considerations in the assessment and care of individuals with limb loss. Being aware of such outcomes in addition to physical sequelae, knowing how to appropriately measure them, and identifying appropriate psychological interventions may enable the MDT to contribute more holistically to the person living well with limb loss.

PSYCHOLOGICAL ADJUSTMENT

Depression and anxiety are commonly associated with limb loss and are more prevalent in this group than in the general population. For example, the presence of depressive symptomatology following amputation has been identified in 12.9% to 32.7% of all cases (Atherton & Robertson, 2006; Desmond & MacLachlan, 2006). In terms of anxiety, Atherton and Robertson (2006) identified 29.9% of individuals with symptoms of anxiety following limb amputation in their sample ($n = 67$), which is much higher than the 12.6% morbidity rate reported in the general adult population (Crawford, Henry, Crombie, & Taylor, 2001). Desmond and MacLachlan (2006) found that 37.5% of the 796 people with LLA in their sample had mild to severe levels of anxiety, while 35.5% of those with ULA ($n = 138$) were affected (Desmond, 2007). A systematic review by Mckechnie and John (2014) concluded that levels of depression and anxiety in those with traumatic limb amputation were higher than in the general population. In one of the relatively few available prospective studies, Singh et al. (2009) followed people with LLA over a 3-year period and found that the incidence of anxiety and depression was high immediately after amputation (23.5% for both depressive and anxiety symptoms using the HADS), decreased during inpatient rehabilitation (2.9%) but increased again after discharge (17.6% and 19.1%, respectively, at follow-up an average of 2.7 years later). They argued that the learning of new skills and reassurance offered by inpatient rehabilitation programs may account for these temporal variations. However, further longitudinal research is warranted.

Although posttraumatic stress disorder (PTSD) has received less focus than depression and anxiety in the literature to date, research indicates that higher rates occur in people with limb loss than in the general population, and symptoms appear to increase across time (Desmond & MacLachlan, 2006; Doukas et al., 2013; Phelps, Williams, Raichle, Turner, & Ehde, 2008). Recently, there has been a growing focus on mental health outcomes of military personnel who sustain limb loss in active service. The Military Extremity Trauma Amputation/Limb Salvage (METALS) study, for example, identified 40.7% of participants with unilateral LLA sustained in the U.S. military with symptoms of depression and 13.3% with possible/probable major depression; 14.8% screened positive for PTSD (Doukas et al., 2013). Finally, given the physical changes to the body following amputation, individuals with acquired limb loss are often reported to express dissatisfaction with their body image (Coffey, Gallagher, Horgan, Desmond, & MacLachlan et al., 2009; Holzer et al., 2014). The experience of depression, anxiety, PTSD, and body image disturbance have been found to be interrelated and linked with other outcomes including poorer quality of life (QoL) and self-esteem, lower levels of perceived social support, reduced prosthesis satisfaction, greater pain, and increased activity limitation. These are discussed in subsequent sections of this chapter. In addition, see Chapter 22, this volume for further discussion of military polytrauma in the post-9/11 period.

While a range of potential negative psychosocial consequences may arise from the loss of a limb, psychological adjustment to amputation is not just about redressing these but also recognizing and promoting positive sequelae. To this end, the research literature includes studies that have determined positive experiences associated with the loss of a limb (Benetato, 2011; Couture, Desrosiers, & Caron, 2011; Gallagher & MacLachlan, 2000a; Livingstone, Van De Mortel, & Taylor, 2011; Oaksford, Frude, & Cuddihy, 2005; Saradjian, Thompson, & Datta, 2008; Stutts, Bills, Erwin, & Good, 2015; Unwin, Kacperek, & Clarke, 2009). This research recognizes the importance of not solely seeing limb loss as a negative life experience. Furthermore, it underscores the importance of exploring predictors of both positive and negative outcomes. In an early study, Dunn (1996) found that people with upper and lower limb loss who found meaning in the loss of a limb had lower levels of depression, while dispositional optimism and perceiving greater control over disability were associated with greater self-esteem and lower levels of depression. Other research has also looked at the impact of adopting different coping strategies. For example, Tuncay and Musabak (2015) reported that problem-focused coping strategies predicted posttraumatic growth in Turkish military veterans with LLA injuries.

A number of recent papers (all based on the same cohort of participants) have examined the role of self-regulatory processes in adjustment to LLA (Coffey, Gallagher, & Desmond, 2014a, 2014b; Coffey, Gallagher, Desmond, & Ryall, 2014; Coffey, Gallagher, Desmond, Ryall, & Wegener, 2014; Dunne, Coffey, Gallagher, & Desmond, 2014). The term *self-regulation* describes a range of theoretical approaches that share the assumption that human behavior is organized around the pursuit of goals, which energize activities and give structure and meaning to people's lives (Carver & Scheier, 1998). The extent to which individuals are able to achieve their goals is thought to have a significant bearing on well-being, as evidenced in several studies of people with chronic illness and disability (Scheier, Carver, & Armstrong, 2012). Self-regulation is relevant to persons with limb amputation, as the impact of limb loss on physical and psychosocial functioning is likely to disrupt the attainment of valued goals in many life domains. A prospective study of 64 individuals with LLA by Coffey et al. (2014a) found that greater disturbance in the attainment of valued goals on admission to an inpatient prosthetic rehabilitation program independently predicted poorer general and social adjustment to amputation 6 months postdischarge.

According to this perspective, to avoid the adverse consequences of failing to attain valued goals and ensure that purpose in life and well-being are maintained, individuals must either overcome their difficulties through continued striving toward goal attainment (goal pursuit), or abandon/scale down threatened goals and manage resulting negative emotions (goal adjustment; Brandtstädter & Renner, 1990). Both cross-sectional (Coffey, Gallagher, Desmond, & Ryall, 2014) and longitudinal (Coffey et al., 2014b) research indicates that stronger goal pursuit and adjustment tendencies are predictive of a range of positive outcomes in people with LLA, including greater QoL and positive affect and lower self-reported disability and negative affect. A longitudinal study of 98 individuals with LLA from admission to rehabilitation up to 15 months postdischarge employed multilevel modelling (Coffey, Gallagher, Desmond, Ryall, & Wegener, 2014) to examine patterns of change in positive affect, self-reported disability, and general adjustment to limb loss. The findings demonstrated that stronger goal pursuit tendencies buffered against decreases in positive affect and promoted decreases in self-reported disability over time, whereas stronger goal adjustment tendencies enhanced increases in general adjustment, indicating that these self-regulatory processes both promote and protect well-being in the face of challenges posed by amputation. A qualitative study by Dunne et al. (2014) set out to explore the types of goal pursuit and adjustment strategies used following amputation in a sample of 30 individuals with LLA 15 months after discharge from inpatient prosthetic rehabilitation. The authors found that goal pursuit strategies centered on internal resource use, planning, technology use, and help use, while goal adjustment strategies focused on interpersonal accommodation, managing limitations, and meaning-making. Although the use of these self-regulatory strategies was adaptive for the most part, some adopted maladaptive strategies such as remaining attached to blocked goals or engaging in cognitive and behavioral avoidance. Overall, these findings indicate the potential value of developing rehabilitation-based interventions to foster adoption of goal pursuit and adjustment strategies in order to promote favorable long-term outcomes for people with LLA.

COGNITIVE FUNCTIONING

The high prevalence of dysvascularity and diabetes as precipitating factors in LLA, combined with the age at which most amputations are carried out (> 65 years and increasing; Ziegler-Graham et al., 2008), means that patients are at greater risk of having or developing impairments in cognitive functioning (Coffey et al., 2012; Marseglia et al., 2014). Such impairments may affect decisional capacity and referral to and delivery of prosthetic rehabilitation services and may lead to variations in prosthetic rehabilitation outcomes (O'Neill & Evans, 2009; Kurichi et al., 2007; Williams et al., 2015). Learning to use a prosthesis is a complex process requiring correct sequencing of a number of novel behaviors and involving memory, attention, and executive functions. Impairments in cognitive functioning could lead to difficulties in learning new skills and ultimately using prostheses optimally and safely (O'Neill & Evans, 2009; Donaghey et al., 2010).

Research evidence in this area is limited by small sample sizes, methodological and measurement variance (Coffey et al., 2012), use of categorical classifications of dementia and/or cognitive impairment (as simply present or absent) often derived from medical chart review (e.g., Carmona et al., 2005; Yu, Lam, Nettel-Aguirre, Donald, & Dukelow, 2010), and reliance on brief cognitive screening tools (e.g., O'Neill, Moran, & Gillespie, 2010; Remes, Isoaho, Vahlberg, Viitanen, & Rautava, 2010; Donaghey, McMillan, & O'Neill, 2010) that may not be sufficiently sensitive to cognitive impairments resulting from cerebrovascular disease (Pendlebury, Mariz, Bull, Mehta, & Rothwell, 2012). These limitations notwithstanding, higher cognitive functioning has been associated with longer hours of prosthesis use and better mobility outcomes (O'Neill & Evans, 2009); while diagnosis of dementia has been associated with greater risk of not using a prosthesis (Taylor et al., 2005) and cognitive impairment has been related to higher numbers of falls (Yu et al., 2010; Pauley, Devlin, & Heslin, 2006). In the only prospective longitudinal study published to date, Williams et al. (2014, 2015) examined cognitive functioning in people with PVD-related LLA ($n = 87$) across three time points (preamputation baseline, 6 weeks postsurgery, and 4 months postsurgery) and assessed functional outcomes 12 months after amputation. Assessments included the Short Portable Mental Status Questionnaire brief cognitive screen (SPMSQ; Pfeiffer, 1975), subtests of the Repeatable Battery for the Assessment of Neuropsychological Status (RBANS; Randolph, Tierney, Mohr, & Chase, 1998) including measures of memory (immediate list recall and delayed list recall) and semantic fluency (which assesses aspects of executive functioning/language), and the Wechsler Adult Intelligence Scale (WAIS III; Wechsler, 1997) digit span measure of working memory. Aggregate and individual scores across all tests ranged from average to impaired at each time point—no persons scored above average. Immediate and delayed recall improved from baseline to 6 weeks and 4 months postsurgery, respectively (Williams et al., 2014). At 12-month follow-up, findings indicated differential associations between domains of cognitive function and functional outcomes. Verbal memory (assessed at 6 weeks) was associated with longer hours of prosthesis use, community integration and participation; higher general mental status (SPMSQ; at 4 months) was associated with greater mobility and social integration; and better working memory (assessed at 6 weeks and 4 months, respectively) was associated with longer hours of prosthesis use and greater mobility. Activity restriction at 12 months was unrelated to immediate, delayed, or working memory; semantic fluency; or general mental status (Williams et al., 2015). The authors highlighted the importance of nuanced neuropsychological assessment to inform rehabilitation and care planning. Given the limitations in research to date, there is clear need for comprehensive examination of the relationships between cognitive functioning and a wide range of rehabilitation outcomes. Greater understanding of which cognitive abilities or limitations are of key importance could inform tailored rehabilitation strategies to support optimal outcomes among patients with cognitive impairments (O'Neill & Evans, 2009; O'Neill et al., 2010). For further discussion regarding assessment, see Chapter 4, this volume.

SEXUAL FUNCTIONING

Changes in the physical body and abilities can lead to negative self-image or interfere with sexual intimacy in some persons with limb loss (PwLL; Holzer et al., 2014). Sexual activity is an important factor contributing to overall QoL, yet few studies have addressed sexual functioning and well-being among individuals with amputations (Geertzen, Van Es, & Dijkstra, 2009; Henderson et al., 2016). Since Geertzen et al.'s 2009 publication of a systematic literature review of sex and sexuality following amputation (which identified just 11 studies published over the preceding 60 years), the topic has garnered increased research attention (Barrera, Teall, Barr, Silva, & Greenberg, 2010; Verschuren, Enzlin, Geertzen, Dijkstra, & Dekker, 2013; Verschuren, Geertzen, Enzlin, Dijkstra, & Dekker, 2016; Verschuren, Geertzen, Enzlin, Dijkstra, & Dekker, 2015; Verschuren, Zhdanova, et al., 2013; Henderson et al., 2016). Recent studies from both the United States and the Netherlands (Verschuren, Zhdanova, et al., 2013; Henderson et al., 2016) suggest that sexuality is rarely broached by patients or discussed by health-care professionals following limb amputation. The perceived competence and comfort levels of health-care professionals in addressing issues of sexual functioning can act as barriers to appropriate assessment and intervention (Verschuren, Enzlin, et al., 2013) and need to be addressed so that a systematic approach to discussion of sexual functioning following amputation, and thus more holistic rehabilitation, can be achieved (Henderson et al., 2016; Wegener, Hofkamp, & Ehde, 2008).

PAIN

Pain is commonly experienced following limb amputation and can be persistent in the long term and difficult to treat (Desmond & MacLachlan, 2010; Gallagher, Franchignoni, Giordano, & MacLachlan, 2010; Alviar, Hale, & Dungca, 2016). Pain can affect multiple sites including the phantom limb (i.e., painful sensation perceived in the amputated body part) and residual limb/stump; areas beyond the amputated limb can also be affected as a result of compensatory movements (e.g., increased forces on the intact limb), secondary musculoskeletal pathologies, and comorbidities (Gailey, Allen, Castles, Kucharik, & Roeder, 2008). Individuals with ULA are at increased risk for pain in the neck/upper back and shoulders (Postema et al., 2016a; Østlie, Franklin, Skjeldal, Skrondal, & Magnus, 2011); overuse syndromes affecting the intact limb—in particular, carpal tunnel syndrome—are also common (Østlie et al., 2011; Burger & Vidmar, 2016). Individuals with LLA are at significantly increased risk for chronic back pain compared with the general population (Ehde et al., 2001).

Pain has been associated with interference in participation in life activities (Amtmann, Morgan, Kim, & Hafner, 2015), restricted prosthesis use (Raichle et al., 2008), poor QoL (Hanley et al., 2009; van der Schans, Geertzen, Schoppen, & Dijkstra, 2002), interference with employment (Pezzin, Dillingham, & MacKenzie, 2000), and negative affect (Darnall et al., 2005). Appropriate pain assessment and multidisciplinary management, incorporating physical, psychological, and social factors, are critical to mitigating these impacts (Ehde & Wegener, 2008). For additional information about pain, assessment, and management, please refer to Chapter 14, this volume.

PARTICIPATION

The majority of research on rehabilitation outcomes following limb loss has centered on physical functioning and activity. According to the World Health Organization (WHO) International Classification of Functioning, Disability and Health (ICF; WHO, 2001), however, disability can also be caused by dysfunction at the level of participation, defined as involvement in life situations. Although amputation is likely to have a considerable influence on participation, few studies have explicitly examined this outcome among persons with limb loss (Gallagher, O'Donovan, Doyle, & Desmond, 2011). The limited evidence available indicates that following amputation, participation restrictions are often experienced in the areas of sports and physical recreation, leisure and cultural activities, family life, and employment (Couture, Caron, & Desrosiers, 2010; Deans, Burns, McGarry, Murray, & Mutrie, 2012; Gallagher, O'Donovan, Doyle, & Desmond, 2011; van Twillert, Stuive, Geertzen, Postema, & Lettinga, 2014). Research on children and adolescents with limb absence/loss indicates few participation restrictions, with the exception of finding suitable work or education and certain social and skill-based activities (de Jong et al., 2012; Lankhorst et al., 2017; Michielsen, van Wijk, & Ketelaar, 2011). Such restrictions appear to be linked with a range of personal limitations (e.g., functional abilities, balance confidence, social discomfort, public self-consciousness, emotional impact of amputation, satisfaction with prosthesis) and environmental constraints (e.g., lack of accessibility, climate, transportation issues; Couture, Caron, & Desrosiers, 2010; Donovan-Hall, Yardley, & Watts, 2002; Dunne, Coffey, Gallagher, Desmond, & Ryall, 2015; Gallagher et al., 2011; Miller, Deathe, Speechley, & Koval, 2001; Murray & Forshaw, 2013). Further research on participation among individuals with limb loss, including children and adolescents, its trajectory over time, and its associations with personal and environmental factors is needed to facilitate improved management and planning in this patient group at an individual, service, and societal level (Gallagher et al., 2011).

EDUCATIONAL AND VOCATIONAL CAPACITIES

Engagement in vocational/educational pursuits is an integral component of participation in life activities for those of working age. Benefits of work following limb loss include economic security, increased opportunities for social interaction, and enhanced psychological well-being (Postema et al., 2016b). Many individuals experience difficulties in rejoining the workforce after limb loss. Amputation is associated with loss of employment and income, lost work time, and reduced opportunities for promotion, hiring, and training (van der Sluis, Hartman, Schoppen, & Dijkstra, 2009). About two thirds of people return to employment following amputation, many working part-time only (Burger, 2009). The vast majority of soldiers who experience combat-related amputation do not remain in military service following limb loss; those who do often have to take on less physically demanding roles (Hurley, Rivera, Wenke, & Krueger, 2015). Success in returning to work is influenced by an extensive range of sociodemographic, amputation/prosthesis-related, functional and employment-related factors (Burger, 2009). Age and preamputation function, prosthesis use, level of education, and support from employers play particularly important roles (Hebert & Burger, 2016; Postema et al., 2016b).

Upper and lower limb amputations present distinct occupational challenges because of the different physical limitations incurred and degree of functionality offered by prostheses. Whereas up to two thirds of individuals who experience LLA are able to return to their previous occupation, those with ULA are often required to seek alternative employment. Such work tends to be more complex and less physically demanding and requires a higher level of education (Burger, 2009). For those who remain in the same workplace, adjustments such as changes in workload or extra training may be required to facilitate their ongoing participation (van der Sluis et al., 2009). Despite these challenges, levels of job satisfaction among people with amputations tend to be very high (Schoppen et al., 2002; van der Sluis et al., 2009). Research indicates that individuals who change their occupation after limb loss integrate more successfully and experience greater job satisfaction than those who remain in their old jobs (Schoppen et al., 2001). These findings indicate the potential value of providing vocational rehabilitation and retraining to all people of working age following amputation. Vocational support services are not widely available at present, however, and represent a significant unmet need in this patient group (Archer, Castillo, MacKenzie, Bosse, & the LEAP Study Group, 2010).

SOCIAL AND BEHAVIORAL FUNCTIONING

The social impact of amputation can be substantial and may require negotiation of evolving roles, relationships, and identities (Hamill, Carson, & Dorahy, 2010; Murray & Forshaw, 2013). Amputation sometimes gives rise to increasing social constraints and feelings of social discomfort, public self-consciousness, and perceived social stigma, which are associated with negative psychosocial sequelae such as activity restriction (Williamson, 1995), poorer general and social adjustment to limb loss (Atherton & Robertson, 2006), and heightened anxiety and depressive symptoms (Atherton & Robertson, 2006; Kratz et al., 2010), but appear to be ameliorated to some extent through appropriate prosthetic prescription (Donovan-Hall et al., 2002; Murray, 2005, 2009).

Social support can be a critical resource in the management of stressful life events. In the case of amputation, individuals with good social resources may benefit not only from the practical support provided by others in terms of renegotiating their physical and social environments following limb loss, but also the emotional support and companionship they offer, which is important in helping them come to terms with this life-changing experience (Williams et al., 2004). However, it appears that amputation poses a risk for social isolation, particularly among those who are older and unmarried, with nontraumatic etiologies (Demet et al., 2003; Williams et al., 2004).

Social support is a broad construct that is usually assessed in terms of either social integration or perceived social support (Cohen, Underwood, & Gottlieb, 2000). *Social integration* is defined as an objective state relating to the number of contacts and interaction a person has with his or her wider social network (Hawkins et al., 2016). Social integration appears to be lower in people with amputations compared with those without a disability (Williams et al., 2004) and is associated with outcomes such as walking ability, occupational function, and QoL (Williams et al., 2004; Hawkins et al., 2016). *Perceived social support* refers to the quality of the social resources a person perceives to be available to her or him and has been linked both cross-sectionally and prospectively with a range of positive physical and psychological outcomes, including lower depressed affect (Rybarczyk et al., 1992; Rybarczyk, Nyenhuis, Nicholas, Cash, & Kaiser, 1995); fewer activity restrictions (Williamson, Schulz, Bridges, & Behan, 1994); better QoL (Asano, Rushton, Miller, & Deathe, 2008); better self-reported health (Bosse et al., 2002); reduced pain interference (Jensen et al., 2002; Williams et al., 2004); increased mobility, life satisfaction, and occupational functioning (Williams et al., 2004); higher positive affect; and greater general adjustment to amputation (Unwin et al., 2009).

ADJUSTMENT TO DISABILITY: FAMILY

The importance of the practical and emotional support provided by family members in helping people to adjust to limb loss is widely recognized (Murray & Forshaw, 2013). Families play a critical role in the postamputation recovery process and often take on the most responsibility for the provision of care, especially partners or spouses who often act as primary caregivers. Providing long-term care to a person with chronic illness or disability can be an all-consuming task that can have significant impacts, both positive and negative, on family members' lives and relationships (Adelman, Tmanova, Delgado, Dion, & Lachs, 2014). Despite this, little attention has been paid to the impact of limb loss on the family (Desmond et al., 2012). Two recent papers examining QoL in caregiver spouses of Iranian veterans with war-related bilateral LLA found poorer outcomes in certain domains (bodily pain, general health) but better in others (role emotion) compared with the general population, despite their spouse's limb loss having occurred more than two decades previously (Ganjparvar, Mousavi, Masumi, Soroush, & Montazeri, 2016; Moradi, Ebrahimzadeh, & Soroush, 2015). Factors associated with poorer QoL among caregivers included having a spouse who is unemployed, experiences mental health difficulties, or was hospitalized within the previous year, while having a job outside the home was associated with a greater QoL.

Although these findings are of limited scope, they provide some indication of the importance and potential value of offering ongoing support not only to the person who undergoes amputation but also to his or her family members, both individually and as a unit. Further research is clearly needed to explore the experiences of family members following a loved one's limb loss, especially those who take on primary caregiving duties, and the impact on family roles and dynamics. The adaptation of existing interventions developed to improve caregiver outcomes in similarly debilitating acquired physical conditions such as stroke or spinal cord injury (Cheng, Chair, & Chau, 2014; Schulz et al., 2009) or development of novel interventions specifically targeting this group should also be considered.

ASSESSMENT

In working with PwLL, psychologists can draw meaningfully on the wide range of generic assessments that are available to them to assess psychological and social issues relevant to the individual. This assessment foregrounds the psychosocial experience of the individual in a field where there is an inevitable emphasis on physical functioning and prosthetic outcomes. Such assessment also plays an important role in screening for at-risk areas (e.g., anxiety, depression, PTSD, body image disturbance, cognitive impairment, perceived social support, participation restrictions), facilitating communication, guiding consultations, informing rehabilitation goals, identifying appropriate and tailoring interventions, monitoring progress, assessing outcomes, and evaluating practice. In addition to the generic assessments available to psychologists, there are some amputation-specific instruments (see Table 16.1); these have predominantly taken a broad adjustment and QoL perspective but play an important role in their particular relevance to target respondents and the specific insight they provide into experiences of amputation and its consequences. All are self-report measures and have been psychometrically evaluated. See Chapter 4, this volume for a review of assessment strategies and instruments.

INTERVENTION

We have noted a range of issues that may arise following limb loss and pointed out that many individuals experience significant psychological distress after amputation. It is equally important to note that most adapt well and do not experience significant distress. Thus, early screening and, where necessary, more comprehensive assessment are needed to determine the treatment needs of the individual. For some, psychological intervention may be used to promote adaptation and growth. For others, who develop significant depression, anxiety, substance use, or other maladaptive responses, psychologists may need to use a range of treatment options.

There are multiple considerations when selecting intervention options. First, with rare exceptions, the efficacy of specific interventions is not well established for PwLL. Rather, the psychologist must utilize clinical judgment to select evidence-based approaches that have been developed and established in other populations. Second, psychologists should include a range of interventions in the treatment plan, expanding the focus from one-on-one treatment to include family, peer support, and

TABLE 16.1

Amputation-Specific Psychosocial Outcome Measures

Name and authors	No. of items	Domains/subscales
Prosthesis Evaluation Questionnaire (Legro et al., 1998)	82	Ambulation Appearance Frustration Perceived response Residual limb health Social burden Sounds Utility Well-being
Trinity Amputation and Prosthesis Experience Scales (TAPES-R; Gallagher & MacLachlan, 2000b; Gallagher et al., 2010)	64	General adjustment Social adjustment Adjustment to limitation Activity restriction Aesthetic satisfaction with prosthesis Functional satisfaction with prosthesis
Orthotic Prosthetic User's Survey (OPUS; Heinemann et al., 2003).	88	The Upper Extremity Functional Status Survey The Lower Extremity Functional Status Survey OPUS-Health Related Quality of Life Index OPUS-Satisfaction With Devices OPUS-Satisfaction With Services
Questionnaire for Persons With a Trans-femoral Amputation (Hagberg, Brånemark, & Hägg, 2004)	70	Prosthetic Use Score (Use) Prosthetic Mobility Score (Mobility) Problem Score (Problem) Global Score (Global)

self-management approaches. Additionally, providers must consider assessment and intervention opportunities across the continuum of care. Finally, competent rehabilitation psychologists provide individual, family, and couples interventions to promote adjustment to disability, behavioral management and team consultation, sexual counseling, and pain management. They are also able to connect PwLL to the peer and self-management resources in the limb loss community.

Early Screening

Early screening can be considered a form of intervention that is appropriate for all persons experiencing amputation. Screening provides an opportunity to provide assurance and affirmation for individuals who are adapting well and to intervene early with those who are experiencing barriers to recovery. Given the high prevalence of rates of emotional distress in PwLL, screening—using established instruments that can be completed by patients with basic reading skills—should be conducted as part of routine postoperative follow-up care.

While persons with traumatic amputation are a minority of PwLL, there is a large literature documenting the multiple factors affecting outcomes after traumatic injury. The American Trauma Society developed the Trauma Survivors Network (Bradford et al., 2011). Part of the suite of services offered by the Trauma Survivors Network is an online recovery assessment tool (see http://www.traumasurvivorsnetwork.org/recovery_assessments) that can be self-administered by patients with either a computer or mobile device and assesses risk factors (pain, PTSD, depression, and alcohol and/or tobacco use) and protective factors (resilience, social support, self-efficacy for return to work, and managing the financial burden of trauma). The recovery assessment tool provides standardized feedback and recommendations for the patient and the provider. The health care professional can review the feedback and make recommendations with the patient to establish the basis for follow-up planning and referral. The online version is a convenient alternative to paper-and-pencil screening.

Psychotherapy

Psychotherapy can take many forms and can utilize a variety of techniques. While data support the beneficial effects of psychotherapy and health and behavior interventions across a variety of patient populations (Chambless, 2005), there are no published controlled trials of psychotherapy specifically focused on PwLL. Most, but not all, of the evidence-based treatments to address psychological difficulties common after limb loss use cognitive–behavioral, behavioral, or interpersonal techniques (Chambless, 2005). Data support specific treatment approaches, as well as suggesting that the therapeutic relationship accounts for much of the treatment benefit (Wampold, 2001). Treatment of depression and PTSD should be guided by evidenced-based approaches that have been established in other populations, as the findings are likely to generalize to PwLL. While there is no specific evidence in persons with limb loss, it is also likely that social problems, such as dealing with social stigma and increasing social skills, may also be addressed effectively with cognitive behavior therapy (CBT; Wegener et al., 2008). Interpersonal psychotherapy (IPT; Klerman, Weissman, Rounsaville, & Chevron, 1994) is appropriate for treatment of acute psychological distress as well as prolonged maintenance of symptoms that are mild to moderate in severity. IPT focuses on relationship issues, but it also takes into account biopsychosocial factors that contribute to the problem.

Coping Skills Training

Coping behaviors that are active and goal-oriented are more helpful to the patient (Desmond & Gallagher, 2008; Elfström, 2007). Interventions focused on building coping skills should include (a) analysis of the situation and current coping techniques, (b) description of the problem, (c) goal setting, and (d) modification of the coping strategies. Catastrophizing, a cognitive response to an event that is marked by exaggerated negative expectations and concerns, has been found to predict both self-reported and objective measures of disability in a variety of chronic pain conditions (Sullivan et al., 2001). Among individuals with limb loss and phantom limb pain, catastrophizing predicts increased pain interference, depressive symptoms, self-reported disability, and psychosocial dysfunction (Hill, Niven, & Knussen, 1995; Jensen et al., 2002). CBT interventions for catastrophizing focus on monitoring, challenging, and changing negative thoughts as well as behavioral activation to increase self-efficacy. Coping strategies such as distraction, positive self-talk, and increasing activity levels are associated with adjustment to chronic pain (Jensen, Turner, Romano, & Karoly, 1991) and may promote psychological health following limb loss.

Recently, there has been increased emphasis on the importance of cognitive processing in adaptation to injury and illness, in PwLL specifically (Phelps et al., 2008). Effective cognitive processing utilizes active meaning-making, revising goals and priorities, and benefit finding. In PwLL, it has been shown that these positive cognitive processing strategies are related to posttraumatic growth (Phelps et al., 2008). This relationship also complements prior research, indicating that disability-related acceptance is important for positive adjustment following amputation (Gallagher & MacLachlan, 2001; Oaksford et al., 2005). Including treatment interventions that assist individuals in revising goals, accepting change, and finding meaning may be of benefit to PwLL.

Based on the dual-process model of adaptive self-regulation (Brandtstädter & Renner, 1990), recent work in PwLL suggests that in early rehabilitation fostering the use of goal pursuit (assimilative efforts to actively change unsatisfactory life circumstances or behavior to correspond with goals/preferences) and, when assimilative efforts become ineffective, utilizing goal adjustment (accommodative mode) may help to promote favorable long-term outcomes (Coffey, Gallagher, Desmond, Ryall, & Wegener, 2014). Recently developed interventions for people with rheumatic diseases (Vriezekolk et al., 2013) and polyarthritis (Arends et al., 2017), including sessions specifically targeted at enhancing goal pursuit and adjustment, have produced positive initial findings and may be useful for PwLL.

Pain Management

PwLL may present with a variety of pain problems. A wide range of psychological pain treatments have been used, ranging from cognitive–behavioral interventions, mindfulness, and hypnosis to biofeedback, imagery, mirror treatment, and virtual reality. With the exception of mirror therapy for phantom limb pain (PLP), there is little data on the efficacy in PwLL, and clinicians must be guided by data from other populations.

Expert panels and meta-analyses have found good evidence for the use of cognitive behavioral interventions for chronic pain management (Ehde, Dillworth, & Turner, 2014). These interventions typically include components of the behavioral model, particularly relaxation training, and some components of operant conditioning. However, an emphasis is also placed on cognitive factors, such as attitudes and beliefs that underlie maladaptive emotional and behavioral responses to pain. Mindfulness interventions have been demonstrated to have small effects on pain intensity, moderate effects on negative affective states such as depression and anxiety, and moderate effects on QoL outcomes (Chiesa & Serretti, 2011; Reiner, Tibi, & Lipsitz, 2013). It should be emphasized that reduction in pain intensity is not the goal of mindfulness interventions. The focus is on appreciation for life in the context of pain (Chiesa & Serretti, 2011; Reiner et al., 2013). Along these lines, acceptance and commitment therapy (ACT; Hayes, Strosahl, & Wilson, 2003) is a form of behavioral therapy that integrates mindfulness with commitment and behavior change strategies (Dahl, Wilson, Luciano, & Hayes, 2005). The past decade has seen an increase in investigation of the utility of ACT in reducing emotional and physical disability related to pain.

Although there is still no treatment for PLP that is reliably effective, other interventions used by psychologists include transcutaneous electrical nerve stimulation, biofeedback, relaxation therapy, and hypnotherapy (Ehde & Wegener, 2008; MacIver & Lloyd, 2010). Recently there has also been considerable interest in the use of mental imagery and virtual and augmented reality (Brodie, Whyte, & Niven, 2007; Cole, Crowle, Austwick, & Henderson Slater, 2009; Desmond, O'Neill, de Paor, Mac Darby, & MacLachlan, 2006). Based on the assumption that PLP may arise because of a conflict between the visual and proprioceptive experience of an amputated limb, Ramachandran and Rogers-Ramachandran (1996) suggested that illusionary movement of an amputated limb might alleviate pain by aligning the experiences or by helping to replace a remembered image of a painfully twisted limb with an image in a more relaxed posture. They were able to demonstrate pain relief for some patients, not for others, but spurred great interest in the area. Although subsequent research has shown some promise (Darnall, 2009), there have also been reports that the procedure is distressing and painful for some (Chan et al., 2007). Based on the same principles, the use of augmented reality (using computer simulation) has also had mixed results (Desmond et al., 2006). Illusory visual representations of the missing limb (through imagery, virtual or augmented reality techniques) can improve the pain experience of at least some people with PLP. There is a dearth of research on PLP treatment in pediatric populations, although at least one case study has reported positive outcomes (Ramsey, Karlson, & Collier, 2017). Larger scale studies in both adults and children that report long-term follow-up are needed; clinicians should be aware of the potential for such interventions to cause distress and increase pain (Moseley, Gallace, & Spence, 2008).

Self-Management

It important to emphasize that most PwLL will not meet the criteria for clinical depression, generalized anxiety disorder, or PTSD. However, even those who have subclinical symptoms of distress and anxiety may benefit from services that address maladaptive coping responses and enhance resilience and positive coping mechanisms. Collaborative, patient-centered models of care emphasize the need for patients and their families to assume greater responsibility for their care and call for providers to support patients and families in these activities (Bodenheimer, Wagner, & Grumbach, 2002; Institute of Medicine Committee on Quality of Health Care in America, 2001). Empowering patients to take charge of their recovery through increasing self-efficacy and activation is a central component to these models. An increasing body of literature suggests that two approaches are particularly helpful in promoting patient activation: cognitive, behavioral-based, self-management programs and peer support programs.

Self-management (SM) interventions incorporate the principles of CBT; key elements include knowledge, self-monitoring, skills acquisition and problem-solving (Lorig & Holman, 2003). SM approaches have gained widespread application with chronic conditions in which pain and disability are common (Wegener et al., 2008). Given secondary conditions such as depression and pain that accompany limb amputation, interventions that specifically focus on preventing or reducing these have been developed.

One such intervention is the Promoting Amputee Life Skills (PALS) self-management course. This intervention consists of eight weekly 90-minute group sessions followed by a booster session 2 weeks later. The groups are led by trained leaders, one of whom is a person with limb loss. The PALS intervention was compared with support group participation in a randomized controlled trial with PwLL (Wegener, Mackenzie, Ephraim, Ehde, & Williams, 2009). Compared with the control group, PALS participants were less likely to report symptoms of depression and were less bothered about limitations of everyday function; they also reported better function, higher levels of general self-efficacy, and more positive mood. The effects were greatest for participants who completed the program, patients younger than 65 years, and those who were less than 3 years postamputation, suggesting that early intervention may be more effective (Wegener et al., 2009). There is the potential to deliver SM interventions using online technologies. The PALS program is available online through the Amputee Coalition (http://www.palsamputeelifeskills.org/). As with other online programs for other populations (Beevers et al., 2017), the PALS program has the potential to reduce symptoms and improve outcomes.

For individuals who experience amputation as a result of trauma, the NextSteps self-management program is available online (http://nextstepsonline.org) and in-person at trauma centers that participate in the Trauma Survivors Network. The online version provides a strategy for connecting trauma survivors throughout the United States and teaches them the essential skills of SM. The SM literature indicates that programs incorporating social support and peer interaction have the greatest effects in changing behavior and maintaining these gains. Thus, delivering the SM program in the context of social interaction and support may enhance an individual's ability to achieve positive outcomes.

Peer Visitation and Support

Peer interactions and support groups are premised on the idea that through exposure to successful individuals with similar illnesses or injuries, less experienced persons can learn and adopt more effective behaviors and improve social support (Wegener et al., 2008). Support groups can form part of formal rehabilitation programs or may be facilitated via patient advocacy/consumer organizations. There has been widespread adoption of these programs; however, the data on efficacy, timing, characteristics of effective peer mentors, and who benefits and who may not, are limited. There is evidence indicating these approaches can be effective for depression (Pfeiffer, Heisler, Piette, Rogers, & Valenstein, 2011), cancer (Helgeson, Cohen, Schulz, & Yasko, 2000), and diabetes (Tang, Ayala, Cherrington, & Rana, 2011). Peer discussion groups may be more helpful for individuals who lack support but may be harmful for those who have high levels of support (Helgeson et al., 2000). When positive outcomes are reported in studies, the most favorable findings are greater self-efficacy, higher QoL, and fewer depressive symptoms (Tang et al., 2011).

The Peer Visitor Program offered by the Amputee Coalition of America (http://www.amputee-coalition.org) is perhaps the most widely used model in the context of amputation. The Amputee Coalition has now trained and certified a network of more than one thousand peer visitors (including patients with amputations and their families) throughout the United States, most of whom are affiliated with one or more health-care facilities (Butcher, 2009). A peer visit may be requested from the organization (Amputee Coalition; U.S. Armed Forces Amputee Patient Care Program). Both the Amputee Coalition of America and the American Trauma Society provide resources for establishing hospital-based peer visitation programs. Peer visitation is an integral part of the U.S. Armed Forces Amputee Patient Program and is highly valued among service members with combat-related amputations. While peer support is often welcomed by PwLL, the specific benefits to amputation patients have yet to be empirically established.

Intervention Across the Continuum of Care

While rehabilitation psychologists have traditionally provided services to PwLL on the inpatient rehabilitation unit and in the outpatient setting, there is a growing recognition that rehabilitation psychology principles and skills may be of use throughout the continuum of care ranging from the preoperative period to postcare community settings. In the United States and other upper-middle-income countries, most amputations are nontraumatic and are planned to address complications of chronic disease. Little attention has been devoted to the period of amputation care preceding surgery, during which there is the opportunity to prepare the individual psychologically for amputation. Providing education, addressing fears, connecting to successful peer role models and the limb loss community, identifying coping and social support resources, and focusing on the individual's enduring characteristics at this juncture have the potential to improve adaptation. Individuals who require care in the intensive care unit (ICU) encounter an environment that may provoke anxiety, helplessness, humiliation due to the hospital procedures, loss of privacy, threat of death or further trauma, or an altered state of consciousness. There is a growing literature (Jackson & Jutte, 2016; Stucky, Jutte, Warren, Jackson, & Merbitz, 2016) that supports the need for rehabilitation psychology services in the ICU environment (also see Chapter 28, this volume). As the individual progresses through the care continuum, it is critical to connect the individual to the limb loss community to access opportunities for peer support, social and leisure pursuits, and advocacy.

CONCLUSION

Rehabilitation psychology research and practice can make a significant contribution to the lives and care of people with limb loss. However, many opportunities for the continued advancement of its scientific base and its application to the development of clinical services for people with limb loss remain. Indeed, when one considers the broader global burden of amputation and the limited formal psychology input in many settings, these needs are considerably magnified.

Throughout this chapter, we have identified pertinent areas in need of further understanding, including the role of cognitive functioning, sexual functioning, substance use, participation in life activities, and peer support on outcomes. The impact of limb loss on family members and carers also requires further research toward a stronger understanding. Developing and examining ways to promote living well with limb loss is an enduring priority for rehabilitation psychologists. In this regard, ongoing efforts to establish the efficacy of specific psychological interventions are paramount. Conversely, where there is an existing evidence base for specific interventions (e.g., PALS, NextSteps), continuing development work, such as investigating ways of extending their reach and impact by making them available online, is required. Recent research also highlights the potential of developing interventions that target self-regulatory strategies (e.g., goal pursuit, adjustment strategies) in promoting favorable long-term outcomes for people living with limb loss.

References

Adelman, R. D., Tmanova, L. L., Delgado, D., Dion, S., & Lachs, M. S. (2014). Caregiver burden: A clinical review. *JAMA, 311*, 1052–1060. http://dx.doi.org/10.1001/jama.2014.304

Alviar, M. J. M., Hale, T., & Dungca, M. (2016). Pharmacologic interventions for treating phantom limb pain. *Cochrane Database of Systematic Reviews, 10*, CD006380.

Alzamora, M. T., Forés, R., Pera, G., Baena-Díez, J. M., Heras, A., Sorribes, M., . . . Torán, P. (2016). Incidence of peripheral arterial disease in the ARTPER population cohort after 5 years of follow-up. *BMC Cardiovascular Disorders, 16*, 8. http://dx.doi.org/10.1186/s12872-015-0170-6

Amtmann, D., Morgan, S. J., Kim, J., & Hafner, B. J. (2015). Health-related profiles of people with lower limb loss. *Archives of Physical Medicine and Rehabilitation, 96*, 1474–1483. http://dx.doi.org/10.1016/j.apmr.2015.03.024

Archer, K. R., Castillo, R. C., MacKenzie, E. J., Bosse, M. J., & the LEAP Study Group. (2010). Perceived need and unmet need for vocational, mental health, and other support services after severe lower-extremity trauma. *Archives of Physical Medicine and Rehabilitation, 91*, 774–780. http://dx.doi.org/10.1016/j.apmr.2010.01.006

Arends, R. Y., Bode, C., Taal, E., & Van de Laar, M. A. (2017). A mixed-methods process evaluation of a goal management intervention for patients with polyarthritis. *Psychology & Health, 32*, 38–60. http://dx.doi.org/10.1080/08870446.2016.1240173

Asano, M., Rushton, P., Miller, W. C., & Deathe, B. A. (2008). Predictors of quality of life among individuals who have a lower limb amputation. *Prosthetics and Orthotics International*, *32*, 231–243. http://dx.doi.org/10.1080/03093640802024955

Atherton, R., & Robertson, N. (2006). Psychological adjustment to lower limb amputation amongst prosthesis users. *Disability and Rehabilitation*, *28*, 1201–1209. http://dx.doi.org/10.1080/09638280600551674

Barrera, M., Teall, T., Barr, R., Silva, M., & Greenberg, M. (2010). Sexual function in adolescent and young adult survivors of lower extremity bone tumors. *Pediatric Blood & Cancer*, *55*, 1370–1376. http://dx.doi.org/10.1002/pbc.22761

Beevers, C. G., Pearson, R., Hoffman, J. S., Foulser, A. A., Shumake, J., & Meyer, B. (2017). Effectiveness of an Internet intervention (Deprexis) for depression in a united states adult sample: A parallel-group pragmatic randomized controlled trial. *Journal of Consulting and Clinical Psychology*, *85*, 367–380. http://dx.doi.org/10.1037/ccp0000171

Benetato, B. B. (2011). Posttraumatic growth among Operation Enduring Freedom and Operation Iraqi Freedom amputees. *Journal of Nursing Scholarship*, *43*, 412–420. http://dx.doi.org/10.1111/j.1547-5069.2011.01421.x

Biddiss, E., & Chau, T. (2007). Upper-limb prosthetics: Critical factors in device abandonment. *American Journal of Physical Medicine & Rehabilitation*, *86*, 977–987. http://dx.doi.org/10.1097/PHM.0b013e3181587f6c

Bodenheimer, T., Wagner, E. H., & Grumbach, K. (2002). Improving primary care for patients with chronic illness. *JAMA*, *288*, 1775–1779. http://dx.doi.org/10.1001/jama.288.14.1775

Bosse, M. J., MacKenzie, E. J., Kellam, J. F., Burgess, A. R., Webb, L. X., Swiontkowski, M. F., . . . Castillo, R. C. (2002). An analysis of outcomes of reconstruction or amputation after leg-threatening injuries. *The New England Journal of Medicine*, *347*, 1924–1931. http://dx.doi.org/10.1056/NEJMoa012604

Boyle, J. P., Thompson, T. J., Gregg, E. W., Barker, L. E., & Williamson, D. F. (2010). Projection of the year 2050 burden of diabetes in the US adult population: Dynamic modeling of incidence, mortality, and prediabetes prevalence. *Population Health Metrics*, *8*, 29. http://dx.doi.org/10.1186/1478-7954-8-29

Bradford, A. N., Castillo, R. C., Carlini, A. R., Wegener, S. T., Teter, H., Jr., & Mackenzie, E. J. (2011). The Trauma Survivors Network: Survive. Connect. Rebuild. *The Journal of Trauma and Acute Care Surgery*, *70*, 1557–1560. http://dx.doi.org/10.1097/TA.0b013e3182196e7e

Brandtstädter, J., & Renner, G. (1990). Tenacious goal pursuit and flexible goal adjustment: Explication and age-related analysis of assimilative and accommodative strategies of coping. *Psychology and Aging*, *5*, 58–67. http://dx.doi.org/10.1037/0882-7974.5.1.58

Brodie, E. E., Whyte, A., & Niven, C. A. (2007). Analgesia through the looking-glass? A randomized controlled trial investigating the effect of viewing a "virtual" limb upon phantom limb pain, sensation and movement. *European Journal of Pain*, *11*, 428–436. http://dx.doi.org/10.1016/j.ejpain.2006.06.002

Burger, H. (2009). Return to work after amputation. In C. Murray (Ed.), *Amputation, prosthesis use, and phantom limb pain* (pp. 101–114). New York, NY: Springer. http://dx.doi.org/10.1007/978-0-387-87462-3_7

Burger, H., & Vidmar, G. (2016). A survey of overuse problems in patients with acquired or congenital upper limb deficiency. *Prosthetics and Orthotics International*, *40*, 497–502. http://dx.doi.org/10.1177/0309364615584658

Butcher, L. (2009). Amputee network provides peer support. *Bulletin of the American College of Surgeons*, *94*(9), 20–23.

Carmona, G. A., Hoffmeyer, P., Herrmann, F. R., Vaucher, J., Tschopp, O., Lacraz, A., & Vischer, U. M. (2005). Major lower limb amputations in the elderly observed over ten years: The role of diabetes and peripheral arterial disease. *Diabetes & Metabolism*, *31*, 449–454. http://dx.doi.org/10.1016/S1262-3636(07)70215-X

Carver, C. S., & Scheier, M. F. (1998). *On the self-regulation of behavior*. New York, NY: Cambridge University Press. http://dx.doi.org/10.1017/CBO9781139174794

Chambless, D. L. (2005). Compendium of empirically supported therapies. In G. P. Koocher, J. Norcross, & S. Hill (Eds.), *Psychologists' desk reference* (2nd ed.; pp. 183–192). New York, NY: Oxford University Press.

Chan, B. L., Witt, R., Charrow, A. P., Magee, A., Howard, R., Pasquina, P. F., . . . Tsao, J. W. (2007). Mirror therapy for phantom limb pain. *The New England Journal of Medicine*, *357*, 2206–2207. http://dx.doi.org/10.1056/NEJMc071927

Cheng, H. Y., Chair, S. Y., & Chau, J. P.-C. (2014). The effectiveness of psychosocial interventions for stroke family caregivers and stroke survivors: A systematic review and meta-analysis. *Patient Education & Counseling*, *95*, 30–44. http://dx.doi.org/10.1016/j.pec.2014.01.005

Chiesa, A., & Serretti, A. (2011). Mindfulness-based interventions for chronic pain: A systematic review of the evidence. *The Journal of Alternative and Complementary Medicine*, *17*, 83–93. http://dx.doi.org/10.1089/acm.2009.0546

Coffey, L., Gallagher, P., & Desmond, D. (2014a). A prospective study of the importance of life goal characteristics and goal adjustment capacities in longer term psychosocial adjustment to lower limb amputation. *Clinical Rehabilitation*, *28*, 196–205. http://dx.doi.org/10.1177/0269215513497736

Coffey, L., Gallagher, P., & Desmond, D. (2014b). Goal pursuit and goal adjustment as predictors of disability and quality of life among individuals with a lower limb amputation: A prospective study. *Archives of Physical Medicine and Rehabilitation*, *95*, 244–252. http://dx.doi.org/10.1016/j.apmr.2013.08.011

Coffey, L., Gallagher, P., Desmond, D., & Ryall, N. (2014). Goal pursuit, goal adjustment, and affective well-being following lower limb amputation. *British Journal of Health Psychology*, *19*, 409–424. http://dx.doi.org/10.1111/bjhp.12051

Coffey, L., Gallagher, P., Desmond, D., Ryall, N., & Wegener, S. T. (2014). Goal management tendencies predict trajectories of adjustment to lower limb amputation up to 15 months post rehabilitation discharge. *Archives of Physical Medicine and Rehabilitation*, *95*, 1895–1902. http://dx.doi.org/10.1016/j.apmr.2014.05.012

Coffey, L., Gallagher, P., Horgan, O., Desmond, D., & MacLachlan, M. (2009). Psychosocial adjustment to diabetes-related lower limb amputation. *Diabetic Medicine*, *26*, 1063–1067. http://dx.doi.org/10.1111/j.1464-5491.2009.02802.x

Coffey, L., O'Keeffe, F., Gallagher, P., Desmond, D., & Lombard-Vance, R. (2012). Cognitive functioning in persons with lower limb amputations: A review. *Disability and Rehabilitation*, *34*, 1950–1964. http://dx.doi.org/10.3109/09638288.2012.667190

Cohen, S., Underwood, L. G., & Gottlieb, B. H. (Eds.). (2000). *Social support measurement and intervention: A guide for health and social scientists*. Oxford, England: Oxford University Press. http://dx.doi.org/10.1093/med:psych/9780195126709.001.0001

Cole, J., Crowle, S., Austwick, G., & Henderson Slater, D. (2009). Exploratory findings with virtual reality for phantom limb pain; from stump motion to agency and analgesia. *Disability and Rehabilitation*, *31*, 846–854. http://dx.doi.org/10.1080/09638280802355197

Couture, M., Caron, C. D., & Desrosiers, J. (2010). Leisure activities following a lower limb amputation. *Disability and Rehabilitation*, *32*, 57–64. http://dx.doi.org/10.3109/09638280902998797

Couture, M., Desrosiers, J., & Caron, C. D. (2011). Cognitive appraisal and perceived benefits of dysvascular lower limb amputation: A longitudinal study. *Archives of Gerontology and Geriatrics*, *52*, 5–11. http://dx.doi.org/10.1016/j.archger.2009.11.002

Crawford, J. R., Henry, J. D., Crombie, C., & Taylor, E. P. (2001). Normative data for the HADS from a large non-clinical sample. *British Journal of Clinical Psychology*, *40*, 429–434. http://dx.doi.org/10.1348/014466501163904

Dahl, J., Wilson, K., Luciano, C., & Hayes, S. C. (2005). *Acceptance and commitment therapy for chronic pain*. Oakland, CA: New Harbinger.

Darnall, B. D. (2009). Self-delivered home-based mirror therapy for lower limb phantom pain. *American Journal of Physical Medicine & Rehabilitation*, *88*, 78–81. http://dx.doi.org/10.1097/PHM.0b013e318191105b

Darnall, B. D., Ephraim, P., Wegener, S. T., Dillingham, T., Pezzin, L., Rossbach, P., & MacKenzie, E. J. (2005). Depressive symptoms and mental health service utilization among persons with limb loss: Results of a national survey. *Archives of Physical Medicine and Rehabilitation*, *86*, 650–658. http://dx.doi.org/10.1016/j.apmr.2004.10.028

Deans, S., Burns, D., McGarry, A., Murray, K., & Mutrie, N. (2012). Motivations and barriers to prosthesis users participation in physical activity, exercise and sport: A review of the literature. *Prosthetics and Orthotics International*, *36*, 260–269. http://dx.doi.org/10.1177/0309364612437905

de Jong, I. G., Reinders-Messelink, H. A., Tates, K., Janssen, W. G., Poelma, M. J., van Wijk, I., & van der Sluis, C. K. (2012). Activity and participation of children and adolescents with unilateral congenital below elbow deficiency: An online focus group study. *Journal of Rehabilitation Medicine*, *44*, 885–892. http://dx.doi.org/10.2340/16501977-1027

Demet, K., Martinet, N., Guillemin, F., Paysant, J., & André, J.-M. (2003). Health related quality of life and related factors in 539 persons with amputation of upper and lower limb. *Disability and Rehabilitation*, *25*, 480–486. http://dx.doi.org/10.1080/0963828031000090434

Desmond, D., & Gallagher, P. (2008). Coping and psychosocial adjustment to amputation. I. In P. Gallagher, D. M. Desmond, & M. MacLachlan (Eds.), *Psychoprosthetics: State of the knowledge* (pp. 11–21). London, England: Springer-Verlag. http://dx.doi.org/10.1007/978-1-84628-980-4_2

Desmond, D. M. (2007). Coping, affective distress, and psychosocial adjustment among people with traumatic upper limb amputations. *Journal of Psychosomatic Research*, *62*, 15–21. http://dx.doi.org/10.1016/j.jpsychores.2006.07.027

Desmond, D. M., Coffey, L., Gallagher, P., MacLachlan, M., Wegener, S. T., & O'Keeffe, F. (2012). Limb amputation. In P. Kennedy (Ed.), *The Oxford handbook of rehabilitation psychology* (pp. 351–367). Oxford, England: Oxford University Press.

Desmond, D. M., & MacLachlan, M. (2006). Coping strategies as predictors of psychosocial adaptation in a sample of elderly veterans with acquired lower limb amputations. *Social Science & Medicine*, *62*, 208–216. http://dx.doi.org/10.1016/j.socscimed.2005.05.011

Desmond, D. M., & MacLachlan, M. (2010). Prevalence and characteristics of phantom limb pain and residual limb pain in the long term after upper limb amputation. *International Journal of Rehabilitation*

Research, *33*, 279–282. http://dx.doi.org/10.1097/MRR.0b013e328336388d

Desmond, D. M., O'Neill, K., de Paor, A., Mac Darby, G., & MacLachlan, M. (2006). Augmenting the reality of phantom limbs: Three case studies using an augmented mirror box procedure. *JPO Journal of Prosthetics and Orthotics*, *18*, 74–79. http://dx.doi.org/10.1097/00008526-200607000-00005

Dillingham, T. R., & Pezzin, L. E. (2008). Rehabilitation setting and associated mortality and medical stability among persons with amputations. *Archives of Physical Medicine and Rehabilitation*, *89*, 1038–1045. http://dx.doi.org/10.1016/j.apmr.2007.11.034

Dillingham, T. R., Pezzin, L. E., & Shore, A. D. (2005). Reamputation, mortality, and health care costs among persons with dysvascular lower-limb amputations. *Archives of Physical Medicine and Rehabilitation*, *86*, 480–486. http://dx.doi.org/10.1016/j.apmr.2004.06.072

Donaghey, C. L., McMillan, T. M., & O'Neill, B. (2010). Errorless learning is superior to trial and error when learning a practical skill in rehabilitation: A randomized controlled trial. *Clinical Rehabilitation*, *24*, 195–201. http://dx.doi.org/10.1177/0269215509353270

Donovan-Hall, M. K., Yardley, L., & Watts, R. J. (2002). Engagement in activities revealing the body and psychosocial adjustment in adults with a trans-tibial prosthesis. *Prosthetics and Orthotics International*, *26*, 15–22. http://dx.doi.org/10.1080/03093640208726617

Doukas, W. C., Hayda, R. A., Frisch, H. M., Andersen, R. C., Mazurek, M. T., Ficke, J. R., . . . MacKenzie, E. J. (2013). The Military Extremity Trauma Amputation/Limb Salvage (METALS) study: Outcomes of amputation versus limb salvage following major lower-extremity trauma. *The Journal of Bone and Joint Surgery: American Volume*, *95*, 138–145. http://dx.doi.org/10.2106/JBJS.K.00734

Dunn, D. S. (1996). Well-being following amputation: Salutary effects of positive meaning, optimism, and control. *Rehabilitation Psychology*, *41*, 285–302. http://dx.doi.org/10.1037/0090-5550.41.4.285

Dunne, S., Coffey, L., Gallagher, P., & Desmond, D. (2014). "If I can do it I will do it, if I can't, I can't": A study of adaptive self-regulatory strategies following lower limb amputation. *Disability and Rehabilitation*, *36*, 1990–1997. http://dx.doi.org/10.3109/09638288.2014.885993

Dunne, S., Coffey, L., Gallagher, P., Desmond, D., & Ryall, N. (2015). Beyond function: Using assistive technologies following lower limb loss. *Journal of Rehabilitation Medicine*, *47*, 561–568. http://dx.doi.org/10.2340/16501977-1962

Edwards, D. S., Guthrie, H. C., Yousaf, S., Cranley, M., Rogers, B. A., & Clasper, J. C. (2016). Trauma-related amputations in war and at a civilian major trauma centre—Comparison of care, outcome and the challenges ahead. *Injury*, *47*, 1806–1810. http://dx.doi.org/10.1016/j.injury.2016.05.029

Ehde, D. M., Dillworth, T. M., & Turner, J. A. (2014). Cognitive–behavioral therapy for individuals with chronic pain: Efficacy, innovations, and directions for research. *American Psychologist*, *69*, 153–166. http://dx.doi.org/10.1037/a0035747

Ehde, D. M., Smith, D. G., Czerniecki, J. M., Campbell, K. M., Malchow, D. M., & Robinson, L. R. (2001). Back pain as a secondary disability in persons with lower limb amputations. *Archives of Physical Medicine and Rehabilitation*, *82*, 731–734. http://dx.doi.org/10.1053/apmr.2001.21962

Ehde, D. M., & Wegener, S. T. (2008). Management of Chronic Pain after Limb Loss. In P. Gallagher, D. M. Desmond, & M. MacLachlan (Eds.), *Psychoprosthetics: State of the knowledge* (pp. 33–51). London, England: Springer-Verlag. http://dx.doi.org/10.1007/978-1-84628-980-4_4

Elfström, M. L. (2007). Coping and cognitive behavioural models in physical and psychological rehabilitation. In P. Kennedy (Ed.), *Psychological management of physical disabilities: A practitioner's guide* (pp. 40–57). New York, NY: Routledge.

Ephraim, P. L., Dillingham, T. R., Sector, M., Pezzin, L. E., & MacKenzie, E. J. (2003). Epidemiology of limb loss and congenital limb deficiency: A review of the literature. *Archives of Physical Medicine and Rehabilitation*, *84*, 747–761.

Fletcher, D. D., Andrews, K. L., Butters, M. A., Jacobsen, S. J., Rowland, C. M., & Hallett, J. W., Jr. (2001). Rehabilitation of the geriatric vascular amputee patient: A population-based study. *Archives of Physical Medicine and Rehabilitation*, *82*, 776–779. http://dx.doi.org/10.1053/apmr.2001.21856

Frengopoulos, C., Burley, J., Viana, R., Payne, M. W., & Hunter, S. W. (2017). Association between Montreal Cognitive Assessment scores and measures of functional mobility in lower extremity amputees after inpatient rehabilitation. *Archives of Physical Medicine and Rehabilitation*, *98*, 450–455. http://dx.doi.org/10.1016/j.apmr.2016.06.012

Gailey, R., Allen, K., Castles, J., Kucharik, J., & Roeder, M. (2008). Review of secondary physical conditions associated with lower-limb amputation and long-term prosthesis use. *Journal of Rehabilitation Research & Development*, *45*, 15–30. http://dx.doi.org/10.1682/JRRD.2006.11.0147

Gallagher, P., Allen, D., & MacLachlan, M. (2001). Phantom limb pain and residual limb pain following lower limb amputation: A descriptive analysis. *Disability and Rehabilitation*, *23*, 522–530. http://dx.doi.org/10.1080/09638280010029859

Gallagher, P., Franchignoni, F., Giordano, A., & MacLachlan, M. (2010). Trinity amputation and prosthesis experience scales: A psychometric assessment using classical test theory and Rasch analysis. *American Journal of Physical Medicine & Rehabilitation*, *89*, 487–496. http://dx.doi.org/10.1097/PHM.0b013e3181dd8cf1

Gallagher, P., & MacLachlan, M. (2000a). Positive meaning in amputation and thoughts about the amputated limb. *Prosthetics and Orthotics International*, *24*, 196–204. http://dx.doi.org/10.1080/03093640008726548

Gallagher, P., & MacLachlan, M. (2000b). Development and psychometric evaluation of the Trinity Amputation and Prosthesis Experience Scales (TAPES). *Rehabilitation Psychology*, *45*, 130–154. http://dx.doi.org/10.1037/0090-5550.45.2.130

Gallagher, P., & MacLachlan, M. (2001). Adjustment to an artificial limb: A qualitative perspective. *Journal of Health Psychology*, *6*, 85–100. http://dx.doi.org/10.1177/135910530100600107

Gallagher, P., O'Donovan, M.-A., Doyle, A., & Desmond, D. (2011). Environmental barriers, activity limitations and participation restrictions experienced by people with major limb amputation. *Prosthetics and Orthotics International*, *35*, 278–284. http://dx.doi.org/10.1177/0309364611407108

Ganjparvar, Z., Mousavi, B., Masumi, M., Soroush, M., & Montazeri, A. (2016). Determinants of quality of life in the caregivers of Iranian war survivors with bilateral lower-limb amputation after more than two decades. *Iranian Journal of Medical Sciences*, *41*, 257–264.

Geertzen, J. H., Van Es, C. G., & Dijkstra, P. U. (2009). Sexuality and amputation: A systematic literature review. *Disability and Rehabilitation*, *31*, 522–527. http://dx.doi.org/10.1080/09638280802240589

Gregg, E. W., Li, Y., Wang, J., Rios Burrows, N. R., Ali, M. K., Rolka, D., . . . Geiss, L. (2014). Changes in diabetes-related complications in the United States, 1990–2010. *The New England Journal of Medicine*, *370*, 1514–1523. http://dx.doi.org/10.1056/NEJMoa1310799

Hagberg, K., Brånemark, R., & Hägg, O. (2004). Questionnaire for Persons with a Transfemoral Amputation (Q-TFA): Initial validity and reliability of a new outcome measure. *Journal of Rehabilitation Research & Development*, *41*, 695–706. http://dx.doi.org/10.1682/JRRD.2003.11.0167

Hall, V., Thomsen, R. W., Henriksen, O., & Lohse, N. (2011). Diabetes in Sub Saharan Africa 1999–2011: Epidemiology and public health implications. A systematic review. *BMC Public Health*, *11*, 564. http://dx.doi.org/10.1186/1471-2458-11-564

Hamill, R., Carson, S., & Dorahy, M. (2010). Experiences of psychosocial adjustment within 18 months of amputation: An interpretative phenomenological analysis. *Disability and Rehabilitation*, *32*, 729–740. http://dx.doi.org/10.3109/09638280903295417

Hanley, M. A., Ehde, D. M., Jensen, M., Czerniecki, J., Smith, D. G., & Robinson, L. R. (2009). Chronic pain associated with upper-limb loss. *American Journal of Physical Medicine & Rehabilitation*, *88*, 742–751. http://dx.doi.org/10.1097/PHM.0b013e3181b306ec

Hawkins, A. T., Pallangyo, A. J., Herman, A. M., Schaumeier, M. J., Smith, A. D., Hevelone, N. D., . . . Nguyen, L. L. (2016). The effect of social integration on outcomes after major lower extremity amputation. *Journal of Vascular Surgery*, *63*, 154–162. http://dx.doi.org/10.1016/j.jvs.2015.07.100

Hayes, S. C., Strosahl, K. D., & Wilson, K. G. (2003). *Acceptance and commitment therapy: An experiential approach to behavior change*. New York, NY: Guilford Press.

Hebert, J. S., & Burger, H. (2016). Return to work following major limb loss. In I. Z. Schultz & R. J. Gatchel (Eds.), *Handbook of return to work: From research to practice* (pp. 505–517). New York, NY: Springer. http://dx.doi.org/10.1007/978-1-4899-7627-7_28

Henderson, A. W., Turner, A. P., Williams, R. M., Norvell, D. C., Hakimi, K. N., & Czerniecki, J. M. (2016). Sexual activity after dysvascular lower extremity amputation. *Rehabilitation Psychology*, *61*, 260–268. http://dx.doi.org/10.1037/rep0000087

Heinemann, A. W., Bode, R. K., & O'Reilly, C. (2003). Development and measurement properties of the Orthotics and Prosthetics Users' Survey (OPUS): A comprehensive set of clinical outcome instruments. *Prosthetics and Orthotics International*, *27*, 191–206. http://dx.doi.org/10.1080/03093640308726682

Helgeson, V. S., Cohen, S., Schulz, R., & Yasko, J. (2000). Group support interventions for women with breast cancer: Who benefits from what? *Health Psychology*, *19*, 107–114. http://dx.doi.org/10.1037/0278-6133.19.2.107

Hill, A., Niven, C. A., & Knussen, C. (1995). The role of coping in adjustment to phantom limb pain. *Pain*, *62*, 79–86. http://dx.doi.org/10.1016/0304-3959(94)00253-B

Holzer, L. A., Sevelda, F., Fraberger, G., Bluder, O., Kickinger, W., & Holzer, G. (2014). Body image and self-esteem in lower-limb amputees. *PLoS One*, *9*, e92943. http://dx.doi.org/10.1371/journal.pone.0092943

Hurley, R. K., Jr., Rivera, J. C., Wenke, J. C., & Krueger, C. A. (2015). Identifying obstacles to return to duty in severely injured combat-related servicemembers with amputation. *Journal of Rehabilitation Research and Development*, *52*, 53–62. http://dx.doi.org/10.1682/JRRD.2014.04.0094

Institute of Medicine Committee on Quality of Health Care in America. (2001). *Crossing the quality chasm: A new health system for the 21st century*. Washington, DC: National Academies Press.

Jackson, J. C., & Jutte, J. E. (2016). Rehabilitating a missed opportunity: Integration of rehabilitation psychology into the care of critically ill patients, survivors, and caregivers. *Rehabilitation Psychology*, *61*, 115–119. http://dx.doi.org/10.1037/rep0000091

Jensen, M. P., Ehde, D. M., Hoffman, A. J., Patterson, D. R., Czerniecki, J. M., & Robinson, L. R. (2002). Cognitions, coping and social environment predict adjustment to phantom limb pain. *Pain*, *95*, 133–142. http://dx.doi.org/10.1016/S0304-3959(01)00390-6

Jensen, M. P., Turner, J. A., Romano, J. M., & Karoly, P. (1991). Coping with chronic pain: A critical review of the literature. *Pain*, *47*, 249–283. http://dx.doi.org/10.1016/0304-3959(91)90216-K

Jones, W. S., Patel, M. R., Dai, D., Subherwal, S., Stafford, J., Calhoun, S., & Peterson, E. D. (2012). Temporal trends and geographic variation of lower-extremity amputation in patients with peripheral artery disease: Results from U.S. Medicare 2000–2008. *Journal of the American College of Cardiology*, *60*, 2230–2236. http://dx.doi.org/10.1016/j.jacc.2012.08.983

Klerman, G. L., Weissman, M. M., Rounsaville, B. J., & Chevron, E. S. (1994). *Interpersonal psychotherapy of depression: A brief, focused, specific strategy*. New York, NY: Rowman & Littlefield.

Kratz, A. L., Williams, R. M., Turner, A. P., Raichle, K. A., Smith, D. G., & Ehde, D. (2010). To lump or to split? Comparing individuals with traumatic and nontraumatic limb loss in the first year after amputation. *Rehabilitation Psychology*, *55*, 126–138. http://dx.doi.org/10.1037/a0019492

Kurichi, J. E., Kwong, P. L., Reker, D. M., Bates, B. E., Marshall, C. R., & Stineman, M. G. (2007). Clinical factors associated with prescription of a prosthetic limb in elderly veterans. *Journal of the American Geriatrics Society*, *55*, 900–906. http://dx.doi.org/10.1111/j.1532-5415.2007.01187.x

Lankhorst, I. M., Baars, E. C., van Wijk, I. V., Janssen, W. G., Poelma, M. J., & van der Sluis, C. K. (2017). Living with transversal upper limb reduction deficiency: limitations experienced by young adults during their transition to adulthood. *Disability and Rehabilitation, 39*, 1623–1630. http://dx.doi.org/10.1080/09638288.2016.1206632

Legro, M. W., Reiber, G. D., Smith, D. G., del Aguila, M., Larsen, J., & Boone, D. (1998). Prosthesis evaluation questionnaire for persons with lower limb amputations: Assessing prosthesis-related quality of life. *Archives of Physical Medicine and Rehabilitation*, *79*, 931–938. http://dx.doi.org/10.1016/S0003-9993(98)90090-9

Livingstone, W., Van De Mortel, T. F., & Taylor, B. (2011). A path of perpetual resilience: Exploring the experience of a diabetes-related amputation through grounded theory. *Contemporary Nurse*, *39*, 20–30. http://dx.doi.org/10.5172/conu.2011.39.1.20

Lorig, K. R., & Holman, H. (2003). Self-management education: History, definition, outcomes, and mechanisms. *Annals of Behavioral Medicine*, *26*, 1–7. http://dx.doi.org/10.1207/S15324796ABM2601_01

MacIver, K., & Lloyd, D. (2010). Management of phantom limb pain. In C. D. Murray (Ed.), *Amputation, prosthesis use, and phantom limb pain: An interdisciplinary perspective* (pp. 157–174). London, England: Springer.

Marseglia, A., Xu, W., Rizzuto, D., Ferrari, C., Whisstock, C., Brocco, E., . . . Maggi, S. (2014). Cognitive functioning among patients with diabetic foot. *Journal of Diabetes and Its Complications*, *28*, 863–868. http://dx.doi.org/10.1016/j.jdiacomp.2014.07.005

Mbanya, J. C. N., Motala, A. A., Sobngwi, E., Assah, F. K., & Enoru, S. T. (2010). Diabetes in sub-Saharan Africa. *The Lancet*, *375*, 2254–2266. http://dx.doi.org/10.1016/S0140-6736(10)60550-8

Mckechnie, P. S., & John, A. (2014). Anxiety and depression following traumatic limb amputation: A systematic review. *Injury*, *45*, 1859–1866. http://dx.doi.org/10.1016/j.injury.2014.09.015

Michielsen, A., van Wijk, I., & Ketelaar, M. (2011). Participation and health-related quality of life of Dutch children and adolescents with congenital lower limb deficiencies. *Journal of Rehabilitation Medicine*, *43*, 584–589. http://dx.doi.org/10.2340/16501977-0825

Miller, W. C., Deathe, A. B., Speechley, M., & Koval, J. (2001). The influence of falling, fear of falling, and balance confidence on prosthetic mobility and social activity among individuals with a lower extremity amputation. *Archives of Physical Medicine and Rehabilitation*, *82*, 1238–1244. http://dx.doi.org/10.1053/apmr.2001.25079

Moradi, A., Ebrahimzadeh, M. H., & Soroush, M. R. (2015). Quality of life of caregiver spouses of veterans with bilateral lower extremity amputations. *Trauma Monthly*, *20*, e21891. http://dx.doi.org/10.5812/traumamon.21891

Moseley, G. L., Gallace, A., & Spence, C. (2008). Is mirror therapy all it is cracked up to be? Current evidence and future directions. *Pain*, *138*, 7–10. http://dx.doi.org/10.1016/j.pain.2008.06.026

Murray, C. D. (2005). The social meanings of prosthesis use. *Journal of Health Psychology*, *10*, 425–441. http://dx.doi.org/10.1177/1359105305051431

Murray, C. D. (2009). Being like everybody else: The personal meanings of being a prosthesis user. *Disability and Rehabilitation*, *31*, 573–581. http://dx.doi.org/10.1080/09638280802240290

Murray, C. D., & Forshaw, M. J. (2013). The experience of amputation and prosthesis use for adults: A meta-synthesis. *Disability and Rehabilitation, 35*, 1133–1142. http://dx.doi.org/10.3109/09638288.2012.723790

National Amputee Statistical Database. (2009). *The amputee statistical database for the United Kingdom 2006/07*. Edinburgh, Scotland: Information Services Division, NHS Scotland.

Oaksford, K., Frude, N., & Cuddihy, R. (2005). Positive coping and stress-related psychological growth following lower limb amputation. *Rehabilitation Psychology, 50*, 266–277. http://dx.doi.org/10.1037/0090-5550.50.3.266

O'Neill, B., Moran, K., & Gillespie, A. (2010). Scaffolding rehabilitation behaviour using a voice-mediated assistive technology for cognition. *Neuropsychological Rehabilitation, 20*, 509–527. http://dx.doi.org/10.1080/09602010903519652

O'Neill, B. F., & Evans, J. J. (2009). Memory and executive function predict mobility rehabilitation outcome after lower-limb amputation. *Disability and Rehabilitation, 31*, 1083–1091. http://dx.doi.org/10.1080/09638280802509579

Østlie, K., Franklin, R. J., Skjeldal, O. H., Skrondal, A., & Magnus, P. (2011). Musculoskeletal pain and overuse syndromes in adult acquired major upper-limb amputees. *Archives of Physical Medicine and Rehabilitation, 92*, 1967–1973. http://dx.doi.org/10.1016/j.apmr.2011.06.026

Pauley, T., Devlin, M., & Heslin, K. (2006). Falls sustained during inpatient rehabilitation after lower limb amputation: Prevalence and predictors. *American Journal of Physical Medicine & Rehabilitation, 85*, 521–532. http://dx.doi.org/10.1097/01.phm.0000219119.58965.8c

Pendlebury, S. T., Mariz, J., Bull, L., Mehta, Z., & Rothwell, P. M. (2012). MoCA, ACE-R, and MMSE versus the National Institute of Neurological Disorders and Stroke-Canadian Stroke Network Vascular Cognitive Impairment Harmonization Standards Neuropsychological Battery after TIA and stroke. *Stroke, 43*, 464–469. http://dx.doi.org/10.1161/STROKEAHA.111.633586

Pezzin, L. E., Dillingham, T. R., & MacKenzie, E. J. (2000). Rehabilitation and the long-term outcomes of persons with trauma-related amputations. *Archives of Physical Medicine and Rehabilitation, 81*, 292–300. http://dx.doi.org/10.1016/S0003-9993(00)90074-1

Pfeiffer, E. (1975). A short portable mental status questionnaire for the assessment of organic brain deficit in elderly patients. *Journal of the American Geriatrics Society, 23*, 433–441. http://dx.doi.org/10.1111/j.1532-5415.1975.tb00927.x

Pfeiffer, P. N., Heisler, M., Piette, J. D., Rogers, M. A., & Valenstein, M. (2011). Efficacy of peer support interventions for depression: A meta-analysis. *General Hospital Psychiatry, 33*, 29–36. http://dx.doi.org/10.1016/j.genhosppsych.2010.10.002

Phelps, L. F., Williams, R. M., Raichle, K. A., Turner, A. P., & Ehde, D. M. (2008). The importance of cognitive processing to adjustment in the 1st year following amputation. *Rehabilitation Psychology, 53*, 28–38. http://dx.doi.org/10.1037/0090-5550.53.1.28

Postema, S. G., Bongers, R. M., Brouwers, M. A., Burger, H., Norling-Hermansson, L. M., Reneman, M. F., . . . van der Sluis, C. K. (2016a). Musculoskeletal complaints in transverse upper limb reduction deficiency and amputation in the Netherlands: Prevalence, predictors, and effect on health. *Archives of Physical Medicine and Rehabilitation, 97*, 1137–1145. http://dx.doi.org/10.1016/j.apmr.2016.01.031

Postema, S. G., Bongers, R. M., Brouwers, M. A., Burger, H., Norling-Hermansson, L. M., Reneman, M. F., . . . van der Sluis, C. K. (2016b). Upper limb absence: Predictors of work participation and work productivity. *Archives of Physical Medicine and Rehabilitation, 97*(6), 892–899. http://dx.doi.org/10.1016/j.apmr.2015.12.022

Raichle, K. A., Hanley, M. A., Molton, I., Kadel, N. J., Campbell, K., Phelps, E., . . . Smith, D. G. (2008). Prosthesis use in persons with lower- and upper-limb amputation. *Journal of Rehabilitation Research and Development, 45*, 961–972. http://dx.doi.org/10.1682/JRRD.2007.09.0151

Ramachandran, V. S., & Rogers-Ramachandran, D. (1996). Synaesthesia in phantom limbs induced with mirrors. *Proceedings of the Royal Society of London B: Biological Sciences, 263*, 377–386. http://dx.doi.org/10.1098/rspb.1996.0058

Ramsey, L. H., Karlson, C. W., & Collier, A. B. (2017). Mirror therapy for phantom limb pain in a 7-year-old male with osteosarcoma. *Journal of Pain and Symptom Management,* online first publication.

Randolph, C., Tierney, M. C., Mohr, E., & Chase, T. N. (1998). The Repeatable Battery for the Assessment of Neuropsychological Status (RBANS): Preliminary clinical validity. *Journal of Clinical and Experimental Neuropsychology, 20*, 310–319. http://dx.doi.org/10.1076/jcen.20.3.310.823

Reiner, K., Tibi, L., & Lipsitz, J. D. (2013). Do mindfulness-based interventions reduce pain intensity? A critical review of the literature. *Pain Medicine, 14*, 230–242. http://dx.doi.org/10.1111/pme.12006

Remes, L., Isoaho, R., Vahlberg, T., Viitanen, M., & Rautava, P. (2010). Quality of life among lower extremity peripheral arterial disease patients who have undergone endovascular or surgical revascularization: A case-control study. *European Journal of Vascular & Endovascular Surgery, 40*, 618–625. http://dx.doi.org/10.1016/j.ejvs.2010.03.028

Robinson, V., Sansam, K., Hirst, L., & Neumann, V. (2010). Major lower limb amputation—What, why and how to achieve the best results. *Orthopaedics and Trauma*, *24*, 276–285. http://dx.doi.org/10.1016/j.mporth.2010.03.017

Rybarczyk, B., Nyenhuis, D. L., Nicholas, J. J., Cash, S. M., & Kaiser, J. (1995). Body image, perceived social stigma, and the prediction of psychosocial adjustment to leg amputation. *Rehabilitation Psychology*, *40*, 95–110. http://dx.doi.org/10.1037/0090-5550.40.2.95

Rybarczyk, B. D., Nyenhuis, D. L., Nicholas, J. J., Schulz, R., Alioto, R. J., & Blair, C. (1992). Social discomfort and depression in a sample of adults with leg amputations. *Archives of Physical Medicine and Rehabilitation*, *73*, 1169–1173.

Salamon, T., Lerner, A., Rothem, D., Altshuler, A., Karmeli, R., Solomonov, E., & Biswas, S. (2016). Retrospective analysis of case series of patients with vascular war injury treated in a district hospital. *Injury*, *47*, 811–817. http://dx.doi.org/10.1016/j.injury.2016.02.008

Saradjian, A., Thompson, A. R., & Datta, D. (2008). The experience of men using an upper limb prosthesis following amputation: Positive coping and minimizing feeling different. *Disability and Rehabilitation*, *30*, 871–883. http://dx.doi.org/10.1080/09638280701427386

Scheier, M. F., Carver, C. S., & Armstrong, G. H. (2012). Behavioral self-regulation, health, and illness. In A. Baum, T. A. Revenson, & J. E. Singer (Eds.), *Handbook of health psychology* (pp. 79–97). New York, NY: Psychology Press.

Schoppen, T., Boonstra, A., Groothoff, J. W., de Vries, J., Göeken, L. N., & Eisma, W. H. (2002). Job satisfaction and health experience of people with a lower-limb amputation in comparison with healthy colleagues. *Archives of Physical Medicine and Rehabilitation*, *83*, 628–634. http://dx.doi.org/10.1053/apmr.2002.32473

Schoppen, T., Boonstra, A., Groothoff, J. W., de Vries, J., Göeken, L. N., & Eisma, W. H. (2003). Physical, mental, and social predictors of functional outcome in unilateral lower-limb amputees. *Archives of Physical Medicine and Rehabilitation*, *84*, 803–811. http://dx.doi.org/10.1016/S0003-9993(02)04952-3

Schoppen, T., Boonstra, A., Groothoff, J. W., van Sonderen, E., Göeken, L. N., & Eisma, W. H. (2001). Factors related to successful job reintegration of people with a lower limb amputation. *Archives of Physical Medicine and Rehabilitation*, *82*, 1425–1431. http://dx.doi.org/10.1053/apmr.2001.26074

Schulz, R., Czaja, S. J., Lustig, A., Zdaniuk, B., Martire, L. M., & Perdomo, D. (2009). Improving the quality of life of caregivers of persons with spinal cord injury: A randomized controlled trial. *Rehabilitation Psychology*, *54*, 1–15. http://dx.doi.org/10.1037/a0014932

Singh, R., Ripley, D., Pentland, B., Todd, I., Hunter, J., Hutton, L., & Philip, A. (2009). Depression and anxiety symptoms after lower limb amputation: The rise and fall. *Clinical Rehabilitation*, *23*, 281–286. http://dx.doi.org/10.1177/0269215508094710

Stucky, K., Jutte, J. E., Warren, A. M., Jackson, J. C., & Merbitz, N. (2016). A survey of psychology practice in critical-care settings. *Rehabilitation Psychology*, *61*, 201–209. http://dx.doi.org/10.1037/rep0000071

Stutts, L. A., Bills, S. E., Erwin, S. R., & Good, J. J. (2015). Coping and posttraumatic growth in women with limb amputations. *Psychology, Health & Medicine*, *20*, 742–752. http://dx.doi.org/10.1080/13548506.2015.1009379

Sullivan, M. J. L., Thorn, B., Haythornthwaite, J. A., Keefe, F., Martin, M., Bradley, L. A., & Lefebvre, J. C. (2001). Theoretical perspectives on the relation between catastrophizing and pain. *The Clinical Journal of Pain*, *17*, 52–64. http://dx.doi.org/10.1097/00002508-200103000-00008

Tang, T. S., Ayala, G. X., Cherrington, A., & Rana, G. (2011). A review of volunteer-based peer support interventions in diabetes. *Diabetes Spectrum*, *24*, 85–98. http://dx.doi.org/10.2337/diaspect.24.2.85

Taylor, S. M., Kalbaugh, C. A., Blackhurst, D. W., Hamontree, S. E., Cull, D. L., Messich, H. S., . . . Youkey, J. R. (2005). Preoperative clinical factors predict postoperative functional outcomes after major lower limb amputation: An analysis of 553 consecutive patients. *Journal of Vascular Surgery*, *42*, 227–234. http://dx.doi.org/10.1016/j.jvs.2005.04.015

Tuncay, T., & Musabak, I. (2015). Problem-focused coping strategies predict posttraumatic growth in veterans with lower-limb amputations. *Journal of Social Service Research*, *41*, 466–483. http://dx.doi.org/10.1080/01488376.2015.1033584

Unwin, J., Kacperek, L., & Clarke, C. (2009). A prospective study of positive adjustment to lower limb amputation. *Clinical Rehabilitation*, *23*, 1044–1050. http://dx.doi.org/10.1177/0269215509339001

van der Schans, C. P., Geertzen, J. H. B., Schoppen, T., & Dijkstra, P. U. (2002). Phantom pain and health-related quality of life in lower limb amputees. *Journal of Pain and Symptom Management*, *24*, 429–436. http://dx.doi.org/10.1016/S0885-3924(02)00511-0

van der Sluis, C. K., Hartman, P. P., Schoppen, T., & Dijkstra, P. U. (2009). Job adjustments, job satisfaction and health experience in upper and lower limb amputees. *Prosthetics and Orthotics International*, *33*, 41–51. http://dx.doi.org/10.1080/03093640802555917

van Twillert, S., Stuive, I., Geertzen, J. H., Postema, K., & Lettinga, A. T. (2014). Functional performance, participation and autonomy after discharge from prosthetic rehabilitation: Barriers, facilitators and outcomes. *Journal of Rehabilitation Medicine*, *46*, 915–923. http://dx.doi.org/10.2340/16501977-1846

Varma, P., Stineman, M. G., & Dillingham, T. R. (2014). Epidemiology of limb loss. *Physical Medicine and Rehabilitation Clinics of North America*, *25*, 1–8. http://dx.doi.org/10.1016/j.pmr.2013.09.001

Verschuren, J. E., Enzlin, P., Geertzen, J. H., Dijkstra, P. U., & Dekker, R. (2013). Sexuality in people with a lower limb amputation: A topic too hot to handle? *Disability and Rehabilitation*, *35*, 1698–1704. http://dx.doi.org/10.3109/09638288.2012.751134

Verschuren, J. E., Geertzen, J. H., Enzlin, P., Dijkstra, P. U., & Dekker, R. (2015). People with lower limb amputation and their sexual functioning and sexual well-being. *Disability and Rehabilitation*, *37*, 187–193. http://dx.doi.org/10.3109/09638288.2014.913704

Verschuren, J. E., Geertzen, J. H., Enzlin, P., Dijkstra, P. U., & Dekker, R. (2016). Sexual functioning and sexual well-being in people with a limb amputation: A cross-sectional study in the Netherlands. *Disability and Rehabilitation*, *38*, 368–373. http://dx.doi.org/10.3109/09638288.2015.1044029

Verschuren, J. E., Zhdanova, M. A., Geertzen, J. H., Enzlin, P., Dijkstra, P. U., & Dekker, R. (2013). Let's talk about sex: lower limb amputation, sexual functioning and sexual well-being: A qualitative study of the partner's perspective. *Journal of Clinical Nursing*, *22*, 3557–3567. http://dx.doi.org/10.1111/jocn.12433

Vriezekolk, J. E., Eijsbouts, A. M., van Lankveld, W. G., Beenackers, H., Geenen, R., & van den Ende, C. H. (2013). An acceptance-oriented cognitive–behavioral therapy in multimodal rehabilitation: A pre-post test evaluation in highly distressed patients with rheumatic diseases. *Patient Education and Counseling*, *91*, 357–363. http://dx.doi.org/10.1016/j.pec.2013.01.018

Wampold, B. E. (2001). *The great psychotherapy debate: Models, methods, and findings*. Mahwah, NJ: Erlbaum.

Wechsler, D. (1997). *Wechsler Adult Intelligence Scale—Third edition (WAIS III)*. San Antonio, TX: Pearson.

Wegener, S. T., Hofkamp, S. E., & Ehde, D. M. (2008). Interventions for psychological issues in amputation. In P. Gallagher, D. M. Desmond, & M. MacLachlan (Eds.), *Psychoprosthetics: State of the knowledge* (pp. 91–106). London, England: Springer-Verlag. http://dx.doi.org/10.1007/978-1-84628-980-4_7

Wegener, S. T., Mackenzie, E. J., Ephraim, P., Ehde, D., & Williams, R. (2009). Self-management improves outcomes in persons with limb loss. *Archives of Physical Medicine and Rehabilitation*, *90*, 373–380. http://dx.doi.org/10.1016/j.apmr.2008.08.222

Williams, R. M., Ehde, D. M., Smith, D. G., Czerniecki, J. M., Hoffman, A. J., & Robinson, L. R. (2004). A two-year longitudinal study of social support following amputation. *Disability and Rehabilitation*, *26*, 862–874. http://dx.doi.org/10.1080/09638280410001708878

Williams, R. M., Turner, A. P., Green, M., Norvell, D. C., Henderson, A. W., Hakimi, K. N., . . . Czerniecki, J. M. (2014). Changes in cognitive function from presurgery to 4 months postsurgery in individuals undergoing dysvascular amputation. *Archives of Physical Medicine and Rehabilitation*, *95*, 663–669. http://dx.doi.org/10.1016/j.apmr.2013.11.013

Williams, R. M., Turner, A. P., Green, M., Norvell, D. C., Henderson, A. W., Hakimi, K. N., . . . Czerniecki, J. M. (2015). Relationship between cognition and functional outcomes after dysvascular lower extremity amputation: A prospective study. *American Journal of Physical Medicine & Rehabilitation*, *94*, 707–717. http://dx.doi.org/10.1097/PHM.0000000000000235

Williamson, G. M. (1995). Restriction of normal activities among older adult amputees: The role of public self-consciousness. *Journal of Clinical Geropsychology*, *1*, 229–242.

Williamson, G. M., Schulz, R., Bridges, M. W., & Behan, A. M. (1994). Social and psychological factors in adjustment to limb amputation. *Journal of Social Behavior & Personality*, *9*, 249–268.

World Health Organization. (2001). *World Health Organization International Classification of Functioning, Disability and Health (ICF)*. Geneva, Switzerland: Author. Available at http://www.who.int/classifications/icf/en/

Yu, J. C., Lam, K., Nettel-Aguirre, A., Donald, M., & Dukelow, S. (2010). Incidence and risk factors of falling in the postoperative lower limb amputee while on the surgical ward. *PM & R*, *2*, 926–934. http://dx.doi.org/10.1016/j.pmrj.2010.06.005

Ziegler-Graham, K., MacKenzie, E. J., Ephraim, P. L., Travison, T. G., & Brookmeyer, R. (2008). Estimating the prevalence of limb loss in the United States: 2005 to 2050. *Archives of Physical Medicine and Rehabilitation*, *89*, 422–429. http://dx.doi.org/10.1016/j.apmr.2007.11.005

CHAPTER 17

SPINAL CORD INJURIES

M. Jan Tackett and Philip M. Ullrich

Spinal cord injury and disorders (SCI/D) encompass a wide range of conditions that impact health, well-being, and community participation. The vast majority of SCI/D occur as the result of sudden trauma, which requires each person to adapt quickly to a new level of physical functioning (St. Andre et al., 2011). Neurological deficits range from mild mobility impairment to complete paralysis of the body from the neck down. Regardless of the degree of impact on physical functioning, SCI/D can drastically change most aspects of a person's life. Adaptation to SCI/D represents a major challenge and places people at greater risk for secondary medical conditions and mental health problems. Physical limitations, chronic pain, architectural barriers, and social marginalization combine to create a formidable challenge toward living a good life (Erosa et al., 2014). That stated, most people with SCI/D adapt to a new level of functioning and continue with rewarding and meaningful lives. Health-care providers can have a powerful impact on each person's response to SCI/D, including the fundamental beliefs they have about life, health, the meaning of injury, and ways to cope with adversity (Trieschmann, 1988).

The goal of this chapter is to provide practical information for providers addressing the psychosocial needs of this population based on empirical studies of people with SCI/D, as well as what can be reasonably generalized from other bodies of research. We first describe common characteristics of people with SCI/D, injury classification methods and rates, as well as common etiologies. Thereafter, we transition to problems that include both physical and psychological components and in which rehabilitation psychologists often play an important role. Next, we identify common psychosocial concerns that arise after SCI/D, and interventions useful for facilitating successful adaptation among all people with SCI/D across the lifespan. Finally, we focus on treatments targeting specific problems for which people with SCI/D are at greater risk compared with the general population.

DESCRIPTIVE CHARACTERISTICS OF THE SCI/D POPULATION

Understanding the context of SCI/D can make a psychologist more effective in working with members of this group. Although every injury is unique, knowing the basics related to demographics, causes, classification, and terminology can improve rapport, preserve therapy time, and provide groundwork for effective intervention in individual cases.

Neurological Classification of Injury and Disorders

SCI/D involve damage to the spinal cord and/or its nerve fibers. Nerves above the level of spinal cord damage continue to work normally while nerve

http://dx.doi.org/10.1037/0000129-018
Handbook of Rehabilitation Psychology, Third Edition, L. A. Brenner, S. A. Reid-Arndt, T. R. Elliott, R. G. Frank, and B. Caplan (Editors-in-Chief)

signal transmission below the level of damage is blocked. *Level of neurological function* is defined as the segment of the spinal cord that corresponds to the lowest part of the body where normal motor and sensory function are preserved. This level is identified by medical examination using the International Standards for Neurological Classification of SCI/D (Kirschblum et al., 2011). The spinal column is divided into four sections: cervical, thoracic, lumbar, and sacral. SCI/D can be generally classified as tetraplegia and paraplegia. Tetraplegia is caused by cervical area damage and involves some degree of paralysis of upper body and lower body. Paraplegia is caused by damage to the spinal cord in the thoracic, lumbar, and sacral areas and involves paralysis in some areas of the chest, abdomen, hips, legs, and feet while upper body functions are preserved. The American Spinal Injury Association (ASIA) Impairment Scale (AIS) system (Kirschblum et al., 2011) is also used to classify severity of spinal cord damage as complete (i.e., no sensory or motor nerve function below the level of damage) or incomplete (i.e., some preserved sensory and/or motor function below the level of damage). This is a critical distinction, as people with incomplete injuries typically have greater neurological recovery and mobility.

Etiology

Damage to the spinal cord can occur from a variety of sources that are generally classified as traumatic or nontraumatic. The term *SCI* is typically used to refer to spinal cord damage sustained from traumatic sources such as motor vehicle accidents or gunshots. The term *spinal cord disorder* usually refers to spinal cord damage that occurs from nontraumatic sources such as diseases or infections. Information on traumatic spinal cord injury etiology rates and other population statistics in the United States primarily comes from routine dissemination of data from the SCI Model System (https://msktc.org/sci/model-system-centers), which is sponsored by the National Institute on Disability, Independent Living, and Rehabilitation Research (NIDILRR; https://acl.gov/about-acl/about-national-institute-disability-independent-living-and-rehabilitation-research) to conduct research and provide information and resources to people with SCI, caregivers, health-care professionals, and the general public. The Department of Veterans Affairs (VA; https://www.va.gov/) is another important source of epidemiological data on persons with SCI, particularly because veterans represent a large proportion of persons with SCI in the United States and tend to experience a greater number of socioeconomic and lifestyle risk factors for disease and disability, such as older age, single marital status, unemployment, lower education, and lower income (National Academies of Sciences, Engineering, and Medicine, 2017). Currently, 14 SCI Model System Centers contribute data to the SCI Model Systems Data Center (https://www.nscisc.uab.edu/). Data accumulated in the United States show that vehicle crashes, falls, and violence are the leading cause of traumatic SCI in both the SCI Model System and the VA (National Spinal Cord Injury Statistical Center, 2016; St. Andre et al., 2011). Most (76%) veterans with SCI/D have traumatic injuries, but the VA cares for a large number of veterans with nontraumatic spinal cord disorders. Among the 24% of veterans with spinal cord damage because of nontraumatic causes, spinal stenosis is by far the leading cause (74.1%) followed by infection (8.6%), tumor (4.6%), syringomyelia (4.4%), spinal column degeneration (4.1%), vascular conditions (3.7%), and other nontraumatic causes (2.8%).

Demographics

Members of racial and ethnic minority groups are overrepresented in SCI/D populations. Within the SCI Model System, 63% of people with SCI are of White ethnicity, and 22% African American, followed by 11% Hispanic, 2% Native American, and 1% Asian (National Spinal Cord Injury Statistical Center, 2016). Veteran samples are 71% to 76% White, 18% to 23% African American, and 5% to 6% Hispanic (St. Andre et al., 2011).

Average age at time of SCI/D differs between veteran (56–64 years; St. Andre et al., 2011) and nonveteran samples (42 years). Veterans with SCI/D are more likely to be married than their counterparts in the Model Systems (42%–48% vs. 33%, respectively; St. Andre et al., 2011; National Spinal Cord Injury Statistical Center, 2016). Gender representation also differs between veteran and nonveteran samples.

Twenty percent of people with new SCI in the Model Systems are women (National Spinal Cord Injury Statistical Center, 2016), as compared with only 2% to 3% of veterans (St. Andre et al., 2011).

COMMON PHYSICAL CONCERNS

People with SCI/D face a complex array of physical challenges directly and indirectly related to paralysis. Chronic pain, sexual issues, high-risk health behaviors, exercise and nutrition all pose challenges for maintaining a healthy active life with SCI/D. In this section we describe recent findings related to addressing these important concerns.

Pain

Pain is a complex, treatment-resistant problem with serious effects on functioning and well-being among people with SCI/D. Pain after SCI/D can be categorized as musculoskeletal versus neuropathic. Musculoskeletal pain is due to damage to tissue or bone. Neuropathic pain (also known as central pain) is due to nervous system damage or disease. Musculoskeletal pain is the more common variety of pain after SCI/D, but neuropathic pains tend to be the more severe (Cardenas, Turner, Warms, & Marshall, 2002; Siddall, McClelland, Rutkowski, & Cousins, 2003). Over 75% of patients with SCI/D report some pain, with severe, disabling pain conditions occurring in about one third (Ullrich, 2007). Longitudinal studies show that pain conditions after SCI/D are likely to assume a chronic course (Cruz-Almeida, Martinez-Arizala, & Widerström-Noga, 2005; Siddall et al., 2003; Ullrich, Lincoln, et al., 2013) with a chance of worsening over time in spite of active treatments (Jensen, Hoffman, & Cardenas, 2005; Rintala, Hart, & Priebe, 2004).

Pain has been shown to reduce the frequency of scheduled rehabilitation therapies (Zanca, Dijkers, Hammond, & Horn, 2013) and is the most frequently cited factor complicating rehabilitation treatment sessions, more so than fatigue, spasticity, or other medical complications (Dijkers & Zanca, 2013). Pain interferes with daily activities and work roles among persons with SCI/D (Ehde & Hanley, 2006; Turner, Cardenas, Warms, & McClellan, 2001; Widerström-Noga, Felipe-Cuervo, & Yezierski, 2001).

Robust associations among pain, psychological distress, and functional disability are very well-documented in people with SCI/D. Pain and depression co-occur in 19% to 27% of patients (Ullrich, Lincoln, et al., 2013). In some studies, co-occurrence rates are elevated such that patients experiencing co-occurring pain and psychological distress outnumber those with individual syndromes (Cairns, Adkins, & Scott, 1996; Ullrich, Lincoln, et al., 2013; Ullrich, Smith, et al., 2013). Pain and distress levels tend to be more severe and enduring when conditions co-occur (Ullrich, Smith, et al., 2013). Psychologists have a central role in interdisciplinary pain treatment. See Chapter 14, this volume for additional discussion of pain assessment and treatment.

Sexual Issues

Sexual functioning issues span physical and psychological functioning considerations in the SCI/D population and represent an important area of intervention for rehabilitation psychologists. Relationships and sexual functioning are critical components of active engagement in the community and hold powerful meaning for all members of our society. People with SCI/D are confronted with challenges in these areas that are connected to the neurological impact of their condition, their own perceptions of sexuality, and the social context of relationships and disability. Each of these areas can benefit from better understanding and effective self-management.

The physical aspects of sexuality are of prime interest to people with any significant change in their health status. Following a diagnosis of SCI/D most people express a great deal of concern about the impact of the injury on their ability to engage in sexual activity (Anderson, 2004). Since neurological impact varies according to the level and degree of injury, capacity for sexual activity will vary widely depending on the level and severity of injury. For men, erections are generally impaired and sperm motility is diminished. Depending on the level and completeness of injury, it is typical for men to lose psychogenic erection while maintaining reflexogenic erections (Rees, Fowler, & Maas, 2007). For women, lubrication and sensation are decreased (Rees et al., 2007). Sexual desire continues after injury, but drive reduces over time for most (Charlifue, Gerhart,

Menter, Whiteneck, & Manley, 1992). Capacity for orgasm is reduced for most people, but individuals with SCI/D should be reminded that it is still possible for intercourse to lead to pregnancy.

Bowel and bladder changes and the potential for other medical complications constitute additional challenges to sexual activity. Most people with SCI/D can overcome these challenges to active intercourse with the assistance of medications, devices, procedures, and lubricants.

Perhaps as important as the neurological impact of SCI/D are the secondary dysfunctions that have roots in perceptions and attitudes (Trieschmann, 1988). These include changes to sexual self-image and thoughts about sexuality in relation to disability. Education can change these perceptions to address fundamental barriers to success in the physical and interpersonal components of sexual functioning.

Another target is related to social perceptions of sexuality and disability. Frank conversations need to acknowledge that individuals with SCI/D will face complex barriers to finding partners because of marginalization of and misconceptions about people with disabilities (Olkin, 1999) while also drawing attention to the fact that many do find success in dating after SCI/D. Directly addressing the social realities facing people with SCI/D can foster success in intimacy and sexuality.

To improve quality of life for people adapting to SCI/D, members of the rehabilitation team need to be willing to introduce discussion of sexuality and be familiar with sufficient information about the topic. The classic P-LI-SS-IT (Permission, Limited Information, Specific Suggestions, Intensive Therapy) model (Annon, 1976) is a helpful method for providers to understand their level of knowledge and their role in the process. It is critical for providers to incorporate information for members of sexual minorities, and make information about healthy sexuality available to all people with SCI/D regardless of age or the presence of a partner. Education can be provided in individual, group, video and written format, depending on patients' personal preference (Hough, Stone, & Buse, 2013). Collaborating with urology and occupational therapy can be helpful in clarifying information for patients, if necessary.

Health Behaviors

People with SCI/D are at increased risk for medical problems because of reduced mobility, nervous system dysfunction, and increased inflammatory responses (Charlifue, Jha, & Lammertse, 2010). Furthermore, they have higher rates of diabetes (Banerjea, Findley, Smith, Findley, & Sambamoorthi, 2009), stroke (LaVela et al., 2012), hypertension, and cardiovascular disease (Groah, Weitzenkamp, Sett, Soni, & Savic, 2001) than the general population. Respiratory illness, pressure injuries, and bowel or bladder problems are leading causes of death and hospitalization for this population. Higher incidence of medical problems contributes to increased mortality rates among people with SCI (Garshick et al., 2005). As such, it is crucial for individuals with SCI/D to maintain healthy behaviors and prevent secondary medical conditions so they can focus on goals like staying active and integrated with their communities. Some interventions (e.g., for weight management) may be most effective if delivered via the entire SCI team to capitalize on the multiple specialized areas of expertise of the interdisciplinary team (Locatelli, Gerber, Goldstein, Weaver, & LaVela, 2014).

People with SCI/D are more likely to be current smokers than people in the general population (Saunders, Krause, Saladin, & Carpenter, 2015; Weaver et al., 2011), and this is concerning, given their vulnerabilities to additional health problems. Smoking after SCI/D may aggravate respiratory problems, pressure injuries, pain, and depression (Davies & McColl, 2002; Krause & Broderick, 2004; Weaver et al., 2011). Krause and Saunders (2011) demonstrated that smoking and alcohol consumption were related to higher mortality rates, and community activity was related to lower mortality rates after SCI. Over half of people with SCI/D who smoke were contemplating quitting in the next 6 to 12 months (Weaver et al., 2011), and had attempted to quit in the past year (Saunders et al., 2015; Weaver et al., 2011). Fortunately, recent findings suggest that smoking is generally decreasing among people with SCI/D, bringing cigarette use approximately in line with the rate in the general population (Saunders, Krause, Carpenter, & Saladin, 2014). Smoking cessation interventions are an important component of rehabilitation, and psychologists play a major role.

Exercise and Nutrition

Weight management is a critical issue for people with SCI/D. More than half of people with SCI/D may be overweight or obese (Weaver et al., 2007). Weight typically increases after rehabilitation for SCI/D (de Groot, Post, Postma, Sluis, & van der Woude, 2010), leading to higher rates of weight-related conditions (Rajan, McNeely, Hammond, Goldstein, & Weaver, 2010) and poorer rehabilitation outcomes (Stenson, Deutsch, Heinemann, & Chen, 2011). Despite numerous barriers to success in this important area, some progress has been made in behavior change programming (Locatelli & LaVela, 2016). It is recommended that providers overcome discomfort with the topic of healthy eating to generate an organized, appealing program for improving weight management in people with SCI/D (Locatelli, Gerber, Goldstein, Weaver, & LaVela, 2014).

Physical exercise is a critical part of health maintenance and has its own set of barriers for this population. One aspect of this problem is the general lack of participation in moderate to heavy leisure time physical activity (Perrier, Stork, & Martin Ginis, 2016). Numerous barriers have been identified, and clinicians are encouraged to target barriers with the greatest opportunity for change: knowledge about exercise and the cost of access to exercise equipment (Cowan, Nash, & Anderson, 2013). Since exercise activities common to most people are not available to people with SCI/D, it takes considerable creative and financial effort to generate functional alternatives. For example, the exercise needs of a person with C4 AIS B tetraplegia would be vastly different from those of someone with T12 AIS C paraplegia. The role of the team is often to connect individuals with adapted community resources if they are available.

A peer support approach has been evaluated to improve leisure time physical activity in SCI with some evidence of success. Effective intervention depends on tailoring intervention to individual readiness to change (i.e., nonintenders vs. intenders; Martin Ginis, Nigg, & Smith, 2013). Several interventions have shown promise for increasing activity: telephone-based motivational counseling, peer in-home intervention, and group cognitive behavior therapy (CBT) (Brawley, Arbour-Nicitopoulos, & Martin Ginis, 2013; Latimer-Cheung et al., 2013).

PSYCHOSOCIAL CONCERNS AFTER SCI/D

As noted previously, most people with SCI/D adapt effectively despite the environmental barriers in their community. On the other hand, this population is at higher risk for a variety of mental health problems. What follows is a review of approaches psychologists can consider when consulted to work with a person with SCI/D experiencing depression, anxiety, pain, or other common mental health problems. Much of what is known about treatment of mental health problems with people with SCI/D has been borrowed from work with the general population, but trials of specific interventions have shown some encouraging outcomes. Interventions need to take place during acute rehabilitation and as part of routine follow-up care as needs arise (Duchnick, Letsch, & Curtiss, 2009).

Clinical teams engage in psychosocial treatment with patients in a variety of contexts. The following section describes some typical approaches, barriers to care, and possible directions for future investigation. At this point we reflect on the fact that the existence of SCI/D does not constitute a psychological problem per se; rather, our efforts facilitate each person's adaptation to the environment with the assets he or she brings to the situation. Although some people with SCI/D require specific treatments for specific mental health problems, the majority of people with SCI/D adapt successfully to their situation (Dunn, Uswatte, & Elliott, 2009) and benefit from interventions that encourage them to capitalize on their strengths.

Psychological Adaptation to Spinal Cord Injury and Dysfunction

Rehabilitation psychologists are often consulted to work with people who are tapping into their preserved strengths to build a meaningful life with SCI/D. Targets of intervention include improving relationships in light of changed physical and possibly social/familial functions; fostering independence in self-care; minimizing secondary medical complications; promoting sleep, exercise, and community participation; and reducing days of hospitalization, health-care utilization, and cost of care.

Adaptation to disability covers a great deal of territory in the research literature related to SCI/D.[1] In the past, a period of severe sadness was considered critical to successful adaptation to SCI/D. For much of the history of research on SCI/D adaptation, the absence of depression or other pathology was seen as the primary indicator of ultimately successful adaptation (Livneh & Martz, 2014), but this paints an incomplete picture. Quality-of-life measures normed with the general population could be ineffective or inaccurate in capturing the important aspects of adaption for people with SCI/D. Recently, greater attention has been paid to measuring positive indicators of quality of life and meaning as a proxy for successful adaptation to disability (Dunn & Dougherty, 2005). Adaptation involves psychological, biological, and environmental resources focused on achieving an optimal level of functioning (McMillen & Cook, 2003; Peter, Müller, Cieza, & Geyh, 2012). Psychologists can explore the impact of personal factors like persistence, faith, courage, community and family connection as part of a comprehensive evaluation. A heartening transition in the study of adaptation to SCI/D has been the growing focus on measuring the positive factors that predict success.

Although important questions remain, several factors have been demonstrated to promote positive adaptation. In their review of the SCI/D quality-of-life literature, van Leeuwen and colleagues (2012) wrote the following:

> The most consistent determinants of QOL in the literature are a person's total perceived degree of control in life; their sense of coherence; positive factors such as hope and purpose in life; feelings of self-worth such as self-efficacy and self-esteem; positive and negative affect; and posttraumatic cognitions. A higher score on each of these determinants is related to greater QOL, except for negative affect and negative posttraumatic cognitions for which the inverse is true. (p. 184)

It is possible to address each of these in psychotherapy.

One critical component of successful adaptation to SCI/D is the appraisal and meaning of the disability for the particular individual. Interpretation of the meaning of the injury as a threat or loss has been linked to difficulties in adaptation, while perceiving SCI/D to be a challenge tends to be connected with more positive outcomes (Kennedy, Lude, Elfström, & Smithson, 2010; Peter, Müller, Cieza, & Geyh, 2012). This is consistent with the predicted importance of "fighting spirit" in response to injury identified in recent findings (Bonanno, Kennedy, Galatzer-Levy, Lude, & Elfström, 2012). Personal appraisals about injury and physical functioning have been linked to life satisfaction, specifically as it affects the selection of coping approaches (Mignogna, Christie, Holmes, & Ames, 2015). Interventions targeting appraisals (which are often based on inaccurate assumptions about future capabilities) have demonstrated some benefits for people with SCI/D.

A second theme in understanding trajectory of adaptation to SCI involves the various approaches to coping. Engagement coping (including planning, active problem-solving, and seeking social support) has been linked with better adaptation. In contrast, avoidance coping (including behavioral disengagement) has been linked with poor outcomes and lower quality of life (Kennedy et al., 2000). This implies that interventions should encourage (possibly through role playing) specific active coping techniques.

Another trend in the adaptation literature is related to the importance of feelings of purpose and meaning after SCI/D. The presence of both higher purpose in life and general self-efficacy have been linked to better adaption and fewer mental health problems (Peter et al., 2012). Spiritual well-being has been connected with higher quality of life in

[1]In this section we use the word *adaptation*, whereas others have opted for *adjustment*, *reaction*, or *response*. In effect, we are all referring to thoughts, emotions, and behaviors that occur as people proceed with a good life after SCI/D.

this population (Wilson, Forchheimer, Heinemann, Warren, & McCullumsmith, 2017). Along the same lines, hope, optimism, and life coherence (i.e., finding purpose in life) have been associated with better performance in rehabilitation and positive evaluations of quality of life (Kortte, Stevenson, Hosey, Castillo, & Wegener, 2012; Krause & Edles, 2014). The critical role of disability-related appraisals has also been demonstrated, providing clues about what kinds of narratives (e.g., facing a challenge, finding meaning) predict better quality of life following SCI/D (van Leeuwen, Hoekstra, van Koppenhagen, de Groot, & Post, 2012). In fact, some efforts have actively helped people identify the positive impacts of SCI/D (McMillen & Cook, 2003).

Adaptation occurs over time following diagnosis and continues over the lifespan, not necessarily proceeding according to any prescribed orderly stages (Elliott & Frank, 1996). Most change occurs in the first year after injury and then stabilizes (Mortenson, Noreau, & Miller, 2010; Pollard & Kennedy, 2007). One critical part of adaptation involves the willingness of the person to consider adapted forms of past meaningful activities and/or adoption of new activities that are consistent with core values and that provide meaning in life. Collaboration with recreation therapists and other team members can be of critical importance in overcoming barriers to community participation and facilitating adaptation.

Vocational and Educational Issues

Employment represents one important aspect of community participation that is particularly salient for many people with SCI/D. The majority of people with SCI sustain their injuries in young adulthood when career development is especially important. However, only between 24% and 32% of people with SCI/D are employed 10 years after injury (Ottomanelli & Lind, 2009). Most persons with SCI do desire to return to work but report barriers such as transportation challenges, poor physical health, and physical limitations such as constraints in wheelchair mobility or poor hand function (Ottomanelli & Lind, 2009). Additionally, there may be financial disincentives to employment, as people with SCI/D may be concerned about potential loss of governmental financial and health benefits.

Educational level may be the most important predictor of return to work after SCI/D, with people having a college degree being more likely to return to work and those with fewer than 12 years of education less likely to do so (Ottomanelli & Lind, 2009). Educational and training opportunities after SCI/D increase the odds of employment. Severity of injury also relates to employment rates: People with paraplegia are twice as likely to be employed as those with tetraplegia (Ottomanelli & Lind, 2009).

Employment has been associated with increased life satisfaction and higher self-esteem. People who are employed after SCI/D show quality-of-life levels comparable to those of noninjured individuals (Westgren & Levi, 1998). Vocational attainments represent important life goals and treatment targets for people with SCI/D, but traditional vocational rehabilitation programs (designed for people with cognitive or mental challenges) are not readily applicable to people with physical disabilities (Ottomanelli & Lind, 2009). As an alternative to traditional programs, the supported employment approach emphasizes rapid and individualized community-based job finding and continuous follow-up to maintain employment (Ottomanelli & Lind, 2009). Supported employment approaches to vocational rehabilitation have recently been successfully applied among people with SCI/D, with program participants achieving employment rates more than twice that of nonparticipants (Ottomanelli et al., 2012).

Pediatrics or Developmental Issues

Important differences can be apparent between patients living with SCI/D at different developmental stages of life, with ramifications for the challenges they are facing in living with SCI/D and how practitioners can best help them. It should be kept in mind that as youth and adult development are highly variable, practitioners should remain observant for individual differences and changes in developmental foci (Rose, 2012). Youth with SCI tend to demonstrate resilience after injury as reflected in levels of anxiety and depression comparable to those of noninjured samples (Anderson et al., 2009). Curiously, parental ratings of the quality of life of injured youth are more closely related to parental mental health than that of their child (Kelly et al., 2011). However, youth with SCI/D do experience lower levels of community participation and quality of life compared with those of their noninjured peers (Garma, Kelly, Daharsh, & Vogel, 2011). A particular challenge for parents of youths with SCI/D and their care providers is to foster developmentally appropriate activity patterns and social roles while also managing the challenges of SCI/D that may be at odds with normal development. In general, dependence upon parents and others because of physical limitations may make it difficult to pursue the independence that typically comes with age.

Older adults with SCI/D often experience amplified effects of aging (Groah et al., 2012) and, as compared with younger people with SCI/D, they may require additional functional assistance and show more rapid onset of functional declines (Charlifue et al., 2010). In spite of age-related problems, people with SCI tend to experience advancing age with low distress and high life satisfaction (Rose, 2012). While older people with SCI have elevated rates of depression compared with those of their noninjured peers, they have lower rates of depression compared with those of younger people with SCI (Bombardier, Richards, Krause, Tulsky, & Tate, 2004).

Positive Psychology Interventions

With an increasing focus on patient strengths and assets, positive psychology interventions appear to be a good fit for people with SCI/D. Positive psychology is the scientific study of human flourishing and the factors that enable and sustain it (Seligman & Csikszentmihalyi, 2000). The emphasis in positive psychology on building strengths and maximizing quality of life is highly consistent with the aims, history, and culture of rehabilitation psychology (Dunn & Dougherty, 2005; Dunn et al., 2009; Ehde, 2010).

Many positive psychology constructs are relevant for individuals with SCI/D. Hope, purpose in life, self-efficacy, and positive affect have been consistently linked to well-being after SCI (Post & van Leeuwen, 2012). In one study, the ability to find meaning and purpose in life was strongly related to well-being after SCI/D, whereas injury severity was not (deRoon-Cassini, de St. Aubin, Valvano, Hastings, & Horn, 2009). Individuals who are hopeful and who experience frequent positive emotions in the early phases of rehabilitation report higher life satisfaction after discharge (Kortte, Gilbert, Gorman, & Wegener, 2010). Hopeful thinking and personal resilience are linked to greater participation and life satisfaction after SCI/D (Chan, Chan, Ditchman, Phillips, & Chou, 2013).

The umbrella term *positive psychology interventions* (PPIs) refers to a diverse group of self-help and clinician-led approaches aimed at cultivating well-being. Although there is some disagreement about what distinguishes PPIs from more traditional clinical strategies, PPIs are "primarily aimed at increasing positive feelings, positive behaviors, or positive cognitions, as opposed to ameliorating pathology or fixing negative thoughts or maladaptive behavior patterns" (Sin & Lyubomirsky, 2009, p. 469). Among the more well-established and empirically supported PPIs are well-being therapy (WBT) and positive psychotherapy (PPT). In WBT, the clinician helps the client to identify previous episodes of well-being, no matter how short lived, and to identify and address the factors that interrupted these episodes (Fava & Ruini, 2003). In PPT, the clinician guides the client through a series of activities focused on identifying one's strengths and using them in new ways; building gratitude and expressing it to others; and fostering engagement, meaning, and other positive experiences (Seligman, Rashid, & Parks, 2006). An array of similar activities has been tested in various self-help formats, Internet-based delivery methods, and combinations/packages (Sin & Lyubomirsky, 2009). On the whole, PPIs significantly enhance well-being and decrease depressive symptoms (Bolier et al., 2013).

Little research has directly tested whether positive psychology interventions help people with SCI/D, but preliminary studies highlight their potential to do so. Müller et al. (2016) reported promising results in a feasibility study of an online positive psychology intervention for people with disabilities, including SCI/D: Intervention participants reported greater benefits for pain control and life satisfaction compared with a control group. Likewise, Migliorini et al. (2015) reported results from a randomized controlled trial (RCT) testing a CBT program with a positive psychology module (which focused on pursuing goals, experiencing more positive events, and building psychological resiliency): Intervention participants, all of whom had SCI/D, reported higher life satisfaction and lower depression after taking part in the program. Nierenberg et al. (2016) made a strong case for the utility of well-being therapy for people with SCI/D.

Psychoeducational Approaches

At its core, rehabilitation is an educational process (Trieschmann, 1988), and psychologists are frequently called upon to provide educational programming and consultation. The challenge for rehabilitation teams is to prepare patients to become lifelong learners when it comes to the complex management of their conditions. At first, people with SCI/D are inundated with new information and learning challenges related to the medical facts about their condition and their implications for the practical requirements of living with a disability. Psychologists can provide input for improving the provision of education programs generally and consultation related to the needs of specific patients. From a content point of view, psychologists often participate in educational sessions related to adaptation to disability, sexuality, and intimacy as well as behavior change concerning substance use, exercise, and diet.

It is critical for educators to take into account the various barriers to learning that exist for people with SCI/D, including possible cognitive impairment, health-care needs, and transportation problems. These barriers are particularly difficult to overcome for people with limited financial resources. Additionally, psychologists should consider the needs of learners in the SCI/D population including age, motivation, and keeping information relevant to their situation (van Wyk, Backwell, & Townson, 2015). Because family members are a critical part of the patient's environment, family involvement in education is also helpful. This is especially true of relatives who are involved with the person's care. Peer instruction can be another component of educational programming, with information coming from a credible expert further ahead in the process of establishing a satisfying and meaningful life after injury. Many components of education in the SCI/D rehabilitation process are amenable to distance learning and Internet communication. There are several off-the-shelf educational programs related to SCI/D, including the *Yes You Can!* manual (http://www.nxtbook.com/nxtbooks/pva/yesyoucan4/index.php).

Self-Management

Rehabilitation is specifically aimed at providing people with SCI/D with the skills necessary for independently managing their complex health-care needs. Psychologists can play an important role in designing, structuring, and evaluating self-management programs so patients derive the benefits over the lifespan. Shorter lengths of stay and long distances between rehabilitation resources contribute to the importance of successful self-management.

The effectiveness of self-management approaches has been demonstrated in a variety of patient populations yielding improved symptom management, enhanced self-efficacy, and greater vigilance about changes to health status (Barlow, Wright, Sheasby, Turner, & Hainsworth, 2002). The usefulness of a self-management approach with people with SCI/D has been explored on a qualitative level. Critical factors leading to improved outcomes included assertiveness, feeling independent, managing caregivers, and attribution of responsibility (Munce et al., 2016).

Virtual Care/Telehealth

Telehealth, videoconferencing, and other distance health-care intervention methods are becoming popular treatment modalities for people with SCI/D. The opportunity exists to improve access to care for this population when transportation barriers and long distances between specialty SCI/D resources present obstacles. Medical monitoring (skin, diabetes, or blood pressure management) and mental health interventions are areas with successful trials via encrypted Internet communication (Dallolio et al., 2008). As technology improves, this resource will likely become critical for providing access to health-care services regardless of the person's location.

Peer Support and Peer Counseling

Peer visitation (PV) provides individuals with injury an opportunity to interact with and learn from successful role models. Also, the opportunity to help newly injured people can provide more experienced people with a structure for making a meaningful social contribution. Peer mentoring relationships have been found to be unique in that mentors are seen as being more equitable, mutual, accepting, credible, and normalizing than other noninjured social supporters (Veith, Sherman, Pellino, & Yasui, 2006). PV has been found to be an effective means of improving long-term adjustment in people with SCI/D (Boschen, Tonack, & Gargaro, 2003). It has also been associated with increased occupational activity and life satisfaction in this population (Sherman, DeVinney, & Sperling, 2004). Because of barriers to transportation and community access, it is critical for peer support to extend beyond visits during hospitalization.

Screening and Assessment Approaches

Most people with SCI/D achieve some degree of successful rehabilitation and integration into the community. Even so, they remain at risk for a variety of problems, and early detection of medical and mental health complications can prevent traumatic negative outcomes. Many SCI/D systems of care use standardized approaches for screening patients and identifying specific mental health concerns (see Table 17.1 for some useful instruments). During acute rehabilitation, everyone should be screened for depression, anxiety, posttraumatic stress disorder (PTSD), pain, substance use, and cognitive impairment. The diversity of preserved physical function in this population can make it difficult to select valid and meaningful assessment tools. Clinicians must balance the need for timely results against the requirements of valid and interpretable data. Although it has grown over the years, the range of usable instruments remains limited. In addition to level of preserved physical function, common problems like pain, medication side effects, fatigue, sleep, mood, vision, and hearing need to be considered when selecting test instruments.

Because SCI/D involves lifelong management of complex health conditions, some health-care systems offer annual evaluations, including screening in the above areas. In addition to asking about medical and mental health problems, psychologists can inquire about healthy functioning in the areas of caregiver management, family relationships, sexuality, community access, transportation, and health behaviors.

TABLE 17.1

Assessment and Intervention With People With Spinal Cord Injury and Disorders (SCI/D)

Topic	Assessment	Intervention options
Adaptation to disability	▪ Satisfaction With Life Scale (Diener, Emmons, Larsen, & Griffin, 1985) ▪ The Craig Handicap Assessment and Reporting Technique (Whiteneck, 1992) ▪ Life Satisfaction Questionnaire—9 (Budh & Österåker, 2007)	▪ Coping effectiveness training* ▪ Acceptance and commitment therapy+ ▪ Positive psychology interventions+ ▪ Well-being therapy+ ▪ Psychoeducation ▪ Peer support*
Sexuality		▪ PLISSIT model
Vocational/ academic	▪ Impact on Participation and Autonomy (Cardol, de Haan, van den Bos, de Jong, & de Groot, 1999)	▪ Supported employment* ▪ Vocational rehabilitation
Health self-management	▪ Assessment of Life Habits (Noreau, Fougeyrollas, & Vincent, 2002)	▪ Peer support* ▪ Psychoeducation ▪ Motivational enhancement+

TABLE 17.1

Assessment and Intervention With People With Spinal Cord Injury and Disorders (SCI/D) (*Continued*)

Topic	Assessment	Intervention options
Family/caregiver therapy		▪ Integrative behavioral family therapy+
Pain	▪ Numerical Pain Scale (Farrar, Young, LaMoreaux, Werth, & Poole, 2001) ▪ McGill Pain Questionnaire (Melzack, 1975) ▪ Brief Pain Inventory (short form; Tan, Jensen, Thornby, & Shanti, 2004)	▪ Cognitive behavior therapy* ▪ Self-hypnosis training* ▪ Mindfulness training ▪ Motivational enhancement ▪ Psychoeducation
Depression	▪ Center for Epidemiological Studies Depression Scale (Radloff, 1977) ▪ Patient Health Questionare-9 (Kroenke, Spitzer, & Williams, 2001) ▪ Beck Depression Inventory—Fast Screen for Medical Patients (Benedict, Fishman, McClellan, Bakshi, & Weinstock-Guttman, 2003)	▪ Coping effectiveness training* ▪ Cognitive behavior therapy* ▪ Behavioral activation+ ▪ Venlafaxine XR*
Anxiety	▪ Hospital Anxiety and Depression Scale (HADS-A anxiety subscale; Woolrich, Kennedy, & Tasiemski, 2006) ▪ State Anxiety Inventory (Form Y; Spielberger, 1983) ▪ Beck Anxiety Inventory (Beck & Steer, 1990) ▪ Generalized Anxiety Disorder 7 Item Scale (Spitzer, Kroenke, Williams, & Löwe, 2006)	▪ Cognitive behavior therapy*
PTSD	▪ Primary Care PTSD Screen (Pains et al., 2003) ▪ Posttraumatic Stress Disorder Checklist (Blanchard, Jones-Alexander, Buckley, & Forneris, 1996)	▪ Prolonged exposure+ ▪ Cognitive processing therapy+
Substance use issues	▪ Alcohol Use Disorders Identification Test (Saunders, Aasland, Babor, de la Fuente, & Grant, 1993) ▪ WHO Alcohol, Smoking, and Substance Involvement Screening Test (WHO ASSIST; WHO ASSIST Working Group, 2002)	▪ Motivational enhancement+

Cognitive impairment	▪ California Verbal Learning Test-II (Delis et al., 2000)
	▪ Brief Test of Attention (Schretlen, 1989)
	▪ Boston Naming Test (Kaplan, Goodglass, & Weintraub, 2001)
	▪ Wechsler Adult Intelligence Scale—4th ed. (Wechsler, Coalson, & Raiford, 2008):
	  ▪ Picture completion
	  ▪ Vocabulary
	  ▪ Similarities
	  ▪ Arithmetic
	  ▪ Digit span
	  ▪ Information
	  ▪ Comprehension
	▪ Wechsler Memory Scale—4th ed. (Wechsler, 2009)
	  ▪ Logical memory I, II
	▪ Continuous Visual Memory Test (Trahan & Larrabee, 1988)
	▪ Benton Judgment of Line Orientation (Benton, Hamsher, Varney, & Spreen, 1983)
	▪ Controlled Oral Word Association Test (Ruff, Light, Parker, & Levin, 1996)
	▪ Category Fluency Test (Animals; Tombaugh, Kozak, & Rees, 1999)
	▪ Trails A & B (Oral Form; Ricker & Axelrod, 1994)
		▪ Cognitive behavior therapy+
		▪ Compensatory interventions+
		▪ Environmental management+

Note. PLISSIT = intervention including Permission, Limited Information, Specific Suggestions, and Intensive Therapy; XR = extended release; PTSD = posttraumatic stress disorder; WHO = World Health Organization. *Empirically supported intervention: SCI/D population. +Empirically supported intervention: other populations.

PSYCHIATRIC COMORBIDITIES

Effective intervention for people with SCI/D depends on accurate and thorough case conceptualization; understanding the prevalence and risk factors for various mental health conditions is critical. This section describes the most common mental health concerns for people with SCI/D: depression, anxiety disorders, posttraumatic stress disorders, and substance use disorders. Rehabilitation psychologists play a central role in identifying these problems during initial rehabilitation and ongoing care as well as tailoring treatments to meet the needs of individual patients.

Depression

Symptoms of depression are very common for people with SCI/D and have been connected with poor quality of life, unsatisfactory health behavior, and greater impact of secondary medical conditions (Krueger, Noonan, Williams, Trenaman, & Rivers, 2013). Rates of depression have been estimated at 23% in Model Systems populations (Fann et al., 2011) and at 27% to 28% in VHA populations (Banerjea et al., 2009; Ullrich, Smith, Blow, Valenstein, & Weaver, 2014). A recent meta-analysis suggested that approximately 22% of people with SCI/D experience depression (Williams & Murray, 2015). Far too often, depression goes undiagnosed (Elliott & Frank, 1996), and many patients have limited access to treatment (Fann et al., 2011) or inadequate courses of antidepressant treatment (Smith, Weaver, & Ullrich, 2007).

People with SCI/D and depression are at very high risk for additional psychiatric comorbidities (Fann et al., 2011). In fact, 70% of veterans diagnosed with depression had at least one additional comorbidity, typically posttraumatic stress disorders or anxiety disorders (Ullrich et al., 2014). This is markedly elevated, considering that only 45% of people with depression in the general population have additional comorbidities. Comorbidity rates should be concerning to clinicians because co-occurring conditions are likely to be more severe and resistant to treatment (Clark, Watson, & Reynolds, 1995; Kessler et al., 2005). Efforts to assess and treat depression after SCI as an isolated disorder may be limited in effectiveness and applicable to few patients.

Health-care providers need to be aware of factors that place a person at greater risk for depression. It appears that people are at highest risk for mental health problems immediately after diagnosis and directly following discharge from rehabilitation (Duchnick et al., 2009; Schönenberg et al., 2014), although symptoms tend to stabilize over time (Kishi, Robinson, & Forrester, 1994). People with SCI/D are also at risk for mood decline when experiencing secondary medical conditions. People with chronic pain are at greater risk for depression (Hoffman, Bombardier, Graves, Kalpakjian, & Krause, 2011). Bombardier, Fann, et al. (2012) found that infrequent meaningful activity and low self-efficacy contributed to risk for depression. Depression has been linked to specific ways of thinking about life and disability. Negative self-appraisal (Huang et al., 2015) and appraisal of the circumstances of the disability (e.g., self-blame, generalization of danger) can contribute to the development of depression and PTSD (Agar, Kennedy, & King, 2006; Hatcher, Whitaker, & Karl, 2009).

People with SCI/D are at greater risk for suicide than other groups (DeVivo, Black, Richards, & Stover, 1991), and efforts are being made to understand this problem and determine how health care providers can reduce deaths by suicide. Because suicide rates are elevated among this population, regular screenings need to be part of any ongoing health care program. All members of a treatment team, including family members, should be comfortable with evaluating suicide risk and identifying suicide prevention resources.

Clinicians should also consider factors that can decrease the risk of developing depression. Across a variety of studies, self-efficacy and self-esteem have been connected with better mental health and better quality of life (meta-analysis; Peter et al., 2012). Another possible protective factor is a sense of coherence, which has been associated with well-being (Lustig, 2005). Active meaning-making is associated with better mental health and well-being and lower mortality (deRoon-Cassini et al., 2009; Krause, Carter, Zhai, & Reed, 2009). Social participation and social support have been connected with lower risk for depression (Müller, Peter, Cieza, & Geyh, 2012). Acceptance and fighting spirit are associated with lower depression (Elfström, Kennedy, Lude, & Taylor, 2007). Hope and optimism are important buffers during rehabilitation, but might not endure in the long run, placing the individual at increasing risk for depression if hoped-for improvement does not occur.

Accurate screening and measurement of depression have been problematic in the SCI/D population because many providers consider depression to be a normal response to SCI/D and have difficulty differentiating certain symptoms of depression from those that are natural consequences of SCI/D (Elliott & Frank, 1996). Also, psychologists should avoid the assumption that a person with SCI/D is in grief response, which seems to happen less than one might think (Klyce et al., 2015). In the service of accurate measurement, strong evidence exists that the Patient Health Questionnaire-9 (PHQ-9) can be effective for screening and tracking depression in this population (Bombardier, Kalpakjian, et al., 2012).

Coping approaches have been linked to positive outcomes following SCI/D, including lower depression (Pollard & Kennedy, 2007). Coping strategies are often new or existing skills that are applied in critical situations such as in response to a decline in physical function. It appears that engagement coping predicts fewer depression symptoms and avoidant coping can be problematic (Livneh & Martz, 2014). This seems particularly important for people who have low life coherence and/or little hope. Coping effectiveness training (CET), based on Lazarus and Folkman's (1984) work, can be implemented with this population in group or individual interventions. Results have been generally positive, although not consistent about who benefits from the training. King and Kennedy (1999) found reductions in depression and anxiety at discharge and six-week follow-up with a seven-session CET group intervention. In an effort to specify the active ingredient of this intervention, Kennedy, Duff, Evans, and Beedie (2003) demonstrated a reduction in depression and anxiety but no change in coping strategies used. A trial with a VA population compared CET with supportive group therapy and found no difference in depression and anxiety between the two groups, both improved (Duchnick et al., 2009).

Research related to the application of CBT with the SCI/D population has included a diverse range of interventions, including "psychoeducation, relaxation training, cognitive restructuring, increased behavioral activation and assertiveness training"; the specific impact of each of these components needs to be investigated independently (Mehta et al., 2011, page 22). One study found that a 10-week group CBT intervention was helpful for people with high levels of depression or anxiety but not for patients with milder mood problems (Craig, Hancock, Chang, & Dickson, 1998).

Behavioral activation should also be considered as a first choice for treatment of depression in the SCI/D population (Bombardier, Fann, et al., 2012). *Behavioral activation* is a behavioral therapy approach that provides structure for increasing participation in rewarding activities. Because participation in the community and physical activity are critical to quality of life and physical health, behavioral activation is a perfect match for people with SCI/D. Psychologists are encouraged to develop tailored approaches that help people address barriers in the local social and architectural environment.

Anxiety Disorders

Anxiety disorders in people with SCI/D are less well understood than depression, but approximately 20% report symptoms reaching the threshold of an anxiety disorder in the 2 years after injury (Galvin & Godfrey, 2001). Generalized anxiety disorder and panic disorder are more common in people with SCI/D than in the general population and can compromise participation in acute rehabilitation and successful community reintegration.

Feelings of helplessness, dependency, and vulnerability can contribute to preexisting anxiety problems following acquired disability. Anxiety related to falling during transfer training can become a barrier to participation in rehabilitation and is often a target for intervention. For many patients, ventilator weaning causes a great deal of anxiety; these patients might respond well to relaxation, mindfulness, and hypnosis-based interventions, although effectiveness has not been demonstrated through controlled trials. Anxiety often contributes to sleep problems for people with SCI/D. CBT approaches can be effective for people with anxiety and panic disorder, although treatment effectiveness with this population also needs further study.

Anxiety symptoms that contribute to lower quality of life and less successful adaptation have been linked to specific ways of interpreting injury. Threat appraisal is the way people evaluate their situation, what dangers exist for them, and what information is relevant to their safety. Unrealistic threat appraisal could lead to higher anxiety and maladaptive coping strategies (Kennedy et al., 2010). As noted previously, CBT (and specifically CET) have been successful in lowering anxiety symptoms for people with SCI. Results are more convincing with people with higher symptom levels compared with those with mild anxiety.

Posttraumatic Stress Disorder

Because damage to the spinal cord is often caused by extreme trauma and threat of death, high rates of PTSD might be expected in SCI/D populations. Data on the prevalence of PTSD after SCI/D support this expectation. Rates of current and lifetime prevalence of PTSD among people with SCI/D are 12% and 29%, respectively (Radnitz et al., 1998). Comparable prevalence rates have been found in studies of people with SCI/D during or shortly after rehabilitation (Kennedy & Duff, 2001; Lude, Kennedy, Evans, Lude, & Beedie, 2005; Nielsen, 2003) or even decades after initial injury (Banerjea et al., 2009; Krause, Saunders, & Newman, 2010).

It is likely that some people with SCI/D are at elevated risk for developing PTSD symptoms. Risk factors include preinjury trauma, cause of injury, feelings of guilt, and methods of coping with trauma. Not surprisingly, avoidance coping has been connected with risk for developing PTSD symptoms in the SCI/D population (Lude et al., 2005). Given that avoidance is a hallmark component of PTSD, and avoidance-based coping is associated with lower quality of life and mental health outcomes for people with SCI/D (Livneh & Martz, 2014), it is critical to successfully identify and treat symptoms of PTSD as early as possible for this population. Negative appraisal has also been connected with PTSD (Agar et al., 2006). As in many other populations, PTSD and depression frequently co-occur.

Cognitive Deficits

Cognitive impairment is a common comorbidity for people with SCI/D, and this can have a profound impact on acute rehabilitation and long-term adaptation to disability (Fortmann et al., 2013). Prevalence estimates for comorbidity of SCI/D and traumatic brain injury (TBI) alone have ranged from 30% to 60% (Craig, Guest, Tran, & Middleton, 2017), and this range belies the problem of inaccurate screening. Severity of TBI in the SCI/D population has been estimated at approximately 34% mild, 10% mild complicated, 6% moderate, and 10% severe (Macciocchi, Seel, Thompson, Byams, & Bowman, 2008). In addition to TBI, typical causes of cognitive impairment in the SCI/D population include anoxia, cerebral vascular accident, dementia, polypharmacy, insomnia, and delirium. Historical factors such as alcohol and drug abuse, prior successive traumatic brain injuries, and medical comorbidities also increase the risk of cognitive problems following SCI/D. Cognitive impairment can contribute to poor outcomes and higher costs in SCI/D rehabilitation (Bradbury et al., 2008).

Rehabilitation programs need to customize interventions to capitalize on the person's preserved strengths to improve chances of success. Additionally, assessment can be helpful in setting realistic goals and making appropriate discharge arrangements (Ricker & Regan, 1999). Neuropsychological assessment and interprofessional treatment coordination are critical for rehabilitation interventions to be effective. Accuracy in detecting TBI in the SCI/D population has been identified as a challenge (Watanabe, Zafonte, & Lairson, 1999). Accurately evaluating a broad spectrum of strengths and weakness for people with minimal upper extremity function can be difficult. Given the current selection of measures available, psychologists need to be flexible and creative in addition to understanding their limitations in this important area. Clinicians and researchers are challenged to develop valid and useful evaluation batteries for assessment of people with various levels of preserved function in order to accurately inform treatment.

Ongoing cognitive impairment can have a negative impact on successful functioning after rehabilitation. The critical tasks related to community reintegration, relationships, medical self-management, and the management of care providers are all likely to suffer. Rehabilitation psychologists working with people with SCI/D are challenged with helping to determine what aspects of independent functioning are most affected by cognitive rather than physical limitations so effective interventions can be implemented. Ongoing monitoring and assessment can detect changes in symptoms over time and allow the rehabilitation team to explore additional resources.

Substance Use Issues

Substance abuse is a critical problem for people managing complex health conditions, and this is especially true for individuals with SCI/D. Successful participation in rehabilitation involves cognitive and motivational challenges, and substance abuse can be a barrier. Unfortunately, alcohol problems are more prevalent in the SCI/D group than in the general population. This is the case for people admitted for rehabilitation (more than 30%) and for people with SCI/D living in the community (14% with alcohol abuse, 11% with prescription or illegal drug use; Elliott, Kurylo, Chen, & Hicken, 2002; Tate, Forchheimer, Krause, Meade, & Bombardier, 2004). Preinjury alcohol problems are acknowledged by 35% to 49% of people with SCI/D (Bombardier & Rimmele, 1998; Tate, 1993), and these may have played in role in causing SCI/D in more than one-third of people with SCI/D (Bombardier & Rimmele, 1998; Heinemann, Keen, Donohue, & Schnoll, 1988; Heinemann, Schnoll, Brandt, Maltz, & Keen, 1988). People with SCI/D and a history of alcohol problems participate less in therapies (Heinemann & Hawkins, 1995), have lower functional gains during rehabilitation, and have longer lengths of stay (Bombardier, Stroud, Esselman, & Rimmele, 2004). Among people with SCI/D, those at greater risk for alcohol and substance misuse after injury are younger, male, less educated, experiencing pain, or have preinjury substance problems (Heinemann, Keen, et al., 1988; Stroud, Bombardier, Dyer, Rimmele, & Esselman, 2011; Tate et al., 2004).

The consequences of substance abuse after SCI/D are grave. Alcohol abuse has also been linked to depression, anger, anxiety, lower satisfaction with life, and other psychosocial problems in this population (Heinemann & Hawkins, 1995). There is also little doubt that excessive use of alcohol or other substances can impair a person's ability to prevent myriad secondary medical conditions such as pressure injuries, urinary tract infections, and respiratory illness (Elliott et al., 2002). Other research has linked substance use disorders to higher mortality rates after SCI/D (Findley, Banerjea, & Sambamoorthi, 2011).

Given the high incidence of substance use (particularly alcohol abuse) contributing to SCI/D, combined with the high frequency of substance use aggravating health and life satisfaction following SCI/D, health care providers need to be vigilant and active in addressing these problems. Facilitating change in substance use behavior is an important component of rehabilitation intervention and often becomes a factor for people with SCI/D living in the community. For some, the diagnosis of SCI/D becomes an opportunity for behavior change; health care providers can support this improvement with motivational interviewing (Bombardier & Rimmele, 1998). Recent findings suggest that patients with the most complications are likely to be the most receptive to intervention, and rehabilitation psychologists should seize these opportunities. Throughout the health care system, providers are encouraged to be assertive in evaluating substance use, and barriers to substance use treatment need to be reduced (Stroud et al., 2011).

Brief intervention by a health care provider can have a powerful impact on alcohol use in medical populations, and SCI/D service providers are encouraged to include such interventions in their work with patients. Motivational enhancement approaches have proven effective with a wide range of populations and are likely a great next step for people with SCI/D (Gentilello et al., 1999).

CONCLUSION

Psychologists can play a critical role in the lives of people with SCI/D, whether that is to encourage adaptation or to respond to the development of mental health syndromes. During acute rehabilitation, psychologists are often involved with providing support to the person and family members, helping them navigate the complex health-care system, and setting the stage for a mindful approach to adaptation. Moreover, psychologists need to be part of ongoing monitoring and health maintenance throughout the lifespan for people with SCI/D. To succeed at this role, psychologists will need to continue to build on the progress in research and practice that has helped inform practice so far. Future work in this area will need to identify the most important targets for intervention and the active components of treatment that can address those targets (Hart & Ehde, 2015). Psychologists need to keep in mind the importance of advocacy and being a conduit for community resources as well as the importance of environmental factors for quality of life. As this chapter should indicate, successful treatment with this population includes consideration of a broad range of factors that contribute to living consistent with one's values, forging meaning, and developing sustainable relationships regardless of the person's level of function.

References

Agar, E., Kennedy, P., & King, N. (2006). The role of negative cognitive appraisals in PTSD symptoms following spinal cord injuries. *Behavioural and Cognitive Psychotherapy*, *34*, 437–452. http://dx.doi.org/10.1017/S1352465806002943

Anderson, C. J., Kelly, E. H., Klaas, S. J., Russell, H., Daharsh, E., & Vogel, L. C. (2009). Anxiety and depression in children and adolescents with spinal cord injuries. *Developmental Medicine & Child Neurology*, *51*, 826–832. http://dx.doi.org/10.1111/j.1469-8749.2009.03268.x

Anderson, K. D. (2004). Targeting recovery: Priorities of the spinal cord–injured population. *Journal of Neurotrauma*, *21*, 1371–1383. http://dx.doi.org/10.1089/neu.2004.21.1371

Annon, J. (1976). *The behavioral treatment of sexual problems: Brief therapy*. Hagerstown, MD: Harper & Row.

Banerjea, R., Findley, P. A., Smith, B., Findley, T., & Sambamoorthi, U. (2009). Co-occurring medical and mental illness and substance use disorders among veteran clinic users with spinal cord injury patients with complexities. *Spinal Cord*, *47*, 789–795. http://dx.doi.org/10.1038/sc.2009.42

Barlow, J., Wright, C., Sheasby, J., Turner, A., & Hainsworth, J. (2002). Self-management approaches for people with chronic conditions: A review. *Patient Education & Counseling*, *48*, 177–187. http://dx.doi.org/10.1016/S0738-3991(02)00032-0

Beck, A. T., & Steer, R. A. (1990). *Manual for the Beck Anxiety Inventory*. San Antonio, TX: Psychological Corporation.

Benedict, R. H., Fishman, I., McClellan, M. M., Bakshi, R., & Weinstock-Guttman, B. (2003). Validity of the Beck Depression Inventory—Fast Screen in multiple sclerosis. *Multiple Sclerosis Journal*, *9*, 393–396. http://dx.doi.org/10.1191/1352458503ms902oa

Benton, A. L., Hamsher, K. D., Varney, N. R., & Spreen, O. (1983). *Judgment of line orientation*. New York, NY: Oxford University Press.

Blanchard, E. B., Jones-Alexander, J., Buckley, T. C., & Forneris, C. A. (1996). Psychometric properties of the PTSD Checklist (PCL). *Behaviour Research and Therapy*, *34*, 669–673.

Bolier, L., Haverman, M., Westerhof, G. J., Riper, H., Smit, F., & Bohlmeijer, E. (2013). Positive psychology interventions: A meta-analysis of randomized controlled studies. *BMC Public Health*, *13*, 119. http://dx.doi.org/10.1186/1471-2458-13-119

Bombardier, C. H., Fann, J. R., Tate, D. G., Richards, J. S., Wilson, C. S., Warren, A. M., . . . the PRISMS Investigators. (2012). An exploration of modifiable risk factors for depression after spinal cord injury: Which factors should we target? *Archives of Physical Medicine and Rehabilitation*, *93*, 775–781. http://dx.doi.org/10.1016/j.apmr.2011.12.020

Bombardier, C. H., Kalpakjian, C. Z., Graves, D. E., Dyer, J. R., Tate, D. G., & Fann, J. R. (2012). Validity of the Patient Health Questionnaire—9 in assessing major depressive disorder during inpatient spinal cord injury rehabilitation. *Archives of Physical Medicine and Rehabilitation*, *93*, 1838–1845. http://dx.doi.org/10.1016/j.apmr.2012.04.019

Bombardier, C. H., Richards, J. S., Krause, J. S., Tulsky, D., & Tate, D. G. (2004). Symptoms of major depression in people with spinal cord injury: Implications for screening. *Archives of Physical Medicine and Rehabilitation*, *85*, 1749–1756. http://dx.doi.org/10.1016/j.apmr.2004.07.348

Bombardier, C. H., & Rimmele, C. T. (1998). Alcohol use and readiness to change after spinal cord injury. *Archives of Physical Medicine and Rehabilitation*, *79*, 1110–1115. http://dx.doi.org/10.1016/S0003-9993(98)90180-0

Bombardier, C. H., Stroud, M. W., Esselman, P. C., & Rimmele, C. T. (2004). Do preinjury alcohol problems predict poorer rehabilitation progress in persons with spinal cord injury? *Archives of Physical Medicine and Rehabilitation*, *85*, 1488–1492. http://dx.doi.org/10.1016/j.apmr.2003.10.010

Bonanno, G. A., Kennedy, P., Galatzer-Levy, I. R., Lude, P., & Elfström, M. L. (2012). Trajectories of resilience, depression, and anxiety following spinal cord injury. *Rehabilitation Psychology*, *57*, 236–247. http://dx.doi.org/10.1037/a0029256

Boschen, K. A., Tonack, M., & Gargaro, J. (2003). Long-term adjustment and community reintegration following spinal cord injury. *International Journal of Rehabilitation Research*, *26*, 157–164. http://dx.doi.org/10.1097/00004356-200309000-00001

Bradbury, C. L., Wodchis, W. P., Mikulis, D. J., Pano, E. G., Hitzig, S. L., McGillivray, C. F., . . . Green, R. E. (2008). Traumatic brain injury in patients with traumatic spinal cord injury: Clinical and economic consequences. *Archives of Physical Medicine and Rehabilitation*, *89*, S77–S84. http://dx.doi.org/10.1016/j.apmr.2008.07.008

Brawley, L. R., Arbour-Nicitopoulos, K. P., & Martin Ginis, K. A. (2013). Developing physical activity interventions for adults with spinal cord injury: Part 3: A pilot feasibility study of an intervention to increase self-managed physical activity. *Rehabilitation Psychology*, *58*, 316–321. http://dx.doi.org/10.1037/a0032814

Budh, C. N., & Österåker, A.-L. (2007). Life satisfaction in individuals with a spinal cord injury and pain. *Clinical Rehabilitation*, *21*, 89–96. http://dx.doi.org/10.1177/0269215506070313

Cairns, D. M., Adkins, R. H., & Scott, M. D. (1996). Pain and depression in acute traumatic spinal cord injury: Origins of chronic problematic pain? *Archives of Physical Medicine and Rehabilitation*, *77*, 329–335. http://dx.doi.org/10.1016/S0003-9993(96)90079-9

Cardenas, D. D., Turner, J. A., Warms, C. A., & Marshall, H. M. (2002). Classification of chronic pain associated with spinal cord injuries. *Archives of Physical Medicine and Rehabilitation*, *83*, 1708–1714. http://dx.doi.org/10.1053/apmr.2002.35651

Cardol, M., de Haan, R. J., van den Bos, G. A., de Jong, B. A., & de Groot, I. J. (1999). The development of a handicap assessment questionnaire: The impact on participation and autonomy (IPA). *Clinical Rehabilitation*, *13*, 411–419. http://dx.doi.org/10.1191/026921599668601325

Chan, J. Y. C., Chan, F., Ditchman, N., Phillips, B., & Chou, C. (2013). Evaluating Snyder's hope theory as a motivational model of participation and life satisfaction for individuals with spinal cord injury: A path analysis. *Rehabilitation Research, Policy, and Education*, *27*, 171–185. http://dx.doi.org/10.1891/2168-6653.27.3.171

Charlifue, S., Jha, A., & Lammertse, D. (2010). Aging with spinal cord injury. *Physical Medicine and Rehabilitation Clinics of North America*, *21*, 383–402. http://dx.doi.org/10.1016/j.pmr.2009.12.002

Charlifue, S. W., Gerhart, K. A., Menter, R. R., Whiteneck, G. G., & Manley, M. S. (1992). Sexual issues of women with spinal cord injuries. *Paraplegia*, *30*, 192–199.

Clark, L. A., Watson, D., & Reynolds, S. (1995). Diagnosis and classification of psychopathology: Challenges to the current system and future directions. *Annual Review of Psychology*, *46*, 121–153. http://dx.doi.org/10.1146/annurev.ps.46.020195.001005

Cowan, R. E., Nash, M. S., & Anderson, K. D. (2013). Exercise participation barrier prevalence and association with exercise participation status in individuals with spinal cord injury. *Spinal Cord*, *51*, 27–32. http://dx.doi.org/10.1038/sc.2012.53

Craig, A., Guest, R., Tran, Y., & Middleton, J. (2017). Cognitive impairment and mood states after spinal cord injury. *Journal of Neurotrauma*, *34*, 1156–1163. http://dx.doi.org/10.1089/neu.2016.4632

Craig, A. R., Hancock, K., Chang, E., & Dickson, H. (1998). Immunizing against depression and anxiety after spinal cord injury. *Archives of Physical Medicine and Rehabilitation*, *79*, 375–377. http://dx.doi.org/10.1016/S0003-9993(98)90136-8

Cruz-Almeida, Y., Martinez-Arizala, A., & Widerström-Noga, E. G. (2005). Chronicity of pain associated with spinal cord injury: A longitudinal analysis. *Journal of Rehabilitation Research & Development*, *42*, 585–594. http://dx.doi.org/10.1682/JRRD.2005.02.0045

Dallolio, L., Menarini, M., China, S., Ventura, M., Stainthorpe, A., Soopramanien, A., . . . the THRIVE Project. (2008). Functional and clinical outcomes of telemedicine in patients with spinal cord injury. *Archives of Physical Medicine and Rehabilitation*, *89*, 2332–2341. http://dx.doi.org/10.1016/j.apmr.2008.06.012

Davies, D. S., & McColl, M. A. (2002). Lifestyle risks for three disease outcomes in spinal cord injury. *Clinical Rehabilitation*, *16*, 96–108. http://dx.doi.org/10.1191/0269215502cr443oa

de Groot, S., Post, M. W. M., Postma, K., Sluis, T. A., & van der Woude, L. H. V. (2010). Prospective analysis of body mass index during and up to 5 years after discharge from inpatient spinal cord injury rehabilitation. *Journal of Rehabilitation Medicine*, *42*, 922–928. http://dx.doi.org/10.2340/16501977-0605

Delis, D. C., Kramer, J. H., Kaplan, E., & Ober, B. A. (2000). *CVLT-II: California Verbal Learning Test: Adult version, manual*. San Antonio, TX: Psychological Corporation.

deRoon-Cassini, T. A., de St. Aubin, E., Valvano, A., Hastings, J., & Horn, P. (2009). Psychological well-being after spinal cord injury: Perception of loss and meaning making. *Rehabilitation Psychology*, *54*, 306–314. http://dx.doi.org/10.1037/a0016545

DeVivo, M. J., Black, K. J., Richards, J. S., & Stover, S. L. (1991). Suicide following spinal cord injury. *Paraplegia, 29*, 620–627.

Diener, E. D., Emmons, R. A., Larsen, R. J., & Griffin, S. (1985). The satisfaction with life scale. *Journal of Personality Assessment, 49*, 71–75. http://dx.doi.org/10.1207/s15327752jpa4901_13

Dijkers, M. P., & Zanca, J. M. (2013). Factors complicating treatment sessions in spinal cord injury rehabilitation: Nature, frequency, and consequences. *Archives of Physical Medicine and Rehabilitation, 94*, S115–S124. http://dx.doi.org/10.1016/j.apmr.2012.11.047

Duchnick, J. J., Letsch, E. A., & Curtiss, G. (2009). Coping effectiveness training during acute rehabilitation of spinal cord injury/dysfunction: A randomized clinical trial. *Rehabilitation Psychology, 54*, 123–132. http://dx.doi.org/10.1037/a0015571

Dunn, D. S., & Dougherty, S. B. (2005). Prospects for a positive psychology of rehabilitation. *Rehabilitation Psychology, 50*, 305–311. http://dx.doi.org/10.1037/0090-5550.50.3.305

Dunn, D. S., Uswatte, G., & Elliott, T. R. (2009). Happiness, resilience, and positive growth following physical disability: Issues for understanding, research, and therapeutic intervention. *Oxford Handbook of Positive Psychology, 2*, 651–664.

Dunn, M., Sommer, N., & Gambina, H. (1992). A practical guide to team functioning. In C. Zejdlik (Ed.), *Management of spinal cord injury* (2nd ed., pp. 229–239). Monterey, CA: Jones and Bartlett.

Ehde, D. M. (2010). Application of positive psychology to rehabilitation psychology. In Frank, R. G., Rosenthal, M., & Caplan, B. (Eds.), *Handbook of rehabilitation psychology* (pp. 417–424). Washington, DC: American Psychological Association. http://dx.doi.org/10.1037/15972-029

Ehde, D. M., & Hanley, M. A. (2006). Pain in patient groups frequently treated by physiatrists. *Physical Medicine and Rehabilitation Clinics of North America, 17*, 275–285. http://dx.doi.org/10.1016/j.pmr.2005.12.009

Elfström, M. L., Kennedy, P., Lude, P., & Taylor, N. (2007). Condition-related coping strategies in persons with spinal cord lesion: A cross-national validation of the Spinal Cord Lesion-Related Coping Strategies Questionnaire in four community samples. *Spinal Cord, 45*, 420–428. http://dx.doi.org/10.1038/sj.sc.3102003

Elliott, T. R., & Frank, R. G. (1996). Depression following spinal cord injury. *Archives of Physical Medicine and Rehabilitation, 77*, 816–823. http://dx.doi.org/10.1016/S0003-9993(96)90263-4

Elliott, T. R., Kurylo, M., Chen, Y., & Hicken, B. (2002). Alcohol abuse history and adjustment following spinal cord injury. *Rehabilitation Psychology, 47*, 278–290. http://dx.doi.org/10.1037/0090-5550.47.3.278

Erosa, N. A., Berry, J. W., Elliott, T. R., Underhill, A. T., & Fine, P. R. (2014). Predicting quality of life 5 years after medical discharge for traumatic spinal cord injury. *British Journal of Health Psychology, 19*, 688–700. http://dx.doi.org/10.1111/bjhp.12063

Fann, J. R., Bombardier, C. H., Richards, J. S., Tate, D. G., Wilson, C. S., Temkin, N., & the PRISMS Investigators. (2011). Depression after spinal cord injury: Comorbidities, mental health service use, and adequacy of treatment. *Archives of Physical Medicine and Rehabilitation, 92*, 352–360. http://dx.doi.org/10.1016/j.apmr.2010.05.016

Farrar, J. T., Young, J. P., Jr., LaMoreaux, L., Werth, J. L., & Poole, R. M. (2001). Clinical importance of changes in chronic pain intensity measured on an 11-point numerical pain rating scale. *Pain, 94*, 149–158.

Fava, G. A., & Ruini, C. (2003). Development and characteristics of a well-being enhancing psychotherapeutic strategy: Well-being therapy. *Journal of Behavior Therapy and Experimental Psychiatry, 34*, 45–63. http://dx.doi.org/10.1016/S0005-7916(03)00019-3

Findley, P. A., Banerjea, R., & Sambamoorthi, U. (2011). Excess mortality associated with mental illness and substance use disorders among veteran clinic users with spinal cord injury. *Disability and Rehabilitation, 33*, 1608–1615. http://dx.doi.org/10.3109/09638288.2010.540294

Fortmann, A. L., Rutledge, T., Corey McCulloch, R., Shivpuri, S., Nisenzon, A. N., & Muse, J. (2013). Satisfaction with life among veterans with spinal cord injuries completing multidisciplinary rehabilitation. *Spinal Cord, 51*, 482–486. http://dx.doi.org/10.1038/sc.2012.172

Galvin, L. R., & Godfrey, H. P. (2001). The impact of coping on emotional adjustment to spinal cord injury (SCI): Review of the literature and application of a stress appraisal and coping formulation. *Spinal Cord, 39*, 615–627. http://dx.doi.org/10.1038/sj.sc.3101221

Garma, S. I., Kelly, E. H., Daharsh, E. Z., & Vogel, L. C. (2011). Health-related quality of life after pediatric spinal cord injury. *Journal of Pediatric Psychology, 36*, 226–236. http://dx.doi.org/10.1093/jpepsy/jsq037

Garshick, E., Kelley, A., Cohen, S. A., Garrison, A., Tun, C. G., Gagnon, D., & Brown, R. (2005). A prospective assessment of mortality in chronic spinal cord injury. *Spinal Cord, 43*, 408–416. http://dx.doi.org/10.1038/sj.sc.3101729

Gentilello, L. M., Rivara, F. P., Donovan, D. M., Jurkovich, G. J., Daranciang, E., Dunn, C. W., . . . Ries, R. R. (1999). Alcohol interventions in a trauma center as a means of reducing the risk of injury recurrence. *Annals of Surgery, 230*, 473–480. http://dx.doi.org/10.1097/00000658-199910000-00003

Groah, S. L., Charlifue, S., Tate, D., Jensen, M. P., Molton, I. R., Forchheimer, M., . . . Campbell, M. (2012).

Spinal cord injury and aging: Challenges and recommendations for future research. *American Journal of Physical Medicine & Rehabilitation*, *91*, 80–93. http://dx.doi.org/10.1097/PHM.0b013e31821f70bc

Groah, S. L., Weitzenkamp, D., Sett, P., Soni, B., & Savic, G. (2001). The relationship between neurological level of injury and symptomatic cardiovascular disease risk in the aging spinal injured. *Spinal Cord*, *39*, 310–317. http://dx.doi.org/10.1038/sj.sc.3101162

Hart, T., & Ehde, D. M. (2015). Defining the treatment targets and active ingredients of rehabilitation: Implications for rehabilitation psychology. *Rehabilitation Psychology*, *60*, 126–135. http://dx.doi.org/10.1037/rep0000031

Hatcher, M. B., Whitaker, C., & Karl, A. (2009). What predicts post-traumatic stress following spinal cord injury? *British Journal of Health Psychology*, *14*, 541–561. http://dx.doi.org/10.1348/135910708X373445

Heinemann, A. W., & Hawkins, D. (1995). Substance abuse and medical complications following spinal cord injury. *Rehabilitation Psychology*, *40*, 125–141. http://dx.doi.org/10.1037/0090-5550.40.2.125

Heinemann, A. W., Keen, M., Donohue, R., & Schnoll, S. (1988). Alcohol use by persons with recent spinal cord injury. *Archives of Physical Medicine and Rehabilitation*, *69*, 619–624.

Heinemann, A. W., Schnoll, S., Brandt, M., Maltz, R., & Keen, M. (1988). Toxicology screening in acute spinal cord injury. *Alcoholism: Clinical and Experimental Research*, *12*, 815–819. http://dx.doi.org/10.1111/j.1530-0277.1988.tb01352.x

Hoffman, J. M., Bombardier, C. H., Graves, D. E., Kalpakjian, C. Z., & Krause, J. S. (2011). A longitudinal study of depression from 1 to 5 years after spinal cord injury. *Archives of Physical Medicine and Rehabilitation*, *92*, 411–418. http://dx.doi.org/10.1016/j.apmr.2010.10.036

Hough, S., Stone, M. T., & Buse, D. C. (2013). Dating and relationship psychoeducational group for veterans with spinal cord injury/Dysfunction: A historical account of an initial clinical course. *Sexuality and Disability*, *31*, 337–359. http://dx.doi.org/10.1007/s11195-013-9330-8

Huang, C.-Y., Chen, W.-K., Lu, C.-Y., Tsai, C.-C., Lai, H.-L., Lin, H.-Y., . . . Chen, C.-I. (2015). Mediating effects of social support and self-concept on depressive symptoms in adults with spinal cord injury. *Spinal Cord*, *53*, 413–416. http://dx.doi.org/10.1038/sc.2014.158

Jensen, M. P., Hoffman, A. J., & Cardenas, D. D. (2005). Chronic pain in individuals with spinal cord injury: A survey and longitudinal study. *Spinal Cord*, *43*, 704–712. http://dx.doi.org/10.1038/sj.sc.3101777

Kaplan, E., Goodglass, H., & Weintraub, S. (2001). *Boston Naming Test*. Austin, TX: Pro-Ed.

Kelly, E. H., Anderson, C. J., Garma, S. I., Russell, H. F., Klaas, S. J., Gorzkowski, J. A., & Vogel, L. C. (2011). Relationships between the psychological characteristics of youth with spinal cord injury and their primary caregivers. *Spinal Cord*, *49*, 200–205. http://dx.doi.org/10.1038/sc.2010.78

Kennedy, P., & Duff, J. (2001). Post traumatic stress disorder and spinal cord injuries. *Spinal Cord*, *39*, 1–10. http://dx.doi.org/10.1038/sj.sc.3101100

Kennedy, P., Duff, J., Evans, M., & Beedie, A. (2003). Coping effectiveness training reduces depression and anxiety following traumatic spinal cord injuries. *British Journal of Clinical Psychology*, *42*, 41–52. http://dx.doi.org/10.1348/014466503762842002

Kennedy, P., Lude, P., Elfström, M. L., & Smithson, E. (2010). Cognitive appraisals, coping and quality of life outcomes: A multi-centre study of spinal cord injury rehabilitation. *Spinal Cord*, *48*, 762–769. http://dx.doi.org/10.1038/sc.2010.20

Kennedy, P., Marsh, N., Lowe, R., Grey, N., Short, E., & Rogers, B. (2000). A longitudinal analysis of psychological impact and coping strategies following spinal cord injury. *British Journal of Health Psychology*, *5*, 157–172. http://dx.doi.org/10.1348/135910700168838

Kessler, R. C., Berglund, P., Demler, O., Jin, R., Merikangas, K. R., & Walters, E. E. (2005). Lifetime prevalence and age-of-onset distributions of *DSM–IV* disorders in the National Comorbidity Survey replication. *Archives of General Psychiatry*, *62*, 593–602. http://dx.doi.org/10.1001/archpsyc.62.6.593

King, C., & Kennedy, P. (1999). Coping effectiveness training for people with spinal cord injury: Preliminary results of a controlled trial. *British Journal of Clinical Psychology*, *38*, 5–14. http://dx.doi.org/10.1348/014466599162629

Kirschblum, S. C., Burns, S. P., Biering-Sorensen, F., Donovan, W., Graves, D. E., Jha, A., . . . Waring, W. (2011). International standards for neurological classification of SCI/D (revised 2011). *Journal of Spinal Cord Medicine*, *34*, 535–546. http://dx.doi.org/10.1179/204577211X13207446293695

Kishi, Y., Robinson, R. G., & Forrester, A. W. (1994). Prospective longitudinal study of depression following spinal cord injury. *The Journal of Neuropsychiatry and Clinical Neurosciences*, *6*, 237–244. http://dx.doi.org/10.1176/jnp.6.3.237

Klyce, D. W., Bombardier, C. H., Davis, T. J., Hartoonian, N., Hoffman, J. M., Fann, J. R., & Kalpakjian, C. Z. (2015). Distinguishing grief from depression during acute recovery from spinal cord injury. *Archives of Physical Medicine and Rehabilitation*, *96*, 1419–1425. http://dx.doi.org/10.1016/j.apmr.2015.02.018

Kortte, K. B., Gilbert, M., Gorman, P., & Wegener, S. T. (2010). Positive psychological variables in the prediction of life satisfaction after spinal cord injury. *Rehabilitation Psychology*, *55*, 40–47. http://dx.doi.org/10.1037/a0018624

Kortte, K. B., Stevenson, J. E., Hosey, M. M., Castillo, R., & Wegener, S. T. (2012). Hope predicts positive functional role outcomes in acute rehabilitation populations. *Rehabilitation Psychology*, *57*, 248–255. http://dx.doi.org/10.1037/a0029004

Krause, J. S., & Broderick, L. (2004). Patterns of recurrent pressure ulcers after spinal cord injury: Identification of risk and protective factors 5 or more years after onset. *Archives of Physical Medicine and Rehabilitation, 85,* 1257–1264. http://dx.doi.org/10.1016/j.apmr.2003.08.108

Krause, J. S., Carter, R., Zhai, Y., & Reed, K. (2009). Psychologic factors and risk of mortality after spinal cord injury. *Archives of Physical Medicine and Rehabilitation*, *90*, 628–633. http://dx.doi.org/10.1016/j.apmr.2008.10.014

Krause, J. S., & Edles, P. A. (2014). Injury perceptions, hope for recovery, and psychological status after spinal cord injury. *Rehabilitation Psychology*, *59*, 176–182. http://dx.doi.org/10.1037/a0035778

Krause, J. S., & Saunders, L. L. (2011). Health, secondary conditions, and life expectancy after spinal cord injury. *Archives of Physical Medicine and Rehabilitation*, *92*, 1770–1775. http://dx.doi.org/10.1016/j.apmr.2011.05.024

Krause, J. S., Saunders, L. L., & Newman, S. (2010). Posttraumatic stress disorder and spinal cord injury. *Archives of Physical Medicine and Rehabilitation*, *91*, 1182–1187. http://dx.doi.org/10.1016/j.apmr.2010.05.012

Kroenke, K., Spitzer, R. L., & Williams, J. B. (2001). The PHQ-9: Validity of a brief depression severity measure. *Journal of General Internal Medicine*, *16*, 606–613. http://dx.doi.org/10.1046/j.1525-1497.2001.016009606.x

Krueger, H., Noonan, V. K., Williams, D., Trenaman, L. M., & Rivers, C. S. (2013). The influence of depression on physical complications in spinal cord injury: Behavioral mechanisms and health-care implications. *Spinal Cord*, *51*, 260–266. http://dx.doi.org/10.1038/sc.2013.3

Latimer-Cheung, A. E., Arbour-Nicitopoulos, K. P., Brawley, L. R., Gray, C., Justine Wilson, A., Prapavessis, H., . . . Martin Ginis, K. A. (2013). Developing physical activity interventions for adults with spinal cord injury: Part 2: Motivational counseling and peer-mediated interventions for people intending to be active. *Rehabilitation Psychology*, *58*, 307–315. http://dx.doi.org/10.1037/a0032816

LaVela, S. L., Evans, C. T., Prohaska, T. R., Miskevics, S., Ganesh, S. P., & Weaver, F. M. (2012). Males aging with a spinal cord injury: Prevalence of cardiovascular and metabolic conditions. *Archives of Physical Medicine and Rehabilitation*, *93*, 90–95. http://dx.doi.org/10.1016/j.apmr.2011.07.201

Lazarus, R., & Folkman, S. (1984). *Stress, appraisal, and coping*. New York, NY: Springer.

Livneh, H., & Martz, E. (2014). Coping strategies and resources as predictors of psychosocial adaptation among people with spinal cord injury. *Rehabilitation Psychology*, *59*, 329–339. http://dx.doi.org/10.1037/a0036733

Locatelli, S. M., Gerber, B. S., Goldstein, B., Weaver, F. M., & LaVela, S. L. (2014). Health care provider practices, barriers, and facilitators for weight management for individuals with spinal cord injuries and disorders. *Topics in Spinal Cord Injury Rehabilitation*, *20*, 329–337. http://dx.doi.org/10.1310/sci2004-329

Locatelli, S. M., & LaVela, S. L. (2016). Documentation of weight management practices for individuals with spinal cord injuries and disorders. *Spinal Cord*, *54*, 1176–1182. http://dx.doi.org/10.1038/sc.2016.59

Lude, P., Kennedy, P., Evans, M., Lude, Y., & Beedie, A. (2005). Post traumatic distress symptoms following spinal cord injury: A comparative review of European samples. *Spinal Cord*, *43*, 102–108. http://dx.doi.org/10.1038/sj.sc.3101688

Lustig, D. C. (2005). The adjustment process for individuals with spinal cord injury: The effect of perceived premorbid sense of coherence. *Rehabilitation Counseling Bulletin*, *48*, 146–156. http://dx.doi.org/10.1177/00343552050480030301

Macciocchi, S., Seel, R. T., Thompson, N., Byams, R., & Bowman, B. (2008). Spinal cord injury and co-occurring traumatic brain injury: Assessment and incidence. *Archives of Physical Medicine and Rehabilitation, 89*, 1350–1357.

Martin Ginis, K. A., Nigg, C. R., & Smith, A. L. (2013). Peer-delivered physical activity interventions: An overlooked opportunity for physical activity promotion. *Translational Behavioral Medicine*, *3*, 434–443. http://dx.doi.org/10.1007/s13142-013-0215-2

McMillen, J. C., & Cook, C. L. (2003). The positive by-products of spinal cord injury and their correlates. *Rehabilitation Psychology*, *48*, 77–85. http://dx.doi.org/10.1037/0090-5550.48.2.77

Mehta, S., Orenczuk, S., Hansen, K. T., Aubut, J.-A., Hitzig, S. L., Legassic, M., . . . the Spinal Cord Injury Rehabilitation Evidence Research Team. (2011). An evidence-based review of the effectiveness of cognitive behavioral therapy for psychosocial issues post-spinal cord injury. *Rehabilitation Psychology*, *56*, 15–25. http://dx.doi.org/10.1037/a0022743

Melzack, R. (1975). The McGill Pain Questionnaire: Major properties and scoring methods. *Pain*, *1*, 277–299.

Migliorini, C., Sinclair, A., Brown, D., Tonge, B., & New, P. (2015). A randomised control trial of an Internet-based cognitive behaviour treatment for mood disorder in adults with chronic spinal cord injury. *Spinal Cord*, *54*, 695–701.

Mignogna, J., Christie, A. J., Holmes, S. A., & Ames, H. (2015). Measuring disability-associated appraisals for veterans with spinal cord injury. *Rehabilitation Psychology*, *60*, 99–104. http://dx.doi.org/10.1037/rep0000022

Mortenson, W. B., Noreau, L., & Miller, W. C. (2010). The relationship between and predictors of quality of life after spinal cord injury at 3 and 15 months after discharge. *Spinal Cord*, *48*, 73–79. http://dx.doi.org/10.1038/sc.2009.92

Müller, R., Gertz, K. J., Molton, I. R., Terrill, A. L., Bombardier, C. H., Ehde, D. M., & Jensen, M. P. (2016). Effects of a tailored positive psychology intervention on well-being and pain in individuals with chronic pain and a physical disability: A feasibility trial. *The Clinical Journal of Pain*, *32*, 32–44. http://dx.doi.org/10.1097/AJP.0000000000000225

Müller, R., Peter, C., Cieza, A., & Geyh, S. (2012). The role of social support and social skills in people with spinal cord injury—A systematic review of the literature. *Spinal Cord*, *50*, 94–106. http://dx.doi.org/10.1038/sc.2011.116

Munce, S. E. P., Webster, F., Fehlings, M. G., Straus, S. E., Jang, E., & Jaglal, S. B. (2016). Meaning of self-management from the perspective of individuals with traumatic spinal cord injury, their caregivers, and acute care and rehabilitation managers: An opportunity for improved care delivery. *BMC Neurology*, *16*, 11. http://dx.doi.org/10.1186/s12883-016-0534-2

National Academies of Sciences, Engineering, and Medicine. (2017). *Communities in action: Pathways to health equity*. Washington, DC: National Academies Press. Retrieved from https://www.ncbi.nlm.nih.gov/books/NBK425844/

National Spinal Cord Injury Statistical Center. (2016). *Spinal cord injury (SCI) facts and figures at a glance*. Birmingham: University of Alabama.

Nielsen, M. S. (2003). Prevalence of posttraumatic stress disorder in people with spinal cord injuries: The mediating effect of social support. *Rehabilitation Psychology*, *48*, 289–295. http://dx.doi.org/10.1037/0090-5550.48.4.289

Nierenberg, B., Mayersohn, G., Serpa, S., Holovatyk, A., Smith, E., & Cooper, S. (2016). Application of well-being therapy to people with disability and chronic illness. *Rehabilitation Psychology*, *61*, 32–43. http://dx.doi.org/10.1037/rep0000060

Noreau, L., Fougeyrollas, P., & Vincent, C. (2002). The LIFE-H: Assessment of the quality of social participation. *Technology and Disability*, *14*, 113–118

Olkin, R. (1999). *What psychotherapists should know about disability*. New York, NY: Guilford Press.

Ottomanelli, L., Goetz, L. L., Suris, A., McGeough, C., Sinnott, P. L., Toscano, R., . . . Thomas, F. P. (2012). Effectiveness of supported employment for veterans with spinal cord injuries: Results from a randomized multisite study. *Archives of Physical Medicine and Rehabilitation*, *93*, 740–747. http://dx.doi.org/10.1016/j.apmr.2012.01.002

Ottomanelli, L., & Lind, L. (2009). Review of critical factors related to employment after spinal cord injury: Implications for research and vocational services. *The Journal of Spinal Cord Medicine*, *32*, 503–531. http://dx.doi.org/10.1080/10790268.2009.11754553

Pains, A., Ouimette, P., Kimerling, R., Cameron, R. P., Hugelshofer, D. S., Shaw-Hegwer, J., . . . Sheikh, J. I. (2003). The Primary Care PTSD Screen (PC-PTSD): Development and operating characteristics. *Primary Care Psychiatry*, *9*, 9–14.

Perrier, M. J., Stork, M. J., & Martin Ginis, K. A. (2016). Type, intensity and duration of daily physical activities performed by adults with spinal cord injury. *Spinal Cord*, *7*, 1–7. http://dx.doi.org/10.1038/sc.2016.86

Peter, C., Müller, R., Cieza, A., & Geyh, S. (2012). Psychological resources in spinal cord injury: A systematic literature review. *Spinal Cord*, *50*, 188–201. http://dx.doi.org/10.1038/sc.2011.125

Pollard, C., & Kennedy, P. (2007). A longitudinal analysis of emotional impact, coping strategies and post-traumatic psychological growth following spinal cord injury: A 10-year review. *British Journal of Health Psychology*, *12*, 347–362. http://dx.doi.org/10.1348/135910707X197046

Post, M. W., & van Leeuwen, C. M. (2012). Psychosocial issues in spinal cord injury: A review. *Spinal Cord*, *50*, 382–389. http://dx.doi.org/10.1038/sc.2011.182

Radloff, L. S. (1977). The CES-D Scale: A self-report depression scale for research in the general population. *Applied Psychological Measurement*, *1*, 385–401 http://dx.doi.org/10.1177/014662167700100306

Radnitz, C. L., Hsu, L., Willard, J., Perez-Strumolo, L., Festa, J., Lillian, L. B., . . . Broderick, C. P. (1998). Posttraumatic stress disorder in veterans with spinal cord injury: Trauma-related risk factors. *Journal of Traumatic Stress*, *11*, 505–520. http://dx.doi.org/10.1023/A:1024404729251

Rajan, S., McNeely, M. J., Hammond, M., Goldstein, B., & Weaver, F. (2010). Association between obesity and diabetes mellitus in veterans with spinal cord injuries and disorders. *American Journal of Physical Medicine & Rehabilitation*, *89*, 353–361. http://dx.doi.org/10.1097/PHM.0b013e3181d896b9

Rees, P. M., Fowler, C. J., & Maas, C. P. (2007). Sexual function in men and women with neurological disorders. *The Lancet, 369*, 512–525. http://dx.doi.org/10.1016/S0140-6736(07)60238-4

Ricker, J., & Regan, T. (1999). Neuropsychological and psychological factors in acute rehabilitation of individuals with both spinal cord injury and traumatic brain injury. *Topics in Spinal Cord Injury Rehabilitation, 5*, 76–82. http://dx.doi.org/10.1310/0YJX-2KYE-VY3Q-9D5V

Ricker, J. H., & Axelrod, B. N. (1994). Analysis of an oral paradigm for the Trail Making Test. *Assessment, 1*, 47–51. http://dx.doi.org/10.1177/107319119400100107

Rintala, D. H., Hart, K. A., & Priebe, M. M. (2004). Predicting consistency of pain over a 10-year period in persons with spinal cord injury. *Journal of Rehabilitation Research and Development, 41*, 75–88. http://dx.doi.org/10.1682/JRRD.2004.01.0075

Rose, J. (2012). Lessons for spinal cord injury rehabilitation taken from adult developmental psychology: 2011 Essie Morgan lecture. *The Journal of Spinal Cord Medicine, 35*, 133–139. http://dx.doi.org/10.1179/2045772312Y.0000000006

Ruff, R. M., Light, R. H., Parker, S. B., & Levin, H. S. (1996). Benton Controlled Oral Word Association Test: Reliability and updated norms. *Archives of Clinical Neuropsychology, 11*, 329–338. http://dx.doi.org/10.1016/0887-6177(95)00033-X

Saunders, J. B., Aasland, O. G., Babor, T. F., de la Fuente, J. R., & Grant, M. (1993). Development of the Alcohol Use Disorders Identification Test (AUDIT): WHO collaborative project on early detection of persons with harmful alcohol consumption—II. *Addiction, 88*, 791–804. http://dx.doi.org/10.1111/j.1360-0443.1993.tb02093.x

Saunders, L. L., Krause, J. S., Carpenter, M. J., & Saladin, M. (2014). Risk behaviors related to cigarette smoking among persons with spinal cord injury. *Nicotine & Tobacco Research, 16*, 224–230. http://dx.doi.org/10.1093/ntr/ntt153

Saunders, L. L., Krause, J. S., Saladin, M., & Carpenter, M. J. (2015). Prevalence of cigarette smoking and attempts to quit in a population-based cohort with spinal cord injury. *Spinal Cord, 53*, 641–645. http://dx.doi.org/10.1038/sc.2015.71

Schönenberg, M., Reimitz, M., Jusyte, A., Maier, D., Badke, A., & Hautzinger, M. (2014). Depression, posttraumatic stress, and risk factors following spinal cord injury. *International Journal of Behavioral Medicine, 21*, 169–176. http://dx.doi.org/10.1007/s12529-012-9284-8

Schretlen, D. (1989). *Brief Test of Attention*. Baltimore, MD: Psychological Assessment Resources.

Seligman, M. E., & Csikszentmihalyi, M. (2000). Positive psychology. An introduction. *American Psychologist, 55*, 5–14. http://dx.doi.org/10.1037/0003-066X.55.1.5

Seligman, M. E. P., Rashid, T., & Parks, A. C. (2006). Positive psychotherapy. *American Psychologist, 61*, 774–788. http://dx.doi.org/10.1037/0003-066X.61.8.774

Sherman, J. E., DeVinney, D. J., & Sperling, K. B. (2004). Social support and adjustment after spinal cord injury: Influence of past peer-mentoring experiences and current live-in partners. *Rehabilitation Psychology, 49*, 140–149. http://dx.doi.org/10.1037/0090-5550.49.2.140

Siddall, P. J., McClelland, J. M., Rutkowski, S. B., & Cousins, M. J. (2003). A longitudinal study of the prevalence and characteristics of pain in the first 5 years following spinal cord injury. *Pain, 103*, 249–257. http://dx.doi.org/10.1016/S0304-3959(02)00452-9

Sin, N. L., & Lyubomirsky, S. (2009). Enhancing well-being and alleviating depressive symptoms with positive psychology interventions: A practice-friendly meta-analysis. *Journal of Clinical Psychology, 65*, 467–487. http://dx.doi.org/10.1002/jclp.20593

Smith, B. M., Weaver, F. M., & Ullrich, P. M. (2007). Prevalence of depression diagnoses and use of antidepressant medications by veterans with spinal cord injury. *American Journal of Physical Medicine & Rehabilitation, 86*, 662–671. http://dx.doi.org/10.1097/PHM.0b013e318114cb6d

Spielberger, C. D. (1983). *Manual for the State-Trait Anxiety Inventory STAI (Form Y) ("Self-Evaluation Questionnaire")*. Palo Alto, CA: Consulting Psychologists Press.

Spitzer, R. L., Kroenke, K., Williams, J. B., & Löwe, B. (2006). A brief measure for assessing generalized anxiety disorder: The GAD-7. *Archives of Internal Medicine, 166*, 1092–1097. http://dx.doi.org/10.1001/archinte.166.10.1092

St. Andre, J. R., Smith, B. M., Stroupe, K. T., Burns, S. P., Evans, C. T., Ripley, D. C., . . . Weaver, F. M. (2011). A comparison of costs and health care utilization for veterans with traumatic and nontraumatic spinal cord injury. *Topics in Spinal Cord Injury Rehabilitation, 16*(4), 27–42. http://dx.doi.org/10.1310/sci1604-27

Stenson, K. W., Deutsch, A., Heinemann, A. W., & Chen, D. (2011). Obesity and inpatient rehabilitation outcomes for patients with a traumatic spinal cord injury. *Archives of Physical Medicine and Rehabilitation, 92*, 384–390. http://dx.doi.org/10.1016/j.apmr.2010.07.235

Stroud, M. W., Bombardier, C. H., Dyer, J. R., Rimmele, C. T., & Esselman, P. C. (2011). Preinjury alcohol and drug use among persons with spinal cord injury: Implications for rehabilitation. *The Journal of Spinal*

Cord Medicine, *34*, 461–472. http://dx.doi.org/10.1179/2045772311Y.0000000033

Tan, G., Jensen, M. P., Thornby, J. I., & Shanti, B. F. (2004). Validation of the Brief Pain Inventory for chronic nonmalignant pain. *The Journal of Pain*, *5*, 133–137. http://dx.doi.org/10.1016/j.jpain.2003.12.005

Tate, D. G. (1993). Alcohol use among spinal cord–injured patients. *American Journal of Physical Medicine & Rehabilitation*, *72*, 192–195. http://dx.doi.org/10.1097/00002060-199308000-00004

Tate, D. G., Forchheimer, M. B., Krause, J. S., Meade, M. A., & Bombardier, C. H. (2004). Patterns of alcohol and substance use and abuse in persons with spinal cord injury: Risk factors and correlates. *Archives of Physical Medicine and Rehabilitation*, *85*, 1837–1847. http://dx.doi.org/10.1016/j.apmr.2004.02.022

Tombaugh, T. N., Kozak, J., & Rees, L. (1999). Normative data stratified by age and education for two measures of verbal fluency: FAS and animal naming. *Archives of Clinical Neuropsychology*, *14*, 167–177. http://dx.doi.org/10.1016/S0887-6177(97)00095-4

Trahan, D. E., & Larrabee, G. J. (1988). *Continuous Visual Memory Test: Professional manual*. Lutz, FL: Psychological Assessment Resources.

Trieschmann, R. (1988). *Spinal cord injuries: Psychological, social, and vocational rehabilitation* (2nd ed.). New York, NY: Demos.

Turner, J. A., Cardenas, D. D., Warms, C. A., & McClellan, C. B. (2001). Chronic pain associated with spinal cord injuries: A community survey. *Archives of Physical Medicine and Rehabilitation*, *82*, 501–508. http://dx.doi.org/10.1053/apmr.2001.21855

Ullrich, P. M. (2007). Pain following spinal cord injury. *Physical Medicine and Rehabilitation Clinics of North America*, *18*, 217–233. http://dx.doi.org/10.1016/j.pmr.2007.03.001

Ullrich, P. M., Lincoln, R. K., Tackett, M. J., Miskevics, S., Smith, B. M., & Weaver, F. M. (2013). Pain, depression, and health care utilization over time after spinal cord injury. *Rehabilitation Psychology*, *58*, 158–165. http://dx.doi.org/10.1037/a0032047

Ullrich, P. M., Smith, B. M., Blow, F. C., Valenstein, M., & Weaver, F. M. (2014). Depression, healthcare utilization, and comorbid psychiatric disorders after spinal cord injury. *Journal of Spinal Cord Medicine*, *37*, 40–45.

Ullrich, P. M., Smith, B. M., Poggensee, L., Evans, C. T., Stroupe, K. T., Weaver, F. M., & Burns, S. P. (2013). Pain and post-traumatic stress disorder symptoms during inpatient rehabilitation among Operation Enduring Freedom/Operation Iraqi Freedom veterans with spinal cord injury. *Archives of Physical Medicine and Rehabilitation*, *94*, 80–85. http://dx.doi.org/10.1016/j.apmr.2012.07.018

van Leeuwen, C. M., Hoekstra, T., van Koppenhagen, C. F., de Groot, S., & Post, M. W. (2012). Trajectories and predictors of the course of mental health after spinal cord injury. *Archives of Physical Medicine and Rehabilitation*, *93*, 2170–2176. http://dx.doi.org/10.1016/j.apmr.2012.07.006

van Wyk, K., Backwell, A., & Townson, A. (2015). A narrative literature review to direct spinal cord injury patient education programming. *Topics in Spinal Cord Injury Rehabilitation*, *21*, 49–60. http://dx.doi.org/10.1310/sci2101-49

Veith, E. M., Sherman, J. E., Pellino, T. A., & Yasui, N. Y. (2006). Qualitative analysis of the peer-mentoring relationship among individuals with spinal cord injury. *Rehabilitation Psychology*, *51*, 289–298. http://dx.doi.org/10.1037/0090-5550.51.4.289

Watanabe, T. K., Zafonte, R. D., & Lairson, E. J. (1999). Traumatic brain injury associated with acute spinal cord injury: Risk factors, evaluation, and outcomes. *Topics in Spinal Cord Injury Rehabilitation*, *5*, 83–90. http://dx.doi.org/10.1310/JDDU-W8FQ-8XQQ-LNT7

Weaver, F. M., Collins, E. G., Kurichi, J., Miskevics, S., Smith, B., Rajan, S., & Gater, D. (2007). Prevalence of obesity and high blood pressure in veterans with spinal cord injuries and disorders: A retrospective review. *American Journal of Physical Medicine & Rehabilitation*, *86*, 22–29. http://dx.doi.org/10.1097/PHM.0b013e31802b8937

Weaver, F. M., Smith, B., LaVela, S. L., Evans, C. T., Ullrich, P., Miskevics, S., . . . Burns, S. P. (2011). Smoking behavior and delivery of evidence-based care for veterans with spinal cord injuries and disorders. *The Journal of Spinal Cord Medicine*, *34*, 35–45. http://dx.doi.org/10.1179/107902610X12911165975061

Wechsler, D. (2009). *Advanced clinical solutions for WAIS-IV and WMS-IV: Administration and scoring manual*. San Antonio, TX: Pearson.

Wechsler, D., Coalson, D. L., & Raiford, S. E. (2008). *WAIS-IV: Wechsler Adult Intelligence Scale*. San Antonio, TX: Pearson.

Westgren, N., & Levi, R. (1998). Quality of life and traumatic spinal cord injury. *Archives of Physical Medicine and Rehabilitation*, *79*, 1433–1439. http://dx.doi.org/10.1016/S0003-9993(98)90240-4

Whiteneck, G. G. (1992). *Craig handicap assessment and reporting technique*. New York, NY: Aspen.

WHO ASSIST Working Group. (2002). The Alcohol, Smoking and Substance Involvement Screening Test (ASSIST): Development, reliability and feasibility. *Addiction*, *97*, 1183–1194.

Widerström-Noga, E. G., Felipe-Cuervo, E., & Yezierski, R. P. (2001). Relationships among clinical characteristics of chronic pain after spinal cord injury. *Archives of Physical Medicine and Rehabilitation*, *82*, 1191–1197. http://dx.doi.org/10.1053/apmr.2001.25077

Williams, R., & Murray, A. (2015). Prevalence of depression after spinal cord injury: A meta-analysis. *Archives of Physical Medicine and Rehabilitation*, *96*, 133–140. http://dx.doi.org/10.1016/j.apmr.2014.08.016

Wilson, C. S., Forchheimer, M., Heinemann, A. W., Warren, A. M., & McCullumsmith, C. (2017). Assessment of the relationship of spiritual well-being to depression and quality of life for persons with spinal cord injury. *Disability and Rehabilitation: An International, Multidisciplinary Journal*, *39*, 491–496. http://dx.doi.org/10.3109/09638288.2016.1152600

Woolrich, R. A., Kennedy, P., & Tasiemski, T. (2006). A preliminary psychometric evaluation of the Hospital Anxiety and Depression Scale (HADS) in 963 people living with a spinal cord injury. *Psychology, Health & Medicine*, *11*, 80–90. http://dx.doi.org/10.1080/13548500500294211

Zanca, J. M., Dijkers, M. P., Hammond, F. M., & Horn, S. D. (2013). Pain and its impact on inpatient rehabilitation for acute traumatic spinal cord injury: Analysis of observational data collected in the SCIRehab study. *Archives of Physical Medicine and Rehabilitation*, *94*, S137–S144. http://dx.doi.org/10.1016/j.apmr.2012.10.035

CHAPTER 18

TRAUMATIC BRAIN INJURY

Suzanne McGarity, Lisa A. Brenner, and John D. Corrigan

Traumatic brain injury (TBI) is a major cause of disability and death worldwide. Although some individuals who sustain a TBI, particularly a mild TBI (mTBI), can return to previous levels of functioning, more severe injuries may result in lifelong impairment and decreased function. In such cases individuals who are injured, as well as families and caregivers, may require long-term services and support. As such, the role of rehabilitation psychologists in the lives of those living with TBI may begin during the acute period of care (e.g., emergency department, intensive care units, medical or rehabilitation inpatient units) and continue for many years postdischarge. In this chapter, we provide foundational information regarding TBI (e.g., operational definition, epidemiology), as well as evidence-informed guidance regarding assessment and treatment practices. It is important to note that research regarding TBI continues to exponentially increase. This growth is in large part due to recent focus on two populations at risk: (a) members of the military who served in Iraq and Afghanistan and (b) individuals engaged in contact sports (e.g., football). As such, those interested in this topic are encouraged to continue to review the literature for emerging, evidence-based practices. Topics addressed here are as follows: (a) criteria for diagnosing and categorizing TBI, (b) epidemiology of TBI, (c) screening and case ascertainment methods, and (d) assessment and treatment approaches.

TBI CRITERIA AND ASSOCIATED KEY TERMS

According to the Centers for Disease Control and Prevention (CDC), TBI "is caused by a bump, blow or jolt to the head or a penetrating head injury that disrupts the normal function of the brain" (Faul, Xu, Wald, & Coronado, 2010, p. 8). Although alternative criteria have been put forth by other organizations (e.g., the World Health Organization), all include the same two key components: an external force that results in an alteration of brain functioning; because a TBI results in damage to the brain caused by an external force, it is distinguished from other sources of acquired brain injury (ABI) such as stroke or anoxia. Thus, a TBI is an ABI, but ABI is a broader category. This distinction is important when considering the characteristic ways in which each kind of ABI damages the brain and the subsequent effects on affect, cognition, and behavior. An external force may result from the head being struck by an object, the head striking an object, the brain undergoing acceleration–deceleration without direct external trauma to the head, a foreign body penetrating the brain, forces generated from events such as a blast or explosion, or some other force yet to be defined (Maas et al., 2010; Menon, Schwab, Wright, Maas, & Demographics and Clinical Assessment Working Group of the International and Interagency Initiative Toward Common Data

http://dx.doi.org/10.1037/0000129-019
Handbook of Rehabilitation Psychology, Third Edition, L. A. Brenner, S. A. Reid-Arndt, T. R. Elliott, R. G. Frank, and B. Caplan (Editors-in-Chief)

Elements for Research on Traumatic Brain Injury and Psychological Health, 2010). The second criterion required to diagnose TBI is the disruption of normal brain functioning, which separates "head trauma" from TBI. These two terms are often mistakenly used interchangeably. The disruption in functioning can be caused by various primary or secondary processes including diffuse axonal injury, wherein axons within the brain are torn by acceleration and/or deceleration forces, contusions (bruises to the brain), and/or penetrating injuries that damage tissue by pushing skull fragments into the brain.

The recently published fifth edition of the American Psychiatric Association's (2013) *Diagnostic and Statistical Manual of Mental Disorders* (*DSM–5*) provides criteria for attributing neurocognitive problems to the injury. TBI and its sequelae are categorized as neurocognitive disorders, conditions in which impaired cognition is present and not the result of congenital or early developmental events. Neurocognitive disorders are classified as either "Mild" or "Major," the difference being whether (a) there have been modest or significant declines in cognitive function compared with preinjury functioning and (b) the impairment interferes with independent performance of everyday activities, often termed *activities of daily living* and *instrumental activities of daily living*. Therefore, the *DSM–5* severity specifiers for neurocognitive disorders do not directly correlate with more commonly used terms to classify TBI severity (described in the next section). *DSM–5* neurocognitive disorder specifiers describe the lasting effects of the injury rather than the immediate degree of alteration of brain functioning. The criteria also stipulate that the cognitive deficits cannot exclusively be related to delirium or better explained by another mental health or physical disorder.

TBI Severity and Symptomatology

Generally, TBIs are classified into three categories of severity: mild (also termed *concussion*), moderate, and severe. TBI severity is determined by the extent of altered brain function arising from the acute impact versus symptom severity in the postinjury period. Several benchmarks are used to classify severity including (a) the alteration of mental state or loss of consciousness (LOC) and its duration, (b) one's ability to process or respond to environmental stimuli (e.g., ability to follow commands), (c) the presence and duration of posttraumatic amnesia (PTA), (d) the presence of neurologic markers (e.g., reflexive and spontaneous behaviors), and (e) imaging results showing structural changes to the brain. Alterations of consciousness can be manifest as confusion, disorientation, or slowed thinking (Menon et al., 2010). More severe injuries can result in LOC, in which the person is unable to respond to any external stimuli. PTA refers to a postinjury confusional state in which the person does not form continuous memories (Sherer, Nakase-Thompson, Yablon, & Gontkovsky, 2005) and may include periods of both altered consciousness and LOC. Common neurological deficits after TBI include muscle weakness, loss of balance and coordination, disruption of vision, change in speech and language, and sensory loss. Finally, coma is the most severe disruption of brain function, during which patients may not display reflexive or spontaneous behavior, such as localizing to pain or opening eyes to the sound of voices. Although many of these signs of altered brain function may improve within seconds, minutes, or hours after the injury, the initial categorical rating of TBI severity describes the worst signs observed at the time of injury, regardless of subsequent change.

The preceding described benchmarks can be used to determine overall level of TBI severity. A commonly used classification system is outlined in Table 18.1. If indices within one contradict another, it is recommended that the injury be classified by the index indicating the greatest level of severity (U.S. Department of Veterans Affairs and Department of Defense, 2016, p. 7).

Injury severity, location of impact, etiology of injury, systems affected by injury, amount of time elapsed, and resources available to aid recovery each contribute to an individual's specific symptom profile after sustaining a TBI. Postinjury symptoms include physical, cognitive, emotional, and behavioral effects, which can occur immediately after injury or develop over time. Symptoms can be experienced for a relatively brief time or be more prolonged. Finally, post-TBI symptoms can be physically observable, experienced subjectively, or both. The person sustaining the injury may notice

TABLE 18.1

Veterans Affairs/Department of Defense Traumatic Brain Injury (TBI) Severity Criteria

Criteria	Mild	Moderate	Severe
Structural imaging	Normal	Normal or abnormal	Normal or abnormal
Loss of consciousness	0–30 minutes	>30 minutes and <24 hours	>24 hours
Alteration of consciousness/mental state*	Up to 24 hours	>24 hours; severity based on other criteria	>24 hours; severity based on other criteria
Posttraumatic amnesia	0–1 day	>1 and <7 days	>7 days
Glasgow Coma Scale (GCS; best available score in first 24 hours)**	13–15	9–12	<9

Note. If a patient meets criteria in more than one category of severity, the higher severity level is assigned. From *VA/DoD Clinical Practice Guideline for the Management of Concussion–Mild Traumatic Brain Injury* (p. 7), by the U.S. Department of Veterans Affairs and Department of Defense, 2016. Retrieved from https://www.healthquality.va.gov/guidelines/Rehab/mtbi/mTBICPGFullCPG50821816.pdf. In the public domain.
*Alteration of mental status must be immediately related to the trauma to the head. Typical symptoms would be looking and feeling dazed and uncertain of what is happening, confusion, and difficulty thinking clearly or responding appropriately to mental status questions, and being unable to describe events immediately before or after the trauma event.
**In April 2015, the Department of Defense released a memorandum recommending against the use of GCS scores to diagnose TBI. See the memorandum for additional information (Assistant Secretary of Defense, 2015).

and report symptoms, or he or she may not be aware of them. Some symptoms are only identified by in-depth assessment and evaluation. Common postinjury symptoms are outlined in Table 18.2.

The anterior portions of the brain including the frontal lobes are most vulnerable to damage as the result of TBI because they are more likely to become contused by contact with the skull or experience shearing during an acceleration–deceleration event. The bones near these parts of the brain have an irregular and rough texture. TBIs involving frontal lobe damage are most common because of

TABLE 18.2

Common Traumatic Brain Injury (TBI) Symptoms by Injury Severity

	Symptoms			
TBI severity	Physical	Cognitive	Emotional	Behavioral
Mild	Headache Dizziness Fatigue Noise/light intolerance	Memory complaints Blurred/double vision Feeling "dazed and confused" Memory gaps	Depression Irritability Anxiety Mood lability	Clumsiness Slowed behavior Agitation
Moderate and severe (in addition to all symptoms for mild TBI)	Observed physical trauma to head Pupillary dilation/asymmetry Seizures Nausea and vomiting Hypoxia Hypotension Cerebral herniation Paralysis Spasticity	Visuospatial problems Problems expressing or understanding language Inability to recognize people, places, or things Problems reading and writing Problems with planning and organizing	Emotional dysregulation Denial Alexithymia	Disruption of motor function Unable to follow commands Pain behaviors Perseveration Aggression Disinhibition Lack of awareness Poor motivation

this structural vulnerability. Additionally, neural networks connecting the frontal lobes with medial structures are vulnerable to stretching and tearing, often called shear injury. The frontal lobes, and the networks they serve, are substantially responsible for organization and regulation of behavior, referred to as *executive functioning*. Persons with frontal lobe damage due to TBI often demonstrate problems with attention, memory, problem-solving, awareness, and adaptability. These deficits result in observable difficulties, such as problems with time management, planning and organizing, remembering details, inhibiting socially undesirable behavior, learning from experience, or acting independently. As a result, persons with frontal lobe injuries are more likely to experience problems returning to or maintaining work and sustaining interpersonal relationships.

TBI as a Chronic Health Condition

In the 2002 Global Report, the World Health Organization expanded the concept of chronic conditions beyond traditional, noncommunicable diseases to encompass any condition following a chronic course that requires lifestyle changes and health care management over time and places considerable demand on patients, families, and health care systems. Symptoms related to a history of TBI, particularly a more severe injury, can meet these criteria, as brain injuries can result in irreversible pathological alterations in physical, cognitive, behavioral, and psychological functioning. History of TBI is also associated with increased incidences of seizures, sleep disorders, neurodegenerative diseases, neuroendocrine dysregulation, and psychiatric diseases, as well as nonneurological disorders such as sexual dysfunction, bladder and bowel incontinence, and systemic metabolic dysregulation that may arise or persist for months to years postinjury. For all these reasons, TBI can increase long-term mortality and reduce life expectancy (Masel & DeWitt, 2010).

EPIDEMIOLOGY

Epidemiological studies of TBI frequency, severity, outcomes, cost, and risk factors have resulted in a body of literature that highlights the significance of TBI as a public health concern. Given the potential for lifelong consequences following TBI, it is important to understand these data to better inform education and prevention efforts, in addition to policies related to treatment and rehabilitation.

Incidence

In 2015, a report to Congress from the CDC indicated that TBI is associated with more than 50,000 deaths annually and accounts for one third of injury-related deaths. In 2010, TBI resulted in approximately 2.5 million emergency department visits. Approximately 87% of individuals returned home, 11% were hospitalized, and 2% died. The causes of TBI, from most to least frequent, include falls, being struck by an object or person, motor vehicle accidents, and self-inflicted injuries. In general, fatal TBIs are most likely to occur in the context of motor vehicle crashes.

Age and gender are two key demographic features associated with higher risk of sustaining a TBI. Adults over age 75 are not only at higher risk for TBI but are most likely to experience a TBI resulting in either hospitalization or death (Faul, Xu, Wald, & Coronado, 2010). Since 2002, there has been a marked increase in documented TBIs requiring acute rehabilitation among older adults due to falls (Cuthbert et al., 2012). Because there are more women in older age groups, females comprise a large proportion of older adult falls. Falls are also the most common cause of TBI among young children, with males and females being equally likely to sustain these injuries. Automobile crashes, violence, and sports-related injuries are more common from adolescence through middle age; males are more likely to incur TBIs from such causes. Overall, males are reported to comprise 59% of TBI-related medical visits (Faul et al., 2010). In addition to demographic risk factors in the general population, certain special populations have elevated risk for TBI.

Veterans and military personnel serving during the Global War on Terrorism are deserving of special consideration when examining incidence rates of TBI. Among those who served in Operation Iraqi Freedom, Operation Enduring Freedom, and Operation New Dawn (OEF/OIF/OND), TBI is one of the “signature injuries” related to deployment. Unique to combat-related TBIs experienced in these conflicts was survival postexposure to a blast wave from an improvised explosive device. However, service members also experienced TBIs from motor vehicle crashes, being struck in the head by shrapnel or other moving objects, and falls. In 2005, the Defense and Veterans Brain Injury Center reported that of the patients treated for injury at Walter Reed Army Medical Center, as many as 30% were diagnosed with TBI, with 56% of these combat-related injuries being categorized as moderate to severe, and 44% as mTBI. In a 2008 RAND report, 19.5% of almost 2,000 returning military personnel reported probable TBI experiences (Tanielian et al., 2008). A later study found that 22.8% of U.S. Army brigade combat soldiers with at least one deployment had a clinician-confirmed TBI (Terrio et al., 2009). It is certain that many TBIs have gone unreported in this population, particularly mTBIs for which the service member may not seek care (McCrea et al., 2008).

Other at-risk populations with a higher incidence of TBI compared with the general population include individuals who are homeless, victims of intimate partner violence, persons with substance use disorders, and individuals involved in the criminal justice system. Among 825 homeless persons in three Canadian cities, 37.2% reported at least 1 incident TBI during a 3-year study period (Nikoo et al., 2017). Among veterans seeking homeless services, 47% were identified as having a probable history of TBI (Russell et al., 2013). Reports have shown that as many as 60% of justice-involved individuals have a history of at least one TBI (Shiroma, Ferguson, & Pickelsimer, 2012). A more recent systematic review of 17 TBI prevalence studies also revealed that a history of TBI is common in prison populations across the United States. The review listed prevalence rates of past TBIs ranging from 36% to 94% in the sample prison populations that were studied (Allely, 2016). Moreover, the CDC (2015) suggested that TBI may influence behavior in such a way that these individuals are more likely to be charged with repeat offenses, resulting in multiple episodes of incarceration. Schofield and colleagues (2006) conducted a retrospective cohort study supporting a modest causal link between TBI and single acts of criminality. Studies such as these not only illustrate the need to account for TBI in managing care in offender populations but also suggest that prevention of TBI may benefit the public by reducing crime rates.

Studies have identified other behavioral and personality characteristics that are risk factors for TBI. Substance use, particularly alcohol use, has been shown to increase risk for TBI. An Australian study of brain injury, mental disorders and substance use found that up to 40% of individuals with a brain injury met *DSM–IV* criteria for substance use disorders before the injury (National Campaign Against Drug Abuse [NCADA], 2009). One recent epidemiological study demonstrated that alcohol use combined with driving accounted for more severe TBIs among individuals younger than 65 years old (Salottolo et al., 2016). As previously mentioned, exposure to intimate partner violence also increases risk of TBI, with early studies finding prevalence rates from 60% to 92% (St. Ivany & Schminkey, 2016). A recent study found that as many as 18.8% of a female veteran sample met screening criteria for intimate partner violence–related TBI history (Iverson & Pogoda, 2015). In addition, traits such as impulsivity and tendency toward self-harm are also associated with increased risk of TBI (NCADA, 2009).

In recent years, much attention has been given to sport-related TBIs. One epidemiological study estimated the annual incidence of sport- and recreation-related concussions to be approximately 3.8 million in the United States (Langlois, Rutland-Brown, & Wald, 2006). Media attention has primarily targeted high-intensity contact sports such as football, boxing, basketball and mixed martial arts. However, risk of TBI is also associated with participation in other sports such as soccer, wrestling, water sports, and equestrian events (Cifu et al., 2016). Furthermore, an athlete who has sustained a brain injury is at higher risk for sustaining additional brain injuries, possibly leading to increased likelihood of long-term consequences. Research in this area has led to the development of "return-to-play" protocols for both youth and adult athletes and improvements in the quality of protective gear for some sports. All 50 states and the District of Columbia have passed legislation addressing concussions in youth sports. In addition, collaboration among universities, health care, and government organizations is continuously improving awareness of and knowledge about sport-related brain injury.

Disability Due to TBI

Each year, 90,000 individuals in the United States experience disability as an immediate and permanent effect of TBI (CDC, 2006). Similar studies have demonstrated that anywhere from 3.5 to 14 million persons are living with TBI-related disabilities (Napolitano, Radecki, & Elovic, 2007; Selassie et al., 2003). Injury severity is, of course, a predictor of long-term disability. Medical comorbidities also predict long-term functional outcomes. Other predictors of greater degree of disability include unemployment at time of injury and lower socioeconomic status. Being married at the time of injury appears to be protective against disability after TBI. Interestingly, the prevalence of persons living with TBI-related disability is higher in rural areas by as much as 24%, a finding believed to be explained by limited transportation and access to treatment centers, leaving primary care physicians as the only source of treatment for those living in these areas (Kaye, 1997; Sample, Tomter, & Johns, 2007). For further discussion of contextual factors that contribute to disability, see Chapter 8, this volume.

Although disability that occurs immediately and continuously postinjury is one aspect of the public burden of TBI, emerging studies indicate that remote TBIs may increase the likelihood of later life morbidity and mortality. A survey study of the association between disability and lifetime history of TBIs, including those that did not result in hospitalization, concluded that the rate of TBI-related disability could easily be three times greater than disability based on hospitalizations only (Whiteneck, Cuthbert, Corrigan, & Bogner, 2016). Others have proposed that the public health concept of "exposure" may be the better way to examine the burden of TBI. That is, each TBI being conceptualized as a potential adverse health event (Corrigan, Yang, Singichetti, Manchester, & Bogner, 2018). Although there are many unanswered questions about delayed consequences of TBI, it is clear that they occur; thus, it is important to detect TBIs regardless of whether they require medical treatment (Institute of Medicine, 2009). Despite the difficulties in obtaining the information, lifetime history of TBI, including both how severe and age at which they occurred, is important for understanding TBI exposure.

SCREENING AND ASSESSMENT

The purpose of screening is to identify a potential history of TBI. Generally, a positive screen results in further evaluation for acute or lifetime history of TBI. As identifying individuals with TBI exposure creates opportunities for education, prevention, and intervention, accurate screening and assessment of TBI history is integral. Researchers have also identified a need for efficient and effective instruments in various settings including nursing homes, prisons, assisted living facilities, shelters for the homeless or victims of domestic abuse, primary care clinics, and substance use disorder programs (Diamond, Harzke, Magaletta, Cummins, & Frankowski, 2007; Gabella, Mangione, Hedegaard, & Kelly, 2007; Walker, Cole, Logan, & Corrigan, 2007; Goldin, Haag, & Trott, 2016). When choosing evidence-based methods, rehabilitation psychologists are encouraged to consider the quality and quantity of existing research that supports a potential method of case ascertainment, as well as whether a standardized protocol for using the tool has been established.

Screening for Lifetime History of TBI

The importance of screening for lifetime history of TBI is illustrated by the substantial body of evidence supporting TBI as a risk factor for an array of negative outcomes. Multiple studies demonstrate a link between TBI and increased risk for posttraumatic stress disorder (PTSD) in both civilian and military populations (Bahraini & Brenner, 2013; Bryant et al., 2010; Hoge et al., 2008). Moreover, Brenner and colleagues (2010) also reported an increased risk for persistent postconcussive symptoms (e.g., headache, dizziness) in veterans with both mTBI and PTSD. Persons with TBI are also at increased risk for depression and substance misuse (Olson-Madden et al., 2010, 2012). In addition to acting as a predictor for psychological problems, TBI is also a risk factor for medical conditions such as epilepsy, neuroinflammation, dementia, and obstructive sleep apnea (Castriotta et al., 2007; Hauser, Annegers, & Kurland, 1991; Wilde et al., 2007). Furthermore, persons with persisting TBI-related disabilities are at risk for other negative events and outcomes. As Reichard, Langlois, Sample, Wald, and Pickelsimer (2007) stated, "Acts of violence and other forms of victimization of persons with disabilities are not uncommon events. These people are 4–10 times more likely to become victims of violence, abuse or neglect than nondisabled persons" (p. 390).

Finally, there is evidence suggesting that TBI increases risk for long-term mortality from multiple causes of death. Harrison-Felix and colleagues have conducted several longitudinal studies using the Traumatic Brain Injury Model Systems National Database, which revealed that persons with TBI are more likely to die from seizures, infections, pneumonia, and circulatory problems (Harrison-Felix, Whiteneck, DeVivo, Hammond, & Jha, 2004, 2006; Harrison-Felix et al., 2009, 2012). Other studies have linked TBI to increased risk for suicide, even many years after injury (Brenner, Ignacio, & Blow, 2011; Fisher et al., 2016). The body of research described in this chapter highlights the potential role of TBI in creating a downward trajectory toward chronic illness, disability, and reduced life expectancy (Brenner, Ignacio, & Blow, 2011). In terms of prevention, identifying history of TBI may help individuals avoid multiple other risk factors (e.g., substance misuse or reinjury) that undermine quality of life.

However, it is important to note that some controversy exists with regard to the utility of screening for TBI. Vanderploeg and Belanger (2013) suggested that the VA system's method of screening for mTBI in OEF/OIF/OND is unnecessary because TBI is a historical event rather than a progressive disease. They further asserted that any persisting symptoms reported after TBI could be addressed in a symptom-specific manner without the need to identify the origin of such symptoms. Other researchers propose that repeated neuropsychological exams that assess for TBI (initiated by these types of screenings) may produce iatrogenic effects—that is, patients may unnecessarily self-identify as "brain injured" or misattribute physical, cognitive, and emotional symptoms to brain injury (Roth & Spencer, 2013), thereby becoming cases of "excess disability." Nevertheless, TBI screening within the VA remains consistent with VA/Department of Defense Clinical Practice Guidelines for the Management of Concussion–Mild Traumatic Brain Injury disseminated in 2016 (U.S. Department of Veterans Affairs and Department of Defense, 2016).

Screening and Assessment Tools

Various tools have been developed for the purpose of screening to determine whether a TBI has occurred; often these tools have been designed for specific settings such as combat zones or athletic competitions. The Military Acute Concussion Evaluation assesses neurological status after potential exposure to concussive events in military settings. The U.S. Department of Defense (2012; see also McCrea et al., 2014) recommends administration as close to the time of injury as possible and requires administration within 24 hours. In both military and civilian settings, emergency medical technicians arriving at an injury scene or emergency department staff are most often tasked with acute assessment of TBI. In these instances, a clinician looks for observable indications of physical trauma to the head and multiple signs of altered brain function, for example, disturbed level of consciousness motor or sensory deficits, slurred speech, or unusual behavior. In emergency medical care, this information is then used to calculate a Glasgow Coma Scale (GCS) score or other injury severity score. An initial severity rating is assigned, and the patient is reevaluated over time. Once in a medical facility, further information about possible structural damage can be obtained with neuroimaging.

In athletic settings, the acute injury event is often observed, and the player is immediately assessed on the sideline for brain injury using "toolkits" developed for coaches, trainers, or other staff. The American Academy of Neurology indicates that the Post-Concussion Symptom Scale/Graded Symptom Checklist and the Standardized Assessment of Concussion when administered early after a suspected concussion have moderate to high sensitivity and specificity in identifying sports concussions relative to those of the reference standard of a clinician-diagnosed concussion (American Academy of Neurology, 2013). If a concussion is suspected, the athlete is typically assessed by medical personnel using the methods already described. The U.S. Food and Drug Administration recognizes the Immediate Post-Concussion Assessment and Cognitive Test as a valid tool used for assessing concussion symptoms. This computerized assessment tool is initially administered preinjury to obtain baseline measurement in areas such as memory, speed, spatial span, and other aspects of cognitive functioning. If an injury occurs, postinjury performance on the same assessments is compared with preinjury performance. The tool can be accessed at https://www.impacttest.com/.

In Department of Defense/VA settings, a "TBI screening reminder" is generated in an individual's medical chart upon return from deployment. The reminder prompts a provider to first ask if the patient has served in OEF/OIF/OND theater of combat and then examine the medical record to determine whether the patient has already been diagnosed with history of TBI. If the answer is yes, the screening is complete. If the answer is no, the clinician is prompted to assess for four criteria to determine whether the patient may have experienced a TBI event. The screening questions query about injury events that may cause TBI, immediate signs of disturbance of consciousness, and persistence of symptoms attributed to the injury events. A positive screen requires a "yes" to all criteria and prompts a consultation for a more thorough evaluation to be conducted by a specialty clinic. Belanger, Vanderploeg, and Sayer's (2016) critical review of brain injury screening in the VA health care system concluded that the screening measures had good internal consistency, variable test–retest reliability and questionable validity. Ultimately, this study demonstrated relatively low sensitivity, as 30% to 60% of TBI cases were missed, but the instrument had adequate specificity. Similarly, Terrio, Nelson, Betthauser, Harwood, and Brenner's (2011) study of sensitivity, specificity, and predictive values of the Post Deployment Health Assessment TBI screening questions (which parallel those used in the VA) found that the screener's sensitivity and specificity were 60% and 90%, respectively, compared with a clinician-confirmed diagnosis. Further analysis revealed that positive responses to the first two questions only resulted in better sensitivity, and only a slight decrease in specificity, compared with results using the tool in its entirety.

The TBI–4 is another standard screening instrument that can be used across most clinical settings (Brenner et al., 2013). The TBI–4 Screener is composed of the following four questions: (a) Have you ever been hospitalized or treated in an emergency room following a head or neck injury? (b) Have you ever been knocked out or unconscious following an accident or injury? (c) Have you ever injured your head or neck in a car accident or from some other moving vehicle accident? and (d) Have you ever injured your head or neck in a fight or fall? These questions elicit information about risky situations and behaviors commonly associated with sustaining a TBI. The second question includes the element of alteration in consciousness that is needed to meet TBI diagnostic criteria. The validity of the screening instrument has been demonstrated with both inpatient and outpatient samples (Brenner et al., 2013; Olson-Madden et al., 2014).

For use in both clinical and research settings, the Ohio State University TBI Identification Method (OSU TBI–ID; Bogner & Corrigan, 2009; Corrigan & Bogner, 2007) is a structured-interview assessment tool that elicits self- or proxy-report of TBI occurring over a person's lifetime. The interview includes initial questions about any past injuries and then focuses on injuries involving a blow to the head or neck or high-velocity forces capable of causing brain injury. Questions about alterations of consciousness follow the elicitation of potential injury events, thus negating the common problem of asking a person to self-diagnose (e.g., "Have you ever had a concussion?"). In a final step, the interviewer queries about times in one's life when there may have been repeated blows to the head. The OSU TBI–ID has demonstrated good reliability, as well as predictive and construct validity (Corrigan & Bogner, 2007; Corrigan et al., 2013; Cuthbert, Whiteneck, Corrigan, & Bogner, 2016; Dams-O'Connor et al., 2013; Whiteneck et al., 2016). The methods of retrospectively identifying a history of TBI via self-report described earlier, as well as others developed for this purpose (Dams-O'Connor et al., 2014; Fortier et al., 2014), vary in sensitivity, specificity, and reliability but share the advantage of not being limited to TBIs that occurred recently or did not receive medical attention. It is also typical in research to ascertain cases of TBI via indirect evidence alone, which includes reviews of medical records for diagnostic or billing codes indicating a history of TBI.

Case ascertainment using codes from medical records also has both strengths and weaknesses. Although this method can be implemented without direct access to the individual who sustained the injury, some studies have suggested that it produces either variable or largely inaccurate results (Bazarian, Veazie, Mookerjee, & Lerner, 2006; Thurman, Alverson, Dunn, Guerrero, & Sniezek, 1999). Major weaknesses lie both in medical provider knowledge regarding TBI and the frequency and variability with which types of electronic codes for medical conditions are used in medical charts. Furthermore, mTBIs may not be recorded when a patient presents to a medical setting for other, more severe injuries or medical comorbidities (Powell, Ferraro, Dikmen, Temkin, & Bell, 2008). These methodological weaknesses can result in underidentification of TBI (i.e., low sensitivity).

Standardized clinical interviews, like the OSU–TBI–ID, are designed to gather information about lifetime history of TBI. This method depends on the accuracy of information being provided by the patient or research participant. For example, studies have shown that the less severe and more remote the injury, the more unreliable the report (Cuthbert et al., 2016). Moreover, individuals may misattribute common physical symptoms such as headache or concentration difficulties to a TBI when those symptoms may not have been caused by the injury. Finally, administering standardized interviews requires time and effort of both the clinician or researcher and the individual providing the self-report. Standardization helps to ensure that ascertainment methods are used consistently, thereby preventing slight methodological change over time and maintaining reliability, which is necessary to preserve validity. Further information regarding specific TBI assessment tools used in rehabilitation settings will be provided in the next section.

INTERVENTION IN REHABILITATION SETTINGS

In 1985, the American Congress of Rehabilitation Medicine developed standards for comprehensive inpatient rehabilitation programs for TBI. These recommendations were later adopted by the Commission on Accreditation of Rehabilitation Facilities (CARF) and expanded to cover an entire spectrum of care to include residential and outpatient settings. CARF's annually published *Standards Manual for Medical Rehabilitation* continues to serve as the gold standard of brain injury treatment (Commission on Accreditation of Rehabilitation Facilities, 2016). The standards call for an interdisciplinary, team-based approach to brain injury rehabilitation in which providers of various disciplines coordinate care by interacting and providing feedback to one another and to the patient and caregiver across all components on the spectrum of care. CARF standards call for psychology services at each level of care, requiring rehabilitation psychologists to demonstrate competency in varying roles, depending upon the patient's progress through rehabilitation and the unique needs.

ACUTE REHABILITATION

When a person experiences a TBI, immediate medical stabilization is the primary focus of care. The immediate goal is to continue life-sustaining treatment and manage primary medical needs or additional acute medical problems that arise. Persons with severe injuries may require continued sedation, intracranial pressure monitoring, evacuation of hematomas, seizure and infection prevention or management, respiratory care, and nutritional support. Once medically stabilized in an emergency department, critical care unit, or other acute care setting, rehabilitation therapies may be initiated until the patient is ready to transition to an acute rehabilitation program. At this stage, the rehabilitation psychologist's role involves assessment and consultation. If the injury has led to a disorder of consciousness, the rehabilitation psychologist may assist in tracking level of consciousness and emergence from posttraumatic amnesia (PTA). Rehabilitation psychologists can assess for level of consciousness using scales such as the GCS (see the TBI Severity and Symptomatology section for a GCS overview), Coma Recovery Scale—Revised (CRS–R; Giacino, Kalmar, & Whyte, 2004), the Rancho Los Amigos Scale (RLAS; Hagen, Malkmus, & Durham, 1972). The CRS was developed to detect subtle changes in arousal and volition among patients with disorders of consciousness particularly coma, vegetative state, and minimally conscious states. It has proven to be highly reliable and valid for use in the early phase of emergence from coma (McDonnell, Giacino, & Kolakowsky-Hayner, 2015). The RLAS was also developed to measure level of consciousness and postinjury cognitive functioning and behavior. Although it does not include the granularity and precision within disorders of consciousness that the CRS–R provides, the RLAS spans a broader spectrum of the initial recovery from coma. Many consider the RLAS to be more of a nomenclature for stages of recovery than an actual assessment device. It does measure degree of disruption of brain functioning, but it is rarely used in the context of describing initial severity of brain injury. One drawback of the RLAS is that it is possible for an injured person to exhibit symptoms and behaviors described by one level and other symptoms and behaviors described by a different level. Each of these measures assists in differentiating between comatose and minimally conscious states, although the CRS–R is the most precise. Rehabilitation psychologists can also bring more precision to tracking acute change after the development of volitional behaviors by using brief assessments such as the Galveston Orientation and Amnesia Test (Levin, O'Donnell, & Grossman, 1979) or the Orientation Log (Jackson, Novack, & Dowler, 1998; Novack, 2000). Continuous monitoring of consciousness and orientation helps to inform treatment plans and to set and modify rehabilitation goals.

Consultation and emotional support services are extremely important in acute rehabilitation settings. Rehabilitation psychologists offer support and education to the patient and family members or caregivers about the patient's expected trajectory of treatment and help them to form appropriate and realistic expectations. Specifically, rehabilitation psychologists, along with social workers and family liaisons, may provide information about the extent of injuries and changes in behavior via discussions with family and provision of educational materials. All those working with the family should be prepared to validate expressed frustration with unstable conditions and uncertain outcomes and help family members to identify their own resources and strengths to draw on and enhance their ability to cope. Rehabilitation psychologists can assist not only by working directly with family members but also by advocating for collaboration between caregivers and providers in developing treatment plans. Family members may benefit from arranging time with staff for daily or weekly briefings. More recent trends in person-centered, holistic approaches to health care highlight the importance of understanding how the relationship between the patient and caregivers, families, and loved ones may affect progress during rehabilitation. Literature informing clinical practice guidelines for working with family and caregivers in acute TBI rehabilitation indicates that family members express four basic needs: (a) need to know, (b) need for consistent information, (c) need for involvement in care, and (d) need to make sense of the experience (Bond, Draeger, Mandleco, & Donnelly, 2003).

Finally, rehabilitation psychologists demonstrate organizational competency in multiple ways. They consult with the rehabilitation team by providing in-service training for staff members, fostering a patient-centered approach to enhance quality of care. Rehabilitation psychologists can help staff to be sensitive to and acknowledge any cultural issues relevant to patient and family. Finally, they can also help to ensure patient's needs and best interests are prioritized in case of any family conflicts.

Postacute Rehabilitation

Patients with less severe injuries or those whose condition no longer requires acute medical management are appropriate for more direct and detailed assessment and intervention. A rehabilitation psychologist continues to have multiple roles at this stage, including providing assessment, intervention, and further consultation and support.

Neuropsychological testing. Rehabilitation psychologists can administer and interpret neuropsychological tests to help identify and describe levels of neurocognitive impairment as well as comorbidities that may complicate the patient's presentation and affect their response to treatment. The goal of the psychologist is to gather information to inform prognosis and treatment goals and help establish a starting point from which to measure progress. Common testing instruments include measures of effort, intelligence, memory, and attention and self-report questionnaires that assess for psychiatric symptoms. This information can be used to provide consultation to the treatment team and to provide further education to both the patient and family. Tools that facilitate assessment of symptom severity and impairment specific to TBI should be included in comprehensive neuropsychological assessments. For those with mTBI, the Neurobehavioral Symptom Inventory (NSI; Cicerone & Kalmar, 1995) is a 22-item self-report measure of postconcussive symptoms. Using a 5-point scale, respondents rate each symptom's degree of severity indicating how much that symptom impairs daily functioning. Items include symptoms across physical, sensory, cognitive, and emotional domains. For those with more severe injury, the Neurobehavioral Functioning Inventory (NFI; Marwitz, 2000) can be used to assess for common daily life problems post-TBI. The measure comprises 76 items across six domains: depression, somatic, memory and attention, communication, aggression, and motor. An additional six "critical items" identify areas that may warrant immediate attention such as blackout spells. Similar to the NSI, a 5-point scale is used to rate frequency of each symptom or problem. The NFI is unique in that it is available in separate patient and family forms that allow the clinician to gather perspectives of both the injured individual and a second-party observer. Both the NSI and NFI are used for assessing specific areas of concern to create and modify treatment plans and track rehabilitation progress. They can also be used in research settings to describe characteristics of specific populations or measure response to treatment.

Neuropsychological testing is crucial to identifying areas of impairment and comparing the patient's cognitive performance to similar cohorts with respect to age and education. Also, current performance is often compared to the individual's presumed premorbid abilities. However, full neuropsychological assessments may not be useful in cases in which there is questionable validity, such as indications of poor test-taking effort or in the presence of severe psychiatric symptoms that diminish performance for reasons that are not reflective of cognitive function. In addition, performance on assessment measures should be interpreted with caution when the patient is taking medications that may affect performance either positively (e.g., psychostimulants) or negatively (e.g., sedatives). Finally, full test batteries may not be possible when aphasia or motor impairment are present. For further discussion of assessment in rehabilitation settings, see Chapter 4, this volume.

Behavior management. Behavioral disturbances such as aggression, disinhibition, and agitation are common among persons who have sustained a TBI. Rehabilitation psychologists can assist the rehabilitation team and family in designing and implementing environmental changes that may mitigate behavioral issues. In addition, rehabilitation psychologists may develop specifically tailored behavior management plans to address dysfunctional behavior. Such plans are most successful when formulated using patient and family input to identify antecedents of the problematic behavior and best methods by which to modify or eliminate it (e.g., reinforcement of desired behavior vs. punishment for undesired behavior).

Psychotherapy for persons with TBI. Persons who have sustained a brain injury may present with a host of psychological problems, some of which may predate the TBI. Common issues targeted in psychotherapy include problems adjusting to disability-related limitations, loss of identity (e.g., role changes in work and family life), chronic pain, depression, grief, substance abuse, and posttraumatic stress. Rehabilitation psychologists may screen for these problems and provide targeted individual or group-based interventions. Treatment should include psychoeducation, symptom management, and evidence-based methods such as cognitive-behavioral approaches and also promote expectations for recovery.

Rehabilitation psychologists demonstrate competency in intervention by implementing evidence-based treatment approaches adapted to the unique needs of their patients. Many well-established treatment protocols for evidence-based therapies have been, or can be, modified to address specific challenges for those coping with symptoms of TBI. For example, research supports the efficacy of prolonged exposure, an evidence-based treatment for PTSD, for persons with TBI when making specific modifications to the protocol, such as allowing for extra time in sessions, promoting use of compensatory strategies to remember key concepts and providing repeated education throughout the treatment protocol (Strom, Wolf, Crawford, Blahnik, & Kretzmer, 2016; Wolf et al., 2015). As Bahraini et al. (2014) summarized,

> Treatment of those with TBI and PTSD should involve a combination of psychoeducation, symptom management, and evidence-based treatments for PTSD and other comorbid behavioral health conditions. Psychoeducation is an important component of any intervention, particularly when delivered early after injury/trauma. (p. 65)

Positive coping strategies for managing emotion dysregulation, self-care strategies, and problem-solving skills should be emphasized in any form of treatment, while maladaptive coping strategies such as isolation and alcohol or other drug use should be identified as barriers to recovery (U.S. Department of Veterans Affairs and Department of Defense, 2009, 2010). Table 18.3 provides a list of evidence-based interventions that have been successfully adapted or developed to fit the needs of persons with TBI in a variety of settings (e.g., inpatient, outpatient, and residential). Studies cited support the use of evidence-based psychological interventions for those with TBIs of all severity level. Also of note, interventions used to treat one specific condition appear to have the potential to reduce disturbances in other areas of emotional or behavioral functioning. For example, treatment for PTSD may also lead to reduced symptoms of depression, and treatment for insomnia may also reduce symptoms of anxiety.

Cognitive remediation. TBI may result in various cognitive deficits affecting attention, memory,

TABLE 18.3

Evidence-Based Psychotherapy Among Those Living With Traumatic Brain Injury (TBI; Exemplars)

Intervention	Condition	Study	Sample	Basic findings
Cognitive behavior therapy (CBT)	Depression	Tiersky et al. (2005)	Mild/moderate TBI Ages 19–62	Experimental group reported significantly lower SCL90–R[a] depression scores compared with control group ($p < .05$).
		Anson and Ponsford (2006)	Moderate/severe TBI Ages 20–81	67%–80% CBT-based coping skills group participants reported increased understanding of use and implementation of coping skills.
		Ponsford et al. (2016)	Mild/moderate/severe TBI Mean age = 42.2 (range not reported)	CBT groups showed significant reduction in depression on DASS,[b] 95% CI [–5.61, –0.12].
	Anxiety	Ponsford et al. (2016)	Mild/moderate/severe TBI Mean age = 42.2 (range not reported)	CBT groups showed significant reduction in anxiety on the HADS,[c] 95% CI [–2.07, –0.06].
		Tiersky et al. (2005)	Mild/moderate TBI Ages 19–62	The experimental group reported significantly lower SCL90–R[a] anxiety subscale scores compared with the control group ($p < .05$).
	Insomnia	Nguyen et al. (2017)	Mild/moderate/severe TBI Ages 16—65	CBT recipients reported better sleep quality on the PSQI,[d] 95% CI [2.56, 7.14], and decreased depression scores on the HADS[c] vs. treatment as usual.

TABLE 18.3

Evidence-Based Psychotherapy Among Those Living With Traumatic Brain Injury (TBI; Exemplars) (*Continued*)

Intervention	Condition	Study	Sample	Basic findings
		Lu, Krellman, and Dijkers (2016)	Mild/moderate/severe TBI Ages 42–60	Participants reported mild reductions in severity of insomnia-related symptoms on the ISI[e] as well as clinically significant reductions in depression and anxiety symptoms on HADS.[c]
Cognitive processing therapy (CPT)	PTSD	Ragsdale and Voss Horrell (2016)	No report of TBI severity ranges Ages 23–57	Veterans in CPT group demonstrated significant reduction in PTSD symptoms on PCL-S[f] and depressive symptoms on BDI–II.[g]
		Chard, Schumm, McIlvain, Bailey, and Parkinson (2011)	Mild/moderate/severe Mean age = 33.9 (no range reported)	Veterans receiving CPT demonstrated reduction in PTSD symptoms on the CAPS[h] and PCL[f] and depressive symptoms on the BDI–II.[g]
Prolonged exposure (PE)	PTSD	Wolf et al. (2015)	Mild/moderate/severe TBI Mean age = 34.01 (no range reported)	Veterans and active duty personnel demonstrated significant decreases in PTSD per PCL[f] scores, B = −3.00, 95% CI [−3.22, −2.78] across both inpatient and outpatient clinical settings. Clinically significant decreases in depressive symptoms were also observed on BDI–II.[g]
		Wolf, Strom, Kehle, and Eftekhari (2012)	Mild/moderate TBI Ages 24–52	Veterans demonstrated significant reductions in pre- to posttreatment PTSD symptoms per PCL[f] scores and depression symptoms per BDI–II[g] scores.
		Ragsdale and Voss Horrell (2016)	No report of severity ranges Ages 23–57	Veterans in PE group demonstrated significant reduction in PTSD symptoms on PCL[f] and depressive symptoms on BDI–II[g].
Problem-solving therapy (PST)	Hopelessness and Suicidality	Matarazzo et al. (2014)	Moderate/severe TBI Ages 28–67	Veterans receiving treatment self-reported benefit in increasing hopefulness and improvement of energy and self-esteem (per qualitative interviews).
Combination CBT and PST		Simpson, Tate, Whiting, and Cotter (2011)	Moderate/severe TBI Ages 18–65	Persons receiving an intervention based on both PST and CBT principles demonstrated decreased levels of hopelessness on the BHS[i] compared with wait-list control group.
		Brenner et al. (2018)	Moderate to severe TBI and moderate to severe hopelessness Ages 26–65	U.S. military veterans receiving an intervention based on both PST and CBT principles demonstrated decreased levels of hopelessness on the BHS[i] compared with wait-list control group.

Note. CI = confidence interval; PCL = PTSD Checklist; PTSD = posttraumatic stress disorder; TBI = traumatic brain injury. [a]Symptom Checklist 90—Revised (Derogatis, 1994). [b]Depression Anxiety and Stress Scale (Lovibond & Lovibond, 1995). [c]Hospital Anxiety and Depression Scale (Zigmond & Snaith, 1983). [d]Pittsburgh Sleep Quality Index (Buysse, Reynolds, Monk, Berman, & Kupfer, 1989). [e]Insomnia Severity Index (Morin, Belleville, Bélanger, & Ivers, 2011). [f]PTSD Checklist-Specific (PCL-S) (Weathers, Litz, Herman, Huska, & Keane, 1993). [g]Beck Depression Inventory (Beck, Steer, & Brown, 1996). [h]Clinician-Administered PTSD Scale (Blake et al., 1995). [i]Beck Hopelessness Scale (Beck & Steer, 1998).

language and communication, executive functioning, and visuoperceptual skills. Deficits in specific areas of function are often addressed through cognitive remediation, which may be offered by speech-language pathologists, occupational therapists, cognitive rehabilitation specialists, or psychologists. Rehabilitation psychologists also often act as adjunct providers who can reinforce cognitive strategies and help patients implement them in their daily activities. Evidence-based clinical protocols may introduce both restorative and compensatory strategies. As the term implies, *restorative approaches* to cognitive remediation aim to regain functions lost or damaged by brain injury. Examples of such strategies include dual task training, memory drills, problem-solving exercises, and conversational skill building (Cicerone et al., 2011). *Compensatory approaches* aim to develop new functions or to use intact functions to compensate for lost functions. Reliance on lost functions is reduced while retained functions are enhanced for adaptation. Examples of compensatory strategies include external memory aids (e.g., smart phone alerts and calendars), visual cues, self-monitoring, and self-regulation techniques.

Research on the general efficacy of cognitive practice after TBI has produced results indistinguishable from spontaneous recovery; however, systematic reviews and clinical practice guidelines have supported the use of specific cognitive remediation strategies for specific goals, including attention training (direct attention training and attention process training), dual-task training, executive functioning training, and memory interventions (Radomski, Anheluk, Bartzen, & Zola, 2016). For example, Rees and colleagues (2007) conducted a systematic review supporting the use of conversational skills training, strategy training for attention deficits, and the use of external cues and memory aids to improve general functioning after TBI. Other systematic reviews have examined evidence supporting the use of various cognitive remediation techniques in TBI populations (Cicerone et al., 2000, 2005, 2011; Rohling, Faust, Beverly, & Demakis, 2009). These reviews included studies published from 2003 to 2008 and found evidence for the efficacy of attention training and errorless learning strategies in memory remediation after TBI. The reviews also suggested that awareness training can improve self-monitoring and self-evaluation after TBI. The authors state that such strategies may be successfully implemented regardless of time since injury. However, there is limited evidence that cognitive remediation strategies result in generalized positive outcomes related to improved social participation or quality of life. These findings lend more support to the use of such strategies as one component of a comprehensive, holistic approach to brain injury rehabilitation.

Psychopharmacological management. Although most psychologists do not prescribe medications, they can offer valuable input and feedback about presenting symptoms and functional status, as well as extent of therapeutic effect, when consulting with prescribers. Rehabilitation psychologists often gather information from self-report measures, observation during clinical care, testing performance, and feedback from family members and treatment team members about the client's functioning. Such information is highly valuable to prescribers when developing an appropriate psychopharmacological treatment plan. Therefore, in addition to more general classes of medications used to treat common psychiatric conditions, psychologists should be familiar with common medications prescribed to patients with TBI. Psychostimulants such as methylphenidate and amantadine are often used to improve arousal, focus, and attention. Antiseizure medications, typical and atypical antipsychotics, and benzodiazepines are often used to control agitation. However, some animal and human studies have shown a negative impact on cognition associated with the use of these medications (Feeney, Gonzalez, & Law, 1982; Massagli, 1991; Smith et al., 1994), which, of course, is counterproductive to rehabilitation goals. Currently, there is no consensus as to which type of medication is best to manage agitation while not interfering with neurological recovery (Williamson et al., 2016).

Facilitation of other postacute rehabilitation services. As previously mentioned, rehabilitation psychologists often operate within an interdisciplinary team. Patients receiving care from multiple providers using various modalities benefit from the assistance of clinicians who can help integrate tools and strategies into their daily routines. For example, a rehabilitation psychologist may assist a patient who is learning memory strategies in cognitive rehabilitation to apply such strategies at home to consistently complete a home-based exercise plan recommended by a physical therapist. Rehabilitation psychologists may also assist patients in communicating with other care providers when questions or concerns arise. Finally, rehabilitation psychologists advocate for TBI patients in the community and help them access resources by making referrals to various rehabilitation center or community programs.

Community Reintegration and Long-Term Management

Upon discharge from inpatient rehabilitation, persons with TBI may transition to various types of settings depending on the level of impairment in daily functioning and available sources of support outside the medical facility. In a study using TBI Model Systems data, Dahdah and colleagues (2014) found that more than 80% of patients receiving inpatient rehabilitation for TBI were discharged back to their home. For patients who require more supervision or lack the resources or family/caregiver support to return home, other possible discharge settings include residential treatment centers, assisted living facilities and nursing homes. Regardless the discharge setting, rehabilitation psychologists assist patients to achieve patient-identified community reintegration goals and master daily management of chronic symptoms. Developing daily structured routines is often an essential component of this goal.

Family reintegration. Rehabilitation psychologists continue to play a vital role in the patient's transition back to home, which typically requires reintegrating into the family unit. Family members can provide feedback to help the patient establish a daily routine comprising tasks that the patient is capable of managing. Roles within the family unit (e.g., parenting obligations, money management) may shift depending on level of disability and may need modification over time. Rehabilitation psychologists assist patients in achieving as much independence as possible but may need to involve family members in helping to administer medications, cueing the patient to continue practicing good self-care skills, and recognizing when rest is needed.

Sexual intimacy is an inherent component of most spousal or partner relationships. Research demonstrates that sexual functioning is a key component of personal happiness and quality of life (Sander, 2013). TBI can hamper sexual functioning in multiple ways, including poor self-image related to changes in physical appearance and limitations, hormonal changes secondary to neuroendocrine conditions, or prolonged use of certain medications. Difficulty interpreting cues or emotional states of others, as well as difficulties expressing emotion and intimacy, can negatively affect personal relationships after a person experiences TBI (Neumann, Malec, & Hammond, 2017; Neumann, Zupan, Malec, & Hammond, 2014). These types of difficulties are significant contributors to problems with sexual intimacy that can further diminish one's self-concept and self-esteem (Sander, 2013). For those individuals who may be seeking out social relationships after brain injury, there may be more general problems affecting interpersonal functioning that limit opportunities for sexual intimacy. For example, speech and communication problems or problems with aggression or impulse control may create barriers to forming intimate relationships with others. These types of problems have been voiced as important concerns by persons with TBI (Gaudet, Crethar, Burger, & Pulos, 2001; National Institutes of Health, 1998). Because these concerns are frequently reported by both patients and partners, addressing sexual problems as a component of reintegration into the family unit and the community should be a priority in rehabilitation practices. Depending on the source of dysfunction, rehabilitation psychologists can assist the patient or partner in communicating accurate messages about sex and intimacy, problem-solving around physical limitations, consulting with prescribers, advocating for additional pharmacological intervention, or helping the individual to develop a more positive self-concept.

Vocational reintegration. Returning to employment after suffering a TBI can be difficult due to chronic physical, cognitive, and emotional effects. Those who were employed at the time of injury may not be able to return to work in the same capacity, or they may have been terminated due to length of absence. Moreover, initial return to work does not guarantee maintenance of employment. Finding new employment after TBI is exponentially more difficult, given changing labor markets (Cuthbert et al., 2015). In 2007, Shames and colleagues examined return to work patterns and reported interaction effects among premorbid characteristics, injury factors, postinjury impairments and personal and environmental factors in TBI patients that influenced return to work outcomes (Shames, Treger, Ring, & Giaquinto, 2007). One major finding was that impaired self-awareness appeared to be a particular barrier to return to work.

It is important to note that military personnel with TBI often face unique challenges to vocational reintegration after TBI. Injuries that are severe enough may warrant medical discharge from military service, ultimately forcing the service member to transition back into the civilian community before he or she had intended. It is common for veterans, with or without brain injury, to experience frustration associated with this transition. Challenges to vocational reintegration for these individuals arise when skills and abilities learned in military service do not translate easily to civilian jobs or are not readily apparent to potential employers. Co-occurring psychiatric issues common to military populations may also present challenges to finding new work, even in cases of mTBI (McGarity et al., 2017).

There are several models of vocational rehabilitation following brain injury (Fadyl & McPherson, 2009; Tyerman, 2012). The model most consistent with clinical practice guidelines for brain injury is a case-coordination approach in which vocational rehabilitation is part of the overall model of care that includes other rehabilitation services (Commission on Accreditation of Rehabilitation Facilities, 2016). In this model, the focus is on early intervention and continuity of care across time. Although vocational rehabilitation specialists serve as primary providers in these programs, rehabilitation psychologists can assist in reinforcing skills and coping strategies learned for managing work-related stress or interpersonal conflict.

CONCLUSION

TBI is a complex injury occurring to the most complicated organ in the body, producing heterogeneous effects and, as a result, multiple and complex challenges. In treating persons with TBI of any severity, rehabilitation psychologists must be prepared to use a host of skills and a breadth of knowledge that encompass both the neurological and neurocognitive aspects of injury to the brain and the psychosocial manifestations of changed functional abilities. Recognition that TBI is a chronic health condition requires additional research to establish evidence-based approaches for proactive management of health and wellness in this population. Future directions in rehabilitative care for persons with TBI will follow trends similar to other fields of health care in adopting more person-centered, holistic approaches to recovery, in consideration of mind, body, and spirit. This modern, holistic approach calls for acknowledging each person's unique combination of symptoms, strengths, and goals and then addressing needs identified as important by patients and families in a way that promotes the highest degree of independence and quality of life. Holistic and person-centered approaches are currently driving research efforts in complementary and alternative medicine, investigating the potential benefits of techniques such as yoga, acupuncture, and dietary supplements for helping those recovering from TBI to maximize their own capacity for self-repair and healing. By emphasizing individual strengths and resources, those living with injuries, as well as those close to them, are encouraged to adopt a stance that is predictive of successful rehabilitation outcomes.

References

Allely, C. S. (2016). Prevalence and assessment of traumatic brain injury in prison inmates: A systematic PRISMA review. *Brain Injury*, *30*, 1161–1180. http://dx.doi.org/10.1080/02699052.2016.1191674

American Academy of Neurology. (2013). Update: Evaluation and management of concussion in sports. *Summary of Evidence-Based Guideline for Clinicians*. Retrieved from https://www.aan.com/siteassets/home-page/tools-and-resources/practicing-neurologist--

administrators/patient-resources/sports-concussion-resources/17emconcussions_tr.pdf

American Psychiatric Association. (2013). *Diagnostic and statistical manual of mental disorders* (5th ed.). Washington, DC: Author.

Anson, K., & Ponsford, J. (2006). Evaluation of a coping skills group following traumatic brain injury. *Brain Injury*, *20*, 167–178. http://dx.doi.org/10.1080/02699050500442956

Assistant Secretary of Defense. (2015). Traumatic brain injury: Updated definition and reporting. Washington, DC: Department of Defense.

Bahraini, N., & Brenner, L. A. (2013). Screening for TBI and persistent symptoms provides opportunities for prevention and intervention. *The Journal of Head Trauma Rehabilitation*, *28*, 223–226. http://dx.doi.org/10.1097/HTR.0b013e318291dab7

Bahraini, N. H., Breshears, R. E., Hernández, T. D., Schneider, A. L., Forster, J. E., & Brenner, L. A. (2014). Traumatic brain injury and posttraumatic stress disorder. *Psychiatric Clinics of North America*, *37*, 55–75. http://dx.doi.org/10.1016/j.psc.2013.11.002

Bazarian, J. J., Veazie, P., Mookerjee, S., & Lerner, E. B. (2006). Accuracy of mild traumatic brain injury case ascertainment using ICD–9 codes. *Academic Emergency Medicine*, *13*, 31–38. http://dx.doi.org/10.1197/j.aem.2005.07.038

Beck, A. T., & Steer, R. A. (1998). *Manual for the Beck Hopelessness Scale*. San Antonio, TX: Psychological Corporation.

Beck, A. T., Steer, R. A., & Brown, G. K. (1996). *Beck Depression Inventory—II manual* (2nd ed.). San Antonio, TX: Psychological Corporation.

Belanger, H. G., Vanderploeg, R. D., & Sayer, N. (2016). Screening for remote history of mild traumatic brain injury in VHA: A critical literature review. *The Journal of Head Trauma Rehabilitation*, *31*, 204–214. http://dx.doi.org/10.1097/HTR.0000000000000168

Blake, D. D., Weathers, F. W., Nagy, L. M., Kaloupek, D. G., Gusman, F. D., Charney, D. S., & Keane, T. M. (1995). The development of a clinician-administered PTSD scale. *Journal of Traumatic Stress*, *8*, 75–90. http://dx.doi.org/10.1002/jts.2490080106

Bogner, J., & Corrigan, J. D. (2009). Reliability and predictive validity of the Ohio State University TBI identification method with prisoners. *The Journal of Head Trauma Rehabilitation*, *24*, 279–291. http://dx.doi.org/10.1097/HTR.0b013e3181a66356

Bond, A. E., Draeger, C. R. L., Mandleco, B., & Donnelly, M. (2003). Needs of family members of patients with severe traumatic brain injury. Implications for evidence-based practice. *Critical Care Nurse*, *23*, 63–72.

Brenner, L. A., Forster, J. E., Hoffberg, A. S., Matarazzo, B. B., Hostetter, T. A., Signoracci, G., & Simpson, G. K. (2018). Window to hope: A randomized controlled trial of a psychological intervention for the treatment of hopelessness among veterans with moderate to severe traumatic brain injury. *The Journal of Head Trauma Rehabilitation*, *33*, E64–E73. http://dx.doi.org/10.1097/HTR.0000000000000351

Brenner, L. A., Homaifar, B. Y., Olson-Madden, J. H., Nagamoto, H. T., Huggins, J., Schneider, A. L., . . . Corrigan, J. D. (2013). Prevalence and screening of traumatic brain injury among veterans seeking mental health services. *The Journal of Head Trauma Rehabilitation*, *28*, 21–30. http://dx.doi.org/10.1097/HTR.0b013e31827df0b5

Brenner, L. A., Ignacio, R. V., & Blow, F. C. (2011). Suicide and traumatic brain injury among individuals seeking Veterans Health Administration services. *The Journal of Head Trauma Rehabilitation*, *26*, 257–264. http://dx.doi.org/10.1097/HTR.0b013e31821fdb6e

Brenner, L. A., Ivins, B. J., Schwab, K., Warden, D., Nelson, L. A., Jaffee, M., & Terrio, H. (2010). Traumatic brain injury, posttraumatic stress disorder, and postconcussive symptom reporting among troops returning from Iraq. *The Journal of Head Trauma Rehabilitation*, *25*, 307–312. http://dx.doi.org/10.1097/HTR.0b013e3181cada03

Bryant, R. A., O'Donnell, M. L., Creamer, M., McFarlane, A. C., Clark, C. R., & Silove, D. (2010). The psychiatric sequelae of traumatic injury. *The American Journal of Psychiatry*, *167*, 312–320. http://dx.doi.org/10.1176/appi.ajp.2009.09050617

Buysse, D. J., Reynolds, C. F., III, Monk, T. H., Berman, S. R., & Kupfer, D. J. (1989). The Pittsburgh Sleep Quality Index: A new instrument for psychiatric practice and research. *Psychiatry Research*, *28*, 193–213. http://dx.doi.org/10.1016/0165-1781(89)90047-4

Castriotta, R. J., Wilde, M. C., Lai, J. M., Atanasov, S., Masel, B. E., & Kuna, S. T. (2007). Prevalence and consequences of sleep disorders in traumatic brain injury. *Journal of Clinical Sleep Medicine*, *3*, 349–356.

Centers for Disease Control and Prevention. (2006). Incidence rates of hospitalization related to traumatic brain injury—12 states, 2002. *Morbidity and Mortality Weekly Report*, *55*, 201–204.

Centers for Disease Control and Prevention, National Center for Injury Prevention and Control, Division of Unintentional Injury Prevention. (2015). *Report to Congress on traumatic brain injury in the United States: Epidemiology and rehabilitation*. Retrieved from https://stacks.cdc.gov/view/cdc/29215

Chard, K. M., Schumm, J. A., McIlvain, S. M., Bailey, G. W., & Parkinson, R. B. (2011). Exploring the efficacy of a residential treatment program incorporating cognitive processing therapy-cognitive for veterans with PTSD and traumatic brain injury. *Journal of Traumatic Stress*, *24*, 347–351. http://dx.doi.org/10.1002/jts.20644

Cicerone, K. D., Dahlberg, C., Kalmar, K., Langenbahn, D. M., Malec, J. F., Bergquist, T. F., . . . Morse, P. A. (2000). Evidence-based cognitive rehabilitation: Recommendations for clinical practice. *Archives of Physical Medicine and Rehabilitation*, *81*, 1596–1615. http://dx.doi.org/10.1053/apmr.2000.19240

Cicerone, K. D., Dahlberg, C., Malec, J. F., Langenbahn, D. M., Felicetti, T., Kneipp, S., . . . Catanese, J. (2005). Evidence-based cognitive rehabilitation: Updated review of the literature from 1998 through 2002. *Archives of Physical Medicine and Rehabilitation*, *86*, 1681–1692. http://dx.doi.org/10.1016/j.apmr.2005.03.024

Cicerone, K. D., & Kalmar, K. (1995). Persistent post-concussion syndrome: The structure of subjective complaints after mTBI. *The Journal of Head Trauma Rehabilitation*, *10*, 1–17. http://dx.doi.org/10.1097/00001199-199510030-00002

Cicerone, K. D., Langenbahn, D. M., Braden, C., Malec, J. F., Kalmar, K., Fraas, M., . . . Ashman, T. (2011). Evidence-based cognitive rehabilitation: Updated review of the literature from 2003 through 2008. *Archives of Physical Medicine and Rehabilitation*, *92*, 519–530. http://dx.doi.org/10.1016/j.apmr.2010.11.015

Cifu, D. X., Uchima, O. K., Davis, A. S., Lower, A. E., Jin, J. L., & Lew, H. L. (2016). Significance of concussions in Hawai'i: From land to sea. *Hawai'i Journal of Medicine & Public Health*, *75*, 262–265.

Commission on Accreditation of Rehabilitation Facilities. (2016). 2016 Medical Program Descriptions. In *Standards Manual for Medical Rehabilitation* (pp. 1–12). Retrieved from http://www.carf.org/programs/

Corrigan, J. D., & Bogner, J. (2007). Initial reliability and validity of the Ohio State University TBI Identification Method. *The Journal of Head Trauma Rehabilitation*, *22*, 318–329. http://dx.doi.org/10.1097/01.HTR.0000300227.67748.77

Corrigan, J. D., Bogner, J., Mellick, D., Bushnik, T., Dams-O'Connor, K., Hammond, F. M., . . . Kolakowsky-Hayner, S. (2013). Prior history of traumatic brain injury among persons in the Traumatic Brain Injury Model Systems National Database. *Archives of Physical Medicine and Rehabilitation*, *94*, 1940–1950. http://dx.doi.org/10.1016/j.apmr.2013.05.018

Corrigan, J. D., Yang, J., Singichetti, B., Manchester, K., & Bogner, J. A. (2018). Lifetime prevalence of TBI with loss of consciousness. *Injury Prevention*, *24*, 396–404. http://dx.doi.org/10.1136/injuryprev-2017-042371

Cuthbert, J. P., Corrigan, J. D., Whiteneck, G. G., Harrison-Felix, C., Graham, J. E., Bell, J. M., & Coronado, V. G. (2012). Extension of the representativeness of the Traumatic Brain Injury Model Systems National Database: 2001 to 2010. *The Journal of Head Trauma Rehabilitation*, *27*, E15–E27. http://dx.doi.org/10.1097/HTR.0b013e31826da983

Cuthbert, J. P., Pretz, C. R., Bushnik, T., Fraser, R. T., Hart, T., Kolakowsky-Hayner, S. A., . . . Sherer, M. (2015). Ten-year employment patterns of working age individuals after moderate to severe traumatic brain injury: A National Institute on Disability and Rehabilitation Research traumatic brain injury model systems study. *Archives of Physical Medicine and Rehabilitation*, *96*, 2128–2136. http://dx.doi.org/10.1016/j.apmr.2015.07.020

Cuthbert, J. P., Whiteneck, G. G., Corrigan, J. D., & Bogner, J. (2016). The reliability of a computer-assisted telephone interview version of the Ohio State University Traumatic Brain Injury Identification Method. *The Journal of Head Trauma Rehabilitation*, *31*, E36–E42. http://dx.doi.org/10.1097/HTR.0000000000000075

Dahdah, M. N., Barisa, M. T., Schmidt, K., Barnes, S. A., Dubiel, R., Dunklin, C., . . . Shafi, S. (2014). Comparative effectiveness of traumatic brain injury rehabilitation: Differential outcomes across TBI model systems centers. *The Journal of Head Trauma Rehabilitation*, *29*, 451–459. http://dx.doi.org/10.1097/HTR.0b013e3182a61983

Dams-O'Connor, K., Cantor, J. B., Brown, M., Dijkers, M. P., Spielman, L. A., & Gordon, W. A. (2014). Screening for traumatic brain injury: Findings and public health implications. *The Journal of Head Trauma Rehabilitation*, *29*, 479–489. http://dx.doi.org/10.1097/HTR.0000000000000099

Dams-O'Connor, K., Spielman, L., Singh, A., Gordon, W. A., Lingsma, H. F., Maas, A. I., . . . Yuh, E. L., & the TRACK–TBI Investigators. (2013). The impact of previous traumatic brain injury on health and functioning: A TRACK–TBI study. *Journal of Neurotrauma*, *30*, 2014–2020. http://dx.doi.org/10.1089/neu.2013.3049

Derogatis, L. (1994). *Administration, scoring and procedures manual for the SCL–90–R; Symptom Checklist–90–R*. Minneapolis, MN: National Computer Systems.

Diamond, P. M., Harzke, A. J., Magaletta, P. R., Cummins, A. G., & Frankowski, R. (2007). Screening for traumatic brain injury in an offender sample: A first look at the reliability and validity of the Traumatic Brain Injury Questionnaire. *The Journal of Head Trauma Rehabilitation*, *22*, 330–338. http://dx.doi.org/10.1097/01.HTR.0000300228.05867.5c

Fadyl, J. K., & McPherson, K. M. (2009). Approaches to vocational rehabilitation after traumatic brain injury: A review of the evidence. *The Journal of Head Trauma Rehabilitation*, *24*, 195–212. http://dx.doi.org/10.1097/HTR.0b013e3181a0d458

Faul, M., Xu, L., Wald, M. M., & Coronado, V. G. (2010). *Traumatic Brain Injury in the United States: Emergency Department Visits, Hospitalizations and Deaths 2002–2006*. Centers for Disease Control and Prevention, National Center for Injury Prevention and Control. Retrieved from https://www.cdc.gov/traumaticbraininjury/pdf/blue_book.pdf

Feeney, D. M., Gonzalez, A., & Law, W. A. (1982). Amphetamine, haloperidol, and experience interact to affect rate of recovery after motor cortex injury. *Science*, *217*, 855–857. http://dx.doi.org/10.1126/science.7100929

Fisher, L. B., Pedrelli, P., Iverson, G. L., Bergquist, T. F., Bombardier, C. H., Hammond, F. M., . . . Zafonte, R. (2016). Prevalence of suicidal behaviour following traumatic brain injury: Longitudinal follow-up data from the NIDRR Traumatic Brain Injury Model Systems. *Brain Injury*, *30*, 1311–1318. http://dx.doi.org/10.1080/02699052.2016.1195517

Fortier, C. B., Amick, M. M., Grande, L., McGlynn, S., Kenna, A., Morra, L., . . . McGlinchey, R. E. (2014). The Boston Assessment of Traumatic Brain Injury-Lifetime (BAT-L) semistructured interview: Evidence of research utility and validity. *The Journal of Head Trauma Rehabilitation*, *29*, 89–98. http://dx.doi.org/10.1097/HTR.0b013e3182865859

Gabella, B. A., Mangione, E. J., Hedegaard, H., & Kelly, J. P. (2007). Comparison of nursing home residents with and without traumatic brain injury: Use of the Minimum Data Set. *The Journal of Head Trauma Rehabilitation*, *22*, 368–376. http://dx.doi.org/10.1097/01.HTR.0000300232.98242.ce

Gaudet, L., Crethar, H. C., Burger, S., & Pulos, S. (2001). Self-reported consequences of traumatic brain injury: A study of contrasting TBI and non-TBI participants. *Sexuality and Disability*, *19*, 111–119. http://dx.doi.org/10.1023/A:1010673722429

Giacino, J. T., Kalmar, K., & Whyte, J. (2004). The JFK Coma Recovery Scale—Revised: Measurement characteristics and diagnostic utility. *Archives of Physical Medicine and Rehabilitation*, *85*, 2020–2029. http://dx.doi.org/10.1016/j.apmr.2004.02.033

Goldin, Y., Haag, H. L., & Trott, C. T. (2016). Screening for history of traumatic brain injury among women exposed to intimate partner violence. *PM & R*, *8*, 1104–1110. http://dx.doi.org/10.1016/j.pmrj.2016.05.006

Hagen, C., Malkmus, D., & Durham, P. (1972). *Levels of cognitive functioning*. Downey, CA: Rancho Los Amigos Hospital.

Harrison-Felix, C., Kreider, S. E., Arango-Lasprilla, J. C., Brown, A. W., Dijkers, M. P., Hammond, F. M., . . . Zasler, N. D. (2012). Life expectancy following rehabilitation: A NIDRR Traumatic Brain Injury Model Systems study. *The Journal of Head Trauma Rehabilitation*, *27*, E69–E80. http://dx.doi.org/10.1097/HTR.0b013e3182738010

Harrison-Felix, C., Whiteneck, G., DeVivo, M., Hammond, F. M., & Jha, A. (2004). Mortality following rehabilitation in the Traumatic Brain Injury Model Systems of Care. *NeuroRehabilitation*, *19*, 45–54.

Harrison-Felix, C., Whiteneck, G., DeVivo, M. J., Hammond, F. M., & Jha, A. (2006). Causes of death following 1 year postinjury among individuals with traumatic brain injury. *The Journal of Head Trauma Rehabilitation*, *21*, 22–33. http://dx.doi.org/10.1097/00001199-200601000-00003

Harrison-Felix, C. L., Whiteneck, G. G., Jha, A., DeVivo, M. J., Hammond, F. M., & Hart, D. M. (2009). Mortality over four decades after traumatic brain injury rehabilitation: A retrospective cohort study. *Archives of Physical Medicine and Rehabilitation*, *90*, 1506–1513. http://dx.doi.org/10.1016/j.apmr.2009.03.015

Hauser, W. A., Annegers, J. F., & Kurland, L. T. (1991). Prevalence of epilepsy in Rochester, Minnesota: 1940–1980. *Epilepsia*, *32*, 429–445. http://dx.doi.org/10.1111/j.1528-1157.1991.tb04675.x

Hoge, C. W., McGurk, D., Thomas, J. L., Cox, A. L., Engel, C. C., & Castro, C. A. (2008). Mild traumatic brain injury in U.S. Soldiers returning from Iraq. *The New England Journal of Medicine*, *358*, 453–463. http://dx.doi.org/10.1056/NEJMoa072972

Institute of Medicine. (2009). *Gulf War and Health: Vol. 7. Long-Term Consequences of Traumatic Brain Injury*. Washington, DC: The National Academies Press.

Iverson, K. M., & Pogoda, T. K. (2015). Traumatic brain injury among women veterans: An invisible wound of intimate partner violence. *Medical Care*, *53*(4, Suppl. 1), S112–S119. http://dx.doi.org/10.1097/MLR.0000000000000263

Jackson, W. T., Novack, T. A., & Dowler, R. N. (1998). Effective serial measurement of cognitive orientation in rehabilitation: The Orientation Log. *Archives of Physical Medicine and Rehabilitation*, *79*, 718–720. http://dx.doi.org/10.1016/S0003-9993(98)90051-X

Kaye, H. S. (1997). *Disability watch: The status of people with disabilities in the United States*. San Francisco: Disability Statistics Center, Institute for Health and Aging, University of California at San Francisco.

Langlois, J. A., Rutland-Brown, W., & Wald, M. M. (2006). The epidemiology and impact of traumatic brain injury: A brief overview. *The Journal of Head Trauma Rehabilitation*, *21*, 375–378. http://dx.doi.org/10.1097/00001199-200609000-00001

Levin, H. S., O'Donnell, V. M., & Grossman, R. G. (1979). The Galveston Orientation and Amnesia Test: A practical scale to assess cognition after head injury. *Journal of Nervous and Mental Disease, 167*, 675–684.

Lovibond, S. H., & Lovibond, P. F. (1995). *Manual for the Depression Anxiety Stress Scales*. Sydney, Australia: Psychology Foundation.

Lu, W., Krellman, J. W., & Dijkers, M. P. (2016). Can Cognitive Behavioral Therapy for Insomnia also treat fatigue, pain, and mood symptoms in individuals with traumatic brain injury? A multiple case report. *NeuroRehabilitation*, *38*, 59–69. http://dx.doi.org/10.3233/NRE-151296

Maas, A. I., Harrison-Felix, C. L., Menon, D., Adelson, P. D., Balkin, T., Bullock, R., . . . Schwab, K. (2010). Common data elements for traumatic brain injury: Recommendations from the interagency working group on demographics and clinical assessment. *Archives of Physical Medicine and Rehabilitation*, *91*, 1641–1649. http://dx.doi.org/10.1016/j.apmr.2010.07.232

Marwitz, J. (2000). *The Neurobehavioral Functioning Inventory*. Retrieved from the Center for Outcome Measurement in Brain Injury: http://www.tbims.org/combi/nfi

Masel, B. E., & DeWitt, D. S. (2010). Traumatic brain injury: A disease process, not an event. *Journal of Neurotrauma*, *27*, 1529–1540. http://dx.doi.org/10.1089/neu.2010.1358

Massagli, T. L. (1991). Neurobehavioral effects of phenytoin, carbamazepine, and valproic acid: Implications for use in traumatic brain injury. *Archives of Physical Medicine and Rehabilitation*, *72*, 219–226.

Matarazzo, B. B., Hoffberg, A. S., Clemans, T. A., Signoracci, G. M., Simpson, G. K., & Brenner, L. A. (2014). Cross-cultural adaptation of the Window to Hope: A psychological intervention to reduce hopelessness among U.S. veterans with traumatic brain injury. *Brain Injury*, *28*, 1238–1247. http://dx.doi.org/10.3109/02699052.2014.916419

McCrea, M., Guskiewicz, K., Doncevic, S., Helmick, K., Kennedy, J., Boyd, C., . . . Jaffee, M. (2014). Day of injury cognitive performance on the Military Acute Concussion Evaluation (MACE) by U.S. military service members in OEF/OIF. *Military Medicine*, *179*, 990–997. http://dx.doi.org/10.7205/MILMED-D-13-00349

McCrea, M., Pliskin, N., Barth, J., Cox, D., Fink, J., French, L., . . . Yoash-Gantz, R. (2008). Official position of the Military TBI Task Force on the role of neuropsychology and rehabilitation psychology in the evaluation, management, and research of military veterans with traumatic brain injury. *Clinical Neuropsychologist*, *22*, 10–26. http://dx.doi.org/10.1080/13854040701760981

McDonnell, E., Giacino, J. T., & Kolakowsky-Hayner, S. A. (2015). A brief overview of the Coma Recovery Scale—Revised: Updates from the COMBI. *The Journal of Head Trauma Rehabilitation*, *30*, 143–145. http://dx.doi.org/10.1097/HTR.0000000000000133

McGarity, S., Barnett, S. D., Lamberty, G., Kretzmer, T., Powell-Cope, G., Patel, N., & Nakase-Richardson, R. (2017). Community reintegration problems among veterans and active duty service members with traumatic brain injury. *The Journal of Head Trauma Rehabilitation*, *32*, 34–45. http://dx.doi.org/10.1097/HTR.0000000000000242

Menon, D. K., Schwab, K., Wright, D. W., Maas, A. I., & Demographics and Clinical Assessment Working Group of the International and Interagency Initiative Toward Common Data Elements for Research on Traumatic Brain Injury and Psychological Health. (2010). Position statement: Definition of traumatic brain injury. *Archives of Physical Medicine and Rehabilitation*, *91*, 1637–1640. Retrieved from http://www.sciencedirect.com/science/article/pii/S0003999310006507

Morin, C. M., Belleville, G., Bélanger, L., & Ivers, H. (2011). The Insomnia Severity Index: Psychometric indicators to detect insomnia cases and evaluate treatment response. *Sleep*, *34*, 601–608. http://dx.doi.org/10.1093/sleep/34.5.601

Napolitano, E., Radecki, J., & Elovic, E. P. (2007). Primary prevention. In N. Zasler, D. Katz, & R. Zafonte (Eds.), *Brain injury medicine: Principles and practice* (p. 57). New York, NY: Demos Medical.

National Campaign Against Drug Abuse, National Drug Strategy. (2009). *Comorbidity of mental disorders and substance use: A brief guide for the primary care clinician*, Chapter 12. Retrieved from http://www.nationaldrugstrategy.gov.au/internet/drugstrategy/publishing.nsf/Content/FE16C454A782A8AFCA2575BE002044D0/

National Institutes of Health. (1998). Rehabilitation of persons with traumatic brain injury. *NIH Consensus Statement*, *16*, 1–41. https://consensus.nih.gov/1998/1998traumaticbraininjury109html.htm

Neumann, D., Malec, J. F., & Hammond, F. M. (2017). The relations of self-reported aggression to alexithymia, depression, and anxiety after traumatic brain injury. *The Journal of Head Trauma Rehabilitation*, *32*, 205–213. http://dx.doi.org/10.1097/HTR.0000000000000261

Neumann, D., Zupan, B., Malec, J. F., & Hammond, F. (2014). Relationships between alexithymia, affect recognition, and empathy after traumatic brain injury. *The Journal of Head Trauma Rehabilitation*, *29*, E18–E27. http://dx.doi.org/10.1097/HTR.0b013e31827fb0b5

Nguyen, S., McKay, A., Wong, D., Rajaratnam, S. M., Spitz, G., Williams, G., . . . Ponsford, J. L. (2017). Cognitive behavior therapy to treat sleep disturbance and fatigue after traumatic brain injury: A pilot randomized controlled trial. *Archives of Physical Medicine and Rehabilitation*, *98*, 1508–1517.e2. http://dx.doi.org/10.1016/j.apmr.2017.02.031

Nikoo, M., Gadermann, A., To, M. J., Krausz, M., Hwang, S. W., & Palepu, A. (2017). Incidence and associated risk factors of traumatic brain injury in a cohort of homeless and vulnerably housed adults in 3 Canadian cities. *The Journal of Head Trauma Rehabilitation*, *32*, E19–E26. http://dx.doi.org/10.1097/HTR.0000000000000262

Novack, T. (2000). *The Orientation Log*. Retrieved from the Center for Outcome Measurement in Brain Injury: http://www.tbims.org/combi/olog

Olson-Madden, J. H., Brenner, L., Harwood, J. E., Emrick, C. D., Corrigan, J. D., & Thompson, C. (2010). Traumatic brain injury and psychiatric diagnoses in veterans seeking outpatient substance abuse treatment. *The Journal of Head Trauma Rehabilitation*, *25*, 470–479. http://dx.doi.org/10.1097/HTR.0b013e3181d717a7

Olson-Madden, J. H., Forster, J. E., Huggins, J., & Schneider, A. (2012). Psychiatric diagnoses, mental health utilization, high-risk behaviors, and self-directed violence among veterans with comorbid history of traumatic brain injury and substance use disorders. *The Journal of Head Trauma Rehabilitation*, *27*, 370–378. http://dx.doi.org/10.1097/HTR.0b013e318268d496

Olson-Madden, J. H., Homaifar, B. Y., Hostetter, T. A., Matarazzo, B. B., Huggins, J., Forster, J. E., . . . Brenner, L. A. (2014). Validating the Traumatic Brain Injury—4 screening measure for veterans seeking mental health treatment with psychiatric inpatient and outpatient service utilization data. *Archives of Physical Medicine and Rehabilitation*, *95*, 925–929. http://dx.doi.org/10.1016/j.apmr.2014.01.008

Ponsford, J., Lee, N. K., Wong, D., McKay, A., Haines, K., Alway, Y., . . . O'Donnell, M. L. (2016). Efficacy of motivational interviewing and cognitive behavioral therapy for anxiety and depression symptoms following traumatic brain injury. *Psychological Medicine*, *46*, 1079–1090. http://dx.doi.org/10.1017/S0033291715002640

Powell, J. M., Ferraro, J. V., Dikmen, S. S., Temkin, N. R., & Bell, K. R. (2008). Accuracy of mild traumatic brain injury diagnosis. *Archives of Physical Medicine and Rehabilitation*, *89*, 1550–1555. http://dx.doi.org/10.1016/j.apmr.2007.12.035

Radomski, M. V., Anheluk, M., Bartzen, M. P., & Zola, J. (2016). Effectiveness of interventions to address cognitive impairments and improve occupational performance after traumatic brain injury: A systematic review. *American Journal of Occupational Therapy*, *70*, 0050p1–9. http://dx.doi.org/10.5014/ajot.2016.020776

Ragsdale, K. A., & Voss Horrell, S. C. (2016). Effectiveness of prolonged exposure and cognitive processing therapy for U.S. veterans with a history of traumatic brain injury. *Journal of Traumatic Stress*, *29*, 474–477. http://dx.doi.org/10.1002/jts.22130

Rees, L., Marshall, S., Hartridge, C., Mackie, D., & Weiser, M. (2007). Cognitive interventions post acquired brain injury. *Brain Injury*, *21*, 161–200. http://dx.doi.org/10.1080/02699050701201813

Reichard, A. A., Langlois, J. A., Sample, P. L., Wald, M. M., & Pickelsimer, E. E. (2007). Violence, abuse, and neglect among people with traumatic brain injuries. *The Journal of Head Trauma Rehabilitation*, *22*, 390–402. http://dx.doi.org/10.1097/01.HTR.0000300234.36361.b1

Rohling, M. L., Faust, M. E., Beverly, B., & Demakis, G. (2009). Effectiveness of cognitive rehabilitation following acquired brain injury: A meta-analytic re-examination of Cicerone et al.'s (2000, 2005) systematic reviews. *Neuropsychology*, *23*, 20–39. http://dx.doi.org/10.1037/a0013659

Roth, R. J., & Spencer, R. J. (2013). Iatrogenic risk in the management of mild traumatic brain injury among combat veterans: A case illustration commentary. *International Journal of Physical Medicine & Rehabilitation*, *1*, 1–7.

Russell, L. M., Devore, M. D., Barnes, S. M., Forster, J. E., Hostetter, T. A., Montgomery, A. E., . . . Brenner, L. A. (2013). Challenges associated with screening for traumatic brain injury among US veterans seeking homeless services. *American Journal of Public Health*, *103*(Suppl. 2), S211–S212. http://dx.doi.org/10.2105/AJPH.2013.301485

Salottolo, K., Carrick, M., Stewart Levy, A., Morgan, B. C., Slone, D. S., & Bar-Or, D. J. (2016). The epidemiology, prognosis, and trends of severe traumatic brain injury with presenting Glasgow Coma Scale of 3. *Journal of Critical Care*, *38*, 197–201. http://dx.doi.org/10.1016/j.jcrc.2016.11.034

Sample, P. L., Tomter, H., & Johns, N. (2007). "The left hand does not know what the right hand is doing": Rural and urban cultures of care for persons with traumatic brain injuries. *Substance Use & Misuse*, *42*, 705–727. http://dx.doi.org/10.1080/10826080701202536

Sander, A. M. (2013). Sexual functioning after traumatic brain injury (Preface). *The Journal of Head Trauma Rehabilitation*, *28*, 161–163. http://dx.doi.org/10.1097/HTR.0b013e318290c109

Schofield, P. W., Butler, T. G., Hollis, S. J., Smith, N. E., Lee, S. J., & Kelso, W. M. (2006). Traumatic brain injury among Australian prisoners: Rates, recurrence and sequelae. *Brain Injury*, *20*, 499–506. http://dx.doi.org/10.1080/02699050600664749

Selassie, A. W., Zaloshnja, E., Langlois, J. A., Miller, T., Jones, P., & Steiner, C. (2003). Incidence of long-term disability following traumatic brain injury hospitalization, United States. *Journal of Head Trauma Rehabilitation*, *23*, 123–131. http://dx.doi.org/10.1097/01.HTR.0000314531.30401.39

Shames, J., Treger, I., Ring, H., & Giaquinto, S. (2007). Return to work following traumatic brain injury: Trends and challenges. *Disability and Rehabilitation, 29*, 1387–1395. http://dx.doi.org/10.1080/09638280701315011

Sherer, M., Nakase-Thompson, R., Yablon, S. A., & Gontkovsky, S. T. (2005). Multidimensional assessment of acute confusion after traumatic brain injury. *Archives of Physical Medicine and Rehabilitation, 86*, 896–904. http://dx.doi.org/10.1016/j.apmr.2004.09.029

Shiroma, E. J., Ferguson, P. L., & Pickelsimer, E. E. (2012). Prevalence of traumatic brain injury in an offender population: A meta-analysis. *The Journal of Head Trauma Rehabilitation, 27*, E1–E10. http://dx.doi.org/10.1097/HTR.0b013e3182571c14

Simpson, G. K., Tate, R. L., Whiting, D. L., & Cotter, R. E. (2011). Suicide prevention after traumatic brain injury: A randomized controlled trial of a program for the psychological treatment of hopelessness. *The Journal of Head Trauma Rehabilitation, 26*, 290–300. http://dx.doi.org/10.1097/HTR.0b013e3182225250

Smith, K. R., Jr., Goulding, P. M., Wilderman, D., Goldfader, P. R., Holterman-Hommes, P., & Wei, F. (1994). Neurobehavioral effects of phenytoin and carbamazepine in patients recovering from brain trauma: A comparative study. *Archives of Neurology, 51*, 653–660. http://dx.doi.org/10.1001/archneur.1994.00540190029012

St. Ivany, A., & Schminkey, D. (2016). Intimate partner violence and traumatic brain injury: State of the science and next steps. *Family & Community Health, 39*, 129–137. http://dx.doi.org/10.1097/FCH.0000000000000094

Strom, T. Q., Wolf, G. K., Crawford, E., Blahnik, M., & Kretzmer, T. (2016). Implementing prolonged exposure for veterans with comorbid PTSD and traumatic brain injury: Two case studies. *Cognitive and Behavioral Practice, 23*, 148–161. http://dx.doi.org/10.1016/j.cbpra.2015.03.003

Tanielian, T., Haycox, L. H., Schell, T. L., Marshall, G. N., Burnam, M. A., Eibner, C., . . . Vaiana, M. E. (2008). *Invisible wounds of war: Summary and recommendations for addressing psychological and cognitive injuries*. Santa Monica, CA: RAND Corporation.

Terrio, H., Brenner, L. A., Ivins, B. J., Cho, J. M., Helmick, K., Schwab, K., . . . Warden, D. (2009). Traumatic brain injury screening: Preliminary findings in a US Army Brigade Combat Team. *The Journal of Head Trauma Rehabilitation, 24*, 14–23. http://dx.doi.org/10.1097/HTR.0b013e31819581d8

Terrio, H. P., Nelson, L. A., Betthauser, L. M., Harwood, J. E., & Brenner, L. A. (2011). Postdeployment traumatic brain injury screening questions: Sensitivity, specificity, and predictive values in returning soldiers. *Rehabilitation Psychology, 56*, 26–31. http://dx.doi.org/10.1037/a0022685

Thurman, D. J., Alverson, C., Dunn, K. A., Guerrero, J., & Sniezek, J. E. (1999). Traumatic brain injury in the United States: A public health perspective. *The Journal of Head Trauma Rehabilitation, 14*, 602–615. http://dx.doi.org/10.1097/00001199-199912000-00009

Tiersky, L. A., Anselmi, V., Johnston, M. V., Kurtyka, J., Roosen, E., Schwartz, T., & Deluca, J. (2005). A trial of neuropsychologic rehabilitation in mild-spectrum traumatic brain injury. *Archives of Physical Medicine and Rehabilitation, 86*, 1565–1574. http://dx.doi.org/10.1016/j.apmr.2005.03.013

Tyerman, A. (2012). Vocational rehabilitation after traumatic brain injury: Models and services. *NeuroRehabilitation, 31*, 51–62.

U.S. Department of Defense. (2012). DoD Policy Guidance for Management of Mild Traumatic Brain Injury/Concussion in the Deployed Setting (Memo No. 6490.11). Retrieved from http://www.dtic.mil/whs/directives/corres/pdf/649011p.pdf

U.S. Department of Veterans Affairs and Department of Defense. (2009). *Clinical practice guideline: Management of concussion/mild traumatic*. Retrieved from https://www.rehab.research.va.gov/jour/09/46/6/pdf/cpg.pdf

U.S. Department of Veterans Affairs and Department of Defense. (2010). *Clinical practice guideline: Management of post-traumatic stress disorder and acute stress reaction*. Retrieved from http://www.healthquality.va.gov/guidelines/MH/ptsd/

U.S. Department of Veterans Affairs and Department of Defense. (2016). *VA/DoD clinical practice guideline for the management of concussion–mild traumatic brain injury*. Retrieved from https://www.healthquality.va.gov/guidelines/Rehab/mtbi/mTBICPGFullCPG50821816.pdf

Vanderploeg, R. D., & Belanger, H. G. (2013). Screening for a remote history of mild traumatic brain injury: When a good idea is bad. *Journal of Head Trauma Rehabilitation, 28*, 211–218.

Walker, R., Cole, J. E., Logan, T. K., & Corrigan, J. D. (2007). Screening substance abuse treatment clients for traumatic brain injury: Prevalence and characteristics. *The Journal of Head Trauma Rehabilitation, 22*, 360–367.

Weathers, F., Litz, B., Herman, D., Huska, J., & Keane, T. (1993). *The PTSD Checklist (PCL): Reliability, validity, and diagnostic utility*. Paper presented at the annual convention of the International Society for Traumatic Stress Studies, San Antonio, TX.

Whiteneck, G. G., Cuthbert, J. P., Corrigan, J. D., & Bogner, J. A. (2016). Prevalence of self-reported lifetime history of traumatic brain injury and associated disability: A statewide population-based survey. *The Journal of Head Trauma Rehabilitation*, *31*, E55–E62. http://dx.doi.org/10.1097/HTR.0000000000000140

Wilde, M. C., Castriotta, R. J., Lai, J. M., Atanasov, S., Masel, B. E., & Kuna, S. T. (2007). Cognitive impairment in patients with traumatic brain injury and obstructive sleep apnea. *Archives of Physical Medicine and Rehabilitation*, *88*, 1284–1288. http://dx.doi.org/10.1016/j.apmr.2007.07.012

Williamson, D. R., Frenette, A. J., Burry, L., Perreault, M. M., Charbonney, E., Lamontagne, F., . . . Bernard, F. (2016). Pharmacological interventions for agitation in patients with traumatic brain injury: Protocol for a systematic review and meta-analysis. *Systematic Reviews*, *5*, 193. http://dx.doi.org/10.1186/s13643-016-0374-6

Wolf, G. K., Kretzmer, T., Crawford, E., Thors, C., Wagner, H. R., Strom, T. Q., . . . Vanderploeg, R. D. (2015). Prolonged exposure therapy with veterans and active duty personnel diagnosed with PTSD and traumatic brain injury. *Journal of Traumatic Stress*, *28*, 339–347. http://dx.doi.org/10.1002/jts.22029

Wolf, G. K., Strom, T. Q., Kehle, S. M., & Eftekhari, A. (2012). A preliminary examination of prolonged exposure therapy with Iraq and Afghanistan veterans with a diagnosis of posttraumatic stress disorder and mild to moderate traumatic brain injury. *The Journal of Head Trauma Rehabilitation*, *27*, 26–32. http://dx.doi.org/10.1097/HTR.0b013e31823cd01f

World Health Organization. (2002). *Innovative care for chronic conditions. Building blocks for action: Global report*. Retrieved from http://www.who.int/chp/knowledge/publications/icccglobalreport.pdf

Zigmond, A. S., & Snaith, R. P. (1983). The hospital anxiety and depression scale. *Acta Psychiatrica Scandinavica*, *67*, 361–370. http://dx.doi.org/10.1111/j.1600-0447.1983.tb09716.x

Chapter 19

NEURODEGENERATIVE DISEASES

Erica Weber and Nancy D. Chiaravalloti

Neurodegenerative diseases often result in myriad symptoms largely relevant to rehabilitation psychologists. Given the nature of such diseases, affected individuals need to be prepared for changes in their cognitive, psychological, and functional abilities as the disease progresses. Oftentimes, family or caregiver support systems will be required. Of note, many diseases discussed herein are diagnosed during an individual's prime middle-age years and involve few premorbid behavioral risk factors, resulting in otherwise healthy individuals rapidly adjusting to life with a chronic illness. Importantly, the prognosis for disability, treatment outcomes, and lifespan considerably vary across diagnoses, requiring that treating professionals are fluent in the specific details regarding these diseases so that they may understand their patient's experience.

In this chapter, we provide psychologists in the rehabilitation field with an overview of relevant factors associated with four major neurodegenerative diseases: multiple sclerosis (MS), Parkinson's disease (PD), amyotrophic lateral sclerosis (ALS, also referred to as motor neuron disease or Lou Gehrig's disease), and Huntington's disease (HD). In each section, we provide basic information regarding the neurological nature of the disease, cognitive and psychological symptoms associated with the diagnosis (as well as impact on everyday life), and current cognitive rehabilitation and psychosocial treatments available.

MULTIPLE SCLEROSIS

Overview

MS is a progressive disease of the central nervous system (CNS) characterized by the production of widespread lesions, or plaques, in the brain and spinal cord These plaques negatively impact the myelin sheath, resulting in the inhibition of axonal transmission. The main disease process in MS has been typically theorized to be inflammatory demyelination. However, axonal damage occurs as well (Trapp et al., 1998). As a result of the widespread development of plaques, MS results in a wide array of symptoms, including motor, cognitive, and neuropsychiatric problems. Individual differences in symptoms and disease course are typical, which hampers understanding of the disease itself, as well as identification of effective treatments for individual symptoms (Chelune, Stott, & Pinkston, 2008).

MS is more prevalent in women (2:1 ratio, female:male) and in specific geographic regions. It is estimated that MS affects more than 2.3 million people worldwide, with diagnosis typically occurring between the ages of 20 and 50 (National Multiple

The preparation of this chapter was supported by the International Progressive MS Alliance (Grant PA0128), the National Multiple Sclerosis Society (Grant RG 4997A5), and the Kessler Foundation.

http://dx.doi.org/10.1037/0000129-020
Handbook of Rehabilitation Psychology, Third Edition, L. A. Brenner, S. A. Reid-Arndt, T. R. Elliott, R. G. Frank, and B. Caplan (Editors-in-Chief)

Sclerosis Society, n.d.). Although the precise cause of MS remains elusive, a combination of immunological, genetic, and viral factors are thought to contribute (Chelune et al., 2008).

Cognitive Changes in MS and Assessment

Cognitive impairment is common in individuals with MS, with estimated prevalence rates ranging from 43% to 70%. MS negatively affects various aspects of cognition, including attention, executive functioning (EF), information processing, and long-term memory (LTM; for a review, see Chiaravalloti & DeLuca, 2008). Overt dementia is rare in MS, with the more common clinical presentation being one of specific and subtle cognitive deficits varying substantially from patient to patient (Fischer, 2001).

The two most common cognitive deficits observed in persons with MS are deficits in LTM and information processing speed (IPS; Chiaravalloti & DeLuca, 2008; Rao, Leo, Bernardin, & Unverzagt, 1991). LTM deficits are seen in 40% to 65% of patients, with the primary source of this deficit being in new learning (NL; DeLuca, Barbieri-Berger, & Johnson, 1994). Individuals with MS require more repetitions of information to learn new information, but once that information has been acquired, recall and recognition are intact (DeLuca et al., 1994). IPS refers to the speed with which one can process information within a circumscribed period of time. Reduced IPS is the most common cognitive deficits in MS (Bergendal, Fredrikson, & Almkvist, 2007), and research has demonstrated that tests of IPS can be used to predict long-term cognitive decline (Bergendal et al., 2007). In some studies, the extent of LTM impairment has been positively correlated with deficits in IPS (e.g., DeLuca, Chelune, Tulsky, Lengenfelder, & Chiaravalloti, 2004), and IPS has been shown to be predictive of performance on everyday tasks (Kalmar, Gaudino, Moore, Halper, & Deluca, 2008). It is thus essential that one be cautious when interpreting deficits in higher order cognition (e.g., learning or executive functioning) in the presence of IPS deficits (MacNiven et al., 2008).

Impairments in working memory (WM) have also been seen in individuals with MS, albeit less commonly than deficits in processing speed (DeLuca et al., 2004). The paced auditory serial addition test (PASAT), a test of working memory with substantial processing speed demands, is a sensitive measure of cognitive dysfunction in MS (Rosti, Hämäläinen, Koivisto, & Hokkanen, 2007). The PASAT serves as the cognitive component of the widely used Multiple Sclerosis Functional Composite (Fischer, Rudick, Cutter, Reingold, & the National MS Society Clinical Outcomes Assessment Task Force, 1999). Basic attention is typically not deficient in MS (Chiaravalloti & DeLuca, 2008), and impairments in sustained and divided attention are more common (McCarthy, Beaumont, Thompson, & Peacock, 2005). Performance on attention tasks is often associated with IPS and WM abilities (Beatty, Paul, Blanco, Hames, & Wilbanks, 1995) and are therefore difficult to parcel out. Deficits in EF (e.g., abstract and conceptual reasoning, fluency, planning, organization) occur in individuals with MS, albeit less frequently than LTM and IPS deficits (Bobholz & Rao, 2003). Roughly 25% of persons with MS may also present with deficits in visual perceptual functions (Vleugels et al., 2000). Difficulties in primary visual processing (e.g., from optic neuritis), which are commonly seen in MS, can negatively impact visual perceptual processing, although perceptual deficits that are independent of primary visual or other cognitive abnormalities can also occur (Vleugels et al., 2000). Primary visual problems can contribute to difficulties on higher order cognitive tasks that have visual demands (Bruce, Bruce, & Arnett, 2007).

Given the prevalence of cognitive dysfunction in individuals with MS, accurate and efficient assessment and diagnosis are essential. Brief screening tools have thus been developed including the Brief Neuropsychological Battery, the Screening Examination for Cognitive Impairment, and the Basso Screening Battery (for a complete review, see R. H. Benedict et al., 2002). The most widely accepted brief screening battery used today is the Brief International Cognitive Assessment in Multiple Sclerosis (Langdon et al., 2012), which assesses only verbal and visuospatial NL and IPS with three tests (California Verbal Learning Test—II, Brief Visual Memory Test—Revised, and the Symbol Digit Modalities Test). When more comprehensive testing is appropriate, a range of batteries have been used, each with their strengths and weaknesses. The most widely accepted battery in use today, the

Minimal Assessment of Cognitive Function in MS, assesses word fluency, visuospatial ability, verbal, and visuospatial LTM, IPS, WM, and EF; it has been shown to be sensitive to the cognitive deficits seen in MS (R. H. Benedict et al., 2006; see Table 19.1). For more information regarding assessment in rehabilitation settings, see Chapter 4, this volume.

Psychological Symptoms and MS

In addition to cognitive deficits, psychological symptoms, including depression and anxiety, are also common in individuals with MS. The lifetime prevalence of depression in MS has been estimated to range from 24% (Marrie et al., 2015) to 60% (Minden et al., 2006), although its exact source remains elusive (Feinstein et al., 2004). It is interesting to note that depression is less common in persons with MS who have predominantly spinal cord lesions, as opposed to brain lesions (Rabins et al., 1986). A relationship has similarly been noted between depression and demyelination (Feinstein et al., 2004), with demyelination in some brain

TABLE 19.1

Recommended Assessments for Specific Neurological Diseases

Disease	Cognitive screening tools and assessments	Psychological assessments
Multiple sclerosis	▪ Brief International Cognitive Assessment in Multiple Sclerosis (BICAMS; R. H. B. Benedict et al., 2012) ▪ Brief Neuropsychological Battery (Rao, Leo, Bernardin, et al., 1991) ▪ Screening Examination for Cognitive Impairment (Beatty, Paul, et al., 1995) ▪ Basso Screening Battery (Basso, Beason-Hazen, Lynn, Rammohan, & Bornstein, 1996) ▪ MS Functional Composite (Fischer, Rudick, Cutter, Reingold, & National MS Society Clinical Outcomes Assessment Task Force, 1999) ▪ Minimal Assessment of Functioning in Multiple Sclerosis (Benedict et al., 2006)	▪ Beck Depression Inventory—II (BDI–II; A. Beck et al., 1996) ▪ Hospital Anxiety and Depression Scale (HADS; Zigmond & Snaith, 1983) ▪ Hamilton Rating Scale for Depression (HAM–D; M. C. Hamilton, 1960) ▪ Center for Epidemiological Studies Depression Scale (CES–D; Radloff, 1977) ▪ Patient Health Questionnaire—9 (PHQ–9; Kroenke, Spitzer, & Williams, 2001) ▪ Profile of Mood States (POMS) ▪ Structured Clinical Interview for DSM–IV (SCID; First, Spitzer, Gibbon, & Williams, 2002)
Parkinson's disease	▪ Unified Parkinson Disease Rating Scale (UPDRS) revision (Movement Disorder Society Task Force on Rating Scales for Parkinson's Disease, 2003) ▪ Penn–UW Recommended Screening and Standard Battery (Watson et al., 2013)	▪ Hamilton Depression Scale (HAM–D; M. C. Hamilton, 1960) ▪ Beck Depression Inventory–II (BDI–II; A. Beck et al., 1996) ▪ Unified Parkinson Disease Rating Scale (UPDRS) revision (Movement Disorder Society Task Force on Rating Scales for Parkinson's Disease, 2003) ▪ Starkstein Apathy Scale (Pedersen et al., 2012) ▪ Hospital Anxiety and Depression Scale (HADS; Zigmond & Snaith, 1983) ▪ Geriatric Depression Scale (GDS; Parmelee & Katz, 1990)
Amyotrophic lateral sclerosis	▪ ALS Cognitive Behavioral Screen (ALS–CBS; Woolley et al., 2010) ▪ Penn State Screening Battery of Frontal and Temporal Dysfunction Syndromes (Flaherty-Craig et al., 2006)	▪ Beck Depression Inventory—II Fast Screen (BDI–II–FS; Kliem, Mößle, Zenger, & Brähler, 2014) ▪ Cambridge Behavior Inventory (Rudnicki & Fewell, 2007) ▪ Frontal Systems Behavior Scale (Stout et al., 2003)
Huntington's disease	▪ Unified Huntington's Disease Rating Scale (UHDRS; Huntington Study Group, 1996) ▪ Huntington's Disease Cognitive Assessment Battery (HD–CAB; Stout et al., 2014)	▪ Beck Depression Inventory—II (BDI–II; Beck et al., 1996) ▪ Hospital Anxiety and Depression Scale (HADS; Zigmond & Snaith, 1983)

regions appearing to contribute more to depression than lesions in other areas. Potentially contributing neuroanatomical factors include cortical–subcortical disconnection in areas essential to limbic system functions (Sabatini et al., 1996) or in frontal and parietal white matter, atrophy (Bakshi et al., 2000), increased lesions in the temporal region (Feinstein et al., 2004), and differences in immunological markers (Foley et al., 1988).

Several studies have shown depression to be associated with neuropsychological functioning in persons with MS (Arnett, 2005). Cognitive domains negatively affected by depression include WM, IPS, NL and memory (NLM), abstract reasoning, EF, and nonverbal intelligence (Gilchrist & Creed, 1994). Although anxiety disorders have been less of a focus of MS research, anxiety is often comorbid with depression and has been shown to have a prevalence as high as 21.9% in MS samples (Marrie et al., 2015). Injection anxiety is a common area of concern as injection has traditionally been the means by which disease-modifying therapies are administered (e.g., D. C. Mohr, Cox, & Merluzzi, 2005). Depression and anxiety have been associated with greater fatigue (Brown et al., 2009), lower quality of life (Fruehwald, Loeffler-Stastka, Eher, Saletu, & Baumhackl, 2001), and reduced adherence to disease-modifying therapies (DiMatteo, Lepper, & Croghan, 2000). The effective treatment of depression could thus lead to substantial improvement in functioning.

Although not an emotional symptom per se, a full discussion of MS symptomatology could not fail to include a brief mention of fatigue. Fatigue is one of the most common symptoms in MS, being reported in more than 90% of patients (Minden et al., 2006) and is often considered to be the worst symptom of disease (Fisk, Pontefract, Ritvo, Archibald, & Murray, 1994). Fatigue has two components—physical and cognitive—and researchers continue to work toward an increased understanding of the relationship between fatigue and cognition in MS (DeLuca, 2005).

Assessment of Psychological Symptoms in MS

Depression and anxiety are traditionally examined using written inventories or clinical interviews. Many research studies use only symptom-based measures, such as the Beck Depression Inventory (Larcombe & Wilson, 1984) or the Hospital Anxiety and Depression Scale (Forman & Lincoln, 2010; see Table 19.1). Researchers may also use clinical interviewing, such as the Structured Clinical Interview for DSM–IV (D. C. Mohr, Boudewyn, Goodkin, Bostrom, & Epstein, 2001) or the Schedule for Affective Disorders and Schizophrenia (Schiffer & Wineman, 1990). There is little agreement regarding the optimal tool to identify depression in MS (Marrie et al., 2015; see Table 19.1). Although fatigue assessment currently relies exclusively on self-report, efforts to develop more objective measurements are ongoing. Subjective reports of fatigue have generally not shown a relationship with cognitive dysfunction (DeLuca, 2005; Johnson, Lange, DeLuca, Korn, & Natelson, 1997), although objective measurements of fatigue have been more successful (DeLuca, Genova, Hillary, & Wylie, 2008).

Role of Cognitive and Psychological Symptoms on Everyday Life in MS

The onset of MS typically occurs between the ages of 20 and 50 years, when individuals are most active and productive in many aspects of their lives (Chelune et al., 2008). The impact of the disease on daily life and employment is thus significant. Functional impairments that are commonly seen in individuals with MS include difficulty shopping independently, completing housework and home repairs, washing clothes, ironing, cooking, driving, and using public transportation (Staples & Lincoln, 1979). Not surprisingly, considerable evidence indicates that quality of life is decreased in individuals diagnosed with MS (Grima et al., 2000). We also have known for many years that cognitive dysfunction is closely associated with functional status in persons with MS (Beatty, Blanco, Wilbanks, Paul, & Hames, 1995). Rao, Leo, Ellington, et al. (1991) found that individuals with MS who were cognitively impaired participated in fewer social and vocational activities, were less likely to be employed, had greater difficulties in carrying out routine household tasks, and were more vulnerable to psychiatric illness than individuals with a purely physical disability. Cognition also affects driving abilities (e.g., Schultheis, Garay, & DeLuca, 2001).

Daily life activities have been shown to be related to specific areas of cognitive dysfunction, including reduced IPS (Goverover, Chiaravalloti, O'Brien, & DeLuca, 2018) and NLM (Nagy et al., 2006). The decreased ability to perform everyday activities similarly correlates with overall quality of life (Gulick, 1997), depression (Wang, Reimer, Metz, & Patten, 2000), increased disability (Henriksson, Fredrikson, Masterman, & Jönsson, 2001), severity and progression of disease (Nortvedt, Riise, Myhr, & Nyland, 2000), disease duration (Pfennings et al., 1999), decreased cerebral integrity on magnetic resonance imaging (Janardhan & Bakshi, 2000), and deficits in cognitive functioning (Cutajar et al., 2000).

Treatment of Cognitive Symptoms in MS

Cognitive rehabilitation (CR) is designed to enhance one's capacity to process and interpret information and improve one's ability to function in all aspects of family and community life (Ragnarsson et al., 1999). CR studies in MS have focused on various aspects of cognition, including attention (e.g., Plohmann et al., 1998), communication skills (Foley et al., 1994), and memory functioning (e.g., Chiaravalloti, Moore, Nikelshpur, & DeLuca, 2013). Treatment protocols have been designed to focus on one aspect of cognition in particular, such as with Attention Process Training (Amato et al., 2014), Fresh Minder 2 (Pusswald, Mildner, Zebenholzer, Auff, & Lehrner, 2014), and BrainStim (Vogt et al., 2009), with clear benefits noted. Other studies focus on multimodal treatment paradigms designed to target several aspects of cognition either simultaneously or consecutively (e.g., Mattioli, Stampatori, Zanotti, Parrinello, & Capra, 2010). A small number of studies have also attempted to improve cognition without focusing on any single or combination of specific skills, with improved psychological symptoms noted (Jønsson, Korfitzen, Heltberg, Ravnborg, & Byskov-Ottosen, 1993; Mendoza, Pittenger, & Weinstein, 2001) but few changes in objectively evaluated cognitive processes (Brenk, Laun, & Haase, 2008). Several standardized, structured treatment protocols are now available to the MS community with various levels of evidence supporting their efficacy.

Although a handful of studies have investigated the CR of the less often impaired domains of EF (e.g., Fink et al., 2010) and WM (Tacchino et al., 2015), the large majority of CR research in MS has focused on the cognitive domains most commonly impaired in this population, NLM and IPS (often referred to as *attention*). Various formats have been tested, including computer-assisted technology (e.g., Chiaravalloti, DeLuca, Moore, & Ricker, 2005), app development (Tacchino et al., 2015), and the application of gaming (Janssen, Boster, Lee, Patterson, & Prakash, 2015). The recent rapid advances in the field highlight the importance of developing effective treatment to minimize the impact of cognitive deficits on the daily life.

The domain of NLM has received the most attention in the MS-related CR literature. Several double-blind, placebo-controlled randomized clinical trials (RCT) have supported the efficacy of the modified Story Memory Technique (mSMT) in MS (Chiaravalloti et al., 2005, 2013), which uses context and imagery to improve NLM via computer-supported CR. Efficacy of the mSMT has been demonstrated across three realms of functioning: objective behavior (Chiaravalloti et al., 2005, 2013), brain functioning (Chiaravalloti, Wylie, Leavitt, & Deluca, 2012; Leavitt, Wylie, Girgis, DeLuca, & Chiaravalloti, 2014), and everyday life (Chiaravalloti et al., 2005, 2013).

RehaCom is a widely used computer-supported CR program that consists of multiple modules addressing several cognitive domains that has been widely applied to persons with MS. Although RehaCom can be used to specifically target isolated cognitive domains such as EF or IPS, many authors (e.g., Parisi et al., 2014) evaluate its impact on multiple cognitive processes simultaneously—namely, attention, IPS, LM, and EF. Positive findings have been noted (Mattioli et al., 2010), with evidence of a maintained treatment effect at 9 months after treatment (Mattioli, Stampatori, Scarpazza, Parrinello, & Capra, 2012) and 2 years posttreatment (Mattioli, Bellomi, Stampatori, Provinciali, et al., 2016). Several studies have shown improvement on objective behavioral measures of attention, IPS and EF, accompanied by changes in patterns of cerebral activation on functional magnetic resonance imaging (Filippi et al., 2012) and resting-state functional connectivity (Parisi et al., 2014). Additional improvements have been noted in regard to depression and QOL after treatment (Parisi et al., 2014). RehaCom has been successfully applied to treat attentional and processing speed deficits in persons with MS, with neuropsychological data, self-reports of daily life functioning, and neuroimaging data all showing substantial support of the RehaCom in MS. Results to date demonstrate that RehaCom leads to changes in objective memory performance, daily life, and neural plasticity.

Multiple authors have additionally supplemented traditional cognitive therapy with other treatment modalities in an attempt to maximize the treatment effect. Such techniques have included transcranial direct current stimulation (Mattioli, Bellomi, Stampatori, Capra, & Miniussi, 2016), cognitive behavior therapy (CBT; Martínez-González & Piqueras, 2015), strategy-oriented neuropsychological rehabilitation (Mäntynen et al., 2014), and physical exercise (e.g., Briken et al., 2013). From these studies, one can conclude that the additive effect of CR and additional therapeutic modalities maximizes benefit.

Treatment of Psychological Symptoms in MS

A recent review of depression treatment in MS (Marrie et al., 2015) reported 13 RCTs published between 1984 and 2014. Most trials examined the effects of psychotherapy (e.g., Forman & Lincoln, 2010; Larcombe & Wilson, 1984), two investigated pharmacotherapy alone (Ehde et al., 2008; Schiffer & Wineman, 1990), and one examined pharmacotherapy and psychotherapy combined (D. C. Mohr et al., 2001). The study of depression has been more common than anxiety, such that 12 of the 13 studies examined depression, with only one examining injection anxiety (D. C. Mohr et al., 2005). In general, this research demonstrates that pharmacologic and psychological interventions for depression in depressed persons with MS are effective in reducing depressive symptoms, with CBT garnering much support (van Straten, Geraedts, Verdonck-de Leeuw, Andersson, & Cuijpers, 2010). However, few studies have investigated pharmacological interventions for depression in MS.

Despite the fact that anxiety has been shown to be fairly common in persons with MS (Korostil & Feinstein, 2007), few studies have examined the efficacy of treatment for anxiety, thus leaving a gap in the literature. D. C. Mohr and colleagues (2005) examined an intervention to reduce anxiety for self-injection in MS, which was the sole method for administration of disease-modifying therapies until recently, noting a nonsignificant improvement in self-injection anxiety after treatment. No controlled studies to our knowledge examined the effectiveness of psychological or pharmacological treatments of common anxiety disorders in persons with MS.

Fatigue has a clear detrimental impact on cognitive functioning in persons with MS, and research is working toward effective treatment. Pharmacological treatments for depression have shown some impact on fatigue in MS samples (Marrie et al., 2015), as fatigue often co-occurs with depression (Marin & Menza, 2004). The effect of depression treatments on fatigue is an area for future study, in addition to the efficacy of new treatments for fatigue specifically. For more information regarding intervention among rehabilitative population, see Chapter 5, this volume.

PARKINSON'S DISEASE

Overview

PD is a hypokinetic movement disorder that largely affects the basal ganglia and frontostriatal circuitry (Troster, Fields, & Koller, 2000). Its primary neuropathological feature is the loss of pigmented cells in the substantia nigra; once depleted to approximately 70% to 80% of its neurons, symptoms begin to emerge and slowly worsen over time (Bernheimer, Birkmayer, Hornykiewicz, Jellinger, & Seitelberger, 1973). Braak and colleagues (2003) developed a neuropathological staging system that chronicles the path of neurodegeneration, with Stages 3 through 6 thought to be more related to cognitive dysfunction (Braak, Rüb, Jansen Steur, Del Tredici, & de Vos, 2005). PD is marked by the presence of four cardinal signs: tremor, rigidity, bradykinesia, and postural instability (Gelb, Oliver, & Gilman, 1999). Risk of PD increases with age, male sex, Caucasian or Hispanic ethnicity, genetic predispositions (both autosomal dominant and recessive), and exposure to specific toxins (e.g., pesticides; Hubble, Cao, Hassanein, Neuberger, & Koller, 1993).

Cognitive Changes in PD

As an individual with PD progresses through the Braak stages, cognitive dysfunction becomes more likely due to increasing pathology in higher order brain regions (Braak et al., 2005). However, one study demonstrated that almost 25% of patients exhibited impairments on three or more scores on a comprehensive neuropsychological battery at time of diagnosis, frequently in EF and LTM (Muslimovic, Post, Speelman, & Schmand, 2005). Findings such as these have led to increasing discussion around the necessity of using criteria for mild cognitive impairment, the syndrome describing the early cognitive stage of Alzheimer's disease marked by laboratory-based cognitive impairments despite intact everyday functioning, for PD (Domellöf, Ekman, Forsgren, & Elgh, 2015).

Ultimately, approximately 20% to 40% of individuals with PD develop dementia before death, with risk for dementia increasing with age (E. Mohr, Mendis, & Grimes, 1995). Given the neuropathological pattern of PD, cognitive domains reliant on frontostriatal pathways are most often affected (Troster & Fields, 2008). Specifically, among the most frequently impaired cognitive domain is EF, including planning, set shifting, set formation, set maintenance, and decision-making (Kudlicka, Clare, & Hindle, 2011). Additional impairments are frequently seen in verbal fluency (Piatt, Fields, Paolo, & Tröster, 1999), psychomotor speed (Peavy et al., 2001), visuoconstruction, and visuoperceptual abilities (even when motor components of the task are removed; Davidsdottir, Cronin-Golomb, & Lee, 2005), NL (Chiaravalloti et al., 2014), prospective memory (Costa, Peppe, Caltagirone, & Carlesimo, 2008), and social cognition (Díez-Cirarda et al., 2015).

Psychological and Behavioral Changes in PD

Individuals living with PD may experience an array of psychological and behavioral symptoms, owing at least in part to the direct impact of monoamine imbalances and frontostriatal system impairment (Weintraub et al., 2005). Specifically, depression is prevalent in PD, with a systematic review citing that more than one third of patients exhibit depressive symptomatology (Reijnders, Ehrt, Weber, Aarsland, & Leentjens, 2008). Julien, Rimes, and Brown (2016) further examined predominant features of depression in this population and demonstrated that behaviors of rumination, avoidance, and symptom focusing were related to greater depressive severity, above and beyond general disability. Often masquerading as depression, apathy is often significant in individuals with PD (Kirsch-Darrow, Fernandez, Marsiske, Okun, & Bowers, 2006). Apathy in this population is most often linked to frontostriatal impairment (Dujardin & Defebvre, 2012), with evidence that it may co-occur with impairments in aspects of social cognition (e.g., emotional facial recognition) due to overlapping neural networks (Robert et al., 2014). Anxiety is also prevalent in this population, with estimates of clinically relevant symptoms in up to 69% of affected individuals (Prediger, Matheus, Schwarzbold, Lima, & Vital, 2012).

Impact of Cognition and Psychological Factors on Everyday Functioning

A number of studies have revealed relationships between cognitive and behavioral sequelae of PD and everyday functioning, which not only indicate poorer outcomes with individuals with dementia or more general cognitive impairment (e.g., cognitive impairment on driving ability; Homann et al., 2003) but also highlight specificity of individual domains or symptoms. For example, EF deficits have been linked to diminished capacity to consent to medical treatment (Dymek, Atchison, Harrell, & Marson, 2001), poorer quality of life (Stegemöller et al., 2014), and increased falls (Mak, Wong, & Pang, 2014), while prospective memory deficits have been linked to greater dependence in activities of daily living (Pirogovsky, Woods, Filoteo, & Gilbert, 2012). Depression and anxiety have additionally been independently linked to diminished health-related quality of life (Fereshtehnejad et al., 2015; Simpson, Lekwuwa, & Crawford, 2014). Importantly, despite the impact of these difficulties on many indices of everyday functioning, research suggests that the presence of cognitive deficits (e.g., executive dysfunction) and depression may not interfere with a comprehensive rehabilitation program and should not serve as contraindications to such treatment (Pierobon et al., 2014).

Cognitive and Psychological Assessment

In general, many providers who work with patient who have PD rely on the Unified Parkinson Disease Rating Scale (UPDRS), which has demonstrated good reliability and validity in detecting PD symptoms and progression (Ramaker, Marinus, Stiggelbout, & Van Hilten, 2002). The UPDRS includes (a) an evaluation of cognition, behavior, and mood; (b) a self-evaluation of activities of daily living; and (c) a clinician-scored motor evaluation, along with notes regarding complications of therapy, the Hoehn and Yahn staging of PD severity, and the clinician-rated Schwab and England Activities of Daily Living Scale (Movement Disorder Society Task Force on Rating Scales for Parkinson's Disease, 2003). Although there is no standardized and widely agreed-on neuropsychological battery for PD, a comprehensive assessment of all potentially impaired domains described earlier (as well as indicators of everyday functioning) is warranted to track risk of dementia (Troster & Fields, 2008). Specific screening batteries have, however, been developed to aid in questions of functional independence, such as driving (Devos et al., 2013). For comprehensive testing, a recent joint venture by the University of Pennsylvania and University of Washington's National Institute of Neurological Disease and Stroke–funded Udall Centers resulted in a consensus battery, called the Penn–UW Recommended Screening and Standard Battery. It allows for supplemental testing as well as adaptations or substitutions for more severely impaired patients.

As with many neurological disorders, assessment of psychological symptoms should take care to limit the impact of vegetative or psychomotor symptoms that may be a manifestation of direct neurological impairments rather than indicative of a mood or anxiety disorder (Bobholz & Rao, 2003; Rosti et al., 2007). Similarly, assessments of frontal behavioral symptoms (e.g., Frontal Systems Behavior Scale; Stout, Ready, Grace, Malloy, & Paulsen, 2003) should be conducted alongside depression inventories to address the role that frontal dysfunction (e.g., presence of apathy) may play in apparent presence of depression (Kirsch-Darrow et al., 2006). Per the Penn–UW recommendations, mood and behavior may be assessed also by using a variety of self-report measures (see Table 19.1).

Treatment of Cognitive Impairments and Psychological Symptoms

A number of studies have begun to demonstrate efficacy for CR programs in PD. For example, a number of well-designed studies (e.g., RCTs) have been conducted using the program REHACOP, a comprehensive structured CR program that trains multiple cognitive domains, including attention, NLM, IPS, language, EF, and social cognition (Sanchez et al., 2014). One such trial (Peña et al., 2014) demonstrated not only improvements across a variety of cognitive domains (i.e., IPS, visual NLM, theory of mind), but also reductions in functional disability. Beyond behavioral change, a study by Díez-Cirarda and colleagues (2017) found that individuals with PD who completed REHACOP had greater resting state functional connectivity relative to a control group (undergoing occupational therapy) as well as greater neural activation on NLM tasks, which were associated with cognitive performance at posttreatment. Similar positive findings have been noted with other CR programs. Specifically, a recent pilot study conducted by Adamski, Adler, Opwis, and Penner (2016) that tested the program BrainStim in individuals with PD and healthy control participants also found improvements on NLM at immediate and delayed (3-month) follow-up. Using more traditional clinician-driven methods of CR, Watermeyer and colleagues (2016) similarly demonstrated that individuals with PD who exhibited symptoms of dementia were able to successfully complete a goal setting semistructured interview, which is helpful to guide rehabilitation efforts toward patient-centered goals.

Given the likelihood of a significant biological contribution to symptoms of depression in PD, much research to date has focused on the efficacy of antidepressants in treating depression in persons with PD. However, a recent meta-analysis (Reijnders et al., 2008) suggested only mild to moderate amelioration of symptoms with antidepressants, thereby paving the way for alternative strategies, such as psychotherapy, to be examined. Indeed, the story of depression in PD may not be entirely biological because these individuals face a degenerative condition that comes with substantial stress and emotional reactions. As a result, a growing body of literature has begun to examine the efficacy of psychosocial interventions, such as CBT, with success both in-person (Dobkin et al., 2011) and via telephone (Dobkin, 2014).

Beyond standard CR and psychotherapy, alternative rehabilitation strategies are gaining traction in PD research and practice. For instance, considerable research has examined the potential impact of physical exercise to improve symptoms (cognitive, emotional, and motor) in PD. For example, Duchesne and colleagues (2015) demonstrated that aerobic exercise (i.e., exercise prescription for stationary bike based on maximal aerobic power) improved inhibition abilities as well as motor learning in a sample of individuals with early-stage PD. Even technologically driven sport-related rehabilitation (i.e., use of Nintendo Wii, or "Wii-hab") has demonstrated short-term benefit for these individuals on motor functioning, performance-based measures of activities of daily living, and quality of life (Herz et al., 2013). Other activity-based rehabilitation methods, such as group singing (Buetow, Talmage, McCann, Fogg, & Purdy, 2014) and boxing (Alves Da Rocha, McClelland, & Morris, 2015), have also received much attention for improving quality of life in PD. Transcranial direct current stimulation is growing in popularity as a technology-based method to improve cognition, with three studies to date reporting enhanced WM (Boggio et al., 2006), phonemic fluency (Pereira et al., 2013), and speeded switching (Doruk, Gray, Bravo, Pascual-Leone, & Fregni, 2014); of note, these benefits may not be universal across all EF because the latter study did not find significant improvement on other tests within this domain.

AMYOTROPHIC LATERAL SCLEROSIS

Overview

First defined by Charcot in 1874, ALS is a neurodegenerative disorder that primarily affects motor neurons, thereby causing dramatic deficits in voluntary motor control (Brooks et al., 1994; Cleveland & Rothstein, 2001).

Clinically, ALS often first presents with difficulty with independent ambulation, limb weakness, increased falls, slurred speech, difficulty swallowing, and muscle cramps and twitching (Cleveland & Rothstein, 2001). Toward the end of life, difficulty breathing and swallowing become prominent features, and individuals often require mechanical assistance. Because there is no definitive diagnostic test for ALS, diagnoses are only made after other potential causes for motor findings, such as myasthenia gravis and spinobulbar muscular atrophy, have been ruled out (Agosta et al., 2015).

Although it is estimated that 5% to 10% of ALS cases are genetically inherited, the vast majority of cases are thought to be due to sporadic gene mutations (Rowland & Shneider, 2001). At the neuronal level, ALS is marked primarily by degeneration and loss of motor neurons with astrocytic gliosis, as well as intraneuronal inclusions (e.g., Lewy-like bodies) within degenerating neurons and glial cells (Ince, Lowe, & Shaw, 1998). Despite better understanding of the disease in recent years, with the notable influence of the "Ice Bucket Challenge" in 2014 that raised more than $115 million in 8 weeks, successful treatments for ALS remain elusive (BBC News, 2015). As of this writing, there is only one U.S. Food and Drug Administration–approved pharmacological treatment (riluzole or Rilutek) that is indicated to slow the progression of the disease, likely by reducing excess glutamate in the brain (Miller, Mitchell, Lyon, & Moore, 2007). However, the median lifespan of patients with ALS after symptom onset is approximately 2 to 3 years, and research suggests that riluzole extends this life expectancy by 2 months (Rowland & Shneider, 2001).

Cognitive Changes in ALS

Although the cardinal symptoms of ALS are related to motor impairment, there has been more recent attention given to cognitive symptoms that co-occur (Ince et al., 1998). In fact, although early estimates suggested that only 1% to 2% of sporadic ALS cases displayed dementia, it is now thought to be a more common finding (upward of 30%), with prevalence of at least mild cognitive deficits occurring in approximately 50% of study samples (Rowland & Shneider, 2001). Most typically, these deficits occur in cognitive domains affected by frontotemporal pathways, particularly EF, recall, WM, and productive language (e.g., verbal fluency; Ringholz et al., 2005). Some research points to bulbar site of symptom onset as a predictor of worse cognitive functioning, but the literature remains mixed (Rippon et al., 2006; Strong et al., 1999). In fact, some genetic mutations resulting in ALS have reliably shown to produce related symptomatology associated with other neurological conditions affecting frontal circuitry, including parkinsonism and frontotemporal dementia (Rowland & Shneider, 2001). More recent studies have begun to highlight the prevalence and ecological relevance of social cognition deficits in this population, which appear to extend beyond frontal behaviors such as apathy and presence of pseudobulbar affect (Merrilees, Klapper, Murphy, Lomen-Hoerth, & Miller, 2010).

Several studies have defined the development and progression of cognitive deficits in individuals with ALS. Kuruvilla, Green, Ayaz, and Murman (2013) demonstrated that, despite normal behavioral WM performance, individuals with ALS exhibited reduced prefrontal activation using functional near infrared spectroscopy. As seen in other neurodegenerative conditions (e.g., MS), this may be viewed as early neurological deficits that predate cognitive deficits seen later in the disease course. Indeed, these findings are echoed in Robinson and colleagues' (2006) 6-month longitudinal study, which compared participants recently diagnosed with ALS and matched caregiver controls on a comprehensive battery of neuropsychological tests. Although there were no group differences at baseline, participants with ALS demonstrated greater cognitive impairment at follow-up, with approximately 37% exhibiting deficits on testing. This suggests that cognitive deficits may rapidly emerge in many patients with ALS, even if not present at initial diagnosis.

Psychological and Behavioral Changes in ALS

Given the poor prognosis for ALS, psychiatric conditions such as depression and anxiety are often prominent in clinicians' minds. However, research suggests that presence of clinically significant mood and anxiety symptoms are not ubiquitous, with estimates varying widely across studies (e.g., 0%–44% for depressive disorders; Averill, Kasarskis, & Segerstrom, 2007; Gould et al., 2015; Taylor, Wicks, Leigh, & Goldstein, 2010). In fact, one study specifically designed to assess depression in the context of wishes to die in end-stage ALS patients showed a 12% rate of depressive disorders (5% with major depressive disorder), a prevalence estimate that the authors noted is much lower than other neurological and medical conditions (e.g., diabetes, MS; Rabkin et al., 2015). Although this may be due to the psychological diversity in a sample for which genetic mutations, and not mood or lifestyle predispositions, choose who develops ALS, another reason for this apparent discrepancy may be the co-occurrence of frontal dysfunction (Mukherjee, 2015). Factors such as presence of apathy, poor awareness, and impaired social cognition may potentially buffer individuals with ALS from classical depressive symptoms (Merrilees et al., 2010). However, these frontal behavioral symptoms tend to yield more problems than benefits. The co-occurrence of frontotemporal dementia–like symptoms, including disinhibition, hyperorality, and irritability, is prevalent among a subset of individuals with ALS (Merrilees et al., 2010; Ringholz et al., 2005).

Impact of Cognition and Psychological Factors on Everyday Functioning

Although cognitive impairment typically receives less attention than the physical aspects of the disease, ALS has been demonstrated to independently impact everyday functioning. In fact, one study demonstrated that cognitive impairment was relatively more detrimental to quality of life than physical functioning in persons with ALS (Goldstein, Atkins, & Leigh, 2002). Cognitive deficits in ALS, particularly early in the disease while the patient can remain largely independent, negatively affects important aspects of daily living, including treatment adherence (Flaherty-Craig, Brothers, Yang, Svoboda, & Simmons, 2011). Beyond the immediate patient, the degree of cognitive impairment in the individuals with ALS also has an impact on the caregiver (Merrilees et al.,

2010; Rabkin, Albert, Rowland, & Mitsumoto, 2009). Indeed, much research has been focused on depression and quality of life in ALS caregivers. Although some studies have indicated the positive impact of caregiving (Rabkin, Wagner, & Del Bene, 2000), caregivers often report increased depression, perceived burden, and poorer quality of life, with indications that a primary basis for these outcomes are secondary to poor communication and insufficient provision of services for the patient (Mockford, Jenkinson, & Fitzpatrick, 2006).

Cognitive and Psychological Assessment

With regard to cognitive assessment, a 2009 practice parameter from the American Association of Neurology noted that there is no established consensus on how to assess cognition in individuals with ALS (Miller et al., 2009). In general, a thorough examination of domains often impaired secondary to frontotemporal system dysfunction is warranted if cognitive impairment is suspected (Ringholz et al., 2005; Strong et al., 1999). However, given the primary motor deficits in this disease, care should be taken when interpreting test results that rely heavily on motor or speech speed. Appropriate testing that minimizes the impact of motor impairment is often necessary, particularly toward suspected late-stage disease (Ringholz et al., 2005). For example, Hicks et al. (2013) developed an eye-tracking version of the Trail-Making Test that has provided good psychometric reliability and validity to assess IPS in individuals with ALS who are unable to write or speak. Additionally, a number of screening batteries have been developed to be sensitive to ALS-related cognitive dysfunction while minimizing motor components (Flaherty-Craig, Eslinger, Stephens, & Simmons, 2006; Woolley et al., 2010; see Table 19.1).

Assessment of psychological symptoms is often similarly affected by disease-related presence of vegetative features that are prevalent in depression (e.g., fatigue, psychomotor slowing; Averill et al., 2007). With this in mind, depression inventories that are specifically designed to circumvent these symptoms of depression are recommended in the ALS population. Such inventories may be those designed for older adult populations who tend to exhibit physical symptoms that may mimic depressive symptoms at higher rates, albeit not due to depression (e.g., Geriatric Depression Scale; Parmelee & Katz, 1990). Alternatively, abridged versions of validated assessments that examine core mood-related symptoms of depression (e.g., Beck Depression Inventory—II Fast Screen) are often used in this population (Averill et al., 2007; Beck, Guth, Steer, & Ball, 1997). Symptoms of frontal dysfunction may be assessed using tools such as the Frontal Systems Behavior Scale or Cambridge Behavior Inventory, both of which have demonstrated validity in ALS (Rudnicki & Fewell, 2007; Tsujimoto et al., 2011).

Treatment of Cognitive Impairments and Psychological Symptoms

As life expectancy following diagnosis is quite short, research endeavors in ALS have largely focused on genetic testing and development of effective medications to cure the disease or alleviate its impact (Rowland & Shneider, 2001). Treatment development focused on improving cognition in ALS is thus rare. However, much has been done to test the efficacy of treatments designed to address psychological symptoms and to alleviate caregiver burden. For example, studies examining the use of eye-tracking communication devices in late-stage disease demonstrate improvements in reducing communication disabilities and improving quality of life for the patient (Caligari, Godi, Guglielmetti, Franchignoni, & Nardone, 2013) as well as the caregiver (Hwang, Weng, Wang, Tsai, & Chang, 2014). The standard of care is treatment via comprehensive, multidisciplinary ALS centers, with the full complement of rehabilitation services to focus on symptom management (Paganoni, Karam, Joyce, Bedlack, & Carter, 2015), which similarly improves quality of life in individuals with ALS (Van den Berg et al., 2005). Particularly for individuals with limited social support, case management has been demonstrated to be important to overall patient and caregiver satisfaction (Bakker et al., 2015). With regard to traditional psychological treatment, few studies have formally evaluated treatment efficacy. A systematic review by Gould and colleagues (2015) revealed only five studies that have evaluated the success of psychotherapy or pharmacotherapy to improve psychological symptoms in ALS, thereby providing insufficient evidence for broad treatment recommendations until additional well-designed research can be conducted.

HUNTINGTON'S DISEASE

Overview

HD is an autosomal-dominant neurodegenerative disorder in which patients exhibit a classic triad of symptoms: motor disturbance, cognitive impairment, and psychiatric symptoms (Walker, 2007). HD is most known for chorea, or involuntary jerking or writing movements, that appear early and throughout the disease presentation. At the neural level, individuals with HD demonstrate substantial loss of neurons and gliosis occurring specifically in the caudate and putamen (Chesselet, Hickey, Zhu, & Levine, 2010). Because the projections to and from these basal ganglia regions are significant, this also results in diffuse brain atrophy, as well as reduced glucose metabolism (Mazziotta et al., 1987). In fact, many such indices of neural damage appear to predate the presence of clinical symptoms (Aylward et al., 1996), perhaps as long as a decade prior (Aylward et al., 2000). Although clinical symptoms can vary across individuals by onset, severity, and progression, the most usual pattern first involves onset of chorea, followed by psychiatric disturbance early, deficits in cognition and everyday functioning, and ultimately more vital motor difficulty (e.g., coordinating breathing, speaking, and swallowing, often resulting in choking) and immobility (Kirkwood, Su, Conneally, & Foroud, 2001).

Cognitive Changes in HD

Cognitive impairment features prominently in the middle and later stages of HD. Given that it represents one third of the classic triad of symptoms in HD (along with motor disturbance and psychiatric symptoms), cognitive impairment occurs in virtually all individuals who progress to these stages of the disease. In fact, one study estimated that approximately 66% of individuals with HD demonstrate global cognitive impairment at least 2 standard deviations below mean control values (Pillon, Dubois, & Agid, 1991). Following a classic "subcortical" disease pattern, the primary deficits in HD involve EF and higher order cognitive abilities (Dumas, van den Bogaard, Middelkoop, & Roos, 2013; Lawrence, Sahakian, & Robbins, 1998). Specific deficits have been evident on tests of concept formation and set switching (Aron et al., 2003; Peinemann et al., 2005), inhibition (Duff et al., 2010; Paulsen et al., 1996), decision-making (Stout, Rodawalt, & Siemers, 2001), and planning (Watkins et al., 2000). Although basic attention abilities are typically spared, more complex aspects of attention (e.g., shifting attention, divided attention) are at greater risk for impairment due to the frontal circuitry required to supervise attentional processes (Lawrence et al., 1996). NLM impairment is often present and is marked by an encoding and retrieval deficit (Delis et al., 1991; Montoya et al., 2006). One major area where HD's cardinal symptoms of cognitive and motor dysfunction intersect is psychomotor speed. Many studies have observed deficits on speeded motor tasks and fine motor coordination (Paulsen et al., 2014; Young et al., 1986). However, due to the overlap in assessment of these constructs, these findings may be due to motor symptoms (e.g., chorea) rather than neurally based IPS. Regardless of mechanism, tests of psychomotor speed are often sensitive to decline in HD (Ho et al., 2003) and help predict transition from prodrome to diagnosis (O'Rourke et al., 2011). With regard to language, although speech production is ultimately impaired due to motor difficulties, language deficits tend to be relatively more subtle. Individuals with HD often experience reduced verbal fluency over the course of their illness as well as an increase in word repetition on fluency tasks (Ho et al., 2002). Similarly, visuospatial impairment is also often seen, particularly as spatial functions become more complex (e.g., assessment of person-centric space, mental rotation; Lineweaver, Salmon, Bondi, & Corey-Bloom, 2005; Potegal, 1971). Of note, longitudinal studies of at-risk individuals suggest that cognitive impairments, particularly inhibitory control and speed of processing, may be evident before motor symptoms (Biglan et al., 2016; Stout et al., 2011).

Psychological and Behavioral Changes in HD

Of the neurodegenerative diseases, HD is the only one featured in this chapter in which psychiatric disturbance is a core feature of the disease. In fact, estimates of psychiatric disturbance in HD have been cited to occur in as many as 79% of patients (Morris, 1991); a recent study in nearly 2,000 individuals with HD reported that only 27% of participants did not evidence any psychiatric symptoms within the previous month (van Duijn et al., 2014). Of these symptoms, depression is the most common, often at its height in middle stages of the disease (Paulsen et al., 2005). Similar to cognitive deficits, depression can predate motor symptoms and HD diagnosis by up to 20 years (Folstein & Folstein, 1983). Evidence for a biological cause of depressive symptomatology is strong (cf. psychosocial stress response to HD diagnosis; Du, Pang, & Hannan, 2013). For example, transgenic mice with genetic code designed to mimic HD exhibit higher levels of depression symptomatology (Pang, Du, Zajac, Howard, & Hannan, 2009; Pouladi et al., 2009). In humans, prodromal gene carriers have higher rates of depression than their gene-negative counterparts (Julien et al., 2007). Moreover, evidence from positron emission tomography studies demonstrates that there is a pathophysiological basis for depression in HD. For example, one study showed greater hypermetabolism in the inferior frontal cortex and thalamus in individuals with HD and depression compared with nondepressed individuals with HD or healthy control participants. Although the neural milieu may be much more compromised relative to individuals with depression but not HD, the mechanisms of depression in this population appear to be comparable to those with clinical depression—specifically, impairments in the serotonin system, brain-derived neurotrophic factor expression, and hypothalamic-pituitary-adrenal axis regulation (Du et al., 2013). Beyond the scope of depression, suicidality is elevated in this clinical population well beyond national suicide rates, as well as rates in other neurological populations (Paulsen et al., 2005). In fact, most studies show at least a fourfold increase in risk for suicide among individuals with HD (Almqvist, Bloch, Brinkman, Craufurd, & Hayden, 1999). Suicidal ideation is most prevalent at time of diagnosis as well as within Stage 2 on the Unified Huntington's Disease Rating Scale, which indicates some degree of functional decline (Paulsen et al., 2005).

Although relatively more rare, psychosis and obsessive–compulsive behaviors also occur at a higher rate in people with HD than the general public (van Duijn et al., 2014; Paulsen, Ready, Hamilton, Mega, & Cummings, 2001). Consistent with other disorders with frontal systems impairment, behavioral apathy is also common in HD (Naarding, Janzing, Eling, van der Werf, & Kremer, 2009; van Duijn et al., 2014). In general, behavioral apathy is associated with cognitive dysfunction and is dissociable from depressive symptoms (Levy et al., 1998). Also potentially related to this neuropathology, behavioral agitation, irritability, and aggressiveness are prevalent, with the latter occurring more frequently in males and individuals with greater incidence of falls (Fisher, Sewell, Brown, & Churchyard, 2014). Lastly, many individuals with HD exhibit anosognosia, or lack of awareness about their illness (Duff et al., 2010; Hoth et al., 2007). Although frequently mistaken by family members as denial or having poor coping skills to deal with their illness, one study demonstrated that anosognosia was correlated with disease severity and duration (Vitale et al., 2001).

Considerations for Genetic Testing

As a dominant genetic disorder, each child of a parent with HD has a 50% chance of inheriting the disease. The genetic code responsible for HD was identified in 1993 (MacDonald et al., 1993), with commercially available genetic testing for private individuals available shortly thereafter. Given the significant clinical presentation, poor prognosis, and lack of disease cure, genetic testing should be undertaken under the careful supervision and monitoring of a genetic counselor (Coustasse, Pekar, Sikula, & Lurie, 2009; Hayes, 1992). A number of important life considerations must be taken into account when choosing to know or reveal one's status as an individual with or at risk for HD, including childbearing, employment, medical documentation, and insurance (Bombard et al., 2009).

With the recent passage of the Genetic Information Nondiscrimination Act and the Affordable Care Act, insurance (for health care specifically) is more protected than in decades past (e.g., health insurance companies may not preclude coverage due to a preexisting condition; Feldman, 2012; Rak & Coffin, 2013; Walcott, Dunn, DeShields, & Baquet, 2014). As risk for depression and suicidality are significantly elevated in this clinical population, decisions to pursue genetic testing should not be undertaken lightly, and support should be provided for those undergoing the process (Licklederer, Wolff, & Barth, 2008).

Impact of Cognitive Changes and Psychological Symptoms on Everyday Life

Impairments in cognition as well as psychiatric disturbance impose a significant impact on the ability of an individual with HD to function in everyday life (Ross, Pantelyat, Kogan, & Brandt, 2014). For instance, cognitive impairment, particularly psychomotor slowing and attention and learning, was revealed to be a strong predictor of cessation of driving in a retrospective study of individuals with HD, although no motor variables remained independently predictive (Beglinger et al., 2012). This finding has borne out in more recent studies examining the impact of cognition on on-road driving evaluation decisions, in which road test performance was significantly correlated with EF, divided attention, IPS, motor functions, and selective attention (Devos et al., 2014). Another facet of functional independence often affected is employment; research suggests that declines in IPS may be a triggering factor in the decision to leave the workforce (Ross et al., 2014).

With regard to psychiatric symptoms, as in other disorders, depressive symptoms show an independent relationship with health-related quality of life, above and beyond what can be explained by disease severity (Ho, Gilbert, Mason, Goodman, & Barker, 2009). Lastly, behavioral symptoms, particularly those of aggression, are often a primary reason for individuals with HD to be placed outside of the home (Shiwach & Patel, 1993), thereby reducing functional independence at a global level. This finding was echoed by J. M. Hamilton and colleagues (2003), who demonstrated that a composite apathy–executive dysfunction behavioral scale predicted decline in independent ability to perform activities of daily living.

Cognitive and Psychological Assessment

In general, many clinicians use the Unified Huntington's Disease Rating Scale (UHDRS; Huntington Study Group, 1996) to quickly and repeatedly assess disease progression across the triad of symptoms (see Table 19.1). Relevant to this audience, it includes a short neuropsychological screening battery of tests thought to be sensitive to HD, including verbal fluency, Symbol Digit Modalities Test, and the Stroop Interference Test. Indeed, the UHDRS cognitive scale demonstrated greater validity in the longitudinal assessment of cognitive decline compared with other commonly used screening tools (i.e., Mini-Mental State Examination and Montreal Cognitive Assessment; Toh et al., 2014). Comprehensive neuropsychological testing should ensure that a battery at least consists of tests that assess various aspects of EF, NLM, IPS, visuospatial functions, verbal fluency, and complex attention, with care taken in the interpretation of scores dependent on motor functioning or rapid speech (Stout, Glikmann-Johnston, & Andrews, 2016). Given the likelihood of fatigue and frustration that may occur during cognitive testing for these individuals, Stout and colleagues devised an efficient six-test battery designed to be sensitive to these domains (Huntington's Disease Cognitive Assessment Battery; Stout et al., 2014). For specific questions of fitness to drive, Devos, Nieuwboer, Tant, De Weerdt, and Vandenberghe (2012) determined that a screening battery of Symbol Digit Modalities Test, Stroop Word Reading Test, and Trail Making Test—Part B could classify individuals who would fail a comprehensive fitness to drive evaluation with 87% accuracy. With regard to behavioral symptoms, a recent comprehensive review by Mestre and colleagues (2016), as part of a working group of the Movement Disorders Society Committee on Rating Scales Development, provided guidelines for "recommended" (higher tier) and "suggested" (lower tier yet still acceptable) rating scales across symptom type for screening purposes. Given the validity and reliability for use in HD, this review recommends use of the Irritability Scale for assessment of irritability (Craig, Hietanen, Markova, & Berrios, 2008), the Beck Depression Inventory—II (Beck, Steer, & Brown, 1996) for depression, and the Hospital Anxiety and Depression Scale (Zigmond & Snaith, 1983) for depression.

Treatment of Cognitive Impairment and Psychological Symptoms in HD

At present, the HD community is largely focused on the promise of new investigational drugs to cure or slow the progression of this "orphan disease." At present, tetrabenazine is the only U.S. Food and Drug Administration–approved drug indicated to treat chorea, although psychiatric medications (e.g., clonazepam) may also help alleviate these symptoms (Roos, 2010). Beyond primary HD treatments, antipsychotic medications such as risperidone have demonstrated efficacy in reducing psychiatric disturbance as well as motor functioning (Duff et al., 2008); antidepressants and antipsychotics are also generally used to treat related symptoms (Roos, 2010).

With regard to treatment of cognitive impairment, a review by Langenbahn, Ashman, Cantor, and Trott (2013) on the use of CR in medical disorders revealed only one published article that met criteria for the review. This single study by Zinzi et al. (2007) used clinician-implemented CR strategies (e.g., metacognitive strategies, external memory aids) in the context of a larger multidisciplinary rehabilitation protocol. Although individuals did not demonstrate cognitive improvement (as measured by the Mini-Mental Status Examination), the authors suggest that the participants' lack of statistically significant cognitive decline over 24 months may be indicative that the protocol helped stave off further decline while in treatment. Since then, one additional study has examined a multidisciplinary rehabilitation program (i.e., comprising physical exercise and occupational therapy tasks) on cognition and brain structure, revealing some evidence for improved recall and increased caudate volume and gray matter in the bilateral dorsolateral prefrontal cortex after 9 months of therapy (Cruickshank et al., 2015). This study is consistent with findings in an HD mouse model, which demonstrated improvements in cognitive and attenuations in neuropathology following exercise (Harrison et al., 2013). Although these studies are promising for improving cognitive functioning in individuals with HD, larger and better controlled studies are warranted to confirm these findings (Andrews, Domínguez, Mercieca, Georgiou-Karistianis, & Stout, 2015).

SYNTHESIS AND FUTURE DIRECTIONS

As can be surmised, despite the overarching umbrella of neurodegeneration, the diseases described herein vary greatly in both prognosis and treatment options. Unfortunately, the collective understanding of cognition and psychological health is relatively behind research on medical advances such as slowing disease progression, genetic testing, or symptom reduction. That said, more recent research within the rehabilitation psychology field has been fruitful in calling attention to the distressing symptoms of cognitive impairment and comorbid psychological symptoms that impact our patients' daily functioning.

Of these diagnoses, it must be acknowledged that the MS field is a prime example of what may be discovered with our rehabilitation expertise and diligent research. The research on the various symptoms associated with MS has expanded considerably over the past 20 years, and researchers are now beginning to understand that MS negatively affects various aspects of functioning, including cognition, emotional functioning, and daily life activities. Despite the identification of the pervasive and influential nature of cognitive deficits in MS, it is only in the past decade that substantial attention is being paid to identifying effective treatments for cognitive impairment in MS. Future research should focus on the identification of effective means of improving cognitive functioning, emotional functioning, and fatigue in MS, with the goal of increasing functional status and overall quality of life. Similar research questions must be examined in PD, ALS, and HD with the same methodological vigor as has been recently seen in MS. Because none of these diseases has a cure as of this writing, it is up to the rehabilitation community to identify means to maximize quality of life and help affected individuals cope with their respective illnesses.

The role of the rehabilitation psychologist is ubiquitous in the assessment and treatment of individuals with these neurodegenerative diseases. Beyond foundational competencies such as knowledge of evidence-based practice and cultural diversity (see Chapters 4, 5, and 10, this volume), it is essential that rehabilitation psychologists working with individuals who are diagnosed with these conditions are strong in both assessment and intervention skills. As described extensively in this chapter, cognitive and psychological assessment is crucial to the appropriate care of these patients and serves a number of purposes. First, repeated assessment of both cognitive abilities and psychological symptoms is often a primary indicator of disease progression and may signal when additional care by the treating neurologist or psychiatrist is necessary. Second, comprehensive assessments are useful for determining how well the person may be functioning independently or if additional supports are needed to help promote optimal daily living. Lastly, communicating assessment results to members of the rehabilitation team and patient's support system can often improve overall rehabilitation outcomes through psychoeducation and adapted treatments (e.g., explaining that a patient may be misunderstanding his or her treatment regimen due to slowed processing speed and impaired encoding).

With regard to intervention-based competencies, rehabilitation psychology is primarily used to promote psychological health in the context of adjusting to disability (in the context of premorbid psychiatric and personality factors). When treating individuals with neurodegenerative conditions, adjustment to disability is a dynamic process due to the inevitable functional decline inherent in these diseases. Additionally, the family and social support system of the identified patient is often included in psychological treatment, whether it is for their own adjustment to the patient's disability or to enlist additional resources to support the patient. In more impaired individuals in this population, rehabilitation psychologists are often called on to assist with devising and implementing strategies for behavior management that may be used across the rehabilitation team and support system. Although at present there are few rehabilitation psychologists performing cognitive interventions, the empirical evidence in support of CR is growing at a rate that suggests increasing incorporation of these protocols in the clinic.

References

Adamski, N., Adler, M., Opwis, K., & Penner, I. K. (2016). A pilot study on the benefit of cognitive rehabilitation in Parkinson's disease. *Therapeutic Advances in Neurological Disorders*, *9*, 153–164. http://dx.doi.org/10.1177/1756285616628765

Agosta, F., Al-Chalabi, A., Filippi, M., Hardiman, O., Kaji, R., Meininger, V., . . . Ludolph, A., & the WFN Research Group on ALS/MND. (2015). The El Escorial criteria: Strengths and weaknesses. *Amyotrophic Lateral Sclerosis & Frontotemporal Degeneration*, *16*, 1–7. http://dx.doi.org/10.3109/21678421.2014.964258

Almqvist, E. W., Bloch, M., Brinkman, R., Craufurd, D., & Hayden, M. R. (1999). A worldwide assessment of the frequency of suicide, suicide attempts, or psychiatric hospitalization after predictive testing for Huntington disease. *American Journal of Human Genetics*, *64*, 1293–1304. http://dx.doi.org/10.1086/302374

Alves Da Rocha, P., McClelland, J., & Morris, M. E. (2015). Complementary physical therapies for movement disorders in Parkinson's disease: A systematic review. *European Journal of Physical and Rehabilitation Medicine*, *51*, 693–704.

Amato, M. P., Goretti, B., Viterbo, R. G., Portaccio, E., Niccolai, C., Hakiki, B., . . . Trojano, M. (2014). Computer-assisted rehabilitation of attention in patients with multiple sclerosis: Results of a randomized, double-blind trial. *Multiple Sclerosis*, *20*, 91–98. http://dx.doi.org/10.1177/1352458513501571

Andrews, S. C., Domínguez, J. F., Mercieca, E.-C., Georgiou-Karistianis, N., & Stout, J. C. (2015). Cognitive interventions to enhance neural compensation in Huntington's disease. *Neurodegenerative Disease Management*, *5*, 155–164. http://dx.doi.org/10.2217/nmt.14.58

Arnett, P. A. (2005). Longitudinal consistency of the relationship between depression symptoms and cognitive functioning in multiple sclerosis. *CNS Spectrums*, *10*, 372–382. http://dx.doi.org/10.1017/S1092852900022744

Aron, A. R., Watkins, L., Sahakian, B. J., Monsell, S., Barker, R. A., & Robbins, T. W. (2003). Task-set switching deficits in early-stage Huntington's disease: Implications for basal ganglia function. *Journal of Cognitive Neuroscience*, *15*, 629–642. http://dx.doi.org/10.1162/jocn.2003.15.5.629

Averill, A. J., Kasarskis, E. J., & Segerstrom, S. C. (2007). Psychological health in patients with amyotrophic lateral sclerosis. *Amyotrophic Lateral Sclerosis, 8*, 243–254. http://dx.doi.org/10.1080/17482960701374643

Aylward, E. H., Codori, A. M., Barta, P. E., Pearlson, G. D., Harris, G. J., & Brandt, J. (1996). Basal ganglia volume and proximity to onset in presymptomatic Huntington disease. *Archives of Neurology, 53*, 1293–1296.

Aylward, E. H., Codori, A. M., Rosenblatt, A., Sherr, M., Brandt, J., Stine, O. C., . . . Ross, C. A. (2000). Rate of caudate atrophy in presymptomatic and symptomatic stages of Huntington's disease. *Movement Disorders, 15*, 552–560. http://dx.doi.org/10.1002/1531-8257(200005)15:3<552::AID-MDS1020>3.0.CO;2-P

Bakker, M., Creemers, H., Schipper, K., Beelen, A., Grupstra, H., Nollet, F., & Abma, T. (2015). Need and value of case management in multidisciplinary ALS care: A qualitative study on the perspectives of patients, spousal caregivers and professionals. *Amyotrophic Lateral Sclerosis & Frontotemporal Degeneration, 16*, 180–186. http://dx.doi.org/10.3109/21678421.2014.971811

Bakshi, R., Czarnecki, D., Shaikh, Z. A., Priore, R. L., Janardhan, V., Kaliszky, Z., & Kinkel, P. R. (2000). Brain MRI lesions and atrophy are related to depression in multiple sclerosis. *NeuroReport, 11*, 1153–1158. http://dx.doi.org/10.1097/00001756-200004270-00003

Basso, M. R., Beason-Hazen, S., Lynn, J., Rammohan, K., & Bornstein, R. A. (1996). Screening for cognitive dysfunction in multiple sclerosis. *Archives of Neurology, 53*, 980–984. http://dx.doi.org/10.1001/archneur.1996.00550100046014

BBC News. (2015, August 19). *Ice bucket challenge helped spur ALS discovery, scientists say*. Retrieved from https://www.bbc.com/news/world-us-canada-33994290

Beatty, W. W., Blanco, C. R., Wilbanks, S. L., Paul, R. H., & Hames, K. A. (1995). Demographic, clinical, and cognitive characteristics of multiple sclerosis patients who continue to work. *Neurorehabilitation and Neural Repair, 9*, 167–173. http://dx.doi.org/10.1177/154596839500900306

Beatty, W. W., Paul, R. H., Blanco, C. R., Hames, K. A., & Wilbanks, S. L. (1995). Attention in multiple sclerosis: Correlates of impairment on the WAIS–R Digit Span Test. *Applied Neuropsychology, 2*, 139–144. http://dx.doi.org/10.1080/09084282.1995.9645351

Beatty, W. W., Paul, R. H., Wilbanks, S. L., Hames, K. A., Blanco, C. R., & Goodkin, D. E. (1995). Identifying multiple sclerosis patients with mild or global cognitive impairment using the Screening Examination for Cognitive Impairment (SEFCI). *Neurology, 45*, 718–723. http://dx.doi.org/10.1212/WNL.45.4.718

Beck, A. T., Guth, D., Steer, R. A., & Ball, R. (1997). Screening for major depression disorders in medical inpatients with the Beck Depression Inventory for Primary Care. *Behaviour Research and Therapy, 35*, 785–791. http://dx.doi.org/10.1016/S0005-7967(97)00025-9

Beck, A. T., Steer, R., & Brown, G. (1996). *Beck Depression Inventory—II*. San Antonio, TX: Psychological Corporation.

Beglinger, L. J., Prest, L., Mills, J. A., Paulsen, J. S., Smith, M. M., Gonzalez-Alegre, P., . . . Uc, E. Y. (2012). Clinical predictors of driving status in Huntington's disease. *Movement Disorders, 27*, 1146–1152. http://dx.doi.org/10.1002/mds.25101

Benedict, R. H., Cookfair, D., Gavett, R., Gunther, M., Munschauer, F., Garg, N., & Weinstock-Guttman, B. (2006). Validity of the minimal assessment of cognitive function in multiple sclerosis (MACFIMS). *Journal of the International Neuropsychological Society, 12*, 549–558. http://dx.doi.org/10.1017/S1355617706060723

Benedict, R. H., Fischer, J. S., Archibald, C. J., Arnett, P. A., Beatty, W. W., Bobholz, J., . . . Munschauer, F. (2002). Minimal neuropsychological assessment of MS patients: A consensus approach. *The Clinical Neuropsychologist, 16*, 381–397. http://dx.doi.org/10.1076/clin.16.3.381.13859

Benedict, R. H. B., Amato, M. P., Boringa, J., Brochet, B., Foley, F., Fredrikson, S., . . . Langdon, D. (2012). Brief International Cognitive Assessment for MS (BICAMS): international standards for validation. *BMC Neurol, 12*, 55. http://dx.doi.org/10.1186/1471-2377-12-55

Bergendal, G., Fredrikson, S., & Almkvist, O. (2007). Selective decline in information processing in subgroups of multiple sclerosis: An 8-year longitudinal study. *European Neurology, 57*, 193–202. http://dx.doi.org/10.1159/000099158

Bernheimer, H., Birkmayer, W., Hornykiewicz, O., Jellinger, K., & Seitelberger, F. (1973). Brain dopamine and the syndromes of Parkinson and Huntington. Clinical, morphological and neurochemical correlations. *Journal of the Neurological Sciences, 20*, 415–455. http://dx.doi.org/10.1016/0022-510X(73)90175-5

Biglan, K. M., Shoulson, I., Kieburtz, K., Oakes, D., Kayson, E., Shinaman, M. A., . . . Shults, C. (2016). Clinical-Genetic Associations in the Prospective Huntington at Risk Observational Study (PHAROS). *JAMA Neurology, 73*, 102–110.

Bobholz, J. A., & Rao, S. M. (2003). Cognitive dysfunction in multiple sclerosis: A review of recent developments. *Current Opinion in Neurology, 16*, 283–288. http://dx.doi.org/10.1097/00019052-200306000-00006

Boggio, P. S., Ferrucci, R., Rigonatti, S. P., Covre, P., Nitsche, M., Pascual-Leone, A., & Fregni, F. (2006). Effects of transcranial direct current stimulation on working memory in patients with Parkinson's disease. *Journal of the Neurological Sciences*, *249*, 31–38. http://dx.doi.org/10.1016/j.jns.2006.05.062

Bombard, Y., Veenstra, G., Friedman, J. M., Creighton, S., Currie, L., Paulsen, J. S., . . . Hayden, M. R. (2009). Perceptions of genetic discrimination among people at risk for Huntington's disease: A cross sectional survey. *BMJ*, *338*, b2175. http://dx.doi.org/10.1136/bmj.b2175

Braak, H., Del Tredici, K., Rüb, U., de Vos, R. A. I., Jansen Steur, E. N. H., & Braak, E. (2003). Staging of brain pathology related to sporadic Parkinson's disease. *Neurobiology of Aging*, *24*, 197–211. http://dx.doi.org/10.1016/S0197-4580(02)00065-9

Braak, H., Rüb, U., Jansen Steur, E. N., Del Tredici, K., & de Vos, R. A. (2005). Cognitive status correlates with neuropathologic stage in Parkinson disease. *Neurology*, *64*, 1404–1410. http://dx.doi.org/10.1212/01.WNL.0000158422.41380.82

Brenk, A., Laun, K., & Haase, C. G. (2008). Short-term cognitive training improves mental efficiency and mood in patients with multiple sclerosis. *European Neurology*, *60*, 304–309. http://dx.doi.org/10.1159/000157885

Briken, S., Gold, S. M., Patra, S., Vettorazzi, E., Harbs, D., Tallner, A., . . . Heesen, C. (2013). Effects of exercise on fitness and cognition in progressive MS: A randomized, controlled pilot trial. *Multiple Sclerosis Journal*, *20*, 382–390.

Brooks, B. R., Antel, J., Bradley, W., Cardy, P., Carpenter, S., Chou, S., . . . Meininger, V. (1994). El escorial World Federation of Neurology criteria for the diagnosis of amyotrophic lateral sclerosis. *Journal of the Neurological Sciences*, *124*(Suppl.), 96–107. http://dx.doi.org/10.1016/0022-510X(94)90191-0

Brown, R. F., Valpiani, E. M., Tennant, C. C., Dunn, S. M., Sharrock, M., Hodgkinson, S., & Pollard, J. D. (2009). Longitudinal assessment of anxiety, depression, and fatigue in people with multiple sclerosis. *Psychology and Psychotherapy: Theory, Research and Practice*, *82*, 41–56. http://dx.doi.org/10.1348/147608308X345614

Bruce, J. M., Bruce, A. S., & Arnett, P. A. (2007). Mild visual acuity disturbances are associated with performance on tests of complex visual attention in MS. *Journal of the International Neuropsychological Society*, *13*, 544–548. http://dx.doi.org/10.1017/S1355617707070658

Buetow, S. A., Talmage, A., McCann, C., Fogg, L., & Purdy, S. (2014). Conceptualizing how group singing may enhance quality of life with Parkinson's disease. *Disability and Rehabilitation*, *36*, 430–433. http://dx.doi.org/10.3109/09638288.2013.793749

Caligari, M., Godi, M., Guglielmetti, S., Franchignoni, F., & Nardone, A. (2013). Eye tracking communication devices in amyotrophic lateral sclerosis: Impact on disability and quality of life. *Amyotrophic Lateral Sclerosis & Frontotemporal Degeneration*, *14*, 546–552. http://dx.doi.org/10.3109/21678421.2013.803576

Chelune, G. J., Stott, H., & Pinkston, J. (2008). Multiple sclerosis. In J. E. Morgan & J. H. Ricker (Eds.), *Textbook of clinical neuropsychology* (pp. 599–615). New York, NY: Taylor and Francis.

Chesselet, M. F., Hickey, M. A., Zhu, C., & Levine, M. S. (2010). Huntington's disease: Neurodegeneration. In L. R. Squire (Ed.), *Encyclopedia of neuroscience* (pp. 39–44). http://dx.doi.org/10.1016/B978-008045046-9.00511-8

Chiaravalloti, N. D., & DeLuca, J. (2008). Cognitive impairment in multiple sclerosis. *The Lancet Neurology*, *7*, 1139–1151. http://dx.doi.org/10.1016/S1474-4422(08)70259-X

Chiaravalloti, N. D., DeLuca, J., Moore, N. B., & Ricker, J. H. (2005). Treating learning impairments improves memory performance in multiple sclerosis: A randomized clinical trial. *Multiple Sclerosis*, *11*, 58–68. http://dx.doi.org/10.1191/1352458505ms1118oa

Chiaravalloti, N. D., Ibarretxe-Bilbao, N., DeLuca, J., Rusu, O., Pena, J., García-Gorostiaga, I., & Ojeda, N. (2014). The source of the memory impairment in Parkinson's disease: Acquisition versus retrieval. *Movement Disorders*, *29*, 765–771. http://dx.doi.org/10.1002/mds.25842

Chiaravalloti, N. D., Moore, N. B., Nikelshpur, O. M., & DeLuca, J. (2013). An RCT to treat learning impairment in multiple sclerosis: The MEMREHAB trial. *Neurology*, *81*, 2066–2072. http://dx.doi.org/10.1212/01.wnl.0000437295.97946.a8

Chiaravalloti, N. D., Wylie, G., Leavitt, V., & Deluca, J. (2012). Increased cerebral activation after behavioral treatment for memory deficits in MS. *Journal of Neurology*, *259*, 1337–1346. http://dx.doi.org/10.1007/s00415-011-6353-x

Cleveland, D. W., & Rothstein, J. D. (2001). From Charcot to Lou Gehrig: Deciphering selective motor neuron death in ALS. *Nature Reviews Neuroscience*, *2*, 806–819. http://dx.doi.org/10.1038/35097565

Costa, A., Peppe, A., Caltagirone, C., & Carlesimo, G. A. (2008). Prospective memory impairment in individuals with Parkinson's disease. *Neuropsychology*, *22*, 283–292. http://dx.doi.org/10.1037/0894-4105.22.3.283

Coustasse, A., Pekar, A., Sikula, A., & Lurie, S. (2009). Ethical considerations of genetic presymptomatic testing for Huntington's disease. *Journal of Hospital Marketing & Public Relations*, *19*, 129–141. http://dx.doi.org/10.1080/15390940903041583

Craig, K. J., Hietanen, H., Markova, I. S., & Berrios, G. E. (2008). The Irritability Questionnaire: A new scale for the measurement of irritability. *Psychiatry Research*, *159*, 367–375. http://dx.doi.org/10.1016/j.psychres.2007.03.002

Cruickshank, T. M., Thompson, J. A., Domínguez D, J. F., Reyes, A. P., Bynevelt, M., Georgiou-Karistianis, N., . . . Ziman, M. R. (2015). The effect of multidisciplinary rehabilitation on brain structure and cognition in Huntington's disease: An exploratory study. *Brain and Behavior*, *5*, e00312. http://dx.doi.org/10.1002/brb3.312

Cutajar, R., Ferriani, E., Scandellari, C., Sabattini, L., Trocino, C., Marchello, L. P., & Stecchi, S. (2000). Cognitive function and quality of life in multiple sclerosis patients. *Journal of Neurovirology*, *6*(Suppl. 2), S186–S190.

Davidsdottir, S., Cronin-Golomb, A., & Lee, A. (2005). Visual and spatial symptoms in Parkinson's disease. *Vision Research*, *45*, 1285–1296. http://dx.doi.org/10.1016/j.visres.2004.11.006

Delis, D. C., Massman, P. J., Butters, N., Salmon, D. P., Cermak, L. S., & Kramer, J. H. (1991). Profiles of demented and amnesic patients on the California Verbal Learning Test: Implications for the assessment of memory disorders. *Psychological Assessment*, *3*, 19–26. http://dx.doi.org/10.1037/1040-3590.3.1.19

DeLuca, J. (2005). Fatigue, cognition and mental effort. In J. DeLuca (Ed.), *Fatigue as a window to the brain* (pp. 37–57). Cambridge, MA: MIT Press.

DeLuca, J., Barbieri-Berger, S., & Johnson, S. K. (1994). The nature of memory impairments in multiple sclerosis: Acquisition versus retrieval. *Journal of Clinical and Experimental Neuropsychology*, *16*, 183–189. http://dx.doi.org/10.1080/01688639408402629

DeLuca, J., Chelune, G. J., Tulsky, D. S., Lengenfelder, J., & Chiaravalloti, N. D. (2004). Is speed of processing or working memory the primary information processing deficit in multiple sclerosis? *Journal of Clinical and Experimental Neuropsychology*, *26*, 550–562. http://dx.doi.org/10.1080/13803390490496641

DeLuca, J., Genova, H. M., Hillary, F. G., & Wylie, G. (2008). Neural correlates of cognitive fatigue in multiple sclerosis using functional MRI. *Journal of the Neurological Sciences*, *270*, 28–39. http://dx.doi.org/10.1016/j.jns.2008.01.018

Devos, H., Nieuwboer, A., Tant, M., De Weerdt, W., & Vandenberghe, W. (2012). Determinants of fitness to drive in Huntington disease. *Neurology*, *79*, 1975–1982. http://dx.doi.org/10.1212/WNL.0b013e3182735d11

Devos, H., Nieuwboer, A., Vandenberghe, W., Tant, M., De Weerdt, W., & Uc, E. Y. (2014). On-road driving impairments in Huntington disease. *Neurology*, *82*, 956–962. http://dx.doi.org/10.1212/WNL.0000000000000220

Devos, H., Vandenberghe, W., Tant, M., Akinwuntan, A. E., De Weerdt, W., Nieuwboer, A., & Uc, E. Y. (2013). Driving and off-road impairments underlying failure on road testing in Parkinson's disease. *Movement Disorders*, *28*, 1949–1956. http://dx.doi.org/10.1002/mds.25701

Díez-Cirarda, M., Ojeda, N., Peña, J., Cabrera-Zubizarreta, A., Gómez-Beldarrain, M. A., Gómez-Esteban, J. C., & Ibarretxe-Bilbao, N. (2015). Neuroanatomical correlates of theory of mind deficit in Parkinson's disease: A multimodal imaging study [erratum available at http://dx.doi.org/10.1371/journal.pone.0144482]. *PLoS One*, *10*, e0142234. http://dx.doi.org/10.1371/journal.pone.0142234

Díez-Cirarda, M., Ojeda, N., Peña, J., Cabrera-Zubizarreta, A., Lucas-Jiménez, O., Gómez-Esteban, J. C., . . . Ibarretxe-Bilbao, N. (2017). Increased brain connectivity and activation after cognitive rehabilitation in Parkinson's disease: A randomized controlled trial. *Brain Imaging and Behavior*, *11*, 1640–1651. http://dx.doi.org/10.1007/s11682-016-9639-x

DiMatteo, M. R., Lepper, H. S., & Croghan, T. W. (2000). Depression is a risk factor for noncompliance with medical treatment: Meta-analysis of the effects of anxiety and depression on patient adherence. *Archives of Internal Medicine*, *160*, 2101–2107. http://dx.doi.org/10.1001/archinte.160.14.2101

Dobkin, R. D. (2014). The relationship between telephone-administered cognitive-behavioral therapy for depression and neuropsychological functioning in Parkinson's disease. *The Journal of Neuropsychiatry and Clinical Neurosciences*, *26*, E10–E11. http://dx.doi.org/10.1176/appi.neuropsych.13030065

Dobkin, R. D., Menza, M., Allen, L. A., Gara, M. A., Mark, M. H., Tiu, J., . . . Friedman, J. (2011). Cognitive-behavioral therapy for depression in Parkinson's disease: A randomized, controlled trial. *The American Journal of Psychiatry*, *168*, 1066–1074. http://dx.doi.org/10.1176/appi.ajp.2011.10111669

Domellöf, M. E., Ekman, U., Forsgren, L., & Elgh, E. (2015). Cognitive function in the early phase of Parkinson's disease, a five-year follow-up. *Acta Neurologica Scandinavica*, *132*, 79–88. http://dx.doi.org/10.1111/ane.12375

Doruk, D., Gray, Z., Bravo, G. L., Pascual-Leone, A., & Fregni, F. (2014). Effects of tDCS on executive function in Parkinson's disease. *Neuroscience Letters*, *582*, 27–31. http://dx.doi.org/10.1016/j.neulet.2014.08.043

Du, X., Pang, T. Y. C., & Hannan, A. J. (2013). A tale of two maladies? Pathogenesis of depression with and without the Huntington's disease gene mutation. *Frontiers in Neurology*, *4*, 1–13. http://dx.doi.org/10.3389/fneur.2013.00081

Duchesne, C., Lungu, O., Nadeau, A., Robillard, M. E., Boré, A., Bobeuf, F., . . . Doyon, J. (2015). Enhancing both motor and cognitive functioning in Parkinson's disease: Aerobic exercise as a rehabilitative intervention. *Brain and Cognition, 99*, 68–77. http://dx.doi.org/10.1016/j.bandc.2015.07.005

Duff, K., Beglinger, L. J., O'Rourke, M. E., Nopoulos, P., Paulson, H. L., & Paulsen, J. S. (2008). Risperidone and the treatment of psychiatric, motor, and cognitive symptoms in Huntington's disease. *Annals of Clinical Psychiatry, 20*, 1–3. http://dx.doi.org/10.1080/10401230701844802

Duff, K., Paulsen, J. S., Beglinger, L. J., Langbehn, D. R., Wang, C., Stout, J. C., . . . Queller, S., & the Predict-HD Investigators of the Huntington Study Group. (2010). "Frontal" behaviors before the diagnosis of Huntington's disease and their relationship to markers of disease progression: Evidence of early lack of awareness. *The Journal of Neuropsychiatry and Clinical Neurosciences, 22*, 196–207. http://dx.doi.org/10.1176/jnp.2010.22.2.196

Dujardin, K., & Defebvre, L. (2012). Apathy in Parkinson disease: What are the underlying mechanisms? *Neurology, 79*, 1082–1083. http://dx.doi.org/10.1212/WNL.0b013e3182698dd4

Dumas, E. M., van den Bogaard, S. J. A., Middelkoop, H. A. M., & Roos, R. A. C. (2013). A review of cognition in Huntington's disease. *Frontiers in Bioscience (Scholar Edition), 5*, 1–18. http://dx.doi.org/10.2741/S355

Dymek, M. P., Atchison, P., Harrell, L., & Marson, D. C. (2001). Competency to consent to medical treatment in cognitively impaired patients with Parkinson's disease. *Neurology, 56*, 17–24. http://dx.doi.org/10.1212/WNL.56.1.17

Ehde, D. M., Kraft, G. H., Chwastiak, L., Sullivan, M. D., Gibbons, L. E., Bombardier, C. H., & Wadhwani, R. (2008). Efficacy of paroxetine in treating major depressive disorder in persons with multiple sclerosis. *General Hospital Psychiatry, 30*, 40–48. http://dx.doi.org/10.1016/j.genhosppsych.2007.08.002

Feinstein, A., Roy, P., Lobaugh, N., Feinstein, K., O'Connor, P., & Black, S. (2004). Structural brain abnormalities in multiple sclerosis patients with major depression. *Neurology, 62*, 586–590. http://dx.doi.org/10.1212/01.WNL.0000110316.12086.0C

Feldman, E. A. (2012). The Genetic Information Nondiscrimination Act (GINA): Public policy and medical practice in the age of personalized medicine. *Journal of General Internal Medicine, 27*, 743–746. http://dx.doi.org/10.1007/s11606-012-1988-6

Fereshtehnejad, S. M., Shafieesabet, M., Farhadi, F., Hadizadeh, H., Rahmani, A., Naderi, N., . . . Lökk, J. (2015). Heterogeneous Determinants of Quality of Life in Different Phenotypes of Parkinson's Disease. *PLoS ONE, 10*, e0137081. http://dx.doi.org/10.1371/journal.pone.0137081

Filippi, M., Riccitelli, G., Mattioli, F., Capra, R., Stampatori, C., Pagani, E., . . . Rocca, M. A. (2012). Multiple sclerosis: Effects of cognitive rehabilitation on structural and functional MR imaging measures—An explorative study. *Radiology, 262*, 932–940. http://dx.doi.org/10.1148/radiol.11111299

Fink, F., Rischkau, E., Butt, M., Klein, J., Eling, P., & Hildebrandt, H. (2010). Efficacy of an executive function intervention programme in MS: A placebo-controlled and pseudo-randomized trial. *Multiple Sclerosis, 16*, 1148–1151. http://dx.doi.org/10.1177/1352458510375440

First, M. B., Spitzer, R. L., Gibbon, M., & Williams, J. B. (2002). *Structured Clinical Interview for DSM–IV–TR Axis I Disorders, Research Version, Patient Edition (SCID-I/P)*. New York: Biometrics Research, New York State Psychiatric Institute.

Fischer, J. S. (2001). Cognitive impairments in multiple sclerosis. In S. D. Cook (Ed.), *Handbook of multiple sclerosis* (pp. 233–256). New York, NY: Marcel Dekker. http://dx.doi.org/10.1201/9780824741846.ch10

Fischer, J. S., Rudick, R. A., Cutter, G. R., Reingold, S. C., & the National MS Society Clinical Outcomes Assessment Task Force. (1999). The Multiple Sclerosis Functional Composite Measure (MSFC): An integrated approach to MS clinical outcome assessment. *Multiple Sclerosis Journal, 5*, 244–250. http://dx.doi.org/10.1177/135245859900500409

Fisher, C. A., Sewell, K., Brown, A., & Churchyard, A. (2014). Aggression in Huntington's disease: A systematic review of rates of aggression and treatment methods. *Journal of Huntington's Disease, 3*, 319–332.

Fisk, J. D., Pontefract, A., Ritvo, P. G., Archibald, C. J., & Murray, T. J. (1994). The impact of fatigue on patients with multiple sclerosis. *The Canadian Journal of Neurological Sciences, 21*, 9–14. http://dx.doi.org/10.1017/S0317167100048691

Flaherty-Craig, C., Eslinger, P., Stephens, B., & Simmons, Z. (2006). A rapid screening battery to identify frontal dysfunction in patients with ALS. *Neurology, 67*, 2070–2072. http://dx.doi.org/10.1212/01.wnl.0000247667.89251.43

Flaherty-Craig, C. V., Brothers, A., Yang, C., Svoboda, R., & Simmons, Z. (2011). Declines in problem solving and anosognosia in amyotrophic lateral sclerosis: Application of Guilford's structure of intellect theory. *Cognitive and Behavioral Neurology, 24*, 26–34. http://dx.doi.org/10.1097/WNN.0b013e3182138454

Foley, F. W., Dince, W. M., Bedell, J. R., LaRocca, N. G., Kalb, R., Caruso, L. S., . . . Shnek, Z. M. (1994). Psychoremediation of communication skills for cognitively impaired persons with multiple sclerosis. *Journal of Neurologic Rehabilitation, 8*(4), 165–176.

Foley, F. W., Miller, A. H., Traugott, U., LaRocca, N. G., Scheinberg, L. C., Bedell, J. R., & Lennox, S. S. (1988). Psychoimmunological dysregulation in multiple sclerosis. *Psychosomatics*, *29*, 398–403. http://dx.doi.org/10.1016/S0033-3182(88)72340-3

Folstein, S. E., & Folstein, M. F. (1983). Psychiatric features of Huntington's disease: Recent approaches and findings. *Psychiatric Developments*, *1*, 193–205.

Forman, A. C., & Lincoln, N. B. (2010). Evaluation of an adjustment group for people with multiple sclerosis: A pilot randomized controlled trial. *Clinical Rehabilitation*, *24*, 211–221. http://dx.doi.org/10.1177/0269215509343492

Fruehwald, S., Loeffler-Stastka, H., Eher, R., Saletu, B., & Baumhackl, U. (2001). Depression and quality of life in multiple sclerosis. *Acta Neurologica Scandinavica*, *104*, 257–261. http://dx.doi.org/10.1034/j.1600-0404.2001.00022.x

Gelb, D. J., Oliver, E., & Gilman, S. (1999). Diagnostic criteria for Parkinson disease. *Archives of Neurology*, *56*, 33–39. http://dx.doi.org/10.1001/archneur.56.1.33

Gilchrist, A. C., & Creed, F. H. (1994). Depression, cognitive impairment and social stress in multiple sclerosis. *Journal of Psychosomatic Research*, *38*, 193–201. http://dx.doi.org/10.1016/0022-3999(94)90115-5

Goldstein, L. H., Atkins, L., & Leigh, P. N. (2002). Correlates of Quality of Life in people with motor neuron disease (MND). *Amyotrophic Lateral Sclerosis and Other Motor Neuron Disorders*, *3*, 123–129. Retrieved from https://www.ncbi.nlm.nih.gov/pubmed/12495573

Gould, R. L., Coulson, M. C., Brown, R. G., Goldstein, L. H., Al-Chalabi, A., & Howard, R. J. (2015). Psychotherapy and pharmacotherapy interventions to reduce distress or improve well-being in people with amyotrophic lateral sclerosis: A systematic review. *Amyotrophic Lateral Sclerosis and Frontotemporal Degeneration*, *16*, 293–302. http://dx.doi.org/10.3109/21678421.2015.1062515

Goverover, Y., Chiaravalloti, N., O'Brien, A., & DeLuca, J. (2018). Evidenced-based cognitive rehabilitation for persons with multiple sclerosis: An updated review of the literature from 2007 to 2016. *Archives of Physical Medicine and Rehabilitation*, *99*, 390–407.

Grima, D. T., Torrance, G. W., Francis, G., Rice, G., Rosner, A. J., & Lafortune, L. (2000). Cost and health related quality of life consequences of multiple sclerosis. *Multiple Sclerosis*, *6*, 91–98. http://dx.doi.org/10.1177/135245850000600207

Gulick, E. E. (1997). Correlates of quality of life among persons with multiple sclerosis. *Nursing Research*, *46*, 305–311. http://dx.doi.org/10.1097/00006199-199711000-00002

Hamilton, J. M., Salmon, D. P., Corey-Bloom, J., Gamst, A., Paulsen, J. S., Jerkins, S., . . . Peavy, G. (2003). Behavioural abnormalities contribute to functional decline in Huntington's disease. *Journal of Neurology, Neurosurgery & Psychiatry*, *74*, 120–122. http://dx.doi.org/10.1136/jnnp.74.1.120

Hamilton, M. C. (1960). Hamilton Depression Rating Scale (HAM–D). *Journal of Neurology, Neurosurgery & Psychiatry*, *23*, 56–62.

Harrison, D. J., Busse, M., Openshaw, R., Rosser, A. E., Dunnett, S. B., & Brooks, S. P. (2013). Exercise attenuates neuropathology and has greater benefit on cognitive than motor deficits in the R6/1 Huntington's disease mouse model. *Experimental Neurology*, *248*, 457–469. http://dx.doi.org/10.1016/j.expneurol.2013.07.014

Hayes, C. V. (1992). Genetic testing for Huntington's disease—A family issue. *The New England Journal of Medicine*, *327*, 1449–1451. http://dx.doi.org/10.1056/NEJM199211123272008

Henriksson, F., Fredrikson, S., Masterman, T., & Jönsson, B. (2001). Costs, quality of life and disease severity in multiple sclerosis: A cross-sectional study in Sweden. *European Journal of Neurology*, *8*, 27–35. http://dx.doi.org/10.1046/j.1468-1331.2001.00169.x

Herz, N. B., Mehta, S. H., Sethi, K. D., Jackson, P., Hall, P., & Morgan, J. C. (2013). Nintendo Wii rehabilitation ("Wii-hab") provides benefits in Parkinson's disease. *Parkinsonism & Related Disorders*, *19*, 1039–1042. http://dx.doi.org/10.1016/j.parkreldis.2013.07.014

Hicks, S. L., Sharma, R., Khan, A. N., Berna, C. M., Waldecker, A., Talbot, K., . . . Turner, M. R. (2013). An eye-tracking version of the trail-making test. *PLoS One*, *8*, e84061. http://dx.doi.org/10.1371/journal.pone.0084061

Ho, A. K., Gilbert, A. S., Mason, S. L., Goodman, A. O., & Barker, R. A. (2009). Health-related quality of life in Huntington's disease: Which factors matter most? *Movement Disorders*, *24*, 574–578. http://dx.doi.org/10.1002/mds.22412

Ho, A. K., Sahakian, B. J., Brown, R. G., Barker, R. A., Hodges, J. R., Ané, M. N., . . . Bodner, T., & the NEST-HD Consortium. (2003). Profile of cognitive progression in early Huntington's disease. *Neurology*, *61*, 1702–1706. http://dx.doi.org/10.1212/01.WNL.0000098878.47789.BD

Ho, A. K., Sahakian, B. J., Robbins, T. W., Barker, R. A., Rosser, A. E., & Hodges, J. R. (2002). Verbal fluency in Huntington's disease: A longitudinal analysis of phonemic and semantic clustering and switching. *Neuropsychologia*, *40*, 1277–1284. http://dx.doi.org/10.1016/S0028-3932(01)00217-2

Homann, C. N., Suppan, K., Homann, B., Crevenna, R., Ivanic, G., & Ruzicka, E. (2003). Driving in Parkinson's disease—A health hazard? *Journal of*

Neurology, *250*, 1439–1446. http://dx.doi.org/10.1007/s00415-003-0239-5

Hoth, K. F., Paulsen, J. S., Moser, D. J., Tranel, D., Clark, L. A., & Bechara, A. (2007). Patients with Huntington's disease have impaired awareness of cognitive, emotional, and functional abilities. *Journal of Clinical and Experimental Neuropsychology*, *29*, 365–376. http://dx.doi.org/10.1080/13803390600718958

Hubble, J. P., Cao, T., Hassanein, R. E., Neuberger, J. S., & Koller, W. C. (1993). Risk factors for Parkinson's disease. *Neurology*, *43*, 1693–1697. http://dx.doi.org/10.1212/WNL.43.9.1693

Huntington Study Group. (1996). Unified Huntington's Disease Rating Scale: Reliability and consistency. *Movement Disorders*, *11*, 136–142. http://dx.doi.org/10.1002/mds.870110204

Hwang, C. S., Weng, H. H., Wang, L. F., Tsai, C. H., & Chang, H. T. (2014). An eye-tracking assistive device improves the quality of life for ALS patients and reduces the caregivers' burden. *Journal of Motor Behavior*, *46*, 233–238. http://dx.doi.org/10.1080/00222895.2014.891970

Ince, P. G., Lowe, J., & Shaw, P. J. (1998). Amyotrophic lateral sclerosis: Current issues in classification, pathogenesis and molecular pathology. *Neuropathology and Applied Neurobiology*, *24*, 104–117. http://dx.doi.org/10.1046/j.1365-2990.1998.00108.x

Janardhan, V., & Bakshi, R. (2000). Quality of life and its relationship to brain lesions and atrophy on magnetic resonance images in 60 patients with multiple sclerosis. *Archives of Neurology*, *57*, 1485–1491. http://dx.doi.org/10.1001/archneur.57.10.1485

Janssen, A., Boster, A., Lee, H., Patterson, B., & Prakash, R. S. (2015). The effects of video-game training on broad cognitive transfer in multiple sclerosis: A pilot randomized controlled trial. *Journal of Clinical and Experimental Neuropsychology*, *37*, 285–302. http://dx.doi.org/10.1080/13803395.2015.1009366

Johnson, S. K., Lange, G., DeLuca, J., Korn, L. R., & Natelson, B. (1997). The effects of fatigue on neuropsychological performance in patients with chronic fatigue syndrome, multiple sclerosis, and depression. *Applied Neuropsychology*, *4*, 145–153. http://dx.doi.org/10.1207/s15324826an0403_1

Jønsson, A., Korfitzen, E. M., Heltberg, A., Ravnborg, M. H., & Byskov-Ottosen, E. (1993). Effects of neuropsychological treatment in patients with multiple sclerosis. *Acta Neurologica Scandinavica*, *88*, 394–400. http://dx.doi.org/10.1111/j.1600-0404.1993.tb05366.x

Julien, C. L., Rimes, K. A., & Brown, R. G. (2016). Rumination and behavioural factors in Parkinson's disease depression. *Journal of Psychosomatic Research*, *82*, 48–53. http://dx.doi.org/10.1016/j.jpsychores.2016.01.008

Julien, C. L., Thompson, J. C., Wild, S., Yardumian, P., Snowden, J. S., Turner, G., & Craufurd, D. (2007). Psychiatric disorders in preclinical Huntington's disease. *Journal of Neurology, Neurosurgery & Psychiatry*, *78*, 939–943. http://dx.doi.org/10.1136/jnnp.2006.103309

Kalmar, J. H., Gaudino, E. A., Moore, N. B., Halper, J., & Deluca, J. (2008). The relationship between cognitive deficits and everyday functional activities in multiple sclerosis. *Neuropsychology*, *22*, 442–449. http://dx.doi.org/10.1037/0894-4105.22.4.442

Kirkwood, S. C., Su, J. L., Conneally, P., & Foroud, T. (2001). Progression of symptoms in the early and middle stages of Huntington disease. *Archives of Neurology*, *58*, 273–278. http://dx.doi.org/10.1001/archneur.58.2.273

Kirsch-Darrow, L., Fernandez, H. H., Marsiske, M., Okun, M. S., & Bowers, D. (2006). Dissociating apathy and depression in Parkinson disease. *Neurology*, *67*, 33–38. http://dx.doi.org/10.1212/01.wnl.0000230572.07791.22

Kliem, S., Mößle, T., Zenger, M., & Brähler, E. (2014). Reliability and validity of the Beck Depression Inventory—Fast Screen for medical patients in the general German population. *Journal of Affective Disorders*, *156*, 236–239. http://dx.doi.org/10.1016/j.jad.2013.11.024

Korostil, M., & Feinstein, A. (2007). Anxiety disorders and their clinical correlates in multiple sclerosis patients. *Multiple Sclerosis*, *13*, 67–72. http://dx.doi.org/10.1177/1352458506071161

Kroenke, K., Spitzer, R. L., & Williams, J. B. W. (2001). The PHQ–9: Validity of a brief depression severity measure. *Journal of General Internal Medicine*, *16*, 606–613. http://dx.doi.org/10.1046/j.1525-1497.2001.016009606.x

Kudlicka, A., Clare, L., & Hindle, J. V. (2011). Executive functions in Parkinson's disease: Systematic review and meta-analysis. *Movement Disorders*, *26*, 2305–2315. http://dx.doi.org/10.1002/mds.23868

Kuruvilla, M. S., Green, J. R., Ayaz, H., & Murman, D. L. (2013). Neural correlates of cognitive decline in ALS: An fNIRS study of the prefrontal cortex. *Cognitive Neuroscience*, *4*, 115–121. http://dx.doi.org/10.1080/17588928.2013.797889

Langdon, D. W., Amato, M. P., Boringa, J., Brochet, B., Foley, F., Fredrikson, S., . . . Benedict, R. H. (2012). Recommendations for a Brief International Cognitive Assessment for Multiple Sclerosis (BICAMS). *Multiple Sclerosis*, *18*, 891–898. http://dx.doi.org/10.1177/1352458511431076

Langenbahn, D. M., Ashman, T., Cantor, J., & Trott, C. (2013). An evidence-based review of cognitive rehabilitation in medical conditions affecting cognitive function. *Archives of Physical Medicine and Rehabilitation*, *94*, 271–286. http://dx.doi.org/10.1016/j.apmr.2012.09.011

Larcombe, N. A., & Wilson, P. H. (1984). An evaluation of cognitive-behaviour therapy for depression in patients with multiple sclerosis. *The British Journal of Psychiatry*, *145*, 366–371. http://dx.doi.org/10.1192/bjp.145.4.366

Lawrence, A. D., Sahakian, B. J., Hodges, J. R., Rosser, A. E., Lange, K. W., & Robbins, T. W. (1996). Executive and mnemonic functions in early Huntington's disease. *Brain: A Journal of Neurology*, *119*, 1633–1645. http://dx.doi.org/10.1093/brain/119.5.1633

Lawrence, A. D., Sahakian, B. J., & Robbins, T. W. (1998). Cognitive functions and corticostriatal circuits: Insights from Huntington's disease. *Trends in Cognitive Sciences*, *2*, 379–388. http://dx.doi.org/10.1016/S1364-6613(98)01231-5

Leavitt, V. M., Wylie, G. R., Girgis, P. A., DeLuca, J., & Chiaravalloti, N. D. (2014). Increased functional connectivity within memory networks following memory rehabilitation in multiple sclerosis. *Brain Imaging and Behavior*, *8*, 394–402. http://dx.doi.org/10.1007/s11682-012-9183-2

Levy, M. L., Cummings, J. L., Fairbanks, L. A., Masterman, D., Miller, B. L., Craig, A. H., . . . Litvan, I. (1998). Apathy is not depression. *The Journal of Neuropsychiatry and Clinical Neurosciences*, *10*, 314–319. http://dx.doi.org/10.1176/jnp.10.3.314

Licklederer, C., Wolff, G., & Barth, J. (2008). Mental health and quality of life after genetic testing for Huntington disease: A long-term effect study in Germany. *American Journal of Medical Genetics. Part A*, *146A*, 2078–2085. http://dx.doi.org/10.1002/ajmg.a.32423

Lineweaver, T. T., Salmon, D. P., Bondi, M. W., & Corey-Bloom, J. (2005). Differential effects of Alzheimer's disease and Huntington's disease on the performance of mental rotation. *Journal of the International Neuropsychological Society*, *11*, 30–39. http://dx.doi.org/10.1017/S1355617705050034

MacDonald, M. E., Ambrose, C. M., Duyao, M. P., Myers, R. H., Lin, C., Srinidhi, L., . . . Harper, P. S. (1993). A novel gene containing a trinucleotide repeat that is expanded and unstable on Huntington's disease chromosomes. *Cell*, *72*, 971–983. http://dx.doi.org/10.1016/0092-8674(93)90585-E

MacNiven, J. A. B., Davis, C., Ho, M. Y., Bradshaw, C. M., Szabadi, E., & Constantinescu, C. S. (2008). Stroop performance in multiple sclerosis: Information processing, selective attention, or executive functioning? *Journal of the International Neuropsychological Society*, *14*, 805–814. http://dx.doi.org/10.1017/S1355617708080946

Mak, M. K., Wong, A., & Pang, M. Y. (2014). Impaired executive function can predict recurrent falls in Parkinson's disease. *Archives of Physical Medicine and Rehabilitation*, *95*, 2390–2395. http://dx.doi.org/10.1016/j.apmr.2014.08.006

Mäntynen, A., Rosti-Otajärvi, E., Koivisto, K., Lilja, A., Huhtala, H., & Hämäläinen, P. (2014). Neuropsychological rehabilitation does not improve cognitive performance but reduces perceived cognitive deficits in patients with multiple sclerosis: A randomised, controlled, multi-centre trial. *Multiple Sclerosis*, *20*, 99–107. http://dx.doi.org/10.1177/1352458513494487

Marin, H., & Menza, M. A. (2004). Specific treatment of residual fatigue in depressed patients. *Psychiatry*, *1*, 12–18. Retrieved from https://www.ncbi.nlm.nih.gov/pmc/articles/PMC3012615/

Marrie, R. A., Reingold, S., Cohen, J., Stuve, O., Trojano, M., Sorensen, P. S., . . . Reider, N. (2015). The incidence and prevalence of psychiatric disorders in multiple sclerosis: A systematic review. *Multiple Sclerosis*, *21*, 305–317. http://dx.doi.org/10.1177/1352458514564487

Martínez-González, A. E., & Piqueras, J. A. (2015). Long-term effectiveness of combined cognitive-behavioral and neuropsychological intervention in a case of multiple sclerosis. *Neurocase*, *21*, 584–591. http://dx.doi.org/10.1080/13554794.2014.960425

Mattioli, F., Bellomi, F., Stampatori, C., Capra, R., & Miniussi, C. (2016). Neuroenhancement through cognitive training and anodal tDCS in multiple sclerosis. *Multiple Sclerosis*, *22*, 222–230. http://dx.doi.org/10.1177/1352458515587597

Mattioli, F., Bellomi, F., Stampatori, C., Provinciali, L., Compagnucci, L., Uccelli, A., . . . Capra, R. (2016). Two years follow up of domain specific cognitive training in relapsing remitting multiple sclerosis: A randomized clinical trial. *Frontiers in Behavioral Neuroscience*, *10*, 28. http://dx.doi.org/10.3389/fnbeh.2016.00028

Mattioli, F., Stampatori, C., Scarpazza, C., Parrinello, G., & Capra, R. (2012). Persistence of the effects of attention and executive functions intensive rehabilitation in relapsing remitting multiple sclerosis. *Multiple Sclerosis and Related Disorders*, *1*, 168–173. http://dx.doi.org/10.1016/j.msard.2012.06.004

Mattioli, F., Stampatori, C., Zanotti, D., Parrinello, G., & Capra, R. (2010). Efficacy and specificity of intensive cognitive rehabilitation of attention and executive functions in multiple sclerosis. *Journal of the Neurological Sciences*, 288, 101–105. http://dx.doi.org/10.1016/j.jns.2009.09.024

Mazziotta, J. C., Phelps, M. E., Pahl, J. J., Huang, S. C., Baxter, L. R., Riege, W. H., . . . Markham, C. H. (1987). Reduced cerebral glucose metabolism in asymptomatic subjects at risk for Huntington's disease. *The New England Journal of Medicine, 316*, 357–362. http://dx.doi.org/10.1056/NEJM198702123160701

McCarthy, M., Beaumont, J. G., Thompson, R., & Peacock, S. (2005). Modality-specific aspects of sustained and divided attentional performance in multiple sclerosis. *Archives of Clinical Neuropsychology, 20*, 705–718. http://dx.doi.org/10.1016/j.acn.2005.04.007

Mendoza, R. J., Pittenger, D. J., & Weinstein, C. S. (2001). Unit management of depression of patients with multiple sclerosis using cognitive remediation strategies: A preliminary study. *Neurorehabilitation and Neural Repair, 15*, 9–14. http://dx.doi.org/10.1177/154596830101500102

Merrilees, J., Klapper, J., Murphy, J., Lomen-Hoerth, C., & Miller, B. L. (2010). Cognitive and behavioral challenges in caring for patients with frontotemporal dementia and amyotrophic lateral sclerosis. *Amyotrophic Lateral Sclerosis, 11*, 298–302. http://dx.doi.org/10.3109/17482961003605788

Mestre, T. A., van Duijn, E., Davis, A. M., Bachoud-Levi, A.-C., Busse, M., Anderson, K. E., . . . Martinez-Martin, P. (2016). Rating scales for behavioral symptoms in Huntington's disease: Critique and recommendations. *Movement Disorders*, 1–13. http://dx.doi.org/10.1002/mds.26675

Miller, R. G., Jackson, C. E., Kasarskis, E. J., England, J. D., Forshew, D., Johnston, W., . . . Woolley, S. C., & the Quality Standards Subcommittee of the American Academy of Neurology. (2009). Practice parameter update: The care of the patient with amyotrophic lateral sclerosis: Multidisciplinary care, symptom management, and cognitive/behavioral impairment (an evidence-based review). *Neurology, 73*, 1227–1233. http://dx.doi.org/10.1212/WNL.0b013e3181bc01a4

Miller, R. G., Mitchell, J. D., Lyon, M., & Moore, D. H. (2007). Riluzole for amyotrophic lateral sclerosis (ALS)/motor neuron disease (MND). *Cochrane Database of Systematic Reviews*, CD001447.

Minden, S. L., Frankel, D., Hadden, L., Perloff, J., Srinath, K. P., & Hoaglin, D. C. (2006). The Sonya Slifka Longitudinal Multiple Sclerosis Study: Methods and sample characteristics. *Multiple Sclerosis, 12*, 24–38. http://dx.doi.org/10.1191/135248506ms1262oa

Mockford, C., Jenkinson, C., & Fitzpatrick, R. (2006). A Review: Carers, MND and service provision. *Amyotrophic Lateral Sclerosis, 7*, 132–141. http://dx.doi.org/10.1080/14660820600601028

Mohr, D. C., Boudewyn, A. C., Goodkin, D. E., Bostrom, A., & Epstein, L. (2001). Comparative outcomes for individual cognitive-behavior therapy, supportive-expressive group psychotherapy, and sertraline for the treatment of depression in multiple sclerosis. *Journal of Consulting and Clinical Psychology, 69*, 942–949. http://dx.doi.org/10.1037/0022-006X.69.6.942

Mohr, D. C., Cox, D., & Merluzzi, N. (2005). Self-injection anxiety training: A treatment for patients unable to self-inject injectable medications. *Multiple Sclerosis, 11*, 182–185. http://dx.doi.org/10.1191/1352458505ms1146oa

Mohr, E., Mendis, T., & Grimes, J. D. (1995). Late cognitive changes in Parkinson's disease with an emphasis on dementia. *Advances in Neurology, 65*, 97–113.

Montoya, A., Pelletier, M., Menear, M., Duplessis, E., Richer, F., & Lepage, M. (2006). Episodic memory impairment in Huntington's disease: A meta-analysis. *Neuropsychologia, 44*, 1984–1994. http://dx.doi.org/10.1016/j.neuropsychologia.2006.01.015

Morris, M. (1991). Psychiatric aspects of Huntington's disease. In P. S. Harper (Ed.), *Huntington's disease* (pp. 81–126). London, England: Saunders.

Movement Disorder Society Task Force on Rating Scales for Parkinson's Disease. (2003). The Unified Parkinson's Disease Rating Scale (UPDRS): Status and recommendations. *Movement Disorders, 18*, 738–750. http://dx.doi.org/10.1002/mds.10473

Mukherjee, D. (2015). Recognizing psychological diversity in people with end-stage amyotrophic lateral sclerosis. *American Medical Association Journal of Ethics, 17*, 530–534. http://dx.doi.org/10.1001/journalofethics.2015.17.6.nlit2-1506

Muslimovic, D., Post, B., Speelman, J. D., & Schmand, B. (2005). Cognitive profile of patients with newly diagnosed Parkinson disease. *Neurology, 65*, 1239–1245. http://dx.doi.org/10.1212/01.wnl.0000180516.69442.95

Naarding, P., Janzing, J. G., Eling, P., van der Werf, S., & Kremer, B. (2009). Apathy is not depression in Huntington's disease. *The Journal of Neuropsychiatry and Clinical Neurosciences, 21*, 266–270.

Nagy, H., Bencsik, K., Rajda, C., Benedek, K., Beniczky, S., Kéri, S., & Vécsei, L. (2006). The effects of reward and punishment contingencies on decision-making in multiple sclerosis. *Journal of the International Neuropsychological Society, 12*, 559–565. http://dx.doi.org/10.1017/S1355617706060644

National Multiple Sclerosis Society. (n.d.). *Multiple sclerosis: Just the facts*. Retrieved from https://www.nationalmssociety.org/nationalmssociety/media/msnationalfiles/brochures/brochure-just-the-facts.pdf

Nortvedt, M. W., Riise, T., Myhr, K. M., & Nyland, H. I. (2000). Performance of the SF-36, SF-12, and RAND-36 summary scales in a multiple sclerosis population. *Medical Care, 38*, 1022–1028. http://dx.doi.org/10.1097/00005650-200010000-00006

O'Rourke, J. J. F., Beglinger, L. J., Smith, M. M., Mills, J., Moser, D. J., Rowe, K. C., . . . the PREDICT-HD Investigators of the Huntington Study Group. (2011). The Trail Making Test in prodromal Huntington disease: Contributions of disease progression to test performance. *Journal of Clinical and Experimental Neuropsychology*, *33*, 567–579. http://dx.doi.org/10.1080/13803395.2010.541228

Paganoni, S., Karam, C., Joyce, N., Bedlack, R., & Carter, G. T. (2015). Comprehensive rehabilitative care across the spectrum of amyotrophic lateral sclerosis. *NeuroRehabilitation*, *37*, 53–68. http://dx.doi.org/10.3233/NRE-151240

Pang, T. Y. C., Du, X., Zajac, M. S., Howard, M. L., & Hannan, A. J. (2009). Altered serotonin receptor expression is associated with depression-related behavior in the R6/1 transgenic mouse model of Huntington's disease. *Human Molecular Genetics*, *18*, 753–766. http://dx.doi.org/10.1093/hmg/ddn385

Parisi, L., Rocca, M. A., Mattioli, F., Copetti, M., Capra, R., Valsasina, P., . . . Filippi, M. (2014). Changes of brain resting state functional connectivity predict the persistence of cognitive rehabilitation effects in patients with multiple sclerosis. *Multiple Sclerosis*, *20*, 686–694. http://dx.doi.org/10.1177/1352458513505692

Parmelee, P. A., & Katz, I. R. (1990). Geriatric depression scale. *Journal of the American Geriatrics Society*, *38*, 1379. http://dx.doi.org/10.1111/j.1532-5415.1990.tb03461.x

Paulsen, J. S., Long, J. D., Ross, C. A., Harrington, D. L., Erwin, C. J., Williams, J. K., . . . Barker, R. A., & the PREDICT-HD Investigators and Coordinators of the Huntington Study Group. (2014). Prediction of manifest Huntington's disease with clinical and imaging measures: A prospective observational study. *The Lancet Neurology*, *13*, 1193–1201. http://dx.doi.org/10.1016/S1474-4422(14)70238-8

Paulsen, J. S., Nehl, C., Hoth, K. F., Kanz, J. E., Benjamin, M., Conybeare, R., . . . Turner, B. (2005). Depression and stages of Huntington's disease. *The Journal of Neuropsychiatry and Clinical Neurosciences*, *17*, 496–502. http://dx.doi.org/10.1176/jnp.17.4.496

Paulsen, J. S., Ready, R. E., Hamilton, J. M., Mega, M. S., & Cummings, J. L. (2001). Neuropsychiatric aspects of Huntington's disease. *Journal of Neurology, Neurosurgery & Psychiatry*, *71*, 310–314. http://dx.doi.org/10.1136/jnnp.71.3.310

Paulsen, J. S., Stout, J. C., DeLaPena, J., Romero, R., Tawfik-Reedy, Z., Swenson, M. R., . . . Malloy, P. F. (1996). Frontal behavioral syndromes in cortical and subcortical dementia. *Assessment*, *3*, 327–337. http://dx.doi.org/10.1177/107319119600300312

Peavy, G. M., Salmon, D., Bear, P. I., Paulsen, J. S., Cahn, D. A., Hofstetter, C. R., . . . Shult, C. W. (2001). Detection of mild cognitive deficits in Parkinson's disease patients with the WAIS–R NI. *Journal of the International Neuropsychological Society*, *7*, 535–543. http://dx.doi.org/10.1017/S1355617701755014

Pedersen, K. F., Alves, G., Larsen, J. P., Tysnes, O.-B., Møller, S. G., & Brønnick, K. (2012). Psychometric properties of the Starkstein Apathy Scale in patients with early untreated Parkinson disease. *The American Journal of Geriatric Psychiatry*, *20*, 142–148. http://dx.doi.org/10.1097/JGP.0b013e31823038f2

Peinemann, A., Schuller, S., Pohl, C., Jahn, T., Weindl, A., & Kassubek, J. (2005). Executive dysfunction in early stages of Huntington's disease is associated with striatal and insular atrophy: A neuropsychological and voxel-based morphometric study. *Journal of the Neurological Sciences*, *239*, 11–19. http://dx.doi.org/10.1016/j.jns.2005.07.007

Peña, J., Ibarretxe-Bilbao, N., García-Gorostiaga, I., Gomez-Beldarrain, M. A., Díez-Cirarda, M., & Ojeda, N. (2014). Improving functional disability and cognition in Parkinson disease: Randomized controlled trial. *Neurology*, *83*, 2167–2174. http://dx.doi.org/10.1212/WNL.0000000000001043

Pereira, J. B., Junqué, C., Bartrés-Faz, D., Martí, M. J., Sala-Llonch, R., Compta, Y., . . . Tolosa, E. (2013). Modulation of verbal fluency networks by transcranial direct current stimulation (tDCS) in Parkinson's disease. *Brain Stimulation*, *6*, 16–24. http://dx.doi.org/10.1016/j.brs.2012.01.006

Pfennings, L., Cohen, L., Adèr, H., Polman, C., Lankhorst, G., Smits, R., & van der Ploeg, H. (1999). Exploring differences between subgroups of multiple sclerosis patients in health-related quality of life. *Journal of Neurology*, *246*, 587–591. http://dx.doi.org/10.1007/s004150050408

Piatt, A. L., Fields, J. A., Paolo, A. M., & Tröster, A. I. (1999). Action (verb naming) fluency as an executive function measure: Convergent and divergent evidence of validity. *Neuropsychologia*, *37*, 1499–1503. http://dx.doi.org/10.1016/S0028-3932(99)00066-4

Pierobon, A., Giardini, A., Maestri, R., Farina, C., Callegari, S., Torlaschi, V., . . . Frazzitta, G. (2014). Disexecutive functions and depression in patients with Parkinson disease: The impact on rehabilitation outcome. *American Journal of Physical Medicine & Rehabilitation*, *93*, 1–10. http://dx.doi.org/10.1097/PHM.0000000000000092

Pillon, B., Dubois, B., & Agid, Y. (1991). Severity and specificity of cognitive impairment in Alzheimer's, Huntington's, and Parkinson's diseases and progressive supranuclear palsy. *Annals of the New York Academy of Sciences*, *640*, 224–227. http://dx.doi.org/10.1111/j.1749-6632.1991.tb00222.x

Pirogovsky, E., Woods, S. P., Filoteo, J. V., & Gilbert, P. E. (2012). Prospective memory deficits are associated with poorer everyday functioning in Parkinson's disease. *Journal of the International Neuropsychological Society*, *18*, 986–995. http://dx.doi.org/10.1017/S1355617712000781

Plohmann, A. M., Kappos, L., Ammann, W., Thordai, A., Wittwer, A., Huber, S., . . . Lechner-Scott, J. (1998). Computer assisted retraining of attentional impairments in patients with multiple sclerosis. *Journal of Neurology, Neurosurgery & Psychiatry*, *64*, 455–462. http://dx.doi.org/10.1136/jnnp.64.4.455

Potegal, M. (1971). A note on spatial-motor deficits in patients with Huntington's disease: A test of a hypothesis. *Neuropsychologia*, *9*, 233–235. http://dx.doi.org/10.1016/0028-3932(71)90047-9

Pouladi, M. A., Graham, R. K., Karasinska, J. M., Xie, Y., Santos, R. D., Petersén, A., & Hayden, M. R. (2009). Prevention of depressive behaviour in the YAC128 mouse model of Huntington disease by mutation at residue 586 of huntingtin. *Brain: A Journal of Neurology*, *132*, 919–932. http://dx.doi.org/10.1093/brain/awp006

Prediger, R. D. S., Matheus, F. C., Schwarzbold, M. L., Lima, M. M. S., & Vital, M. A. B. F. (2012). Anxiety in Parkinson's disease: A critical review of experimental and clinical studies. *Neuropharmacology*, *62*, 115–124.

Pusswald, G., Mildner, C., Zebenholzer, K., Auff, E., & Lehrner, J. (2014). A neuropsychological rehabilitation program for patients with multiple sclerosis based on the model of the ICF. *NeuroRehabilitation*, *35*, 519–527.

Rabins, P. V., Brooks, B. R., O'Donnell, P., Pearlson, G. D., Moberg, P., Jubelt, B., . . . Folstein, M. F. (1986). Structural brain correlates of emotional disorder in multiple sclerosis. *Brain*, *109*, 585–597. http://dx.doi.org/10.1093/brain/109.4.585

Rabkin, J. G., Albert, S. M., Rowland, L. P., & Mitsumoto, H. (2009). How common is depression among ALS caregivers? A longitudinal study. *Amyotrophic Lateral Sclerosis*, *10*, 448–455. http://dx.doi.org/10.3109/17482960802459889

Rabkin, J. G., Goetz, R., Factor-Litvak, P., Hupf, J., McElhiney, M., Singleton, J., Mitsumoto, H., & the Als Cosmos Study Group. (2015). Depression and wish to die in a multicenter cohort of ALS patients. *Amyotrophic Lateral Sclerosis and Frontotemporal Degeneration*, *16*, 265–273. http://dx.doi.org/10.3109/21678421.2014.980428

Rabkin, J. G., Wagner, G. J., & Del Bene, M. (2000). Resilience and distress among amyotrophic lateral sclerosis patients and caregivers. *Psychosomatic Medicine*, *62*, 271–279. http://dx.doi.org/10.1097/00006842-200003000-00020

Radloff, L. S. (1977). The CES–D Scale: A self-report depression scale for research in the general population. *Applied Psychological Measurement*, *1*, 385–401. http://dx.doi.org/10.1177/014662167700100306

Ragnarsson, K. T., Clarke, W. R., Daling, J. R., Garber, S. L., Gustafson, C. F., Holland, A. L., & the NIH Consensus Development Panel on Rehabilitation of Persons With Traumatic Brain Injury. (1999). Consensus conference. Rehabilitation of persons with traumatic brain injury. *JAMA*, *282*, 974–983. http://dx.doi.org/10.1001/jama.282.10.974

Rak, S., & Coffin, J. (2013). Affordable Care Act. *The Journal of Medical Practice Management*, *28*, 317–319.

Ramaker, C., Marinus, J., Stiggelbout, A. M., & Van Hilten, B. J. (2002). Systematic evaluation of rating scales for impairment and disability in Parkinson's disease. *Movement Disorders*, *17*, 867–876. http://dx.doi.org/10.1002/mds.10248

Rao, S. M., Leo, G. J., Bernardin, L., & Unverzagt, F. (1991). Cognitive dysfunction in multiple sclerosis. I. Frequency, patterns, and prediction. *Neurology*, *41*, 685–691. http://dx.doi.org/10.1212/WNL.41.5.685

Rao, S. M., Leo, G. J., Ellington, L., Nauertz, T., Bernardin, L., & Unverzagt, F. (1991). Cognitive dysfunction in multiple sclerosis. II. Impact on employment and social functioning. *Neurology*, *41*, 692–696. http://dx.doi.org/10.1212/WNL.41.5.692

Reijnders, J. S., Ehrt, U., Weber, W. E., Aarsland, D., & Leentjens, A. F. (2008). A systematic review of prevalence studies of depression in Parkinson's disease. *Movement Disorders*, *23*, 183–189. http://dx.doi.org/10.1002/mds.21803

Ringholz, G. M., Appel, S. H., Bradshaw, M., Cooke, N. A., Mosnik, D. M., & Schulz, P. E. (2005). Prevalence and patterns of cognitive impairment in sporadic ALS. *Neurology*, *65*, 586–590. http://dx.doi.org/10.1212/01.wnl.0000172911.39167.b6

Rippon, G. A., Scarmeas, N., Gordon, P. H., Murphy, P. L., Albert, S. M., Mitsumoto, H., . . . Stern, Y. (2006). An observational study of cognitive impairment in amyotrophic lateral sclerosis. *Archives of Neurology*, *63*, 345–352. http://dx.doi.org/10.1001/archneur.63.3.345

Robert, G., Le Jeune, F., Dondaine, T., Drapier, S., Péron, J., Lozachmeur, C., . . . Drapier, D. (2014). Apathy and impaired emotional facial recognition networks overlap in Parkinson's disease: A PET study with conjunction analyses. *Journal of Neurology, Neurosurgery & Psychiatry*, *85*, 1153–1158. http://dx.doi.org/10.1136/jnnp-2013-307025

Robinson, K. M., Lacey, S. C., Grugan, P., Glosser, G., Grossman, M., & McCluskey, L. F. (2006). Cognitive functioning in sporadic amyotrophic lateral sclerosis: A six-month longitudinal study. *Journal of Neurology,*

Neurosurgery & Psychiatry, *77*, 668–670. http://dx.doi.org/10.1136/jnnp.2005.073403

Roos, R. A. C. (2010). Huntington's disease: A clinical review. *Orphanet Journal of Rare Diseases*, *5*, 40. http://dx.doi.org/10.1186/1750-1172-5-40

Ross, C. A., Pantelyat, A., Kogan, J., & Brandt, J. (2014). Determinants of functional disability in Huntington's disease: Role of cognitive and motor dysfunction. *Movement Disorders*, *29*, 1351–1358. http://dx.doi.org/10.1002/mds.26012

Rosti, E., Hämäläinen, P., Koivisto, K., & Hokkanen, L. (2007). PASAT in detecting cognitive impairment in relapsing-remitting MS. *Applied Neuropsychology*, *14*, 101–112. http://dx.doi.org/10.1080/09084280701319938

Rowland, L. P., & Shneider, N. A. (2001). Amyotrophic lateral sclerosis. *The New England Journal of Medicine*, *344*, 1688–1700. http://dx.doi.org/10.1056/NEJM200105313442207

Rudnicki, S. A., & Fewell, D. (2007). The Cambridge Behavior Inventory in evaluating frontotemporal function in patients with motor neuron disease. *Amyotrophic Lateral Sclerosis*, *8*(Suppl. 1), 27–28.

Sabatini, U., Pozzilli, C., Pantano, P., Koudriavtseva, T., Padovani, A., Millefiorini, E., . . . Lenzi, G. L. (1996). Involvement of the limbic system in multiple sclerosis patients with depressive disorders. *Biological Psychiatry*, *39*, 970–975.

Sanchez, P., Pena, J., Bengoetxea, E., Ojeda, N., Elizagarate, E., Ezcurra, J., & Gutierrez, M. (2014). Improvements in negative symptoms and functional outcome after a new generation cognitive remediation program: A randomized controlled trial. *Schizophrenia Bulletin*, *40*, 707–715. http://dx.doi.org/10.1093/schbul/sbt057

Schiffer, R. B., & Wineman, N. M. (1990). Antidepressant pharmacotherapy of depression associated with multiple sclerosis. *The American Journal of Psychiatry*, *147*, 1493–1497. http://dx.doi.org/10.1176/ajp.147.11.1493

Schultheis, M. T., Garay, E., & DeLuca, J. (2001). The influence of cognitive impairment on driving performance in multiple sclerosis. *Neurology*, *56*, 1089–1094. http://dx.doi.org/10.1212/WNL.56.8.1089

Shiwach, R. S., & Patel, V. (1993). Aggressive behaviour in Huntington's disease: A cross-sectional study in a nursing home population. *Behavioural Neurology*, *6*, 43–47. http://dx.doi.org/10.1155/1993/424032

Simpson, J., Lekwuwa, G., & Crawford, T. (2014). Predictors of quality of life in people with Parkinson's disease: Evidence for both domain specific and general relationships. *Disability and Rehabilitation*, *36*, 1964–1970. http://dx.doi.org/10.3109/09638288.2014.883442

Staples, D., & Lincoln, N. B. (1979). Intellectual impairment in multiple sclerosis and its relation to functional abilities. *Rheumatology and Rehabilitation*, *18*, 153–160. http://dx.doi.org/10.1093/rheumatology/18.3.153

Stegemöller, E. L., Nocera, J., Malaty, I., Shelley, M., Okun, M. S., Hass, C. J., & the NPF Quality Improvement Initiative Investigators. (2014). Timed up and go, cognitive, and quality-of-life correlates in Parkinson's disease. *Archives of Physical Medicine and Rehabilitation*, *95*, 649–655. http://dx.doi.org/10.1016/j.apmr.2013.10.031

Stout, J. C., Glikmann-Johnston, Y., & Andrews, S. (2016). Cognitive assessment strategies in Huntington's disease research. *Journal of Neuroscience Methods*, *265*, 19–24. Retrieved from https://www.ncbi.nlm.nih.gov/pubmed/26719240

Stout, J. C., Paulsen, J. S., Queller, S., Solomon, A. C., Whitlock, K. B., Campbell, J. C., . . . Aylward, E. H. (2011). Neurocognitive signs in prodromal Huntington disease. *Neuropsychology*, *25*, 1–14. http://dx.doi.org/10.1037/a0020937

Stout, J. C., Queller, S., Baker, K. N., Cowlishaw, S., Sampaio, C., Fitzer-Attas, C., Borowsky, B., & the HD-CAB Investigators. (2014). HD–CAB: A cognitive assessment battery for clinical trials in Huntington's disease. *Movement Disorders*, *29*, 1281–1288. http://dx.doi.org/10.1002/mds.25964

Stout, J. C., Ready, R. E., Grace, J., Malloy, P. F., & Paulsen, J. S. (2003). Factor analysis of the Frontal Systems Behavior Scale (FrSBe). *Assessment*, *10*, 79–85. http://dx.doi.org/10.1177/1073191102250339

Stout, J. C., Rodawalt, W. C., & Siemers, E. R. (2001). Risky decision making in Huntington's disease. *Journal of the International Neuropsychological Society*, *7*, 92–101. http://dx.doi.org/10.1017/S1355617701711095

Strong, M. J., Grace, G. M., Orange, J. B., Leeper, H. A., Menon, R. S., & Aere, C. (1999). A prospective study of cognitive impairment in ALS. *Neurology*, *53*, 1665–1670. http://dx.doi.org/10.1212/WNL.53.8.1665

Tacchino, A., Pedullà, L., Bonzano, L., Vassallo, C., Battaglia, M. A., Mancardi, G., . . . Brichetto, G. (2015). A new app for at-home cognitive training: Description and pilot testing on patients with multiple sclerosis. *JMIR mHealth and uHealth*, *3*, e85. http://dx.doi.org/10.2196/mhealth.4269

Taylor, L., Wicks, P., Leigh, P. N., & Goldstein, L. H. (2010). Prevalence of depression in amyotrophic lateral sclerosis and other motor disorders. *European Journal of Neurology*, *17*, 1047–1053. http://dx.doi.org/10.1111/j.1468-1331.2010.02960.x

Toh, E. A., MacAskill, M. R., Dalrymple-Alford, J. C., Myall, D. J., Livingston, L., Macleod, S. A. D., & Anderson, T. J. (2014). Comparison of cognitive and UHDRS measures in monitoring disease progression in Huntington's disease: A 12-month longitudinal study. *Translational Neurodegeneration*, *3*, 15. http://dx.doi.org/10.1186/2047-9158-3-15

Trapp, B. D., Peterson, J., Ransohoff, R. M., Rudick, R., Mörk, S., & Bö, L. (1998). Axonal transection in the lesions of multiple sclerosis. *The New England Journal of Medicine*, *338*, 278–285. http://dx.doi.org/10.1056/NEJM199801293380502

Troster, A. I., & Fields, J. A. (2008). Parkinson's disease and related disorders of a frontostriatal system (pp. 536–577). In J. Morgan & J. Ricker (Eds.), *Textbook of clinical neuropsychology*. New York, NY: Taylor & Francis.

Troster, A. I., Fields, J. A., & Koller, W. C. (2000). Parkinson's disease and Parkinsonism. In C. E. Coffey & J. L. Cummings (Eds.), *Textbook of geriatric neuropsychiatry* (2nd ed., pp. 559–600). Washington, DC: American Psychiatric Press.

Tsujimoto, M., Senda, J., Ishihara, T., Niimi, Y., Kawai, Y., Atsuta, N., . . . Sobue, G. (2011). Behavioral changes in early ALS correlate with voxel-based morphometry and diffusion tensor imaging. *Journal of the Neurological Sciences*, *307*, 34–40. http://dx.doi.org/10.1016/j.jns.2011.05.025

Van den Berg, J. P., Kalmijn, S., Lindeman, E., Veldink, J. H., de Visser, M., Van der Graaff, M. M., . . . Van den Berg, L. H. (2005). Multidisciplinary ALS care improves quality of life in patients with ALS. *Neurology*, *65*, 1264–1267. http://dx.doi.org/10.1212/01.wnl.0000180717.29273.12

van Duijn, E., Craufurd, D., Hubers, A. A., Giltay, E. J., Bonelli, R., Rickards, H., . . . Landwehrmeyer, G. B., & the European Huntington's Disease Network Behavioural Phenotype Working Group. (2014). Neuropsychiatric symptoms in a European Huntington's disease cohort (REGISTRY). *Journal of Neurology, Neurosurgery & Psychiatry*, *85*, 1411–1418. http://dx.doi.org/10.1136/jnnp-2013-307343

van Straten, A., Geraedts, A., Verdonck-de Leeuw, I., Andersson, G., & Cuijpers, P. (2010). Psychological treatment of depressive symptoms in patients with medical disorders: A meta-analysis. *Journal of Psychosomatic Research*, *69*, 23–32. http://dx.doi.org/10.1016/j.jpsychores.2010.01.019

Vitale, C., Pellecchia, M. T., Grossi, D., Fragassi, N., Cuomo, T., Di Maio, L., & Barone, P. (2001). Unawareness of dyskinesias in Parkinson's and Huntington's diseases. *Neurological Sciences*, *22*, 105–106. http://dx.doi.org/10.1007/s100720170066

Vleugels, L., Lafosse, C., van Nunen, A., Nachtergaele, S., Ketelaer, P., Charlier, M., & Vandenbussche, E. (2000). Visuoperceptual impairment in multiple sclerosis patients diagnosed with neuropsychological tasks. *Multiple Sclerosis*, *6*, 241–254. http://dx.doi.org/10.1177/135245850000600406

Vogt, A., Kappos, L., Calabrese, P., Stöcklin, M., Gschwind, L., Opwis, K., & Penner, I. K. (2009). Working memory training in patients with multiple sclerosis—Comparison of two different training schedules. *Restorative Neurology and Neuroscience*, *27*, 225–235.

Walcott, F. L., Dunn, B. K., DeShields, M., & Baquet, C. (2014). The Affordable Care Act and genetic testing for inheritable cancer syndromes: Impact on high-risk underserved minorities. *Journal of Health Care for the Poor and Underserved*, *25*(Suppl.), 46–62. http://dx.doi.org/10.1353/hpu.2014.0070

Walker, F. O. (2007). Huntington's disease. *The Lancet*, *369*, 218–228. http://dx.doi.org/10.1016/S0140-6736(07)60111-1

Wang, J. L., Reimer, M. A., Metz, L. M., & Patten, S. B. (2000). Major depression and quality of life in individuals with multiple sclerosis. *International Journal of Psychiatry in Medicine*, *30*, 309–317. http://dx.doi.org/10.2190/PGWT-UXJ0-7UEH-LGRY

Watermeyer, T. J., Hindle, J. V., Roberts, J., Lawrence, C. L., Martyr, A., Lloyd-Williams, H., . . . Clare, L. (2016). Goal setting for cognitive rehabilitation in mild to moderate Parkinson's disease dementia and dementia with Lewy bodies. *Parkinson's Disease*, *2016*, 8285041. http://dx.doi.org/10.1155/2016/8285041

Watkins, L. H. A., Rogers, R. D., Lawrence, A. D., Sahakian, B. J., Rosser, A. E., & Robbins, T. W. (2000). Impaired planning but intact decision making in early Huntington's disease: Implications for specific fronto-striatal pathology. *Neuropsychologia*, *38*, 1112–1125. http://dx.doi.org/10.1016/S0028-3932(00)00028-2

Watson, G. S., Cholerton, B. A., Gross, R. G., Weintraub, D., Zabetian, C. P., Trojanowski, J. Q., . . . Leverenz, J. B., & the Udall Centers of Excellence for Parkinson's Disease Research at the University of Pennsylvania and the University of Washington. (2013). Neuropsychologic assessment in collaborative Parkinson's disease research: A proposal from the National Institute of Neurological Disorders and Stroke Morris K. *Alzheimer's & Dementia*, *9*, 609–614. http://dx.doi.org/10.1016/j.jalz.2012.07.006

Weintraub, D., Newberg, A. B., Cary, M. S., Siderowf, A. D., Moberg, P. J., Kleiner-Fisman, G., . . . Katz, I. R. (2005). Striatal dopamine transporter imaging correlates with anxiety and depression symptoms in Parkinson's disease. *Journal of Nuclear Medicine*, *46*, 227–232.

Woolley, S. C., York, M. K., Moore, D. H., Strutt, A. M., Murphy, J., Schulz, P. E., & Katz, J. S. (2010). Detecting frontotemporal dysfunction in ALS: Utility of the ALS Cognitive Behavioral Screen (ALS–CBS). *Amyotrophic Lateral Sclerosis*, *11*, 303–311. http://dx.doi.org/10.3109/17482961003727954

Young, A. B., Penney, J. B., Starosta-Rubinstein, S., Markel, D. S., Berent, S., Giordani, B., . . . Hichwa, R. (1986). PET scan investigations of Huntington's disease: Cerebral metabolic correlates of neurological features and functional decline. *Annals of Neurology*, *20*, 296–303. http://dx.doi.org/10.1002/ana.410200305

Zigmond, A. S., & Snaith, R. P. (1983). The hospital anxiety and depression scale (HADS). *Acta Psychiatrica Scandinavica*, *67*, 361–370.

Zinzi, P., Salmaso, D., De Grandis, R., Graziani, G., Maceroni, S., Bentivoglio, A., . . . Jacopini, G. (2007). Effects of an intensive rehabilitation programme on patients with Huntington's disease: A pilot study. *Clinical Rehabilitation*, *21*, 603–613. http://dx.doi.org/10.1177/0269215507075495

CHAPTER 20

NEURODEVELOPMENTAL DISORDERS

Kerri P. Nowell, Kimberly E. Bodner, Michael D. Mohrland, and Stephen M. Kanne

Neurodevelopmental disorders comprise a broad spectrum of conditions that affect a child's brain and nervous system and are similar in that they present in early development. Although symptom presentation may certainly change and even remit to varying degrees over the lifespan, all neurodevelopmental disorders are characterized by developmental deficits that impact functioning in personal, social, academic, and occupational arenas.

By some estimates, neurodevelopmental disorders affect approximately 15% of individuals aged 3 to 17 years in the United States (Boyle et al., 2011); therefore, it is important for rehabilitation psychologists to understand core symptoms and co-occurring difficulties associated with neurodevelopmental disabilities. The overarching goal of this chapter is to increase rehabilitation psychologists' awareness of various considerations when working with individuals who have neurodevelopmental disabilities, using autism spectrum disorder (ASD) as a model. An illustrative case study involving an individual with ASD is provided at the end of the chapter. Although not specifically in a rehabilitation setting, this case study demonstrates how ASD affects both evaluation and treatment planning.

The *Diagnostic and Statistical Manual of Mental Disorders* (fifth edition [*DSM–5*]; American Psychiatric Association, 2013) identifies seven categories of neurodevelopmental disorders including intellectual disabilities, communication disorders, ASD, attention-deficit/hyperactivity disorder (ADHD), specific learning disorders, motor disorders, and "other neurodevelopmental disorders." Generally, neurodevelopmental disorders interfere with development in areas such as communication, social interactions, learning, executive functioning, and motor skills beginning in childhood. Difficulties associated with neurodevelopmental disorders may persist into adulthood. An in-depth study of each category of neurodevelopmental disorders is beyond the scope of this chapter; however, the *DSM–5* provides thorough descriptions of these disorders for reference. For further discussion of developmental perspectives in rehabilitation psychology, see Chapter 11, this volume.

NEURODEVELOPMENTAL DISORDERS IN REHABILITATION PSYCHOLOGY: AUTISM SPECTRUM DISORDER AS A MODEL

The primary focus of this chapter is ASD, a neurodevelopmental disorder characterized by deficits in social-communication and restricted, repetitive behaviors. Specifically, an individual with ASD may have deficits in general problem-solving, adaptive skills, and communication. Deficits in executive functioning, difficulties maintaining attention, and high levels of impulsivity and hyperactivity are also commonly encountered. A diagnosis of ASD is also often accompanied by developmental motor coordination difficulties, stereotyped movements, and academic difficulties. Given the multidimensional

http://dx.doi.org/10.1037/0000129-021
Handbook of Rehabilitation Psychology, Third Edition, L. A. Brenner, S. A. Reid-Arndt, T. R. Elliott, R. G. Frank, and B. Caplan (Editors-in-Chief)

symptoms, ASD presents an ideal model to consider how neurodevelopmental disorders may influence an individual's functioning and, in particular, the work of rehabilitation psychologists.

Rehabilitation psychologists are highly likely to encounter individuals with ASD in their practice. ASD is an increasingly common disorder and currently estimated to occur in one in 59 individuals (Baio et al., 2018). The increase in ASD is thought to be a reflection of improved methods of identification, increased availability of diagnostic services, and changes in conceptualization of the ASD over time (for an in-depth discussion see Saracino et al., 2010).

ASD also illustrates the costs, barriers, and burden of care to individuals and families that often accompany neurodevelopmental disorders. The costs, both emotional and financial, associated with caring for an individual with ASD are significant (Johnson & Rodriguez, 2013; Murphy et al., 2016). ASD is a lifelong disorder, and individuals with ASD face substantial needs related to core symptoms and associated difficulties across their lifespan. Children with ASD attend more health care visits, need more time during visits, are more likely to be hospitalized, and have longer hospital stays than typically developing individuals (see the systematic review by Johnson & Rodriguez, 2013).

INDIVIDUAL-BASED CONSIDERATIONS

For an individual, ASD-related symptoms and comorbidities often create challenges in providing and receiving care, which may be further exacerbated in rehabilitation settings. The core symptoms of ASD include communication challenges and behavioral difficulties that often impact the evaluation, identification, and treatment of rehabilitation needs. Furthermore, at the individual level, several additional areas may interfere with outcomes and need to be considered in development of appropriate acute and long-term treatment plans. These include sensory differences, wandering and elopement, problems with sleep, and family dynamics.

Core ASD Symptoms

Conceptualized as a single disorder, ASD is diagnosed based on the presence of behavioral characteristics occurring in two domains: social communication and restricted repetitive behaviors and interests (American Psychiatric Association, 2013). Deficits in social communication may include a deficit in social-emotional reciprocity (e.g., failure to share interests, emotions, or affect with others), a deficit in nonverbal behaviors in social interactions (e.g., poor modulation of eye contact or gestures with verbal communication), or deficits in relationships (e.g., absence of interest in peers, difficulties adjusting behaviors across social contexts). Restrictive, repetitive behavioral symptoms include repetitive movements, unusual/circumscribed interests, insistence on sameness, and sensory concerns.

Best practice evaluations for diagnosis consist of interviews with caregivers, review of records, and careful consideration of developmental information. Interviews may be informal or standardized, but regardless of the format (i.e., informal or standardized), interviews should be structured to address key areas specific to ASD including past and current behaviors related to social-communication and restricted, repetitive behaviors and developmental history. In addition, observation of and interaction with the individual should occur with particular attention to social-communication and restricted, repetitive behaviors. Although observation can be completed without the use of a formal observation measure, use of such a measure increases diagnostic accuracy. Examples of screening measures, formal interview and observation measures are included in Table 20.1.

Associated Medical Conditions

Some medical conditions are more commonly experienced in individuals with ASD. A high percentage of individuals with ASD have associated medical concerns, including seizures and gastrointestinal difficulties. Of note, between 11% and 39% of individuals develop epilepsy, with an age of onset in the early teenage years (Kohane et al., 2012). If the underlying genetic etiology can be identified, there are often other phenotypic factors associated with a syndrome that should be taken into account. Obviously, these conditions can have a large impact on any rehabilitation program because they can directly affect health and ability to participate, as well as have implications if not addressed appropriately.

TABLE 20.1

Examples of Commonly Used Diagnostic and Assessment Instruments

Category	Instrument	Age range
Screening	Modified Checklist for Autism in Toddlers, Revised, With Follow-Up (Robins, Fein, & Barton, 2009)	16–30 months
	Social Communication Questionnaire (Rutter, Bailey, & Lord, 2003)	4 years–adult
	Social Responsiveness Scale (2nd ed; Constantino & Gruber, 2012)	2 years, 6 months–adult
Diagnosis	Autism Diagnostic Interview—Revised (Rutter, LeCouteur, & Lord, 2003)	2 years–adult
	Autism Diagnostic Observation Schedule (2nd ed.; Lord et al., 2012)	2 years–adult
	Childhood Autism Rating Scale (2nd ed.; Schopler & Bourgondien, 2010)	2 years–adult
Cognitive/developmental	Mullen Scales of Early Learning (Mullen, 1995)	Birth–68 months
	Bayley Scales of Infant Development (3rd ed.; Bayley, 2005)	1–42 months
	Differential Abilities Scale (2nd ed.; Elliott, 2007)	2 years, 6 months–17 years, 11 months
	Wechsler Preschool and Primary Scale of Intelligence (4th ed.; Wechsler, 2014)	2 years, 6 months–7 years, 7 months
	Leiter International Performance Scale (3rd ed.; Roid, Miller, Pomplun, & Koch, 2013)	3 years–adult
Language	Clinical Evaluation of Language Fundamentals (5th ed.; Wiig, Semel, & Secord, 2013)	5–21 years
	Peabody Picture Vocabulary Test (4th ed.; Dunn & Dunn, 2007)	2 years, 6 months–adult
	Expressive One Word Picture Vocabulary Test (4th ed.; Martin & Brownell, 2011)	2–18 years
Adaptive skills	Vineland Adaptive Behavior Scales (3rd ed.; Sparrow, Cicchetti, & Saulnier, 2016)	Birth–adult
	Adaptive Behavior Assessment System (3rd ed.; Harrison & Oakland, 2015)	Birth–adult
Executive functioning	Delis–Kaplan Executive Function System (Delis, Kaplan, & Kramer, 2001)	8 years–adult
	Behavior Rating Inventory of Executive Function (Gioia, Isquith, Guy, & Kenworthy, 2013)	5–18 years
Emotional-behavioral	Behavior Assessment System for Children (3rd ed.; Reynolds & Kamphaus, 2015)	2 years–college age
	Achenbach Child Behavior Checklist (Achenbach, 1991)	6–18 years

Intellectual Functioning

Rehabilitation psychologists should consider the level of intellectual functioning for an individual with ASD because core symptoms are interpreted in the context of the individual's developmental level, and ASD frequently co-occurs with intellectual disability. ASD is a remarkably heterogeneous disorder, and individuals may present with superior intellectual functioning skills or have significant intellectual functioning deficits. In the past, the majority of those with ASD were thought to have overall intellectual functioning (IQ) abilities in the impaired range, but this is no longer considered to be true. Currently, it is estimated that intellectual disability occurs in approximately 50% of individuals with ASD (Volkmar et al., 2014). Specific assessment of intellectual functioning is considered essential to acute and long-term intervention planning because intellectual functioning is a strong predictor of long-term functioning (cf. Howlin, Goode, Hutton, & Rutter, 2004). However, given the impact on social interaction, language, and motor skills in ASD, results from an IQ test often need to be interpreted with some caution. In particular, the presence of a language disorder may create a significant discrepancy that clouds the interpretation of the full-scale IQ, suggesting that the nonverbal IQ may be the better estimate. Examples of evidence-based intellectual assessment instruments are listed in Table 20.1.

Language and Communication

Rehabilitation psychologists should also consider barriers related to language and communication when working with an individual with ASD. Delays and difficulties in communication are a core feature of ASD. These deficits transcend receptive and expressive language difficulties and include nonverbal communication (e.g., gestures, eye contact, facial expressions) as well as the social nuances of language often referred to as *language pragmatics* (e.g., inferences, meaning). Language abilities may range from a complete lack of verbal–vocal communication abilities to intact conversational speech and may include atypical language characteristics such as stereotyped, idiosyncratic, and repetitive speech (e.g., echolalia, scripted speech; American Psychiatric Association, 2013). In addition to exhibiting characteristic social-communication symptoms, individuals may also meet criteria for language disorder or speech sound disorder. Although language may be delayed, recent studies have shown that the majority of individuals with ASD achieve some functional language (Wodka, Mathy, & Kalb, 2013).

There are several tools commonly used to assess language that range from comprehensive to brief assessments that supply a snapshot of functioning (see Table 20.1). Individuals with ASD may also have difficulties making inferences, especially those related to emotional understanding (Bodner, Engelhardt, Minshew, & Williams, 2015) and may be quite literal in interpretation of language (Loukusa et al., 2007). Rehabilitation psychologists should be aware of clients' language abilities to facilitate the best methods of conducting interviews, interventions, and providing recommendations for future treatments. Furthermore, rehabilitation psychologists should adjust their own communication style to meet the needs of clients and families and confirm understanding by clients and caregivers. In cases of more severe language impairments, the use of assistive communication devices, such as an iPad with supporting applications (e.g., Proloquo2Go) or the Picture Exchange Communication System, may be necessary to effectively communicate with clients (Hill & Flores, 2014).

Adaptive Skills

Adaptive skills have obvious relevance to rehabilitation, as this is typically an area of focus with regard to specific programs. Standardized measures of adaptive behavior (see Table 20.1) have several benefits over a functional interview or observation alone because they offer standardized documentation of impairment and disability, objective strengths and weaknesses profiles, data that meets requirements for eligibility of some services, and objective means of developing treatment goals.

Several researchers have demonstrated that adaptive skills in individuals with ASD, although strongly associated with assessed level of IQ, vary independently (Kanne et al., 2011). That is, a very bright individual with ASD as assessed through IQ may still have significant difficulty with everyday living skills. It would not be uncommon for an individual with ASD to have significant adaptive deficits that are preexisting and associated with his or her diagnosis of ASD. Consequently, rehabilitation psychologists may find that typical interventions used to increase adaptive skills are less effective than with other populations of individuals, and as such, modifications to interventions may be necessary.

Executive Functioning

Executive functioning encompasses processes such as response selection, initiation, execution, and monitoring and is often significant area of weakness for individuals with ASD. These deficits are evident to the degree that some researchers have posited this as one of the underlying core deficits and suggest that these deficits account for many of the functional difficulties observed (Happé, Booth, Charlton, & Hughes, 2006; Pellicano, 2012). Individuals with ASD often have difficulty with aspects of mental flexibility, inhibition, working memory, and planning. Further, two foundational constructs have been proposed that place executive dysfunction as a core component of ASD including *central coherence* (contextual information processing) and *theory of mind* (attribution of mental states; Beaumont & Newcombe, 2006; Happé et al., 2006; Pellicano, 2012). Deficits in executive functioning can also result in difficulties related to transitions, organization, engagement, and following multistep instructions.

As rehabilitation psychologists are aware, performance-based testing (see examples in Table 20.1) compared to real-world demonstration of executive functions are often not as strongly related as one would think. Using both assessment methods is preferred. Also, collaborative information (e.g., self, parent, and teacher checklists) provides a more comprehensive picture of executive function skills. Similar to adaptive functioning, rehabilitation designed to address executive deficits may be less effective due to preexisting challenges in this area. With regard to treatment and intervention, there is minimal research assessing intervention specific to executive dysfunction in ASD. A school-based research curriculum has been published targeting flexibility and goal-focused executive functions, and results of that program appear promising (Cannon, Kenworthy, Alexander, Werner, & Anthony, 2011). Also, visual supports are considered to meet evidence-based criteria and can be used to address many difficulties associated with executive functioning deficits (Knight, Sartini, & Spriggs, 2015).

Challenging Behaviors

Individuals with ASD often have concomitant behaviors that are either part of the core features or ancillary and are impactful to a rehabilitation program. An individual with ASD may exhibit a range of problematic behaviors, including aggression, self-injurious behaviors, or self-stimulatory and repetitive behaviors. Those with ASD often have extremely rigid behaviors that may also be problematic to a rehabilitation program. In addition, behavioral symptoms associated with deficits in attention, executive functioning, and activity level commonly co-occur, with 30% to 80% of children with ASD also meeting the diagnostic criteria for ADHD (Rommelse, Franke, Geurts, Hartman, & Buitelaar, 2010). In their systematic review, Johnson and Rodriguez (2013) highlighted four behavioral domains that were noted to be barriers to medical treatment of children with ASD: noncompliance, hyperactive, self-stimulatory, and self-injurious behaviors. Such challenging behaviors may be associated with multiple factors, such as difficulties with change, communication difficulties, and medical factors, among others. For example, difficulties with change or transitions may lead to client anxiety, noncompliance, aggression, and inattention.

Interventions based on behavioral principles (i.e., applied behavior analysis [ABA]) are supported by significant scientific evidence in the treatment of behavioral difficulties for individuals with ASD (cf. Missouri Autism Guidelines Initiative, 2012). Such interventions can range from environmental modifications (i.e., antecedent modifications), such as visual schedules, timers, warnings before transitions, and increased structure in the environment, to intensive, individualized approaches, such as discrete trial training or functional communication training. Recommendations for behavioral intervention may include the development of a behavioral intervention plan to be implemented by providers across settings. Teaching caregivers how to structure the environment, issue commands, and follow through with appropriate consequences (designed to increase appropriate behaviors and decrease inappropriate, problematic behaviors) is particularly important for individuals with ASD.

Internalizing Behaviors and Emotional Concerns

Mental health needs are greater in individuals with ASD compared with the general population, with many individuals experiencing comorbid emotional difficulties (Strang et al., 2012). Symptoms of anxiety and depression are the most commonly experienced emotional comorbidities (Mayes, Calhoun, Murray, Ahuja, & Smith, 2011; Strang et al., 2012). Subclinical-to-clinical levels of anxious symptoms are estimated to occur in approximately 50% to 80% of children with ASD (Mayes et al., 2011; Strang et al., 2012), depressive symptoms are estimated to occur in 40% to 55%, and suicidal ideation is estimated to occur in 14% of children with ASD (Mayes, Gorman, Hillwig-Garcia, & Syed, 2013). Importantly, emotional comorbidities are thought to impact life functioning and exacerbate existing core ASD symptoms (Strang et al., 2012), and they are likely to persist into adulthood.

Rehabilitation psychologists working with individuals with ASD should be aware of the high base rate of mental health needs, particularly anxiety and depression, compared with the general population. Screening for anxiety and depression is important because if symptoms are present, they will affect outcomes and will need to be considered when developing treatment plans. Factors such as an individual's age and level of insight may help or hinder identification of needs related to such difficulties. Depending on the results of broadband measures (see Table 20.1), follow-up assessment using narrow-band measures (e.g., Multidimensional Anxiety Scale for Children, second edition [March, 2013]; Children's Depression Inventory 2 [Kovacs, 2011]) may be warranted.

Evidence-based treatment approaches to emotional difficulties such as depression or anxiety are dependent on the individual's age and level of functioning. For example, cognitive behavior therapy with direct instruction of social skills can be effective in the treatment of anxiety and depression for higher functioning individuals (Sukhodolsky, Bloch, Panza, & Reichow, 2013). Modifications to traditional cognitive behavior therapy approaches (e.g., using concrete, visual strategies; incorporating the individual's interests) may result in more positive outcomes (Wood et al., 2009).

Sensory

Hyper- or hyporeactivity to sensory input is quite prevalent in individuals with ASD, affecting more than 90% of diagnosed individuals to some degree (Marco, Hinkley, Hill, & Nagarajan, 2011). Sensory abnormalities may manifest in diverse ways, including seeking out sensory input (e.g., smelling, licking, and visual inspection) or avoiding sensory input (e.g., overwhelmed by touch, noise, or motion). Sensory processing abnormalities may exacerbate social-communication deficits, and contribute to challenging behaviors, distress, anxiety, avoidance, and even self-injury exhibited by individuals with ASD. Rehabilitation psychologists should explore potential sensory barriers because they may have a profound impact on their clients' abilities to receive treatments (Leekam, Nieto, Libby, Wing, & Gould, 2007; Marco et al., 2011) and how they react to their environment.

Some controversy exists with regard to how best to address behavioral difficulties (e.g., self-injury, stereotyped behaviors, sensory aversions) that appear to be associated with sensory interests or aversions. In particular, sensory integration therapy (SIT) is commonly recommended and used by occupational therapists. The goal of SIT is to improve the individual's ability to process sensory information and, thus, exhibit decreased rates of behavioral difficulties (Devlin, Leader, & Healy, 2009; Lang et al., 2012). Although therapists frequently use this approach, there is minimal evidence supporting it as an efficacious treatment, and in fact, implementing such an approach may result in increased rates of problem behavior (Lang et al., 2012). Consequently, behavioral approaches and treatments that involve modification of the individual's environment (e.g., providing noise-cancelling headphones, minimizing the use of fluorescent lights) appear to be most appropriate.

Safety

Individuals with ASD are at risk of physical harm due to elopement behaviors (Anderson et al., 2012; Kiely, Migdal, Vettam, & Adesman, 2016), with 30% to 50% of children with ASD exhibiting these behaviors. Thus, rehabilitation psychologists may encounter clients entering their care as a result of injuries sustained from elopement (e.g., wandered into traffic, near-drowning), or clients may be an acute elopement risk while under their care (Anderson et al., 2012; McIlwain & Fournier, 2010). Consequently, the frequency of elopement behaviors should be systematically assessed. Preventative programming is an important first step for an individual at risk of elopement. In addition to ensuring that the environment is secure (e.g., appropriate locks on doors and windows) plans may include wearing of alarms or monitoring devices.

Sleep Difficulties

Sleep concerns (e.g., trouble falling and staying asleep) are common, as approximately 40% to 80% of individuals with ASD have co-occurring sleep difficulties (cf. Cohen, Conduit, Lockley, Rajaratnam, & Cornish, 2014; Reynolds & Malow, 2011). Lack of quality sleep can lead to an increase in challenging behaviors, such as inattentiveness, aggression, and noncompliance (Cohen et al., 2014; Mazurek & Sohl, 2016) and may be associated with difficulties in daytime cognitive and adaptive functioning (Taylor, Schreck, & Mulick, 2012). Rehabilitation psychologists may facilitate recovery by identifying and treating underlying sleep disorders in clients with ASD in conjunction with the primary focus of treatment (Vriend, Corkum, Moon, & Smith, 2011).

SYSTEMS-LEVEL CONSIDERATIONS

Beyond the level of the individual, rehabilitation psychologists should consider systems-level factors that may impact their client's acute and long-term functioning. Some of the most relevant systems-level issues include family-dynamics, transition, advocacy, and vocational goals for individuals with ASD.

Family Dynamics

Family members of individuals with ASD play a large role in their care, especially if the clients have cognitive or language impairments. In addition to the typical responsibilities associated with parenting, caregivers of people with ASD are a vital resource to inform clinical interviews, complete questionnaires, and assist in executing treatment recommendations for clients. The emotional and financial burden associated with caring for a person with ASD results in significant stress and challenges (Vogan et al., 2014), and parents of children with ASD are at increased risk for mental health problems (Ingersoll & Hambrick, 2011). Family quality of life may be particularly affected when an individual has more significant deficits in daily living skills (Gardiner & Iarocci, 2015). Providers working with families should consider the supports available to caregivers including availability of respite services and make recommendations to address those needs as appropriate.

Biological parents of individuals with ASD are more likely to present with subclinical symptoms associated with ASD as a result of the high heritability of ASD, often termed the broader autism phenotype. The etiology of ASD is most often considered to be multifactorial and is thought to be the result of a complex interaction between genes (i.e., gene–gene interactions) and between genes and the environment (Murphy et al., 2016). Although no single gene has been identified as causal or relevant for all cases of ASD, the disorder has an estimated heritability of about 50% (De Rubeis & Buxbaum, 2015), and parents of individuals with ASD are more likely to exhibit mild features of ASD associated with rigidity, aloofness, few friendships, and oversensitivity to criticism (Piven et al., 1997). Consequently, providers may need to adjust their communication style or make accommodations for family members who show these features.

Education

Individuals with ASD are protected under several federal legislative statutes over the course of their lifespan, and, consistent with the competencies outlined for rehabilitation psychologists (see Chapter 1, this volume), understanding those statutes is an essential component of providing effective care. Children between 3 and 21 years of age with a diagnosis of ASD may be eligible to receive supports and services via special education under the eligibility category of autism.

Importantly, a medical diagnosis of ASD is neither necessary nor sufficient to meet special education eligibility criteria, a fact that can be confusing for families who are attempting to secure appropriate services for their child. Furthermore, although schools are required to consider outside evaluations and recommendations that may be relevant to establishing an individualized education program (IEP), there is considerable variation across school districts as to how much weight is given to evaluations completed by outside professionals. Diagnoses that are completed using best practice procedures and are accompanied by an evaluation report detailing how final diagnostic decisions were made will likely be most helpful to schools. If a school determines that a student is not eligible for special education service, he or she may still be eligible for accommodations with a medical diagnosis as protected by the Americans With Disabilities Act (ADA) under Section 504, which requires that all individuals have equal access to the general education curriculum (34 C.F.R. Part 104).

Transition Planning

For individuals with ASD, similar to many other conditions treated by rehabilitation psychologists, the process of transition from adolescent to adulthood spans years and can involve layers of varied agencies and service providers. From a systems perspective, individuals with ASD transition from a system of accommodations and services through the school system (as mandated and funded through the Individuals With Disabilities Education Act [IDEA]) where parents and school professionals play a primary role in advocacy, to a system of request, where vocational accommodations and services often rely more on the advocacy of the individual with ASD or delegates (supported through ADA and the Rehabilitation Act).

Effective transition planning takes into account adaptive functioning, degrees of independent living, and person-centered planning, and it informs vocational, postsecondary educational, medical, legal (e.g., guardianship), and financial planning arrangements. An updated neuropsychological evaluation before graduating high school is suggested to inform this process and document the needs required for optimal transitioning. It has been recommended that the transition process start by age 14, but this is not mandated under IDEA until age 16. There are several toolkits available to assist in this process (e.g., http://www.autismspeaks.org).

Vocational Preparation

Individuals with ASD are employed at lower rates compared with many other disabilities (Roux et al., 2013). The social-communication skill challenges and deficits in self-awareness (e.g., difficulties identifying personal strengths) make job selection and job interviews difficult for individuals with ASD. The odds of being employed with a disability are highest if there are strong parental expectations, a previous history of household responsibilities, stronger social skills, stronger self-care skills, and male gender (Carter et al., 2012).

Despite these challenges, individuals with ASD often have strengths that are desirable to employers, such as following rules, consistency, and attention to detail. As opposed to the traditional interview–hire–work timeline, various techniques and modifications (e.g., job training software, job previews, traveling interviews, trial work periods) have also shown promise with those who have ASD (Chen, Sung, & Pi, 2015; Seaman & Cannella-Malone, 2016). Vocational supports with individuals who have ASD have also shown benefit including job coaching and use of technology for teaching or training and cuing (Nicholas et al., 2015). Many other resources are available for both employees and employers supporting the hiring and supporting of individuals with ASD in the workforce (e.g., Autism Speaks, Job Accommodation Network website, National Governors Association).

Individuals with ASD, once identified, are afforded "reasonable accommodations" in the workplace as mandated through ADA. Recent ADA revisions require contractors to invite applicants to self-identify as an individual with a disability (in addition to inviting their present employees to self-identify every 5 years). These revisions emphasize self-disclosure because ASD and other conditions, such as traumatic brain injury, can present as "invisible disabilities." The issue of whether and when to disclose a disability is a dynamic process that takes various forms throughout one's lifetime and in different settings. For assistance in this process, the 411 on Disability Disclosure was developed (http://www.ncwd-youth.info).

CASE EXAMPLE: MATTHEW—ASD AND TRANSITION PLANNING

A case example is included in this section. Although the case was not seen in a formal rehabilitation setting, it illustrates the heterogeneous nature of ASD and demonstrates how a rehabilitation psychologist may consider each of the factors described in the preceding sections as they conceptualize a case, make recommendations, and design a treatment plan.

This case depicts Matthew, an 18-year-old Caucasian man, diagnosed with ASD, who had recently graduated from high school. Matthew was referred for a psychological evaluation by his primary care physician to assist with diagnostic clarification and transition planning. Matthew's case provides an example of a young adult with ASD, without significant intellectual functioning deficits but with myriad factors that must be considered.

Medical

Matthew's medical history includes a remote history of childhood epilepsy, since resolved. His history of ASD was thought to be the primary determinate in his current presentation and prognosis. Matthew was not taking any prescription medications at the time of the evaluation. Medication for ADHD had been prescribed in the past but Matthew preferred not to take medications.

Core ASD Symptoms

Matthew was first diagnosed with ASD in early childhood. His interpersonal presentation (verbal and nonverbal communication skills) for the present evaluation continued to be consistent with a diagnosis of ASD. In particular, he preferred staying at home playing video games rather than socializing, conversation topics would predictably gravitate toward his interest in particular television shows or movies, and he had great difficulty gauging the interest level of others in his interactions. This deficit in social perception was especially evident in interactions with female peers. Therefore, Matthew's established diagnosis of ASD continued to be evident, and core symptoms of ASD remained a barrier to social functioning.

Intellectual Functioning

Matthew's cognitive profile was mostly intact. When he was first diagnosed with ASD, his nonverbal intellect was assessed to be above average. At the present evaluation, the nonverbal domain remained above average. Working memory was a relative weakness, while academic skills and memory were within normal limits. Overall, given Matthew's relatively intact cognitive profile, the treating psychologists concluded that it was likely he would be able to learn new functional skills.

Language and Communication

Although language was not formally assessed, Matthew's functional use of language was below expected levels as conveyed via an adaptive behavior measure. Matthew did not appear to have deficits in word finding, vocabulary, articulation, or basic understanding of what he heard. Rather, his communication challenges were indicative of deficits in higher level conversational skills, social insight, and language pragmatics. As a result of his pragmatic language difficulties, recommendations accommodations in the vocational setting (e.g., provision of social scripts for communication with customers). Language therapy targeting social communication skills was also recommended.

Adaptive Skills

Consistent with his ASD diagnosis, Matthew had a history of adaptive skill deficits. At the time of the evaluation, his ability to complete everyday living tasks was quite low. He wanted a driver's license, but there was an agreement with his parents that he would first show them greater responsibility. Matthew participated in chores at home, and his father was working with him on money management, such as using a debit card; encouragingly, at the time of the evaluation, Matthew had not purchased more than he should. Standardized assessment revealed continued deficits in adaptive skills. In particular, he demonstrated weaknesses with inaccuracy in following a recipe, incorrectly calculating small change, and forgetfulness on a practical short-term memory task. Overall, Matthew exhibited underdeveloped functional life skills for his age and neurocognitive profile. To develop his functional adaptive life skills, occupational therapy and a life skills group, tailored to higher functioning young adults with ASD, was recommended.

Executive Functioning

Matthew exhibited deficits in aspects of attention and executive functioning, per parent-completed checklists. Cognitive flexibility was the most problematic executive function domain. Therefore, recommendations were provided for vocational accommodations (e.g., consistent workday schedule, advanced preparation for inevitable changes) and postsecondary educational accommodations (e.g., advanced provision of notes, assistance in understanding major concepts and big picture themes).

Problem Behaviors

In addition to ASD, Matthew had a prior diagnosis of ADHD. As noted earlier, Matthew had an intense interest in playing on his computer. Whenever his parents would tell him to take a break from the computer, Matthew would erupt, although this never came to the point of physical aggression. The results of psychological checklists completed by Matthew and his father were widely discrepant.

Matthew denied all symptoms of emotional distress and behavior dysregulation, while his father endorsed global clinical elevations in the mild–moderate clinical range.

Counseling was recommended for several treatment goals, including family communication, social skills, goal setting, and frustration tolerance. Specifically, therapy was recommended to improve Matthew's ability to communicate effectively with his parents regarding his own psychological state, to build his self-advocacy skills, and to help Matthew's parents understand Matthew's perspective. Counseling was also recommended as a means to clarify and implement Matthew's personal goals (e.g., driver's license) as well as problem solve alongside Matthew in negotiating with his parents regarding an appropriate balance of computer and other sedative activities.

Family Dynamics

Matthew lived at home with his parents. Although the evaluation revealed ineffective communication between Matthew and his parents, Matthew's parents were supportive and appropriately involved. Despite some disagreement, he and his parents shared the same overarching goal for Matthew, that of optimal functional independence. The team discussed specific family-related supports that Matthew would need as he transitioned into adulthood and provided the family with resources specific to transitioning, such as the Autism Transition Toolkit (http://www.autismspeaks.org/family-services/tool-kits/transition-tool-kit).

Vocational Preparation

Matthew's personal goals included obtaining a full-time job, and he had completed supervised custodial work while a senior in high school through the transition services offered via his IEP. Matthew was connected with the Division of Vocational Rehabilitation (DVR) and receiving Social Security benefits. However, since graduating high school, Matthew had remained at home, mostly playing games on the computer.

Matthew's parents reported that he had demonstrated a strong work ethic while completing his high school work experience. He enjoyed manual work, was interested in learning a particular trade, and had completed a preliminary course offered through a local vocational program. This vocational interest seemed a good fit given the minimal social interaction required, the ordering and arranging nature of the job, the methodical routine, the step-wise procedures, and the fact that it capitalized on his relative strength in visual reasoning. His parents were supportive of Matthew pursuing his trade interest.

The team recommended several services and accommodations that are provided through DVR, including provision of a job coach, communication assistance (e.g., provision of written and verbal communication, provision of scripts, minimization of communication demands in conflict situations), active monitoring of Matthew's stress level and environmental stimulation, a written schedule (e.g., consistent workday schedule, advanced preparation for schedule changes), assistance in learning new policies and procedures, small chunks of verbal information presented at a time, and minimization of distractions and multitasking. A list of vocational accommodations for individuals with ASD is provided at http://askjan.org.

Summary

The issues raised in Matthew's case primarily relate to transition and are common with many clients served by rehabilitation psychologists. The varied services required for optimal functional outcomes in ASD are similar to those required of many young adults with disabilities during the transition years. In addition, Matthew's case illustrates the impact of executive functioning and social skill impairments in an individual with ASD whose overall level of intellectual functioning is within normal limits. Rehabilitation psychologists are well situated to assist in identifying executive dysfunction deficits and recommend interventions or accommodations to maximize functioning. As a result of their training, they also recognize that individuals like Matthew often struggle as they attempt to develop a healthy identity while navigating a complex social world.

CONCLUSION

Rehabilitation psychologists will likely encounter individuals with neurodevelopmental disorders, and it is highly likely they will encounter an individual with an ASD diagnosis. An individual with a neurodevelopmental disorder has preexisting deficits that require consideration when developing a rehabilitation treatment plan, even though those deficits may not be a specific target of rehabilitation. Given the unique preexisting challenges for individuals with ASD, future research focusing on outcomes for rehabilitation clients with comorbid neurodevelopmental disorders is important. In particular, research investigating outcomes including rate of recovering and discharge, rates of reinjury, and resources devoted to rehabilitation is essential.

A rehabilitation psychologist is likely familiar with and received training in the use of the majority of assessment instruments described in this chapter. The exceptions are the ASD diagnostic tools. In particular, evidence-based instruments such as the Autism Diagnostic Observation Schedule—2 and Autism Diagnostic Interview—Revised (Rutter, LeCouteur, & Lord, 2003) require specific and sophisticated training in administration and interpretation. Similarly, best practice treatment recommendations overlap considerably with best practice treatments recommended for neurotypical individuals. However, for individuals with ASD, there is an emphasis on behaviorally based approaches. In particular, when developing interventions designed to target problem behaviors that manifest as a result of ASD symptoms, approaches based on ABA principles have the most evidential support.

Neurodevelopmental disorders result in specialized assessment and treatment planning considerations. As noted earlier, understanding how an individual presented before needing rehabilitation will be essential in the development of an appropriate treatment plan. Special considerations in ASD that also impact assessment and treatment planning include difficulties associated with core symptoms (e.g., social-communication deficits, restricted interests) as well as co-occurring difficulties (e.g., language deficits, sleeping difficulties) and require the rehabilitation psychologist to systematically consider how each of the domains described in this chapter might influence acute intervention as well as long-term goals.

Finally, working with individuals who are diagnosed with a neurodevelopmental disorder requires effective consultation skills. Rehabilitation psychologists need to communicate with experts in a variety of disciplines and across various systems of care to ensure that a client receives the most appropriate acute and long-term treatment. Developing the level of expertise required to understand the nuanced and idiosyncratic needs associated with all neurodevelopmental disorders is perhaps an unrealistic goal for most rehabilitation psychologists. However, as outlined in the standards of training of rehabilitation psychologists, developing expertise in the use of effective consultation, including cross-discipline consultation, is an expectation (Stiers et al., 2015; see also Chapter 6, this volume). The field of neurodevelopmental disabilities clearly highlights why this is an important expectation and an essential skill for rehabilitation psychologists.

References

Achenbach, T. M. (1991). *Achenbach Child Behavior Checklist and Teacher Report Form*. Burlington, VT: ASEBA.

American Psychiatric Association. (2013). *Diagnostic and statistical manual of mental disorders* (5th ed.). Washington, DC: Author.

Anderson, C., Law, J. K., Daniels, A., Rice, C., Mandell, D. S., Hagopian, L., & Law, P. A. (2012). Occurrence and family impact of elopement in children with autism spectrum disorders. *Pediatrics*, *130*, 870–877. http://dx.doi.org/10.1542/peds.2012-0762

Baio, J., Wiggins, L., Christensen, D. L., Maenner, M. J., Daniels, J., Warren, Z., . . . Dowling, N. F., & the Centers for Disease Control. (2018). Prevalence of autism spectrum disorder among children aged 8 years—Autism and developmental disabilities monitoring network, 11 sites, United States 2014, *MMWR. Surveillance Summaries: Morbidity and Mortality Weekly Report. Surveillance Summaries*, *67*, 1–23. http://dx.doi.org/10.15585/mmwr.ss6706a1

Bayley, N. (2005). *Bayley Scales of Infant and Toddler Development—Third Edition*. San Antonio, TX: Pearson Assessment.

Beaumont, R., & Newcombe, P. (2006). Theory of mind and central coherence in adults with high-functioning autism or Asperger syndrome. *Autism*, *10*, 365–382. http://dx.doi.org/10.1177/1362361306064416

Bodner, K. E., Engelhardt, C. R., Minshew, N. J., & Williams, D. L. (2015). Making inferences: Comprehension of physical causality, intentionality, and emotions in discourse by high-functioning older children, adolescents, and adults with autism. *Journal of Autism and Developmental Disorders*, *45*, 2721–2733. http://dx.doi.org/10.1007/s10803-015-2436-3

Boyle, C. A., Boulet, S., Schieve, L. A., Cohen, R. A., Blumberg, S. J., Yeargin-Allsopp, M., . . . Kogan, M. D. (2011). Trends in the prevalence of developmental disabilities in US children, 1997–2008. *Pediatrics, 127*, 1034–1042. http://dx.doi.org/10.1542/peds.2010-2989

Cannon, L., Kenworthy, L., Alexander, K. C., Werner, M. A., & Anthony, L. G. (2011). *Unstuck and on target! An executive function curriculum to improve flexibility for children with autism spectrum disorders*. Baltimore, MD: Paul H. Brookes.

Carter, E. W., Austin, D., & Trainor, A. A. (2012). Predictors of postschool employment outcomes for young adults with severe disabilities. *Journal of Disability Policy Studies, 23*, 50–63. http://dx.doi.org/10.1177/1044207311414680

Chen, J. L., Sung, C., & Pi, S. (2015). Vocational rehabilitation service patterns and outcomes for individuals with autism of different ages. *Journal of Autism and Developmental Disorders, 45*, 3015–3029. http://dx.doi.org/10.1007/s10803-015-2465-y

Cohen, S., Conduit, R., Lockley, S. W., Rajaratnam, S. M. W., & Cornish, K. M. (2014). The relationship between sleep and behavior in autism spectrum disorder (ASD): A review. *Journal of Neurodevelopmental Disorders, 6*, 44. http://dx.doi.org/10.1186/1866-1955-6-44

Constantino, J. N., & Gruber, C. P. (2012). *Social Responsiveness Scale Manual, Second Edition (SRS–2)*. Los Angeles, CA: Western Psychologic Services.

Delis, D. C., Kaplan, E., & Kramer, J. H. (2001). *Delis–Kaplan Executive Function System Manual*. San Antonio, TX: The Psychological Corporation.

De Rubeis, S., & Buxbaum, J. D. (2015). Recent advances in the genetics of autism spectrum disorder. *Current Neurology and Neuroscience Reports, 15*, 36. http://dx.doi.org/10.1007/s11910-015-0553-1

Devlin, S., Leader, G., & Healy, O. (2009). Comparison of behavioral intervention and sensory-integration therapy in the treatment of self-injurious behavior. *Research in Autism Spectrum Disorders, 3*, 223–231. http://dx.doi.org/10.1016/j.rasd.2008.06.004

Dunn, L. M., & Dunn, D. M. (2007). *Peabody Picture Vocabulary Test, Fourth Edition (PPVT–IV)*. San Antonio, TX: Pearson.

Elliott, C. D. (2007). *Differential Abilities Scale—Second Edition (DAS-II)*. San Antonio, TX: Harcourt Assessment.

Gardiner, E., & Iarocci, G. (2015). Family quality of life and ASD: The role of child adaptive functioning and behavior problems. *Autism Research, 8*, 199–213. http://dx.doi.org/10.1002/aur.1442

Gioia, G. A., Isquith, P. K., Guy, S. C., & Kenworthy, L. (2013). *Behavior Rating Inventory of Executive Function, Second Edition (BRIEF–2)*. Los Angeles, CA: Western Psychological Services.

Happé, F., Booth, R., Charlton, R., & Hughes, C. (2006). Executive function deficits in autism spectrum disorders and attention-deficit/hyperactivity disorder: Examining profiles across domains and ages. *Brain and Cognition, 61*, 25–39. http://dx.doi.org/10.1016/j.bandc.2006.03.004

Harrison, P., & Oakland, T. (2015). *Adaptive Behavior Assessment System—Second Edition (ABAS–II)*. Los Angeles, CA: Western Psychological Services.

Hill, D. A., & Flores, M. M. (2014). Comparing the picture exchange communication system and the iPad™ for communication of students with autism spectrum disorder and developmental delay. *TechTrends, 58*, 45–53. http://dx.doi.org/10.1007/s11528-014-0751-8

Howlin, P., Goode, S., Hutton, J., & Rutter, M. (2004). Adult outcome for children with autism. *Journal of Child Psychology and Psychiatry, 45*, 212–229. http://dx.doi.org/10.1111/j.1469-7610.2004.00215.x

Ingersoll, B., & Hambrick, D. Z. (2011). The relationship between the broader autism phenotype, child severity, and stress and depression in parents of children with autism spectrum disorders. *Research in Autism Spectrum Disorders, 5*, 337–344. http://dx.doi.org/10.1016/j.rasd.2010.04.017

Johnson, N. L., & Rodriguez, D. (2013). Children with autism spectrum disorder at a pediatric hospital: A systematic review of the literature. *Pediatric Nursing, 39*, 131–141.

Kanne, S. M., Gerber, A. J., Quirmbach, L. M., Sparrow, S. S., Cicchetti, D. V., & Saulnier, C. A. (2011). The role of adaptive behavior in autism spectrum disorders: Implications for functional outcome. *Journal of Autism and Developmental Disorders, 41*, 1007–1018. http://dx.doi.org/10.1007/s10803-010-1126-4

Kiely, B., Migdal, T. R., Vettam, S., & Adesman, A. (2016). Prevalence and correlates of elopement in a nationally representative sample of children with developmental Disabilities in the United States. *PLoS ONE, 11*, e0148337. http://dx.doi.org/10.1371/journal.pone.0148337

Knight, V., Sartini, E., & Spriggs, A. D. (2015). Evaluating visual activity schedules as evidence-based practice for individuals with autism spectrum disorders. *Journal of Autism and Developmental Disorders, 45*, 157–178. http://dx.doi.org/10.1007/s10803-014-2201-z

Kohane, I. S., McMurry, A., Weber, G., MacFadden, D., Rappaport, L., Kunkel, L., . . . Churchill, S. (2012). The co-morbidity burden of children and young adults with autism spectrum disorders. *PLoS One, 7*, e33224. http://dx.doi.org/10.1371/journal.pone.0033224

Kovacs, M. (2011). *Children's Depression Inventory 2 (CDI 2)*. North Tonawanda, NY: Multi-Health Systems.

Lang, R., O'Reilly, M., Healy, O., Rispoli, M., Lydon, H., Streusand, W., . . . Giesbers, S. (2012). Sensory integration therapy for autism spectrum disorders: A systematic review. *Research in Autism Spectrum Disorders*, *6*, 1004–1018. http://dx.doi.org/10.1016/j.rasd.2012.01.006

Leekam, S. R., Nieto, C., Libby, S. J., Wing, L., & Gould, J. (2007). Describing the sensory abnormalities of children and adults with autism. *Journal of Autism and Developmental Disorders*, *37*, 894–910. http://dx.doi.org/10.1007/s10803-006-0218-7

Lord, C., Rutter, M., DiLavore, P. C., Risi, S., Gotham, K., & Bishop, S. L. (2012). *Autism Diagnostic Observation Schedule—Second Edition Manual*. Torrance, CA: Western Psychological Services.

Loukusa, S., Leinonen, E., Kuusikko, S., Jussila, K., Mattila, M. L., Ryder, N., . . . Moilanen, I. (2007). Use of context in pragmatic language comprehension by children with Asperger syndrome or high-functioning autism. *Journal of Autism and Developmental Disorders*, *37*, 1049–1059. http://dx.doi.org/10.1007/s10803-006-0247-2

Marco, E. J., Hinkley, L. B. N., Hill, S. S., & Nagarajan, S. S. (2011). Sensory processing in autism: A review of neurophysiologic findings. *Pediatric Research*, *69*, 48R–54R. http://dx.doi.org/10.1203/PDR.0b013e3182130c54

Martin, N. A., & Brownell, R. (2011). *Expressive One Word Picture Vocabulary Test, Fourth Edition (EOWPVT–4)*. Novato, CA: ATP Assessments.

Mayes, S. D., Calhoun, S. L., Murray, M. J., Ahuja, M., & Smith, L. A. (2011). Anxiety, depression, and irritability in children with autism relative to other neuropsychiatric disorders and typical development. *Research in Autism Spectrum Disorders*, *5*, 474–485. http://dx.doi.org/10.1016/j.rasd.2010.06.012

Mayes, S. D., Gorman, A. A., Hillwig-Garcia, J., & Syed, E. (2013). Suicide ideation and attempts in children with autism. *Research in Autism Spectrum Disorders*, *7*, 109–119. http://dx.doi.org/10.1016/j.rasd.2012.07.009

Mcllwain, L., & Fournier, W. (2010). Wandering and autism: The need for data and resources. *Interagency Autism Coordinating Committee Meeting*. Retrieved from https://iacc.hhs.gov/meetings/iacc-meetings/2010/full-committee-meeting/october22/slides_fournier_mcilwain_102210.pdf

Mazurek, M. O., & Sohl, K. (2016). Sleep and behavioral problems in children with autism spectrum disorder. *Journal of Autism and Developmental Disorders*, *46*, 1906–1915. http://dx.doi.org/10.1007/s10803-016-2723-7

Missouri Autism Guidelines Initiative. (2012). *Autism spectrum disorders: Guide to evidence-based interventions: A 2012 consensus publication*. Jefferson City, MO: Author.

Mullen, E. M. (1995). *Mullen Scales of Early Learning*. Circle Pines, MN: American Guidance Service.

Murphy, C. M., Wilson, C. E., Robertson, D. M., Ecker, C., Daly, E. M., Hammond, N., . . . McAlonan, G. M. (2016). Autism spectrum disorder in adults: Diagnosis, management, and health services development. *Neuropsychiatric Disease and Treatment*, *12*, 1669–1686. http://dx.doi.org/10.2147/NDT.S65455

Nicholas, D. B., Attridge, M., Zwaigenbaum, L., & Clarke, M. (2015). Vocational support approaches in autism spectrum disorder: A synthesis review of the literature. *Autism*, *19*, 235–245. http://dx.doi.org/10.1177/1362361313516548

Pellicano, E. (2012). The development of executive function in autism. *Autism Research and Treatment*, *2012*, 146132. http://dx.doi.org/10.1155/2012/146132

Piven, J., Palmer, P., Landa, R., Santangelo, S., Jacobi, D., & Childress, D. (1997). Personality and language characteristics in parents from multiple-incidence autism families. *American Journal of Medical Genetics*, *74*, 398–411. http://dx.doi.org/10.1002/(SICI)1096-8628(19970725)74:4<398::AID-AJMG11>3.0.CO;2-D

Reynolds, A. M., & Malow, B. A. (2011). Sleep and autism spectrum disorders. *Pediatric Clinics of North America*, *58*, 685–698. http://dx.doi.org/10.1016/j.pcl.2011.03.009

Reynolds, C. R., & Kamphaus, R. W. (2015). *Behavior Assessment System for Children—Second Edition (BASC–2)*. San Antonio, TX: Pearson.

Robins, D. L., Fein, D., & Barton, M. (2009). *Modified Checklist for Autism in Toddlers, Revised, With Follow-Up (M-CHAT-R/F)*™. Storrs, CT: Self-published. Retrieved from https://mchatscreen.com/wp-content/uploads/2015/09/M-CHAT-R_F_Rev_Aug2018.pdf

Roid, G. H., Miller, L. J., Pomplun, M., & Koch, C. (2013). *Leiter International Performance Scale, Third Edition*. Wood Dale, IL: Stoelting.

Rommelse, N. N., Franke, B., Geurts, H. M., Hartman, C. A., & Buitelaar, J. K. (2010). Shared heritability of attention-deficit/hyperactivity disorder and autism spectrum disorder. *European Child & Adolescent Psychiatry*, *19*, 281–295. http://dx.doi.org/10.1007/s00787-010-0092-x

Roux, A. M., Shattuck, P. T., Cooper, B. P., Anderson, K. A., Wagner, M., & Narendorf, S. C. (2013). Postsecondary employment experiences among young adults with an autism spectrum disorder. *Journal of the American Academy of Child & Adolescent Psychiatry*, *52*, 931–939. http://dx.doi.org/10.1016/j.jaac.2013.05.019

Rutter, M., Bailey, A., & Lord, C. (2003). *The Social Communication Questionnaire (SCQ) manual*. Los Angeles, CA: Western Psychological Services.

Rutter, M., LeCouteur, A., & Lord, C. (2003). *Autism Diagnostic Interview—Revised*. Los Angeles, CA: Western Psychological Services.

Saracino, J., Noseworthy, J., Steiman, M., Reisinger, L., & Fombonne, E. (2010). Diagnostic and assessment issues in autism surveillance and prevalence. *Journal of Developmental and Physical Disabilities*, *22*, 317–330. http://dx.doi.org/10.1007/s10882-010-9205-1

Schopler, E., & Bourgondien, M. E. (2010). *Childhood Autism Rating Scale, Second Edition*. Los Angeles, CA: Western Psychological Services.

Seaman, R. L., & Cannella-Malone, H. I. (2016). Vocational skills interventions for adults with autism spectrum disorder: A review of the literature. *Journal of Developmental and Physical Disabilities*, *28*, 479–494. http://dx.doi.org/10.1007/s10882-016-9479-z

Section 504 of the Rehabilitation Act of 1973, 34 C.F.R. Part 104.

Sparrow, S. S., Cicchetti, D. V., & Saulnier, C. (2016). *Vineland Adaptive Behavior Scales, Third Edition*. San Antonio, TX: Pearson.

Stiers, W., Barisa, M., Stucky, K., Pawlowski, C., Van Tubbergen, M., Turner, A. P., . . . Caplan, B. (2015). Guidelines for competency development and measurement in rehabilitation psychology postdoctoral training. *Rehabilitation Psychology*, *60*, 111–122. http://dx.doi.org/10.1037/a0038353

Strang, J. F., Kenworthy, L., Daniolos, P., Case, L., Wills, M. C., Martin, A., & Wallace, G. L. (2012). Depression and anxiety symptoms in children and adolescents with autism spectrum disorders without intellectual disability. *Research in Autism Spectrum Disorders*, *6*, 406–412. http://dx.doi.org/10.1016/j.rasd.2011.06.015

Sukhodolsky, D. G., Bloch, M. H., Panza, K. E., & Reichow, B. (2013). Cognitive-behavioral therapy for anxiety in children with high-functioning autism: A meta-analysis. *Pediatrics*, *132*, E1341–E1350. http://dx.doi.org/10.1542/peds.2013-1193

Taylor, M. A., Schreck, K. A., & Mulick, J. A. (2012). Sleep disruption as a correlate to cognitive and adaptive behavior problems in autism spectrum disorders. *Research in Developmental Disabilities*, *33*, 1408–1417. http://dx.doi.org/10.1016/j.ridd.2012.03.013

Vogan, V., Lake, J. K., Weiss, J. A., Robinson, S., Tint, A., & Lunsky, Y. (2014). Factors associated with caregiver burden among parents of individuals with ASD: Differences across intellectual functioning. *Family Relations*, *63*, 554–567. http://dx.doi.org/10.1111/fare.12081

Volkmar, F., Siegel, M., Woodbury-Smith, M., King, B., McCracken, J., State, M., & the American Academy of Child and Adolescent Psychiatry (AACAP) Committee on Quality Issues (CQI). (2014). Practice parameter for the assessment and treatment of children and adolescents with autism spectrum disorder. *Journal of the American Academy of Child & Adolescent Psychiatry*, *53*, 237–257. http://dx.doi.org/10.1016/j.jaac.2013.10.013

Vriend, J. L., Corkum, P. V., Moon, E. C., & Smith, I. M. (2011). Behavioral interventions for sleep problems in children with autism spectrum disorders: Current findings and future directions. *Journal of Pediatric Psychology*, *36*, 1017–1029. http://dx.doi.org/10.1093/jpepsy/jsr044

Wechsler, D. (2014). *Wechsler Preschool and Primary Scale of Intelligence—4th Edition (WPPSI–IV)*. San Antonio, TX: The Psychological Corporation.

Wiig, E. H., Semel, E., & Secord, W. A. (2013). *Clinical Evaluation of Language Fundamentals, Fifth Edition (CELF–5)*. San Antonio, TX: Pearson Assessment.

Wodka, E. L., Mathy, P., & Kalb, L. (2013). Predictors of phrase and fluent speech in children with autism and severe language delay. *Pediatrics*, *131*, 1128–1134. http://dx.doi.org/10.1542/peds.2012-2221

Wood, J. J., Drahota, A., Sze, K., Har, K., Chiu, A., & Langer, D. A. (2009). Cognitive behavioral therapy for anxiety in children with autism spectrum disorders: A randomized, controlled trial. *Journal of Child Psychology and Psychiatry, and Allied Disciplines*, *50*, 224–234. http://dx.doi.org/10.1111/j.1469-7610.2008.01948.x

CHAPTER 21

CEREBROVASCULAR ACCIDENTS

Michelle M. Haddad, Gitendra Uswatte, Victor W. Mark, and Kathleen T. Bechtold

Stroke compels study and care by psychologists because it damages the organ responsible for producing thought, emotion, and behavior. Depending on the location of damage in the brain, survivors of stroke experience difficulty with controlling their movement, perceiving their world, processing and remembering information, and regulating their emotions and behavior. Impairments of these abilities affect how survivors of stroke engage in work, recreation, and relationships with others. Family and friends are also affected; care and support for their loved one with stroke sometimes require marked changes in their lives. In this chapter, we discuss the rehabilitation psychology care of adults with stroke, including (a) briefly describing the epidemiology and pathophysiology of stroke, (b) introducing the roles of rehabilitation psychologists in stroke care, (c) discussing the sequelae of stroke and their assessment and treatment by type of impairment (i.e., motor, somatosensory, cognitive, affective, and behavioral), and (d) discussing the impact of stroke on the interpersonal, vocational, and social roles of the individual. In the last section, we discuss future directions for research and care.

DEFINING STROKE

Stroke is typically diagnosed by reviewing the patient's clinical presentation and neuroimaging data. The two most common stroke syndromes are ischemic stroke and hemorrhagic stroke. The American Heart Association/American Stroke Association (AHA/ASA) defines *ischemic stroke* as an episode of neurological dysfunction caused by focal cerebral, spinal, or retinal infarction (Sacco et al., 2013). Infarction reflects focal cell death from prolonged lack of oxygenation. When brain cells are deprived of oxygen, they are unable to function properly but often may be salvaged if rapid reperfusion with oxygenated blood occurs. Pharmacological agents that promote tissue reperfusion are preferred, if diagnosis and intervention occur quickly (Jauch et al., 2013). Ischemic infarction is generally associated with lower mortality and better outcomes compared with hemorrhagic (Mozaffarian et al., 2016).

Hemorrhagic stroke refers to bleeding that occurs due to the rupture of cerebral vasculature, most commonly occurring in the intracerebral and subarachnoid spaces. Cell death due to hemorrhagic stroke may result from increased pressure by buildup of blood volume, reduced blood flow from areas downstream of the hemorrhage, or neurotoxic metabolic changes resulting from the bleed. Unlike ischemic stroke, hemorrhagic stroke has no standard pharmacological treatment. Typically, supportive care is given. Surgical intervention may be warranted when blood volume significantly compresses the surrounding structures, although the efficacy of this procedure has been controversial (Hemphill et al., 2015). Although persons with

http://dx.doi.org/10.1037/0000129-022
Handbook of Rehabilitation Psychology, Third Edition, L. A. Brenner, S. A. Reid-Arndt, T. R. Elliott, R. G. Frank, and B. Caplan (Editors-in-Chief)

hemorrhagic stroke have initially worse disability than those with ischemic stroke, such individuals also have greater functional gains during inpatient rehabilitation (Katrak, Black, & Peeva, 2009).

EPIDEMIOLOGY

Recent epidemiological data suggest the global prevalence of stroke is approximately 33 million, with an annual incidence of approximately 17 million (Feigin et al., 2014). In the United States, approximately 795,000 people experience a stroke each year, of which 610,000 are first strokes (Mozaffarian et al., 2016). Of these, an estimated 87% are ischemic and 13% are hemorrhagic. However, it is important to note that stroke incidence varies significantly with age, gender, race, and socioeconomic status, so general population statistics must be interpreted with caution. Stroke incidence increases with age. Women have a higher lifetime prevalence of stroke than men because women live longer than men (Seshadri et al., 2006). African Americans have a significantly higher incidence of stroke than European Americans; the risk is more than double in some age groups (Howard et al., 2013; White et al., 2005). Stroke mortality varies geographically in the United States, with higher rates in the southeastern area known as the "stroke belt" (Howard et al., 1995). Globally, there is a higher prevalence of stroke in lower and middle-income countries (Feigin et al., 2014).

Stroke mortality has declined over the past decade, and stroke (considered separately from other cardiovascular diseases) has fallen from the third leading cause of death in the United States to the fifth (Mozaffarian et al., 2016). Nonetheless, stroke remains a leading cause of serious long-term disability. Recent studies suggest that greater than 70% of individuals discharged from the hospital following acute medical management of stroke received some type of rehabilitation services (Mozaffarian et al., 2016).

RISK FACTORS AND PREVENTION

Although some risk factors for stroke are not modifiable (e.g., age, sex, race/ethnicity, genetic predisposition), many others are and should be targets for health care providers. Of these, high blood pressure is one of the most significant, present in the majority of individuals who have had a first stroke (Lackland et al., 2014). Comorbid medical conditions including diabetes mellitus, disorders of heart rhythm, chronic kidney disease, and obstructive sleep apnea, among others, are also associated with an increased risk of stroke. Increased control of these disorders could reduce the risk of stroke, although further studies are needed. Of behavioral risk factors, tobacco use and physical inactivity are two of the most significant (McDonnell et al., 2013; Shah & Cole, 2010). Although frequently thought to be associated with stroke risk, there is inconsistent evidence for a link between cholesterol and other lipids and stroke. However, a Mediterranean-style diet that is high in proteins, healthy fats, fruits, and vegetables and low in carbohydrates has been found to be protective against stroke (Estruch et al., 2013). Management of these factors could also prevent recurrent stroke.

ROLES OF THE REHABILITATION PSYCHOLOGIST IN STROKE CARE: AN OVERVIEW

From the critical care service through acute care, acute rehabilitation, subacute care, and postacute community reentry, the rehabilitation psychologist provides assessment, intervention, and consultation services that assist the patient, family, and care team through the process of recovery and rehabilitation. The rehabilitation psychologist must tailor assessment and interventions to address the particular needs of a given patient, family, and care team and given the treatment setting. Unlike in clinical psychology, in which individual psychotherapy is the dominant mode of care, the rehabilitation psychologist has an important role in assisting the care team (Karol, 2014). The rehabilitation psychologist's interventions in this capacity range from (a) coaching a physical therapist on how to motivate a patient to engage in physical therapy sessions, (b) to providing guidelines to nursing staff on how to respond to a patient who is perceived as belligerent, (c) to addressing care team dynamics that interfere with treatment. Two areas of growing interest are implementing procedures to generalize rehabilitation gains to settings outside of the rehabilitation facility (Taub et al., 2013) and using technology to extend therapy beyond the rehabilitation facility (Lum, Uswatte, Taub, Hardin, & Mark, 2006; see also Chapter 30, this volume). These team-focused roles for the rehabilitation psychologist facilitate the success of overall rehabilitation for each patient.

For patient-focused care, the focus of rehabilitation evolves over the course of care (see Table 21.1), and so does the focus of the rehabilitation psychologist. In the critical care setting, the psychologist focuses on the environment, patient, and family. Structuring the clinical environment to facilitate patients' orientation to situation and time of day is critical for reducing confusion and managing anxiety. Interventions with patients, depending on their cognitive status, aim to provide stimulation structured to promote progressively higher levels of alertness, manage anxiety that can arise from a reduced sense of personal control, and address confusion that can arise from cognitive impairment. Family and friends can be taught to assist in raising the level of arousal and awareness of the patient as well as adjusting to the change in circumstances. Volume 61, Issue 2, of *Rehabilitation Psychology* contains an in-depth discussion of rehabilitation psychology in the critical care setting (see also Chapter 28, this volume).

For patients who are medically stable and engaging in initial rehabilitation activities on the acute medical floor or within a more comprehensive acute, inpatient rehabilitation setting, the focus shifts to assisting patients to understand their impairments, adopt new strategies and skills for self-care and life management, and adjust emotionally to the effects of impairments on functioning. Because awareness of impairments and their impact on daily life functioning can be poor in individuals with stroke (Kortte & Wegener, 2004), the rehabilitation psychologist should not only understand the difference between anosognosia, which is neurologically based, and denial of illness, which is psychologically based, but also have strong therapeutic skills for addressing these problems (Kortte & Wegener, 2004). Integration through education and training of family and friends who are to serve as caregivers is ramped up during this phase.

In the postacute setting, the foregoing skills, strategies, and knowledge are built on as the patient continues to recover, regaining function in daily life activities. The rehabilitation psychologist develops interventions during this phase to address more complex aspects of function such as social competence in interpersonal and professional relationships and significant emotional adjustment difficulties as well as the more chronic problems, such as pain, fatigue, and cognitive impairments that can disrupt daily life engagement. The caregiver's role evolves as well, and interventions are targeted on assisting the caregiver to adapt and adjust to those role changes. Supporting the caregivers through ongoing education, training, and encouragement to engage in their

TABLE 21.1

Phases of Rehabilitation

Setting	Critical care/medical stabilization	Nursing facility/ subacute rehab facility	Inpatient acute rehabilitation unit/ inpatient medical unit	Residential program/ day treatment program/outpatient program	Outpatient program/ community-based services
Focus	Medical stabilization and recovery of very basic life function	Basic self-care and self-management; reintroduction to basic life management (low intensity) *or* skill maintenance	Basic self-care and self-management; reintroduction to basic life management and community-access (high intensity)	Life task reengagement with habitual integration of skills and equipment use	Life management, community integration, social integration

own self-care during this postacute phase helps to ensure that there is a healthy system for the patient. Additionally, the rehabilitation psychologist helps patients understand their role in reducing their risk for stroke recurrence and otherwise improving their overall health.

Regardless of the setting or phase of recovery, the rehabilitation psychologist must address key cross-cutting issues that can become barriers to patients' engagement in the recovery and rehabilitation process. These include pain, fatigue, cognitive dysfunction, emotional dysregulation, and adjustment difficulties (see Table 21.2). However, the rehabilitation psychologist also must hone in on patients' assets, such as positive affective states and hopefulness, because these strengths have been found to be related to level of rehabilitation engagement and positive outcomes (Kortte, Stevenson, Hosey, Castillo, & Wegener, 2012; Ramanathan-Elion, McWhorter, Wegener, & Bechtold, 2016). Understanding the interplay among an individual's impairments, assets, and environmental barriers is the foundation on which the rehabilitation psychologist builds suitable interventions to maximize patient engagement. Thus, the rehabilitation psychologist must be well versed in the physical, cognitive, emotional, and behavioral sequelae of stroke and how recovery is affected as much by the "who" of the brain that was injured as the brain injury itself.

AREAS OF IMPAIRMENT AFTER STROKE: ASSESSMENT AND INTERVENTION

The sequelae of stroke depend on its type, location, and severity. It behooves the rehabilitation psychologist to have a solid understanding of the possible impairments in function that can occur, with the goal of (a) assessing and providing interventions for these impairments when appropriate; (b) providing education to the patient and family about the constellation of impairments, how these impairments will impact functioning now and in the future, and how these impairments will be addressed by the rehabilitation team; and (c) collaborating with the rest of the rehabilitation team to develop and implement the assessment and intervention plan. Impairments following stroke fall broadly into the domains of motor, somatosensory, cognitive, affective, and behavioral. Given that the effects of individual impairments on daily life function are complex and interact, the rehabilitation psychologist can play a key role in assisting the patient, the family, and the rehabilitation team in understanding how changes in cognition, affective regulation, emotional adjustment, and behavioral control can affect the patient's motor and sensory function during task completion and activity engagement. Furthermore, the rehabilitation psychologist is uniquely positioned to help integrate understanding the person within the design of the rehabilitation plan so that treatment is tailored to meet the individual needs of patients. The review of poststroke impairments that follows is not meant to be comprehensive. Rather, the review aims to provide the rehabilitation psychologist with an overview of the areas of impairment to consider in the care of individuals who are poststroke.

Hemiparesis

Of all physical sequelae of stroke, hemiparesis (i.e., weakness of the extremities) is the most common, affecting about 80% of patients (Lawrence et al., 2001). Marked unilateral motor impairments occur mainly contralateral to the lesion in the brain; lesions in the lower brainstem can affect the body on the same side. Impairment of the upper limb is generally more common than impairment of the lower limb (Duncan et al., 1994). The degree of motor impairment is similar between the upper and lower limbs in most patients (Tyson, Chillala, Hanley, Selley, & Tallis, 2006). Initially, most individuals experience hypotonic weakness of the more affected extremities but later may develop spasticity (discussed in the next subsection; see also Ward, 2012). There is no clear consensus in the research literature regarding predictors of motor recovery after stroke, although patients with milder impairment immediately after stroke tend to have better functional outcomes than those whose motor abilities are more significantly affected (Coupar, Pollock, Rowe, Weir, & Langhorne, 2012). As many as two thirds of patients may still experience significant hemiparesis at 6 months poststroke (Lai, Studenski, Duncan, & Perera, 2002). It is recommended that treatment for poststroke hemiparesis begin as soon

TABLE 21.2

Key Goals of the Rehabilitation Psychologist and Corresponding Competencies and Evidence-Based Assessment and Treatment Methods

Competencies required	Assessment and treatment methods
Goal A: Help patient to manage pain	
Pain assessment	VAS, NRS, McGill Pain Questionnaire, clinical interview (Turk & Melzack, 2001)
Functional analysis of pain behaviors and their antecedents and consequents	See Gachtel, 2005
Behavioral management of pain, including teaching professional and family caregivers not to reinforce pain behaviors	See Gachtel, 2005
Relaxation training or mindfulness meditation	PMR, diaphragmatic breathing, and guided imagery (Gachtel, 2005), MBSR (McCracken & Vowles, 2014)
Hypnosis	See Jensen & Patterson, 2014
Cognitive reframing	CBT (Ehde, Dillworth, & Turner, 2014)
Acceptance	ACT (McCracken & Vowles, 2014)
Goal B: Help patient to manage fatigue	
Fatigue assessment	Fatigue Assessment Scale (Michielsen, De Vries, & Van Heck, 2003), Fatigue Impact Scale (J. D. Fisk et al., 1994), Fatigue Scale for Motor and Cognitive Functions (Hubacher et al., 2012)
Relaxation training or mindfulness meditation	PMR, diaphragmatic breathing, and guided imagery (Davis, Robbins Eshelman, & McKay, 2008), MBSR (Crane et al., 2017)
Activity modification, including teaching professional and family caregivers to pace the activity of the patient	Behavioral Activation/Pleasant Events Scheduling (Kanter, Puspitasari, Santos, & Nagy, 2012), Activity Pacing (Goudsmit, Nijs, Jason, & Wallman, 2012)
Goal C: Help patient to manage cognitive impairment	
Executive function assessment	D–KEFS (Homack, Lee, & Riccio, 2005)
Memory assessment	Everyday Memory Questionnaire (Royle & Lincoln, 2008), Subjective Memory Questionnaire (Bennett-Levy & Powell, 1980), Wechsler Memory Scale (Wechsler, 2009)
Aphasia assessment	WAB–R (Kertesz, 2007), Token Test—Short Form (Spellacy & Spreen, 1969), Verbal Activity Log (Haddad et al., 2017)
Spatial neglect assessment	Star Cancellation Test from the Behavioral Inattention Test battery (Wilson, Cockburn, & Halligan, 1987)
Treatment of executive dysfunction, memory disorders, aphasia, and spatial neglect	Several promising methods to treat these impairments have been developed (see text), but none are available yet with rigorous evidence of efficacy
	Clinicians can consult the Cognitive Rehabilitation Manual (Haskins et al., 2014) for compensatory strategies for addressing impairments in executive function

(*continues*)

TABLE 21.2

Key Goals of the Rehabilitation Psychologist and Corresponding Competencies and Evidence-Based Assessment and Treatment Methods (*Continued*)

Competencies required	Assessment and treatment methods
Goal D: Help patient with psychological adjustment to injury	
Affective assessment	BDI–II, CES–D, PHQ-2, PHQ-9, GAD–7, HADS, PCL (Ferro et al., 2016)
Personality assessment	MMPI–2 (Butcher et al., 2001), PAI (Morey, 2007)
Identification of strengths	The Trait Hope Scale (Snyder et al., 1991); COPE Inventory (Carver, Scheier, & Weintraub, 1989), The Positive and Negative Affect Scale (Watson, Clark, & Tellegen, 1988) Also see Ramanathan-Elion, McWhorter, Wegener, & Bechtold, 2016
Promotion of positive affective states	Coaching individuals on using solution-focused approaches (A. M. Grant, 2012; Green, Oades, & Grant, 2006), writing about intensely positive experiences (Burton & King, 2004; Lyubomirsky, Sousa, & Dickerhoof, 2006), noting blessings to increase gratitude (Emmons & McCullough, 2003; Seligman, Steen, Park, & Peterson, 2005), using signature character strengths in new ways (Seligman et al., 2005).
Relaxation training or mindfulness meditation	PMR, diaphragmatic breathing, guided imagery, MBSR
Activity modification	Behavioral Activation/Pleasant Events Scheduling
Promoting change	Motivational Interviewing (Watkins et al., 2011)
Cognitive reframing	CBT (Broomfield et al., 2011)

Note. VAS = Visual Analog Scale; NRS = numerical rating scale; PMR = progressive muscle relaxation; MBSR = mindfulness-based stress reduction; CBT = cognitive behavior therapy; ACT = Acceptance and commitment therapy; D–KEFS = Delis–Kaplan Executive Function System; WAB–R = Western Aphasia Battery—Revised; BDI–II = Beck Depression Inventory II; CES–D = Center for Epidemiological Studies Depression Scale; PHQ-2, PHQ-9 = two-item and nine-item Patient Health Questionnaire; GAD–7 = seven-item Generalized Anxiety Disorder scale; HADS = Hospital Anxiety and Depression Scale; PCL = Post-Traumatic Stress Checklist; MMPI–2 = Minnesota Multiphasic Personality Inventory—2; PAI = Personality Assessment Inventory.

as the patient is medically stable enough to tolerate therapies (Winstein et al., 2016).

Interventions to treat poststroke hemiparesis are nearly as many and varied as are patients' clinical presentations and needs after a stroke. In general, AHA/ASA guidelines indicate that stroke patients should be treated by a specialized interdisciplinary team, as previously described. Treatment may take place in an inpatient rehabilitation facility during the acute and subacute phase of recovery or in an outpatient setting in the subacute to chronic phases. Most commonly, rehabilitation of motor deficits is accomplished through a combination of medication management, physical therapy (PT), and occupational therapy (OT).

The most common and standard interventions provided by these disciplines are broadly termed *motor practice*. They consist of repetitive practice with the impaired limb(s) in the context of tasks involving either a specific movement or a functional one (i.e., activities of daily living [ADLs] training). Although repetitive motor practice is the most common treatment, there is mixed evidence regarding its efficacy, particularly in the acute care inpatient setting (E. L. Miller et al., 2010). Constraint-induced movement therapy (CIMT) is an efficacious intervention for chronic poststroke hemiparesis that focuses primarily on reversing "learned nonuse" by shaping use of the more affected limb while restraining the less affected limb with a cloth mitt. CIMT also involves a set of behavioral techniques collectively termed the *Transfer Package* that are used to facilitate transfer gains made in the clinic to the real-world life situation (Taub, Uswatte, King, et al., 2006; Taub, Uswatte, Mark, & Morris, 2006). For a comprehensive overview and recommendations for treatment of poststroke motor impairment, see E. L. Miller et al. (2010) and Winstein et al. (2016).

Spasticity

Poststroke spasticity, or hypertonicity, is thought to arise from the disconnection of sensory and motor information in the brain from lower motor areas of the spinal cord and is characterized by abnormally increased muscle tone and involuntary muscle activation. About 25% to 50% of patients experience spasticity at some point during their recovery from stroke, most commonly within the first 6 months (Ward, 2012). Poststroke spasticity is a significant source of disability and can also be associated with chronic pain (Winstein et al., 2016). Management of spasticity is multimodal, including muscle stretching exercises and medications. Conditions that can aggravate spasticity, including infection, should also be ruled out (E. L. Miller et al., 2010).

Ataxia

Ataxia is characterized by impaired movement coordination that can result from stroke damage to the cerebellum or cerebellar connections to other parts of the brain. It is relatively uncommon but has a significant impact on functional ability. There is currently no standard treatment for poststroke ataxia (Winstein et al., 2016).

Apraxia

Apraxia manifests as the selective impairment of learned purposive movements (Winstein et al., 2016). Less common than the other sequelae discussed in this section, limb apraxia results from deficits either in the spatial-temporal control of goal-directed movement (Dovern, Fink, & Weiss, 2012) or in generating the movement pattern and bodily part orientation that are specific for a particular gesture or object's use (Hoeren et al., 2014). There is currently no standard treatment for limb apraxia, but several interventions aimed at retraining skilled movements necessary for the performance of ADLs have shown some efficacy in randomized controlled trials under laboratory conditions (Winstein et al., 2016).

Somatosensory Impairment

More than half of all patients who have experienced a stroke have somatosensory impairment of some type. Astereognosis, or loss of the ability to perceive and recognize objects through touch, has been identified as the most common somatosensory impairment, with up to 89% of patients affected to some degree. Exteroception (the ability to process stimuli from the environment) and proprioception (ability to discern movement of part of the body in relation to the rest of the body) are impaired in approximately 60% of people. Other impairments in tactile sensation have been found to affect about half of all patients who have had a stroke (Connell, Lincoln, & Radford, 2008; Kessner, Bingel, & Thomalla, 2016).

Somatosensory impairments may affect quality of life by causing discomfort but may also have more significant effects. Somatosensory impairment can complicate motor recovery and can be associated with increased fall risk, particularly in patients who have diminished balance as a result of exteroceptive or proprioceptive deficits. Somatosensory loss is associated with decreased spontaneous use of an affected limb, which can lead to the development of learned nonuse and greater disability. Finally, patients with somatosensory deficits may be unable to perform ADLs and may therefore be unable to live independently.

Assessment of somatosensory function is complicated because it requires the report of the patient and may therefore be difficult to test in a systematic, objective way. As a result, clinical test protocols often have poor reliability and validity. More frequently, evaluation is informal and based on self-report. Standardized scales that assess sensory modalities and have shown favorable psychometric properties include the Fugl-Meyer Sensory Scale (Fugl-Meyer, Jääskö, Leyman, Olsson, & Steglind, 1975), the Nottingham Sensory Assessment (Stolk-Hornsveld, Crow, Hendriks, van der Baan, & Harmeling-van der Wel, 2006), and the Rivermead Assessment of Somatosensory

Perception (Winward, Halligan, & Wade, 2002). Although treatment of somatosensory deficits has received less attention in both research literature and clinical practice than has been devoted to motor recovery, several evidence-based interventions are available (see Kessner et al., 2016).

Visual Impairment

Visual impairment commonly follows stroke, affecting up to 30% of patients. Hemianopia (i.e., reduction or loss of half the visual field) is the most common visual syndrome in patients with stroke (Sand et al., 2013). Other impairments include diplopia (double vision), ptosis (drooping of the eyelid), and eye movement disorders. In the most extreme cases, patients may experience cortical blindness—the inability to process visual information as a result of profound bilateral damage to the visual cortex.

Although visual impairment may seem less dramatic than the classic motor deficits that follow stroke, it can be associated with significant disability and diminished quality of life. Patients with visual impairments experience difficulty with a variety of daily activities, from navigation and orientation to instrumental ADLs such as driving, reading, and managing finances secondary to the challenges of visually processing the information in their environment. Even simple, pleasant activities, such as watching television, may become difficult. Finally, poststroke visual impairment limits rehabilitation potential and may inhibit living independently (Sand et al., 2013).

To address these impairments, neurovisual rehabilitation focuses on maximizing spared function and implementing compensatory strategies. This type of therapy has three elements: restitution, compensation, and substitution (Kerkhoff, 2000). Therapies targeted toward restitution are founded on the idea that areas of residual vision can be strengthened and maximized, likely through processes of neuroplasticity (Sabel, 2008). Compensation- and substitution-focused therapies teach patients to use visual aids and behavioral strategies, such as head turning, to ameliorate the functional difficulties that come with reduced vision.

Poststroke Pain

Approximately half of patients experience chronic pain following stroke, many on a daily basis (Harrison & Field, 2015). Poststroke pain is associated with multiple negative outcomes, including increased cognitive dysfunction and general disability, worse quality of life, increased fatigue, and a higher incidence of depression. Following stroke, patients may develop complex regional pain syndrome, which includes pain, edema, vasomotor dysfunction, and bone demineralization (O'Donnell et al., 2013). Poststroke headache also occurs in a subset of patients. Mechanisms of poststroke pain may include lesions affecting areas of the brain associated with the processing of pain, spasticity or muscle tension, and musculoskeletal pain from altered motor function. In some cases, the specific etiology of poststroke pain is unknown (Harrison & Field, 2015).

Management of poststroke pain is often multimodal and may include multiple disciplines. Medications are often the primary approach with physician oversight. OT and PT may be important for treating musculoskeletal and spasticity-related pain. There is also a crucial role for psychology in the management of poststroke pain including nonpharmacological pain management strategies, such as guided imagery, progressive muscle relaxation, and hypnosis. Cognitive behavior therapy and acceptance and commitment therapy have both been shown to be effective in the long-term treatment of chronic pain (Ehde, Dillworth, & Turner, 2014; McCracken & Vowles, 2014). See Chapter 14, this volume for additional discussion of pain assessment and intervention.

Executive Dysfunction

One of the most often described cognitive impairments following stroke is executive dysfunction (Mark, 2016). The executive functions include planning (which requires abstraction), initiation, staying mindful of task objectives (termed *working memory*), modifying behavior based on feedback, prioritizing goals, sequencing activities, and inhibiting attention to irrelevant stimuli (Keil & Kaszniak, 2002; Lesniak, Bak, Czepiel, Seniów, & Członkowska, 2008). Speed of information processing can be included within the executive function domain because it assesses the time-related efficiency of cognitive operations. Among the most widely used assessments of executive function are tests of language fluency, inhibition of well-learned associations, and maintaining alternation of attention to different kinds of stimuli. The Delis-Kaplan Executive Functioning Scale (Homack, Lee, & Riccio, 2005) is a common battery that includes each of the aforementioned types of assessments.

The treatment of executive disorders is still in its nascence because this complex set of cognitive functions has no singular mechanism and relies on well-orchestrated integration of information. Overall, interventions for impaired executive function poststroke have been directed at *remediating* underlying disruption of information processing and integration. A variety of techniques have been applied, with most rooted in computer-based tasks to "strengthen" attention or working memory. However, to date, meta-analytic reviews of the literature have not found strong support for overall improvements in executive function with different types of computer-based interventions (Bogdanova, Yee, Ho, & Cicerone, 2016; van de Ven, Murre, Veltman, & Schmand, 2016).

In the past decade, there has been a burgeoning of brain-stimulation approaches that hold some promise for improving cognition. Recent explorations have found forms of noninvasive brain stimulation (transcranial direct current stimulation [tDCS] and transcranial magnetic stimulation [TMS]) can improve executive function as well as other cognitive domains (Andrade et al., 2015; Martin-Trias et al., 2016). However, the improvements have not persisted, so further research is needed to identify methods that will foster maintenance. Although the bulk of the research has been on remedial interventions for poststroke executive function, clinicians are encouraged to extrapolate from the broader acquired brain injury literature and consider compensatory-based interventions when designing interventions for executive dysfunction. The interested reader may consult the *Cognitive Rehabilitation Manual* (Haskins et al., 2014) for compensatory strategies that are effective for executive dysfunction.

In addition to cognitive rehabilitative approaches, there is some evidence that certain medications may bolster executive function by augmenting attention. Medications, such as modafinil, can improve initiation and benefit rehabilitation participation following cerebral hemorrhage (Sugden & Bourgeois, 2004). A randomized, placebo-controlled trial found that selegiline can benefit a variety of executive functions in stroke patients (Bartolo, Zucchella, Capone, Sandrini, & Pierelli, 2015).

Memory Disorders

Depending on the method of assessment, among other factors, the incidence of memory impairment following stroke has been reported to range from 23% to 55% at the subacute phase, which declines to 11% to 33% by 1 year (Snaphaan & de Leeuw, 2007). Memory is not one unitary function but rather a complex system that includes semantic memory, episodic memory, and procedural memory. In brief, the semantic (declarative) memory is a complex multimodal process capable of fast single-trial encoding (Squire, 1992). The information can be declared, has truth value, is accessible, and can form the basis for inferences about other objects and events in the world (Tulving, 2005). Episodic memory relates semantic knowledge (e.g., knowledge of ourselves and the world) to time and place (Tulving, 1985). Finally, procedural memory is a form of implicit memory regarding task performance as it becomes habitual with practice (Squire, 2004). It holds the "procedures" for performing tasks, which become habitual with practice. Procedural memory is only rarely impaired. It can be relied on for patients following stroke to relearn self-care skills (e.g., steps to completing a transfer from bed to chair).

During assessment, it can help to understand the patient's experience of memory dysfunction with self-report instruments, such as the Everyday Memory Questionnaire—Revised (Royle & Lincoln, 2008) or the Subjective Memory Questionnaire (Bennett-Levy & Powell, 1980). However, given that individuals can have impaired awareness of cognitive changes following stroke, it is also important to objectively memory. Assessing semantic memory has been traditionally structured to capture the encoding of verbal information (rote or within a context) or visual information and the subsequent retrieval of that information within cued and uncued formats. Two frequently used instruments are the Wechsler Memory Scale—IV (Wechsler, 2009) and the California Verbal Learning Test—II (Delis, Kramer, & Kaplan, 2000).

Although short-term gains with memory training have been reported in patients following strokes, thus far clinical trials have not shown sustained improvements 3 months or longer afterward (das Nair, Cogger, Worthington, & Lincoln, 2016). Given the relative lack of evidence supporting efficacy over the longer term, remediation approaches are not the goal of rehabilitation. The core interventions for memory impairments have focused on using external strategies and equipment to compensate for the impairment to promote effective life management. Patients are encouraged to learn strategies to document scheduled activities and tasks to be completed so that the individual can follow a written schedule rather than rely on impaired memory to recall what needs to be done. However, the patient must also consider what did not get accomplished yesterday, any changes in schedule given unexpected life situations, and planning for more infrequent life activities that may disrupt the routines of day-to-day life for such a system to be effective. It should be noted that success in daily life management is highly reliant on accurate episodic memory to understand the consequences of past behavior and anticipate, think about, and plan for the personal future (Atance & O'Neill, 2001; Kwan et al., 2013). Thus, patients with impaired memory will be hindered in their ability to act on the basis of their knowledge of the past and their expectations for the future, leading to impaired predicting of what is to come, planning and goal-setting, and differentiating right from wrong (Tulving, 2005). Interventions need to increase the patient's awareness of the memory impairments to incorporate the impact of the impairment on ability to predict, plan, set goals, and make decisions. Thus, a multifaceted approach that addresses the breakdowns that occur because of the memory impairment as well as the awareness of the effects of the impairment on function in daily life is essential. For a synopsis of cognitive rehabilitation strategies and approaches to address these types of breakdowns in cognitive functioning, see the *Cognitive Rehabilitation Manual* (Haskins et al., 2014) or *Ecologically Oriented Neurorehabilitation of Memory* (Stringer, 2007).

Agnosia

Agnosia is the inability to recognize a previously familiar person, object, or other stimulus despite adequate sensation. The sudden feeling of familiarity during sensation, the "knowing of knowing" (Hanczakowski, Zawadzka, Collie, & Macken, 2017), is a prerequisite for recognizing a specific face or thing. When agnosic patients are asked to report their perception of a stimulus, they can describe its elementary sensory qualities, such as its shade, sound volume, or weight, but they lack the sense of familiarity for the specific entity itself.

In visual agnosia, the patient cannot identify a viewed object despite being able to describe its size and shape. For example, when a patient with visually agnosia looks at a tape dispenser, the patient can correctly say that it is round and small but would be unable to integrate the parts to recognize the whole tape dispenser. Prosopagnosia is the inability to recognize a specific person's face, despite being able to describe the person's general appearance, age, ethnicity, or age. About half of patients with right hemisphere stroke can have prosopagnosia (Hier, Mondlock, & Caplan, 1983). Patients with prosopagnosia typically also have visual agnosia (Assal, Favre, & Anderes, 1984). Despite its common occurrence, prosopagnosia is not routinely tested in stroke care, and strategies for its management have not been well developed (Cousins, 2013).

Aphasia

Aphasia is the disturbance of the use of symbolic information (primarily language), and it appears in about one third of patients in the acute phase. Aphasia assessment batteries assess conversational skills, grammar use, fluency, comprehension, repetition, and naming. Several systems are widely used to classify subtypes of aphasia, often without consensus on their criteria. However, it is generally recognized that aphasia can be classified into either "fluent" or "nonfluent" main subtypes, reflecting whether the individual can either speak fluidly or with considerable effort (Boller, 1981). Aphasias may include paraphasias (inadvertently producing incorrect words, or substituting incorrect speech sounds), or jargon aphasia, which is rife with completely new words that nonetheless retain the

Gestalt of speech sounds that resemble the patient's native language. *Alexia*, the inability to read despite seeing letters or other symbolic characters, is not unusual following posterior left hemisphere stroke and has been found in 2% of a large registry of stroke patients (Hoffmann, 2009).

A number of speech-language pathology interventions have been found to improve performance on tests of language in the laboratory (Brady, Kelly, Godwin, Enderby, & Campbell, 2016), yet few have been shown to influence actual use of language outside the treatment setting. A widely used approach, melodic intonation therapy, in which patients sing when practicing sentences, is not consistently successful (Van Der Meulen, Van de Sandt-Koenderman, Heijenbrok, Visch-Brink, & Ribbers, 2016). Interventions for alexia have not been well developed (Starrfelt et al., 2013). However, recent attention has been directed to ameliorate learned nonuse of verbal communication in aphasia. Accordingly, the adaptation of the CIMT approach to aphasia, hence termed constraint-induced aphasia therapy II (CIAT II), has preliminarily been shown to improve the spontaneous production of speech outside of the clinic (Johnson et al., 2014). Novel therapeutic approaches with technological advances are also being explored. Treating aphasia with either a computer or a smart tablet could allow increased task practice and save treatment expense but at a cost of reduced interaction with a therapist, and thus this is not supported as clinical practice guidelines for treatment of aphasia. Studies using such devices to date (Lavoie, Macoir, & Bier, 2017) have evaluated only small patient samples; follow-up was seldom as long as 1 year, and language outcomes were examined only under controlled circumstances. Considerable growth in recent years has been shown in supplementing speech-language therapy with noninvasive brain electrical or magnetic stimulation (Norise & Hamilton, 2017). Preliminary results with these modalities (tDCS, TMS) have shown benefit with a variety of language functions, with improvements in some cases lasting as much as a year. Extension of benefits to real-world spontaneous speech has not yet been evaluated.

Rehabilitation psychologists can play a role in aphasia treatment by assisting patients in practicing communication skills that have been taught to them by the speech-language pathologist (SLP). Rehabilitation psychologists can focus interventions on helping the patient to understand their aphasia and the key role that communicating with others plays in recovery of language function. Additionally, patients with aphasia face a world in which verbal communication is critical for maintenance of relationships with others and completing multiple life tasks and activities. Many patients avoid communicating with others outside of the SLP treatment room because of the frustration and embarrassment that can accompany the communication challenges. Rehabilitation psychology interventions can help to facilitate the patient's emotional adjustment and motivation to use communication strategies and skills more readily in daily life. Cotreatment sessions with the SLP can help the patient to manage any frustration or emotional upset during the treatment session so the patient can more readily engage in therapy with the SLP.

Unilateral Spatial Neglect

Many stroke patients exhibit an attentional bias to the visual space opposite the involved hemisphere. This condition—unilateral spatial neglect—disrupts many ADLs, as patients may read from only one half of a page, eat from one side of a plate, groom one side of their face, and risk collisions during mobility (Mark, 2003). In its acute presentation, neglect occurs in about half of stroke patients and is about equally common following left versus right hemisphere damage (Kleinman et al., 2007; Stone, Halligan, & Greenwood, 1993), but generally right unilateral neglect is milder and resolves more rapidly than does left neglect. By 3 months, 70% of neglect patients have recovered (Cassidy, Lewis, & Gray, 1998).

Neglect is tested by either informally assessing the patient's interaction with the environment or by formal testing, mostly using pen-and-paper tests, such as the cancellation test. Neglect, as reflected by impaired performance on cancellation tasks, can predict dependency on ADLs after stroke (Agrell, Dehlin, & Dahlgren, 1997).

Despite many decades of testing treatments of neglect, consistent outcomes have not been found (Yang, Zhou, Chung, Li-Tsang, & Fong, 2013), and there has been little attention paid to impact on real-world activities. Currently, research largely focuses on prism adaptation treatment, in which patients practice reaching while wearing goggles that displace their view to the nonneglected side. When the goggles are removed after the practice, patients improve on common laboratory tests by attending more adequately toward the neglect side. However, sustained or consistent benefits have not been found (Azouvi, Jacquin-Courtois, & Luauté, 2017).

EMOTIONAL ADJUSTMENT AND CHANGES IN AFFECT AND EMOTIONAL REGULATION POSTSTROKE

Stroke is a significant, life-changing, often traumatic event. It is common, and even appropriate, for patients to experience a wide variety of emotions as they work to accommodate to what has happened to them, cope with the changes to their functional abilities, and anticipate their lives after hospital discharge. Following a stroke, some individuals have reported feeling a loss of their former self, as if a part of them had actually died (Alaszewski, Alaszewski, & Potter, 2004). Patients may feel a sense of diminished self-worth and may lose trust in their own abilities or in the judgment of those evaluating their progress, particularly if communication regarding goals and expectations has not been sufficiently clear. Recovering from a stroke is also a period of great uncertainty for many patients because it is often not possible to accurately predict specific functional outcomes in the long term. Even when patients are able to resume many of their formerly valued life activities, they may feel that their new level of function is fundamentally different and less satisfying compared with that before the stroke. As patients work toward accommodating to their condition, they may make efforts to find meaning in what has happened to them.

One approach to understanding the course of motional adjustment to stroke is through the bereavement model of coping with loss (Alaszewski et al., 2004). This model posits that although patients may experience the common reactions of denial, anger, bargaining, depression, and acceptance as they might after the death of a loved one, patients may not experience stages in this order, may not pass through all stages, and may not make linear progress from one stage to another. Rehabilitation psychologists must acknowledge the uniqueness of how each stroke survivor and his or her family come to terms with the impact on their lives. This model nevertheless may help to conceptualize the emotions and thoughts experienced by individuals coping with stroke.

Rehabilitation psychologists have a unique role within the clinical team to assist patients in emotionally adjusting to their personal experience of stroke and how it has affected their bodies, self-concepts, and life goals. Providing patients with opportunities to process their thoughts and feelings since having the stroke will assist patients in coming to terms with the changes in themselves and their lives, and help to promote their engagement in the rehabilitation process. To augment the patient's sense of personal control, the entire clinical team should work to create a therapeutic environment where the patient can voice his or her needs and contribute to the identification of rehabilitation goals. Family members can best aid in the process of adjustment by establishing clear communication with the patient and allowing the individual to voice needs, define goals, and discuss expectations.

Poststroke Depression

Depression is the most common poststroke mood disorder, with a prevalence of 20% to 30%, depending on the assessment tools used (Robinson & Jorge, 2016). Depressed mood and anhedonia are the most frequently reported symptoms, but other features of depression may be present as well, including fatigue, changes in sleep and appetite, feelings of guilt or worthlessness, and suicidality (Ferro, Caeiro, & Figueira, 2016). Less commonly, depression symptoms may be accompanied by mania (Santos, Caeiro, Ferro, & Figueira, 2011). Depression may develop shortly after stroke or later in recovery and may be long-lasting. Poststroke depression is associated with increased mortality, poorer functional outcomes, and less efficient use of rehabilitation services (Hadidi, Treat-Jacobson, & Lindquist, 2009). Prestroke mood disorder is the primary risk factor for poststroke depression, along with severity of cognitive and physical disability following the stroke (Ferro et al., 2016).

Poststroke depression is most commonly assessed through a combination of clinical interview and self-report questionnaires. Widely used questionnaires include the Beck Depression Inventory—II (BDI–II; Beck, Steer, Ball, & Ranieri, 1996) and the Patient Health Questionnaire (Kroenke, Spitzer, & Williams, 2001). It should be noted that these instruments are primarily used to screen for depression in the general population and are not specific to poststroke depression. Caution should be used with some instruments (e.g., the BDI–II) because they have not been developed specifically to detect depression in medical populations, and some items overlap with illness-related symptoms the patient may be experiencing (e.g., sleep disturbance, changes in sexual function, appetite changes), leading to a false-positive diagnosis. Poststroke depression is typically treated with antidepressant medication, psychotherapy, or a combination of both (Mead et al., 2012).

Anxiety Disorders

Prevalence rates for poststroke anxiety are similar to those of poststroke depression at 20% to 25% (Campbell Burton et al., 2013). Generalized anxiety is the most common anxiety disorder seen after a stroke, but panic disorder and specific phobias may also occur. Risk factors for poststroke anxiety include prestroke mood disorders, comorbid poststroke depression, and cognitive impairment (Morrison, Pollard, Johnston, & MacWalter, 2005). Unlike depression, poststroke anxiety does not appear to impede physical recovery from stroke, but it is associated with poorer quality of life (Tang, Lau, Mok, Ungvari, & Wong, 2013).

Anxiety is commonly assessed with a combination of clinical interview and self-report measures. Common screening tools include the Generalized Anxiety Disorder seven-item scale (Spitzer, Kroenke, Williams, & Löwe, 2006) and the Hospital Anxiety and Depression Scale (Zigmond & Snaith, 1983). Common treatment approaches include a combination of medication, psychotherapy, and relaxation training (Ferro et al., 2016).

Posttraumatic stress disorder (PTSD) in rehabilitation populations is an area of relatively new and growing interest. Stroke meets the *Diagnostic and Statistical Manual of Mental Disorders* (fifth edition; American Psychiatric Association, 2013) criteria for a precipitating event with the potential to be life-threatening and to be associated with significant feelings of helplessness and loss of control. Prevalence of PTSD in stroke patients varies depending on the assessment measure used but is estimated to be between 10% and 31% (Ferro et al., 2016). Patients who experience delirium or other cognitive impairment may be especially susceptible to PTSD associated with their hospital stay. Additional risk factors include prestroke history of trauma, psychiatric comorbidities, and lower education level (Favrole et al., 2013; Goldfinger et al., 2014). Poststroke PTSD is associated with lower adherence to medication and other follow-up and preventative care (Kronish, Edmondson, Goldfinger, Fei, & Horowitz, 2012).

Screening measures including the Post-Traumatic Stress Checklist have been used to detect PTSD in patients with critical illness. However, evidence suggests that the use of screening measures may lead to a high rate of false positives; therefore, a concurrent interview is recommended (Favrole et al., 2013). Although not specific to stroke, research on critical illness PTSD supports combining pharmacological treatment and psychotherapy, particularly cognitive behavior therapy and exposure-based interventions (Jackson et al., 2016). In addition, providing education on psychological responses to trauma and taking steps to maximize the patient's sense of control over their care can help reduce the risk and impact of PTSD in critical illness populations, including stroke.

Pseudobulbar Affect

Sometimes called *pathological affect*, *pseudobulbar affect* (PBA) is a disorder of emotional lability characterized by uncontrollable laughing or crying in the absence of the patient feeling amusement or sadness, respectively. Prevalence is approximately 17% immediately after stroke, decreasing to about half of this over time. PBA has a detrimental effect on quality of life, especially with regard to social participation. Patients are commonly distressed by their symptoms, may limit their activities, and become isolated as a result. Poststroke depression is a common comorbidity of PBA. Treatment with antidepressants has shown some benefit for patients with PBA (Gillespie, Cadden, Lees, West, & Broomfield, 2016). The compound of dextromethorphan with quinidine is also effective and has been the only medication approved by the U.S. Food and Drug Administration for treating PBA (A. Miller, Pratt, & Schiffer, 2011).

CHANGES IN BEHAVIOR POSTSTROKE

After stroke, individuals may experience changes in behavior, such as apathy, anger, and aggression, and be characterized as having a personality change. Additionally, symptoms such as poststroke fatigue may have a significant effect on behavior. Rehabilitation psychologists have a notable role in characterizing the patient's behavior and understanding it within the context of the illness experience, the stroke sequelae, the emotional response, and the prestroke behavior pattern. Such understanding facilitates designing interventions that truly can address the behaviors that may be maladaptive and disruptive, while respecting the person with all of his or her values, beliefs, foibles, and idiosyncrasies. Additionally, promoting the patient's engaging in healthy behaviors for impacting overall health as well as reducing the stroke risk are key areas for behavioral interventions.

Personality Changes

It is well understood that stroke affects an individual's brain functioning in many ways, forcing an individual to face daily life tasks with a revised set of skills and abilities. In addition, the individual must cope, adapt, and adjust to the constellation of impairments as well as their impact on daily life and the roles he or she has had in all realms of life. Many individuals approach and react to life experiences and challenges differently than they did prestroke, and that is interpreted as a change in personality. However, the behavioral changes that are interpreted as changes to the patient's personality are not necessarily linked to that person's lifelong style and approach to coping. The overall finding is that following stroke, patients tend to engage in more negative, maladaptive behaviors. Whether this tendency is rooted in a true change in "personality" or is better understood as changes in cognitive functioning or emotional regulation, the impact is the same with detrimental effects on interpersonal relationships. The role of the rehabilitation psychologist is to help the patient understand the increase in maladaptive behaviors and the impact on his or her relationship with others. Helping the individual to improve his or her awareness and self-monitoring of behavior and adopt strategies to manage behavior so that it does not affect relationships is the goal. Two of the most common forms of "personality change" that have been recognized poststroke are apathy and aggression.

Apathy is characterized by low motivation, difficulty with initiating spontaneous activity, and a sense of decreased emotional responsiveness or interest in valued activities and relationships (Caeiro, Ferro, & Figueira, 2012). Patients with poststroke apathy are able to perform tasks and activities when instructed or cued to do so but are less likely to do so on their own. Apathetic personality change differs from poststroke depression in that patients do not experience sadness and are not distressed by their lack of interest in daily activities (Ferro et al., 2016). However, depression is a common comorbidity of apathy (Caeiro, Ferro, Pinho E Melo, Canhão, & Figueira, 2013). The Apathy Scale (Marin, Biedrzycki, & Firinciogullari, 1991) may be used to rate the severity of poststroke apathy symptoms. Medications, including dopaminergic agents, antidepressants, and stimulants, can sometimes diminish the symptoms of poststroke apathy. Although limited research has been done on treatments for poststroke apathy, some evidence supports the use of coping-strategy training and problem-solving therapy (Ferro et al., 2016). Family education and behavioral strategies are also important for management.

Approximately 15% to 57% of patients may experience anger after stroke, with estimates varying greatly between studies (Ramos-Perdigués, Mané-Santacana, & Pintor-Pérez, 2015). Although this may be a common reaction to a life-changing event and adjustment to new-onset disability, it may also give rise to behavioral problems that can interfere with the rehabilitation process or significantly damage relationships. Aggression in persons with stroke may occur as a result of behaviorally dysregulated anger but may have other causes as well, including disinhibition, confusion due to cognitive impairment, or delirium (Ferro et al., 2016). Patients who have difficulty with comprehension may be especially susceptible to anger, hostility, and aggressive behavior. There is limited research on assessment and treatment of poststroke aggression, although evidence supports using selective serotonin reuptake inhibitors. Behavioral management strategies may center on education of the family or caregiver, with an effort toward identifying and limiting triggers of aggressive behavior. In some cases, psychotherapy and coping-skills training of the patient may also be beneficial (Ferro et al., 2016).

Fatigue

After stroke, many individuals complain of not having enough energy to complete daily tasks and engage in activities. Poststroke fatigue was previously thought to be a behavioral symptom of poststroke depression, but it has since been found to exist as an independent phenomenon. However, poststroke fatigue remains poorly defined, and there is no consensus on specific diagnostic criteria. In general, *poststroke fatigue* is characterized by chronic lack of energy or feeling of exhaustion, independent of exertion, and not improved by rest. Due to variation in the definition of poststroke fatigue, estimates of prevalence vary widely but may be as high as 74% (Ponchel, Bombois, Bordet, & Hénon, 2015). Poststroke fatigue is frequently reported by patients as one of their most bothersome symptoms and can have a significant impact on cognitive function, social participation, and ADLs. Poststroke fatigue may also be associated with more negative patient views of their own recovery from stroke (Ingles, Eskes, & Phillips, 1999). The etiology of poststroke fatigue is also not entirely clear, although it may be multifactorial, and the research literature suggests associations with mood symptoms, cognitive impairment, inflammatory processes, pain, and sleep disorders (Ponchel et al., 2015).

Although not specific to stroke, several scales are available for the assessment of fatigue including the Fatigue Assessment Scale (Michielsen, De Vries, & Van Heck, 2003), Fatigue Impact Scale (J. D. Fisk et al., 1994), and Fatigue Severity Scale (Lerdal & Kottorp, 2011). In terms of management, it is important to rule out medical comorbidities and side effects of medications. Pharmacological agents used to treat hypersomnia may be beneficial. A behavioral fatigue management program may also be developed that may include elements such as behavioral activation and pleasant events scheduling, increasing physical activity, activity pacing, and mindfulness techniques. There is also support for the value of cognitive behavior therapy in the comprehensive management of poststroke fatigue (Choi-Kwon, Mitchell, & Kim, 2015).

Healthy Behaviors and Secondary Stroke Prevention

Unhealthy behaviors before a stroke likely contributed to the event and, if maintained, risk recurrent stroke. Individuals with a stroke have an increased risk of further stroke compared with the general population: Approximately 3% to 4% will have another stroke. The risk varies with characteristics of the initial stroke, age, comorbid conditions, and adherence to preventative strategies among other factors (Kernan et al., 2014). Rehabilitation psychologists can play a key role in health behavior change to reduce the chance of another stroke and improve patients' overall health.

Comprehensive recommendations for prevention of subsequent stroke are provided by the AHA/ASA (Kernan et al., 2014), foremost among which is management of comorbid medical conditions such as hypertension, hyperlipidemia, obstructive sleep apnea, and atrial fibrillation. Second, it is recommended that patients eat a balanced diet, with the consideration of nutrition consultation for individuals who have particularly complex needs or poor habits in this area. Physical activity is also important for promoting long-term health of individuals who have experienced stroke. This may be a particular challenge for persons who were previously sedentary or who may have new physical limitations resulting from stroke. Nevertheless, physical activity has been shown to benefit both recovery and long-term health maintenance as well as emotional and cognitive function (Saunders et al., 2016). Finally, it is important that patients abstain from substance abuse, most commonly tobacco and alcohol. Rehabilitation psychologists can provide interventions to assist patients in reducing unhealthy behaviors and encourage engagement in healthy activities. These might include goal-setting, problem-solving, and activity scheduling. Use of motivational interviewing during interventions may help to promote healthy behavior change (Watkins et al., 2011).

IMPACT OF STROKE IMPAIRMENTS ON SELF-CARE AND LIFE MANAGEMENT

The ability to live independently and participate in valued activities is often viewed as the most important outcome by patients undergoing rehabilitation from stroke as well as by their family members. Studies have found that patients commonly report feeling a loss of independence, decreased ability to be spontaneous, and a decline in ability to carry out valued activities. Stroke patients experience a wide variety of barriers to participation in these activities, many of which have been discussed in the previous sections of this chapter. With regard to identifying and characterizing these barriers, a recent review of the literature divides them into two categories: (a) visible barriers (e.g., motor difficulties) and (b) invisible barriers (e.g., depression, cognitive impairment). The impact of each specific barrier varies greatly for different individuals; therefore, it is important to fully assess each patient's perceptions, values, and goals (Woodman, Riazi, Pereira, & Jones, 2014).

Multiple standardized scales have been developed for the evaluation of patients' ability to engage in activities of daily living following stroke or other acquired brain injury. Some of the more common measures include the Index of Independence in Activities of Daily Living (Katz, Downs, Cash, & Grotz, 1970), Stroke Impact Scale (Duncan et al., 1999), the Functional Independence Measure (Dodds, Martin, Stolov, & Deyo, 1993), and the Fugl-Meyer Assessment (Fugl-Meyer et al., 1975). However, although these scales may be useful in quantifying and identifying areas of difficulty or advising patients and families making decisions about the ability to return to independent living, they may not capture individual values and therefore may fail to identify the challenges most salient to a specific patient. Standardized assessment measures in this area should be used in conjunction with clinical interview to identify targets for intervention and rehabilitation in individual instances.

When coping with these changes, patients may choose to either resume or discontinue a previously valued activity, to pursue an adapted activity, or to try new activities entirely. In making these decisions, patients must evaluate the personal value placed on a given activity against the barriers to that activity. Assisting in this process can be crucial for the rehabilitation psychologist, both early in the recovery process and over the longer term. Foci of interventions may include building patients' confidence in their ability to adapt to their current level of function, problem-solving real and perceived barriers to such adaptation, and helping patients identify personal meaning to promote values-based life choices.

THE IMPACT ON INTERPERSONAL RELATIONSHIPS

Patients who have experienced a stroke frequently report changes in interpersonal relationships. This may manifest as an increase in perceived stress and anxiety within the relationship, or individuals may simply feel that their social role has changed (e.g., "patient and caregiver" rather than "husband and wife"). Relationships may shift as a result of the patient's need for physical assistance, such as help with transfers or dressing and bathing. Dynamics may also change due to cognitive or emotional sequelae. For example, when patients are unable to drive, make financial decisions, or engage in other previously shared activities, a sense of grief and loss may be experienced by both parties in the relationship. Family and friends of stroke survivors may have to cope with behavioral changes. Cognitive and emotional changes may be particularly difficult for patients, families, and friends to adjust to and thus may be more challenging than physical impairments (Camak, 2015).

Assessment and interventions focused on the constellation and quality of the interpersonal relationships that a patient has in his or her life are important parts of psychological care. Understanding the patient's social environment and support system is based in the patient's views on the various people in his or her life and the roles they have played, are currently playing, and will be playing in the future. Rehabilitation interventions need to consider the amount and type of support from family and friends that can be provided when designing the intervention plan. Additionally, the process of recovery from stroke, given the inherent stressors with illness, hospitalization, impact on finances, and changes in roles, for example, can lead to relationship problems. Rehabilitation psychologists are well poised to provide interventions that can aid the patient and key family and friends in maintaining or even bolstering these relationships during this stressful process.

Caregivers

Families and friends can facilitate the adjustment of stroke survivors and also can serve in important caregiving roles. The physical and mental health of these family members and friends can affect the adjustment and well-being of individuals recovering from stroke (Klinedinst et al., 2009). Although there are positive aspects to caregiving, it is often associated with significant declines in overall quality of life. Caregiving is associated with depressive symptoms and anxiety, stress-related health problems, loss of ability to work, and social isolation. Thus, the adaptation and adjustment of caregivers needs to be a parallel intervention goal to help caregivers maintain their physical and emotional health and foster the resiliency to provide needed care.

The rehabilitation psychologist can facilitate this process by first assessing the role of family and friends in the recovery process as sources of emotional and instrumental social support. Then the psychologist can assist the team in incorporating caregivers throughout the rehabilitation process, which will help to minimize the stress of transition back into the home and community environment for both the patient and the caregiver. The psychologist can assist with education and training of caregivers so that they know best how to provide the optimal level of assistance and support to their loved ones. In addition, the rehabilitation psychologist may take an active part in promoting clear communication between patient and family members as new boundaries and roles are negotiated. Psychoeducation regarding caregiver burden itself may be equally important because caregivers often feel isolated by their own negative responses to assisting loved ones. Social support and caregiver problem-solving skills have been identified as independent predictors of caregiver burden (J. S. Grant et al., 2006). Therefore, therapeutic interventions such as family systems therapy, social problem-solving training, or coping skills training that aim to improve these factors may be beneficial. Given that caregivers engaging in their own self-care is an important and often-overlooked aspect of rehabilitation (Loh, Tan, Zhang, & Ho, 2017), giving permission for and emphasizing the importance of caregiver self-care engagement is an important role for the rehabilitation psychologist.

Sexuality

For many individuals, sexual activities are of high personal value and contribute to overall quality of life. Although stroke can have significant effects on sex for both men and women, this area is often overlooked by medical teams during rehabilitation and recovery. A recent review of the literature found that more than half of patients reported a decrease in sex after stroke, although over time many individuals were able to resume sexual participation. This same analysis found that even in patients who resume sex following stroke, a significant number (as high as 90% in one study) reported decreased sexual satisfaction compared with before stroke (Rosenbaum, Vadas, & Kalichman, 2014). Barriers to sex following stroke may include physical challenges (e.g., comorbid medical conditions, sensorimotor impairment) as well as neurobehavioral difficulties such as cognitive impairment or emotional sequelae. Difficulty may also arise from changes in the nature of the relationship and patients' sense of identity. Psychoeducation regarding poststroke sex should be offered before discharge from the hospital or rehabilitation unit, and sexuality may become an important intervention target for longer term outpatient interventions.

IMPACT OF STROKE IMPAIRMENTS ON KEY LIFE ACTIVITIES

The meaning of life is intertwined with the activities in which a person engages. The key life activities vary from individual to individual, although they all appear to be related to some degree to experiencing self-reliance, self-determination, and self-expression. The most common activities are living in the community, driving, and working. The impairments that are associated with stroke can dramatically impact engagement in such activities, thus altering the meaning of life for that individual. Understanding these key life activities and how engaging in them is affected by the poststroke impairments is critical for designing appropriate interventions to assist the individual in returning to the activity or, when return is not possible, in adapting and adjusting to the "loss" of or changes to those activities.

Independent Living

There is surprisingly little scientific literature available regarding either the percentage of patients who are able to return to independent living after stroke or the determinants of the ability to do so. This likely results from the fact that the goal of inpatient rehabilitation programs is not to discharge patients at a completely independent level, but rather to promote a combination of recovery and compensation that allows individuals to leave the hospital with the assistance of a family member or other caregiver. Notably, however, international practices vary considerably with regard to the average length of stay for inpatient rehabilitation. In the United States, the typical length of hospitalization for stroke rehabilitation is fewer than 20 days (Rinere O'Brien, 2010). In contrast, lengths of stay in many European countries may be several times longer (Geschwindner, Rettke, van den Heuvel, Halfens, & Dassen, 2007; Morone, Paolucci, & Iosa, 2015; Schnitzler, Woimant, Nicolau, Tuppin, & de Peretti, 2014). Thus, cultural standards with regard to the objectives of stroke inpatient rehabilitation may vary considerably. The possible contributions of the duration of hospital stays to stroke rehabilitation outcomes have not been comprehensively studied.

Most stroke patients who are discharged from inpatient care go on to outpatient therapies, and the majority report some level of long-term disability (Mozaffarian et al., 2016). Although standardized assessments such as the Functional Independence Measure (Dodds et al., 1993), Barthel Index (Collin, Wade, Davies, & Horne, 1988), and Modified Rankin Scale (van Swieten, Koudstaal, Visser, Schouten, & van Gijn, 1988) may capture strengths and weaknesses in performing ADLs, these tools alone are not sufficient to plan for the patient's need for assistance upon discharge. Likewise, neuropsychological assessment may elucidate areas of cognitive difficulty that could limit function in the home (e.g., patients with memory deficits may need assistance with medication management), but the findings have limited ecological validity. Ultimately, the treatment team should work in conjunction with the patient and family to determine how much and what kinds of assistance will be needed after discharge from the inpatient unit, recognizing the need to continue to adapt the intervention program during the outpatient programming in light of the patient's evolving needs for assistance. The rehabilitation psychologist may help facilitate this communication and may assist the patient in coping with the strong emotions that are often associated with planning for the future, taking into account changes in functional status.

A number of assistive devices, technologies, and home modifications can assist in making patients more mobile, interactive, and self-reliant within the world around them. The majority of patients discharged from the hospital after stroke will use assistive technology devices (ATDs) and implement environmental modifications within the home. The most common ATDs are mobility aids, which include wheelchairs, walkers, and canes, and bathroom equipment, such as bath seats and commode chairs. Common environmental modifications to the home include the installation of grab bars in the bathroom, alterations to entryways, and changes to floor surfaces to reduce the risk of falls (Sørensen, Lendal, Schultz-Larsen, & Uhrskov, 2003). A wide variety of ATDs are available, and care should ensure that the devices chosen for a given patient align with that individual's psychosocial context and personal values. The Assistive Technology Device

Predisposition Assessment is an evidence-based assessment aimed at facilitating this match (Scherer, Craddock, & Mackeogh, 2011). The goal with the devices, equipment, and modification is to facilitate the patient's access to the home and community so that she or he may engage in self-care, home care, and community-based activities.

Driving

The ability to drive after stroke is important for some patients, particularly younger individuals. Although more studies are needed, the literature suggests that approximately 30% of persons who were fit to drive before stroke return to driving afterward (G. D. Fisk, Owsley, & Pulley, 1997). Common protocols for deciding fitness for driving poststroke have not yet been established, and many patients who return to the road do not undergo any formal evaluation at all. Although road tests are the gold standard for driving fitness, with favorable clinimetric properties (Akinwuntan et al., 2005), they can be costly and time-intensive and therefore may not be suitable for first-line evaluation of all patients interested in returning to driving. A systematic review of screening measures for predicting driving safety identified cognitive tests of executive functioning as the most accurate tools. These included the Trail Making Test, the Rey–Osterreith Complex Figure, and the Useful Field of View Test (Marshall et al., 2007). Although a rehabilitation psychologist should not independently clear a patient for driving, administering a neuropsychological assessment battery may help to determine which patients should be referred for additional assessment including medical clearance and on-road evaluation.

Return to Work

The rate of return to employment following stroke varies greatly, with estimates ranging from 20% to 70% depending on the study (Mennemeyer, Taub, Uswatte, & Pearson, 2006). The strongest predictors of return to employment are younger age and lesser severity of stroke-related disability. Economic factors also play a role, with patients who have greater financial incentive returning to work at higher rates. As with returning to other ADLs, barriers to employment may be either physical or neurobehavioral, with patients who experience cognitive and emotional dysfunction following stroke having a more difficult time returning to work compared with those with only physical impairments (Mennemeyer et al., 2006; Wolfenden & Grace, 2009). Likewise, it is important to assess the value and personal meaning patients ascribe to returning to work because some may have little incentive to do so.

When patients do wish to return to work, this should be addressed early in rehabilitation, as behavioral and problem-solving strategies may help to negotiate a variety of challenges during this transition. Assisting the patient and family in providing education for the patient's employer and colleagues may be beneficial. Patients often benefit from a gradual return-to-work process that includes reduced hours and responsibilities at first while learning and incorporating strategies such as activity-type and -level pacing and cognitive compensation. A comprehensive neuropsychological evaluation is particularly helpful for patients who are attempting a return to work, as the results of this assessment provide key objective information about cognitive and behavioral strengths and weaknesses that can then become therapeutic targets for cognitive rehabilitation, the use of compensatory strategies, or collaborative problem-solving. Psychotherapy may also be of benefit for managing the emotional aspects of returning to work or adjusting to the inability to do so.

One seldom-discussed aspect of this area is the ability of caregivers to return to work as patients progress in their recovery. A study of patients who had received CIMT revealed that, although few of them returned to work despite significant functional gains, many of their caregivers did so. This suggested that patients had improved sufficiently in their functional independence for caregivers to be able and willing to resume their own employment. This may be an important outcome in cases where caregivers have significant incentive to return to work, while patients may view their own ability to work as having less personal value (Mennemeyer et al., 2006).

CONCLUSION

Rehabilitation psychologists play a vital role in the care of stroke survivors. As outlined in this chapter, they assess and provide interventions for stroke-related impairments and changes in function; promote adaptation and adjustment; provide education to the patient and family about the constellation of impairments, how these impairments will affect function now and in the future, and how these impairments will be addressed by the rehabilitation team; and collaborate with the rest of the rehabilitation team to develop and implement the assessment and intervention plan. However, as a field, further work is needed to develop additional interventions to address poststroke sequelae, emotional adjustment, and the impact on engagement in meaningful life activities. For example, empirically supported brief psychotherapy interventions for poststroke depression and anxiety disorders should be made available. Instruments that capture the impact of cognitive impairments on daily life functioning so that clinicians have ecologically valid tools for predicting daily life functioning need to be developed. Cognitive rehabilitation techniques that take advantage of recent findings on neuroplasticity after brain injury need to be developed and tested (Merzenich, Nahum, & Van Vleet, 2014; Uswatte & Taub, 2013). Cultural circumstances that require tailored care need to be identified, and culturally appropriate assessments and therapies need to be developed. Although there are already some investigators studying these areas of stroke care, establishment of centers for research and training, along the lines of the model systems centers for traumatic brain injury and spinal cord injury care, would provide resources for the engagement of a greater number of rehabilitation psychologists in stroke research and thereby catapult the field of stroke care forward.

References

Agrell, B. M., Dehlin, O. I., & Dahlgren, C. J. (1997). Neglect in elderly stroke patients: A comparison of five tests. *Psychiatry and Clinical Neurosciences*, *51*, 295–300. http://dx.doi.org/10.1111/j.1440-1819.1997.tb03201.x

Akinwuntan, A. E., De Weerdt, W., Feys, H., Baten, G., Arno, P., & Kiekens, C. (2005). The validity of a road test after stroke. *Archives of Physical Medicine and Rehabilitation*, *86*, 421–426. http://dx.doi.org/10.1016/j.apmr.2004.04.047

Alaszewski, A., Alaszewski, H., & Potter, J. (2004). The bereavement model, stroke and rehabilitation: A critical analysis of the use of a psychological model in professional practice. *Disability and Rehabilitation*, *26*, 1067–1078. http://dx.doi.org/10.1080/09638280410001703521

American Psychiatric Association. (2013). *Diagnostic and statistical manual of mental disorders* (5th ed.). Washington, DC: Author.

Andrade, S. M., Fernández-Calvo, B., Boggio, P. S., de Oliveira, E. A., Gomes, L. F., Pinheiro Júnior, J. E., . . . Alves, N. T. (2015). Neurostimulation for cognitive rehabilitation in stroke (NeuroCog): Study protocol for a randomized controlled trial. *Trials*, *16*, 435. http://dx.doi.org/10.1186/s13063-015-0945-1

Assal, G., Favre, C., & Anderes, J. P. (1984). Non-reconnaissance d'animaux familiers chez un paysan. Zoo-agnosie ou prosopagnosie pour les animaux [Nonrecognition of familiar animals by a farmer. Zooagnosia or prosopagnosia for animals]. *Revue Neurologique*, *140*, 580–584.

Atance, C. M., & O'Neill, D. K. (2001). Episodic future thinking. *Trends in Cognitive Sciences*, *5*, 533–539. http://dx.doi.org/10.1016/S1364-6613(00)01804-0

Azouvi, P., Jacquin-Courtois, S., & Luauté, J. (2017). Rehabilitation of unilateral neglect: Evidence-based medicine. *Annals of Physical and Rehabilitation Medicine*, *60*, 191–197. http://dx.doi.org/10.1016/j.rehab.2016.10.006

Bartolo, M., Zucchella, C., Capone, A., Sandrini, G., & Pierelli, F. (2015). An explorative study regarding the effect of l-deprenyl on cognitive and functional recovery in patients after stroke. *Journal of the Neurological Sciences*, *349*, 117–123. http://dx.doi.org/10.1016/j.jns.2014.12.039

Beck, A. T., Steer, R. A., Ball, R., & Ranieri, W. (1996). Comparison of Beck Depression Inventories–IA and –II in psychiatric outpatients. *Journal of Personality Assessment*, *67*, 588–597. http://dx.doi.org/10.1207/s15327752jpa6703_13

Bennett-Levy, J., & Powell, G. E. (1980). The Subjective Memory Questionnaire (SMQ). An investigation into the self-reporting of "real-life" memory skills. *British Journal of Social & Clinical Psychology*, *19*, 177–188. http://dx.doi.org/10.1111/j.2044-8260.1980.tb00946.x

Bogdanova, Y., Yee, M. K., Ho, V. T., & Cicerone, K. D. (2016). Computerized cognitive rehabilitation of attention and executive function in acquired brain injury: A systematic review. *The Journal of Head Trauma Rehabilitation*, *31*, 419–433. http://dx.doi.org/10.1097/HTR.0000000000000203

Boller, F. (1981). Strokes and behavior: Disorders of higher cortical functions following cerebral disease. Disorders of language and related function. *Stroke*, *12*, 532–534. http://dx.doi.org/10.1161/01.STR.12.4.532

Brady, M. C., Kelly, H., Godwin, J., Enderby, P., & Campbell, P. (2016). Speech and language therapy for aphasia following stroke. *Cochrane Database of Systematic Reviews*, *6*, CD000425.

Broomfield, N. M., Laidlaw, K., Hickabottom, E., Murray, M. F., Pendrey, R., Whittick, J. E., & Gillespie, D. C. (2011). Post-stroke depression: The case for augmented, individually tailored cognitive behavioural therapy. *Clinical Psychology & Psychotherapy*, *18*, 202–217. http://dx.doi.org/10.1002/cpp.711

Burton, C. M., & King, L. A. (2004). The health benefits of writing about intensely positive experiences. *Journal of Research in Personality*, *38*, 150–163. http://dx.doi.org/10.1016/S0092-6566(03)00058-8

Butcher, J. N., Graham, J. R., Ben-Porath, Y. S., Tellegen, A., Dahlstrom, W. G., & Kaemmer, B. (2001). *MMPI–2: Manual for administration and scoring* (rev. ed.). Minneapolis: University of Minnesota Press.

Caeiro, L., Ferro, J. M., & Figueira, M. L. (2012). Apathy in acute stroke patients. *European Journal of Neurology*, *19*, 291–297. http://dx.doi.org/10.1111/j.1468-1331.2011.03508.x

Caeiro, L., Ferro, J. M., Pinho E Melo, T., Canhão, P., & Figueira, M. L. (2013). Post-stroke apathy: An exploratory longitudinal study. *Cerebrovascular Diseases*, *35*, 507–513. http://dx.doi.org/10.1159/000350202

Camak, D. J. (2015). Addressing the burden of stroke caregivers: A literature review. *Journal of Clinical Nursing*, *24*, 2376–2382. http://dx.doi.org/10.1111/jocn.12884

Campbell Burton, C. A., Murray, J., Holmes, J., Astin, F., Greenwood, D., & Knapp, P. (2013). Frequency of anxiety after stroke: A systematic review and meta-analysis of observational studies. *International Journal of Stroke*, *8*, 545–559. http://dx.doi.org/10.1111/j.1747-4949.2012.00906.x

Carver, C. S., Scheier, M. F., & Weintraub, J. K. (1989). Assessing coping strategies: A theoretically based approach. *Journal of Personality and Social Psychology*, *56*, 267–283. http://dx.doi.org/10.1037/0022-3514.56.2.267

Cassidy, T. P., Lewis, S., & Gray, C. S. (1998). Recovery from visuospatial neglect in stroke patients. *Journal of Neurology, Neurosurgery, and Psychiatry*, *64*, 555–557. http://dx.doi.org/10.1136/jnnp.64.4.555

Choi-Kwon, S., Mitchell, P. H., & Kim, J. S. (2015). Nursing interventions for poststroke fatigue. *Stroke*, *46*, e224–e227. http://dx.doi.org/10.1161/STROKEAHA.115.009534

Collin, C., Wade, D. T., Davies, S., & Horne, V. (1988). The Barthel ADL Index: A reliability study. *International Disability Studies*, *10*, 61–63. http://dx.doi.org/10.3109/09638288809164103

Connell, L. A., Lincoln, N. B., & Radford, K. A. (2008). Somatosensory impairment after stroke: Frequency of different deficits and their recovery. *Clinical Rehabilitation*, *22*, 758–767. http://dx.doi.org/10.1177/0269215508090674

Coupar, F., Pollock, A., Rowe, P., Weir, C., & Langhorne, P. (2012). Predictors of upper limb recovery after stroke: A systematic review and meta-analysis. *Clinical Rehabilitation*, *26*, 291–313. http://dx.doi.org/10.1177/0269215511420305

Cousins, R. (2013). Prosopagnosia after stroke: Potentials for impairment and treatment. *Topics in Stroke Rehabilitation*, *20*, 471–477. http://dx.doi.org/10.1310/tsr2006-471

Crane, R. S., Brewer, J., Feldman, C., Kabat-Zinn, J., Santorelli, S., Williams, J. M., & Kuyken, W. (2017). What defines mindfulness-based programs? The warp and the weft. *Psychological Medicine*, *47*, 990–999. http://dx.doi.org/10.1017/S0033291716003317

das Nair, R., Cogger, H., Worthington, E., & Lincoln, N. B. (2016). Cognitive rehabilitation for memory deficits after stroke. *Cochrane Database Systematic Reviews*, *9*, CD002293.

Davis, M., Robbins Eshelman, E., & McKay, M. (2008). *The relaxation and stress reduction workbook* (6th ed.). Oakland, CA: New Harbinger.

Delis, D. C., Kramer, J. H., & Kaplan, E. (2000). *California Verbal Learning Test—Second edition (CvLT–II)*. Indianapolis, IN: Pearson.

Dodds, T. A., Martin, D. P., Stolov, W. C., & Deyo, R. A. (1993). A validation of the functional independence measurement and its performance among rehabilitation inpatients. *Archives of Physical Medicine and Rehabilitation*, *74*, 531–536. http://dx.doi.org/10.1016/0003-9993(93)90119-U

Dovern, A., Fink, G. R., & Weiss, P. H. (2012). Diagnosis and treatment of upper limb apraxia. *Journal of Neurology*, *259*, 1269–1283. http://dx.doi.org/10.1007/s00415-011-6336-y

Duncan, P. W., Goldstein, L. B., Horner, R. D., Landsman, P. B., Samsa, G. P., & Matchar, D. B. (1994). Similar motor recovery of upper and lower extremities after stroke. *Stroke*, *25*, 1181–1188. http://dx.doi.org/10.1161/01.STR.25.6.1181

Duncan, P. W., Wallace, D., Lai, S. M., Johnson, D., Embretson, S., & Laster, L. J. (1999). The stroke impact scale version 2.0. Evaluation of reliability, validity, and sensitivity to change. *Stroke*, *30*, 2131–2140. http://dx.doi.org/10.1161/01.STR.30.10.2131

Ehde, D. M., Dillworth, T. M., & Turner, J. A. (2014). Cognitive-behavioral therapy for individuals with chronic pain: Efficacy, innovations, and directions for research. *American Psychologist*, *69*, 153–166. http://dx.doi.org/10.1037/a0035747

Emmons, R. A., & McCullough, M. E. (2003). Counting blessings versus burdens: An experimental investigation of gratitude and subjective well-being in daily life. *Journal of Personality and Social Psychology*, *84*, 377–389. http://dx.doi.org/10.1037/0022-3514.84.2.377

Estruch, R., Ros, E., Salas-Salvadó, J., Covas, M. I., Corella, D., Arós, F., . . . Martínez-González, M. A., & the PREDIMED Study Investigators. (2013). Primary prevention of cardiovascular disease with a Mediterranean diet [retracted and republished; see https://www.ncbi.nlm.nih.gov/pubmed/29897867]. *The New England Journal of Medicine*, *368*, 1279–1290. http://dx.doi.org/10.1056/NEJMoa1200303

Favrole, P., Jehel, L., Levy, P., Descombes, S., Muresan, I. P., Manifacier, M. J., & Alamowitch, S. (2013). Frequency and predictors of post-traumatic stress disorder after stroke: A pilot study. *Journal of the Neurological Sciences*, *327*, 35–40. http://dx.doi.org/10.1016/j.jns.2013.02.001

Feigin, V. L., Forouzanfar, M. H., Krishnamurthi, R., Mensah, G. A., Connor, M., Bennett, D. A., . . . Murray, C., & the Global Burden of Diseases, Injuries, and Risk Factors Study 2010 (GBD 2010) and the GBD Stroke Experts Group. (2014). Global and regional burden of stroke during 1990–2010: Findings from the Global Burden of Disease Study 2010. *The Lancet*, *383*, 245–254. http://dx.doi.org/10.1016/S0140-6736(13)61953-4

Ferro, J. M., Caeiro, L., & Figueira, M. L. (2016). Neuropsychiatric sequelae of stroke. *Nature Reviews. Neurology*, *12*, 269–280. http://dx.doi.org/10.1038/nrneurol.2016.46

Fisk, G. D., Owsley, C., & Pulley, L. V. (1997). Driving after stroke: Driving exposure, advice, and evaluations. *Archives of Physical Medicine and Rehabilitation*, *78*, 1338–1345. http://dx.doi.org/10.1016/S0003-9993(97)90307-5

Fisk, J. D., Ritvo, P. G., Ross, L., Haase, D. A., Marrie, T. J., & Schlech, W. F. (1994). Measuring the functional impact of fatigue: Initial validation of the fatigue impact scale. *Clinical Infectious Diseases*, *18*(Suppl. 1), S79–S83. http://dx.doi.org/10.1093/clinids/18.Supplement_1.S79

Fugl-Meyer, A. R., Jääskö, L., Leyman, I., Olsson, S., & Steglind, S. (1975). The post-stroke hemiplegic patient. 1. A method for evaluation of physical performance. *Scandinavian Journal of Rehabilitation Medicine*, *7*, 13–31.

Gachtel, R. J. (2005). *Clinical essentials of pain management*. Washington, DC: American Psychological Association.

Geschwindner, H. M., Rettke, H., van den Heuvel, W. J. A., Halfens, R. J., & Dassen, T. (2007). Rehabilitation in acute stroke patients in German-speaking Switzerland. *Swiss Medical Weekly*, *137*, 205–211.

Gillespie, D. C., Cadden, A. P., Lees, R., West, R. M., & Broomfield, N. M. (2016). Prevalence of pseudobulbar affect following stroke: A systematic review and meta-analysis. *Journal of Stroke and Cerebrovascular Diseases*, *25*, 688–694. http://dx.doi.org/10.1016/j.jstrokecerebrovasdis.2015.11.038

Goldfinger, J. Z., Edmondson, D., Kronish, I. M., Fei, K., Balakrishnan, R., Tuhrim, S., & Horowitz, C. R. (2014). Correlates of post-traumatic stress disorder in stroke survivors. *Journal of Stroke and Cerebrovascular Diseases*, *25*, 1099–1105. http://dx.doi.org/10.1016/j.jstrokecerebrovasdis.2013.09.019

Goudsmit, E. M., Nijs, J., Jason, L. A., & Wallman, K. E. (2012). Pacing as a strategy to improve energy management in myalgic encephalomyelitis/chronic fatigue syndrome: A consensus document. *Disability and Rehabilitation*, *34*, 1140–1147. http://dx.doi.org/10.3109/09638288.2011.635746

Grant, A. M. (2012). Making positive change: A randomized study comparing solution-focused vs. problem-focused coaching questions. *Journal of Systemic Therapies*, *31*, 21–35. http://dx.doi.org/10.1521/jsyt.2012.31.2.21

Grant, J. S., Elliott, T. R., Weaver, M., Glandon, G. L., Raper, J. L., & Giger, J. N. (2006). Social support, social problem-solving abilities, and adjustment of family caregivers of stroke survivors. *Archives of Physical Medicine and Rehabilitation*, *87*, 343–350. http://dx.doi.org/10.1016/j.apmr.2005.09.019

Green, L. S., Oades, L. G., & Grant, A. M. (2006). Cognitive-behavioral, solution-focused life coaching: Enhancing goal striving, well-being, and hope. *The Journal of Positive Psychology*, *1*, 142–149. http://dx.doi.org/10.1080/17439760600619849

Haddad, M. M., Taub, E., Uswatte, G., Johnson, M. L., Mark, V. W., Barghi, A., . . . Rodriguez, C. M. (2017). Assessing the amount of spontaneous real-world spoken language in aphasia: Validation of two methods. *American Journal of Speech-Language Pathology*, *26*, 316–326. http://dx.doi.org/10.1044/2016_AJSLP-15-0115

Hadidi, N., Treat-Jacobson, D. J., & Lindquist, R. (2009). Poststroke depression and functional outcome: A critical review of literature. *Heart & Lung*, *38*, 151–162. http://dx.doi.org/10.1016/j.hrtlng.2008.05.002

Hanczakowski, M., Zawadzka, K., Collie, H., & Macken, B. (2017). Metamemory in a familiar place: The effects of environmental context on feeling of knowing. *Journal of Experimental Psychology: Learning, Memory, and Cognition*, *43*, 59–71. http://dx.doi.org/10.1037/xlm0000292

Harrison, R. A., & Field, T. S. (2015). Post stroke pain: Identification, assessment, and therapy. *Cerebrovascular Diseases*, *39*, 190–201. http://dx.doi.org/10.1159/000375397

Haskins, E. C., Cicerone, K., Dams-O'Conner, K., Eberle, R., Langenbahn, D., Shapiro-Rosenbaum, A., & Trexler, L. E. (2014). *Cognitive Rehabilitation Manual: Translating Evidenced-Based Recommendations into Practice*. Reston, VA: ACRM.

Hemphill, J. C., III, Greenberg, S. M., Anderson, C. S., Becker, K., Bendok, B. R., Cushman, M., . . . Woo, D., the American Heart Association Stroke Council, the Council on Cardiovascular and Stroke Nursing, & the Council on Clinical Cardiology. (2015). Guidelines for the Management of Spontaneous Intracerebral Hemorrhage: A Guideline for Healthcare Professionals From the American Heart Association/American Stroke Association. *Stroke*, *46*, 2032–2060. http://dx.doi.org/10.1161/STR.0000000000000069

Hier, D. B., Mondlock, J., & Caplan, L. R. (1983). Behavioral abnormalities after right hemisphere stroke. *Neurology*, *33*, 337–344. http://dx.doi.org/10.1212/WNL.33.3.337

Hoeren, M., Kümmerer, D., Bormann, T., Beume, L., Ludwig, V. M., Vry, M. S., . . . Weiller, C. (2014). Neural bases of imitation and pantomime in acute stroke patients: Distinct streams for praxis. *Brain: A Journal of Neurology*, *137*, 2796–2810. http://dx.doi.org/10.1093/brain/awu203

Hoffmann, M. (2009). Higher cortical function deficits after stroke: An analysis of 1,000 patients from a dedicated cognitive stroke registry. *Neurorehabilitation and Neural Repair*, *15*, 113–127. http://dx.doi.org/10.1177/154596830101500205

Homack, S., Lee, D., & Riccio, C. A. (2005). Test review: Delis–Kaplan Executive Function System. *Journal of Clinical and Experimental Neuropsychology*, 27, 599–609. http://dx.doi.org/10.1080/13803390490918444

Howard, G., Cushman, M., Howard, V. J., Kissela, B. M., Kleindorfer, D. O., Moy, C. S., . . . Woo, D. (2013). Risk factors for intracerebral hemorrhage: The Reasons for Geographic And Racial Differences in Stroke (REGARDS) study [see erratum at https://www.ahajournals.org/doi/10.1161/STR.0b013e3182964389]. *Stroke*, *44*, 1282–1287. http://dx.doi.org/10.1161/STROKEAHA.111.000529

Howard, G., Evans, G. W., Pearce, K., Howard, V. J., Bell, R. A., Mayer, E. J., & Burke, G. L. (1995). Is the stroke belt disappearing? An analysis of racial, temporal, and age effects. *Stroke*, *26*, 1153–1158. http://dx.doi.org/10.1161/01.STR.26.7.1153

Hubacher, M., Calabrese, P., Bassetti, C., Carota, A., Stöcklin, M., & Penner, I. K. (2012). Assessment of post-stroke fatigue: The fatigue scale for motor and cognitive functions. *European Neurology*, *67*, 377–384. http://dx.doi.org/10.1159/000336736

Ingles, J. L., Eskes, G. A., & Phillips, S. J. (1999). Fatigue after stroke. *Archives of Physical Medicine and Rehabilitation*, *80*, 173–178. http://dx.doi.org/10.1016/S0003-9993(99)90116-8

Jackson, J. C., Jutte, J. E., Hunter, C. H., Ciccolella, N., Warrington, H., Sevin, C., & Bienvenu, O. J. (2016). Posttraumatic stress disorder (PTSD) after critical illness: A conceptual review of distinct clinical issues and their implications. *Rehabilitation Psychology*, *61*, 132–140. http://dx.doi.org/10.1037/rep0000085

Jauch, E. C., Saver, J. L., Adams, H. P., Jr., Bruno, A., Connors, J. J., Demaerschalk, B. M., . . . Yonas, H., the American Heart Association Stroke Council, the Council on Cardiovascular Nursing, the Council on Peripheral Vascular Disease, & the Council on Clinical Cardiology. (2013). Guidelines for the early management of patients with acute ischemic stroke: A guideline for healthcare professionals from the American Heart Association/American Stroke Association. *Stroke*, *44*, 870–947. http://dx.doi.org/10.1161/STR.0b013e318284056a

Jensen, M. P., & Patterson, D. R. (2014). Hypnotic approaches for chronic pain management: Clinical implications of recent research findings. *American Psychologist*, *69*, 167–177. http://dx.doi.org/10.1037/a0035644

Johnson, M. L., Taub, E., Harper, L. H., Wade, J. T., Bowman, M. H., Bishop-McKay, S., . . . Uswatte, G. (2014). An enhanced protocol for CI Aphasia Therapy II: A case series. *American Journal of Speech-Language Pathology*, 23, 60–72. http://dx.doi.org/10.1044/1058-0360(2013/12-0168)

Kanter, J. W., Puspitasari, A. J., Santos, M. M., & Nagy, G. A. (2012). Behavioural activation: History, evidence and promise. *The British Journal of Psychiatry*, *200*, 361–363. http://dx.doi.org/10.1192/bjp.bp.111.103390

Karol, R. L. (2014). Team models in neurorehabilitation: Structure, function, and culture change. *NeuroRehabilitation*, *34*, 655–669.

Katrak, P. H., Black, D., & Peeva, V. (2009). Do stroke patients with intracerebral hemorrhage have a better functional outcome than patients with cerebral infarction? *PM & R*, *1*, 427–433. http://dx.doi.org/10.1016/j.pmrj.2009.03.002

Katz, S., Downs, T. D., Cash, H. R., & Grotz, R. C. (1970). Progress in development of the index of ADL. *The Gerontologist*, *10*, 20–30. http://dx.doi.org/10.1093/geront/10.1_Part_1.20

Keil, K., & Kaszniak, A. W. (2002). Examining executive function in individuals with brain injury: A review. *Aphasiology*, *16*, 305–335. http://dx.doi.org/10.1080/02687030143000654

Kerkhoff, G. (2000). Neurovisual rehabilitation: Recent developments and future directions. *Journal of Neurology, Neurosurgery, and Psychiatry*, *68*, 691–706. http://dx.doi.org/10.1136/jnnp.68.6.691

Kernan, W. N., Ovbiagele, B., Black, H. R., Bravata, D. M., Chimowitz, M. I., Ezekowitz, M. D., . . . Wilson, J. A., & the American Heart Association Stroke Council, Council on Cardiovascular and Stroke Nursing, Council on Clinical Cardiology, and Council on Peripheral Vascular Disease. (2014). Guidelines for the prevention of stroke in patients with stroke and transient ischemic attack: A guideline for healthcare professionals from the American Heart Association/American Stroke Association [see erratum at http://dx.doi.org/10.1161/STR.0000000000000034]. *Stroke*, *45*, 2160–2236. http://dx.doi.org/10.1161/STR.0000000000000024

Kertesz, A. (2007). *Western Aphasia Battery—Revised*. New York, NY: Grune & Stratton.

Kessner, S. S., Bingel, U., & Thomalla, G. (2016). Somatosensory deficits after stroke: A scoping review. *Topics in Stroke Rehabilitation*, *23*, 136–146. http://dx.doi.org/10.1080/10749357.2015.1116822

Kleinman, J. T., Newhart, M., Davis, C., Heidler-Gary, J., Gottesman, R. F., & Hillis, A. E. (2007). Right hemispatial neglect: Frequency and characterization following acute left hemisphere stroke. *Brain and Cognition*, *64*, 50–59. http://dx.doi.org/10.1016/j.bandc.2006.10.005

Klinedinst, N. J., Gebhardt, M. C., Aycock, D. M., Nichols-Larsen, D. S., Uswatte, G., Wolf, S. L., & Clark, P. C. (2009). Caregiver characteristics predict stroke survivor quality of life at 4 months and 1 year. *Research in Nursing & Health*, *32*, 592–605. http://dx.doi.org/10.1002/nur.20348

Kortte, K. B., Stevenson, J. E., Hosey, M. M., Castillo, R., & Wegener, S. T. (2012). Hope predicts positive functional role outcomes in acute rehabilitation populations. *Rehabilitation Psychology*, *57*, 248–255. http://dx.doi.org/10.1037/a0029004

Kortte, K. B., & Wegener, S. T. (2004). Denial of illness in medical rehabilitation populations: Theory, research, and definition. *Rehabilitation Psychology*, *49*, 187–199. http://dx.doi.org/10.1037/0090-5550.49.3.187

Kroenke, K., Spitzer, R. L., & Williams, J. B. (2001). The PHQ-9: Validity of a brief depression severity measure. *Journal of General Internal Medicine*, *16*, 606–613. http://dx.doi.org/10.1046/j.1525-1497.2001.016009606.x

Kronish, I. M., Edmondson, D., Goldfinger, J. Z., Fei, K., & Horowitz, C. R. (2012). Posttraumatic stress disorder and adherence to medications in survivors of strokes and transient ischemic attacks. *Stroke*, *43*, 2192–2197. http://dx.doi.org/10.1161/STROKEAHA.112.655209

Kwan, D., Craver, C. F., Green, L., Myerson, J., & Rosenbaum, R. S. (2013). Dissociations in future thinking following hippocampal damage: Evidence from discounting and time perspective in episodic amnesia. *Journal of Experimental Psychology: General*, *142*, 1355–1369. http://dx.doi.org/10.1037/a0034001

Lackland, D. T., Roccella, E. J., Deutsch, A. F., Fornage, M., George, M. G., Howard, G., . . . Towfighi, A., the American Heart Association Stroke Council, the Council on Cardiovascular and Stroke Nursing, the Council on Quality of Care and Outcomes Research, & the Council on Functional Genomics and Translational Biology. (2014). Factors influencing the decline in stroke mortality: A statement from the American Heart Association/American Stroke Association. *Stroke*, *45*, 315–353. http://dx.doi.org/10.1161/01.str.0000437068.30550.cf

Lai, S. M., Studenski, S., Duncan, P. W., & Perera, S. (2002). Persisting consequences of stroke measured by the Stroke Impact Scale. *Stroke*, *33*, 1840–1844. http://dx.doi.org/10.1161/01.STR.0000019289.15440.F2

Lavoie, M., Macoir, J., & Bier, N. (2017). Effectiveness of technologies in the treatment of post-stroke anomia: A systematic review. *Journal of Communication Disorders*, *65*, 43–53. http://dx.doi.org/10.1016/j.jcomdis.2017.01.001

Lawrence, E. S., Coshall, C., Dundas, R., Stewart, J., Rudd, A. G., Howard, R., & Wolfe, C. D. (2001). Estimates of the prevalence of acute stroke impairments and disability in a multiethnic population. *Stroke*, *32*, 1279–1284. http://dx.doi.org/10.1161/01.STR.32.6.1279

Lerdal, A., & Kottorp, A. (2011). Psychometric properties of the Fatigue Severity Scale—Rasch analyses of individual responses in a Norwegian stroke cohort. *International Journal of Nursing Studies*, *48*, 1258–1265. http://dx.doi.org/10.1016/j.ijnurstu.2011.02.019

Lesniak, M., Bak, T., Czepiel, W., Seniów, J., & Członkowska, A. (2008). Frequency and prognostic value of cognitive disorders in stroke patients. *Dementia and Geriatric Cognitive Disorders*, *26*, 356–363. http://dx.doi.org/10.1159/000162262

Loh, A. Z., Tan, J. S., Zhang, M. W., & Ho, R. C. (2017). The global prevalence of anxiety and depressive symptoms among caregivers of stroke survivors. *Journal of the American Medical Directors Association*, *18*, 111–116. http://dx.doi.org/10.1016/j.jamda.2016.08.014

Lum, P. S., Uswatte, G., Taub, E., Hardin, P., & Mark, V. W. (2006). A telerehabilitation approach to delivery of constraint-induced movement therapy. *Journal of Rehabilitation Research and Development*, *43*, 391–400. http://dx.doi.org/10.1682/JRRD.2005.02.0042

Lyubomirsky, S., Sousa, L., & Dickerhoof, R. (2006). The costs and benefits of writing, talking, and thinking about life's triumphs and defeats. *Journal of Personality and Social Psychology*, *90*, 692–708. http://dx.doi.org/10.1037/0022-3514.90.4.692

Marin, R. S., Biedrzycki, R. C., & Firinciogullari, S. (1991). Reliability and validity of the Apathy Evaluation Scale. *Psychiatry Research*, *38*, 143–162. http://dx.doi.org/10.1016/0165-1781(91)90040-V

Mark, V. W. (2003). Acute versus chronic functional aspects of unilateral spatial neglect. *Frontiers in Bioscience*, *8*, e172–e189. http://dx.doi.org/10.2741/973

Mark, V. W. (2016). Stroke and Behavior. *Neurologic Clinics*, *34*, 205–234. http://dx.doi.org/10.1016/j.ncl.2015.08.009

Marshall, S. C., Molnar, F., Man-Son-Hing, M., Blair, R., Brosseau, L., Finestone, H. M., . . . Wilson, K. G. (2007). Predictors of driving ability following stroke: A systematic review. *Topics in Stroke Rehabilitation*, *14*, 98–114. http://dx.doi.org/10.1310/tsr1401-98

Martin-Trias, P., Bragulat, V., Peña-Gómez, C., Sala-Llonch, R., Lanteaume, L., Cassé-Perrot, C., . . . Bartrés-Faz, D. (2016). Translational challenge models in support of efficacy studies: Neurobehavioral and cognitive changes induced by transcranial magnetic stimulation in healthy volunteers. *CNS & Neurological Disorders—Drug Targets*, *15*, 802–815.

McCracken, L. M., & Vowles, K. E. (2014). Acceptance and commitment therapy and mindfulness for chronic pain: Model, process, and progress. *American Psychologist*, *69*, 178–187. http://dx.doi.org/10.1037/a0035623

McDonnell, M. N., Hillier, S. L., Hooker, S. P., Le, A., Judd, S. E., & Howard, V. J. (2013). Physical activity frequency and risk of incident stroke in a national US study of Blacks and Whites. *Stroke*, *44*, 2519–2524. http://dx.doi.org/10.1161/STROKEAHA.113.001538

Mead, G. E., Hsieh, C. F., Lee, R., Kutlubaev, M. A., Claxton, A., Hankey, G. J., & Hackett, M. L. (2012). Selective serotonin reuptake inhibitors (SSRIs) for stroke recovery. *Cochrane Database of Systematic Reviews*, *11*, CD009286.

Mennemeyer, S. T., Taub, E., Uswatte, G., & Pearson, S. (2006). Employment in households with stroke after Constraint-Induced Movement Therapy. *NeuroRehabilitation*, *21*, 157–165.

Merzenich, M., Nahum, M., & Van Vleet, T. (Eds.). (2014). *Progress in brain research*: Vol. 207. *Changing brains—Applying brain plasticity to advance and recover human ability* (pp. 379–401). Amsterdam, The Netherlands: Elsevier.

Michielsen, H. J., De Vries, J., & Van Heck, G. L. (2003). Psychometric qualities of a brief self-rated fatigue measure: The Fatigue Assessment Scale. *Journal of Psychosomatic Research*, *54*, 345–352. http://dx.doi.org/10.1016/S0022-3999(02)00392-6

Miller, A., Pratt, H., & Schiffer, R. B. (2011). Pseudobulbar affect: The spectrum of clinical presentations, etiologies and treatments [review]. *Expert Review of Neurotherapeutics*, *11*, 1077–1088. http://dx.doi.org/10.1586/ern.11.68

Miller, E. L., Murray, L., Richards, L., Zorowitz, R. D., Bakas, T., Clark, P., Billinger, S. A., & the American Heart Association Council on Cardiovascular Nursing and the Stroke Council. (2010). Comprehensive overview of nursing and interdisciplinary rehabilitation care of the stroke patient: A scientific statement from the American Heart Association. *Stroke*, *41*, 2402–2448. http://dx.doi.org/10.1161/STR.0b013e3181e7512b

Morey, L. C. (2007). *The Personality Assessment Inventory professional manual*. Lutz, FL: Psychological Assessment Resources.

Morone, G., Paolucci, S., & Iosa, M. (2015). In what daily activities do patients achieve independence after stroke? *Journal of Stroke and Cerebrovascular Diseases*, *24*, 1931–1937. http://dx.doi.org/10.1016/j.jstrokecerebrovasdis.2015.05.006

Morrison, V., Pollard, B., Johnston, M., & MacWalter, R. (2005). Anxiety and depression 3 years following stroke: Demographic, clinical, and psychological predictors. *Journal of Psychosomatic Research*, *59*, 209–213. http://dx.doi.org/10.1016/j.jpsychores.2005.02.019

Mozaffarian, D., Benjamin, E. J., Go, A. S., Arnett, D. K., Blaha, M. J., Cushman, M., . . . Turner, M. B., the Writing Group Members, the American Heart Association Statistics Committee, the Stroke Statistics Subcommittee. (2016). Heart Disease and Stroke Statistics—2016 Update: A Report From the American Heart Association. *Circulation*, *133*, e38–e360.

Norise, C., & Hamilton, R. H. (2017). Non-invasive brain stimulation in the treatment of post-stroke and neurodegenerative aphasia: Parallels, differences, and lessons learned. *Frontiers in Human Neuroscience*, *10*, 1–16. http://dx.doi.org/10.3389/fnhum.2016.00675

O'Donnell, M. J., Diener, H. C., Sacco, R. L., Panju, A. A., Vinisko, R., Yusuf, S., & the PRoFESS Investigators. (2013). Chronic pain syndromes after ischemic stroke: PRoFESS trial. *Stroke*, *44*, 1238–1243. http://dx.doi.org/10.1161/STROKEAHA.111.671008

Ponchel, A., Bombois, S., Bordet, R., & Hénon, H. (2015). Factors associated with poststroke fatigue: A systematic review. *Stroke Research and Treatment*, *2015*, 347920. http://dx.doi.org/10.1155/2015/347920

Ramanathan-Elion, D. M., McWhorter, J. W., Wegener, S. T., & Bechtold, K. T. (2016). The role of psychological facilitators and barriers to therapeutic engagement in acute, inpatient rehabilitation. *Rehabilitation Psychology*, *61*, 277–287. http://dx.doi.org/10.1037/rep0000095

Ramos-Perdigués, S., Mané-Santacana, A., & Pintor-Pérez, L. (2015). Prevalence and associated factors of anger post stroke: A systematic review [in Spanish]. *Revista de Neurología*, *60*, 481–489.

Rinere O'Brien, S. (2010). Trends in inpatient rehabilitation stroke outcomes before and after advent of the prospective payment system: A systematic review. *Journal of Neurologic Physical Therapy; JNPT*, *34*, 17–23. http://dx.doi.org/10.1097/NPT.0b013e3181cfd3ac

Robinson, R. G., & Jorge, R. E. (2016). Post-stroke depression: A review. *The American Journal of Psychiatry*, *173*, 221–231. http://dx.doi.org/10.1176/appi.ajp.2015.15030363

Rosenbaum, T., Vadas, D., & Kalichman, L. (2014). Sexual function in post-stroke patients: Considerations for rehabilitation. *Journal of Sexual Medicine*, *11*, 15–21. http://dx.doi.org/10.1111/jsm.12343

Royle, J., & Lincoln, N. B. (2008). The Everyday Memory Questionnaire—Revised: Development of a 13-item scale. *Disability and Rehabilitation*, *30*, 114–121. http://dx.doi.org/10.1080/09638280701223876

Sabel, B. A. (2008). Plasticity and restoration of vision after visual system damage: An update. *Restorative Neurology and Neuroscience*, *26*, 243–247.

Sacco, R. L., Kasner, S. E., Broderick, J. P., Caplan, L. R., Connors, J. J., Culebras, A., . . . the American Heart Association Stroke Council, Council on Cardiovascular Surgery and Anesthesia, the Council on Cardiovascular Radiology and Intervention, the Council on Cardiovascular and Stroke Nursing, the Council on Epidemiology and Prevention, the Council on Peripheral Vascular Disease, & the Council on Nutrition, Physical Activity and Metabolism. (2013). An updated definition of stroke for the 21st century: A statement for healthcare professionals from the American Heart Association/American Stroke Association. *Stroke*, *44*, 2064–2089. http://dx.doi.org/10.1161/STR.0b013e318296aeca

Sand, K. M., Midelfart, A., Thomassen, L., Melms, A., Wilhelm, H., & Hoff, J. M. (2013). Visual impairment in stroke patients—A review. *Acta Neurologica Scandinavica*, *127*(s196), 52–56. http://dx.doi.org/10.1111/ane.12050

Santos, C. O., Caeiro, L., Ferro, J. M., & Figueira, M. L. (2011). Mania and stroke: A systematic review. *Cerebrovascular Diseases*, *32*, 11–21. http://dx.doi.org/10.1159/000327032

Saunders, D. H., Sanderson, M., Hayes, S., Kilrane, M., Greig, C. A., Brazzelli, M., & Mead, G. E. (2016). Physical fitness training for stroke patients. *Cochrane Database of Systematic Reviews*, *3*, CD003316.

Scherer, M. J., Craddock, G., & Mackeogh, T. (2011). The relationship of personal factors and subjective well-being to the use of assistive technology devices. *Disability and Rehabilitation*, *33*, 811–817. http://dx.doi.org/10.3109/09638288.2010.511418

Schnitzler, A., Woimant, F., Nicolau, J., Tuppin, P., & de Peretti, C. (2014). Effect of rehabilitation setting on dependence following stroke: An analysis of the French inpatient database. *Neurorehabilitation and Neural Repair*, *28*, 36–44. http://dx.doi.org/10.1177/1545968313497828

Seligman, M. E., Steen, T. A., Park, N., & Peterson, C. (2005). Positive psychology progress: Empirical validation of interventions. *American Psychologist*, *60*, 410–421. http://dx.doi.org/10.1037/0003-066X.60.5.410

Seshadri, S., Beiser, A., Kelly-Hayes, M., Kase, C. S., Au, R., Kannel, W. B., & Wolf, P. A. (2006). The lifetime risk of stroke: Estimates from the Framingham Study. *Stroke*, *37*, 345–350. http://dx.doi.org/10.1161/01.STR.0000199613.38911.b2

Shah, R. S., & Cole, J. W. (2010). Smoking and stroke: The more you smoke the more you stroke. *Expert Review of Cardiovascular Therapy*, *8*, 917–932. http://dx.doi.org/10.1586/erc.10.56

Snaphaan, L., & de Leeuw, F. E. (2007). Poststroke memory function in nondemented patients: A systematic review on frequency and neuroimaging correlates. *Stroke*, *38*, 198–203. http://dx.doi.org/10.1161/01.STR.0000251842.34322.8f

Snyder, C. R., Harris, C., Anderson, J. R., Holleran, S. A., Irving, L. M., Sigmon, S. T., . . . Harney, P. (1991). The will and the ways: Development and validation of an individual-differences measure of hope. *Journal of Personality and Social Psychology*, *60*, 570–585. http://dx.doi.org/10.1037/0022-3514.60.4.570

Sørensen, H. V., Lendal, S., Schultz-Larsen, K., & Uhrskov, T. (2003). Stroke rehabilitation: Assistive technology devices and environmental modifications following primary rehabilitation in hospital—A therapeutic perspective. *Assistive Technology*, *15*, 39–48. http://dx.doi.org/10.1080/10400435.2003.10131888

Spellacy, F. J., & Spreen, O. (1969). A short form of the token test. *Cortex*, *5*, 391–397. http://dx.doi.org/10.1016/S0010-9452(69)80015-8

Spitzer, R. L., Kroenke, K., Williams, J. B., & Löwe, B. (2006). A brief measure for assessing generalized anxiety disorder: The GAD-7. *Archives of Internal Medicine*, *166*, 1092–1097. http://dx.doi.org/10.1001/archinte.166.10.1092

Squire, L. R. (1992). Memory and the hippocampus: A synthesis from findings with rats, monkeys, and humans. *Psychological Review*, *99*, 195–231. http://dx.doi.org/10.1037/0033-295X.99.2.195

Squire, L. R. (2004). Memory systems of the brain: A brief history and current perspective. *Neurobiology of Learning and Memory*, *82*, 171–177. http://dx.doi.org/10.1016/j.nlm.2004.06.005

Starrfelt, R., Olafsdóttir, R. R., & Arendt, I. M. (2013). Rehabilitation of pure alexia: A review. *Neuropsychological Rehabilitation*, *23*, 755–779. http://dx.doi.org/10.1080/09602011.2013.809661

Stolk-Hornsveld, F., Crow, J. L., Hendriks, E. P., van der Baan, R., & Harmeling-van der Wel, B. C. (2006). The Erasmus MC modifications to the (revised) Nottingham Sensory Assessment: A reliable somatosensory assessment measure for patients with intracranial disorders. *Clinical Rehabilitation*, *20*, 160–172. http://dx.doi.org/10.1191/0269215506cr932oa

Stone, S. P., Halligan, P. W., & Greenwood, R. J. (1993). The incidence of neglect phenomena and related disorders in patients with an acute right or left hemisphere stroke. *Age and Ageing*, *22*, 46–52. http://dx.doi.org/10.1093/ageing/22.1.46

Stringer, A. Y. (2007). *EON-MEM™: Ecologically Oriented Neurorehabilitation of Memory*. Torrance, CA: WPS.

Sugden, S. G., & Bourgeois, J. A. (2004). Modafinil monotherapy in poststroke depression. *Psychosomatics*, *45*, 80–81. http://dx.doi.org/10.1176/appi.psy.45.1.80

Tang, W. K., Lau, C. G., Mok, V., Ungvari, G. S., & Wong, K. S. (2013). Impact of anxiety on health-related quality of life after stroke: A cross-sectional study. *Archives of Physical Medicine and Rehabilitation*, *94*, 2535–2541. http://dx.doi.org/10.1016/j.apmr.2013.07.012

Taub, E., Uswatte, G., King, D. K., Morris, D., Crago, J. E., & Chatterjee, A. (2006). A placebo-controlled trial of constraint-induced movement therapy for upper extremity after stroke. *Stroke*, *37*, 1045–1049. http://dx.doi.org/10.1161/01.STR.0000206463.66461.97

Taub, E., Uswatte, G., Mark, V. W., & Morris, D. M. (2006). The learned nonuse phenomenon: Implications for rehabilitation. *Europa Medicophysica*, *42*, 241–256.

Taub, E., Uswatte, G., Mark, V. W., Morris, D. M., Barman, J., Bowman, M. H., . . . Bishop-McKay, S. (2013). Method for enhancing real-world use of a more affected arm in chronic stroke: Transfer package of constraint-induced movement therapy. *Stroke*, *44*, 1383–1388. http://dx.doi.org/10.1161/STROKEAHA.111.000559

Tulving, E. (1985). *Elements of episodic memory*. New York, NY: Oxford University Press.

Tulving, E. (2005). Episodic memory and autonoesis: Uniquely human? In H. S. Terrace & J. Metcalf (Eds.), *The missing link in cognition: Origins of self-reflective consciousness* (pp. 4–56). New York, NY: Oxford University Press.

Turk, D. C., & Melzack, R. (2001). *Handbook of pain assessment*. New York, NY: Guilford Press.

Tyson, S. F., Chillala, J., Hanley, M., Selley, A. B., & Tallis, R. C. (2006). Distribution of weakness in the upper and lower limbs post-stroke. *Disability and Rehabilitation*, *28*, 715–719. http://dx.doi.org/10.1080/09638280500301584

Uswatte, G., & Taub, E. (2013). Constraint-induced movement therapy: A method for harnessing neuroplasticity to treat motor disorders. *Progress in Brain Research*, *207*, 379–401. http://dx.doi.org/10.1016/B978-0-444-63327-9.00015-1

Van Der Meulen, I., Van De Sandt-Koenderman, M. W., Heijenbrok, M. H., Visch-Brink, E., & Ribbers, G. M. (2016). Melodic intonation therapy in chronic aphasia: Evidence from a pilot randomized controlled trial. *Frontiers in Human Neuroscience*, *10*, 533. http://dx.doi.org/10.3389/fnhum.2016.00533

van de Ven, R. M., Murre, J. M., Veltman, D. J., & Schmand, B. A. (2016). Computer-based cognitive training for executive functions after stroke: A systematic review. *Frontiers in Human Neuroscience*, *10*, 150. http://dx.doi.org/10.3389/fnhum.2016.00150

van Swieten, J. C., Koudstaal, P. J., Visser, M. C., Schouten, H. J. A., & van Gijn, J. (1988). Interobserver agreement for the assessment of handicap in stroke patients. *Stroke*, *19*, 604–607. http://dx.doi.org/10.1161/01.STR.19.5.604

Ward, A. B. (2012). A literature review of the pathophysiology and onset of post-stroke spasticity. *European Journal of Neurology*, *19*, 21–27. http://dx.doi.org/10.1111/j.1468-1331.2011.03448.x

Watkins, C. L., Wathan, J. V., Leathley, M. J., Auton, M. F., Deans, C. F., Dickinson, H. A., . . . Lightbody, C. E. (2011). The 12-month effects of early motivational interviewing after acute stroke: A randomized controlled trial. *Stroke*, *42*, 1956–1961. http://dx.doi.org/10.1161/STROKEAHA.110.602227

Watson, D., Clark, L. A., & Tellegen, A. (1988). Development and validation of brief measures of positive and negative affect: The PANAS scales. *Journal of Personality and Social Psychology*, *54*, 1063–1070. http://dx.doi.org/10.1037/0022-3514.54.6.1063

Wechsler, D. (2009). *WMS–IV administration and scoring manual*. San Antonio, TX: Pearson.

White, H., Boden-Albala, B., Wang, C., Elkind, M. S., Rundek, T., Wright, C. B., & Sacco, R. L. (2005). Ischemic stroke subtype incidence among Whites, Blacks, and Hispanics: The Northern Manhattan Study. *Circulation*, *111*, 1327–1331. http://dx.doi.org/10.1161/01.CIR.0000157736.19739.D0

Wilson, B. A., Cockburn, J., & Halligan, P. W. (1987). *Behavioural Inattention Test*. San Antonio, TX: Pearson.

Winstein, C. J., Stein, J., Arena, R., Bates, B., Cherney, L. R., Cramer, S. C., . . . Zorowitz, R. D., & the American Heart Association Stroke Council, Council on Cardiovascular and Stroke Nursing, Council on Clinical Cardiology, and Council on Quality of Care and Outcomes Research. (2016). Guidelines for Adult Stroke Rehabilitation and Recovery: A Guideline for Healthcare Professionals From the American Heart Association/American Stroke Association [see erratum at http://dx.doi.org/10.1161/STR.0000000000000156]. *Stroke*, *47*, e98–e169. http://dx.doi.org/10.1161/STR.0000000000000098

Winward, C. E., Halligan, P. W., & Wade, D. T. (2002). The Rivermead Assessment of Somatosensory Performance (RASP): Standardization and reliability data. *Clinical Rehabilitation*, *16*, 523–533. http://dx.doi.org/10.1191/0269215502cr522oa

Wolfenden, B., & Grace, M. (2009). Returning to work after stroke: A review. *International Journal of Rehabilitation Research*, *32*, 93–97. http://dx.doi.org/10.1097/MRR.0b013e328325a358

Woodman, P., Riazi, A., Pereira, C., & Jones, F. (2014). Social participation post stroke: A meta-ethnographic review of the experiences and views of community-dwelling stroke survivors. *Disability and Rehabilitation*, *36*, 2031–2043. http://dx.doi.org/10.3109/09638288.2014.887796

Yang, N. Y. H., Zhou, D., Chung, R. C. K., Li-Tsang, C. W. P., & Fong, K. N. K. (2013). Rehabilitation interventions for unilateral neglect after stroke: A systematic review from 1997 through 2012. *Frontiers in Human Neuroscience*, *7*, 187. http://dx.doi.org/10.3389/fnhum.2013.00187

Zigmond, A. S., & Snaith, R. P. (1983). The hospital anxiety and depression scale. *Acta Psychiatrica Scandinavica*, *67*, 361–370. http://dx.doi.org/10.1111/j.1600-0447.1983.tb09716.x

CHAPTER 22

POLYTRAUMA IN THE POST-9/11 ERA: DEFINING CHARACTERISTICS AND POSTACUTE REHABILITATION

Jennifer H. Olson-Madden and Nazanin H. Bahraini

The origin of the term *polytrauma* dates to approximately half a century ago (Border, LaDuca, & Seibel, 1975) when survival rates for patients sustaining multiple traumatic injuries began improving (Butcher & Balogh, 2014). Since then, a variety of definitions have been used to describe the elements of polytrauma. Although there is yet no uniform definition for polytrauma, the most widely used definitions rely on the basic concept of a combination of injuries that cause a life-threatening condition (Pape et al., 2014).

It is important to consider the historical context in which polytrauma has emerged and how that affects how it is defined and conceptualized. As seen throughout history, military conflicts often shape the field of rehabilitation (Uomoto & Williams, 2009). For example, the fields of physical medicine and rehabilitation evolved considerably after World War II because conventional medicine was not meeting the treatment needs of those injured during combat. Similarly, in recent years, the term *polytrauma* has received considerable attention, in part because of the conflicts in Iraq and Afghanistan. The high incidence of blast exposures characteristic of these conflicts combined with significant advances in protective gear and trauma medicine has increased the survival rates of combat deployed U.S. service members who sustain multiple severe injuries (i.e., polytrauma). Thus, military service members must often live with a variety of complications associated with their injuries. Consequently, the Veterans Health Administration (VHA) adopted the term *polytrauma*, which they defined as "injury to the brain in addition to other body parts or systems, resulting in physical, cognitive, psychological, or psychosocial impairments and functional disability" (Department of Veterans Affairs, 2005, p. 3). The definition was revised in 2009 to reflect any combination of multiple bodily systems injured in a single event, which may or may not include brain injury (Department of Veterans Affairs, 2009).

In this chapter, we review polytrauma in the post-9/11 era. Although much of the existing literature in this area is related to injuries sustained by military personnel and veterans during recent conflicts, the impact of findings is relevant to civilian injury as well, particularly in light of the growing threat of terrorist attacks in civilian settings. Specifically, we provide an overview of the characteristics and prevalence of polytrauma, describe some of the most common comorbidities, and discuss current best practices in postacute polytrauma rehabilitation. We also discuss how rehabilitation psychologists are uniquely poised to meet the treatment needs of those with polytraumatic injuries. In such settings, the rehabilitation psychologist serves as a key provider on the multidisciplinary team and facilitates identifying, conceptualizing, and treating the mental, emotional, behavioral, and physical concerns that affect an

http://dx.doi.org/10.1037/0000129-023
Handbook of Rehabilitation Psychology, Third Edition, L. A. Brenner, S. A. Reid-Arndt, T. R. Elliott, R. G. Frank, and B. Caplan (Editors-in-Chief)

individual's adjustment to polytraumatic disability. We also address the important role that the field of rehabilitation psychology serves in conducting polytrauma research, establishing best clinical practices, and engaging in advocacy.

ETIOLOGY AND DEFINING CHARACTERISTICS

Polytraumatic injuries are complex and may impact individuals in a variety of ways depending on the mechanism of injury. In this section, we focus on combat-related incidents whereby polytrauma may occur as a result of explosive devices and shrapnel.

Blast Injury

The U.S. Armed Forces are sustaining new and complex injuries—the majority of which are blast related. The sources of blast injury, which are characteristic of a new era in modern warfare, include improvised explosive devices, artillery, rocket and mortar shells, mines, and rocket-propelled grenades. Four categories of injuries are associated with a blast: primary—the impact from the overpressurization wave with body surfaces, secondary—results from flying debris and bomb fragments, tertiary—results from an individual thrown by a blast, and quaternary—injuries not otherwise caused by the preceding mechanisms (Centers for Disease Control, 2018). As just noted, although the severity and pattern of blast injuries depend on a number of variables (e.g., type of explosive material, surrounding environment, delivery method, distance between the victim and the blast), more individuals are surviving beyond the acute phase of these injuries because of improvements in body armor and advances in trauma care (French, 2010). As a result, the Departments of Defense (DoD) and Veterans Affairs (VA) are providing medical care to individuals sustaining multiple serious injuries, who might have died in previous conflicts.

Given the possible effects of explosions on the human body, it is not surprising that blast injuries are often polytraumatic. Blast-related injuries, which are the most common cause of polytrauma seen among Operation Enduring Freedom and Operation Iraqi Freedom (OEF/OIF) service members, have also been described as often more clinically complex than the injuries seen in civilian rehabilitation settings or those acquired through other mechanisms (Friedemann-Sánchez, Sayer, & Pickett, 2008), such as from a fight or fall. Injured body systems and structures include auditory/vestibular, eye, orbit, face, respiratory, digestive, circulatory, central nervous system, renal/urinary tract, extremity, and soft tissue. Reported symptoms often include mental health concerns and chronic pain.

A number of studies have demonstrated that the pattern of injuries differs among those injured because of blasts compared with other mechanisms. Specifically, injuries to the face, penetrating brain injuries, symptoms of posttraumatic stress, and auditory impairments are more common in blast-injured patients than in those with combat injuries of other etiologies (Sayer et al., 2008). In another sample, those with a traumatic brain injury (TBI) related to a blast were significantly more likely to have had a skull fracture, seizure, or lower limb amputation than those not injured in a blast. These individuals were also more likely to have acute stress symptoms than those who sustained TBI through other mechanisms (Warden, 2006). Similar patterns have been observed in civilian victims of terror attacks, with those injured in a blast having more affected body regions than those injured through other mechanisms and being more severely injured overall (Peleg, Aharonson-Daniel, Michael, Shapira, & Israel Trauma Group, 2003).

COMMON POST-9/11 POLYTRAUMA CONDITIONS

Although an exhaustive list of potential blast-related polytrauma injuries is beyond the scope of this chapter, we describe some of the most common polytrauma conditions in service members and veterans serving in the post-9/11 era.

Traumatic Brain Injury

A TBI is defined as an alteration in brain function caused by an external force (i.e., objects penetrating the brain, the head striking or being struck by an object, acceleration or deceleration of the brain, or exposure to forces associated with blasts;

Menon, Schwab, Wright, Maas, & Demographics and Clinical Assessment Working Group of the International and Interagency Initiative Toward Common Data Elements for Research on Traumatic Brain Injury and Psychological Health, 2010). Signs of alteration in brain function may include loss of consciousness; alteration in mental status, such as being dazed or confused; loss of memory for the event; or focal neurological deficits. A TBI can be further classified into the following severity levels: mild, complicated mild, moderate, and severe. For additional information regarding TBI, see Chapter 18, this volume.

A TBI is one of the most common types of polytrauma injuries sustained by current service members. Pickett, Bender, and Gourley (2010) estimated that up to 60% of blast injuries result in TBI. Deployed service members are at particular risk for *mild* TBI (mTBI) and may experience a range of postinjury symptoms, including headaches, dizziness, fatigue, problems concentrating and remembering, irritability, difficulties managing stress, and sensory deficits. For most individuals who sustain mTBI, postconcussive (PC) symptoms resolve within 3 months postinjury. However, a subset of service members continue to endorse PC symptoms long after the injury event (Hoge et al., 2008; Schneiderman, Braver, & Kang, 2008; Terrio et al., 2009). The severity of TBI sequelae and the extent to which they persist are not linearly associated with injury severity (Saltapidas & Ponsford, 2007; Whittaker, Kemp, & House, 2007). Outcomes may depend on a variety of factors, including psychological/psychiatric sequelae, barriers to returning to work or activities, and litigation/financial incentives.

Depending on the underlying mechanism of trauma, a significant number of TBI patients may present with other concomitant injuries such as limb fractures, amputation, burns, spinal cord injury, hearing loss, visual impairment, posttraumatic stress disorder (PTSD), and other mental health conditions (Friedemann-Sánchez et al., 2008). As described next, the presence of secondary injuries and high-frequency comorbidities (e.g., chronic pain and PTSD) associated with polytrauma can further complicate recovery from TBI, even among those injuries that were mild in nature.

The Polytrauma Clinical Triad and Other Associated Comorbidity Clusters

A high prevalence of OEF/OIF veterans are returning with what is termed the *polytrauma clinical triad* (PCT). The PCT consists of three specific co-occurring conditions: *chronic pain, PTSD*, and *persistent post-concussive symptoms* (PPCS). In a sample of 340 OEF/OIF veterans seen at a Department of Veterans Affairs Polytrauma Network Site, chronic pain, PTSD, and PPCS were simultaneously present in 42.1% of the sample (Lew et al., 2009).

A recent report by the VA Polytrauma and Blast Related Injuries Quality Enhancement Research Initiative showed that the vast majority of patients with a TBI diagnosis also had a mental health disorder, and half of those with TBI had both PTSD and pain diagnoses. Specifically, 55% of veterans with a TBI diagnosis had received both PTSD and pain diagnoses, compared with 13% in veterans without a TBI diagnosis. Furthermore, VA health care use and associated costs were higher in veterans with a diagnosis of TBI compared with those without a TBI diagnosis. A substantial portion of this higher use was due to mental health and rehabilitation health care (Taylor et al., 2015).

Studies have also shown that veterans who screen positive for TBI have higher rates of PTSD, depression, and substance abuse disorder (Carlson et al., 2010; Polusny et al., 2011). Pugh et al. (2014) recently examined distinct patterns of co-occurring physical and mental health conditions among OEF/OIF veterans to identify *other comorbidity clusters beyond the PCT* (TBI, PTSD, and pain). Using latent class analysis, they discovered six distinct comorbidity clusters. For example, one cluster reflected the typical PCT of TBI, PTSD and pain, and another included the PCT *plus* depression and chronic disease (e.g., hypertension, osteoarthritis).

Together these findings highlight the complex and heterogeneous nature of polytrauma and the sequela that often follows. Although clinical presentations vary from one individual to another, the presence of co-occurring physical and psychological conditions are common, and the compounding effects of these conditions can present distinct challenges for recovery. This complexity requires interventions that can address overlapping conditions and associated symptoms that take place within systems of care with a high level of integration and coordination of clinical care and other support services.

POLYTRAUMA REHABILITATION: A MODEL OF CARE

Although acute, emergency-based medical care for patients with traumatic injuries, including blast-related trauma, and associated comorbidities is well described and coordinated, the postacute clinical management of polytrauma patients has been less prescribed and researched (Scott, Belanger, Vanderploeg, Massengale, & Scholten, 2006). Even less attention is paid to long-term recovery, including community reintegration, return to work or school, and a focus on overall wellness. Despite these limitations, there does appear to be expert consensus that a comprehensive, patient-centered interdisciplinary approach is essential for the evaluation and treatment of patients with polytrauma to minimize the consequences of TBI and associated concomitant conditions.

The VHA has been a leader in the development of an integrated network of specialty rehabilitation programs treating military personnel and veterans with polytrauma and TBI. Recognition of an increased incidence of polytrauma/TBI led the VA health care system to formally establish the VA Polytrauma System of Care (PSC) to meet the complex and specialized rehabilitation needs of returning veterans with TBI and polytrauma (Department of Veterans Affairs, n.d.-b). Specialized care is provided at facilities that address the patient's particular rehabilitation, medical, surgical, and/or mental health needs across the life span. The VA PSC is composed of four levels of care that reflect a continuum of services for veterans and service members with polytrauma and TBI ranging from trauma care to acute and postacute rehabilitation, community reintegration, and lifetime community care. As described next, this tiered system integrates specialized services at the regional level, among network sites, and at local VA medical centers.

Level 1 Polytrauma Rehabilitation Centers (PRCs) are five regional referral centers for acute inpatient medical and rehabilitation care for those who have experienced severe injuries. Level 2 Polytrauma Network Sites (PNSs) provide post-acute rehabilitation and coordinate polytrauma services within the Veterans Integrated Service Networks. These nationwide specialized rehabilitation programs offer continued medical care and rehabilitation services for individuals who are transitioning closer to home following discharge from a PRC, and they serve as the entry point for rehabilitation services for those who have experienced a mild-to-moderate TBI or polytraumatic injury. Level 3 Polytrauma Support Clinic Teams (PSCTs) are located in 87 VA medical centers providing outpatient interdisciplinary rehabilitation evaluation and treatment services closer to the patient's home community. PSCT programs may also be the outpatient entry point for those who have experienced a mild-to-moderate TBI or polytraumatic injury. Finally, Level 4 Polytrauma Points of Contact (41 VA medical centers) are at VA medical centers without specialized rehabilitation teams. These Points of Contact coordinate case management and referrals throughout the system and may provide a more limited range of rehabilitation services.

Screening and Evaluation

In this section, we focus specifically on the role of rehabilitation psychologist as part of a larger multidisciplinary team in the VA, primarily in the post-acute levels of the PSC.

In the postacute setting, specialized PNSs and PSCTs that are part of the VA PSC provide assessment of veterans with complex co-occurring problems. This assessment is accomplished by an interdisciplinary team consisting of a physician, rehabilitation therapist, audiologist, speech pathologist, neuropsychologist/rehabilitation psychologist, social worker, and other health care professionals, providing patients with access to the full range of medical and support services within the hospital.

The assessment and evaluation framework adopted by the VA PSC is based on the mechanism of injury approach (Scott et al., 2006). Using this approach, all VA health care facilities screen all veterans from OEF/OIF for possible TBI upon initial contact with the VA health system (Department of

Veterans Affairs, 2007; i.e., case manager screening). Those who screen positive are referred for follow-up evaluations that include a detailed history of the patient's injury, assessment of common symptoms or sequelae of TBI, and physical examination targeted to the veteran's reported symptoms and physical impairments. Following this, patients are referred to specialty care (e.g., behavioral/mental health, audiology, neuropsychological testing) as needed for further evaluation and development of a treatment plan that is focused on their specific needs. In regard to assessment, the rehabilitation psychologist plays an integral role in evaluating and conceptualizing various areas of functioning—cognitive, physical, emotional—using specialized psychological and neuropsychological assessments. In this vein, they can also help identify cross-cutting/transdiagnostic issues that are impacting the course of recovery (e.g., sleep disturbance, poor pain management), which can help the team prioritize treatment goals.

Intervention

Because each TBI and polytrauma is unique and recovery is multifaceted, it is often difficult to predict a person's final level of recovery. Patients respond differently to rehabilitation. Some patients have lengthy stays in an acute, inpatient program, and others receive their care through outpatient services. Some patients treated in the polytrauma programs are able to return to active duty, pursue school, or return to work, whereas others will continue to need more intense supportive services and care (e.g., Department of Veterans Affairs). In this sense, the PSC is designed to meet the changing needs of patients with TBI and polytrauma upon point of entry and throughout the course of their recovery and life span. For those with mTBI, full return to normal functioning is generally expected and conveyed to patients and their families. Individuals receiving rehabilitation for moderate to severe TBI and polytraumatic injuries in the acute phase receive various intensive therapies each day, relearning and developing new compensatory strategies. Rehabilitation psychologists work with the individual to assess and coordinate treatment of symptoms that can affect functional independence, including physical mobility, communication and language skills, thinking/executive functioning, strength/endurance, dizziness/balance, pain, activities of daily living, behavioral and emotional changes, sexuality, body image, and coping. As possible, family or other supportive involvement is highly encouraged.

Posthospitalization, individuals may require any number of ongoing services. It is critical that continuity of medical and psychosocial support is maintained. The role of the rehabilitation psychologist is instrumental in addressing the complexities associated with an individual's adjustment to life with polytraumatic injuries. For example, logistical supports such as housing, transportation, and community reintegration may be required. During the transition phase, rehabilitation psychologists may focus on providing individuals and their families with the opportunity to continue developing and enhancing their lives, including self-management of life skills, coping strategies and psychological adjustment, cognitive remediation, and facilitating a return to school/work. At the outpatient level, ideally individuals have been referred to specialized polytrauma outpatient clinics as described earlier, where treatment emphasizes improvement in symptoms such as headache, sleep, and pain and training in assistive technology designed to support performance of activities of daily living.

Psychoeducation

Psychoeducation, defined as an intervention with systematic, structured, and didactic knowledge transfer for an illness and its treatment—integrating emotional and motivational aspects to enable patients to cope with the illness and to improve its treatment adherence and efficacy (Ekhtiari, Rezapour, Aupperle, & Paulus, 2017)—is a critical component of polytrauma rehabilitation. Moreover, rehabilitation psychologists play an important role in providing psychoeducation either by itself or in the context of other psychotherapies or behavioral interventions.

Psychoeducation can facilitate risk reduction by educating patients about how various lifestyle behaviors can impact recovery. For example, individuals with histories of TBI and polytrauma may be more sensitive to the effects of alcohol and may be at risk for developing a substance use problem (Corrigan, 1995). This, in turn, may place the individual at risk for further injury or worsen the effects of the TBI (Bombardier, Temkin, Machamer, & Dikmen, 2003). Individuals are encouraged to avoid alcohol in the acute phase of injury and rehabilitation and to carefully monitor alcohol intake thereafter. Providing such education to patients and their families may help mitigate risky behavior that may develop as a means of coping with different sequelae related to polytrauma.

Psychoeducation can be particularly effective when combined with or incorporated into other illness self-management strategies, such as cognitive behavioral interventions (for insomnia and pain management). Other strategies to maximize the effects of psychoeducation include tailoring the content so that patients clearly understand the information; incorporating handouts, articles, videos, and other methods to make the information more accessible and salient; not overloading patients with too much information in a single session; and presenting the information in a way that is relevant to patients' goals (Pratt, Gill, Barrett, & Roberts, 2014).

Improved Functioning Through Symptom Management

Emergency medical service and in-hospital guidelines are available to guide the treatment of adults with severe TBI (Centers for Disease Control, 2009; Faul, Wald, Rutland-Brown, Sullivent, & Sattin, 2007), but evidence-based strategies for postacute, chronic moderate-to-severe TBI are lacking. For those with a diagnosis of mTBI, treatment often focuses on symptom management and education emphasizing recovery and gradual resumption of daily responsibilities (e.g., work). This approach is consistent with that outlined in the VA/DOD Clinical Practice Guideline for the Management of Concussion–Mild TBI (Departments of Veterans Affairs and Defense, 2016). The primary goals of symptom management are to decrease symptoms and improve functioning. Therefore, addressing symptoms that are reported by patients as being most impactful is likely to increase treatment engagement and buy-in. Along these lines, targeting issues that are likely contributing to a host of symptoms (e.g., sleep disturbance) may be another way of focusing and prioritizing treatment.

Frequently, individuals with mTBI are managed successfully in primary care settings and do not require specialty intervention. For those with histories of more severe TBI, Cicerone et al. (2005) found that neuropsychological rehabilitation therapies involving cognitive, emotional, interpersonal, and motivational therapies are most commonly used. Such rehabilitation efforts were found to be beneficial for community/work reintegration for those with moderate to severe TBI; however, such evidence is not available for those with milder injuries.

As outlined in the VA/DOD Clinical Practice Guideline (Departments of Veterans Affairs and Defense, 2016), a significant number of the interventions designed to manage symptoms and conditions associated with polytrauma among veterans and service members are behavioral or cognitive-behavioral. Thus, the rehabilitation psychologist can play an integral role in symptom management. For example, relaxation techniques such as controlled breathing or progressive muscle relaxation may reduce irritability and mood swings. Moreover, for mTBI symptoms such as sleep disturbance, cognitive deficits, mood difficulties, and headache, it is likely that improvement in one symptom leads to improvement in other symptoms. Medications to facilitate pain management, promote sleep, and reduce anxiety may also be appropriate and may be considered after thorough evaluation. They are most effective when used in conjunction with other evidence-based behavioral therapies.

Another effective tool that can be used to monitor and manage many symptoms associated with TBI, specifically mTBI, is the use of a smartphone. Features on these devices such as a calendar application can facilitate memory for items such as important dates or appointments and medication reminders. The Concussion Coach is a mobile phone app for military personnel and veterans with histories of mild to moderate TBI (Department of Veterans Affairs, n.d.-a). The app incorporates portable tools that assess symptoms to help individuals develop and use adaptive coping strategies. The Concussion Coach and apps similar to it are intended to conveniently support existing treatments.

Sleep Disturbance

Identifying key treatment targets that cut across conditions or contribute to multiple symptoms is also critical to effectively and efficiently improving rehabilitation outcomes. Take, for instance, the polytrauma clinical triad and its impact on sleep. Lew et al. (2010) showed that when TBI or pain coexisted with PTSD, sleep problems worsened. This finding is not surprising, as sleep problems can reduce pain tolerance and exacerbate other symptoms, such as cognitive deficits and irritability (Lang, Veazey-Morris, & Andrasik, 2014). Moreover, sleep disturbance may be underrecognized and undertreated because patients may be more focused on other symptoms such as cognitive difficulties or pain without recognizing the role that sleep can play in maintaining or exacerbating these symptoms. Given that adequate sleep is essential to maximizing rehabilitation outcomes, incorporating sleep-specific interventions early in treatment may help optimize recovery, particularly among those presenting with multiple co-occurring conditions in which sleep disturbance is a core feature (Lang et al., 2014). Considering that first-line interventions for conditions that are part of the PCT and associated issues, such as sleep disturbance, are largely behavioral, rehabilitation psychologists are well positioned to recognize and treat these issues as part of a larger interdisciplinary approach to treatment.

Pain Management

There is a paucity of evidence to help guide pain assessment and management in patients with polytrauma (Dobscha et al., 2009). Pharmacologic and nonpharmacologic interventions are frequently used to manage the complex rehabilitation needs of an individual with polytrauma and pain. Models of care suggest the addition of a rehabilitation psychologist with a focus on pain (Clark, Scholten, Walker, & Gironda, 2009) to treat behavioral and psychological issues that may be affecting pain experience or treatment while other rehabilitation staff provide additional targeted interventions to assist in pain relief. Evidence-based treatments of chronic pain (e.g., cognitive behavior therapy [CBT]) may be implemented in polytrauma populations, though more rigorous research is needed to establish an evidence base of CBT for pain in individuals with brain injury (Dobscha et al., 2009). Future research should consider the complexity of this population given that many have suffered both polytrauma and psychological trauma (Gironda et al., 2009).

Complementary alternative medicine (CAM) has been used increasingly by individuals with chronic pain as an adjunctive modality to standard treatment (Denneson, Corson, & Dobscha, 2011). Evidence-based CAM techniques such as acupuncture, chiropractic treatments, and biofeedback are commonly used by rehabilitation psychologists to treat individuals with TBI and polytraumatic injuries. Mind–body therapies using meditation, guided imagery, relaxation techniques, and hypnosis may also help to alleviate discomfort caused by chronic pain.

Treatment of Mental Health Disorders

Treatment of comorbid mental health conditions (e.g., depression, PTSD, anxiety) is indicated regardless of whether these are caused by mTBI (Olson-Madden, Brenner, Matarazzo, Signoracci, & the Expert Consensus Collaborators, 2013). Those with mTBI may benefit from any number of empirically based treatments that were initially developed for those without a history of TBI without significant modifications to treatment delivery. For individuals with a history of moderate or severe TBI, modifications to evidence-based interventions can be accomplished (Olson-Madden et al., 2013). CBTs, including traditional and third-wave CBT interventions, have been applied widely to a range of conditions in those with TBI (mild to moderate) with positive findings. For example, there is some support for the position that posttraumatic stress symptomatology following mTBI is treated effectively via CBT (Bryant, Moulds, Guthrie, Dang, & Nixon, 2003; Soo & Tate, 2007). There is also some emerging evidence for third-wave cognitive behavioral interventions, such as mindfulness-based cognitive therapy, in reducing depressive symptoms in those with a history of moderate TBI (Bedard et al., 2014) and acceptance and commitment therapy for psychological adjustment after severe TBI (Kangas & McDonald, 2011). Window to Hope (Brenner et al., 2018) is another CBT-based intervention that was developed specifically for individuals with moderate to severe TBI and hopelessness. Results from two trials show efficacy of this intervention for reducing hopelessness among individuals with moderate to severe TBI, which has important clinical implications given that hopelessness and TBI are both risk factors for suicide (Brenner et al., 2018; Simpson, Tate, Whiting, & Cotter, 2011).

Technological Advances in Treatment Delivery

An impressive advance in the polytrauma system of care is the use of telerehabilitation. This modality of care uses electronic information and telecommunication technology (e.g., videoconferencing) to assist individuals and providers who are separated geographically. The advantages of monitoring an individual's functional status and equipment needs are that access to care is optimized, clinical communication and continuity of care are facilitated, and the need for travel is eliminated. The VHA suggests that telerehabilitation services have increased substantially over the past several years, with more than 20 times more veterans with polytrauma and TBI receiving rehabilitation care by way of video teleconferencing.

Within the PRCs, assistive technology (AT) labs have been created to facilitate the evaluation, development, and implementation of effective AT services, strategies, or devices to improve the function of individuals with polytrauma. The areas of AT evaluation or training include powered mobility and seating, augmentative and alternative communication, adaptive driving vehicles, specialized computer access, electronic cognitive devices and electronic aids to daily living, adaptive sports, learning technologies, and rehabilitation engineering (Department of Veterans Affairs, 2009).

IMPLICATIONS FOR THE FIELD

A priority in the field of rehabilitation psychology should be the identification or development and implementation of strategies that address the complex needs of polytrauma patients and their families. Advanced study regarding special polytrauma patient populations is indicated. For example, in injured geriatric patients, emerging findings suggest poorer functional outcomes, increased mortality, and higher morbidity rates (Dimitriou, Calori, & Giannoudis, 2011). Furthermore, women with TBI and polytrauma tend to fare worse than men with respect to psychiatric and neurobehavioral symptoms post TBI (Colvin et al., 2009; Iverson et al., 2011). As such, additional research regarding these individuals and optimal management strategies that meet their needs is crucial.

Given that there is limited established evidence for mTBI interventions, further research in this area is indicated. For example, more information regarding novel or unconventional therapies (e.g., hyperbaric oxygen, nutritional supplementation) is needed to establish an empirical base. Also, future investigations that employ systematic observational and controlled intervention designs for pain management in patients with polytrauma are vital. Along these lines, stepped care models that target transdiagnostic/cross-cutting symptoms and optimal timing of interventions targeting different symptoms need to be tested further to examine impact on trajectory of recovery.

Although this chapter focused on models that primarily exist in the military and veteran sector, it is important to note that what has been identified is transferable to civilian settings. Terrorist attacks directed against civilian populations remain a significant threat in the United States, yet the civilian medical community has limited training and experience in the diagnosis and treatment of blast-related injuries (Burgess et al., 2010). In such instances, the injuries sustained by civilian survivors share many characteristics found in military polytrauma. For both populations, it is important to consider the compounding effects of multiple injuries as well as the emotional context in which these injuries are sustained. Moreover, these injury characteristics highlight the need for a multidisciplinary approach to treatment, and the role of the rehabilitation psychologist as part of the treatment team in both military and civilian settings cannot be overemphasized.

One challenge that rehabilitation psychologists must address is the implementation of relevant programming. This includes traditional, evidence-based rehabilitation and mental health treatment as well as interventions that may have less empirical support (but that are consistent with recommendations from the American Congress of Rehabilitation Medicine; Haskins et al., 2012). Over the next decade, significant effort by rehabilitation psychologists is needed to gather supportive evidence for various patient populations services as technology advances and patient needs are better understood. As Duchnick, Ropacki, Yutsis, Petska, and Pawlowski (2015) pointed out, implementation of systemwide practices may be difficult (and contraindicated), given the patient- and treatment-focused nature of interventions provided in the current models of care. Further research is also needed to establish suitable assessment tools for long-term functional outcomes in this population and for program evaluation. Rehabilitation psychologists must continue to advocate for the evolution of services to accommodate the needs and promote positive outcomes of patients with polytraumatic injuries.

References

Bedard, M., Felteau, M., Marshall, S., Cullen, N., Gibbons, C., Dubois, S., . . . Moustgaard, A. (2014). Mindfulness-based cognitive therapy reduces symptoms of depression in people with a traumatic brain injury: Results from a randomized controlled trial. *Journal of Head Trauma Rehabilitation*, *29*, E13–E22.

Bombardier, C. H., Temkin, N. R., Machamer, J., & Dikmen, S. S. (2003). The natural history of drinking and alcohol-related problems after traumatic brain injury. *Archives of Physical Medicine and Rehabilitation*, *84*, 185–191. http://dx.doi.org/10.1053/apmr.2003.50002

Border, J. R., LaDuca, J., & Seibel, R. (1975). Priorities in the management of the patient with polytrauma. *Progress in Surgery*, *14*, 84–120. http://dx.doi.org/10.1159/000398211

Brenner, L. A., Forster, J. E., Hoffberg, A. S., Matarazzo, B. B., Hostetter, T. A., Signoracci, G., & Simpson, G. K. (2018). Window to Hope: A randomized controlled trial of a psychological intervention for the treatment of hopelessness among veterans with moderate to severe traumatic brain injury. *The Journal of Head Trauma Rehabilitation*, *33*(2), E64–E73.

Bryant, R. A., Moulds, M. L., Guthrie, R. M., Dang, S. T., & Nixon, R. D. (2003). Imaginal exposure alone and imaginal exposure with cognitive restructuring in treatment of posttraumatic stress disorder. *Journal of Consulting and Clinical Psychology*, *71*, 706–712. http://dx.doi.org/10.1037/0022-006X.71.4.706

Burgess, P., Sullivent, E. E., Sasser, S. M., Wald, M. M., Ossmann, E., & Kapil, V. (2010). Managing traumatic brain injury secondary to explosions. *Journal of Emergencies, Trauma, and Shock*, *3*, 164–172. http://dx.doi.org/10.4103/0974-2700.62120

Butcher, N. E., & Balogh, Z. J. (2014). Update on the definition of polytrauma. *European Journal of Trauma and Emergency Surgery*, *40*, 107–111. http://dx.doi.org/10.1007/s00068-014-0391-x

Carlson, K. F., Nelson, D., Orazem, R. J., Nugent, S., Cifu, D. X., & Sayer, N. A. (2010). Psychiatric diagnoses among Iraq and Afghanistan war veterans screened for deployment-related traumatic brain injury. *Journal of Traumatic Stress*, *23*, 17–24.

Centers for Disease Control. (2009, January 23). Guidelines for field triage of injured patients: Recommendations of the National Expert Panel on Field Triage. *Morbidity and Mortality Weekly Report, 58*(No. RR-1).

Centers for Disease Control. (2018, June). *Explosions and blast injuries: A primer for clinicians*. Retrieved from https://www.cdc.gov/masstrauma/preparedness/primer.pdf

Cicerone, K. D., Dahlberg, C., Malec, J. F., Langenbahn, D. M., Felicetti, T., Kneipp, S., . . . Catanese, J. (2005). Evidence-based cognitive rehabilitation: Updated review of the literature from 1998 through 2002. *Archives of Physical Medicine and Rehabilitation*, *86*, 1681–1692. http://dx.doi.org/10.1016/j.apmr.2005.03.024

Clark, M. E., Scholten, J. D., Walker, R. L., & Gironda, R. J. (2009). Assessment and treatment of pain associated with combat-related polytrauma. *Pain Medicine*, *10*, 456–469.

Colvin, A. C., Mullen, J., Lovell, M. R., West, R. V., Collins, M. W., & Groh, M. (2009). The role of concussion history and gender in recovery from soccer-related concussion. *The American Journal of Sports Medicine*, *37*, 1699–1704. http://dx.doi.org/10.1177/0363546509332497

Corrigan, J. D. (1995). Substance abuse as a mediating factor in outcome from traumatic brain injury. *Archives of Physical Medicine and Rehabilitation*, *76*, 302–309. http://dx.doi.org/10.1016/S0003-9993(95)80654-7

Denneson, L. M., Corson, K., & Dobscha, S. K. (2011). Complementary and alternative medicine use among veterans with chronic noncancer pain. *Journal of Rehabilitation Research and Development*,

48, 1119–1128. http://dx.doi.org/10.1682/JRRD.2010.12.0243

Department of Veterans Affairs. (n.d.-a). Concussion coach (Mobile app). Retrieved from https://www.polytrauma.va.gov/ConcussionCoach.asp

Department of Veterans Affairs. (n.d.-b). *Polytrauma/TBI system of care*. Retrieved from https://www.polytrauma.va.gov/system-of-care/index.asp

Department of Veterans Affairs. (2005). *Polytrauma rehabilitation procedures* (VHA Handbook 1172.1). Washington, DC: Author.

Department of Veterans Affairs. (2007, April 13). *Screening and evaluation of possible traumatic brain injury in Operation Enduring Freedom (OEF) and Operation Iraqi Freedom (OIF) veterans* (Veterans Health Administration Directive 2007-013). Retrieved from https://www.va.gov/optometry/docs/VHA_Directive_2007-013_Screening_Possible_TBI.pdf

Department of Veterans Affairs. (2009, June 9). *Polytrauma—traumatic brain injury (TBI) system of care* (Veterans Health Administration Directive 2009-028). Retrieved from https://www.va.gov/optometry/docs/vha_directive_2009-028_polytrauma_system_of_care.pdf

Departments of Veterans Affairs and Defense. (2016). VA/DOD Clinical Practice Guidelines. Management of Concussion-Mild TBI. Retrieved from https://www.healthquality.va.gov/guidelines/rehab/mtbi/

Dimitriou, R., Calori, G. M., & Giannoudis, P. V. (2011). Polytrauma in the elderly: Specific considerations and current concepts of management. *European Journal of Trauma and Emergency Surgery*, *37*, 539–548. http://dx.doi.org/10.1007/s00068-011-0137-y

Dobscha, S. K., Clark, M. E., Morasco, B. J., Freeman, M., Campbell, R., & Helfand, M. (2009). Systematic review of the literature on pain in patients with polytrauma including traumatic brain injury. *Pain Medicine*, *10*, 1200–1217. http://dx.doi.org/10.1111/j.1526-4637.2009.00721.x

Duchnick, J. J., Ropacki, S., Yutsis, M., Petska, K., & Pawlowski, C. (2015). Polytrauma transitional rehabilitation programs: Comprehensive rehabilitation for community integration after brain injury. *Psychological Services*, *12*, 313–321.

Ekhtiari, H., Rezapour, T., Aupperle, R. L., & Paulus, M. P. (2017). Neuroscience-informed psychoeducation for addiction medicine: A neurocognitive perspective. In T. Calvey & W. M. U. Daniels (Eds.), *Progress in brain research* (Vol. 235, pp. 239–264). New York, NY: Elsevier.

Faul, M., Wald, M. M., Rutland-Brown, W., Sullivent, E. E., & Sattin, R. W. (2007, December). Using a cost-benefit analysis to estimate outcomes of a clinical treatment guideline: Testing the Brain Trauma Foundation guidelines for the treatment of severe traumatic brain injury. *The Journal of Trauma*, *63*, 1271–1278. http://dx.doi.org/10.1097/TA.0b013e3181493080

French, L. M. (2010). Military traumatic brain injury: An examination of important differences. *Annals of the New York Academy of Sciences*, *1208*, 38–45. http://dx.doi.org/10.1111/j.1749-6632.2010.05696.x

Friedemann-Sánchez, G., Sayer, N. A., & Pickett, T. (2008). Provider perspectives on rehabilitation of patients with polytrauma. *Archives of Physical Medicine and Rehabilitation*, *89*, 171–178. http://dx.doi.org/10.1016/j.apmr.2007.10.017

Gironda, R. J., Clark, M. E., Ruff, R. L., Chait, S., Craine, M., Walker, R., & Scholten, J. (2009). Traumatic brain injury, polytrauma, and pain: Challenges and treatment strategies for the polytrauma rehabilitation. *Rehabilitation Psychology*, *54*, 247–258. http://dx.doi.org/10.1037/a0016906

Haskins, E., Cicerone, K., Dams-O'Connor, K., Eberle, R., Langenbahn, D., & Shapiro-Rosenbaum, A. (2012). *Cognitive rehabilitation manual: Translating evidence-based recommendations into practice.* Reston, VA: American Congress of Rehabilitation Medicine.

Hoge, C. W., McGurk, D., Thomas, J. L., Cox, A. L., Engel, C. C., & Castro, C. A. (2008). Mild traumatic brain injury in U.S. soldiers returning from Iraq. *The New England Journal of Medicine*, *358*, 453–463. http://dx.doi.org/10.1056/NEJMoa072972

Iverson, K. M., Hendricks, A. M., Kimerling, R., Krengel, M., Meterko, M., Stolzmann, K. L., . . . Lew, H. L. (2011). Psychiatric diagnoses and neurobehavioral symptom severity among OEF/OIF VA patients with deployment-related traumatic brain injury: A gender comparison. *Women's Health Issues*, *21*(4, Suppl.), S210–S217. http://dx.doi.org/10.1016/j.whi.2011.04.019

Kangas, M., & McDonald, S. (2011). Is it time to act? The potential of acceptance and commitment therapy for psychological problems following acquired brain injury. *Neuropsychological Rehabilitation*, *21*, 250–276. http://dx.doi.org/10.1080/09602011.2010.540920

Lang, K. P., Veazey-Morris, K., & Andrasik, F. (2014). Exploring the role of insomnia in the relation between PTSD and pain in veterans with polytrauma injuries. *The Journal of Head Trauma*

Rehabilitation, *29*, 44–53. http://dx.doi.org/10.1097/HTR.0b013e31829c85d0

Lew, H. L., Otis, J. D., Tun, C., Kerns, R. D., Clark, M. E., & Cifu, D. X. (2009). Prevalence of chronic pain, posttraumatic stress disorder, and persistent postconcussive symptoms in OIF/OEF veterans: Polytrauma clinical triad. *Journal of Rehabilitation Research and Development*, *46*, 697–702. http://dx.doi.org/10.1682/JRRD.2009.01.0006

Lew, H. L., Pogoda, T. K., Hsu, P. T., Cohen, S., Amick, M. M., Baker, E., . . . Vanderploeg, R. D. (2010). Impact of the "polytrauma clinical triad" on sleep disturbance in a department of veterans affairs outpatient rehabilitation setting. *American Journal of Physical Medicine & Rehabilitation*, *89*, 437–445. http://dx.doi.org/10.1097/PHM.0b013e3181ddd301

Menon, D. K., Schwab, K., Wright, D. W., Maas, A. I., & the Demographics and Clinical Assessment Working Group of the International and Interagency Initiative Toward Common Data Elements for Research on Traumatic Brain Injury and Psychological Health. (2010). Position statement: Definition of traumatic rain injury. *Archives of Physical Medicine and Rehabilitation*, *91*, 1637–1640. http://dx.doi.org/10.1016/j.apmr.2010.05.017

Olson-Madden, J. H., Brenner, L. A., Matarazzo, B. B., Signoracci, G. M., & the Expert Consensus Collaborators. (2013). Identification and treatment of TBI and co-occurring psychiatric symptoms among OEF/OIF/OND veterans seeking mental health services within the State of Colorado: Establishing consensus for best practices. *Community Mental Health Journal*, *49*, 220–229. http://dx.doi.org/10.1007/s10597-012-9572-4

Pape, H. C., Lefering, R., Butcher, N., Peitzman, A., Leenen, L., Marzi, I., . . . Balogh, Z. (2014). The definition of polytrauma revisited: An international consensus process and proposal of the new "Berlin definition." *The Journal of Trauma and Acute Care Surgery*, *77*, 780–786. http://dx.doi.org/10.1097/TA.0000000000000453

Peleg, K., Aharonson-Daniel, L., Michael, M., Shapira, S. C., & Israel Trauma Group. (2003). Patterns of injury in hospitalized terrorist victims. *The American Journal of Emergency Medicine*, *21*, 258–262. http://dx.doi.org/10.1016/S0735-6757(03)00043-3

Pickett, T. C., Bender, M. C., & Gourley, E. (2010). Head injury rehabilitation of military members. In C. H. Kennedy & J. L. Moore (Eds.), *Military neuropsychology* (pp. 175–198). New York, NY: Springer.

Polusny, M. A., Kehle, S. M., Nelson, N. W., Erbes, C. R., Arbisi, P. A., & Thuras, P. (2011). Longitudinal effects of mild traumatic brain injury and posttraumatic stress disorder comorbidity on postdeployment outcomes in National Guard soldiers deployed to Iraq. *Archives of General Psychiatry*, *68*, 79–89. http://dx.doi.org/10.1001/archgenpsychiatry.2010.172

Pratt, C. W., Gill, K. J., Barrett, N. M., & Roberts, M. M. (2014). Course, treatment, and outcome of severe mental illnesses. In C. W. Pratt, K. J. Gill, N. M. Barrett, & M. M. Roberts (Eds.), *Psychiatric rehabilitation* (3rd ed., pp. 75–102). New York, NY: Academic Press. http://dx.doi.org/10.1016/B978-0-12-387002-5.00003-2

Pugh, M. J. V., Finley, E. P., Copeland, L. A., Wang, C. P., Noel, P. H., Amuan, M. E., . . . Pugh, J. A. (2014). Complex comorbidity clusters in OEF/OIF veterans: The polytrauma clinical triad and beyond. *Medical Care*, *52*, 172–181. http://dx.doi.org/10.1097/MLR.0000000000000059

Saltapidas, H., & Ponsford, J. (2007). The influence of cultural background on motivation for and participation in rehabilitation and outcome following traumatic brain injury. *The Journal of Head Trauma Rehabilitation*, *22*, 132–139. http://dx.doi.org/10.1097/01.HTR.0000265101.75177.8d

Sayer, N. A., Chiros, C. E., Sigford, B., Scott, S., Clothier, B., Pickett, T., & Lew, H. L. (2008). Characteristics and rehabilitation outcomes among patients with blast and other injuries sustained during the Global War on Terror. *Archives of Physical Medicine and Rehabilitation*, *89*, 163–170. http://dx.doi.org/10.1016/j.apmr.2007.05.025

Schneiderman, A. I., Braver, E. R., & Kang, H. K. (2008). Understanding sequelae of injury mechanisms and mild traumatic brain injury incurred during the conflicts in Iraq and Afghanistan: Persistent postconcussive symptoms and posttraumatic stress disorder. *American Journal of Epidemiology*, *167*, 1446–1452. http://dx.doi.org/10.1093/aje/kwn068

Scott, S. G., Belanger, H. G., Vanderploeg, R. D., Massengale, J., & Scholten, J. (2006). Mechanism-of-injury approach to evaluating patients with blast-related polytrauma. *The Journal of the American Osteopathic Association*, *106*, 265–270.

Simpson, G. K., Tate, R. L., Whiting, D. L., & Cotter, R. E. (2011). Suicide prevention after traumatic brain injury: A randomized controlled trial of a program for the psychological treatment of hopelessness. *The Journal of Head Trauma Rehabilitation*, *26*, 290–300. http://dx.doi.org/10.1097/HTR.0b013e3182225250

Soo, C., & Tate, R. (2007). Psychological treatment for anxiety in people with traumatic brain injury. *Cochrane Database of Systematic Reviews*, *2*, CD005239.

Taylor, B. C., Campbell, E., Nugent, S., Fletcher, L., Bidelspach, D. E., Kehle-Forbes, S. M., . . . Sayer, N. A. (2015, November). *Fiscal Year 2013 VA utili-*

zation report for Iraq and Afghanistan War veterans diagnosed with TBI (PLY 05-2010-2). Retrieved from http://www.polytrauma.va.gov/TBIReports/FY13-TBI-Diagnosis-HCU-Report.pdf

Terrio, H., Brenner, L. A., Ivins, B. J., Cho, J. M., Helmick, K., Schwab, K., . . . Warden, D. (2009). Traumatic brain injury screening: Preliminary findings in a US Army Brigade Combat Team. *The Journal of Head Trauma Rehabilitation*, *24*, 14–23. http://dx.doi.org/10.1097/HTR.0b013e31819581d8

Uomoto, J. M., & Williams, R. M. (2009). Post-acute polytrauma rehabilitation and integrated care of returning veterans: Toward a holistic approach. *Rehabilitation Psychology*, *54*, 259–269. http://dx.doi.org/10.1037/a0016907

Warden, D. (2006). Military TBI during the Iraq and Afghanistan wars. *The Journal of Head Trauma Rehabilitation*, *21*, 398–402. http://dx.doi.org/10.1097/00001199-200609000-00004

Whittaker, R., Kemp, S., & House, A. (2007). Illness perceptions and outcome in mild head injury: A longitudinal study. *Journal of Neurology, Neurosurgery, and Psychiatry*, *78*, 644–646. http://dx.doi.org/10.1136/jnnp.2006.101105

CHAPTER 23

PEDIATRIC ACQUIRED CONDITIONS: BRAIN AND SPINAL CORD INJURIES

Beth S. Slomine and Kelly Jones

Children with brain injuries and spinal cord injuries (SCIs) often require rehabilitation services. As such, rehabilitation psychologists working in pediatric rehabilitation settings should be familiar with these disorders. In this chapter, an overview of acquired brain injury (ABI) and SCI in children is provided. For discussion of adult SCI or traumatic brain injury (TBI), see Chapters 17 and 18, this volume.

ACQUIRED BRAIN INJURY

Children experience ABI resulting from events such as head trauma, hypoxic injuries, stroke, brain tumor, and infectious disease processes. In this section, we focus on children with TBI. Relative to other etiologies of ABI, TBI represents the most common etiology of pediatric ABI. In addition, this section focuses on moderate to severe TBI, as these children are more likely to receive services in a rehabilitation setting.

Epidemiology of Traumatic Brain Injury

TBI is the most common cause of morbidity and mortality in children and adolescents. According to the Centers for Disease Control and Prevention, the rate of TBI is highest in children 0 to 4 years of age (1,256 per 100,000) and adolescents 15 to 19 years of age (757 per 100,000) in the United States, with somewhat lower rates in children 5 to 14 years of age (Faul, Xu, Wald, & Coronado, 2010). Children with TBI are most often evaluated in the emergency department or other outpatient settings and do not require hospitalization. A recent review of population-based epidemiologic studies of pediatric TBI in developed countries revealed that the annual incidence of childhood TBI is 691 per 100,000 in the emergency department, 74 per 100,000 treated in the hospital, and 9 per 100,000 resulting in death (Thurman, 2016). For children who present to the emergency department with blunt head trauma, the vast majority of these injuries are mild (98%), with moderate and severe injuries occurring much less frequently (Quayle et al., 2014).

Risk Factors

Among presentation to the hospital for pediatric TBI, the highest proportion of presentations is for infants and toddlers (49%; Crowe, Babl, Anderson, & Catroppa, 2009). Across all ages, males are at a higher risk of sustaining a TBI than females (Faul et al., 2010). Children with behavioral difficulties (e.g., attention-deficit/hyperactivity disorder [ADHD], conduct disorder) and/or a learning disability are more likely to sustain a TBI (e.g., Max et al., 1997). Family factors such as lower socioeconomic status (SES), higher parental stress, and poor parenting practices are also related to an increased risk for TBI (McKinlay et al., 2010).

The cause of TBI varies across infancy, childhood, and adolescence. A TBI in children younger than 5 years of age is most likely secondary to a fall or nonaccidental trauma (Keenan & Bratton, 2006).

http://dx.doi.org/10.1037/0000129-024
Handbook of Rehabilitation Psychology, Third Edition, L. A. Brenner, S. A. Reid-Arndt, T. R. Elliott, R. G. Frank, and B. Caplan (Editors-in-Chief)

These types of injuries are typically different from other TBIs in that injury is diffuse and has a poorer outcome (related to hypoxia and hypotension). Between 5 and 10 years of age, the most common cause of TBI is sport or transport related (e.g., motor vehicle passenger, pedestrian vs. car, bicycle). Adolescents are at the greatest risk to be injured in a motor vehicle crash.

Outcome

TBI outcome has a dose response with greater impairment associated with the severity of the initial injury (McCarthy et al., 2006). Children with moderate to severe injuries display long-term cognitive and behavioral impairment relative to orthopedic controls (e.g., Taylor et al., 2002). In contrast, mild TBI is often associated with fewer long-term consequences (Cassidy et al., 2004). Given that children with moderate to severe TBIs are much more likely than children with mild TBI to have persisting physical, cognitive, emotional, academic, and functional consequences warranting rehabilitation services, the remainder of this chapter focuses on moderate and severe TBI.

In addition to the severity of the injury based on the initial level of consciousness (e.g., Glasgow Coma Scale; Teasdale & Jennett, 1974), the duration of the impaired level of consciousness predicts the outcome. Time to follow commands (TFC) and duration of posttraumatic amnesia (PTA) are important predictors of functional independence at discharge from inpatient rehabilitation (Suskauer et al., 2009) and at 1-year follow up (Austin, Slomine, Dematt, Salorio, & Suskauer, 2013). At 1- to 2-year follow-up, TFC and PTA significantly predicted global functional outcome above and beyond the Glasgow Coma Scale scores (Davis, Slomine, Salorio, & Suskauer, 2016).

Neuroimaging findings are helpful in predicting outcome. According to a model of TBI severity effects described by Ommaya and Gennarelli (1974), the depth of focal brain lesions is predictive of functional outcome. Injuries resulting from less rotational acceleration tend to involve cortical structures and functional disconnections. Injuries resulting from more severe traumatic forces (i.e., rotational components of accelerative trauma to the head) produce deeper lesions involving subcortical white matter and deep central gray matter. In children with TBI who require inpatient rehabilitation, a greater level of diffuse axonal injury (e.g., corpus callosum, basal ganglia, thalamus, cerebellum, and brain stem) has been associated with a poorer outcome 1 year after injury (Grados et al., 2001).

The effects of age at injury in children and adolescents differ from those in adults, as there is an interruption to the typical trajectory of brain development. Because the injury occurs during a dynamic brain maturation process, children and adolescents are often considered to be "moving targets" due to ongoing recovery as well as continued development and neurological maturation. It was previously thought that recovery from TBI sustained in childhood was more favorable than those sustained in adulthood; however, there is growing evidence to suggest that children who sustain a TBI before 2 years of age demonstrate more global neurobehavioral impairments than those who sustain a TBI after 7 years of age (V. Anderson et al., 2010). Research also suggests better recovery with increasing age at injury (e.g., Donders & Warschausky, 2007). However, it is difficult to interpret age at injury effects, as they are typically confounded by other factors including time since injury and age at evaluation of outcome (Taylor & Alden, 1997), as well as mechanism of injury, which, as previously mentioned, is related to age at injury.

Preinjury intellectual ability, academic achievement, and psychological symptoms are also predictive of outcome after TBI. Specifically, preinjury cognitive disability and parent ratings of behavioral difficulties have been associated with poorer outcome (Johnson, DeMatt, & Salorio, 2009). In addition to child preinjury factors, family factors are related to outcome (Kinsella, Ong, Murtagh, Prior, & Sawyer, 1999). Lower SES has been associated with slower rates of recovery (Yeates et al., 2004). In addition, more favorable family circumstances (e.g., less family burden, less parental psychological distress, and less family dysfunction) were associated with better child outcomes, even after controlling for sociodemographic status and race (Taylor et al., 1999).

Assessment

Because impairments in cognitive, emotional, and behavioral functioning are common following moderate to severe TBI, rehabilitation psychologists should be prepared to conduct broad-based assessments. In addition, specific goals of assessment are often dependent on the setting in which the child is being assessed. Prior to any assessment, it is important to obtain school records and parents' reports and ratings of the child's preinjury behavioral and emotional functioning to determine what changes have occurred after the TBI. At each stage of recovery following TBI, rehabilitation psychologists select specific assessment tools based on the existing evidence about the psychometric properties of these measures, including utility of the tools for treatment planning and informing long-term prognosis. Approaches to assessment at each stage of recovery are provided next.

Acute stage of recovery. After a child is medically stable, he or she may transfer to an inpatient rehabilitation setting. Given the likelihood of ongoing cognitive recovery during an inpatient rehabilitation admission, it is important to monitor recovery throughout that stage. One measure designed to monitor cognitive recovery over time in a pediatric inpatient rehabilitation setting is the Cognitive and Linguistic Scale (CALS; Slomine et al., 2008; Slomine, Grasmick, Suskauer, & Salorio, 2016). The CALS can be used with children as young as 2 years of age through young adulthood and is appropriate for children with the range of cognitive impairments present during inpatient rehabilitation. Other repeatable measures are provided in Table 23.1.

During this acute phase of recovery, assessment of a child's functioning is dependent on his or her presentation (i.e., level of cognitive, behavioral, and physical impairments). If a child presents in a disorder of consciousness at admission (i.e., coma, vegetative/unresponsive wakefulness state, minimally conscious state; see Giacino, Katz, & Whyte, 2013), accurate diagnostic characterization using standardized rating scales is essential to provide an accurate prognostication regarding recovery (see Table 23.1 for commonly used measures to assess level of consciousness). Measures to assess level of consciousness have been developed for use only in adult populations, and the psychometric properties have not been examined in children. At this stage of recovery, the rehabilitation psychologist may assess responses to stimulation and to the environment across different sensory modalities (visual threat, visual tracking, vocalizations, response to noxious

TABLE 23.1

Common Screening and Recovery Tracking Measures for Children With Traumatic Brain Injury

Domain	Measures	Age range
Premorbid functioning	School Records	5–18 years
	Behavior Rating Inventory of Executive Function, Second Edition (Gioia et al., 2015)	2 years and older
	Behavior Rating Inventory of Executive Function—Preschool (Gioia et al., 2003)	
	Behavior Rating Inventory of Executive Function—Adult (Roth et al., 2005)	
	Behavior Assessment System for Children, Third Edition—Parent Report (Reynolds & Kamphaus, 2015)	
Level of consciousness	JFK Coma Recovery Scale—Revised (Giacino et al., 2004)	Not validated with children
	Coma/Near Coma Scale (Rappaport et al., 1992)	Not validated with children
Posttraumatic amnesia	Children's Orientation and Amnesia Test (Ewing-Cobbs et al., 1990)	3–15 years
Global functioning	Functional Independence Measure for Children (Msall et al., 1994)	6 months to 21 years
	Pediatric Evaluation of Disability Inventory (Haley et al., 1992)	6 months to 20 years
Cognitive recovery	Cognitive and Linguistic Scale (Slomine et al., 2008, 2016)	2–21 years
	Repeatable Battery for the Assessment of Neuropsychological Status Update (Randolph, 2012)	12 years and older

olfactory and tactile stimulation) and the presence of higher level, cortical functions (e.g., purposeful/voluntary movements, command following) by eliciting and distinguishing behaviors that are reflexive/automatic from those that represent some level of awareness or purposeful intent. There are several points to consider when conducting these types of evaluation to ensure accurate diagnosis of consciousness:

- Adequate stimulation (e.g., deep pressure stimulation, positioning) is required prior to the evaluation to ensure arousal.
- Sedating medications may dampen arousal and responsiveness.
- Requested responses should not be reflexive (e.g., squeeze my hand, open your eyes) to ensure that reflexive behavior is not misinterpreted as purposeful intent.
- Assessment of command following should incorporate motor behaviors that the child is physically able to perform and use simple, declarative language, one request at a time.
- A long-enough interval should be provided before the next presentation of a stimulus to allow the child adequate time to respond.
- A number of behavioral responses should be trialed (e.g., limb and eye commands), using a broad range of stimuli, at during different times of the day.
- Serial reassessment using reliable measurement strategies should be used, including specialized measurement tools, to establish response consistency.
- Observations of others (e.g., families, nurses, therapists) who spend time with the child should be considered.

As a child develops a means of functional communication, the rehabilitation psychologist typically shifts his or her assessment to monitoring of PTA, which is a stage of recovery marked by confusion, disorientation, and inability to lay down new memories. Assessment of PTA is important because length of PTA is predictive of outcome (Davis et al., 2016) and specific interventions should be employed to minimize confusion and promote orientation and new learning (Slomine & Locascio, 2009). Tools assessing PTA require serial administration over several days and typically include general orientation, temporal orientation, and memory questions (see Table 23.1 for commonly used measures).

Postacute stage of recovery. A more comprehensive neuropsychological evaluation is typically conducted toward the end of a child's inpatient rehabilitation stay or within the first few months following discharge. When planning for school reintegration, assessment should occur as close to the date of the return to school as possible to capture the child's most recent level of cognitive function and provide appropriate recommendations. The goal of a comprehensive neuropsychological evaluation in the rehabilitation setting generally follows the framework of typical pediatric neuropsychological evaluations in that the goals are to provide information regarding the integrity of brain functioning; detect any cognitive impairments; identify emotional or behavioral concerns; and provide appropriate recommendations for home, educational, and community functioning. In the evaluation report, the psychologist should also note whether ongoing recovery is expected and when an updated evaluation should occur. There are many standardized measures available to assess a variety of domains (see Table 23.2).

In addition to standardized, performance-based measures, a comprehensive evaluation should also collect information from parents and consider environmental influences. Comprehensive evaluation generally includes a clinical interview with parents to obtain the child's history and premorbid functioning, as well as formal assessment across the following domains: intellectual functioning, language, visuospatial/visuoconstructional skills, attention, learning and memory, executive functioning, and motor functioning. It is also important to evaluate behavioral, emotional, and adaptive functioning, usually through caregiver reports. Self-report is also useful for older children and those who are higher functioning.

Children with TBI require periodic neuropsychological evaluation to delineate strengths and weaknesses within the context of ongoing development and increasing demands for independence. Reevaluation is typically recommended 1 year postinjury (or sooner

TABLE 23.2

Common Neuropsychological Assessment Measures for Children With Traumatic Brain Injury

Domain	Measures	Method of administration	Age range
Developmental	Mullen Scales of Early Learning (Mullen, 1995)	Performance-based	Birth to 68 months
	Bayley Scales of Infant and Toddler Development, Third Edition (Bayley, 2006)	Performance-based	1–42 months
Intellectual functioning	Wechsler Abbreviated Scale of Intelligence (Wechsler, 2011)	Performance-based	6 years and older
Language	Boston Naming Test, Second Edition (Kaplan et al., 2001)	Performance-based	5 years and older
	Peabody Picture Vocabulary Test, Fourth Edition (Dunn & Dunn, 2007)	Performance-based	30 months and older
Visuospatial and visuoconstructional	Judgment of Line Orientation (Benton et al., 1994)	Performance-based	7 years and older
	Beery–Buktenica Developmental Test of Visual-Motor Integration, Sixth Edition (Beery & Beery, 2010)	Performance-based	2 years and older
Attention	Test of Everyday Attention (TEA and TEA–Ch2; Manly et al., 2016; Robertson, Ward, Ridgeway, & Nimmo-Smith, 1994)	Performance-based	6 years and older
	Wechsler Digit Span Tests (WISC–V, WAIS–IV; Wechsler, 2009, 2014)	Performance-based	6 years and older
	Conners' Continuous Performance Test—3 (Conners, 2015)	Performance-based	4 years and older
Memory	California Verbal Learning Test (CVLT–C, CVLT–3; Delis et al., 1994, 2017)	Performance-based	5 years and older
	Wide Range Assessment of Memory and Learning, Second Edition (Sheslow & Adams, 2003)	Performance-based	5 years and older
	Children's Memory Scale (Cohen, 1997)	Performance-based	5–16 years
Executive functioning	NEPSY–II (Korkman et al., 2007)	Performance-based	3–16 years
	Delis–Kaplan Executive Functioning System (Delis et al., 2001)	Performance-based	8 years and older
	Behavior Rating Inventory of Executive Function, Second Edition (Gioia et al., 2015)	Parent-report	2 years and older
	Behavior Rating Inventory of Executive Function—Preschool (Gioia et al., 2003)		
	Behavior Rating Inventory of Executive Function—Adult (Roth et al., 2005)		
Fine motor	Purdue Pegboard (Tiffin, 1968)	Performance-based	5 years and older
	Grooved Pegboard (Trites, 1977)	Performance-based	5 years and older
Behavioral and emotional	Behavior Assessment System for Children, Third Edition (Reynolds & Kamphaus, 2015)	2–21 years	Parent-, self-report
	Conners, Third Edition (Conners, 2008)	Parent-report	6–18 years
Adaptive functioning	Adaptive Behavior Assessment System, Third Edition (Harrison & Oakland, 2015)	Parent-report	0 years and older
	Vineland Adaptive Behavior Scales, Third Edition (Sparrow et al., 2016)	Parent-report	0 years and older

Note. TEA–Ch = Test of Everyday Attention for Children; WISC–V = Wechsler Intelligence Scale for Children, Fifth Edition; WAIS–IV = Wechsler Adult Intelligence Scale, Fourth Edition; CVLT–C = California Verbal Learning Test for Children; CVLT–3 = California Verbal Learning Test, Third Edition.

if there is a change in neurological status). Further evaluations should occur during critical periods throughout childhood, such as when academic expectations increase (e.g., transition to middle and high school) and when an adolescent prepares to transition to secondary education (e.g., college) or employment. To ensure that these evaluations occur when needed, ongoing consultation with individuals and agencies invested in helping children with TBI to reach their potential is needed.

Intervention

Acute stage of recovery. Both pharmacological and behavioral interventions are available to treat common sequelae of TBI. Pharmacological intervention, including dopamine agonists (e.g., methylphenidate, levodopa, bromocriptine, amantadine) and GABA agonists (e.g., zolpidem, baclofen), may be implemented in the acute stage of recovery to promote wakefulness and arousal and to improve basic attentional functioning (Suskauer & Trovato, 2013). Once a child has emerged from a coma, he or she may demonstrate restlessness, agitation, disinhibition, and/or destructive behaviors commonly due to confusion and/or disorientation. In addition to pharmacological intervention (e.g., methylphenidate, antidepressants, amantadine; Suskauer & Trovato, 2013), behavioral interventions are also useful to manage these symptoms. Following TBI, children may not respond well to traditional reinforcement schedules (rewards for appropriate behavior), as contingency learning is often difficult. Alternatively, antecedent management should be used to provide as much environmental control as possible. The child's environment (i.e., more controlled and safe, less distressing) and physiological state (e.g., medications to reduce agitation) should be modified to minimize the likelihood of problematic behavior (Slifer & Amari, 2009). Some examples of environmental control include minimizing sensory stimulation (e.g., limited number of people during interactions), avoiding use of restraints (instead, using a one-to-one aide or net bed), and using external organization aides (e.g., written schedule, memory book). In addition, a structured and consistent routine should be implemented, and the child should be spoken to with clear and concise language. Once a child becomes more stable, greater stimulation and/or challenging environmental conditions can be gradually reintroduced in combination with teaching coping strategies and other skills for self-regulation.

Although psychoeducation should be provided at all stages of recovery, it is particularly important in the acute phase to help normalize the child's recovery process. In a review of family intervention following pediatric TBI, Boschen, Gargaro, Gan, Gerber, and Brandys (2007) found that the leading interventions in increasing caregiver knowledge and decreasing caregiver anxiety included educational and informational components. One role of the pediatric rehabilitation psychologist during the acute phase of recovery is to provide families with information about the child's injury including anticipated recovery of function, impact of the injury on siblings, and realistic expectations and goals for the child (Cole, Paulos, Cole, & Tankard, 2009). The rehabilitation psychologist can also provide the family information about community resources and organizations. It is important to note, however, that psychoeducation is most beneficial when provided over an extended period (e.g., several months) to meet the family's stage of acceptance of and readiness for change.

Postacute stage of recovery. Once a child is medically stable and no longer in a state of PTA, intervention often shifts to providing cognitive rehabilitation, which is broadly described as a systematic intervention designed to compensate for or ameliorate the impact of cognitive and/or behavioral difficulties following TBI, with the ultimate goal to improve daily functioning (Ylvisaker, Szekeres, & Haarbauer-Krupa, 1998). Although there are multiple studies in the adult TBI literature that examines the efficacy of cognitive rehabilitation interventions (for review, see Cicerone et al., 2011), few studies have examined efficacy of intervention for children with TBI (Slomine & Locascio, 2009). Ylvisaker and colleagues (1998), however, presented a theoretical framework for providing environmental scaffolding by "everyday people" such as teachers, parents, and other caregivers to promote daily functioning. This theoretical model has been incorporated into family-based interventions for children with brain injury.

For example, in a controlled trial, children with moderate to severe TBI were randomly assigned to receive routine rehabilitation interventions delivered by clinicians or by family members under the supervision of a clinician for 1 year (Braga, Da Paz, & Ylvisaker, 2005). Results indicated that although both groups demonstrated improvements on outcome measures (intellectual functioning, general functioning), only the family intervention group showed statistically significant gains on both outcome measures. In addition, Wade and colleagues developed and evaluated the efficacy of several family-based problem-solving programs using rigorous randomized controlled trials (Wade et al., 2010, 2015). These interventions proved to be most efficacious for adolescents and their families (Wade, Walz, Carey, & Williams, 2008). In contrast, younger children were found to benefit from more parent skills training (Raj et al., 2015), with particular benefit noted for lower income parents.

Attention and working memory training has also received considerable focus in the literature. Although there is support for clinician-assisted attention training in children with an emphasis on developing metacognitive skills, the research on solely computer-based training is mixed. Specifically, several studies of attention training that also involved teaching metacognitive skills in children with TBI (Galbiati et al., 2009), central nervous system disease (e.g., Butler et al., 2008; Conklin et al., 2015), and ABI (Catroppa, Stone, Rosema, Soo, & Anderson, 2014; Van't Hoof et al., 2005) have been found to be efficacious. For example, in the one study of children with TBI that examined attention-specific neuropsychological training (and included interactive involvement with a therapist at each session), the treatment group showed more improvement than the control group on measures of attention and adaptive functioning at 1-year follow-up (Galbiati et al., 2009).

Over the past 10 years, a number of studies have examined computer-based working memory training in pediatric brain injury, although not TBI specific. The findings from these studies are mixed (for reviews, see Morrison & Chein, 2011; Shipstead, Redick, & Engle, 2012). Most recently, in a population-based study, first-grade children with poor working memory performance were randomly assigned to a working memory training or control group. Working memory training was associated with improved visuospatial working memory at 6 and 12 months but not 24 months after training. In addition, there was no impact on academic achievement. These results suggest that the impact of working memory training is temporary and not generalizable (Roberts et al., 2016).

Educational Planning

Following TBI, children often require educational supports to address cognitive, motor, behavioral, and emotional concerns. Psychologists should work with families and school systems to ensure that the child's learning and psychosocial needs are met. Education services are often a necessary component of the continuum of care for youth with moderate to severe TBI. Several federal laws uphold a child's right to receive accommodations and modifications at school for difficulties related to ABI. In 1990, TBI was added to the list of qualifying conditions for special education services under the federal Individuals With Disabilities Education Act (IDEA; Federal Register, 1990). This law mandates that school systems are responsible for identifying and evaluating children with disabilities who are in need of special education and related services, as well as informing and involving caregivers in this process. Under IDEA, a child whose TBI affects academic achievement and school performance is eligible for special education services (i.e., specially designed instruction) provided by public schools at no cost to the parents. To receive these services, children must first be found eligible for special education services by having one or more eligible educational disabilities *and* the disability must have an impact on the child's ability to learn (Carney & Porter, 2001).

If a child is found eligible for special education services, an individualized education program (IEP) is generated by the child's educational team. In some cases, the rehabilitation psychologist serves as a liaison to the school system or provides a report that is used to develop the IEP. The IEP includes the child's academic services as well as the related services (e.g., physical therapy, occupational therapy, speech/language therapy, counseling services, transportation services), program accommodations (i.e., changes that do not alter the content, expectations of the student, or the level of material), and program modifications (i.e., changes that alter what the child is expected to learn) that the child is to receive. Related services are provided only if the child needs the service to access or benefit from his or her educational program. Given the range of outcomes following TBI, settings and accommodations vary greatly.

Children with TBI receive education in a variety of placements. If a child has difficulties with endurance and stamina, he or she may receive homebound instruction before returning to school full-time. Typically, homebound instruction is provided when the student will not be attending school for a minimum number of weeks. A student may also attend school for part of the day and receive homebound instruction a few hours per week. Within the school setting, there is a wide range of placement, depending on the student's needs. Some examples include a special education school, a self-contained classroom within a special education wing or school, a self-contained classroom for the entire day within a regular school, a self-contained classroom for core subjects and regular education classrooms for electives, a regular education classroom with "pull-out" support for specific areas, a regular education classroom with a special education coteacher, and a regular education classroom with a special educator who consults with the classroom teacher. Per the IDEA, the student should receive his or her special education services in the "least restrictive environment" possible. Students with TBI may also qualify for Extended School Year services if they are considered to likely regress significantly in one or more "critical life skills" as a result of an extended school break, typically the summer. If eligible, the student will receive an extension of special education and/or related services beyond the school year.

Although an IEP is needed for children receiving special education or related services, children who do not require that level of support (those with milder impairments) may receive assistance under Section 504 of the Rehabilitation Act of 1973 (Federal Register, 1973). Under this law, children with TBI are eligible for accommodations through a Section 504 Plan so that they can participate in educational programs provided to other students. Common accommodations that can be included in a 504 Plan include extra time on class assignments and testing, copies of teachers' notes, preferential seating, an extra set of books at home, and scheduled rest breaks.

SPINAL CORD INJURY

Children sustain an acquired SCI from events such as trauma to the spine (e.g., falls, gunshot wounds) and other processes, including infections, tumors, and demyelinating disease processes. In this section, we focus on trauma-related SCI.

Epidemiology and Risk Factors

In contrast to TBI, pediatric SCI is uncommon. An SCI before 15 years of age represents less than 4% of the overall incidence of traumatic SCI each year (National Spinal Cord Injury Statistical Center, 2004). An SCI is more common in older adolescents than in other age groups, as greater than 30% of all injuries occur between 17 and 23 years of age. In 2009, the incidence of traumatic SCI up to age 21 was 24 per 1 million (Piatt, 2015). Mechanism and severity of injury is strongly associated with race and economic factors. For example, SCIs as the result of gunshot injuries are more common in African American children. Lower SES has been associated with injures due to firearms or abuse, whereas higher SES has been associated with injuries due to bicycles, horses, and water activities (Piatt, 2015). Violent etiologies (e.g., gunshot wounds) are also slightly more common in preadolescents than in adults (Parent, Mac-Thiong, Roy-Beaudry, Sosa, & Labelle, 2011).

Outcome

Children with SCI often experience significant motor impairments, which are typically classified into two categories. Tetraplegia (i.e., sensory and/or motor loss throughout the body including upper and lower limbs) results from a cervical spine lesion. Paraplegia (sensory and/or motor loss in the lower limbs and possibly trunk but preserved function in upper limbs) results from injury to the thoracic spine or lower. Motor outcome depends on the level of the lesion and the completeness of the injury; higher lesions and more complete injury of the spinal cord are associated with greater motor impairment. In addition, the higher the lesion, the more likely that respiratory function (e.g., breathing, coughing) is impacted by the injury. Little or no voluntary control of bowel and bladder functioning (i.e., neurogenic bowel and bladder) are often a result of SCI, regardless of the level of lesion. These impairments lead to increased self-care demands (e.g., ventilator, tracheostomy tube, catheter, bowel program), which are often difficult for children to independently manage and complete given not only the associated motor impairments but also the level of organization, planning, and problem-solving needed for many of these tasks.

The neurological level and degree of completeness varies with age. Within those with tetraplegia, infants and younger children are more likely to have C1–3 injuries because of their relatively large heads and underdeveloped neck musculature, whereas adolescents are more likely to have C4–8 injuries (DeVivo & Vogel, 2004). Recovery of motor functioning is similar in children compared to adults with similar levels of injury, although there is some evidence to suggest that children may have a slightly better neurological recovery than adults (Parent et al., 2011).

The increased self-care demands and loss of functional independence associated with SCI are expected to place children at high risk for psychosocial distress. In adults with SCI, there is a higher rate of depression and anxiety compared to the general population. In children with SCI, rates of depression and anxiety are comparable to the general population (C. J. Anderson et al., 2009; Klaas, Kelly, Anderson, & Vogel, 2014). According to C. J. Anderson and colleagues (2009), when anxiety and depression are present in children with SCI, they are usually associated with reduced quality of life (QOL). Older age (adolescents vs. children) was also associated with higher rates of depression, and female adolescents had a higher rate of anxiety (Klaas et al., 2014).

Other studies of psychological outcome following pediatric SCI have focused on QOL and community participation. QOL varies based on a number of factors. Higher QOL is associated with younger age at time of injury, lower level injuries, and fewer symptoms of anxiety and depression in the child and/or the caregiver (Garma, Kelly, Daharsh, & Vogel, 2011). In a study of youth with SCI, the relationship between QOL and community participation was stronger in children (6–12 years of age) than in adolescents (13–18 years of age). In addition, among children, greater participation in activities outside the home setting (e.g., school, community, outside the community) was associated with higher QOL. In contrast, being male, having paraplegia, and participating with a more diverse group of others were related to higher QOL among adolescents (Kelly, Klaas, Garma, Russell, & Vogel, 2012).

Coping style in adolescents with SCI is also associated with QOL and mood. Specifically, in a group of adolescents who sustained an SCI at least 1 year prior, escape-oriented coping (e.g., distraction, social withdrawal, self-criticism, blaming others, wishful thinking) was associated with lower QOL and higher levels of depression and anxiety (Smith et al., 2013). In that same study, cognitive restructuring and resignation were identified as the most used coping strategies; however, social support and emotional regulation (strategies for calming) were perceived by the adolescents as most effective.

Assessment

When assessing psychological functioning of children with SCI, like any other acquired injury, it is essential to consider the timing of the assessment. SCI is typically a sudden, often traumatic event that results in significant changes in physical functioning and independence. As a result, within the first months to year after injury, the child and family are adjusting to injury, including the loss of function, increased need for assistance with basic cares (dressing, bathing), and new medical cares (catheterization, ventilation). During this time, assessment should focus on the child and the family's understanding of injury and prognosis as well as adjustment and coping.

SCI results in long-lasting physical, emotional, and social challenges. Coping with these challenges varies over time based on individual and situational factors. In addition, for children, these stressors also change across development. Psychological assessment should focus on psychological well-being within the context of the individual, situation, and developmental factors. Although anxiety and depression may not be higher than the general population (C. J. Anderson et al., 2009; Klaas et al., 2014), it is important to consider assessment of these areas, especially in older adolescents. In addition, rehabilitation psychologists should consider assessment of coping styles, quality of life, and participation in the community. Common assessment measures for children with SCI are listed in Table 23.3.

Given that SCI alone is not expected to impact cognitive functioning, assessment of cognitive functioning is not typically the focus of the rehabilitation psychologist. That said, children with SCI may have preexisting cognitive difficulties that need to be addressed. In addition, children who sustain a traumatic SCI are at high risk for a co-occurring brain injury. In the National Trauma Data Bank, 39% of children with SCI were also coded for TBI (Piatt, 2015). As such, postinjury neuropsychological evaluation, similar to that described in the TBI section, may be useful to better understand the child's cognitive strengths and weaknesses to support the child's learning needs. More details about assessment and treatment of this unique group are provided in the Dual Diagnosis section.

Intervention

Psychoeducation about injury and cognitive behavior therapy (CBT) to promote adjustment and coping are often employed early after injury. When children with SCI present with psychiatric diagnoses such as depression, anxiety, or posttraumatic stress disorder, psychotropic medications may be considered; however, there is no literature describing use of these medications in children with SCI. In addition, although some promising interventions have been used to treat adults with SCI, there are no evidence-based studies of psychosocial interventions for children with SCI.

In adults, CBT-focused treatments have proven to be beneficial, although results are mixed. Most of these studies have focused on group interventions within the first few months after injury. For example, Craig, Hancock, Dickson, and Chang (1997) examined the efficacy of a 10-week protocol of group therapy targeting a range of topics during inpatient rehabilitation admission. Individuals with

TABLE 23.3

Common Assessment Measures for Children With Spinal Cord Injury

Content areas	Measures	Age range (years)	Informant
Depression	Children's Depression Inventory, Second Edition (Kovacs, 2011)	7–17	Parent Self
Anxiety	Revised Children's Manifest Anxiety Scale, Second Edition (Reynolds & Richmond, 2008)	6–19	Self
Personality	Personality Inventory for Children, Second Edition (Lachar & Gruber, 2002)	5–19	Parent
	Minnesota Multiphasic Personality Inventory—Adolescent (Butcher et al., 1992)	14–18	Self
Coping	Kidcope (Spirito et al., 1988)	7–18	Self
Disability and health	Pediatric Quality of Life Inventory (Varni et al., 1999)	All ages	Parent Self (ages 8 and older)
Participation	Children's Assessment of Participation and Enjoyment (King et al., 2004)	6–21	Self

high levels of depression and anxiety at the start of treatment experienced a reduction in symptoms, and those benefits were maintained at 1 year after injury. Similarly, coping-effectiveness training in a group setting was associated with reductions in anxiety and depression in adults with SCI (Kennedy, Duff, Evans, & Beedie, 2003). Guest and colleagues (2015) explored the effects of CBT in a group setting in addition to routine psychosocial rehabilitation on resiliency. Group therapy did not improve resiliency above and beyond routine individual CBT. In addition, a recent Internet-based CBT intervention for individuals with chronic SCI (sustained at least 6 months prior) was associated with lower anxiety, depression, and stress, as well as higher satisfaction with life (Migliorini, Sinclair, Brown, Tonge, & New, 2016). These improvements in mood were maintained in a small group that was examined 6 months after intervention.

Although evidence for psychological treatments following pediatric SCI is limited, cognitive and behavioral techniques have been found to be efficacious in children with a range of psychiatric and medical conditions, including social anxiety (Scaini, Belotti, Ogliari, & Battaglia, 2016), fibromyalgia (Kashikar-Zuck, King, Ting, & Arnold, 2016), and functional abdominal pain disorders (Rutten, Korterink, Venmans, Benninga, & Tabbers, 2015). In addition, based on the findings of Smith and colleagues (2013), which revealed that escape-oriented coping was associated with lower QOL and higher levels of depression and anxiety, interventions designed to reduce escape-oriented coping strategies and to increase the use of other, more adaptive coping strategies may help decrease distress in adolescents with SCI. This example highlights the use of a theory-based approach to intervention when there is no literature to form a basis for appropriate intervention. To plan an appropriate intervention with children and their families, rehabilitation psychologists should be familiar with both theoretical and evidence-based approaches to planning and implementing recommendations.

Educational Planning

Following SCI, children require educational supports to address motor concerns. Pediatric rehabilitation psychologists should work with families and school systems to ensure that the child's learning and psychosocial needs are met. When serving as a liaison for children with SCI, rehabilitation psychologists need to be familiar with relevant federal law and have an adequate understanding of each child's specific needs as well as disability issues more broadly to work with the school system as an effective advocate. As just stated in the section on educational planning for children with ABI, children with disabilities are entitled to a free and appropriate public education. By understanding the educational system and the child's needs, the pediatric rehabilitation psychologist can serve to promote the child's independence and adjustment upon return to the school system, as well as help prepare the child's school team to promote acceptance and social interactions among staff and other students. Helping the child to feel comfortable returning to school and providing information about the child's disability are particularly important.

Independence in the school system is based on the level of lesion, the accessibility of the school environment, and the environmental supports provided. Before the child is able to learn in school, logistics regarding the child's basic transport and medical needs must be considered. For example, for children with all levels of motor impairment, consider transportation to and from school as well as transportation throughout the school building. In addition, a plan for care needs (e.g., ventilators, catheterization) in the school system will need to be developed.

Independence in learning is particularly important to consider for children with higher lesions who have limited upper extremity movement. These children will need modifications both to access materials (e.g., holding books, turning pages) and to demonstrate what they have learned (e.g., answering questions on tests, completing assignments). For children with significant motor needs, a one-to-one aide may be necessary to allow for optimal accessibility.

DUAL DIAGNOSIS

In adults, the incidence of dual diagnosis (SCI and co-occurring TBI) is estimated to be between 25% and 60%, with mild and moderate TBI the most common (Kushner & Alvarez, 2014). In the pediatric population, there are fewer studies. As mentioned earlier, in the National Trauma Data Bank, 39% of children with SCI were also coded for TBI (Piatt, 2015). Regardless of the age of individuals with SCI, the presence of a severe TBI is usually established in acute care because of alterations in consciousness or obvious findings on neuroimaging. In contrast, the subtle initial symptoms of TBI may be overlooked because of often negative initial CT scans and the life-threatening medical issues associated with SCI being treated in the acute care setting. After the acute medical issues associated with SCI are stabilized, diagnosis remains challenging, as there can be an overlap of symptoms associated with SCI and TBI.

To screen for the presence of TBI, careful review of medical records is necessary to determine the initial level of consciousness, any early changes in mental status, and neuroimaging findings. A caregiver report of the child's mental status in the moments to days following an injury can be helpful, although acute changes in mental status can be difficult to discern if the child required emergent intubation and/or early surgical interventions. Depending on the age of the child and the events surrounding the SCI, it is helpful to obtain an understanding of the child's memory surrounding the event to determine if there was a period of PTA at the time of the SCI. Younger children may not be able to describe their recollection of events or separate their recollection of events from what they have been told by others. If concerns arise based on the screening, a more thorough neuropsychological evaluation may be necessary. Identifying the ongoing impact of TBI is essential when determining appropriate interventions and educational accommodations.

Children with SCI who also have cognitive weaknesses may have greater difficulties learning self-care skills following an injury. Specifically, although older children with age-appropriate executive functioning skills and adequate motor abilities may be able to independently perform many aspects of self-care such as dressing or catheterization for bladder control, those with executive dysfunction due to TBI (or preexisting cognitive problems) will likely have more difficulty learning these challenging self-care tasks. As such, the relationship between cognitive functioning and the level of self-care needs is important to consider. For instance, as described by Tarazi, Mahone, and Zabel (2007), a child with executive dysfunction (e.g., a child with ADHD) may not have any difficulty with day-to-day functioning when demands for self-care are minimal; however, the same child may struggle to learn and consistently perform the more intensive self-care demands (e.g., self-catheterization, bowel program). As a result, if a child with an SCI is having difficulty learning self-care skills, the possibility of a co-occurring TBI or preexisting cognitive difficulties (such as ADHD or learning disability) should be considered. In addition to obtaining relevant details from medical records, the child, and the caregiver about the injury and to completing neuropsychological testing, careful examination of preinjury school records or preinjury educational testing can be very informative when attempting to tease apart the contribution of a coexisting TBI and preexisting learning difficulties. Understanding the etiology of cognitive difficulties is important for treatment planning, especially early after SCI, as cognitive difficulties due to TBI may improve over time, whereas difficulties associated with preexisting conditions are not expected to improve.

CONCLUSION

In sum, brain injuries and SCIs have many similarities in adults and children; however, rehabilitation psychologists working in pediatric settings should be familiar with the unique challenges involved in assessment and intervention with children with acquired disorders. Special consideration should be provided to varying etiologies by age, differences in outcome, developmental concerns, and educational planning.

References

Anderson, C. J., Kelly, E. H., Klaas, S. J., Russell, H., Daharsh, E., & Vogel, L. C. (2009). Anxiety and depression in children and adolescents with spinal cord injuries. *Developmental Medicine & Child Neurology*, *51*, 826–832. http://dx.doi.org/10.1111/j.1469-8749.2009.03268.x

Anderson, V., Jacobs, R., Spencer-Smith, M., Coleman, L., Anderson, P., Williams, J., . . . Leventer, R. (2010).

Does early age at brain insult predict worse outcome? Neuropsychological implications. *Journal of Pediatric Psychology*, *35*, 716–727. http://dx.doi.org/10.1093/jpepsy/jsp100

Austin, C. A., Slomine, B. S., Dematt, E. J., Salorio, C. F., & Suskauer, S. J. (2013). Time to follow commands remains the most useful injury severity variable for predicting WeeFIM® scores 1 year after paediatric TBI. *Brain Injury*, *27*, 1056–1062. http://dx.doi.org/10.3109/02699052.2013.794964

Bayley, N. (2006). *Bayley Scales of Infant and Toddler Development* (3rd ed.). San Antonio, TX: Pearson.

Beery, K., & Beery, N. (2010). *Beery-Buktenica Developmental Test of Visual-Motor Integration* (6th ed.). San Antonio, TX: Pearson.

Benton, A., Sivan, A., Hamsher, K., Varney, N., & Spreen, O. (1994). *Contributions to neuropsychological assessment: A clinical manual* (2nd ed.). New York, NY: Oxford University Press.

Boschen, K., Gargaro, J., Gan, C., Gerber, G., & Brandys, C. (2007). Family interventions after acquired brain injury and other chronic conditions: A critical appraisal of the quality of the evidence. *NeuroRehabilitation*, *22*, 19–41.

Braga, L. W., Da Paz, A. C., & Ylvisaker, M. (2005). Direct clinician-delivered versus indirect family-supported rehabilitation of children with traumatic brain injury: A randomized controlled trial. *Brain Injury*, *19*, 819–831. http://dx.doi.org/10.1080/02699050500110165

Butcher, J., Williams, C., Graham, J., Archer, R. P., Tellegen, A., Ben-Porath, Y. S., & Kaemmer, B. (1992). *Minnesota Multiphasic Personality Inventory for Adolescents*. Minneapolis: University of Minnesota Press.

Butler, R. W., Copeland, D. R., Fairclough, D. L., Mulhern, R. K., Katz, E. R., Kazak, A. E., . . . Sahler, O. J. (2008). A multicenter, randomized clinical trial of a cognitive remediation program for childhood survivors of a pediatric malignancy. *Journal of Consulting and Clinical Psychology*, *76*, 367–378. http://dx.doi.org/10.1037/0022-006X.76.3.367

Carney, J., & Porter, P. (2001). The educational needs of children with traumatic brain injury. In L. Schoembrodt (Ed.), *Children with traumatic brain injury: A parents' guide* (pp. 293–349). Bethesda, MD: Woodbine House.

Cassidy, J. D., Carroll, L. J., Peloso, P. M., Borg, J., von Holst, H., Holm, L., . . . the WHO Collaborating Centre Task Force on Mild Traumatic Brain Injury. (2004). Incidence, risk factors and prevention of mild traumatic brain injury: Results of the WHO Collaborating Centre Task Force on Mild Traumatic Brain Injury. *Journal of Rehabilitation Medicine*, *36*(43, Suppl.), 28–60. http://dx.doi.org/10.1080/16501960410023732

Catroppa, C., Stone, K., Rosema, S., Soo, C., & Anderson, V. (2014). Preliminary efficacy of an attention and memory intervention post-childhood brain injury. *Brain Injury*, *28*, 252–260. http://dx.doi.org/10.3109/02699052.2013.860471

Cicerone, K. D., Langenbahn, D. M., Braden, C., Malec, J. F., Kalmar, K., Fraas, M., . . . Ashman, T. (2011). Evidence-based cognitive rehabilitation: Updated review of the literature from 2003 through 2008. *Archives of Physical Medicine and Rehabilitation*, *92*, 519–530. http://dx.doi.org/10.1016/j.apmr.2010.11.015

Cohen, M. (1997). *Children's memory scale*. San Antonio, TX: The Psychological Corporation.

Cole, W. R., Paulos, S. K., Cole, C. A., & Tankard, C. (2009). A review of family intervention guidelines for pediatric acquired brain injuries. *Developmental Disabilities Research Reviews*, *15*, 159–166. http://dx.doi.org/10.1002/ddrr.58

Conklin, H. M., Ogg, R. J., Ashford, J. M., Scoggins, M. A., Zou, P., Clark, K. N., . . . Zhang, H. (2015). Computerized cognitive training for amelioration of cognitive late effects among childhood cancer survivors: A randomized controlled trial. *Journal of Clinical Oncology*, *33*, 3894–3902. http://dx.doi.org/10.1200/JCO.2015.61.6672

Conners, K. (2008). *Conners* (3rd ed.). North Tonawanda, NY: Multi-Health Systems.

Conners, K. (2015). *Conners' Continuous Performance Test, third edition (Conners CPT 3)*. North Tonawanda, NY: Multi-Health Systems.

Craig, A. R., Hancock, K., Dickson, H., & Chang, E. (1997). Long-term psychological outcomes in spinal cord injured persons: Results of a controlled trial using cognitive behavior therapy. *Archives of Physical Medicine and Rehabilitation*, *78*, 33–38. http://dx.doi.org/10.1016/S0003-9993(97)90006-X

Crowe, L., Babl, F., Anderson, V., & Catroppa, C. (2009). The epidemiology of paediatric head injuries: Data from a referral centre in Victoria, Australia. *Journal of Paediatrics and Child Health*, *45*, 346–350. http://dx.doi.org/10.1111/j.1440-1754.2009.01499.x

Davis, K. C., Slomine, B. S., Salorio, C. F., & Suskauer, S. J. (2016). Time to follow commands and duration of posttraumatic amnesia predict GOS-E peds scores 1 to 2 years after TBI in children requiring inpatient rehabilitation. *The Journal of Head Trauma Rehabilitation*, *31*, E39–E47. http://dx.doi.org/10.1097/HTR.0000000000000159

Delis, D., Kaplan, E., & Kramer, J. (2001). *Delis-Kaplan Executive Functioning System*. San Antonio, TX: Pearson.

Delis, D., Kramer, J., Kaplan, E., & Ober, B. (1994). *California Verbal Learning Test*. San Antonio, TX: Pearson.

Delis, D., Kramer, J., Kaplan, E., & Ober, B. (2017). *California verbal learning test (CVLT-3)*. Bloomington, MN: NCS Pearson.

DeVivo, M. J., & Vogel, L. C. (2004). Epidemiology of spinal cord injury in children and adolescents. *The Journal of Spinal Cord Medicine*, *27*(Suppl. 1), S4–S10. http://dx.doi.org/10.1080/10790268.2004.11753778

Donders, J., & Warschausky, S. (2007). Neurobehavioral outcomes after early versus late childhood traumatic brain injury. *The Journal of Head Trauma Rehabilitation*, *22*, 296–302. http://dx.doi.org/10.1097/01.HTR.0000290974.01872.82

Dunn, L., & Dunn, D. (2007). *Peabody Picture Vocabulary Test* (4th ed.). San Antonio, TX: Pearson.

Ewing-Cobbs, L., Levin, H. S., Fletcher, J. M., Miner, M. E., & Eisenberg, H. M. (1990). The Children's Orientation and Amnesia Test: Relationship to severity of acute head injury and to recovery of memory. *Neurosurgery*, *27*, 683–691. http://dx.doi.org/10.1227/00006123-199011000-00003

Faul, M., Xu, L., Wald, M., & Coronado, V. (2010). *Traumatic brain injury in the United States: Emergency department visits, hospitalizations, and deaths 2002–2006*. Atlanta, GA: Centers for Disease Control and Prevention, National Center for Injury Prevention and Control. http://dx.doi.org/10.15620/cdc.5571

Federal Register. (1973). Rehabilitation Act of 1973, as amended, 29 U.S.C. §794, section 504.

Federal Register. (1990). Americans with Disabilities Act of 1990, Public Law 101–336.

Galbiati, S., Recla, M., Pastore, V., Liscio, M., Bardoni, A., Castelli, E., & Strazzer, S. (2009). Attention remediation following traumatic brain injury in childhood and adolescence. *Neuropsychology*, *23*, 40–49. http://dx.doi.org/10.1037/a0013409

Garma, S. I., Kelly, E. H., Daharsh, E. Z., & Vogel, L. C. (2011). Health-related quality of life after pediatric spinal cord injury. *Journal of Pediatric Psychology*, *36*, 226–236. http://dx.doi.org/10.1093/jpepsy/jsq037

Giacino, J. T., Kalmar, K., & Whyte, J. (2004). The JFK Coma Recovery Scale–Revised: Measurement characteristics and diagnostic utility. *Archives of Physical Medicine and Rehabilitation*, *85*, 2020–2029. http://dx.doi.org/10.1016/j.apmr.2004.02.033

Giacino, J. T., Katz, D. I., & Whyte, J. (2013). Neurorehabilitation in disorders of consciousness. *Seminars in Neurology*, *33*, 142–156. http://dx.doi.org/10.1055/s-0033-1348960

Gioia, G., Isquith, P., Guy, S., & Kenworthy, L. (2015). *Behavior Rating Inventory of Executive Function* (2nd ed.). Lutz, FL: Psychological Assessment Resources.

Gioia, G. A., Espy, K. A., & Isquith, P. K. (2003). *Behavioral Rating Inventory of Executive Function–Preschool Version*. Lutz, FL: Psychological Assessment Resources.

Grados, M. A., Slomine, B. S., Gerring, J. P., Vasa, R., Bryan, N., & Denckla, M. B. (2001). Depth of lesion model in children and adolescents with moderate to severe traumatic brain injury: Use of SPGR MRI to predict severity and outcome. *Journal of Neurology, Neurosurgery, & Psychiatry*, *70*, 350–358. http://dx.doi.org/10.1136/jnnp.70.3.350

Guest, R., Craig, A., Nicholson Perry, K., Tran, Y., Ephraums, C., Hales, A., . . . Middleton, J. (2015). Resilience following spinal cord injury: A prospective controlled study investigating the influence of the provision of group cognitive behavior therapy during inpatient rehabilitation. *Rehabilitation Psychology*, *60*, 311–321. http://dx.doi.org/10.1037/rep0000052

Haley, S., Coster, W., Ludlow, L., Haltiwanger, J., & Andrellos, P. (1992). *Pediatric Evaluation of Disability Inventory*. San Antonio, TX: Pearson.

Harrison, P., & Oakland, T. (2015). *Adaptive Behavior Assessment System* (3rd ed.). San Antonio, TX: Pearson.

Johnson, A. R., DeMatt, E., & Salorio, C. F. (2009). Predictors of outcome following acquired brain injury in children. *Developmental Disabilities Research Reviews*, *15*, 124–132. http://dx.doi.org/10.1002/ddrr.63

Kaplan, E., Goodglass, H., & Weintraub, S. (2001). *Boston Naming Test* (2nd ed.). Austin, TX: Pro-Ed.

Kashikar-Zuck, S., King, C., Ting, T. V., & Arnold, L. M. (2016). Juvenile fibromyalgia: Different from the adult chronic pain syndrome? *Current Rheumatology Reports*, *18*, 19. http://dx.doi.org/10.1007/s11926-016-0569-9

Keenan, H. T., & Bratton, S. L. (2006). Epidemiology and outcomes of pediatric traumatic brain injury. *Developmental Neuroscience*, *28*, 256–263. http://dx.doi.org/10.1159/000094152

Kelly, E. H., Klaas, S. J., Garma, S., Russell, H. F., & Vogel, L. C. (2012). Participation and quality of life among youth with spinal cord injury. *Journal of Pediatric Rehabilitation Medicine*, *5*, 315–325.

Kennedy, P., Duff, J., Evans, M., & Beedie, A. (2003). Coping effectiveness training reduces depression and anxiety following traumatic spinal cord injuries. *British Journal of Clinical Psychology*, *42*(Pt. 1), 41–52. http://dx.doi.org/10.1348/014466503762842002

King, G., Law, M., King, S., Hurley, P., Rosenbaum, P., Hanna, S., . . . Young, N. (2004). *Children's Assessment of Participation and Enjoyment (CAPE) and preferences for activities in children*. San Antonio, TX: PsychCorp.

Kinsella, G., Ong, B., Murtagh, D., Prior, M., & Sawyer, M. (1999). The role of the family for behavioral outcome in children and adolescents following traumatic brain injury. *Journal of Consulting and Clinical Psychology*, *67*, 116–123. http://dx.doi.org/10.1037/0022-006X.67.1.116

Klaas, S. J., Kelly, E. H., Anderson, C. J., & Vogel, L. C. (2014). Depression and anxiety in adolescents with pediatric-onset spinal cord injury. *Topics in Spinal Cord Injury Rehabilitation*, *20*, 13–22. http://dx.doi.org/10.1310/sci2001-13

Korkman, M., Kirk, U., & Kemp, S. L. (2007). *NEPSY II. Administrative manual*. San Antonio, TX: Psychological Corporation.

Kovacs, M. (2011). *Children's Depression Inventory* (2nd ed.). North Tonawanda, NY: Multi-Health Systems.

Kushner, D. S., & Alvarez, G. (2014). Dual diagnosis: Traumatic brain injury with spinal cord injury. *Physical Medicine and Rehabilitation Clinics of North America*, *25*, 681–696, ix–x. http://dx.doi.org/10.1016/j.pmr.2014.04.005

Lachar, D., & Gruber, C. P. (2002). *Personality Assessment Inventory for Children* (2nd ed.). North Tonawanda, NY: Multi-Health Systems.

Manly, T., Anderson, V., Crawford, J., George, M., & Robertson, I. H. (2016). *Test of Everyday Attention for Children, second edition*. San Antonio, TX: Pearson.

Max, J. E., Lindgren, S. D., Knutson, C., Pearson, C. S., Ihrig, D., & Welborn, A. (1997). Child and adolescent traumatic brain injury: Psychiatric findings from a paediatric outpatient specialty clinic. *Brain Injury*, *11*, 699–711. http://dx.doi.org/10.1080/026990597123070

McCarthy, M. L., MacKenzie, E. J., Durbin, D. R., Aitken, M. E., Jaffe, K. M., Paidas, C. N., . . . the Children's Health After Trauma Study Group. (2006). Health-related quality of life during the first year after traumatic brain injury. *Archives of Pediatrics & Adolescent Medicine*, *160*, 252–260. http://dx.doi.org/10.1001/archpedi.160.3.252

McKinlay, A., Kyonka, E. G., Grace, R. C., Horwood, L. J., Fergusson, D. M., & MacFarlane, M. R. (2010). An investigation of the pre-injury risk factors associated with children who experience traumatic brain injury. *Injury Prevention*, *16*, 31–35. http://dx.doi.org/10.1136/ip.2009.022483

Migliorini, C., Sinclair, A., Brown, D., Tonge, B., & New, P. (2016). A randomised control trial of an Internet-based cognitive behaviour treatment for mood disorder in adults with chronic spinal cord injury. *Spinal Cord*, *54*, 695–701. http://dx.doi.org/10.1038/sc.2015.221

Morrison, A. B., & Chein, J. M. (2011). Does working memory training work? The promise and challenges of enhancing cognition by training working memory. *Psychonomic Bulletin & Review*, *18*, 46–60. http://dx.doi.org/10.3758/s13423-010-0034-0

Msall, M. E., DiGaudio, K., Rogers, B. T., LaForest, S., Catanzaro, N. L., Campbell, J., . . . Duffy, L. C. (1994). The Functional Independence Measure for Children (WeeFIM). Conceptual basis and pilot use in children with developmental disabilities. *Clinical Pediatrics*, *33*, 421–430. http://dx.doi.org/10.1177/000992289403300708

Mullen, E. (1995). *Mullen Scales of Early Learning: AGS edition*. Circle Pines, MN: American Guidance Service.

National Spinal Cord Injury Statistical Center. (2004, June). *2004 annual statistical report*. University of Alabama at Birmingham, Birmingham, AL.

Ommaya, A. K., & Gennarelli, T. A. (1974). Cerebral concussion and traumatic unconsciousness. Correlation of experimental and clinical observations of blunt head injuries. *Brain: A Journal of Neurology*, *97*, 633–654. http://dx.doi.org/10.1093/brain/97.1.633

Parent, S., Mac-Thiong, J. M., Roy-Beaudry, M., Sosa, J. F., & Labelle, H. (2011). Spinal cord injury in the pediatric population: A systematic review of the literature. *Journal of Neurotrauma*, *28*, 1515–1524. http://dx.doi.org/10.1089/neu.2009.1153

Piatt, J. H., Jr. (2015). Pediatric spinal injury in the US: Epidemiology and disparities. *Journal of Neurosurgery. Pediatrics*, *16*, 463–471. http://dx.doi.org/10.3171/2015.2.PEDS1515

Quayle, K. S., Powell, E. C., Mahajan, P., Hoyle, J. D., Jr., Nadel, F. M., Badawy, M. K., . . . Kuppermann, N. (2014). Epidemiology of blunt head trauma in children in U.S. emergency departments. *The New England Journal of Medicine*, *371*, 1945–1947. http://dx.doi.org/10.1056/NEJMc1407902

Raj, S. P., Antonini, T. N., Oberjohn, K. S., Cassedy, A., Makoroff, K. L., & Wade, S. L. (2015). Web-based parenting skills program for pediatric traumatic brain injury reduces psychological distress among lower-income parents. *The Journal of Head Trauma Rehabilitation*, *30*, 347–356. http://dx.doi.org/10.1097/HTR.0000000000000052

Randolph, C. (2012). *Repeatable Battery for the Assessment of Neuropsychological Status update*. San Antonio, TX: Pearson.

Rappaport, M., Dougherty, A. M., & Kelting, D. L. (1992). Evaluation of coma and vegetative states. *Archives of Physical Medicine and Rehabilitation*, *73*, 628–634.

Reynolds, C., & Kamphaus, R. (2015). *Behavior Assessment System for Children* (3rd ed.). San Antonio, TX: Pearson.

Reynolds, C., & Richmond, B. (2008). *Revised Children's Manifest Anxiety Scale* (2nd ed.). North Tonawanda, NY: Multi-Health Systems.

Roberts, G., Quach, J., Spencer-Smith, M., Anderson, P. J., Gathercole, S., Gold, L., . . . Wake, M. (2016). Academic outcomes 2 years after working memory training for children with low working memory: A randomized clinical trial. *JAMA Pediatrics*, *170*, e154568. http://dx.doi.org/10.1001/jamapediatrics.2015.4568

Robertson, I. H., Ward, T., Ridgeway, V., & Nimmo-Smith, I. (1994). *Test of Everyday Attention*. San Antonio, TX: Pearson.

Roth, R., Isquith, P., & Gioia, G. (2005). *Behavior Rating Inventory of Executive Function–Adult version*. Lutz, FL: Psychological Assessment Resources.

Rutten, J. M., Korterink, J. J., Venmans, L. M., Benninga, M. A., & Tabbers, M. M. (2015). Nonpharmacologic treatment of functional abdominal pain disorders: A systematic review. *Pediatrics*, *135*, 522–535. http://dx.doi.org/10.1542/peds.2014-2123

Scaini, S., Belotti, R., Ogliari, A., & Battaglia, M. (2016). A comprehensive meta-analysis of cognitive-behavioral interventions for social anxiety disorder in children and adolescents. *Journal of Anxiety Disorders*, *42*, 105–112. http://dx.doi.org/10.1016/j.janxdis.2016.05.008

Sheslow, D., & Adams, W. (2003). *Wide range assessment of memory and learning* (2nd ed.). Lutz, FL: Psychological Assessment Resources.

Shipstead, Z., Redick, T. S., & Engle, R. W. (2012). Is working memory training effective? *Psychological Bulletin*, *138*, 628–654. http://dx.doi.org/10.1037/a0027473

Slifer, K. J., & Amari, A. (2009). Behavior management for children and adolescents with acquired brain injury. *Developmental Disabilities Research Reviews*, *15*, 144–151. http://dx.doi.org/10.1002/ddrr.60

Slomine, B., Eikenberg, J., Salorio, C., Suskauer, S., Trovato, M., & Christensen, J. (2008). Preliminary evaluation of the Cognitive and Linguistic Scale: A measure to assess recovery in inpatient rehabilitation following pediatric brain injury. *The Journal of Head Trauma Rehabilitation*, *23*, 286–293. http://dx.doi.org/10.1097/01.HTR.0000336841.53338.2f

Slomine, B., & Locascio, G. (2009). Cognitive rehabilitation for children with acquired brain injury. *Developmental Disabilities Research Reviews*, *15*, 133–143. http://dx.doi.org/10.1002/ddrr.56

Slomine, B. S., Grasmick, P. H., Suskauer, S. J., & Salorio, C. F. (2016). Psychometric properties of the Cognitive and Linguistic Scale: A follow-up study. *Rehabilitation Psychology*, *61*, 328–335. http://dx.doi.org/10.1037/rep0000096

Smith, T. F., Russell, H. F., Kelly, E. H., Mulcahey, M. J., Betz, R. R., & Vogel, L. C. (2013). Examination and measurement of coping among adolescents with spinal cord injury. *Spinal Cord*, *51*, 710–714. http://dx.doi.org/10.1038/sc.2013.65

Sparrow, S., Cicchetti, D., & Saulnier, C. (2016). *Vineland Adaptive Behaviors Scales* (3rd ed.). San Antonio, TX: Pearson.

Spirito, A., Stark, L. J., & Williams, C. (1988). Development of a brief coping checklist for use with pediatric populations. *Journal of Pediatric Psychology*, *13*, 555–574. http://dx.doi.org/10.1093/jpepsy/13.4.555

Suskauer, S. J., Slomine, B. S., Inscore, A. B., Lewelt, A. J., Kirk, J. W., & Salorio, C. F. (2009). Injury severity variables as predictors of WeeFIM scores in pediatric TBI: Time to follow commands is best. *Journal of Pediatric Rehabilitation Medicine*, *2*, 297–307.

Suskauer, S. J., & Trovato, M. K. (2013). Update on pharmaceutical intervention for disorders of consciousness and agitation after traumatic brain injury in children. *PM & R*, *5*, 142–147. http://dx.doi.org/10.1016/j.pmrj.2012.08.021

Tarazi, R., Mahone, E., & Zabel, T. (2007). Self-care independence in children with neurological disorders: An interactional model of adaptive demands and executive dysfunction. *Rehabilitation Psychology*, *52*, 196–205. http://dx.doi.org/10.1037/0090-5550.52.2.196

Taylor, H. G., & Alden, J. (1997). Age-related differences in outcomes following childhood brain insults: An introduction and overview. *Journal of the International Neuropsychological Society*, *3*, 555–567.

Taylor, H. G., Yeates, K. O., Wade, S. L., Drotar, D., Klein, S. K., & Stancin, T. (1999). Influences on first-year recovery from traumatic brain injury in children. *Neuropsychology*, *13*, 76–89. http://dx.doi.org/10.1037/0894-4105.13.1.76

Taylor, H. G., Yeates, K. O., Wade, S. L., Drotar, D., Stancin, T., & Minich, N. (2002). A prospective study of short- and long-term outcomes after traumatic brain injury in children: Behavior and achievement. *Neuropsychology*, *16*, 15–27. http://dx.doi.org/10.1037/0894-4105.16.1.15

Teasdale, G., & Jennett, B. (1974). Assessment of coma and impaired consciousness. A practical scale. *The Lancet*, *2*, 81–84. http://dx.doi.org/10.1016/S0140-6736(74)91639-0

Thurman, D. J. (2016). The epidemiology of traumatic brain injury in children and youths: A review of research since 1990. *Journal of Child Neurology*, *31*, 20–27. http://dx.doi.org/10.1177/0883073814544363

Tiffin, J. (1968). *Purdue pegboard examiners manual*. Rosemont, IL: London House.

Trites, R. (1977). *Neuropsychological test manual*. Ontario, Canada: Royal Ottawa Hospital.

Van't Hooft, I., Andersson, K., Bergman, B., Sejersen, T., Von Wendt, L., & Bartfai, A. (2005). Beneficial effect from a cognitive training programme on children with acquired brain injuries demonstrated in a controlled study. *Brain Injury*, *19*, 511–518. http://dx.doi.org/10.1080/02699050400025224

Varni, J. W., Seid, M., & Rode, C. A. (1999). The PedsQL™: Measurement model for the pediatric quality of life inventory. *Medical Care*, *37*, 126–139. http://dx.doi.org/10.1097/00005650-199902000-00003

Wade, S., Walz, N., Carey, J., & Williams, K. (2008). Preliminary efficacy of a web-based family problem solving treatment program for adolescents with traumatic brain injury. *Journal of Head Trauma Rehabilitation*, 23, 369–377.

Wade, S. L., Kurowski, B. G., Kirkwood, M. W., Zhang, N., Cassedy, A., Brown, T. M., . . . Taylor, H. G. (2015). Online problem-solving therapy after traumatic brain injury: A randomized controlled trial. *Pediatrics*, *135*, e487–e495. http://dx.doi.org/10.1542/peds.2014-1386

Wade, S. L., Walz, N. C., Carey, J., Williams, K. M., Cass, J., Herren, L., . . . Yeates, K. O. (2010). A randomized trial of teen online problem solving for improving executive function deficits following pediatric traumatic brain injury. *The Journal of Head Trauma Rehabilitation*, *25*, 409–415. http://dx.doi.org/10.1097/HTR.0b013e3181fb900d

Wechsler, D. (2009). *Wechsler Adult Intelligence Scale* (3rd ed.). San Antonio, TX: Pearson.

Wechsler, D. (2011). *Wechsler Abbreviated Scale of Intelligence* (2nd ed.). San Antonio, TX: Pearson.

Wechsler, D. (2014). *Wechsler Intelligence Scale for Children* (5th ed.). San Antonio, TX: Pearson.

Yeates, K. O., Swift, E., Taylor, H. G., Wade, S. L., Drotar, D., Stancin, T., & Minich, N. (2004). Short- and long-term social outcomes following pediatric traumatic brain injury. *Journal of the International Neuropsychological Society*, *10*, 412–426. http://dx.doi.org/10.1017/S1355617704103093

Ylvisaker, M., Szekeres, S., & Haarbauer-Krupa, J. (1998). Cognitive rehabilitation: Organization, memory, and language. In M. Ylvisaker (Ed.), *Traumatic brain injury rehabilitation: Children and adolescents* (Rev. ed., pp. 181–220). Boston, MA: Butterworth-Heinemann.

Part III

TOPICS IN PRACTICE AND PUBLIC HEALTH

CHAPTER 24

HEALTH POLICY IMPLICATIONS FOR REHABILITATION PSYCHOLOGY

Kristofer J. Hagglund and Robert G. Frank

Health care in the United States is a complex, ever-changing, and enigmatic system that accounts for nearly 20% of the nation's gross domestic product. In many respects, it is unparalleled. The health care system provides some of the most sophisticated patient care available in the world, produces life-extending and life-enhancing research and technology, and has highly regarded education and training systems. In other respects, this system does not provide care to all who need it and is inefficient, extremely costly, and inconsistent in quality. To its critics, the U.S. health care system is not a system at all but a highly politicized aggregation of providers, insurers, payers, government officials, lobbyists, and other stakeholders who have a common mission but different agendas. Both views are defensible, which makes studying and working in U.S. health care interesting and rewarding, if also confounding and frustrating.

Rehabilitation psychology is modestly represented in the U.S. health care system. Its aggregated expenditures for clinical services and research barely register in the accounting of health care costs. Research in the field of rehabilitation psychology, although clinically applicable and valuable, is not a major focus of federal research spending. The discipline, however, changes lives for the better, advancing the health, well-being, and participation of those with chronic illnesses and disabling conditions. With this societal benefit as leverage, rehabilitation psychology has the opportunity to become a more engaged and active participant in health policy development. A foundational element of successful policy engagement is understanding the underlying structure and mechanics of this confusing system.

Being familiar with the history of the U.S. health care system and its major components is essential to an informed deliberation of the proposals to change it. Eliminating, altering, or replacing any major program of the health care system will affect thousands or millions of people and is likely to have both intended and unintended consequences. Nearly every new Congress and presidential administration has proposed a major change to the health care system during the past 50 years. A few of these succeeded. For example, the Children's Health Insurance Program (CHIP; Social Security Act, 1997) was signed into law by President Bill Clinton, expanding health care access to low-income children. President George Bush signed into law the Medicare Prescription Drug, Improvement, and Modernization Act of 2003, thereby expanding prescription drugs for seniors and others eligible for Medicare.

President Barack Obama, with the help of a Democrat-controlled Congress, signed the Patient Protection and Affordable Care Act (ACA) into law in 2010, beginning an overhaul of the U.S. health care system. Since the passage of the ACA, there have been more than 50 attempts to repeal most or all of it. To date, none of these repeal attempts have

http://dx.doi.org/10.1037/0000129-025
Handbook of Rehabilitation Psychology, Third Edition, L. A. Brenner, S. A. Reid-Arndt, T. R. Elliott, R. G. Frank, and B. Caplan (Editors-in-Chief)

succeeded. This does not mean that the ACA will remain intact indefinitely. In fact, like almost all comprehensive federal laws, there are many components that could be improved with subsequent legislation. Rehabilitation psychologists will benefit from remaining informed and monitoring the legislative proposals.

This chapter provides an overview of the structure and the function of the health care system. It provides a summary of the ACA and major health care programs. Health system legislation is reviewed, along with the potential effects on access to insurance and health care, quality of care, and health care costs. The chapter also focuses on the health care system's components most related to rehabilitation psychology and its stakeholders (e.g., patients, students).

PATIENT PROTECTION AND AFFORDABLE CARE ACT

On March 23, 2010, President Barack Obama signed the ACA into law. This law is arguably the most significant domestic policy legislation since 1965. At that time, President Lyndon Johnson signed into law the Medicare and Medicaid Acts, the social insurance programs that were part of his larger Great Society initiative. The ACA made significant changes to insurance regulation, established health insurance exchanges and encouraged state Medicaid expansion. In addition, the ACA created pilot programs to improve quality and experiment with different payment mechanisms and initiated modest initiatives in wellness and public health. The ACA was implemented incrementally, and its most significant effect was to reduce the number of uninsured Americans, thereby increasing access to health care. Indeed, 20 million Americans gained insurance with the implementation of the ACA. According to the National Health Insurance Survey, the number of uninsured declined from 16.0% (48 million individuals) in 2010 to 9.1% (28.4 million) in 2016 (Graves & Nikpay, 2017). Arguably, the ACA also slowed the rate of rising health care costs, although the great recession also had a suppressive effect on health care spending.

The ACA is a massive law that influenced nearly every component of the health care system. The key features of the law that affected individuals with chronic illnesses or disabilities included a ban on denial of insurance for persons with preexisting conditions, a ban on annual and lifetime benefit limits, and subsidized public exchanges. The law also called for automatic nationwide expansion of Medicaid with higher income allowances—138% of the federal poverty limit (FPL)—making health care insurance and care more accessible to those with chronic conditions and disabilities who previously exceeded income or asset limits. The U.S. Supreme Court later overturned that component of the law, stating essentially that states were not obligated to expand their Medicaid programs (Liptak, 2012).

Much of the rhetoric during and after the 2016 national elections concerned the repeal of the ACA. Repeal of a law as complicated as the ACA is not a simple task, as was seen during the 115th Congress. Even before the 115th Congress, many aspects of the ACA had come under fire from the legislation's opponents. In particular, the ACA's tax penalty on individuals who fail to buy insurance as required by the individual mandate and the tax penalties on large employers who do not offer coverage to their employees have been criticized by political conservatives as having limited effectiveness (Pear, 2017). The individual mandate and the large-employer mandate were included in the ACA to force younger, healthier individuals to obtain coverage to improve the risk pool for insurers and to ensure that individuals do not enroll for insurance only when they become sick (called *moral hazard* by economists). In December 2017, the Congress passed and President Trump signed the Tax Cuts and Jobs Act of 2017. Although primarily a tax bill, the Tax Cuts and Jobs Act eliminated the individual mandate in the ACA effective 2019.

Separate from the Medicaid expansion, refundable health insurance premium tax credits were made available to individuals and families whose income was between 100% and 400% of poverty. To obtain these credits, the individual or family must purchase coverage through a state or federal exchange and then receive credit on their federal tax form. Additional cost-sharing subsidies for people with low incomes from 100% to 250% of the FPL were made possible through lower deductibles and copays. The exchanges offered four plans named for metals. The premium plan—a platinum plan—costs the most and covers 90% of health costs. The least expensive plan—the bronze plan—covers 60% of health costs. To qualify for cost-sharing subsidies for low-income individuals (100%–250% FPL), individuals had to purchase the silver plan—referring to the third richest insurance plan of four (Cox, Claxton, & Levitt, 2017). In addition, ACA banned "red-lining" for previous health conditions, the practice of denying coverage for services related to a prior or existing illness or disability. The ACA also allowed children to enroll in their parents' health plan until the age of 26. Both changes proved popular with consumers while ensuring a fairer health market.

Both the ACA and many health reform bills rely on refundable tax credits to help enrollees obtain health insurance. Understanding the nature of refundable tax credits and tax deductions can be critical to estimating the benefit of legislation. Tax credits are the amount a taxpayer can reduce his or her federal income tax. An advanceable tax is made available when the premium payment is due. That is, the taxpayer can be forwarded the anticipated credit when the insurance premium is due rather than wait for the tax return to be completed. Tax credits reduce the amount of income tax charged. Advanceable tax credits have the added advantage of increasing access to insurance by providing a financial resource when it is needed.

FEDERAL AND STATE SOCIAL HEALTH INSURANCE PROGRAMS

One of the most striking features of the structure of the health system is the nearly equal involvement of both the public sector and the private sector. This kind of dual arrangement is unique among the nations in the Organisation for Economic Co-operation and Development (OECD),[1] which tend to have health systems that are dominated by the public sector. In the U.S. health care system, the public sector is best known for Medicare and Medicaid.

Medicare is the federal social insurance program for individuals 65 years of age and older, persons with disabilities, and persons with end-stage renal disease. It was signed into law in 1965 and has generally received broad bipartisan support. The two original programs of Medicare, known as Part A and Part B, cover hospital care and related services and physician services, respectively. Part D, the Medicare Prescription Drug Program, was added in 2003 with the passage of the Medicare Prescription Drug, Improvement, and Modernization Act. The ACA enhanced much of Medicare, including closing the "donut hole" in Part D, the portion of the Medicare prescription drug plan where the Medicare beneficiary was 100% responsible for the medication costs (The Washington Post, 2010). Part C, also known as Medicare Advantage, is a program whereby insurance companies construct health care plans from Parts A, B, and D and market these inclusive plans to Medicare-eligible beneficiaries. The insurance companies receive funding from Medicare taxes and, most often, premiums.

For Part A ("Hospital Insurance"), eligible beneficiaries are automatically "opted in," resulting in nearly all-eligible individuals participating in this component of Medicare. The rates of enrollment for the other parts of Medicare are also very high. In total, 55 million Americans have Medicare (Henry J. Kaiser Family Foundation, 2016b), including 9 million individuals with disabilities (The Boards of Trustees of the Federal Hospital Insurance and Federal Supplemental Medical Insurance Trust Funds, 2016). Medicare is funded by a specific payroll tax on both wage earners and their employers, by premiums, and by modest cost sharing. With both the baby boom generation reaching retirement and health care cost inflation, Medicare is not collecting revenues at the same rates as its expenditures. The Medicare Trustees report of 2016 stated that Part A of Medicare is financially solvent through 2028; after that, without changes, the collected and current revenue will fail to meet its costs (The Boards of Trustees of the Federal Hospital

[1]The OECD (2018) is an organization of 35 advanced and emerging nations with the mission to "promote policies that will improve the economic and social well-being of people around the world" (para. 1). It uses data and expert analyses to provide governments with strong policy recommendations to facilitate progress toward accomplishing its mission. The cross-nation data are useful for comparing and contrasting the nations' various infrastructure programs and policies.

Insurance and Federal Supplemental Medical Insurance Trust Funds, 2016). Medicare is considered a mandatory program by statute, meaning that its funding is mostly not subject to the annual appropriations process in Congress. Medicare will benefit financially from any policy or programming that "bends the cost curve" downward, such as allowing Medicare, as an entity, to negotiate with pharmaceutical companies for lower prescription drug prices. If nothing is done, Medicare will eventually require restructuring to reduce benefits, limit eligibility, reduce payments to providers, and increase cost sharing or taxes.

Psychologists are eligible providers for Medicare and may receive payment for both inpatient and outpatient services, including services delivered via telehealth (American Psychological Association, 2017a). Medicare, like many other payers, is moving toward value-based payments that include performance metrics for providers that will determine enhanced payments or penalties. The metrics will address quality of care, as outlined in the Merit-Based Incentive Payment System (MIPS; American Psychological Association, 2017a).

The MIPS program was authorized under the Medicare Access and CHIP Reauthorization Act of 2015 (MACRA), which encourages physicians and others to participate in alternative payment models that incentivize cost control, quality, and efficiency (Hussey, Liu, & White, 2017). It is likely that the MACRA-authorized reimbursement systems will slow provider and hospital spending, but long-term effects are still being studied (Hussey et al., 2017). Rehabilitation psychologists could play an important role in slowing Medicare spending while maintaining high-quality care for individuals with disabilities as part of the programs authorized by MACRA, including accountable care organizations or health care quality demonstrations. In general, psychologists participating in Medicare and with other public and private payers will want to stay informed about these payment system changes.

Medicaid is a shared federal–state social insurance program for nearly 69 million individuals with low incomes, including pregnant women, children and their parents, the elderly, and those with disabilities (U.S. Government Accountability Office, 2017). Upwards of 10 million individuals are dually enrolled in Medicare and Medicaid (Henry J. Kaiser Family Foundation, 2016b). For these low-income individuals, Medicaid helps pay Medicare premiums and cost-sharing charges. Means testing is the principal method to determine Medicaid eligibility, but there are other categorical criteria. For example, the Medicaid Home and Community Based Services program provides long-term care services for many children and adults with intellectual, developmental, and physical disabilities and/or mental/emotional disorders (Elliott et al., 2011). Home and Community Based Services can be a huge support to individuals with disability, but each state must apply to the Centers for Medicare and Medicaid Services for a waiver (a variation from the prescribed Medicaid program) to implement the program. In most states, working-age adults without disabilities or dependents do not qualify for Medicaid regardless of their income, leaving millions of low-income individuals without consistent access to health care.

States manage their own Medicaid programs within broad federal guidelines, including establishing income criteria for eligibility and determining the optional services to be provided (e.g., prescriptions and psychological services). Medicaid is funded by federal and state taxes. Federal funding is provided by a complicated matching formula mostly tied to per capita income in each state, such that the states with the lowest per capita income receive more federal support than states with higher per capita income. With the ACA, states had the option of expanding their Medicaid programs to cover more people and receive nearly full funding from the federal government for a defined period. As of 2018, 34 states plus the District of Columbia expanded their Medicaid programs.

The CHIP is similar to Medicaid and is focused on children. Whereas Medicare is under federal control, states and territories manage their own Medicaid and CHIP programs within broad parameters set by the federal government. Rehabilitation psychologists' participation in Medicaid and CHIP programs is more limited than with Medicare, depending upon the state's Medicaid plan.

Other well-known government health programs include the Veterans Health Care Program and related health care programs (e.g., TRICARE, CHAMPVA). Other shared programs include the programs of the Health Resources and Services Administration, such as the Community Health Centers and the National Health Service Corps; the Centers for Disease Control and Prevention; and the public health system (services focusing on the health of the population, such as monitoring disease and health status in communities).

PRIVATE SECTOR HEALTH PROGRAMS

Insurance companies, hospitals and clinics, psychologists, physicians, and other providers; pharmaceutical companies; medical device manufacturers; and a myriad of associated producers and services represent the private sector. Nearly all of the private sector is involved with the public health care sector, not the least because the private sector often depends on government programs and has to abide by state and federal policies and laws. There is often overlap in the two sectors. The individuals and institutions in both public and private sectors, arguably, have a common mission to improve and protect the health of the people of the nation.

The public and private sectors often have different agendas, however, producing innovation and creating tension. For example, most new life-saving and life-extending technologies, devices, and pharmaceuticals are the product of research and development in universities and private industry. Relative to the rest of the world, the United States has produced a substantial amount of the new technology, making it one of the best places to receive sophisticated care and treatment for the most serious and complicated diseases. Because the technology and pharmaceuticals are produced in the private, free-market sector, they are often quite expensive when first released for use under patent protection, thereby limiting their access to many people who do not have insurance that covers these therapeutic entities. Many people in the United States do not have reasonable access to basic care and treatment, due to the conflicting agendas of the public and private sector. The tension among the public and private health care sectors often impedes efficient delivery of health care (Berwick, Nolan, & Whittington, 2008).

Arguably the best way to understand the U.S. health care system's function is to consider Don Berwick and colleagues' (2008) "Triple Aim" approach, the goals of which are "improving the experience of care; improving the health of populations; and reducing per capita costs of care for populations" (p. 760). The perfect health system for the United States would strive for universal access to high-quality care provided in a cost-effective manner. Of course, these are aspirational goals and are far from the current state of the system. Much of the health policy debate centers on the push and pull of these three aims.

CONTROLLING HEALTH CARE SYSTEM COSTS

Health care spending in the United States has grown relentlessly for decades, typically outpacing the rates of growth in gross domestic product (GDP) and workers' wages. Health care expenditures surpassed $3.2 trillion in 2015 and reached 17.8% of GDP (Martin, Hartman, Washington, Catlin, & National Health Expenditure Accounts Team, 2016). This growth is a weighty topic because health spending adds to the annual deficit and impinges on spending in other important areas, such as wages, education, transportation, and other infrastructure needs. At the same time, even with the substantial reduction in the uninsured with the ACA, there are millions of people in the United States who even now do not receive needed care or high-quality care because of a lack of insurance and the prohibitive costs of services (Henry J. Kaiser Family Foundation, 2016a).

Individuals with disabilities often present complex health care problems requiring more frequent primary care and specialist visits and long-term support services. Because of the complexity and breadth of services needed, individuals with disabilities account for a larger percentage of health care spending than their proportion of the population. In the Medicaid program, for example, 14% of the recipients have disabilities, and they account for 40% of the spending in Medicaid (Centers for Medicare and Medicaid Services, n.d.). Health policy experts have frequently called for evaluating different models of care and payment to moderate spending for persons with disabilities and the elderly. The challenge is to subtract inefficient or wasteful spending while maintaining high-quality care and promoting health and participation.

The importance of "wraparound" services, such as accessible transportation or delivered meals, as a means of preventing more costly expenditures is becoming increasingly recognized. Yet the integration of these services into conventional health care systems is far from universal. Similarly, the delivery of services in alternative formats is becoming more widely used and appreciated. For example, telehealth for providing individual or family therapy and similar "talking" interventions has demonstrated effectiveness (McCord, Saenz, Armstrong, & Elliott, 2015) and is becoming more widely reimbursed.

Long-term projections indicate that the prevalence of disabling conditions will increase with the aging U.S. population even while disability rates are holding steady among the working-age population and the elderly (Kaye, 2013). Although disability rates are not generally increasing, Kaye (2013) reported that the elderly with cognitive impairments are likely to continue living in the community. If this trend holds, innovative home-based or telehealth/telemonitoring programs may be necessary to meet the needs of this population. Kaye also reported a large increase in mental health–related disabilities among the working-age population. Programs to help individuals maintain independence and employment could have a large effect on health, participation, and cost outcomes for this population. Overall, however, the increased prevalence of disability among baby boomers will create further demand for services and higher health and long-term support costs (Kaye, 2013).

As rehabilitation psychologists know, patient outcomes can be improved and inefficient health spending reduced with coordinated, team-based care. The team model continues to be appreciated and applied in rehabilitation settings (Butt & Caplan, 2010). In most other health care settings, there remains uncoordinated care that is exacerbated by a segmentation of mental and physical health providers, health organizations, and the larger health care system.

For example, insurance for mental/behavioral health is still often a "carve out" from medical and surgical benefits, even if the benefits have to be uniform, as prescribed by the Mental Health Parity and Addiction Equity Act of 2008 and related laws (Centers for Medicare and Medicaid Services, n.d.). Reimbursements to providers for mental and behavioral health services are low relative to other medical/surgical services. In addition, there is inconsistent mental health coverage across state Medicaid programs (American Psychological Association, 2017b), even though Medicaid is a critical source for care for those with mental health conditions (Henry J. Kaiser Family Foundation, 2017). Absent or inadequate mental health care is linked to poorer health outcomes and greater use of medical/surgical services (Clarke et al., 2016). The solution to the vicious cycle of limited state budgets resulting in the inadequate provision of mental health services, causing poorer health outcomes and higher health care and social program use, has mostly eluded state and federal policymakers. Continued advocacy and research documenting the value of integrated care is essential if this social problem is to be remedied.

Existing examples of effective interdisciplinary care document improved outcomes and reduced unnecessary costs. For example, Clarke and colleagues established and evaluated a program that they called Behavioral Health Associates in the UCLA accountable care organization (ACO). By embedding psychologists and other mental health providers in the primary care setting, patients had a substantive reduction in emergency department use (Clarke et al., 2016).

IMPROVING ACCESS TO HEALTH CARE

Providing Americans with access to health care has been a challenge for decades and the primary reason for current and historical calls to overhaul the U.S. health care system. Substantial research has demonstrated that people without health insurance have higher rates of preventable morbidity and mortality. For persons with disabilities, who often have a "thinner margin of health" (Dejong et al., 2002, p. 267), lack of access to appropriate care can quickly become devastating. Unfortunately, from 1995 to 2007 the number of people without health insurance hovered at about 16% of the population (Henry J. Kaiser Family Foundation, 2016a). The ACA successfully reversed this trend. At the end of 2015, the number of uninsured nonelderly Americans stood at 28.5 million, a decrease of nearly 13 million since 2013 (Henry J. Kaiser Family Foundation, 2016a). The ACA's components that caused this reduction included the following:

- Allowing young adults to remain on their parents' health insurance plan until 26 years of age. Approximately 2.9 million young adults gained insurance through this mechanism, dramatically reducing their uninsured rate (Porterfield & Huang, 2016).
- Highly subsidizing expansion of state Medicaid programs. Thirty-four states and the District of Columbia expanded eligibility to 138% of the FPL.
- Federal and state-based health insurance marketplaces (exchanges) for individuals and families to purchase health insurance that included subsidies for the purchase costs based on incomes of up to 400% of the FPL. The exchanges are available, in general, to individuals who do not have existing employer-based insurance and who do not qualify for another federal program (e.g., Medicaid). The marketplaces offer (mostly) private health insurance products.
- The elimination of denial of insurance based on preexisting conditions.
- Not allowing premium costs to be based on health history or previous health care use (Goodell, 2016).

Even with the ACA, substantive population disparities in access to health insurance and health care persist. The populations that have poor access and/or experience less-than-adequate care include racial and ethnic minority groups, those who live in rural areas, and adults with low incomes (Purnell et al., 2016). Persons with disabilities have also had historical difficulty accessing high-quality care. Hanson, Neuman, Dutwin, and Kasper (2003) used a national telephone survey of nonelderly adults with disabilities and found that individuals with disabilities have lower incomes, higher unemployment, and poorer health. Because of these disadvantages, they are more likely to have ADL limitations and higher health care use and to experience cost barriers to receiving needed care. Persons with disabilities without insurance were found to be at a particular disadvantage in obtaining appropriate care. They frequently delayed or went without needed care, even primary care by providers that were sensitive to the particular needs of persons with disabilities (Hanson et al., 2003).

Young adults with disabilities are at risk because they are likely to lose insurance when transitioning to adulthood (Krahn, Walker, & Correa-De-Araujo, 2015; Porterfield & Huang, 2016). Young adults with disabilities may be on their parents' policies or in a CHIP program and lose coverage if they are unable to work and gain employer-based care or qualify for Medicaid. It is typical that the qualifying definition of a work-limiting disability for Medicaid as an adult is more restrictive than definitions of disabilities for children (Krahn et al., 2015). Previous research has shown that Medicaid provides adequate, but uneven, access to health care services most needed by individuals with disabilities (Beatty et al., 2003).

QUALITY

Rehabilitation psychology has long known that integrated, interdisciplinary, patient-centered care provides the best outcomes for patients, including increased participation in desired roles (Butt & Caplan, 2010). This type of care is most commonly used in inpatient rehabilitation settings; it is less common in outpatient settings, although model programs have been established throughout the nation. Certainly, the historical fee-for-service payment systems have impeded the development of high-quality integrated care. Under fee-for-service models, providers are rewarded for piecemeal work. Little attention is given to more inclusive definitions of health or well-being and to long-term outcomes. The decade-long emphasis on implementing value-based payment systems is beginning to shift the focus of providers to more holistic care models because they are being held accountable for outcomes (Szanton, Leff, Wolff, Roberts, & Gitlin, 2016).

Rehabilitation psychology uses an interdisciplinary practice approach—important to ACOs and other types of integrated care entities that are striving to improve health and lower costs. ACOs and demonstration projects focused on integrated care are beginning to understand the need to address issues that are outside of the clinic and hospital walls. For example, Szanton and colleagues (2016) described a structured, home-based program for elderly persons with limitations in performing basic activities of daily living (ADLs), such as dressing, eating, and bathing. The program involves structured interventions delivered by an occupational therapist, a nurse, and a handyman. Participants experienced meaningful improvement in ADL performance, Instrumental ADLs (more advanced ADLs, such cleaning, managing money), performance, and depressive symptoms. Their homes were also made safer (Szanton et al., 2016).

LOOKING TO THE FUTURE

Future legal and policy-driven changes to health care delivery and financing will largely, but not wholly, influence who gets access to care, how good that care will be, and how much it will cost. The question of who pays the additional costs, however, remains unaddressed. Beyond the forces of Congress and the state houses are other influences driven by consumers, providers, insurers, and other stakeholders. Rehabilitation psychologists may be active participants in shaping these forces because of their long history of working on interdisciplinary teams with complex clients for the purposes of promoting health, well-being, and participation. Looking forward, rehabilitation psychologists will be able to contribute to the discussion and effective policy and health care model development. For example, the patient-centered care approach, a long-standing staple of rehabilitation, is increasingly involving patient-reported outcomes. Patient-reported outcome measures may even become part of the value-based payments (Lavallee et al., 2016).

Cost pressures will modify the landscape of our health care system in the future. The aging of the American and global population will impact health care systems. Since 2015, there have been more people older than 65 than children age 5 and younger (World Health Organization, 2011). The use of health services increases with age, and older people have higher health expenses per capita. The aging of the population does not promise an increase in disabilities but does indicate differences in chronic conditions (World Health Organization, 2011). Aged Americans have more disability and chronic health conditions than their European peers (World Health Organization, 2011). In addition, the American propensity to readily adopt new technologies for health care interventions will continue as a major cost driver. Taken together, these trends suggest significant health policy debates over health care costs and priorities.

Demographic changes and ever-increasing cost pressures in health care are overlaid upon fundamental changes in a society driven by machine intelligence. The rapid adoption of advanced machines to perform many routine activities will impact health care and health policy. These advances may bring efficiencies to health care that were not possible previously because of a reliance upon expensive labor. These changes will also modify rehabilitation as smart machines are integrated into the human body and robots provide routine care activities (Frank, 2017). (Refer to Chapters 30 and 31 and the Afterword, this handbook, for additional discussion of future changes in care secondary to technological advances.)

The ACA, through multiple mechanisms, pushed our health care system to a greater emphasis on prevention with requirements to monitor the health status of the population, not just an individual. Regardless of modifications in the ACA, it is likely there will continue to be an emphasis on population health with incentives paid to providers according to contractual benchmarks. This trend will enhance pressures toward truly integrated primary and specialty care.

CHANGING THE SYSTEM

Addressing the problems in the American health care system has been a frequent topic of discussion for the U.S. Congress. Despite numerous discussions and proposals for change, few major pieces of legislation have altered the current system. Presidents Truman, Johnson, Nixon, Clinton, Bush,

Obama, and Trump have all proposed significant legislation to modify health care, but only Johnson and Obama have succeeded in shepherding major change (though one could argue that President Bush sponsored significant legislation by the addition of prescription drugs to Medicare in 2003).

Oliver, Lee, and Lipton (2004) discussed the conditions necessary to pass legislation to improve the health care system. They noted John Kingdon (1995) proposed that issues rise to the top of the policy agenda when two conditions are met:

> First, an abrupt shift in how a problem is perceived or in who controls the levers of governmental power opens a "window of opportunity" for policy innovation. Second, three relatively independent "streams" in the policy process—problems, policies, and politics—must converge. If advocates are able to couple their preferred policy alternative with the prevailing definition of the problem and the priorities of political leaders, organized interests, and public opinion, then the resulting alternative is likely to rise on the policy agenda and may lead to significant action within a short period of time. (Oliver et al., 2004, p. 310)

The convergence of Kingdon's "problems, policies, and politics" means that the opportunity to pass legislation is quite challenging and requires constant effort on behalf of advocates. Successful advocacy requires highly educated proponents of legislation who appreciate the importance of these different vectors merging to create a moment where change is possible. Too often, advocacy is viewed a one-time visit to a member of Congress. Effective advocacy requires constant effort and awareness of opportunity and the process of legislation. Not only is it necessary to understand the nuances of the proposed issue but it is important to understand how legislation is created by Congress. Although there have been a few significant pieces of legislation that have radically changed the American health care system, most changes occur through incremental legislation.

Ashkanazi, Hagglund, Lee, Swaine, and Frank (2010) cited Lynn Etheredge's (2007) observation that changes in national health policy required sustained development across several election cycles. Kingdon (1995) said, "Creative activity usually involves the recombination of old elements more than fresh invention of new ones" (p. 124). Opportunity as an advocate can rest upon the ability to incorporate proposed legislation into the reworking of historic proposals or ideas.

Many advocates for health reform focus on federal issues and opportunities, which is understandable given the size of federal health expenditures and the consequences of psychologists being omitted from critical legislation. However, the importance of engagement in healthy policy at the state level should not be ignored. Over the past 20 years, psychologists have enjoyed significant progress in state legislatures that have advanced the profession. Psychologists with appropriate training have the ability to prescribe medications in five states. Other key advances are enhanced practice rights and insurance reform. State psychological associations drive state health reform, and they often do so in collaboration with other professional organizations. Participating in the state association is vital to the future of psychology practice.

CONCLUSION

Federal health policy is as complex as its impact on the federal budget is huge. Because so much money is affected by changes in health policy, the process is complicated by the involvement of many stakeholders who have divergent interests. Psychology, and specifically rehabilitation psychology, is a tiny part of the health policy dialog. Accordingly, psychologists must be sensitive to the opportunity to work within coalitions that serve our agenda. One of the biggest drivers in health care is the aging of the American population. With aging, the prevalence of disabling conditions increases creating the need for rehabilitation psychology services. The growing number of older Americans increases the frequency and impact of costly chronic diseases such heart disease, diabetes, cancer, dementing conditions, obesity, and arthritis. These conditions pull for more intensive medical interventions and technological evaluations. Psychology treatments tend to be lost in this process. Psychologists offer many services that are critical to preventing or slowing the advancement of chronic conditions. Under the ACA, ACOs will be responsible for the overall health of the population, which is advantageous to psychology services, if they are appreciated. It is vital to support the advancement of psychological interventions through careful evaluation of the effectiveness of treatments. Of importance, actions that increase access to health care, improve quality, and decrease costs are generally compatible with the inclusion of psychology services.

References

American Psychological Association. (2017a). *Complete guide to Medicare for psychologists*. Retrieved from https://www.apaservices.org/practice/medicare

American Psychological Association. (2017b). *Medicaid and psychology*. Retrieved from http://www.apa.org/helpcenter/medicaid.aspx

Ashkanazi, G. S., Hagglund, K. J., Lee, A., Swaine, Z., & Frank, R. G. (2010). Health policy 101: Fundamental issues in health care reform. In R. G. Frank, M. Rosenthal, & B. Caplan (Eds.), *Handbook of rehabilitation psychology* (2nd ed., pp. 439–449). Washington, DC: American Psychological Association. http://dx.doi.org/10.1037/15972-031

Beatty, P. W., Hagglund, K. J., Neri, M. T., Dhont, K. R., Clark, M. J., & Hilton, S. A. (2003). Access to health care services among people with chronic or disabling conditions: Patterns and predictors. *Archives of Physical Medicine and Rehabilitation*, *84*, 1417–1425. http://dx.doi.org/10.1016/S0003-9993(03)00268-5

Berwick, D. M., Nolan, T. W., & Whittington, J. (2008). The triple aim: Care, health, and cost. *Health Affairs*, *27*, 759–769. http://dx.doi.org/10.1377/hlthaff.27.3.759

The Boards of Trustees of the Federal Hospital Insurance and Federal Supplemental Medical Insurance Trust Funds. (2016, June 22). *The 2016 annual report of the Boards of Trustees of the Federal Hospital Insurance and Federal Supplemental Medical Insurance Trust Funds*. Retrieved from https://www.cms.gov/Research-Statistics-Data-and-Systems/Statistics-Trends-and-Reports/ReportsTrustFunds/Downloads/TR2016.pdf

Butt, L., & Caplan, B. (2010). The rehabilitation team. In R. G. Frank, M. Rosenthal, & B. Caplan (Eds.), *Handbook of rehabilitation psychology* (2nd ed., pp. 451–457). Washington, DC: American Psychological Association. http://dx.doi.org/10.1037/15972-032

Centers for Medicare and Medicaid Services. (n.d.). *July 2018 Medicaid and CHIP enrollment data highlights*. Retrieved from https://wayback.archive-it.org/2651/20181001140224/https://www.medicaid.gov/medicaid/program-information/medicaid-and-chip-enrollment-data/report-highlights/index.html

Clarke, R. M., Jeffrey, J., Grossman, M., Strouse, T., Gitlin, M., & Skootsky, S. A. (2016). Delivering on accountable care: Lessons from a behavioral health program to improve access and outcomes. *Health Affairs*, *35*, 1487–1493. http://dx.doi.org/10.1377/hlthaff.2015.1263

Cox, C., Claxton, G., & Levitt, L. (2017, March 10). *How Affordable Care Act repeal and replace plans might shift health insurance tax credits*. Retrieved from https://www.kff.org/health-reform/issue-brief/how-affordable-care-act-repeal-and-replace-plans-might-shift-health-insurance-tax-credits/

Dejong, G., Palsbo, S. E., Beatty, P. W., Jones, G. C., Knoll, T., & Neri, M. T. (2002). The organization and financing of health services for persons with disabilities. *The Milbank Quarterly*, *80*, 261–301. http://dx.doi.org/10.1111/1468-0009.t01-1-00004

Elliott, T. R., Phillips, C. D., Patnaik, A., Naiser, E., Booth, E. A., Fournier, C. J., . . . Dyer, J. A. (2011). Medicaid Personal Care Services and caregivers' reports of children's health: The dynamics of a relationship. *Health Services Research*, *46*(6, Pt. 1), 1803–1821. http://dx.doi.org/10.1111/j.1475-6773.2011.01284.x

Etheredge, L. M. (2007). Technologies of health policy. *Health Affairs*, *26*, 1537–1538. http://dx.doi.org/10.1377/hlthaff.26.6.1537

Frank, R. G. (2017). Hither and thither: How do we innovate? *Rehabilitation Psychology*, *62*, 1–6. http://dx.doi.org/10.1037/rep0000114

Goodell, S. (2016). Uninsurance rates and the Affordable Care Act: What does recent research show about the changes in uninsurance rates since 2010? *Health Policy Brief*. Retrieved from https://www.healthaffairs.org/healthpolicybriefs/brief.php?brief_id8157

Graves, J. A., & Nikpay, S. S. (2017). The changing dynamics of US health insurance and implications for the future of the Affordable Care Act. *Health Affairs*, *36*, 297–305. http://dx.doi.org/10.1377/hlthaff.2016.1165

Hanson, K. W., Neuman, P., Dutwin, D., & Kasper, J. D. (2003). Uncovering the health challenges facing people with disabilities: The role of health insurance. *Health Affairs, Suppl. Web Exclusives*, W3-552–65.

Henry J. Kaiser Family Foundation. (2016a). *Key facts about the uninsured population*. Retrieved from https://www.kff.org/uninsured/fact-sheet/key-facts-about-the-uninsured-population/

Henry J. Kaiser Family Foundation. (2016b). *An overview of Medicare*. Retrieved from https://www.kff.org/medicare/issue-brief/an-overview-of-medicare/

Henry J. Kaiser Family Foundation. (2017, May). *Medicaid's role in behavioral health*. Retrieved from https://www.kff.org/infographic/medicaids-role-in-behavioral-health/

Hussey, P. S., Liu, J. L., & White, C. (2017). The Medicare Access and CHIP Reauthorization Act: Effects on Medicare payment policy and spending. *Health Affairs, 36*, 697–705. http://dx.doi.org/10.1377/hlthaff.2016.0559

Kaye, H. S. (2013). Disability rates for working-age adults and for the elderly have stabilized, but trends for each mean different results for costs. *Health Affairs, 32*, 127–134. http://dx.doi.org/10.1377/hlthaff.2012.0533

Kingdon, J. W. (1995). *Agendas, alternatives, and public policies* (2nd ed.). Boston, MA: Addison-Wesley Educational.

Krahn, G. L., Walker, D. K., & Correa-De-Araujo, R. (2015). Persons with disabilities as an unrecognized health disparity population. *American Journal of Public Health, 105*(Suppl. 2), S198–S206. http://dx.doi.org/10.2105/AJPH.2014.302182

Lavallee, D. C., Chenok, K. E., Love, R. M., Petersen, C., Holve, E., Segal, C. D., & Franklin, P. D. (2016). Incorporating patient-reported outcomes into health care to engage patients and enhance care. *Health Affairs, 35*, 575–582. http://dx.doi.org/10.1377/hlthaff.2015.1362

Liptak, A. (2012, June 28). Supreme Court upholds health care law, 5–4, in victory for Obama. *The New York Times*. Retrieved from https://www.nytimes.com/2012/06/29/us/supreme-court-lets-health-law-largely-stand.html

Martin, A. B., Hartman, M., Washington, B., Catlin, A., & National Health Expenditure Accounts Team. (2016). National health spending: Faster growth in 2015 as coverage expands and utilization increases. *Health Affairs, 36*, 166–176. http://dx.doi.org/10.1377/hlthaff.2016.1330

McCord, C. E., Saenz, J. J., Armstrong, T. W., & Elliott, T. R. (2015). Training the next generation of counseling psychologists in the practice of telepsychology. *Counselling Psychology Quarterly, 28*, 324–344. http://dx.doi.org/10.1080/09515070.2015.1053433

Medicare Access and CHIP Reauthorization Act of 2015, Pub. L. No. 114-10, 129 Stat. 87 (2015).

Medicare Prescription Drug, Improvement, and Modernization Act of 2003, Pub. L. No. 108-173, 117 Stat. 2066 (2003).

Mental Health Parity and Addiction Equity Act of 2008, Pub. L. No. 110-343, 122 Stat. 3765 (2010).

Oliver, T. R., Lee, P. R., & Lipton, H. L. (2004). A political history of Medicare and prescription drug coverage. *The Milbank Quarterly, 82*, 283–354. http://dx.doi.org/10.1111/j.0887-378X.2004.00311.x

Organisation for Economic Co-operation and Development. (2018). *About the OECD*. Retrieved from http://www.oecd.org/about/

Patient Protection and Affordable Care Act of 2010, Pub. L. No. 111-148, 124 Stat. 119 (2010).

Pear, R. (2017, January 4). Republicans' 4-step plan to repeal the affordable care act. *The New York Times*. Retrieved from https://www.nytimes.com/2017/01/04/us/affordable-care-act-congress-repeal-plan.html

Porterfield, S. L., & Huang, J. (2016). Affordable care act provision had similar, positive impacts for young adults with and without disabilities. *Health Affairs, 35*, 873–879. http://dx.doi.org/10.1377/hlthaff.2015.1262

Purnell, T. S., Calhoun, E. A., Golden, S. H., Halladay, J. R., Krok-Schoen, J. L., Appelhans, B. M., & Cooper, L. A. (2016). Achieving health equity: Closing the gaps in health care disparities, interventions, and research. *Health Affairs, 35*, 1410–1415. http://dx.doi.org/10.1377/hlthaff.2016.0158

Social Security Act, Title XXI, 42 U.S.C. 7, §§1397aa–1397mm (1997).

Szanton, S. L., Leff, B., Wolff, J. L., Roberts, L., & Gitlin, L. N. (2016). Home-based care program reduces disability and promotes aging in place. *Health Affairs, 35*, 1558–1563. http://dx.doi.org/10.1377/hlthaff.2016.0140

Tax Cuts and Jobs Act of 2017, Pub. L. No. 115-97, 131 Stat. 2054 (2017).

U.S. Government Accountability Office. (2017, June). *Federal low-income programs: Eligibility and benefits differ for selected programs due to complex and varied rules* (Report to the Chairman, Committee on the Budget, U.S. Senate). Retrieved from http://www.gao.gov/assets/690/685641.pdf

The Washington Post. (2010). *Landmark: The inside story of America's new health-care law—The Affordable Care Act—and what it means for us all*. New York, NY: Perseus.

World Health Organization. (2011, October). *Global health and aging* (NIH Publication No. 11-7737). Washington, DC: U.S. Department of Health and Human Services.

Chapter 25

DISABILITY-RELATED GLOBAL HEALTH NEEDS

Jacob Bentley, Malcolm MacLachlan, Priscille Geiser, Hasheem Mannan, and Haibin Zou

The World Report on Disability (World Health Organization [WHO] & World Bank, 2011) has major implications for rehabilitation psychology (MacLachlan & Mannan, 2014). The report noted a paradigm shift away from the "medical" model and toward a social and rights-based approach. It also provided a summary of evidence to suggest that disability is highly prevalent and is increasing, is extremely diverse, and disproportionately affects vulnerable populations and poor people. Moreover, the report has highlighted that people with disabilities face widespread barriers to accessing services and have worse health and socioeconomic outcomes than the general population. Findings associated with disability occur globally; however, the nature and extent of disability may differ across contexts. Disability varies in relation to contextual factors, but several patterns of influential social factors that determine their occurrence are similar (see Chapter 26, this volume).

Recognition of social and contextual factors influencing functional status and outcomes is one of the distinguishing features of global health. Indian psychologists Awasthi, Yadava, and Pandey (2016) recognized that disability is a global health concern. They argued that "the prevalence of disability, rehabilitation awareness, education, accessibility and availability of rehabilitation services are the greatest challenge for the development of society as well as the country" (p. 196). Although context is integral to understanding disability, this chapter focuses on common factors relevant to disability and its intersection with global health.

According to the global health movement, disorder and disability are seen as being similarly patterned with distinct local settings and living conditions that influence how such disabilities are experienced and expressed (MacLachlan, 2006). The idea of the "right to health" (i.e., the right to access health care appropriate to one's needs) is consistent with another hallmark of the global health movement: a focus on social justice. As the social determinants of health are broadly distributed, this approach also sees a broad range of stakeholders as having a legitimate stake in global health (Commission on Social Determinants of Health, 2008; Koplan et al., 2009).

The Commission on Social Determinants of Health (2008) has stated that a society should be judged by "how fairly health is distributed across the social spectrum" and how it protects people from disadvantage. The commission has recommended three broad action areas to achieve these goals: (a) improving the conditions of daily life—the circumstances under which people are born, grow, live, work, and age; (b) tackling the inequitable distribution of power, money, and resources; and (c) increasing resources to allow better measurement of the problem and evaluation of actions taken. Although psychology has certainly made important contributions to rehabilitation and global health, it often has done

http://dx.doi.org/10.1037/0000129-026
Handbook of Rehabilitation Psychology, Third Edition, L. A. Brenner, S. A. Reid-Arndt, T. R. Elliott, R. G. Frank, and B. Caplan (Editors-in-Chief)

so disease by disease and problem by problem rather than in a systemic manner that reflects the patterning of health determinants.

This chapter focuses on themes that challenge and provide opportunities for rehabilitation psychology at a global level rather than on contextual or cultural factors specific to any individual environment. We first consider a variety of global health stakeholder perspectives relevant to disability in low- and middle-income countries (LMICs), where approximately 80% of individuals with disabilities around the world reside (WHO & World Bank, 2011). We then focus on the theoretical implications of a global health perspective for rehabilitation psychology. We also explore different but related micro-, meso- and macrolevels at which a "globally minded" rehabilitation psychologist can work. We conclude the chapter by illustrating contributions that rehabilitation psychologists could make to address challenges in resource-limited environments.

GLOBAL HEALTH STAKEHOLDER PERSPECTIVES

A Civil Society Perspective: Inclusion of Persons With Disabilities

Global health needs and priorities often are identified in confined expert discussions among health professionals, researchers, or public health specialists. Although these opinions are essential to identify and analyze trends, global health, by nature, concerns everyone; therefore, the perspective of people themselves, especially groups that are most at risk of discrimination, should not be overlooked. In general, people's participation in health has seen much progress in past decades, from user-centered to community-based approaches. These approaches have played a major role in ensuring that services are tailored to users' needs and are informed by insightful methods of listening, and that users' voices are at the center of health care services from planning to delivery. Unfortunately, however, such service approaches are not yet a reality for many people with disabilities, especially in low-income regions (Geiser & Boersma, 2013). In addition, seeing disability as a medical issue and/or difference in an individual's capacities as a deficit has disempowered the participation of persons with disabilities in society (see Chapter 9, this volume). Such basic assumptions of the medical model continue to persist in rehabilitative care efforts, a perspective that civil society and especially disabled people's organizations have opposed for many years. This opposition perhaps has its clearest expression in the Convention on the Rights of Persons with Disabilities, which has asserted that disability is fundamentally a human rights issue. This is not to deny that people with certain types of impairments may have enhanced needs for health services (Boot, Dinsmore, Khasnabis, & MacLachlan, 2017) but, rather, that many people with disabilities do not, and that disability is not fundamentally defined by a health problem (MacLachlan & Mannan, 2013). The experience that people with disabilities have with health services may be a useful probe for exploring the overall accessibility and equity of health care provision in a society (MacLachlan, Mannan, & McAuliffe, 2011a; see Chapter 12, this volume).

People with intellectual and psychosocial disabilities are particularly at risk of being discriminated against in health due to stigma and denial of the capacity to decide for themselves (Flynn, 2011), which sometimes results in forced treatment (Boot et al., 2017). In contrast, lack of access to relevant and necessary services among people with disabilities can be observed in data that have demonstrated that, compared with the general population, people with disabilities are twice as likely to find health care providers' skills and facilities inadequate, 3 times more likely to be denied health care, and 4 times more likely to report being be treated badly in the health care system (WHO, 2013).

Despite global commitments from the health-for-all objective of the Alma-Ata Declaration of 1978 (WHO, 1978) to more recent aspirations for universal health coverage, the health sector often remains unconcerned with disability. The Alma-Ata Declaration, for example, represented the first international statement recognizing primary health care as a basic human right. Based on 10 core premises, the declaration has been adopted by all WHO member states. However, more than 40 years later, much progress is needed to realize such benefits for the majority of persons with disability globally. Indeed, rehabilitation in the context of an overall poorly delivered health service is naturally problematic. Broader change therefore is needed using a rights-based approach and closely linking with disabled people's organizations to channel the voices of persons with disabilities in health.

Through civil society consultations (e.g., inclusion of formative input from persons with disabilities) that have contributed to shape the sustainable development goals (SDGs; see the United Nations' [UN; 2015] resolution "Transforming Our World: The 2030 Agenda for Sustainable Development" [2030 Agenda]; see also UN, 2016), the disability community has advocated for accessible, affordable, adaptable, quality, and accountable health services that promote meaningful lives. With a renewed pledge to leave no one behind, including in health, the SDGs provide a new path toward greater equity in health. Four features of the 2030 Agenda offer hope for greater success and opportunities for rehabilitation psychology to make a meaningful and strong contribution: (a) a deliberate focus on fighting inequalities, (b) broader ownership, (c) human rights underpinning the agenda, and (d) an interconnected vision of social, environmental, and economic dimensions of health. Equally, these opportunities may challenge and indeed change professional disciplines that are molded in conventional Western-style health assumptions (e.g., primary focus on the individual instead of the communal) and systems (e.g., access to a hospital-based continuum of rehabilitative care rather than community-based care provision). Professions such as rehabilitation psychology may need to reflect on if and how they will change their positioning, their role, the type of work they do, and fundamentally their relationship with people with disabilities (including power dynamics or differentials).

The realization of the preceding four aspirations in low-income contexts often will depend on working through service provision and targeted lobbying that has been developed by civil society over many decades. Therefore, there is great need for rehabilitation psychology as a profession to develop not only relevant clinical skills but also alternative models of service provision (e.g., through community-based rehabilitation workers; see further discussion later in this chapter), and to become activists in lobbying for the resources and policy change to help people with disabilities live full and productive lives.

A United Nations Perspective: Poverty and Employment Equity

The International Labour Organization (ILO) is the UN body that is responsible for promoting "decent work." Despite the significant contribution of psychology as a discipline to work/industrial/organizational issues, including those related to poverty reduction (Carr & Sloan, 2003; MacLachlan, Carr, & McAuliffe, 2010), rehabilitation psychology perhaps has not fully grasped the opportunities that work presents for rehabilitation and well-being, or indeed the idea that it is a right to be advocated for. Consistent with the overarching mission and vision of rehabilitation psychology, the specialty should continue to seek to address the need for inclusive employment for several reasons described in the following paragraphs (ILO, Gender, Equality and Diversity Branch, 2015).

The first reason is that people with disabilities are at a higher risk of poverty than the population at large, and a vicious reinforcing negative cycle exists between poverty and disability. Responsible factors include lack of access to education, skills development, and decent, productive employment. Job-seekers and entrepreneurs with disabilities are at a disadvantage in their search for decent, productive work, as reflected in the lower employment rates, higher unemployment rates, and significantly lower labor force participation rates (B. Murray, 2013).

Second, once in employment, people with disabilities may continue to face discrimination. A number of factors affect the employability of people with disabilities (Vornholt, Uitdewilligen, & Nijhuis, 2013), and they often are in part-time, low-paid work with poor career prospects, or they work in poor-quality subsistence jobs in the informal economy. It is evident that people with certain types of disabilities face greater difficulties than others in their search for jobs, and women with disabilities are less likely to have a decent job than either nondisabled women or men with disabilities; special attention therefore needs to be given to developing viable career paths for women with disabilities (Lindstrom, Doren, Post,

& Lombardi, 2013). The intersectionality of disability and diversity (Yoshida, Hanass-Hancock, Nixon, & Bond, 2014) is a challenge that rehabilitation psychology has not fully grasped, but with its combination of clinical, organizational, and social psychology techniques, it is in a good position to do so.

Third, it is likely that segregation from inclusive employment is discriminatory and damaging to the longer term self-development of people with disabilities. As a result of their marginal status, many persons with disabilities may become discouraged, have low self-confidence, and be unwilling to take risks that could gain them employment. They may prefer to stay in more familiar and protected environments, avoiding negative experiences of stereotype and living with many constraints that they experience as a result (Silverman & Cohen, 2014).

There are clear examples of continuing labor challenges to be observed in the international community. China, for example, has an estimated 85 million persons with disabilities. Less than a quarter of them (about 22 million) are employed; of that number, 40% of are women and 60% are men. However, only one third of those individuals are in inclusive employment (i.e., employed in the same sort of jobs that nondisabled people do), whereas the remainder are in some form of sheltered employment or self-entrepreneurship (Wang, Chen, Guo, Pang, & Zheng, 2016). Even though, for instance, China has a quota-levy system requiring companies to employ a proportion of people with disabilities, companies often seek to avoid doing so and/or are lacking in the appropriate human resources knowledge to facilitate the employment of people with disabilities. To address that situation, the ILO over the past 10 years has promoted initiatives to support inclusive employment and initiatives to tackle the discrimination faced by people with disabilities in China. Funded by Irish Aid, this work has supported the China Disabled Persons' Federation to improve the legal and policy environment for the employment of persons with disabilities (Sanchez, 2015). The ILO also has sought to establish a business and disability network to propel knowledge sharing through collaboration with Disabled People's Organizations and the use of peer-to-peer support in working contexts. These initiatives have meant that more persons with disabilities have found and stayed in work than previously was the case (ILO, 2015).

There is a clear need for rehabilitation psychology to reach out beyond the clinic setting into the community, and beyond that into the employment, education, and justice settings, which present new and exciting opportunities for rehabilitation psychology in a wide range of high-, middle-, and low-income contexts. Fundamentally, therefore, rehabilitation psychology needs to orientate itself toward a greater cross-section of working and to engage with the intersectionality of impairment and empowerment.

A Measurement Perspective

To better understand the relationship between disability and poverty, valid and reliable metrics are needed. The UN (2015) resolution 70/1 entitled "Transforming Our World: The 2030 Agenda for Sustainable Development" represents one attempt at better understanding poverty–disability relationships as one of a host of focus areas. The resolution established an interagency expert group on SDG indicators, and, during a recent annual meeting, the final list of 229 proposed indicators was been presented to the United Nations Statistical Commission for their consideration; for example, Goal 16 seeks to "promote peaceful and inclusive societies for sustainable development, provide access to justice for all and build effective, accountable and inclusive institutions at all levels" (UN, 2018, p. 18). Within that goal, one of the specified targets (i.e., 16.7) is to ensure responsive, inclusive, participatory, and representative decision making at all levels. As a result, reducing discrepancies in the proportions of positions (i.e., by sex, age, persons with disabilities, and population groups) in public institutions (i.e., national and local legislatures, public service, and judiciary) compared with national distributions is among the subordinate indicators of progress toward the overarching goal (i.e., 16.7.1). Based on these proposed indicators, the Sustainable Development Solutions Network (2016), a global initiative of the UN, created a preliminary SDG Index and Dashboard using only indicators with significant country coverage, technically sound methodologies, and frequent updates. A final list of indicators was agreed on by the Statistical Commission in 2016 and then adopted by the Economic and Social Council and the General Assembly ("Global Indicator Framework," n.d.). Furthermore, the Statistical Commission created the High-Level Group for Partnership, Coordination and Capacity-Building for Statistics for the 2030 Agenda for Sustainable Development with the aim of establishing a global partnership for sustainable development data.

The High-Level Group comprises member states, including regional and international agencies, as observers and reports annually to the Statistical Commission. In terms of useful measurement for health-related indicators C. J. L. Murray (2015) recommended the *Global Burden of Disease* (note that the terminology of *burden* regretfully is negative and deficit focused), a big data approach highlighting the need for "pluralistic data synthesis and analysis" that is inclusive of national statistical authorities and nongovernmental organizations. Although Murray's commentary noted that not all indicators can be met by the Global Burden of Disease indices and some require 'considerable work to develop and refine data systems and analytics,' he did not provide full details of how and what these data systems and analytics may constitute.

The indicator framework seeks to create an evidence-informed environment for achievement of the SDGs; the environment should be one familiar for rehabilitation research and practice. It may offer rehabilitation psychology the opportunity to broaden its scope by aligning indicators across diverse sectors—health, education, employment, justice—with the effects of targeted programs. In this way, rehabilitation psychologists may be able to assess, for instance, their contribution to employment, justice, or partnership-building with civil society and government because all of these have indicators associated with them. Momentum for this sort of work also will be gathered by rehabilitation psychology to develop a deliberate focus on the implementation of relevant health and rehabilitation articles of the Convention on the Rights of Persons with Disabilities.

We have reviewed a number of different perspectives that challenge and provide opportunities to rehabilitation psychology within the realm of global health. To address these perspectives, we also contend that we need to think of rehabilitation psychology operating in a number of different ways and at different levels.

A REHABILITATION PSYCHOLOGY THEORY PERSPECTIVE

Theory and conceptual modeling contributions are two of rehabilitation psychology's greatest assets that can be exported for use in disability-focused global health initiatives. The influence of basic rehabilitation psychology tenets and foundational principles can be readily identified (Bentley, Bruyère, LeBlanc, & MacLachlan, 2016) in the WHO's widely adopted International Classification of Functioning, Disability and Health (ICF; WHO, 2001). However, it is incumbent on the discipline to extend the influential work of founders such as Beatrice Wright and Tamera Dembo to current challenges encountered by persons with disabilities worldwide. Indeed, "thinking globally" brings into focus several opportunities for continued evolution of psychological theory and its practical application to disability-related dilemmas facing the international community. Current considerations for rehabilitation psychology include ongoing needs for (a) integration of psychological theory with other disciplines; (b) reconceptualization of environmental factors, particularly those salient to LMIC settings; and (c) optimization of service delivery strategies focused on increasing uptake among particularly vulnerable populations.

Maintaining awareness of and connection to global health initiatives provide the specialty with an ever-evolving road map for how to contribute. The *World Report on Disability* (WHO & World Bank, 2011) and international summits, such as the Bamako Call for Action on Research for Health (WHO, 2008), for example, highlight the need for an interdisciplinary coordination of efforts in the international community. The Bamako Call, for example, brought together constituents from the ministries of 53 countries who concluded that "the nature of research and innovation for health improvement . . . is not sufficiently inter-disciplinary and inter-sectoral" (WHO, 2008). Being rooted in an interdisciplinary philosophy has numerous implications for the field of rehabilitation psychology. One clear implication resides in the need for the ongoing development of integrated, interdisciplinary theory that can be translated into targeted services for persons with disabilities in low-resource settings.

Integrating Rehabilitation Psychology and Global Health From a Systems Perspective

If rehabilitation psychology is to contribute meaningfully to global rehabilitation challenges, then it must simultaneously meet the aforementioned needs at different levels and do so in an interconnected manner. To illustrate, we draw on some of our own previous research in this regard. Exhibit 25.1 outlines features of what can be termed *micro-*, *meso-*, and *macroperspectives* within psychology. Each level of rehabilitation psychology—micro, meso, and macro—interact and may use overlapping approaches and techniques. It is important to recognize that each level can achieve different benefits for people with disabilities, and each is a legitimate outlet for the skills and enthusiasm of rehabilitation psychologists.

EXHIBIT 25.1

Features of Micro-, Meso-, and Macroperspectives Within Rehabilitation Psychology

Micropsychology perspective **Within and about the individual**
Genetic (e.g., inheritance, polygenetic, epigenetic) Nervous system (e.g., central and peripheral: brain and nerve functioning) Bodily functioning (e.g., anatomy and physiology: endocrine, immune, cardiovascular, respiratory) Individual (e.g., cognition, perception, motivation)
Mesopsychology perspective **Relations between people in groups**
Group (e.g., identity, prejudice, facilitation) Organization (e.g., teamwork, achievement, identity) Community (e.g., empowerment, participation, advocacy)
Macropsychology perspective **Societal processes within and between countries**
Systems (e.g., interdependence, complexity, changing) Structures (e.g., institutions, political power, environment) National (e.g., laws, policies, governance) Global (e.g., declarations, alliances, treaties)

Macropsychology. At macrolevel, which is greatly underdeveloped in psychology in general and in rehabilitation psychology in particular, the concern is with the settings and conditions in which people live. Contextual factors not only strongly influence an individual's behavior but also the provision of services and opportunities for people with disabilities (McVeigh et al., 2016). McVeigh and colleagues explored the context-mechanism-outcome configurations (CMOCs) that are most likely to promote good policy and governance in how health and rehabilitation services can effectively interact, especially in poorly resourced settings. Differences in culture, contexts, training, presentation, or related supports means that no one set of actions is universally applicable. Rather, in line with the realist approach adopted by McVeigh et al., the settings and conditions represent a series of contingencies through which certain actions must take traction. This often is a rather messy and changing dynamic, so research and interventions may have to be rather less positivist (e.g., reliant on empirical methods and data) than the scientist–practitioner ethos common within rehabilitation psychology.

An important part of addressing the macrolevel is policy development and implementation. Policies determine what resources flow to whom—who should get what and why (MacLachlan, 2014). We have demonstrated that social, health, and rehabilitation policies often are inequitable: Those most in need of resources often have the least access to them. *EquiFrame*, our instrument for assessing the inclusion of vulnerable and marginalized groups in health policies (Amin et al., 2011; Mannan et al., 2012), assists policymakers in developing and analyzing public policies within a human rights framework. It comprises 21 core concepts of human rights, and identifies 12 vulnerable groups based on a series of consultations, UN declarations, and research evidence. These core concepts of human rights relate "to principles underlying the provision of universal, equitable and accessible health services" (Amin et al., 2011, p. 13).

EquiFrame now has been used to assess a variety of international health documents (Eide, Amin, MacLachlan, Mannan, & Schneider, 2013), regional policies on health priorities in Africa (Schneider,

Eide, Amin, MacLachlan, & Mannan, 2013), European policies on disability and development cooperation (Andersen & Mannan, 2012), India's disability policy (O'Dowd, Mannan, & McVeigh, 2013), and three South African policies on Black economic empowerment, employment, and cooperation (O'Donnell, 2008). It has been used to develop new, or revise existing, policies in South Africa (i.e., disability and rehabilitation polices), Malawi (i.e., national health policy and national health research policy), and Sudan (to guide the future development of all health policies). In the Lao People's Democratic Republic, EquiFrame has been used with Handicap International to support the process of developing a policy/strategy/action plan on disability. In Europe, it has been used it to analyze inclusion in the sexual and reproductive health policies of Ukraine, Scotland, Moldova, and Spain. Inspired by the psychological theory of social dominance (Sidanius & Pratto, 2001), it implicitly addresses the extent to which some groups have greater power and more resources than others.

However, inclusion in policy "on the books" does not necessarily mean EquiFrame has been fairly developed or subsequently implemented. We therefore have developed the policy tool *EquIPP* (Equity and Inclusion in Policy Processes; Huss & MacLachlan, 2016) to foster and assess the extent of equity and inclusion in the process of policy development and implementation. EquIPP identifies 17 key actions to support the development, implementation, and evaluation of inclusive policies in a highly participative and inclusive manner. Policy is a notoriously messy and nonlinear process, and much policy analysis is discursive and reflective. All of this is vital, but one of the unique contributions of EquiFrame and EquIPP resides in the combination of quantitative and qualitative data they produce. We recently completed a project—Inclusive Asia—using these measures with the governments of Malaysia, Timor-Leste, and Cambodia (see, e.g., Timor-Leste National Commission for the United Nations Educational, Scientific and Cultural Organization [UNESCO], 2016) as part of a pilot for UNESCO's management of social transformations program, which resulted in the development of the Inclusive Policy Lab. All resources in the lab are open access, and reports will share results from different countries and identify best practices.

Although policy is one aspect of macrolevel change, social structures are another target. Several of us also are involved in the Knowledge Management Programme of the United Nations Partnerships on the Rights of Persons with Disabilities, which has produced structural changes that have improved the lives of people with disabilities (United Partnership to Promote the Rights of Persons with Disabilities, 2016). Such changes include advancing the rights of persons with mental and intellectual disabilities in Moldova through introduction of justice oversight of existing psychiatric institutions, adoption of an adult deinstitutionalization strategy, and reform of the legal guardianship system. Another example is the creation of a network of Inclusive Cities in Indonesia that has brought together municipalities committed to promoting disability rights. In Costa Rica, a network of inclusive businesses is now better more supported so that it has been able to double its capacity, which is leading to a broader and deeper private sector commitment to the employment of people with disabilities. Although these changes have occurred at the structural level, they have been instituted through the development of a theory of change that has involved many behavior intervention principles well known to rehabilitation psychologists.

The dominant, underlying theories and foundational principles of rehabilitation can be applied to macropsychological challenges to inclusion for persons with disabilities (Bentley et al., 2016). The international literature outlined in this section provides examples across varied contexts. At a global level, evaluating the degree to which macrolevel movements toward health system accessibility and equitability likely can be most effective when concentrating on the experiences of persons with disabilities. For rehabilitation psychologists interested in initiating this work, the process may begin with a needs assessment that identifies a population (e.g., people experiencing disability secondary to spinal cord injury), measures that population's access to care on parameters of interest, and compares those findings with accessibility for individuals without activity limitations. Such a comparison would begin to identify broad health system considerations (e.g., disproportionate health care coverage limitations, transportation barriers, inaccessibility of the physical environment) and potential modes of additional assessment or intervention. Tools such as EquiFrame and EquIPP then could be used to identify policy-level barriers and corresponding opportunities to promote the human right to access and inclusion of people with disabilities at multiple levels.

Mesopsychology. The mesolevel of rehabilitation psychology is concerned with human interaction within groups, organizations, and the community. The "othering" of disability (Mik-Meyer, 2016) is psychological but also physical. Park, Faulkner, and Schaller (2003) argued that although humans developed a disease-avoidance system, that system operates to include many false positives:

> Anomalous features that are not due to disease (e.g., limb amputation due to accident) may also activate it, contributing to prejudicial attitudes and behaviors directed toward people with disabilities . . . linking chronic and temporary concerns about disease to implicit negative attitudes toward and behavioral avoidance of disabled others. (p. 65)

Such distancing and the associated lack of exposure to how the "othered" differ from each other therefore results in stereotyping, often prejudicially, in which the target is feared, leaving negative attitudes about, for instance, competence to learn, work, and even live in the community setting (Bowman, 1986). Here are the workings of stigma (Goffman, 1969).

Indeed, many of the greatest barriers that people with disabilities experience are due to stigma at the mesorelational level (MacLachlan & Swartz, 2009). Thus, even when people received adequate or excellent services within the realm of health, their lack of access to education, employment, or justice may mean that good rehabilitation practice at the individual level fails to work its way through to meaningful changes in their life. Where resources are scarce, the relational aspects of rehabilitation psychology (e.g., advocacy for inclusion of individuals with disabilities in all decision making, interdisciplinary focus, consultation-related competencies, comfort with conceptualizing and intervening on relationships between and within systems) may be even more important and less expensive than individual focused interventions. This is therefore one of several challenges to rehabilitation psychology: to become more community focused and more accessible, and perhaps to innovate its delivery mechanisms. For example, one strategy for partially addressing these challenges would be to use *train-the-trainer*—training members of the lay community in a health behavior intervention with the intention that they subsequently will train others—and similar methodologies that deemphasize dependence on direct access to health care professionals (e.g., rehabilitation psychologists). Train-the-trainer approaches shift tasks from health care providers to "consumers," caregivers, and others from the lay community. These approaches may be particularly applicable in low-resource environments with known human resources limitations and in scenarios in which stigma or attitudinal barriers are concerns. Such programs have yielded promising results across an array of disability-related challenges (Delaney et al., 2011; Marks, Sisirak, & Chang, 2013).

Micropsychology. The micropsychological focus on the individual in rehabilitation psychology has produced considerable insights into and improvements in the treatment and quality of life of many individuals across a range of conditions. One example of a microperspective in rehabilitation psychology would be the work on amputation and the fitting of prosthetics limbs, and their associated psychological factors (Desmond & MacLachlan, 2002). Research at the microlevel includes neuroscience perspectives from experimental manipulation of transitory bodily experience (MacLachlan, Desmond, & Horgan, 2003) to the application of neuromatrix theory (Melzack, 1990) to explain phantom experiences in terms of genetically inherited prewiring of the motor and sensory cortex, to how amputation disrupts genetic/inherited sensorimotor mapping and the associated neural plasticity that has been shown to occur (Flor et al., 1995). At the level of the individual organism, there has been a considerable focus on an individual's coping with the challenges of amputation (Desmond & MacLachlan,

2005). This area of research has grown in the past 20 years as conditions associated with amputation, such as diabetes, have become more prevalent, and with greater numbers of people surviving serious accidents and illnesses. The aging population can be expected to experiences more disorders resulting in amputation, such as peripheral vascular disease (Pell, Donnan, Fowkes, & Ruckley, 1993). The microfocus clearly needs to continue but also blended to take account of the different settings and conditions in which people experience such problems.

The ICF model of disability (WHO, 2001) presents disability as an experience and not a personal attribute. The ICF conceptualizes disability as a dynamic person-task-environment interaction. Someone with a bodily or mental impairment experiences limitations in his or her activities to the extent that the person encounter barriers in society—both physical and psychosocial. For instance, where universal design is adopted in public spaces (Crews & Zavotka, 2006) or where people have access to technologies that allow them to keep living at home (Cho, MacLachlan, Clarke, & Mannan, 2016), they may have fewer activity restrictions and therefore experience less disability. However, the experiences of disability at an individual level clearly are a combination of impairment, activity restriction, social exclusion, and disempowerment form participation; these additional factors point toward a relational level beyond the individual.

Addressing Challenges in Resource-Limited Environments

One of the foremost opportunities for contribution by rehabilitation psychology pertains to the evaluation of person–environment relationship factors influencing the functioning of individuals with disabilities in LMICs. The quality and relative influence of environmental barriers undoubtedly varies according to local context. Additional data are needed to identify physical and attitudinal environmental barriers experienced in LMICs. Several instruments have been developed to quantify the various environmental factors described by the ICF (Alvarelhão et al., 2012). Although assessments of environmental factors have been used in LMICs (Dijkers, Yavuzer, Ergin, Weitzenkamp, & Whiteneck, 2002; Sekaran et al., 2010), few instruments have been developed or validated for use in these contexts. Additional theory development is needed to better conceptualize the unique environmental barriers encountered by persons with disabilities in LMICs. It likely will require fundamental reconsideration of how environmental factors are assessed through collaborative development with local stakeholders and individuals with disabilities living in varied LMIC settings. Integration of rehabilitation psychology's expertise in person–environment interactions is essential to public health models focused on planning and implementing disability-related population health programs (see, e.g., the PRECEDE-PROCEED model in Green & Kreuter, 2005).

CONCLUSION

We have illustrated only a few of the ways in which rehabilitation psychology can contribute to global rehabilitation needs. Rehabilitation psychologists can contribute in many areas: They are influencing cultural factors on rehabilitation (Uomoto & Wong, 2015) and developing new community-based models of service delivery using innovative approaches, such as task-shifting (MacLachlan, Mannan, & McAuliffe, 2011b) or people with disabilities acting as their own "therapists" with peer support (Wegener, Mackenzie, Ephraim, Ehde, & Williams, 2009). They also are developing assistive technology provision at the individual, group, national, and global levels through initiatives, such as the Global Collaboration on Assistive Technology. Assistive technology can be seen as the mediator of human rights for many people, and, as it has been argued, is critical for achieving every one of the 17 SDGs (Tebbutt et al., 2016).

A primary challenge faced by rehabilitation psychology is nested in a broader challenge to psychology in general. The replicability of some key findings of experimental psychology has been called into question (Open Science Collaboration, 2015), even when the conditions for replication have been quite similar to the original findings—similar settings, countries, and participants. Where these basic conditions differ—different sociopolitical systems, different cultural beliefs, different interpersonal norms, or younger, older, or a greater representation of marginalized groups—we may expect even less success at replicating "classic" findings. This idea is neatly encapsulated in the assertion that most people in the world are not WEIRD; that is, they are not Western educated in Western ways and living in industrialized settings, and are neither rich nor part of democratic political systems (Henrich, Heine, & Norenzayan, 2010). There are many different ways in which psychology and rehabilitation psychology in particular can respond. One such approach is to narrow down focus on very specific intervention techniques—behavioral change techniques—for which there is evidence for their efficacy (albeit usually from WEIRD settings) and to build programmatic interventions based on an cumulation of components that work (somewhere).

A contrasting but not necessarily incompatible approach is to see the techniques of intervention as only a part (and not necessarily the most important part) of a process of behavioral change that places behavioral change techniques in a chain of CMOCs (Pawson & Tilley, 1997). Here, the nexus of action is how people use the techniques—or what works, for whom, in what circumstances, and why?—rather than the prescription of such techniques in environments that often seemed are assumed to be sterile of culture, context, or resource constraints. This approach offers a fertile environment in which to develop psychological theory (often so-called middle-range theories) based on what works in greatly differing settings and for perhaps greatly differing people rather than assuming we can accumulate a set of techniques that will work for most people in most places. The intricacies and complexities of these CMOCs may benefit greatly from the sort of sophisticated behavioral analysis that psychologists are trained to offer. In complex environments, however, we should not expect that a simple accumulation of techniques is going to be the central component of behavioral change (McVeigh et al., 2016).

In this chapter, we have sought to convey some challenges that are arising from taking a global perspective on disability and rehabilitation. We have argued that rehabilitation psychology needs to infuse some outside perspectives, including from civil society agencies and UN organizations, as well as the need to measure progress toward the SDGs. There are other perspectives that we have not had the space to cover: those from professional organizations, the global south and the global north, employers and entrepreneurs, and perhaps most especially people with disabilities and those providing community-based rehabilitation services. This is a broad scope, but it can be embraced by conceiving of rehabilitation psychology as working at different but interacting levels—at the micro-, meso- and macrolevels. Rehabilitation psychology must continue to strengthen its bedrock of contributions at the microlevel, but it now also must develop greater commitment to the meso- and macrolevels. We should enhance our contribution to a systems thinking perspective, linking different parts of the community-based rehabilitation matrix, and embrace a more activist position to advance the rights and opportunities of people with disabilities, thus allowing individuals to benefit more fully from the provision of rehabilitation services.

References

Alvarelhão, J., Silva, A., Martins, A., Queirós, A., Amaro, A., Rocha, N., & Lains, J. (2012). Comparing the content of instruments assessing environmental factors using the International Classification of Functioning, Disability and Health. *Journal of Rehabilitation Medicine*, *44*, 1–6. http://dx.doi.org/10.2340/16501977-0905

Amin, M., MacLachlan, M., Mannan, H., El Tayeb, S., El Khatim, A., Swartz, L., . . . Schneider, M. (2011). EquiFrame: A framework for analysis of the inclusion of human rights and vulnerable groups in health policies. *Health and Human Rights*, *13*, 1–20.

Andersen, A., & Mannan, H. (2012). Assessing the quality of European policies on disability and development cooperation: A discussion of core concepts of human rights and coherence. *Disability and International Development*, *1*, 16–24.

Awasthi, P., Yadava, V., & Pandey, R. P. (2016). Disability, rehabilitation and rehabilitation psychology: An overview. *Indian Journal of Community Psychology*, *12*, 196–210.

Bentley, J. A., Bruyère, S. M., LeBlanc, J., & MacLachlan, M. (2016). Globalizing rehabilitation psychology: Application of foundational principles to global health and rehabilitation challenges. *Rehabilitation Psychology*, *61*, 65–73. http://dx.doi.org/10.1037/rep0000068

Boot, F. H., Dinsmore, J., Khasnabis, C., & MacLachlan, M. (2017). Intellectual disability and assistive technology: Opening the GATE wider. *Frontiers in Public Health, 5*. http://dx.doi.org/10.3389/fpubh.2017.00010

Bowman, I. (1986). Teacher training and the integration of handicapped pupils: Some findings from a fourteen nation UNESCO study. *European Journal of Special Needs Education, 1*, 29–38. http://dx.doi.org/10.1080/0885625860010105

Carr, S. C., & Sloan, T. S. (Eds.). (2003). *Poverty and psychology: From global perspective to local practice*. Boston, MA: Springer. http://dx.doi.org/10.1007/978-1-4615-0029-2

Cho, H. Y., MacLachlan, M., Clarke, M., & Mannan, H. (2016). Accessible home environments for people with functional limitations: A systematic review. *International Journal of Environmental Research and Public Health, 13*, 826. http://dx.doi.org/10.3390/ijerph13080826

Commission on Social Determinants of Health. (2008). *Closing the gap in a generation: Health equity through action on the social determinants of health* [Final Report]. Geneva, Switzerland: World Health Organization. Retrieved from http://apps.who.int/iris/bitstream/handle/10665/43943/9789241563703_eng.pdf;jsessionid=23B9790014A9428A804563120007C262?sequence=1

Crews, D. E., & Zavotka, S. (2006). Aging, disability, and frailty: Implications for universal design. *Journal of Physiological Anthropology, 25*, 113–118. http://dx.doi.org/10.2114/jpa2.25.113

Delaney, C., Fortinsky, R., Doonan, L., Grimes, R. L., Terra-Lee, P., Rosenberg, S., & Bruce, M. L. (2011). Depression screening and interventions for older home health care patients: Program design and training outcomes for a train-the-trainer model. *Home Health Care Management & Practice, 23*, 435–445. http://dx.doi.org/10.1177/1084822311405459

Desmond, D., & MacLachlan, M. (2002). Psychological issues in prosthetic and orthotic practice: A 25 year review of psychology in *Prosthetics and Orthotics International*. *Prosthetics and Orthotics International, 26*, 182–188. http://dx.doi.org/10.1080/03093640208726646

Desmond, D. M., & MacLachlan, M. (2005). Factor structure of the Trinity Amputation and Prosthesis Experience Scales (TAPES) with individuals with acquired upper limb amputations. *American Journal of Physical Medicine & Rehabilitation, 84*, 506–513. http://dx.doi.org/10.1097/01.phm.0000166885.16180.63

Dijkers, M. P., Yavuzer, G., Ergin, S., Weitzenkamp, D., & Whiteneck, G. G. (2002). A tale of two countries: Environmental impacts on social participation after spinal cord injury. *Spinal Cord, 40*, 351–362. http://dx.doi.org/10.1038/sj.sc.3101310

Eide, A. H., Amin, M., MacLachlan, M., Mannan, H., & Schneider, M. (2013). Addressing equitable health of vulnerable groups in international health documents. *ALTER-European Journal of Disability Research/Revue Européenne de Recherche sur le Handicap, 7*, 153–162.

Flor, H., Elbert, T., Knecht, S., Wienbruch, C., Pantev, C., Birbaumers, N., . . . Taub, E. (1995). Phantom-limb pain as a perceptual correlate of cortical reorganization following arm amputation. *Nature, 375*, 482–484. http://dx.doi.org/10.1038/375482a0

Flynn, E. (2011). *From rhetoric to action: Implementing the UN Convention on the Rights of Persons with Disabilities*. Cambridge, England: Cambridge University Press.

Geiser, P., & Boersma, M. (2013). The role of the community in CBR. In G. Musoke & P. Geiser (Eds.), *Linking CBR: Disability and rehabilitation* (pp. 24–35). Kyambogo, Uganda: CBR Africa Network.

Global indicator framework for the sustainable development goals and targets of the 2030 Agenda for Sustainable Development. (n.d.). Retrieved from https://unstats.un.org/sdgs/indicators/Global%20Indicator%20Framework%20after%20refinement_Eng.pdf

Goffman, E. (1969). The insanity of place. *Psychiatry: Interpersonal and biological processes, 32*, 357–388. http://dx.doi.org/10.1080/00332747.1969.11023600

Green, L. W., & Kreuter, M. W. (2005). *Health program planning: An educational and ecological approach* (4th ed.). New York, NY: McGraw-Hill.

Henrich, J., Heine, S. J., & Norenzayan, A. (2010). The weirdest people in the world? *Behavioral and Brain Sciences, 33*, 61–83. http://dx.doi.org/10.1017/S0140525X0999152X

Huss, T., & MacLachlan, M. (2016). *Equity and Inclusion in Policy Processes (EquIPP): A framework to support equity & inclusion in the process of policy development, implementation and evaluation*. Dublin, Ireland: Global Health Press.

International Labour Organization, Gender, Equality and Diversity Branch. (2015). *Decent work for persons with disabilities: Promoting rights in the global development agenda* (3rd ed.). Geneva, Switzerland: Author.

Koplan, J. P., Bond, T. C., Merson, M. H., Reddy, K. S., Rodriguez, M. H., Sewankambo, N. K., . . . & the Consortium of Universities for Global Health Executive Board. (2009). Towards a common definition of global health. *The Lancet, 373*, 1993–1995. http://dx.doi.org/10.1016/S0140-6736(09)60332-9

Lindstrom, L., Doren, B., Post, C., & Lombardi, A. (2013). Building career PATHS (postschool achievement through higher skills) for young women with disabilities. *Career Development Quarterly, 61*, 330–338. http://dx.doi.org/10.1002/j.2161-0045.2013.00059.x

MacLachlan, M. (2006). *Culture and health: A critical perspective towards global health*. Hoboken, NJ: Wiley.

MacLachlan, M. (2014). Macropsychology, policy, and global health. *American Psychologist*, *69*, 851–863. http://dx.doi.org/10.1037/a0037852

MacLachlan, M., Carr, S. C., & McAuliffe, E. (2010). *The aid triangle: Recognizing the human dynamics of dominance, justice and identity*. Halifax, Nova Scotia: Fernwood.

MacLachlan, M., Desmond, D., & Horgan, O. (2003). Psychological correlates of illusory body experiences. *Journal of Rehabilitation Research and Development*, *40*, 59–66.

MacLachlan, M., & Mannan, H. (2013). Is disability a health problem? *Social Inclusion*, *1*, 139–141. http://dx.doi.org/10.17645/si.v1i2.110

MacLachlan, M., & Mannan, H. (2014). The *World Report on Disability* and its implications for rehabilitation psychology. *Rehabilitation Psychology*, *59*, 117–124. http://dx.doi.org/10.1037/a0036715

MacLachlan, M., Mannan, H., & McAuliffe, E. (2011a). Access to health care of persons with disabilities as an indicator of equity in health systems. *Open Medicine*, *5*, e10–e12.

MacLachlan, M., Mannan, H., & McAuliffe, E. (2011b). Staff skills not staff types for community-based rehabilitation. *The Lancet*, *377*, 1988–1989. http://dx.doi.org/10.1016/S0140-6736(10)61925-3

MacLachlan, M., & Swartz, L. (Eds.). (2009). *Disability & international development: Towards inclusive global health*. New York, NY: Springer. http://dx.doi.org/10.1007/978-0-387-93840-0

Mannan, H., McVeigh, J., Amin, M., MacLachlan, M., Swartz, L., Munthali, A., & Van Rooy, G. (2012). Core concepts of human rights and inclusion of vulnerable groups in the disability and rehabilitation policies of Malawi, Namibia, Sudan, and South Africa. *Journal of Disability Policy Studies*, *23*, 67–81. http://dx.doi.org/10.1177/1044207312439103

Marks, B., Sisirak, J., & Chang, Y. C. (2013). Efficacy of the HealthMatters program train-the-trainer model. *Journal of Applied Research in Intellectual Disabilities*, *26*, 319–334. http://dx.doi.org/10.1111/jar.12045

McVeigh, J., MacLachlan, M., Gilmore, B., McClean, C., Eide, A. H., Mannan, H., . . . Normand, C. (2016). Promoting good policy for leadership and governance of health related rehabilitation: A realist synthesis. *Globalization and Health*, *12*, 1–18. http://dx.doi.org/10.1186/s12992-016-0182-8

Melzack, R. (1990). Phantom limbs and the concept of a neuromatrix. *Trends in Neurosciences*, *13*, 88–92. http://dx.doi.org/10.1016/0166-2236(90)90179-E

Mik-Meyer, N. (2016). Othering, ableism and disability: A discursive analysis of co-workers' construction of colleagues with visible impairments. *Human Relations*, *69*, 1341–1363. http://dx.doi.org/10.1177/0018726715618454

Murray, B. (2013, 17–19 July). *Economic empowerment of persons with disabilities through social protection and poverty reduction*. Presentation at the panel discussion at the 6th Conference of States Parties to the Convention on the Rights of Persons with Disabilities, New York, NY.

Murray, C. J. L. (2015). Choosing indicators for the health-related SDG targets. *Lancet*, *386*, 1314–1317. http://dx.doi.org/10.1016/S0140-6736(15)00382-7

O'Donnell, R. (2008). *An examination of the economic empowerment of people with disabilities in South Africa*. Dublin, Ireland: Centre for Global Health, Trinity College Dublin, University of Dublin.

O'Dowd, J., Mannan, H., & McVeigh, J. (2013). India's disability policy—Analysis of core concepts of human rights. *Disability, CBR and Inclusive Development*, *24*, 69–90.

Open Science Collaboration. (2015). Estimating the reproducibility of psychological science. *Science*, *349*, aac4716. http://dx.doi.org/10.1126/science.aac4716

Park, J. H., Faulkner, J., & Schaller, M. (2003). Evolved disease-avoidance processes and contemporary anti-social behavior: Prejudicial attitudes and avoidance of people with physical disabilities. *Journal of Nonverbal Behavior*, *27*, 65–87. http://dx.doi.org/10.1023/A:1023910408854

Pawson, R., & Tilley, N. (1997). *Realistic evaluation*. London, England: Sage.

Pell, J. P., Donnan, P. T., Fowkes, F. G. R., & Ruckley, C. V. (1993). Quality of life following lower limb amputation for peripheral arterial disease. *European Journal of Vascular Surgery*, *7*, 448–451. http://dx.doi.org/10.1016/S0950-821X(05)80265-8

Sanchez, J. (2015). *Moving towards disability inclusion: Stories of change*. Geneva, Switzerland: International Labour Office.

Schneider, M., Eide, A. H., Amin, M., MacLachlan, M., & Mannan, H. (2013). Inclusion of vulnerable groups in health policies: Regional policies on health priorities in Africa. *African Journal of Disability*, 2, a40. http://dx.doi.org/10.4102/ajod.v2i1.40

Sekaran, P., Vijayakumari, F., Hariharan, R., Zachariah, K., Joseph, S. E., & Senthil Kumar, R. K. (2010). Community reintegration of spinal cord-injured patients in rural south India. *Spinal Cord*, *48*, 628–632. http://dx.doi.org/10.1038/sc.2010.6

Sidanius, J., & Pratto, F. (2001). *Social dominance: An intergroup theory of social hierarchy and oppression*. New York, NY: Cambridge University Press.

Silverman, A. M., & Cohen, G. L. (2014). Stereotypes as stumbling-blocks: How coping with stereotype threat affects life outcomes for people with physical disabilities. *Personality and Social Psychology Bulletin, 40*, 1330–1340. http://dx.doi.org/10.1177/0146167214542800

Sustainable Development Solutions Network. (2016, February 15). *Preliminary sustainable development goal index and dashboard* [Draft Paper]. Retrieved from http://unsdsn.org/resources/publications/sdg-index/

Tebbutt, E., Brodmann, R., Borg, J., MacLachlan, M., Khasnabis, C., & Horvath, R. (2016). Assistive products and the sustainable development goals (SDGs). *Globalization and Health, 12*, 79. http://dx.doi.org/10.1186/s12992-016-0220-6

Timor-Leste National Commission for the United Nations Educational, Scientific and Cultural Organization. (2016). *Promoting Social Inclusion in Timor-Leste: Analysis of national disability policy framework in Timor-Leste* [Report]. Retrieved from http://www.unesco.or.id/download/Report_Social_Inclusion_PwD_TimorLeste.pdf

United Nations. (2008, May 3). *Convention on the Rights of Persons with Disabilities: Optional protocol.* Retrieved from http://www.un.org/disabilities/documents/convention/convoptprot-e.pdf

United Nations. (2015). *Transforming our world: The 2030 agenda for sustainable development.* Retrieved from https://sustainabledevelopment.un.org/content/documents/21252030%20Agenda%20for%20Sustainable%20Development%20web.pdf

United Nations. (2016, 22 November). *Mainstreaming disability in the implementation of the 2030 Agenda for Sustainable Development* (Report of the Secretary-General). New York, NY: Author. Retrieved from http://www.un.org/ga/search/view_doc.asp?symbol=E/CN.5/2017/4

United Nations. (2018). *Global indicator framework for the sustainable development goals and targets of the 2030 agenda for sustainable development.* Retrieved from https://unstats.un.org/sdgs/indicators/Global%20Indicator%20Framework%20after%20refinement_Eng.pdf

United Partnership to Promote the Rights of Persons with Disabilities. (2016). *Connections: Building partnerships for disability rights* [Report]. New York, NY: United Nations Development Programme. Retrieved from file:///C:/Users/laure/Downloads/UNPRPD-REPORT-SPREADS-WEB.pdf

Uomoto, J. M., & Wong, T. M. (2015). *Multicultural neurorehabilitation: Clinical principles for rehabilitation professionals.* New York, NY: Springer.

Vornholt, K., Uitdewilligen, S., & Nijhuis, F. J. (2013). Factors affecting the acceptance of people with disabilities at work: A literature review. *Journal of Occupational Rehabilitation, 23*, 463–475. http://dx.doi.org/10.1007/s10926-013-9426-0

Wang, Z., Chen, G., Guo, C., Pang, L., & Zheng, X. (2016). Socioeconomic inequalities and multi-disability among the population aged 15–64 years from 1987 to 2006 in China. *International Journal of Environmental Research and Public Health, 13*, 1033. http://dx.doi.org/10.3390/ijerph13101033

Wegener, S. T., Mackenzie, E. J., Ephraim, P., Ehde, D., & Williams, R. (2009). Self-management improves outcomes in persons with limb loss. *Archives of Physical Medicine and Rehabilitation, 90*, 373–380. http://dx.doi.org/10.1016/j.apmr.2008.08.222

World Health Organization. (1978). *Declaration of Alma-Ata.* Retrieved from http://www.who.int/publications/almaata_declaration_en.pdf

World Health Organization. (2001). *International Classification of Functioning, Disability and Health: ICF.* Geneva, Switzerland: Author.

World Health Organization. (2008). *The Bamako call to action on research for health.* Retrieved from http://www.who.int/rpc/news/BAMAKOCALLTOACTIONFinalNov24.pdf

World Health Organization. (2013). *WHO global disability action plan 2014–2021: Better health for all people with disability.* Retrieved from http://apps.who.int/iris/bitstream/10665/199544/1/9789241509619_eng.pdf

World Health Organization & World Bank. (2011). *World report on disability*. Geneva, Switzerland: Author. Retrieved from http://whqlibdoc.who.int/publications/2011/9789240685215_eng.pdf

Yoshida, K., Hanass-Hancock, J., Nixon, S., & Bond, V. (2014). Using intersectionality to explore experiences of disability and HIV among women and men in Zambia. *Disability and Rehabilitation, 36*, 2161–2168. http://dx.doi.org/10.3109/09638288.2014.894144

CHAPTER 26

PUBLIC HEALTH MODELS OF CARE

Jacob Bentley and Stephen T. Wegener

The 21st-century health care system has expanded its focus from individual health to initiatives that promote health for larger groups and populations (for additional distinctions, see the Afterword, this handbook). There are many reasons for this shift, including a move toward health care systems' assuming responsibility and risk for populations of individuals whom they insure and for whom they provide care. Understanding the principles of public health is essential for rehabilitation psychologists who want to take a leadership role in health care, as well as for those looking to expand the impact of their care to groups of individuals. It often is at the intersection of two fields of study that new insights are developed and changes in paradigms occur. As such, this chapter is designed to partially fill a gap regarding public health knowledge among many rehabilitation psychologists. It is hoped that the information presented will inspire rehabilitation psychologists to consider a broader application of their specialized knowledge and skills, and facilitate the application of public health principles to expand the impact of their work. For the occasional public health scholars who happen upon this work, it may be helpful to consider how the field of rehabilitation psychology offers insights that may shape their work in improving the lives of persons with disability and with chronic health conditions. Specifically, the information presented builds on previous work (Frank, 1999; Lollar, 2008; Winett, King, & Altman, 1989). We summarize key public health principles relevant to rehabilitation psychology and conclude with opportunities to contribute through assessment, intervention, and advocacy.

KEY PRINCIPLES IN PUBLIC HEALTH

The Centers for Disease Control and Prevention (CDC) Foundation defines *public health* as "the science of protecting and improving the health of [families and communities through promotion of healthy lifestyles, research for disease and injury prevention, and detection and control of] infectious diseases" (CDC Foundation, n.d., "Public Health Connects Us All"). Public health as a discipline has been marked by an emphasis on the health of populations using epidemiological and data driven approaches while focusing on social and environmental factors related to health. As such, social justice themes of equity and inclusion often are at the forefront of public health work.

For training and education purposes, the Association of Schools & Programs of Public Health (2006) developed a core competency model to be used by all master of public health degree programs accredited by the Council on Education for Public Health. The model defines five discipline-specific areas of knowledge thought to be at the core of public health—Biostatistics, Environmental Health Sciences, Epidemiology, Health Policy Management, and Social and Behavioral Sciences—as well as

http://dx.doi.org/10.1037/0000129-027
Handbook of Rehabilitation Psychology, Third Edition, L. A. Brenner, S. A. Reid-Arndt, T. R. Elliott, R. G. Frank, and B. Caplan (Editors-in-Chief)

seven shared but relevant interdisciplinary domains: Communication and Informatics, Diversity and Culture, Leadership, Professionalism, Program Planning, Public Health Biology, and Systems Thinking. Traditionally, public health professionals have focused their efforts on any one of the five discipline-specific domains; however, many ultimately have pursued expertise on specific populations or subspecialty content areas, such as International Health, Human Nutrition, Health Systems, Mental Health, or Maternal Health.

Epidemiology

Epidemiology can be defined as the scientific, systematic, and data-driven study of the frequency, pattern, and determinants (e.g., causes, risk factors) of health-related states in a specified population (U.S. Department of Health and Human Services, 2012). Using the epidemiological tools, public health scientists provide data to select targets for prevention and care, guide evidence-based practices, and shape policy. At its core, epidemiology is focused on concepts of population and comparison. Epidemiologists examine and describe health events by following a process analogous to that of the five *W*s of journalism: (a) what (health issue of concern), (b) who (person), (c) where (place), (d) when (time), and (e) why/how (causes, risk factors, modes of transmission). Epidemiologists count cases or health events and describe them in terms of time, place, and person; divide the number of cases by an appropriate denominator to calculate rates; and compare those rates over time or for different groups of people. They often use cohort or case-control studies to evaluate differences in disease and injury occurrence across populations while generating hypotheses about risk. To test hypotheses, they use analytic methodologies that fall into broad categories of experimental and observational. Five major tasks of epidemiology in public health practice have been identified as follows: (a) surveillance, (b) field investigation, (c) analytic studies, (d) evaluation (effectiveness and efficiency research), and (e) interdisciplinary linkages.

Looking at the concepts of incidence and prevalence provides a way to illustrate the epidemiological principles just described. Before counting cases, the epidemiologist must decide what to count, that is, what to call a case. For that, the epidemiologist uses a case definition. A *case definition* is a set of standard criteria for classifying whether a person has a particular disease, syndrome, or other health condition. Some case definitions, particularly those used for national surveillance, have been developed and adopted as national standards that ensure comparability. Use of an agreed on standard case definition ensures that every case is equivalent, regardless of when or where it occurred, or who identified it (see Chapter 24, this volume). *Incidence* is a measure of disease that allows us to determine a person's probability of being diagnosed with a disease during a given period. Therefore, incidence is the number of newly diagnosed cases of a disease. An *incidence rate* is the number of new cases of a disease divided by the number of persons at risk for the disease. For example, overall, approximately 800,000 first-time or recurrent strokes occur in the United States each year (Ovbiagele & Nguyen-Huynh, 2011). In terms of incidence, age is a major factor in determining risk. Among adults aged 35 to 44 years, the incidence is 30 to 120 per 100,000 each year. For those aged 65 to 74 years, the incidence is 670 to 970 over the course of 1 year per every 100,000. *Prevalence*, in contrast, is a measure of disease that allows us to determine a person's likelihood of having a disease. Therefore, the number of prevalent cases is the total number of cases of disease existing in a population. A is the total number of cases of a disease existing in a population divided by the total population. Returning to the example of stroke, the estimated prevalence would be described as approximately 7 million individuals (or 3% of the adult population) either recently diagnosed or otherwise known to be living following stroke. Themes from the major epidemiological tasks and their interaction with rehabilitation psychology principles are described later in this chapter.

Prevention

Efforts for disease and injury prevention rest at the forefront of activities in many public health sectors. Prevention activities and programs are organized to interact with illness processes on a continuum that extends from before an injury or disease incident occurs to well into the management phases. These efforts often are discussed in terms of primary, secondary, tertiary, and quaternary prevention. Each of these prevention concepts are briefly discussed as follows.

Primary prevention looks to reduce risk for the onset of an injury or disease, or to bolster resistance to an identified harmful agent. Efforts may be focused on ameliorating environmental causes of a disease or promoting adaptive health behavior change. Some primary prevention programs require active participation from members of the target population (e.g., attending smoking cessation classes), whereas others do not (e.g., taxes that fund statewide tobacco reduction programs). Due to their influence on injury prevalence and severity, examples of particular relevance to rehabilitation providers include policy and legislative initiatives to mandate the use of seatbelts or bicycle helmets.

Secondary prevention focuses on early detection and treatment of subclinical pathology. These procedures typically begin with screening tests conducted by a health care provider followed by early cost-efficient interventions. Examples include routine mammograms to detect early stage breast cancer and nutrition or exercise programs to reduce stroke risk. For rehabilitation psychologists, secondary prevention efforts may take the form of advocating for and facilitating the development of concussion screening procedures for athletes or early detection procedures to identify those demonstrating risk for problematic opioid use in the context of chronic pain.

Tertiary prevention occurs in the context of an already developed clinical condition and seeks to reduce burden of disease, as well as associated secondary complications. Examples that reflect the core traditional responsibilities of rehabilitation psychologists include spinal cord injury (SCI) rehabilitation that focuses on improved functional capacity, disease management skill development, and psychosocial interventions and efforts to maximize quality of life. In this way, tertiary prevention includes interventions aimed at modifying behaviors that place a person with spinal cord impairments at risk for autonomic dysreflexia or pressure ulcers. Remediation, rehabilitation, and improved quality of life are the underlying goals of prevention at this level.

Jamoulle and Roland (1995) first proposed the concept of *quaternary prevention*. Its definition has evolved slightly over the years to refer to an "action taken to identify a patient or a population at risk of over-medicalization, to protect them from invasive medical interventions, and provide for them procedures which are ethically acceptable" (Jamoulle, 2015, p. 62). This level of prevention focuses on harm-reduction activities in the provision of health care and shared clinical decision making with the patient's necessarily serving as an active agent. Quaternary prevention brings into focus instances in which "not doing" may be more beneficial or preventive than "doing." Providing psychological/behavioral interventions that reduce prescriptions of narcotic pain medication in the chronic management of low back pain is one example of quaternary prevention in rehabilitation psychology practice. The quaternary prevention literature has begun to explore whether the typically negative valenced concept of *clinical inertia*, that is, the "failure of health care providers to initiate or intensify therapy when indicated" (Reach, Pechtner, Gentilella, Corcos, & Ceriello, 2017, p. 501), may represent a safeguard for patients in certain situations. Giugliano and Esposito (2011), for example, have reviewed evidence in the management of cardiovascular disease identifying potential rationales for a provider's going against current practice guidelines due to uncertainty as to whether those guidelines apply to the individual person.

Surveillance and Screening

Concepts of testing, screening, case finding, and surveillance are important when attempting to understand methodologies used in pursuing prevention initiatives in public health. As in clinical practice settings, *testing* in the public health definition refers to procedures used to identify cases of a diagnosis or medical condition. A sample from a population may be selected for testing in the presence of identifiable risk factors. *Screening* occurs when a testing procedure is applied to all individuals in an identified population. Screening may be implemented for *case finding*, that is, the identification of individuals who are asymptomatic or presymptomatic but who are suspected to be at risk for a condition, or *surveillance* purposes, such as monitoring illness incidence or prevalence over time. Surveillance is integral because it provides a means for monitoring effectiveness of prevention and intervention programs while also assisting in the process of deciding where to allocate resources.

Insights into population-level health can be obtained through national health behavior agendas and data surveillance systems. The Behavioral Risk Factor Surveillance System (BRFSS) is a collaborative project between all 50 U.S. states, participating U.S. territories, and the CDC. It is an ongoing telephone-based interview surveillance system designed to measure behavioral risk factors among adults residing in the United States. The interview has three components: a core set of questions, optional modules on specific topics, and state-added questions. The overall objective is "to collect uniform, state-specific data on preventive health practices and risk behaviors that are linked to chronic diseases, injuries, and preventable infectious diseases" (CDC, 2014, p. 1). The BRFSS datasets are readily accessible through the CDC website to enable scholars to conduct population-based health behavior research at the state or national levels. Although practical limitations associated with population surveying restrict the breadth of disability-related research questions to be addressed through the BRFSS to some extent (Mann et al., 2015), as one example, researchers have used the database to evaluate trends in socioeconomic-, racial- and gender-based factors in disability (Courtney-Long, Romano, Carroll, & Fox, 2017; Randolph & Andresen, 2004). Additional information about opportunities for rehabilitation psychology researchers to use source databases like the BRFSS is provided in the Opportunities in Assessment, Intervention, and Advocacy at the Population Level section later in this chapter.

Person–Environment Focus

Public health has long focused on the creation of environments that facilitate health (Winett et al., 1989). This creation can be accomplished through community-based initiatives, policy development, and recognition of the importance of environmental factors. In recent years, advancements have been seen in each of these initiative domains. At the community level, there is growing evidence off the wide-ranging potential of targeted public health environmental modifications in the promotion of adaptive health behaviors. There is strong evidence, for example, that creating and increasing access to settings conducive to physical activity are effective in increasing levels of physical activity when combined with informational outreach (Kahn et al., 2002). Another specific example of public health community-based interventions is a Seattle, Washington-based housing authority project targeting increased use of asthma-reduction building materials when developing low-income public housing (Takaro, Krieger, Song, Sharify, & Beaudet, 2011). The cost of changes in housing design, building materials and construction ranged from $5,000 to $7,000 and resulted in reduced asthma triggers, symptoms, and exacerbations. Children in these homes ($n = 34$) had a 70% increase in symptom-free days than in their previous homes and a 67% reduction in the need for asthma-related urgent health services.

With regard to policy, the Americans With Disabilities Act of 1990 (ADA) served as a milestone advancement in the United States by increasing access and equal opportunity for persons with disabilities across domains of public life. Similarly, appreciation of the influence of the environment on personal functioning in the context of a chronic illness in the international community has been enhanced since the adoption of the International Classification of Functioning, Disability and Health (ICF; WHO, 2001). The ICF has been adopted by 191 nations around the world and represents an important conceptual shift by moving the focus from cause to impact and recognizing disability as a universal human experience. The focus on the environment seen in the ICF, in many respects, represents the actualization of behavioral psychologist and Kurt Lewin's work on person–environment interaction.

Multisystemic Intervention

Public health initiatives span multiple social–ecological system levels. As described earlier, these efforts often focus on environmental factors and policy development or revision. Concepts of universal design, accessibility, barrier-free design, and inclusive design all are products of an increased appreciation of environmental barriers and facilitators

(Iwarsson & Ståhl, 2003). Architect Ronald Mace (1985) defined *universal design* as "a way of designing a building or facility . . . so it is both attractive and functional for all people disabled or not" (p. 147).

Since then, seven principles of universal design (Story, Mueller, & Mace, 1998) have been developed and widely adopted internationally. Broadly, principles of universal design can be applied from the microlevel to macrolevel. As such, the focus of universal design initiatives may be to reduce mobility barriers in the built physical neighborhood environment or on measures to increase physical activity, safety, and social capital for persons with disabilities. Universal design is not just another term for accessibility, although an ADA mandate often involves a post hoc revision to correct an exclusive environment. Rather, universal design is focused on social inclusion from the very earliest stage of development for product designs or built environments. "Design for all," commonly used in Europe, represents an apt synonym in that captures universal design's broader potential for promoting social inclusion by shifting the focus of formative development processes (Iwarsson & Ståhl, 2003; Sanford, 2012).

Policy Influence

Health policy development and implementation through the use of research data and advocacy are key to public health intervention. There are several prominent examples of such public health initiatives in the United States over the past several decades; those initiatives have spanned efforts involving either passive (e.g., policies requiring manufacturers to include airbags in automobiles) or active participation by the population (e.g., policies requiring drivers and passengers to fasten seatbelts). Policy development and revision occur through a recursive feedback loop among empirical study, evaluation of population-based goals, and advocacy to policymakers. The Healthy People Project (Office of Disease Prevention and Health Promotion [ODPHP], 2017) has provided a framework for organizing decade-long national health initiatives that influence this feedback loop in the United States. A federal interagency work group, including representation from the National Institutes of Health, was commissioned to organize the effort to develop measurable health objectives for the 2010–2020 decade. The initiative, called Healthy People 2020, covers 1,200 objectives across 42 topic areas. Perhaps most pertinent to rehabilitation psychologists is the Disability and Health topic. There are 21 measurable objectives identified within this topic that spans the domains of Systems and Policies, Barriers to Health Care, Environment, and Activities and Participation. Objectives of interest include "increase the proportion of adults with disabilities who report sufficient social and emotional support" (objective DH-17; Office of Disease Prevention and Health Promotion, n.d.) and "reduce the proportion of adults with disabilities aged 18 years and older who experience delays in receiving primary and periodic preventive care due to specific barriers" (objective DH-4; Office of Disease Prevention and Health Promotion, n.d.). These objectives reflect rehabilitation practice on an individual level; however, population-based initiatives such as Healthy People provide additional value by establishing common goals and targets for public health activities. A midcourse review of progress toward Disability and Health objectives found that 28.6% ($n = 6$) of the objectives had been met, 23.8% ($n = 5$) demonstrated little or no detectable change, 14.3% ($n = 3$) were improving, 14.3% ($n = 3$) were getting worse, and 19% ($n = 4$) only had baseline data available (Office of Disease Prevention and Health Promotion, 2017).

Healthy People assists with identifying nationwide health improvement priorities, increasing public awareness of chronic illness and disability determinants, providing measurable public health objectives and goals, promoting actions to strengthen policies. Ultimately, it identifies best practices based on available empirical evidence.

OPPORTUNITIES IN ASSESSMENT, INTERVENTION, AND ADVOCACY AT THE POPULATION LEVEL

Public health as a discipline has been marked by an emphasis on the health of populations resulting a strong focus on social and environmental factors in health and social justice. We see many of these same themes when we explore the roots and current activities in rehabilitation psychology. Greater attention to the principles of public health in the discipline and practice of rehabilitation psychology may improve the reach and impact of our work. Moreover, infusion of rehabilitation psychological expertise and principles can be to the benefit of public health work in varied respects as described in this section.

Epidemiology

National databases likely are underused because rehabilitation psychologists have focused on clinical research databases. The Model Systems of Care databases are perhaps the most accessed by rehabilitation psychology researchers. The three primary Model Systems of Care provide national databases for SCI, traumatic brain injury (TBI), and burn injury populations. Funded by the National Institute on Disability, Independent Living, and Rehabilitation Research, these Model Systems collect data across multiple collaborating sites around the United States with the goal of enhancing knowledge about the long-term consequences of injury and factors associated with improved long-term clinical outcomes. The TBI Model Systems of Care (TBIMS), for example, consists of 16 rehabilitation centers that provide comprehensive specialty services across the continuum of care (e.g., from the acute injury phase through to community reintegration). Each center contributes data to what has become the largest longitudinal TBI database in existence. As of 2016, 14,633 cases have been included in the database ("The Traumatic Brain Injury Model Systems," 2016). More than 400 peer-reviewed publications have been produced based on TBI Model Systems of Care research, and an additional 155 peer-reviewed manuscripts using the national database have been published.

Rehabilitation psychology has underappreciated and used the larger administrative data sets to explore population-based issues of impairment, activity restriction, and participation using primarily self-report measures that match well with the ICF model. Several databases that bear greater attention from the rehabilitation psychology community include (a) the BRFSS, the nation's premier system of health-related telephone surveys that collect state data about U.S. residents regarding their health-related risk behaviors, chronic health conditions, and use of preventive services; (b) the Disability and Health Data System, an online source of state-level data on adults with disabilities; (c) the U.S. Census Bureau American Community Survey, an ongoing national survey of U.S. households that includes information on demographic, socioeconomic, and housing information, and disability; (d) the National Health Interview Survey, a household survey of children and adults using personal interviews to collects information on a broad range of health topics, such as health insurance, doctor's office visits, physical activity, and other health behaviors, and includes disability questions; and (e) the National Health and Nutrition Examination Survey, an ongoing survey of adults and children that uses face-to-face interviews and physical examinations to assess health status, and includes disability questions.

Prevention

Although, as health service providers, rehabilitation psychologists have focused primarily on the health of individuals and their families, there have been efforts to embrace the public health principle of prevention. These efforts usually have focused on tertiary prevention, the prevention of secondary health conditions once an injury or illness has occurred (e.g., pressure sores following SCI) or the prevention of more severe disability (e.g., by providing assessment and advocacy to obtain workplace accommodations following the onset of multiple sclerosis). The data are still accumulating regarding the efficacy of these efforts across rehabilitation populations. However, promising studies have suggested that programs working in a secondary prevention model can have meaningful impact on both improving outcomes and controlling health care costs (Ravesloot, Seekins, & White, 2005; Wegener, Mackenzie, Ephraim, Ehde, & Williams, 2009). Significant work in field of occupational rehabilitation, partially inspired by the pioneering work of Fordyce (1995), has suggested that secondary prevention programs following the onset of acute pain can prevent transition to chronic pain and disability (Linton & van Tulder, 2001; Sullivan & Stanish, 2003).

With the growing use of opioids for chronic noncancer pain and the related abuse and mortality, there is an opportunity for rehabilitation psychologists to work in the quaternary prevention model to prevent opioid overtreatment and resulting health problems. Several classes of intervention have demonstrated initial efficacy in reducing opioid overuse, and all have a potential role for rehabilitation psychologists (Atluri, Akbik, & Sudarshan, 2012). Prescription monitoring programs (PMPs) are statewide databases being implemented in most states; they contain prescriber and patient-level prescription data on select drugs of abuse. Health professionals can use these databases to monitor patients' drug use and identify patients with prescription drug use patterns indicative of abuse. Law enforcement can use PMPs to identify providers with unusual prescription patterns who may be engaging in illegal activities. The use of PMPs requires behavior change on the part of providers. Several studies have suggested that the use of the databases can impact opioid abuse and misuse (Reifler et al., 2012). Rehabilitation psychologists recognize the difficulty in changing behavior and can contribute to these efforts by contributing to the development and testing of interventions to modify prescriber behavior. Another approach to mitigating opioid misuse and abuse is the use of risk stratification tools to screen patients into high-, medium-, and low-risk categories (Manchikanti, Atluri, Trescot, & Giordano, 2008; Passik, Kirsh, & Casper, 2008). Although there is significant variation in the psychometric data regarding individual tools, several instruments have adequate psychometric properties, sensitivity, and specificity for use in clinical work. Here, rehabilitation psychologists can contribute at the health system level by designing and implementing integrated screening programs and assist at the patient care level by assisting in clinical decision making.

The expertise of rehabilitation psychologists in assessing disability has the potential to enrich public health policy-relevant activities (e.g., developing new instruments to determine a child's disability/impairments and family resources to be eligible for the state's Medicaid home-based personal care services program). Rehabilitation psychologists will need to demonstrate their value by applying their principles, knowledge, and skills to focus on population health. These examples provide a notion of the scope of activity that rehabilitation psychologists can engage in when working in a public health prevention mode. Rehabilitation psychologists have behavior change, program management and evaluation, and advocacy skills that assist in the primary prevention of injury, secondary and tertiary prevention following illness or injury, and quaternary prevention in areas ranging from chronic pain (Sullivan & Stanish, 2003) to brain injury (Brenner, Homaifar, Adler, Wolfman, & Kemp, 2009).

Surveillance and Screening

Screening procedures intended to capture the scope of disability have evolved in recent years. Rehabilitation psychologists are well positioned to ensure a sound underlying theoretical basis for population-level disability screening tools and participate in the development and psychometric evaluation of screening procedures. The Washington Group on Disability Statistics (2006), established by the United Nations in 2001, endorsed an impairment-based set of questions intended to be used in capturing census-level screening data about disability. The Washington Group questions assess difficulties across six functional domains: vision, hearing, mobility, self-care, cognition, and communication. The benefit of this approach lies in its conciseness and the ability to identify potential cases warranting additional assessment. However, census data captured in this way have the limitation of being incomplete with regard to disability as a complex person-task-environment interaction. As a result, public health researchers often will follow up on positive screening results with a more detailed instrument, such as the 36-item interviewer-administered WHO Disability Assessment Schedule 2.0 (WHODAS 2.0; Ustun, Kostanjsek, Chatterji, & Rehm, 2010).

Collaborations between public health and rehabilitation psychology researchers can evaluate population-level surveillance and screening procedures by integrating the macrolevel focus of population-level surveillance with the foundational principles of screening procedures (Bentley, Bruyère,

LeBlanc, & MacLachlan, 2016). For example, the authors of this chapter collaborated with public health colleagues to evaluate the utility of population-level disability screening (e.g., Washington Group questions; Bachani et al., 2014) and surveillance procedures (e.g., WHO Disability Assessment Schedule 2.0; Bachani et al., 2016; Ustun et al., 2010) in rural Uganda, as well as to assess medical rehabilitation capacity in Ghana (Christian et al., 2016) Moreover, beyond screening and surveillance, rehabilitation psychologists have developed measures subsequently used in large-scale public health studies that elucidate the role of the physical and social environment in determining role participation (Gray, Gould, & Bickenbach, 2003; Simeonsson, Carlson, Huntington, McMillen, & Brent, 2001; Whiteneck et al., 2004).

Person–Environment Focus

Principles of public health highlight the importance of environmental interventions in the context of a person's chronic health condition, a concept that has been apparent to rehabilitation psychologists for decades (Lewin, 1935; Wright, 1983). Perhaps most notably, Kurt Lewin (1935) provided a now classic framework for understanding person–environment interactions through the heuristic quasimathematical formula $B = f(P, E)$ in which B represents an observable behavior, P represents all within-person factors influencing behavior (e.g., states and traits), and E represents external environmental factors in the surrounding physical and the social ecology. As described elsewhere (Bentley et al., 2016), Lewin's legacy at the intersection of rehabilitation psychology and public health is apparent in WHO's ICF model of disability. If rehabilitation psychologists are to take a more active role in community-based intervention and policy formation, they will need move beyond the medical model and clinical role, and integrate a public health perspective. Rather than focus on the individual and aspects of the medical diagnosis, a contemporary public health approach takes an ecological view that evaluates for disparities to access to care, disparities in the type and quality of services offered, and disparities in subsequent outcomes that affect the health and well-being of persons with disabilities (McLeroy, Bibeau, Steckler, & Glanz, 1988). As Meyerson (1988) observed, "If . . . psychologists, like their counterparts in public health, orient themselves toward person environment interactions, so central to the Lewinian tradition, a new and even more favorable Zeitgeist for people with disabilities may be in the offing" (pp. 186–187; see Chapter 9, this volume).

Multisystemic Intervention

In considering possible points of contact between rehabilitation psychology and public health, there are opportunities to use frameworks provided by each discipline for understanding the life cycle of health programs and basic principles of outcome evaluation at various systemic levels. For example, Green and Kreuter (2005) developed the PRECEDE-PROCEED model for planning, implementing, and evaluating public health programs. The model has been used across a variety of health disciplines but remains underused in rehabilitation psychology research and practice. The name of the model is an acronym that describes its purpose: predisposing, reinforcing, and enabling constructs in educational/ecological diagnosis, and evaluation policy, regulatory, and organizational constructs in educational and environmental development. Put together, the elements of the PRECEDE-PROCEED model help to identify a target problem, screen for risks, and give direction to create change.

The model first identifies the main focus and the desirable outcome, and then lists potential factors, such as behavioral, lifestyle, or environmental, that may influence the outcomes. In turn, these factors are seen as being influenced by predisposing, enabling, and reinforcing factors. The model comprises eight phases: four program planning phases (e.g., PRECEDE) and four program evaluation phases (e.g., PROCEED). This model was developed to be flexible so that it can be applied from individual hospital program planning to the development of community-based interventions. As a result, it has diverse applications in health behavior research (Gielen, McDonald, Gary, & Bone, 2008) and has been used widely to develop community-based interventions, which is important because many publicly funded community-based interventions have shown to be both successful and cost-effective. The Trust for America's Health (2009) conducted a study in which it found that investing $10 per person per year in evidence-based community health programs that target specific health behaviors (e.g., increased physical activity, improved nutrition, tobacco use prevention and cessation) resulted in an excess of $16 billion saved within 5 years.

An example from the early psychotherapy literature serves to illustrate the consideration of health outcomes from a perspective relevant to an integrative view of public health and rehabilitation psychology. Strupp and Hadley (1977) provided a tripartite view of a mental health and model for evaluating therapeutic outcomes. One distinctive element of the model pertained to identifying stakeholders in defining mental health: society, individual health care consumers, and mental health professionals. Each of these stakeholders has distinct value assumptions that influence whether an outcome is viewed as successful or not. Society often values "behavioral stability, predictability, and conformity to the social code" (p. 188). Individuals receiving mental health care services value improvement in their own sense of personal well-being. Mental health care providers are focused most on the application of procedures designed to influence a problematic behavior/experience or some unobservable psychological target. (Of historical note, Strupp & Hadley, 1977, used the term *personality structure* as a reflection of their psychodynamic orientation.) Of course, providers also value adaptation to the social environment and enhancement of subjective well-being but are focused primarily on assisting people to conform to a theory-driven view of health. Conflict can emerge based on the extent that each of these perspectives is in alignment or in tension with one another. For Strupp and Hadley, resolution occurs when each of these perspectives is considered simultaneously and when the inherent limitations of each perspective are acknowledged.

A more recent model of having a multidimensional view of health outcomes is the "Triple Aim" championed by the Institute for Healthcare Improvement (n.d.). The model calls for simultaneous pursuit of high-quality patient experience, improved patient outcomes, and reduced costs. Some have extended this model to add a fourth aim-improved provider satisfaction (Bodenheimer & Sinsky, 2014).

Both Strupp and Hadley (1977) and the Institute for Healthcare Improvement's (n.d.) Triple Aim capture a key principle of public health: that health care outcomes need to be considered from multiple perspectives and that both individual and societal impacts of health care decisions need to be considered. This multidimensional view of health outcomes is important in two ways. The model reminds us that individuals seeking care, providers, and society have different outcomes of interest and all need to be considered when planning treatment and assessing outcome. Recent shifts in health care toward patient-centered treatment have heightened the attention to patients' values and goals, which have been lost in a provider-driven health care system. The patient is becoming to be seen as the key stakeholder whose needs and wishes take precedent whenever possible. The shift in policy toward patient-centered approaches has contributed to health systemwide reflection on basic value assumptions and their interface with the individual's right to guide effective health care practices. The contemporary care provider now assumes the role of expert advisor with perhaps less emphasis on the power/influence denoted by the term *expert* than in the past. At the societal level, the drive toward evidence-based practices influences the redefinition of illness and, by extension, the evaluation of treatment efficacy.

Policy Influence

Rehabilitation psychology has a long history of policy influence that can be observed at the local, national, and international levels (see Chapter 24, this volume). Contributions of principles inherent to the field can be seen in the development of the ADA in the United States, ICF model of disability (WHO, 2001), and *World Report on Disability* (World Health Organization & World Bank, 2011). Social justice themes of advocacy and activism are central to the mission of rehabilitation psychology. Indeed, the current vision statement of the American

Psychological Association (APA) Division of Rehabilitation Psychology includes aspirations to

- be the premier source of psychological knowledge regarding disability and chronic health conditions for health care professionals, policymakers, the public, and the media; and
- champion disability as a human rights and social justice issue (see http://www.div22.org/mission-and-vision-statements/).

Opportunities for policy intervention abound in this era of health care reform. Major questions remain in the United States regarding insurance plan availability, structure of disability payments, infrastructure, and access to services among marginalized and minority populations with chronic illness and disability. Contribution to these large-scale areas of need can take many forms. For example, in describing the implications of the *World Report* for rehabilitation psychology, MacLachlan and Mannan (2014) identified promotion of research utilization as a means to assist people with disabilities in advocating to have their own needs met. From this perspective, research use that directly includes persons with disabilities creates a reciprocal process for empirical study to inform policy. Advocacy becomes evidence based, research findings extend to the practical end of policy development/revision, and policy has a data-driven foundation that gives rise to emerging research in needed topic areas. International examples of this process highlight the potential for such an approach (Mannan, Amin, MacLachlan, & the EquitAble Consortium, 2011).

From a broader perspective, rehabilitation psychologists have a number of pathways to contribution. Advocacy for policies that provide coverage of mental health and substance use disorders, as outlined in the Paul Wellstone and Pete Domenici Mental Health Parity and Addiction Equity Act of 2008, prohibit preexisting medical conditions as health insurance policy exclusionary criteria and disallow lifetime or annual dollar limits on coverage. These policies are particularly salient to the populations served in rehabilitation psychology. This advocacy can be done through any number of grassroots mechanisms, including sending signed letters to local and national representatives or service on professional organization councils and committees. The American Public Health Association, for example, has a disability section that for years has advocated for topics that parallel rehabilitation psychology interests. Within APA, there are three government relations offices (i.e., Education, Public Interest, and Science) and two APA-affiliated organizations (i.e., APA Practice Organization and Education Advocacy Trust) that engage in advocacy activities. APA members interested in advocacy can sign up to receive federal updates and action alerts through the APA Federal Action Network (see http://cqrcengage.com/apapolicy/home). APA has published *A Psychologist's Guide to Federal Advocacy* (APA, 2014) and organized advocacy initiatives to reflect several core issues, including disability (http://www.apa.org/about/gr/issues/disability/index.aspx) and health disparities (http://www.apa.org/about/gr/issues/health-disparities/index.aspx).

CONCLUSION

The largest challenges rehabilitation psychology faces in U.S. health care today are not those of infectious disease but rather prevention and management of complex health conditions, chronic disease, and disability. Such prevention and management will require interdisciplinary perspectives and collaboration. It is clear from the material presented in this chapter and in other earlier writings (Frank, 1999; Lollar, 2008; Winett et al., 1989) that additional emphasis in rehabilitation psychology on the principles and tools of public health will broaden the impact of the field. Public health helps rehabilitation psychology to recognize the important environmental, social, and economic factors in health and health care (see Chapter 25, this volume). It reminds us of the value of data and epidemiological approaches in understanding health problems and tracking progress of individuals and populations. Furthermore, it reinforces the importance of social justice in practice and policy.

Although threads of population- and policy-level intervention clearly are present in the historical roots of rehabilitation psychology, many of the daily activities of rehabilitation psychologists focus primarily on assessment, intervention, and consultation at the individual or family levels. Efforts to balance this important work with attention to macrolevel prevention and intervention will enable rehabilitation psychology to more fully realize its potential and sphere of influence. Rehabilitation psychology like much of health care (and indeed recapitulating the evolution of public health over time) has moved from doing things for people to doing things to people, and now doing things with people. Infusing rehabilitation psychology teaching, research, practice, and advocacy with the spirit and tools of public health will help the field to stay in touch with its roots and expand its reach.

References

American Psychological Association. (2014). *A psychologist's guide to federal advocacy*. Washington, DC: American Psychological Association, Education Government Relations Office & Public Interest Government Relations Office.

Americans With Disabilities Act of 1990, 42 U.S.C.A. § 1201 *et seq.* (West 1993).

Association of Schools & Programs of Public Health, Education Committee. (2006). *Master's degree in public health core competency development project (Version 2.3)*. Retrieved from https://s3.amazonaws.com/aspph-wp-production/app/uploads/2014/04/Version2.31_FINAL.pdf

Atluri, S., Akbik, H., & Sudarshan, G. (2012). Prevention of opioid abuse in chronic non-cancer pain: An algorithmic, evidence based approach. *Pain Physician, 15*, ES177–ES189.

Bachani, A. M., Galiwango, E., Kadobera, D., Bentley, J. A., Bishai, D., Wegener, S., & Hyder, A. A. (2014). A new screening instrument for disability in low-income and middle-income settings: Application at the Iganga-Mayuge Demographic Surveillance System (IM-DSS), Uganda. *BMJ Open*, *4*, e005795. http://dx.doi.org/10.1136/bmjopen-2014-005795

Bachani, A. M., Galiwango, E., Kadobera, D., Bentley, J. A., Bishai, D., Wegener, S., . . . Hyder, A. A. (2016). Characterizing disability at the Iganga-Mayuge Demographic Surveillance System (IM-DSS), Uganda. *Disability and Rehabilitation*, *38*, 1291–1299. http://dx.doi.org/10.3109/09638288.2015.1079928

Bentley, J. A., Bruyère, S. M., LeBlanc, J., & MacLachlan, M. (2016). Globalizing rehabilitation psychology: Application of foundational principles to global health and rehabilitation challenges. *Rehabilitation Psychology*, *61*, 65–73. http://dx.doi.org/10.1037/rep0000068

Bodenheimer, T., & Sinsky, C. (2014). From triple to quadruple aim: Care of the patient requires care of the provider. *Annals of Family Medicine*, *12*, 573–576. http://dx.doi.org/10.1370/afm.1713

Brenner, L. A., Homaifar, B. Y., Adler, L. E., Wolfman, J. H., & Kemp, J. (2009). Suicidality and veterans with a history of traumatic brain injury: Precipitating events, protective factors, and prevention strategies. *Rehabilitation Psychology*, *54*, 390–397.

CDC Foundation. (n.d.). What is public health? Retrieved from http://www.cdcfoundation.org/content/what-public-health

Centers for Disease Control and Prevention. (2014). *Behavioral Risk Factor Surveillance System. Overview: BRFSS 2013*. Atlanta, GA: Author. Retrieved from https://www.cdc.gov/brfss/annual_data/2013/pdf/overview_2013.pdf

Christian, A., Bentley, J. A., Aryeetey, R., Ackuaku, D., Mayer, R., & Wegener, S. (2016). Assessment of rehabilitation capacity in Ghana. *Disability, CBR and Inclusive Development*, *27*, 33–60. http://dx.doi.org/10.5463/dcid.v1i1.494

Courtney-Long, E. A., Romano, S. D., Carroll, D. D., & Fox, M. H. (2017). Socioeconomic factors at the intersection of race and ethnicity influencing health risks for people with disabilities. *Journal of Racial and Ethnic Health Disparities*, *4*, 213–222.

Fordyce, W. E. (Ed.). (1995). *Back pain in the workplace: Management of disability in nonspecific conditions. A report of the Task Force on Pain in the Workplace of the International Association for the Study of Pain*. Seattle, WA: International Association for the Study of Pain.

Frank, R. G. (1999). Rehabilitation psychology: We zigged when we should have zagged. *Rehabilitation Psychology*, *44*, 36–51. http://dx.doi.org/10.1037/0090-5550.44.1.36

Gielen, A. C., McDonald, E. M., Gary, T. L., & Bone, L. R. (2008). Using the precede-proceed model to apply health behavior theories. In K. Glanz, B. K. Rimer, K. Viswanath, K. Glanz, B. K. Rimer, & K. Viswanath (Eds.), *Health behavior and health education: Theory, research, and practice* (4th ed., pp. 407–433). San Francisco, CA: Jossey-Bass.

Giugliano, D., & Esposito, K. (2011). Clinical inertia as a clinical safeguard. *JAMA*, *305*, 1591–1592. http://dx.doi.org/10.1001/jama.2011.490

Gray, D. B., Gould, M., & Bickenbach, J. E. (2003). Environmental barriers and disability. *Journal of Architectural and Planning Research*, *20*, 29–37.

Green, L. W., & Kreuter, M. W. (2005). *Health program planning: An educational and ecological approach*. Columbus, OH: McGraw-Hill.

Institute for Healthcare Improvement. (n.d.). *IHI Triple Aim initiative: Better care for individuals, better health for populations, lower per capita costs*. Retrieved from http://www.ihi.org/Engage/Initiatives/TripleAim/Pages/default.aspx

Iwarsson, S., & Ståhl, A. (2003). Accessibility, usability and universal design—Positioning and definition of concepts describing person–environment relationships. *Disability and Rehabilitation, 25*, 57–66. http://dx.doi.org/10.1080/dre.25.2.57.66

Jamoulle, M. (2015). Quaternary prevention, an answer of family doctors to overmedicalization. *International Journal of Health Policy and Management, 4*, 61–64. http://dx.doi.org/10.15171/ijhpm.2015.24

Jamoulle, M., & Roland, M. (1995). *Quaternary prevention* [Unpublished manuscript for Wonca International Classification Committee annual workshop, Hong Kong, China]. Retrieved from http://hdl.handle.net/2268/173994

Kahn, E. B., Ramsey, L. T., Brownson, R. C., Heath, G. W., Howze, E. H., Powell, K. E., . . . Corso, P. (2002). The effectiveness of interventions to increase physical activity. A systematic review. *American Journal of Preventive Medicine, 22*, 73–107. http://dx.doi.org/10.1016/S0749-3797(02)00434-8

Lewin, K. (1935). *A dynamic theory of personality*. New York, NY: McGraw-Hill.

Linton, S. J., & van Tulder, M. W. (2001). Preventive interventions for back and neck pain problems: What is the evidence? *Spine, 26*, 778–787. http://dx.doi.org/10.1097/00007632-200104010-00019

Lollar, D. (2008). Rehabilitation psychology and public health: Commonalities, barriers, and bridges. *Rehabilitation Psychology, 53*, 122–127. http://dx.doi.org/10.1037/0090-5550.53.2.122

Mace, R. (1985). Universal design, barrier-free environments for everyone. *Designers West, 33*, 147–152.

MacLachlan, M., & Mannan, H. (2014). The *World Report on Disability* and its implications for rehabilitation psychology. *Rehabilitation Psychology, 59*, 117–124. http://dx.doi.org/10.1037/a0036715

Manchikanti, L., Atluri, S., Trescot, A. M., & Giordano, J. (2008). Monitoring opioid adherence in chronic pain patients: Tools, techniques, and utility. *Pain Physician, 11*, S155–S180.

Mann, J., Balte, P., Clarkson, J., Nitcheva, D., Graham, C. L., & McDermott, S. (2015). What are the specific disability and limitation types underlying responses to the BRFSS disability questions? *Disability and Health Journal, 8*, 17–28. http://dx.doi.org/10.1016/j.dhjo.2014.06.007

Mannan, H., Amin, M., MacLachlan, M., & the EquitAble Consortium. (2011). *The EquiFrame manual: A tool for evaluating and promoting the inclusion of vulnerable groups and core concepts of human rights in health policy documents*. Dublin, Ireland: Global Health Press.

McLeroy, K. R., Bibeau, D., Steckler, A., & Glanz, K. (1988). An ecological perspective on health promotion programs. *Health Education Quarterly, 15*, 351–377. http://dx.doi.org/10.1177/109019818801500401

Meyerson, L. (1988). The social psychology of the physical disability: 1948 and 1988. *Journal of Social Issues, 44*, 173–188. http://dx.doi.org/10.1111/j.1540-4560.1988.tb02056.x

Office of Disease Prevention and Health Promotion. (n.d.). Disability and health. Retrieved from https://www.healthypeople.gov/2020/topics-objectives/topic/disability-and-health/objectives

Office of Disease Prevention and Health Promotion. (2017). Disability and health. In *Healthy People 2020: Midcourse review*. Retrieved from https://www.cdc.gov/nchs/data/hpdata2020/HP2020MCR-C09-DH.pdf

Ovbiagele, B., & Nguyen-Huynh, M. N. (2011). Stroke epidemiology: Advancing our understanding of disease mechanism and therapy. *Neurotherapeutics, 8*, 319–329. http://dx.doi.org/10.1007/s13311-011-0053-1

Passik, S. D., Kirsh, K. L., & Casper, D. (2008). Addiction-related assessment tools and pain management: Instruments for screening, treatment planning, and monitoring compliance. *Pain Medicine, 9*, S145–S166. http://dx.doi.org/10.1111/j.1526-4637.2008.00486.x

Paul Wellstone and Pete Domenici Mental Health Parity and Addiction Equity Act of 2008. P.L. No. 110-343, 122 Stat. 3765 (2008).

Randolph, D. S., & Andresen, E. M. (2004). Disability, gender, and unemployment relationships in the United States from the Behavioral Risk Factor Surveillance System. *Disability & Society, 19*, 403–414. http://dx.doi.org/10.1080/0968759041000168949

Ravesloot, C., Seekins, T., & White, G. (2005). Living well with a disability health promotion intervention: Improved health status for consumers and lower costs for health care policymakers. *Rehabilitation Psychology, 50*, 239–245. http://dx.doi.org/10.1037/0090-5550.50.3.239

Reach, G., Pechtner, V., Gentilella, R., Corcos, A., & Ceriello, A. (2017). Clinical inertia and its impact on treatment intensification in people with type 2 diabetes mellitus. *Diabetes & Metabolism, 43*, 501–511. http://dx.doi.org/10.1016/j.diabet.2017.06.003

Reifler, L. M., Droz, D., Bailey, J. E., Schnoll, S. H., Fant, R., Dart, R. C., & Bucher Bartelson, B. (2012). Do prescription monitoring programs impact state trends in opioid abuse/misuse? *Pain Medicine, 13*, 434–442. http://dx.doi.org/10.1111/j.1526-4637.2012.01327.x

Sanford, J. A. (2012). *Universal design as a rehabilitation strategy: Design for the ages*. New York, NY: Springer.

Simeonsson, R. J., Carlson, D., Huntington, G. S., McMillen, J. S., & Brent, J. L. (2001). Students with disabilities: A national survey of participation in school activities. *Disability and Rehabilitation*, *23*, 49–63. http://dx.doi.org/10.1080/09638280175005 8134

Story, M. F., Mueller, J. L., & Mace, R. L. (1998). *The universal design file: Designing for people of all ages and abilities*. Raleigh, NC: Center for Universal Design, North Carolina State University. Retrieved from http://files.eric.ed.gov/fulltext/ED460554.pdf

Strupp, H. H., & Hadley, S. W. (1977). A tripartite model of mental health and therapeutic outcomes. With special reference to negative effects in psychotherapy. *American Psychologist*, *32*, 187–196. http://dx.doi.org/10.1037/0003-066X.32.3.187

Sullivan, M. J., & Stanish, W. D. (2003). Psychologically based occupational rehabilitation: The pain–disability prevention program. *Clinical Journal of Pain*, *19*, 97–104. http://dx.doi.org/10.1097/00002508-200303000-00004

Takaro, T. K., Krieger, J., Song, L., Sharify, D., & Beaudet, N. (2011). The breathe-easy home: The impact of asthma-friendly home construction on clinical outcomes and trigger exposure. *American Journal of Public Health*, *101*, 55–62. http://dx.doi.org/10.2105/AJPH.2010.300008

The Traumatic Brain Injury Model Systems [Slides of National Database Update]. (2016). Retrieved from https://www.tbindsc.org/StaticFiles/Documents/2016%20TBIMS%20Slide%20Presentation.pdf

The Trust for America's Health. (2009). *Prevention for a Healthier America: Investments in disease prevention yield significant savings, stronger communities*. Retrieved from https://www.tfah.org/report-details/prevention-for-a-healthier-america/

U.S. Department of Health and Human Services. (2012). *Principles of epidemiology in public health practice: An introduction to applied epidemiology and biostatistics* (3rd ed.). Atlanta, GA: Centers for Disease Control and Prevention. Retrieved from https://www.cdc.gov/ophss/csels/dsepd/ss1978/ss1978.pdf

Ustun, T. B., Kostanjsek, N., Chatterji, S., & Rehm, J. (2010). *Measuring health and disability: Manual for WHO Disability Assessment Schedule (WHODAS 2.0)*. Geneva, Switzerland: World Health Organization; Retrieved from http://whqlibdoc.who.int/publications/2010/97892 41547598_eng.pdf

Washington Group on Disability Statistics. (2006). *Overview of implementation protocols for testing the Washington Group Short Set of Questions on Disability*. Hyattsville, MD: Centers for Disease Control National Center for Health Statistics.

Wegener, S. T., Mackenzie, E. J., Ephraim, P., Ehde, D., & Williams, R. (2009). Self-management improves outcomes in persons with limb loss. *Archives of Physical Medicine and Rehabilitation*, *90*, 373–380. http://dx.doi.org/10.1016/j.apmr.2008.08.222

Whiteneck, G. G., Harrison-Felix, C. L., Mellick, D. C., Brooks, C. A., Charlifue, S. B., & Gerhart, K. A. (2004). Quantifying environmental factors: A measure of physical, attitudinal, service, productivity, and policy barriers. *Archives of Physical Medicine and Rehabilitation*, *85*, 1324–1335. http://dx.doi.org/10.1016/j.apmr.2003.09.027

Winett, R. A., King, A. C., & Altman, D. G. (1989). *Health psychology and public health: An integrative approach*. New York, NY: Pergamon Press.

World Health Organization. (2001). *International Classification of Functioning, Disability and Health: ICF*. Geneva, Switzerland: Author.

World Health Organization & World Bank. (2011). *World report on disability*. Geneva, Switzerland: Author. Retrieved from http://whqlibdoc.who.int/publications/2011/9789240685215_eng.pdf

Wright, B. A. (1983). *Physical disability: A psychosocial approach* (2nd ed.). New York, NY: HarperCollins. http://dx.doi.org/10.1037/10589-000

CHAPTER 27

REHABILITATION PSYCHOLOGISTS IN PUBLIC SERVICE

Kathleen S. Brown, Hannah R. Martinez, and Patrick H. DeLeon

Over the past 70 years, the practice of rehabilitation has undergone dramatic changes secondary to medical and technological advancements. At the same time, work done for the *World Report on Disability* (World Health Organization [WHO], 2011a) suggests that the prevalence of disability is increasing, with the population of those living with disabilities being more diverse and vulnerable. Individuals with disabilities have been shown to have worse health and socioeconomic outcomes and face widespread barriers in accessing services (WHO, 2011a). Moreover, because of the gradual rise of debilitating chronic health conditions and costs of health care, as well as increases in combat- and work-related disabilities, how and where rehabilitation services are delivered has also evolved. In turn, resources needed to facilitate the care for those with disability and chronic health conditions often outstrip allocated resources. High cost and limited coverage for acute and post-acute care for co-occurring physical, neurological, sensory, and psychological symptoms contribute to this problem (Gutenbrunner, Blumenthal, Geng, & Egen, 2017). Moreover, costly yet necessary services, such as "dental care, hearing and vision services, and long-term services and supports," are often not covered, resulting in missed opportunities for prevention and maintaining/facilitating function (Willink, Davis, Schoen, & Wolff, 2016, p. 849).

Nearly 27% of working-age people with disabilities were employed in 2013, and an additional 15% were unemployed but actively seeking work (U.S. Department of Labor, Bureau of Labor Statistics, 2014). Psychosocial challenges are associated with the reality that people with disabilities are more often unemployed or greatly underemployed compared with their peers without disabilities, creating a significant loss of income, social and economic participation, and equality for people with disabilities (Theis, Roblin, Helmick, & Luo, 2017). The purpose of the Americans With Disabilities Act (ADA, 1990) was to change the culture of the United States to one of full inclusion of people with all types of disabilities. The law consists of five titles: employment, public services, transportation, public accommodations, and telecommunications. To date, it is the most comprehensive law concerning disability rights, requiring compliance by employers, business owners, and providers of goods. Americans with disabilities report having greater access to goods and services from businesses, state and local governments, and their local communities since the inception of the ADA (National Council on Disability, 2007). However, there is much progress yet to be made given the complex array of demographic, fiscal, medical, technological, and other developments that continue to unfold nationally. A continuing catch-22 for many individuals with disabilities is that, despite often being well enough

http://dx.doi.org/10.1037/0000129-028
Handbook of Rehabilitation Psychology, Third Edition, L. A. Brenner, S. A. Reid-Arndt, T. R. Elliott, R. G. Frank, and B. Caplan (Editors-in-Chief)

to work at least part time, part-time work does not come with the benefits they need (Hastings, 2010). As people with chronic illnesses have higher medical costs than healthy individuals, economic disincentives to engage in the workforce remain.

In response to these changes, rehabilitation psychologists have the opportunity to assume leadership roles in clinical, administrative, academic, and public service settings. In these roles, they can advance service provision, resource allocation, education, and research and policy development, as well as the implementation of innovations. In this chapter, we discuss (a) the concept of "public service," and (b) the roles and activities that rehabilitation psychologists provide across public service authorities, with a specific emphasis on military, veteran, and criminal justice settings. We then highlight training opportunities available within the Veterans Health Administration (VHA). Finally, we discuss employment challenges faced by psychologists within public service settings, as well as opportunities they are afforded (e.g., publicly funded research, innovations).

REHABILITATION PSYCHOLOGISTS IN PUBLIC SERVICE

The American Psychological Association (APA) defined *public service psychology* as that which serves the needs of the general public, and specifically identifies the following authorities: (a) community and state hospitals, (b) the criminal justice systems, (c) police and public safety services, (d) American Indian country and Native American communities, and (e) the Departments of Defense and Veterans Affairs (Anderson, 2003). Services within these settings are provided within a network of psychological, biological, social, environmental, and political contexts. Rehabilitation psychologists who work in the public sector educate and train, as well as provide clinical care to and advocate for individuals experiencing disability and chronic health conditions (WHO, 2011b). They also conduct and disseminate research. As in other settings, assistance may be provided to aid individuals, their families, and caregivers within the social and community network to achieve rehabilitation goals through intervention. Individuals with a disability seeking care within the public sector who are working to increase access and participation may also benefit from the assistance of rehabilitation psychologists to address systemic inequalities related to accessing quality care in rural and/or indigenous communities. Rehabilitation psychologists are also called up to ensure that those in the criminal justice system received necessary accommodations and treatment. These efforts often include engaging in discourses regarding public policy.

Individuals with disabilities often seek public-sector resources to address basic physical, emotional, social, and job-related needs. Frequently, however, there is a lack of fit between individuals' health needs and the resources provided by the public health care and medical financing systems designed to provide and pay for acute and postacute care (Gutenbrunner et al., 2017). Funding systems and payment criteria can influence what services are provided, and specialty providers are available to provide rehabilitative care, resulting in inequalities in rehabilitation service delivery. Variations in the provision of rehabilitation services can also result from who owns such services (e.g., states, insurance companies, private sector, nongovernmental organizations), payment systems (e.g., per diem, per intervention, per case), specialization and roles of team members, and referral and case management systems (Gutenbrunner et al., 2017).

For example, suitable services for the long-term rehabilitation care for individuals with spinal cord injury (SCI) in a rural community ideally should be available within the communities in which they live. Frequent complications of SCI, such as neurogenic bladder and bowel, urinary tract infections, pressure ulcers, orthostatic hypotension, spasticity and autonomic dysreflexia, would be handled in the community hospital, which may be the only source of medical care. This often results in the individual with SCI seeking urgent or emergency care, which drives up costs for both the patients and the facility. Such services are primarily biomedically focused and can make it difficult for patients to get regular and more comprehensive biopsychosocial follow-up care to enhance their long-term adaptation and integration into the community. Without consistent specialized care, potential complications such as depression, substance abuse, and suicidal thoughts or behaviors may be overlooked or negatively impacted by professional biases (Nas, Yazmalar, Şah, Aydin, & Öneş, 2015). Moreover, adequate personal care, or access to specialized equipment or resources that could facilitate independent functioning and community participation, may be either unavailable or unaffordable (for further discussion of community participation, see Chapter 8, this volume).

Gutenbrunner and colleagues (2015) proposed an international classification framework of health-related rehabilitation service delivery to classify and compare service organizations at the regional, national, and international levels. Such a classification system facilitates comparisons between disciplines, services, and funding sources, independent of geography, to identify the critical elements of effectiveness and impact in the delivery of rehabilitation care within the public domain. The framework uses three dimensions divided into 20 categories: first, the service provider (location, organization, context, facility, human resources, technical resources and equipment, quality assurance, profit orientation, and other categories of provider); second, the funding of the service (source of money, criteria of cost refund, and other criteria of funding); and third, the service delivery (strategy, target groups, service goals, aspects of time, intensity, team structure, mode of production, and other categories of service delivery). Rehabilitation psychologists must be a part of a consensus process, in collaboration with other professionals, to develop a comprehensive rehabilitation classification system that can then be used to develop health care policy for necessary rehabilitative services, compare rehabilitation services worldwide, and identify gaps in rehabilitation systems.

REHABILITATION PSYCHOLOGY PRACTICE WITHIN THE DEPARTMENT OF DEFENSE'S MILITARY HEALTH SYSTEM AND THE DEPARTMENT OF VETERANS AFFAIRS' VETERANS HEALTH ADMINISTRATION

The mission of the Department of Defense's (DoD) Military Health System (MHS) is to maintain the health of military personnel so they can carry out their military missions. These include delivering health care during wartime and providing support to military families and retirees entrusted to its care (MHS, Defense Health Agency, 2017). The MHS relies on approximately 2,000 military and civilian psychologists to provide programs vital to the health and well-being of the members of the U.S. Armed Forces and their families (MHS, Defense Health Agency, 2017). These programs include behavioral health care for posttraumatic stress, suicide prevention, substance abuse, and domestic violence, as well as programs that address the specialized needs of children. Psychologists in the DoD are often required to function both as generalists and specialists (Cronin, 1998). They are expected to provide a wide range of nontraditional services in nontraditional contexts. Settings are varied, with psychologists serving in medical hospitals and clinics, teaching within service training schools on military bases, supporting counterintelligence investigations and operations, and conducting administrative duties while stationed in headquarter command posts.

Fitness for duty is the primary criterion for active-duty service. With advances in medical technology and improved prosthetics, the trend in military culture is to keep seriously wounded soldiers or soldiers with disability on active duty. There are a variety of specialized programs and services designed by the military and the Department of Veterans Affairs (VA) to help severely injured service members transition back to duty or, post–military discharge, to transition back to civilian life. For those in wounded-warrior programs, the delivery of psychosocial rehabilitation is grounded in theories of learning and the building of character to cope with community (Penk & Little, 2013). Psychosocial rehabilitation focuses on the functioning of the person as he or she interacts with family, friends, coworkers, and the community. Such programs are designed to help wounded warriors overcome barriers and access resources to improve quality of living for themselves, for families and friends, with peers and coworkers, and with their community in order to requalify as fit for duty.

Whereas psychologists in the DoD are focused on keeping a workforce healthy, the Veterans Health Administration (VHA) mission is to provide America's veterans with high-quality health care post–military service. The VHA implements the medical benefits program of VA through the administration and operation of numerous VA medical centers, outpatient clinics, community-based outpatient clinics, and community living centers (nursing homes), as well as non-VA medical facilities. The VHA employs approximately 1,200 psychologists. Within the APA, Veterans' Affairs Psychologists is the largest section of its Division 18 (Public Service). VA behavioral health care uses a recovery-oriented model based on principles of psychosocial rehabilitation, with goals defined by the veteran in collaboration with the treatment team.

Many veterans, particularly those who have been recently deployed, experience comorbid physical, psychological, and neurocognitive problems that significantly impact their functioning (Holdeman, 2009; Lew et al., 2009; Thomas et al., 2010). In response, the VHA has expanded services across outpatient, residential, and inpatient settings; and provides multiple entry points for care, including 300 Veteran Centers that provide readjustment counseling, the Military and Veterans Crisis Line (call, text, chart), and VHA staff on college and university campuses (U.S. Department of Veterans Affairs, 2015). Proactive screening—to identify veterans who have symptoms of depression, have posttraumatic stress disorder (PTSD), have problem use of alcohol, are at risk for suicide, or have experienced military sexual trauma—facilitates engagement in care. The number of veterans receiving specialized mental health services continues to rise, with 900,000 in FY 2006 to more than 1.6 million in FY 2015 (U.S. Department of Veterans Affairs, 2017).

REHABILITATION PSYCHOLOGY PRACTICE WITHIN THE CRIMINAL JUSTICE SYSTEM

Within the criminal justice system, the purpose of rehabilitation is to prepare an individual to successfully reintegrate into society. To accomplish this, corrections systems provide professional services and programs aimed at restoring the individual to useful life functioning, while reducing the risk of recidivism. As with medical rehabilitation programs, the success of rehabilitation programs in the criminal justice system depends largely on the ability to identify and address specific inmate needs. The fit between an inmate's need and the service provided appears to be an important determinant of successful reentry (Gill & Wilson, 2017).

The Bureau of Justice Statistics is the primary source for statistics in the United States on crime, criminal offenders, victims of crime, and the operations of criminal justice systems at all levels of government. The National Inmate Survey-3 (NIS-3; U.S. Department of Justice, Bureau of Justice Statistics, 2015) was conducted in 233 state and federal prisons, 358 local jails, and 15 special confinement facilities operated by Immigration and Customs Enforcement (ICE), the U.S. military, and correctional authorities in American Indian country. As a part of the 2011–2012 survey, the NIS-3 assessed the prevalence of disabilities with other health problems, such as a current chronic condition, obesity, ever having an infectious disease, and past-30-day serious psychological distress (Maruschak, Berzofsky, & Unangst, 2015). To increase understanding regarding the number of individuals living with disabilities among incarcerated populations versus members of the noninstitutionalized general population, Maruschak, Berzofsky, and Unangst (2015) compared the NIS-3 data with the 2012 American Community Survey and 2009–2012 National Survey on Drug Use and Health (U.S. Department of Health and Human Services, Substance Abuse and Mental Health Services Administration, 2013, 2015). Prisoners were nearly 3 times more likely and jail inmates were more than 4 times more likely than members of the general population to report having at least one disability. An estimated 32% of prisoners and 40% of jail inmates reported having at least one disability. About two in 10 prisoners and three in 10 jail inmates reported having a cognitive disability, the most common reported disability in both populations. Prisoners who have had traumatic brain injuries (TBI) may experience mental health problems such as severe depression and anxiety, substance use disorders (Slaughter, Fann, & Ehde, 2003), difficulty controlling anger, or suicidal thoughts and/or attempts (Blaauw, Arensman, Kraaij, Winkel, & Bout, 2002). At the time of their arrest, 41% of male offenders and 52% of female offenders are under the influence of drugs, alcohol, or both (U.S. Department of Justice, Bureau of Justice Statistics, 2005). Women convicted of a violent crime are more likely to have sustained a precrime TBI and/or incurred some other form of physical abuse (Brewer-Smyth, Burgess, & Shults, 2004). Slaughter et al. (2003) highlighted the need for more research to tease out the role of TBI sequelae of anger, aggression, impulsivity, and memory loss in initial and recidivism rates in the criminal justice system. Recently, there has been an increase in research examining the relationship between TBI and involvement in the criminal justice system. However, much of this research remains largely retrospective and descriptive, such as by comparing rates of TBI in the offending population with the rates of TBI in the general population (Ray & Richardson, 2017). For further information regarding TBI, see Chapter 18, this volume.

There are limited data related to the prevalence of, impact on imprisonment, and available services for inmates with physical disabilities in state prisons. This is in part due to differences in definitions and screening tools used by different departments of corrections, along with the lack of reporting to obtain baselines for this population (Prins, 2014). Inmates with a physical disability may require greater resources, including special equipment (e.g., hearing aids, wheelchairs) and services (e.g., handicapped-accessible living areas and interpreters). Krienert, Henderson, and Vandiver (2003) found little consistency across states in the collection and maintenance of information pertaining to the number and types of disabilities found within institutional populations. At least half of the state departments of corrections that responded to their survey revealed that they did not keep figures with respect to how many inmates had disabilities. The results imply that many state departments of corrections might not be in full compliance with the mandates issued by Title II of the ADA, which requires government entities, including state and local correctional institutions, to make their facilities, programs, services, and activities accessible to both inmates and their visitors.

Although deserving of the same high standards of care as those in traditional mental health facilities, individuals with serious mental illnesses who are incarcerated pose major treatment challenges for both correctional personnel and health care providers. Approximately 20% of inmates in jails and 15% of inmates in state prisons are now estimated to have a serious mental illness (Kaeble, Glaze, Tsoutis, & Minton, 2016). James and Glaze (2006) reported that currently there are 10 times as many mentally ill people in prisons and jails in America than are in U.S. state hospitals. Individuals with mental illness who are incarcerated range from violent to nonviolent offenders, and from those who were born with disabilities to those who have been adversely impacted by circumstances and environment.

The punitive nature of imprisonment and social control inherent in the U.S. criminal justice system is incompatible with the supportive therapeutic milieus that the mentally ill need to rehabilitate. Imprisonment often causes punishing conditions, such as severe material deprivations, highly restricted movement and liberty, lack of meaningful activity, a nearly total absence of personal privacy, and high levels of interpersonal mistrust, danger, and fear. Such conditions can be powerful psychological stressors that can adversely impact a prisoner's well-being, even more so for those with premorbid mental health conditions. In many states, inmates with mental illness were found to be incarcerated longer than other prisoners due either to requiring a pretrial evaluation or restoration of competency to stand trial, or to having more difficulty following jail and prison rules secondary to impaired thinking (Council of State Governments, 2002). For example, in a study in Washington State prisons, mentally ill inmates accounted for 41% of infractions even though they constituted only 19% of the prison population. Inmates with mental illness are also disproportionately locked down in segregation, where they remain isolated in their cells and experience severely restricted access to programs and activities, including mental health treatment (Beck, 2015). Those inmates housed in segregation found their way there due to behaviors associated with a mental illness, or they developed symptoms of mental illness due to their prolonged isolation (Grassian, 2006).

Individuals with disabilities in the criminal justice system are underserved by rehabilitation psychologists. The foundational principles of rehabilitation psychology (Wright, 1983) can inform successful rehabilitation efforts toward lower recidivism and successful reentry into society (see Chapter 9, this volume). Promoting access to services such as attaining a basic education, entry-level job training through vocational rehabilitation, and life-skills programs (e.g., communication skills, household skills, budgeting, parenting techniques) for the development of prosocial behaviors to cope with emotions and develop alternative ways of thinking and acting have been shown to reduce rates of recidivism (Jensen & Reed, 2006).

Lack of treatment and rehabilitation for persons with TBI, physical disabilities, and mental health and substance abuse problems while incarcerated increases the probability that they will again abuse alcohol and/or drugs when released (U.S. Department of Health and Human Services, Substance Abuse and Mental Health Services Administration, 1998). Rehabilitation psychologists must continue to correctly identify the prevalence of TBI, as well as other disabilities and health conditions, in correctional populations; improve methods of screening in incarcerated populations; and develop efficacious treatment approaches, such as cognitive and behavioral therapies, pharmacotherapy, and vocational rehabilitation, in jail settings (Bogner & Corrigan, 2009; Slaughter et al., 2003). This could decrease the frequency and severity of mood and behavioral problems and potentially reduce recidivism rates. More involvement of rehabilitation psychologists at the state and federal levels would also add a disability perspective to the ongoing conversation about prison conditions, and inform national policymakers about the unique issues faced by inmates with disabilities and mental illness.

TRAINING REHABILITATION PSYCHOLOGISTS IN THE PUBLIC SECTOR

Marketplace changes in health care have reduced the number of opportunities for psychology internships and postdoctoral fellowships nationally, resulting in growing concerns about how psychology will ensure access to high-quality clinical training. Given the variability found in rehabilitation psychology training sites in a survey of U.S. and Canadian training programs, Stiers and Stucky (2008) urged the field to advocate for increased structure in and funding of training programs for rehabilitation psychology practice. A national conference was convened in 2011 to develop training guidelines for rehabilitation psychology designed to promote quality, consistency, and excellence in the education and training of rehabilitation psychologist practitioners, and to promote competence in their practice (Stiers et al., 2012). The Council of Rehabilitation Psychology Postdoctoral Training Programs was also established at that time to promote the adoption and implementation of these guidelines by training programs, and to formally recognize programs in compliance with the guidelines. A revised set of competencies for rehabilitation psychology that differs in both content and structure now guides the profession (see Chapter 1, this volume).

Nationally, VA has been the leader in advancing training for health professionals. Education and training of health care professionals for VA and for the nation is one of four statutory core missions of the Department of Veterans Affairs (formally, until 1989, the Veterans Administration) and one that VA has historically taken very seriously. As World War II was winding down, the nation was faced with a massive demobilization and return of veteran soldiers to the U.S. Lacking both capacity and staffing, VA initiated a program of academic affiliations with the nation's medical schools. This both brought health care professionals to VA and provided a vibrant training ground for medical students and residents. Simultaneously, psychology staffing was required to deal with the mental health and rehabilitation needs of returning veterans, and VA began to develop close affiliations with academic departments of psychology. It was largely as a result of VA's need to determine which psychology graduate programs were of high quality that the APA developed its initial accreditation program (Fowler, 2002). Currently, VA training opportunities are overseen by its Office of Academic Affiliations. Funding is allocated largely according to perceived employment needs. Thus, because psychology has been identified as a discipline with unfilled vacancies, VA psychology training programs have expanded substantially in recent years. Fifty percent (50%)

of U.S. psychologists and 70% of VA psychologists have had VA training prior to employment (U.S. Department of Veterans Affairs, VA Office of Academic Affiliations, 2017).

In the face of lengthy U.S. wars in Afghanistan and Iraq, there has been a national focus on the special needs of returning veterans with regard to mental and behavioral health issues as well as to rehabilitation (Sayer et al., 2009; Seal, Bertenthal, Miner, Sen, & Marmar, 2007; Seal et al., 2009). In response, VA committed to greatly enhanced mental health staffing and services nationally (Burnam, Meredith, Tanielian, & Jaycox, 2009). VA has long supported internship-level training in psychology, with 679 positions nationally. Psychology postdoctoral training was approved in 1992; however, it did not truly expand until the 2000–2001 academic year, when the number of funded postdoctoral residency positions expanded from five to 38. Numbers have since grown substantially: in 2016 there were approximately 440 positions at 67 VA sites in 32 states, Puerto Rico, and Washington, DC.

Because of the strength of psychology staff across the nation, psychology as a discipline was particularly poised to develop new internship and postdoctoral programs and to enhance existing ones (Baker & Pickren, 2007). In recent years, VA has increased its focus on developing training opportunities in smaller and more rural VA health care settings. These programs provide the same kinds of opportunities as do larger, more traditional programs; they are also intended to generate a cadre of health care professionals eager to remain in and serve in those smaller and more rural settings. It is the expectation of VA that each training program will achieve full accreditation within 3 years of its initial funding.

Postdoctoral training in VA ensures that these new professionals have the skills relevant and necessary for providing quality care for veterans but is also able to facilitate their recruitment into staffing vacancies. Continued efforts to increase federal funding for psychology graduate training will help ensure that psychology will be among those health care professions recognized and reimbursed appropriately under federal and state health care initiatives, and that it will remain relevant in the evolving health care environment.

Though training programs are overseen nationally, they are proposed and developed locally, depending largely on the particular skills and programs available at the specific site. Emphasis areas of postdoctoral residencies are broad and range from the traditional mental-health-focused, to behavioral health, SCI, TBI and polytrauma, PTSD, substance use disorders, homelessness, and rehabilitation for blindness. Though many of VA's postdoctoral residency programs offer training in various rehabilitation areas and settings, three of the six APA-accredited programs in the Rehabilitation Psychology Specialty are located in VA settings. All such accredited residencies are 2-year programs, in accord with standards for specialty accreditation in Rehabilitation Psychology.

EMPLOYMENT CHALLENGES IN PUBLIC SERVICE

In current federal and state legislation, psychologists are now viewed as "optional" rather than "mandatory" service providers (National Conference of State Legislatures, 2015). Therefore, as a profession, psychologists are often targets for personnel budget cuts. Psychologists must therefore learn to think in terms of both the costs incurred and the benefits derived from their employment. In human service settings, the bottom line for employment becomes, "Who can provide the most services at the lowest cost?" Rehabilitation psychologists must therefore learn how to market their profession by measuring outcomes, productivity, and cost-efficacy. In the public service sector, programs should empower individuals to become productive members of the community. Rehabilitation psychologists offer invaluable services, such as vocational assessments and vocational rehabilitation, that ensure individuals with disabilities do not become casualties of society (Rall, Reed, & Essex, 2016). To maintain funding, however, rehabilitation psychologists must identify what they are doing that is truly distinctive, necessary, income-generating, and/or cost-effective for their employers, in order to best advocate for those that they serve.

PUBLICLY FUNDED REHABILITATION RESEARCH

The National Institute on Disability, Independent Living and Rehabilitation Research (NIDILRR) is designed to promote knowledge that helps increase opportunities and appropriate support in communities for individuals with disabilities. The NDILRR has shifted its priorities to address innovative and emerging health delivery systems for those with severe disabilities. Such individuals remain a hard-to-serve population due to low provider-reimbursement rates that result in little financial incentive to serve this population well. Community-based interventions, services, and supports have not typically been reimbursable as they do not technically meet the definition of medical necessity (Kaye & Harrington, 2015). This mismatch between need and current financing models results in fragmented and duplicative care, preventable secondary conditions, and poorer health outcomes, all of which compromise cost containment and quality-of-life goals (Iglehart, 2011). The shift to new ways of providing health services across the continuum of care and of financing creates an exciting opportunity for rehabilitation psychologists to identify and investigate innovation occurring at the provider, program, and community levels.

INNOVATIONS IN PUBLIC SECTOR REHABILITATION PSYCHOLOGY

Health care as a whole is moving toward a new and exciting era that focuses not only on the collaboration of patient and provider but also on the integration of all facets of life in the healing process. Rehabilitation psychology has been instrumental in the shift of health care from a commodity to a way of life. The National Intrepid Center of Excellence (NICoE) at Walter Reed in Bethesda, Maryland, is tackling this merger in a number of ways. One important way is the use of service dogs in both the physical and emotional rehabilitation of veterans and military service members (Owen, Finton, Gibbons, & DeLeon, 2016). Rehabilitation psychology efforts at the NICoE focus on service members living with TBI, many of whom have a comorbid diagnosis of PTSD. Service dogs are trained to aid the veteran diagnosed with PTSD by patrolling the perimeter of a room to confirm its safety; turning on the lights to interrupt a veteran's nightmare; alerting the veteran to take medication at the proper times; or nudging the veteran when someone is unexpectedly approaching to prevent a startle response (Esnayra & Love, 2005). Service dogs are also trained to perform specific tasks for individuals with limited mobility, such as those who are blind or use wheelchairs. Psychologists can incorporate such alternative modes of treatment delivery and assess the impact on functional independence. Further research is needed to support the use of service dogs for symptom reduction and to optimize quality of life, particularly among those with PTSD. Such empirical evidence is needed to support policy changes for the use of this intervention (Marston & Kopicki, 2015).

In addition to their rigorous training for specific disability accommodations, service dogs have "pet" qualities that can increase positive social interactions for individuals restricted to wheelchairs who might be avoided in public places more often than those who are not. They are also used for individuals with less physically apparent conditions, such as diabetes or panic attacks. Rehabilitation psychologists are charged with efficiently using available resources in creative ways, such as recommending the use of a service dog and other adaptations to extend the safety and independence of an individual with a disability.

Innovative programs are not limited to the federal sector, however. States have launched and expanded programs to help veterans transition; to ensure them meaningful employment and access to proper physical and mental health services; and to support families in adjusting to their loved one's transition. Recent state initiatives have focused on the transfer of technical skills; access to higher education, housing, and career guidance and support; and hiring incentives for employers (Cook & Kim, 2009; Kidder & Carter, 2013; Montgomery, Hill, Kane, & Culhane, 2013). Rehabilitation services are being specifically addressed as well. For example, New Jersey launched an impressive initiative to tailor rehabilitation services to veterans who have been mandated to the criminal justice system (State of New Jersey, 2018). Rehabilitation psychologists work in and consult with state agencies to address needed programs and regulatory changes to further the missions of health departments and human services and their intersections with the criminal justice system to ensure that individuals with disabilities receive necessary care.

The growing accessibility of computer-assisted technology will change rehabilitation programs through the use of virtual-reality environments to enhance motor, cognitive, and psychological functioning. Increased survival rates following stroke or other traumas, and the increased lifespan of people living with diseases such as dementia and Parkinson's, have led to a growing prevalence of individuals with long-term conditions and long-term rehabilitation needs. As these long-term needs extend beyond the initial acute treatment phase, the need for interventions greatly exceeds therapy time available on an individual basis. Developing cost-effective and efficient therapeutic tools that allow individuals to engage in long-term home-based rehabilitation is increasingly important to meet rehabilitation demands. Research is needed to demonstrate whether virtual-reality technology extends the ability to influence the nervous system, or whether moving within a virtual environment simply motivates the individual to perform more optimally (Keshner, 2004). Technological advances in other platforms, such as implantable electromyographic (EMG) electrodes, EMG pattern recognition, targeted reinnervation, and powered exoskeletons that change restoration of function lost after a stroke or SCI, also raise questions about the implications of the increasing integration of technologies in the human body that need to be addressed at both conceptual and methodological levels (Gaggioli, 2017). As significant advancements occur in the fields of electronics, computing, and communications technologies at more affordable costs, research must address how best to integrate such technologies to meet the needs of patients, therapists, and other caregivers (see Chapters 30 and 31, this volume).

CONCLUSION

Serving in critical roles within the public sector, rehabilitation psychologists focus on rehabilitation and chronic disease management across the lifespan. Incorporating the opinions and values of the consumers is of upmost import. The nation's changing attitude toward health care is fostering an open-minded, creative environment for solving problems and improving outdated methods of delivering care. To make progress in how services are delivered in the public sector, however, will require institutions and government to think differently and be willing to relinquish techniques and tools that no longer work. Farrell and Goodman (2013) suggested four principles that public sector leaders should consider: the use of better evidence for decision making; greater engagement and empowerment of citizens; thoughtful investments in expertise and skill building; and closer collaboration with the private and social sectors. Each of these principles is important for creating more effective yet affordable systems and government. Innovations in rehabilitation psychology arise from resources already being used, consumer input and feedback, and new theoretical and technological advancements. Rehabilitation psychology has proven useful not only as a single component in the new configuration of health care, but as a contributor, an inspiration, and a partner across public systems of care. *Health*, defined as "a state of complete physical, mental, and social well-being and not merely the absence of disease or infirmity" (WHO, 1946), for the entire nation is ever growing within reach. During this evolution, rehabilitation psychologists serving within the public sector have the exciting opportunity to continue to lead the way in developing the highest possible quality of health care.

References

Americans With Disabilities Act of 1990, 42 U.S.C. § 12101 et seq.

Anderson, N. B. (2003, June). Division 18: A dedication to public service. *Monitor on Psychology, 34*(6). Retrieved from http://www.apa.org/monitor/jun03/rc.aspx

Baker, R. R., & Pickren, W. E. (2007). *Psychology and the Department of Veterans Affairs: A historical analysis of training, research, practice, and advocacy*. Washington, DC: American Psychological Association.

Beck, A. J. (2015). *Use of restrictive housing in U.S. prisons and jails, 2011–12*. United States Department of Justice, Bureau of Justice Statistics. Retrieved from https://www.bjs.gov/content/pub/pdf/urhuspj1112.pdf

Blaauw, E., Arensman, E., Kraaij, V., Winkel, F. W., & Bout, R. (2002). Traumatic life events and suicide risk among jail inmates: The influence of types of events, time period and significant others. *Journal of Traumatic Stress*, *15*, 9–16. http://dx.doi.org/10.1023/A:1014323009493

Bogner, J., & Corrigan, J. D. (2009). Reliability and predictive validity of the Ohio State University TBI identification method with prisoners. *Journal of Head Trauma Rehabilitation*, *24*, 279–291. http://dx.doi.org/10.1097/HTR.0b013e3181a66356

Brewer-Smyth, K., Burgess, A. W., & Shults, J. (2004). Physical and sexual abuse, salivary cortisol, and neurologic correlates of violent criminal behavior in female prison inmates. *Biological Psychiatry*, *55*, 21–31. http://dx.doi.org/10.1016/S0006-3223(03)00705-4

Burnam, M. A., Meredith, L. S., Tanielian, T., & Jaycox, L. H. (2009). Mental health care for Iraq and Afghanistan war veterans. *Health Affairs*, *28*, 771–782. http://dx.doi.org/10.1377/hlthaff.28.3.771

Cook, B. J., & Kim, Y. (2009). *From soldier to student: Easing the transition of service members on campus*. Washington, DC: American Association of State Colleges and Universities. Retrieved from https://www.acenet.edu/news-room/Documents/From-Soldier-to-Student-Easing-the-Transition-of-Service-Members-on-Campus.pdf

Council of State Governments. (2002). *Criminal justice/mental health consensus project*. Retrieved from https://www.ncjrs.gov/pdffiles1/nij/grants/197103.pdf

Cronin, C. (Ed.). (1998). *Military psychology: An introduction*. Needham Heights, MA: Ginn Press.

Esnayra, J., & Love, C. (2005). *A survey of mental health patients utilizing psychiatric service dogs*. Arlington, VA: Psychiatric Service Dog Society.

Farrell, D., & Goodman, A. (2013). *Government by design: Four principles for a better public sector*. Retrieved from https://www.mckinsey.com/industries/public-sector/our-insights/government-by-design-four-principles-for-a-better-public-sector

Fowler, R. D. (2002). APA and the VA: An enduring partnership. *Monitor on Psychology*, *33*(8), 9. Retrieved from http://www.apa.org/monitor/sep02/rc.aspx

Gaggioli, A. (2017). Cyborg-psychology. *Cyberpsychology, Behavior, and Social Networking*, *20*, 458. http://dx.doi.org/10.1089/cyber.2017.29078.csi

Gill, C., & Wilson, D. B. (2017). Improving the success of reentry programs: Identifying the impact of service–need fit on recidivism. *Criminal Justice and Behavior*, *44*, 336–359. http://dx.doi.org/10.1177/0093854816682048

Grassian, S. (2006). Psychiatric effects of solitary confinement. *Washington University Journal of Law & Policy*, *22*, 325–383. Retrieved from https://openscholarship.wustl.edu/cgi/viewcontent.cgi?article81362&context8law_journal_law_policy

Gutenbrunner, C., Bickenbach, J., Kiekens, C., Meyer, T., Skempes, D., Nugraha, B., . . . Stucki, G. (2015). ISPRM discussion paper: Proposing dimensions for an international classification system for service organization in health-related rehabilitation. *Journal of Rehabilitation Medicine*, *47*, 809–815. http://dx.doi.org/10.2340/16501977-2002

Gutenbrunner, C., Blumenthal, M., Geng, V., & Egen, C. (2017). Rehabilitation services provision and payment. *American Journal of Physical Medicine & Rehabilitation*, *96*(2, Suppl. 1), S35–S40. http://dx.doi.org/10.1097/PHM.0000000000000668

Hastings, R. R. (2010). *Has the Americans with Disability Act made a difference?* Society for Human Resource Management. Retrieved from https://www.shrm.org/resourcesand tools/hr-topics/behavioral-competencies/global-and-culturaleffectiveness/pages/hastheadamadeadifference.aspx

Holdeman, T. C. (2009). Review of Invisible wounds of war: Psychological and cognitive injuries, their consequences, and services to assist recovery. *Psychiatric Services*, *60*, 273. http://dx.doi.org/10.1176/ps.2009.60.2.273

Iglehart, J. K. (2011). Desperately seeking savings: States shift more Medicaid enrollees to managed care. *Health Affairs*, *30*, 1627–1629. http://dx.doi.org/10.1377/hlthaff.2011.0836

James, D. J., & Glaze, L. E. (2006). *Mental health problems of prison and jail inmates*. U.S. Department of Justice, Bureau of Justice Statistics. Retrieved from https://www.bjs.gov/content/pub/pdf/mhppji.pdf

Jensen, E. L., & Reed, G. E. (2006). Adult correctional education programs: An update on current status based on recent studies. *Journal of Offender Rehabilitation*, *44*, 81–98. http://dx.doi.org/10.1300/J076v44n01_05

Kaeble, D., Glaze, L., Tsoutis, A., & Minton, T. (2016). *Correctional populations in the United States, 2014*. U.S. Department of Justice, Bureau of Justice Statistics. Retrieved from https://www.bjs.gov/content/pub/pdf/cpus14.pdf

Kaye, H. S., & Harrington, C. (2015). Long-term services and supports in the community: Toward a research agenda. *Disability and Health Journal*, *8*(1), 3–8.

Keshner, E. A. (2004). Virtual reality and physical rehabilitation: A new toy or a new research and rehabilitation tool? *Journal of NeuroEngineering and Rehabilitation*, *1*, 8. http://dx.doi.org/10.1186/1743-0003-1-8

Kidder, K., & Carter, P. (2013). *Needs assessment: Veterans in the western United States*. Washington, DC: Center for a New American Security. Retrieved from https://

www.cnas.org/publications/reports/needs-assessment-veterans-in-the-western-united-states

Krienert, J. L., Henderson, M. L., & Vandiver, D. M. (2003). Inmates with physical disabilities: Establishing a knowledge base. *Southwest Journal of Criminal Justice, 1*, 13–23.

Lew, H. L., Otis, J. D., Tun, C., Kerns, R. D., Clark, M. E., & Cifu, D. X. (2009). Prevalence of chronic pain, posttraumatic stress disorder, and persistent post-concussive symptoms in OIF/OEF veterans: Polytrauma clinical triad. *Journal of Rehabilitation Research & Development, 46*, 697–702. http://dx.doi.org/10.1682/JRRD.2009.01.0006

Marston, H., & Kopicki, A. (2015). The impact of service dogs on post-traumatic stress disorder in the veteran population. *The Military Psychologist, 30*, 16–21. Retrieved from https://www.militarypsych.org/uploads/8/5/4/5/85456500/military_psychologist_30-1.pdf

Maruschak, L. M., Berzofsky, M., & Unangst, J. (2015). *Medical problems of state and federal prisoners and jail inmates, 2011–12*. Washington, DC: U.S. Department of Justice, Office of Justice Programs, Bureau of Justice Statistics. Retrieved from https://www.bjs.gov/content/pub/pdf/mpsfpji1112.pdf

Military Health System, Defense Health Agency. (2017). *Access to health care*. Retrieved from https://health.mil/Military-Health-Topics/Access-Cost-Quality-and-Safety/Access-to-Healthcare

Montgomery, A. E., Hill, L. L., Kane, V., & Culhane, D. P. (2013). Housing chronically homeless veterans: Evaluating the efficacy of a housing first approach to HUD-VASH. *Journal of Community Psychology, 41*, 505–514. http://dx.doi.org/10.1002/jcop.21554

Nas, K., Yazmalar, L., Şah, V., Aydin, A., & Öneş, K. (2015). Rehabilitation of spinal cord injuries. *World Journal of Orthopedics, 6*, 8–16. http://dx.doi.org/10.5312/wjo.v6.i1.8

National Conference of State Legislatures. (2015). *Mental health benefits: State laws mandating and regulating*. Retrieved from http://www.ncsl.org/research/health/mental-health-benefits-state-mandates.aspx

National Council on Disability. (2007). *The impact of the Americans with Disabilities Act: Assessing the progress toward achieving the goals of the ADA*. Retrieved from https://ncd.gov/rawmedia_repository/f493e262_8a9e_49c8_ad84_404a1b91d7c3.pdf

Owen, R. P., Finton, B. J., Gibbons, S. W., & DeLeon, P. H. (2016). Canine-assisted adjunct therapy in the military: An intriguing alternative modality. *The Journal for Nurse Practitioners, 12*, 95–101. http://dx.doi.org/10.1016/j.nurpra.2015.09.014

Penk, W. E., & Little, D. (2013). Psychosocial rehabilitation of physically and psychologically wounded. In B. A. Moore & J. E. Barnett (Eds.), *Military psychologists' desk reference*, (pp. 274–278). New York, NY: Oxford University Press. http://dx.doi.org/10.1093/med:psych/9780199928262.003.0056

Prins, S. J. (2014). Prevalence of mental illnesses in U.S. state prisons: A systematic review. *Psychiatric Services, 65*, 862–872. http://dx.doi.org/10.1176/appi.ps.201300166

Rall, J., Reed, J. B., & Essex, A. (2016, December 15). *Employing people with disabilities*. National Conference of State Legislatures. Retrieved from http://www.ncsl.org/research/labor-and-employment/employing-people-with-disabilities.aspx

Ray, B., & Richardson, N. J. (2017). Traumatic brain injury and recidivism among returning inmates. *Criminal Justice and Behavior, 44*, 472–486. http://dx.doi.org/10.1177/0093854816686631

Sayer, N. A., Cifu, D. X., McNamee, S., Chiros, C. E., Sigford, B. J., Scott, S., & Lew, H. L. (2009). Rehabilitation needs of combat-injured service members admitted to the VA polytrauma rehabilitation centers: The role of PM&R in the care of wounded warriors. *PM & R, 1*, 23–28. http://dx.doi.org/10.1016/j.pmrj.2008.10.003

Seal, K. H., Bertenthal, D., Miner, C. R., Sen, S., & Marmar, C. (2007). Bringing the war back home: Mental health disorders among 103,788 US veterans returning from Iraq and Afghanistan seen at Department of Veterans Affairs facilities. *Archives of Internal Medicine, 167*, 476–482. http://dx.doi.org/10.1001/archinte.167.5.476

Seal, K. H., Metzler, T. J., Gima, K. S., Bertenthal, D., Maguen, S., & Marmar, C. R. (2009). Trends and risk factors for mental health diagnoses among Iraq and Afghanistan veterans using Department of Veterans Affairs health care, 2002–2008. *American Journal of Public Health, 99*, 1651–1658. http://dx.doi.org/10.2105/AJPH.2008.150284

Slaughter, B., Fann, J. R., & Ehde, D. (2003). Traumatic brain injury in a county jail population: Prevalence, neuropsychological functioning and psychiatric disorders. *Brain Injury, 17*, 731–741. http://dx.doi.org/10.1080/0269905031000088649

State of New Jersey. (2018). Veterans diversion program. Department of Military and Veterans Affairs. Retrieved from https://www.nj.gov/military/veterans/diversion-program/#intro

Stiers, W., Hanson, S., Turner, A. P., Stucky, K., Barisa, M., Brownsberger, M., . . . Kuemmel, A. (2012). Guidelines for postdoctoral training in rehabilitation psychology. *Rehabilitation Psychology, 57*, 267–279. http://dx.doi.org/10.1037/a0030774

Stiers, W., & Stucky, K. (2008). A survey of training in rehabilitation psychology practice in the United States and Canada: 2007. *Rehabilitation Psychology, 53*, 536–543. http://dx.doi.org/10.1037/a0013827

Theis, K. A., Roblin, D. W., Helmick, C. G., & Luo, R. (2017). Prevalence and causes of work disability among working-age U.S. adults, 2011–2013, NHIS. *Disability and Health Journal, 11*, 108–115.

Thomas, J. L., Wilk, J. E., Riviere, L. A., McGurk, D., Castro, C. A., & Hoge, C. W. (2010). Prevalence of mental health problems and functional impairment among active component and National Guard soldiers 3 and 12 months following combat in Iraq. *Archives of General Psychiatry, 67*, 614–623. http://dx.doi.org/10.1001/archgenpsychiatry.2010.54

U.S. Department of Health and Human Services, Substance Abuse and Mental Health Services Administration. (1998). *Substance use disorder treatment for people with physical and cognitive disabilities* (Treatment Improvement Protocol [TIP] Series 29, DHHS Publication No. [SMA] 98-3249). Retrieved from https://www.ncbi.nlm.nih.gov/books/NBK64881/

U.S. Department of Health and Human Services, Substance Abuse and Mental Health Services Administration. (2013). *Results from the 2012 National Survey on Drug Use and Health: Summary of National Findings*, NSDUH Series H-46, HHS Publication No. (SMA) 13-4795. Rockville, MD: Substance Abuse and Mental Health Services Administration.

U.S. Department of Health and Human Services, Substance Abuse and Mental Health Services Administration. (2015). *National Survey on Drug Use and Health, 2009*. Retrieved from http://dx.doi.org/10.3886/ICPSR29621.v6

U.S. Department of Justice, Bureau of Justice Statistics. (2005). *Substance dependence, abuse, and treatment of jail inmates*. Retrieved from https://www.bjs.gov/content/pub/pdf/sdatji02.pdf

U.S. Department of Justice, Bureau of Justice Statistics. (2015). *National Inmate Survey, 2011–2012*. http://dx.doi.org/10.3886/ICPSR35009.v1

U.S. Department of Justice, Bureau of Justice Statistics. (2017). *Indicators of mental health problems reported by prisoners and jail inmates, 2011–2012*. Retrieved from https://www.bjs.gov/content/pub/pdf/imhprpji1112.pdf

U.S. Department of Labor, Bureau of Labor Statistics. (2014). *Persons with a disability: Labor force characteristics summary*, Table A (includes noninstitutionalized people ages 16–64). Retrieved from https://www.bls.gov/news.release/disabl.a.htm

U.S. Department of Veterans Affairs. (2015). *Department of Veterans Affairs (VA)/community mental health (CMH) partnership pilots*. Section 3(a) of Executive Order #13625, Summary Report, February 2015. Retrieved from https://www.mentalhealth.va.gov/docs/VA_Community_MH_Partnership_Pilots-Lessons_Learned_FINAL.pdf

U.S. Department of Veterans Affairs. (2017). *Analysis of VA health care utilization among Operation Enduring Freedom (OEF), Operation Iraqi Freedom (OIF), and Operation New Dawn (OND) veterans: Cumulative from 1st Qtr FY 2002 through 3rd Qtr FY 2015 (October 1, 2001–June 30, 2015)*. Retrieved from https://www.publichealth.va.gov/docs/epidemiology/healthcare-utilization-report-fy2015-qtr3.pdf

U.S. Department of Veterans Affairs, VA Office of Academic Affiliations. (2017). *Associated Health Education Program*. Retrieved from https://www.va.gov/oaa/ahe_default.asp

Willink, A., Davis, K., Schoen, C., & Wolff, J. (2016). Physical and/or cognitive impairment, out-of-pocket spending, and Medicaid entry among older adults. *Journal of Urban Health, 93*, 840–850. http://dx.doi.org/10.1007/s11524-016-0078-1

World Health Organization. (1946). *Preamble to the Constitution of the World Health Organization as adopted by the International Health Conference*, New York.

World Health Organization. (2011a). Ch. 1: Understanding disability. *World report on disability*. Retrieved from http://www.who.int/disabilities/world_report/2011/chapter1.pdf

World Health Organization. (2011b). Ch. 4: Rehabilitation. *World report on disability*. Retrieved from http://www.who.int/disabilities/world_report/2011/chapter4.pdf

Wright, B. A. (1983). *Physical disability: A psychosocial approach* (2nd ed.). New York, NY: Harper & Row. http://dx.doi.org/10.1037/10589-000

CHAPTER 28

REHABILITATION PSYCHOLOGISTS IN CRITICAL CARE SETTINGS

Kirk Stucky and Ann Marie Warren

Hospital-based, health service psychology practice has steadily evolved thanks to the ingenuity, perseverance, and quality care provided by countless pioneering clinicians. Relative to their early involvement in traditional mental health settings, psychologists have steadily expanded their scope of practice and now provide clinical services, conduct research, and maintain leadership roles in a wide variety of medical settings. The success of health service psychology in these endeavors is reflected by the multiple outpatient and inpatient practice settings that now require or recommend that a psychologist be part of the interdisciplinary or multidisciplinary team (e.g., transplant team, pediatric clinics, rehabilitation settings, memory disorders clinics). Many of these recommendations or requirements, or both, were not present more than 20 years ago when the first author started his professional career.

In line with a long tradition of branching out into new hospital-based settings, psychologists now also provide services in both intensive and critical care environments.[1] In the United Kingdom and other European countries, psychologists are routinely members of the critical care team (Agarwala, Ahmed, & Patil, 2011; Sukantarat, Greer, Brett, & Williamson, 2007; Tan, Brett, Stokes, & Guideline Development Group, 2009). Conversely, in the United States, this practice model is not as common, although there has been increasing interest in and growing appreciation that a sizable cohort of psychologists in the United States have been practicing quietly in these settings for many years. Furthermore, several well-received symposia have addressed this subject at national conferences, including the 2015 and 2016 American Psychological Association Division 22 midwinter conferences. These events inspired the creation of a special section in the journal of *Rehabilitation Psychology* entitled "The Role of Rehabilitation Psychology in Critical Care and Acute Medical Settings" (Jackson & Jutte, 2016). That journal contains articles addressing such issues as caregiver strain, posttraumatic stress disorder (PTSD), and the integration of rehabilitation psychology principles into the care of patients and families in critical care settings. Readers who are familiar with that publication will recognize that we have relied on it heavily in writing this chapter.

This chapter is designed to provide a brief but broad overview of psychology practice in critical care settings and its relevance to contemporary rehabilitation practice and research. A comprehensive review of this topic would far exceed space limitations; therefore, the focus is on brief summarizations

[1]There are many different types of intensive and critical care units (e.g., cardiac, neurologic, medical, pediatric) that often are described or labeled more specifically (e.g., coronary care unit, surgical intensive care unit, medical intensive care unit, neonatal intensive care unit). Essentially, the concept of *critical* or *intensive care* refers to care in which the patient's life is threatened and without such care death would be imminent. Although some might define *intensive* and *critical care* differently, for the purposes of this chapter *intensive* and *critical care* are used interchangeably.

http://dx.doi.org/10.1037/0000129-029
Handbook of Rehabilitation Psychology, Third Edition, L. A. Brenner, S. A. Reid-Arndt, T. R. Elliott, R. G. Frank, and B. Caplan (Editors-in-Chief)

designed to point the way to a more directed and in-depth study for the interested reader. Although we are aware that a survey recently demonstrated that psychologists from several specialty backgrounds (i.e., health, rehabilitation, and neuropsychology) are involved in critical care settings (Stucky, Jutte, Warren, Jackson, & Merbitz, 2016), for the purposes of this chapter, we have elected to focus on a discussion of specific implications for rehabilitation psychologists with hope that it might stimulate critical thinking about evolving roles, activities, opportunities, and issues for that specialty. Admittedly, the foundational principles of health, rehabilitation, and neuropsychology are similar in that they all emphasize the application of the biopsychosocial model in medical settings. However, rehabilitation psychologists have a unique set of skills and specific competencies that, in our opinion, make them especially well suited for practice in critical care environments.

CRITICAL CARE TRENDS

In the following subsections, we highlight some likely influences on psychology's expanded role, including increased survivorship; recognition of postintensive care complications for patients, family members, and caregivers; more stringent criteria for admission to inpatient rehabilitation; and the development and expansion of Level I trauma centers.

Increased Survivorship

In North America, 6 million people are admitted to a general medical or general surgical intensive care unit (ICU) each year with life threatening conditions, such as sepsis, acute respiratory distress syndrome, and multisystem organ failure (Deutschman, Ahrens, Cairns, Sessler, & Parsons, 2012; Society of Critical Care Medicine, 2011). In addition, in the United States, more than 1 million patients are hospitalized at Level I or Level II trauma centers each year with varying levels of consequent disability (Hall, DeFrances, Williams, Golosinskiy, & Schwartzman, 2010; National Center for Injury Prevention and Control, n.d.; Prin & Li, 2016). Over the past 2 decades, advances in critical care medicine have resulted in decreased mortality rates, thus increasing the number of ICU survivors. Not surprisingly, many of these survivors experience chronic physical, cognitive, and emotional residuals that place them at risk for recurrent rehospitalization, debility, and premature death (Davydow, Gifford et al., 2008; Desai, Law, & Needham, 2011). A growing body of evidence indicates that psychologists can assist in early identification or intervention, or both, targeting those at risk with desirable influences on outcomes and quality of life (Andreoli, Novaes, Karam, & Knobel, 2001; Archer, Castillo, Wegener, Abraham, & Obremskey, 2012; Davidson, Jones, & Bienvenu, 2012; Jackson et al., 2016; Merbitz, Westie, Dammeyer, Butt, & Schneider, 2016; van der Schaaf, Beelen, Dongelmans, Vroom, & Nollet, 2009a).

Postintensive Care Complications

Survivors of critical illness can experience chronic issues sometimes years beyond the original hospitalization, which not only impact them but family members and caregivers as well. This experience has been referred to in varying terms as "the burden of survivorship" (Iwashyna & Netzer, 2012), caregiver burden, and caregiver strain (Thornton & Travis, 2003). Recognizing these trends, experts in the field outlined and proposed criteria for postintensive care syndrome (PICS), which included impairments in three realms of function—physical, cognitive, and mental health—and PICS-Family (PICS-F), which primarily impacts the mental health of the caregiver (Needham et al., 2012; Society of Critical Care Medicine, 2011). With regard to the development of PICS, Jackson and Jutte (2016) wrote,

> While this syndrome is yet to be found in the pages of diagnostic manuals it deserves further study for many reasons not least of all because it reflects the beginning of the development of a common language and because it may prove to be a valuable way to conceptualize cases. (p. 116)

Despite an increased understanding and attention to PICS and PICS-F, many of these individuals are lost to follow-up after discharge from the ICU (Dowdy et al., 2005; Griffiths, Barber, Cuthbertson, & Young, 2006; Needham et al., 2012). To address this issue, some hospital systems in the United Kingdom, Europe, and the United States have established outpatient treatment centers specifically designed to address survivor needs (Jackson & Jutte, 2016; van den Born-van Zanten, Dongelmans, Dettling-Ihnenfeldt, Vink, & van der Schaaf, 2016). In some of these settings, psychologists have been at the forefront of the identification, treatment, and prevention of psychological complications frequently seen during or following critical illness.

More Stringent Criteria for Admission to Inpatient Rehabilitation

Today, large sections of the patient population that received intensive inpatient rehabilitation in the past are no longer admitted secondary to more stringent criteria and numerous restrictions created by new Medicare guidelines, private insurance limitations, discharge planning requirements, reduced length of stay, and the prioritization of cost savings or cost cutting (Ottenbacher et al., 2004). As a consequence of changes in health care and health care financing, a higher proportion of patients are being discharged from the acute medical setting with little to no exposure to rehabilitative interventions (van der Schaaf, Beelen, Dongelmans, Vroom, & Nollet, 2009b). In the authors' experience and based on conversations with other hospital-based rehabilitation psychologists, this trend has resulted in increased requests for psychology consultation during the patient's acute care admission, as well as requests to regularly attend rounds with the trauma team. These requests originally were based in a desire to facilitate transition to the inpatient unit for qualified patients. However, in some settings with increased exposure to rehabilitation psychology services, the critical and intensive care teams also not only request but expect intervention-oriented services (e.g., behavioral management, family education and support, nonpharmacologic pain management, psychotherapy). Also, due to shortened length of stay and increased barriers to inpatient rehabilitation admission, the team also often recognizes that if these services are not requested early, they might never be received (Nancy Merbitz, personal communication, November 23, 2016; Merbitz, Merbitz, & Ripsch, 2012).

The Development and Expansion of Level I Trauma Centers

In 1987, the American College of Surgeons Committee on Trauma developed standards that outlined the resources necessary to provide optimal care for patients who have sustained life-threatening injuries. The result was the development and formal verification of Level I trauma centers throughout the United States. As a consequence of adopting and embracing advanced standards of care, admission to a Level I trauma center relative to other hospitals increases by 25% the survival rate of individuals with serious injury (MacKenzie et al., 2006). Trauma centers maintain a sophisticated interdisciplinary team that works collaboratively to save lives and spearhead efforts to reduce recidivism and promote trauma prevention. In addition to these services, a Level I trauma center is required to have active research, educational, prevention, and public outreach programs. In 2013, Warren, Stucky, and Sherman argued that rehabilitation psychologists' unique training prepared them to assist in these endeavors. This paper is now referenced as a supplemental reading in the chapter on rehabilitation in *Resources for Optimal Care of the Injured Patient* published by the American College of Surgeons Committee on Trauma (2014, p. 93). It also is interesting to note that in a recent survey, psychologists who worked in critical care settings at least monthly were more likely to be at a Level I or pediatric trauma center, and a higher proportion of rehabilitation-oriented providers provided intensive care, critical care, and neurointensive care services relative to nonrehabilitation-oriented providers (Stucky et al., 2016). This trend may be related to the unique skills that rehabilitation-oriented psychologists possess. For example, rehabilitation psychologist competencies, such as interprofessional collaboration and consultation, adaptation to disability, and facilitation of continuity of care, are a natural fit in the critical care environment. However, the trend also is likely related to new legislative mandates or accreditation requirements, or both, such as those in Florida that at designated trauma centers require a psychologist to evaluate all patients with brain or spinal cord injury within 72 hours of admission (Florida Department of Health, 2013).

COMMON PATIENT, FAMILY, AND CAREGIVER ISSUES: TREATMENT IMPLICATIONS

A plethora of life-threatening medical events can precipitate ICU admission, and each of these conditions has unique medical features and comorbidities that increase the risk for specific complications. The differences and complexities notwithstanding, studies have shown that survivors of critical illness are at risk for a variety of physical, cognitive, and mental health issues. A brief discussion of common conditions is provided in the proceeding subsections, followed by a discussion of implications and suggestions as to how the rehabilitation psychologist's unique expertise can be used to improve patient care and the overall effectiveness of the critical care program. Then, we briefly touch on concepts and future directions that require further exploration.

Delirium and Cognitive Impairment

Delirium is estimated to occur in up to 80% of patients on the medical ICU at some point during their hospitalization (Ely et al., 2001) and has been associated with poor physical and psychological recovery as well as persistent cognitive impairment (Girard et al., 2010; Hopkins & Jackson, 2006; Hopkins et al., 1999; Ouimet, Kavanagh, Gottfried, & Skrobik, 2007). Furthermore, these persistent cognitive impairments often continue to impact personal and advanced activities of daily living, quality of life, and return to work (Iwashyna, Ely, Smith, & Langa, 2010; Needham et al., 2013).

Rehabilitation psychologists are trained to provide brief and expedient bedside assessments of mental and behavioral status (e.g., cognitive-log, Mini mental status exam) and can convert those findings into meaningful recommendations for the staff and family members. Furthermore, there a wide range of predisposing (e.g., reduced cognitive or cerebral reserve) and precipitating (e.g., drugs, toxins, trauma) factors can contribute to the development of delirium that members of the critical care team, including the psychologist, must remain mindful of and attentive to throughout the ICU admission (Stucky & Liff, 2014). In concert with these medical interventions, a well-integrated rehabilitation psychologist can ensure that the team remains attentive to other factors that may be promoting persistent cognitive compromise while also encouraging or directing interventions aimed at reducing confusion or reducing preventable cognitive, emotional, or behavioral complications (e.g., low stimulation environment, sleep hygiene, behavioral management plans). In addition, rehabilitation psychologists and neuropsychologists typically have the expertise necessary to provide cognitive assessment that can track progress and inform treatment planning. For example, accurately tracking the length of coma (i.e., time to follow commands) and length of posttraumatic confusion, especially following traumatic brain injury, is valuable in determining injury severity and making predictions regarding short- and long-term outcomes (Roebuck-Spencer & Sherer, 2018; Stucky, Kirkwood, & Donders, 2014).

Anxiety and Trauma- and Stressor-Related Disorders

Estimates regarding the rates of anxiety disorders, as well as the trauma- and stressor-related disorders (e.g., ASD, PTSD, adjustment disorders) in the trauma population and in ICU survivors have varied widely (Davydow, Desai, et al., 2008; Davydow, Gifford, et al., 2008; Hopkins, Key, Suchyta, Weaver, & Orme, 2010; Kapfhammer, Rothenhäusler, Krauseneck, Stoll, & Schelling, 2004; Schelling et al., 1998; Ursano et al., 2004). Following traumatic injury, PTSD rates range from 20% to 40% (Wiseman, Foster, & Curtis, 2013). The fear of serious injury or death invoked by an inability to breathe (e.g., severe asthma attack, acute respiratory distress syndrome), move or feel one's body (e.g., spinal cord injury, traumatic amputation), or unrelenting pain (e.g., burn injury, orthopedic trauma) are possible contributors to these types of disorders. Although many survivors experience steady emotional recovery, a sizable percentage will continue to report symptoms and eventually meet full criteria for PTSD (Kress et al., 2003; Ursano et al., 2004).

It also is interesting that some critical care survivors who report vague or no recollection of the actual time spent in the critical care environment still develop ASD or PTSD during or after ICU admission. Amnesia for the ICU admission may be due to the severity of the condition itself (e.g., traumatic brain injury, delirium) or the administration of various medications that disrupt memory acquisition (Granja et al., 2005, 2008). Understandably, sedation, subsequent paralysis, and the intentional induction of amnestic states is often necessary to ensure that lifesaving procedures or treatments can be administered properly. In addition, these agents can prevent patients from unintentionally hurting themselves or developing harmful levels of agitation in which their health might be further compromised (e.g., increased intracranial pressure, removal of tubes and lines, falls; Kress et al., 2003). However, empirical studies in the mid-1990s began to show that excessive sedation resulted in a prolonged length of mechanical ventilation and a higher risk for respiratory infections as well as delirium (Kress et al., 2003). Furthermore, multiple studies have found that patients with delusional memories regarding their ICU admission were at greater risk for developing PTSD-like symptoms (Jones, Bäckman, & Griffiths, 2012; Weinert & Sprenkle, 2008).

The factors that contribute to the development or maintenance of anxiety disorders or trauma-and stressor-related disorders in critical care survivors and their loved ones remain an open area of study. A number of provoking fundamental questions remain unanswered and study results are somewhat contradictory. For example, O'Donnell et al. (2010) concluded that ICU admission was an independent risk factor for the development of PTSD even when controlling for other important disease related factors. That finding would seem to suggest that increased exposure to the critical care environment should likely increase the risk for PTSD in an incremental or dose–response type fashion. However, other researchers have not verified that relationship (McGiffin, Galatzer-Levy, & Bonanno, 2016). Increasingly, research has suggested that evidence-based treatments for PTSD, such as prolonged exposure, can be applied to acute medical settings such as minimal sessions of prolonged exposure used in the emergency room setting following trauma (Rothbaum et al., 2012). Clinically, in working with survivors of traumatic injury, the authors have found that an initial evaluation that includes validation of normal responses to trauma along with psychoeducation on the importance of not avoiding traumatic memories can result in symptom improvement. However, more research must be implemented to determine if prolonged exposure and other evidence-based strategies, such as cognitive processing therapy, can be adapted for use in acute care settings, including the ICU and trauma recovery units.

Preexisting Psychopathology and Depression

Patients in the ICU often have a preexisting history of substance abuse, psychiatric treatment, or untreated psychological and psychosocial problems, which also may be a direct contributor to their admission. Alternatively, individuals with no psychiatric history are likely to experience normal and, in some cases, debilitating emotional adjustment issues following life threatening events, surgical procedures, and new onset disability. Numerous studies have demonstrated that psychiatric conditions have a negative impact on overall quality of life (Dowdy et al., 2005; Stevenson et al., 2013; Weinert, Gross, Kangas, Bury, & Marinelli, 1997), depressive symptoms (Bienvenu et al., 2012; Davydow et al., 2009; Dowdy et al., 2006, 2008, 2009; Kessler, Chiu, Demler, Merikangas, & Walters, 2005), and mental health issues after physical injury (Wiseman et al., 2013).

After medical stabilization, individuals with preexisting psychopathology, substance abuse issues, or both, often require transition to other programs (e.g., inpatient psychiatric admission, day treatment programs). Given the decline of psychiatric resources (Rubin & Zorumski, 2012), psychologists who are embedded in the critical care team often are positioned in a manner that allows them to work collaboratively with case management and social work services, thus optimizing triage decisions and placement. The psychologists' expertise in maximizing or minimizing the impact of premorbid coping strategies and personality characteristics can make a unique contribution that facilitates the team's overall effectiveness in caring for the patient and the patient's family. Researchers also have become increasingly interested in resilience or factors that are protective for individuals exposed to stressful events. Interventions designed to improve an individual's healthy emotional expression and regulation, stress management, and use of active coping strategies may be helpful. Although this work has been implemented in other patient populations, including those with cancer (Zainal, Booth, & Huppert, 2013), cardiovascular disease (Klainin-Yobas, Ng, Stephen, & Lau, 2016) and diabetes (Gonzalez, Tanenbaum, & Commissariat, 2016), this area of study remains largely unexplored in critical care survivors.

Family and Caregiver Strain

The psychological impact of a critical care admission on family members and loved ones is sometimes overlooked (Azoulay et al., 2005; Kross et al., 2011; van den Born-van Zanten et al., 2016). In some cases, loved ones face the emotional impact of critical illness more so than patients, especially when patients are unaware or even oblivious regarding the severity of their condition (e.g., those in coma or heavily sedated; Warren et al., 2016). Simultaneously, family members have to face a host of emotionally taxing challenges, including but not limited to the initial shock of ICU admission and prospect of losing their loved one. They must make difficult and often unanticipated decisions regarding the person's care (e.g., surgical options, do not resuscitate options) and handle the person's affairs in and outside of the hospital (McAdam, Dracup, White, Fontaine, & Puntillo, 2010). Furthermore, family members are bombarded with visits from a variety of hospital staff and specialists, all of whom may deliver important bits of information pertaining to the patient's situation. Consequently, family members often feel overwhelmed or confused, sometimes because they are having a hard time keeping up with, understanding, or organizing the information delivered. At times, this difficulty is more related to the way in which the information is being delivered, especially when medical language is being used to explain something to an audience that is naive to that type of terminology. Moreover, following ICU discharge, family members may have to act as a primary caregiver; they sometimes must reduce work hours or stop working altogether, often with real financial consequences, which only adds to the overall stress load (Finkelstein, Corso, & Miller, 2006). Considering these issues, it is not surprising that multiple studies have shown that family members, caregivers, and loved ones are at increased risk for developing depression, anxiety, and PTSD during or following the critical care experience (Davidson et al., 2012; Paul & Rattray, 2008; Pochard et al., 2001; Schmidt & Azoulay, 2012).

Psychologists have to remain vigilant to the above-mentioned issues secondary to awareness that caregiver burnout and problematic family dynamics can have a negative impact on the patient's care. Consequently, psychologists often prioritize and spend more time with the family than with the patient, especially during the early ICU admission. As regular members of the critical care team, it is not unusual for physicians and other staff to ask psychologists to meet privately with the family to discuss or explore sensitive issues. More specific requests often occur after the physician and critical care team have had contact with the family, and emotional or psychosocial issues have been revealed or suspected. Rehabilitation psychologists are quite familiar with this model of family-centered and interdisciplinary care through specific competencies that stress collaboration with diverse professionals (Cox, Cox, & Caplan, 2013; Stiers et al., 2015; see Chapter 1, this volume). Not surprisingly, with regard to communication consistency, it also has been suggested that a rehabilitation psychologist can play an instrumental role as liaison between the patient, family, and various medical teams by crafting a unified and understandable message (Warren et al., 2013). To function competently in this capacity, a psychologist must have mastery of critical care lingo and knowledge, which most mental health professionals are not exposed to during training. Before talking with families, we have learned that, whenever possible, the psychologist should communicate directly with the critical care team to ensure that the information delivered is accurate and consistent. As a member of the critical care team, the rehabilitation psychologist can be a leader who continuously reminds and facilitates the team's inclusion of loved ones in decision making and patient care, provides frequent updates and consistent information, and allows team members to be actively involved in patient care at a level that feels comfortable.

Care Transition and Continuity

Despite the stressful nature of the ICU environment, families and patients can develop close ties and become quite comfortable over time with the staff. Although there often is relief as the patient improves and no longer needs to be on the ICU, there also is real and palpable anxiety regarding discharge. Patients and their families may be concerned about experiencing illness recurrence or complications, having to learn a whole new set of providers, going to an environment in which they will not receive the same level of attention, and facing the prospect of having to take on new caregiving tasks.

Rehabilitation psychologists often are uniquely positioned to act as a liaison between the ICU, step-down surgical units, and inpatient or outpatient rehabilitation programs, thus facilitating continuity of care. When rehabilitation psychologists are able to follow patients closely, they often develop therapeutic relationships that can be valuable during transition and transfer, even if they do not provide services in both settings. In 2016, Stucky et al. offered an opinion that health service psychologists may be instrumental in providing value-added services during early critical time points in recovery as well as facilitating patient transfer by (a) asking open-ended questions for patients/family members to describe their thoughts pertaining to transfer, (b) ascertaining what type of information might be helpful to them, (c) providing imaginal exposure to the acute care medical floor, (d) introducing one of their providers before transition, (e) and meeting with them immediately following the transition (and beyond, if necessary).

PROMISING INTERVENTIONS AND FUTURE DIRECTIONS

ICU Diaries

Intensive care unit diaries are written documents created by families during the patient's critical care admission. They often are kept in the patient's room and may contain such sections as daily events, questions for physicians, staff names and specialty, information regarding the condition itself, or treatment options. Some recent studies have suggested that the implementation of ICU diaries can be helpful in ameliorating not only patient distress but also that of their family members (Garrouste-Orgeas et al., 2012; Jones et al., 2010, 2012). Some useful websites allow a family to set up a web page dedicated to the patient; there, daily updates can be posted to allow others to access the information—as long as they have a password or permission from the family—thus reducing the burden on the family to provide multiple individual updates daily to concerned parties.

Rehabilitation psychologists often act as educators who support patients and family members by translating complex medical information into more understandable terms. Rehabilitation psychologists also are familiar with helping patients and families to "write their own story" as a method of helping them adjust to or move toward the acceptance of disability or their "new normal." These skills translate easily into teaching adaptive coping and organizational strategies, including the creation of daily notes or diaries. Later, survivors may be curious about their ICU admission (because they often do not remember it), and the diary can be used as an educational tool or in therapy as the family is adjusting to life postcritical care. Currently, a number of useful online resources are available to professionals, patients, and families (see Chapter 12, this volume). A comprehensive list has not been provided because of space limitations and given that website addresses tend to change over time. Interested readers should consider perusal of the following sites, which are likely to remain active long term: http://www.icudelirium.org (Vanderbilt University) and http://www.myicucare.org/Pages/default.aspx (Society of Critical Care Medicine).

Outpatient Follow-Up

Follow-up ICU clinics have been established with increasing frequency in the United Kingdom (30%; Griffiths et al., 2006) and Netherlands (40%; van der Schaaf, Bakhshi-Raiez, van der Steen, Dongelmans, & de Keizer, 2015). In the United States, this model is less common, although some larger medical centers have begun to establish the practice (Jackson & Jutte, 2016). Although these are exciting clinical developments, little evidence has indicated how effective they are in addressing caregiver strain or diminishing the impact of PICS or PICS-F on quality of life or meaningful functional variables (van den Born-van Zanten et al., 2016). In line with this philosophy of care, other programs are exploring the development of formal community- and home-based programs for patients who do not receive or have access to traditional rehabilitation programs (Jackson & Jutte, 2016).

Ideally, ICU follow-up clinics would have a rehabilitation psychologist embedded in the team. Even if this were the case, however, the embedded psychologist would not be able to meet all clinical demands and thus would benefit from a number of community-based practitioners capable of meeting the population's needs. Psychologists in the community with little to no hospital-based experience may struggle to understand the nuances of a critical care survivor or family's experience. Thus, we also foresee a role for the rehabilitation psychologist in educating colleagues and developing networks of diverse providers who can adequately meet the various needs of this population (e.g., psychotherapy, cognitive rehabilitation, neuropsychological assessment, integrated primary care, risk factor modification).

Training Requirements

In medical settings, there is always a risk of providing or being asked to provide services beyond one's training or scope of practice. In the critical care environment, these risks are possibly even greater, and psychologists can do real harm by providing unnecessary or ineffective services, relaying improper or confusing information, or ineffectively communicating results and recommendations from the critical care team to the patient or family member. Admittedly, both authors of this chapter and the majority of our colleagues involved with critical care did not complete a formal internship or fellowship that specifically focused on the delivery of psychological services in the critical care setting. Because this is a relatively new area of interest compared with other hospital practice settings, it makes sense that most of today's practitioners have learned by doing and perhaps applying a commonsense trial-and-error-type approach, slowly determining what interventions and assessment techniques work best. However, it is apparent that, in addition to a solid foundation in the biopsychosocial model, there is a specific knowledge and skill set necessary to function competently in these environments, especially when branching out into services beyond traditional consultation or answering restricted referral questions (e.g., capacity assessment, suicide risk assessment). In the future, we foresee the development of guidelines or suggestions regarding how a psychologist can be properly prepared to work in these unique and challenging settings.

THE PSYCHOLOGIST'S ROLE IN PROGRAM DEVELOPMENT, RESEARCH, AND ADMINISTRATION

Ideally, critical care teams should be interdisciplinary in that each member understands the other's primary role(s) and how each optimally interfaces with and complements one another. In turn, this knowledge and philosophical approach allows the team to more fully take advantage of its strengths while minimizing weaknesses or gaps in service delivery. Once they have become regular members of the critical care team, psychologists also can make unique contributions to the program that extend beyond patient care. Some of these potential benefits and value-added services are discussed as follows.

Staff Support

Repeated exposure to trauma, critical illness, death and dying, and other highly charged emotional situations will steadily increase the odds of eventual exposure to a situation that uniquely affects and remains with the provider. When emotional residuals mount, the result can be burnout, secondary traumatic stress, and compassion fatigue (Figley, 1995). (Of course, as a member of the critical care team, the psychologist faces these same risks.) Depending on the individual circumstances, psychologists may provide a range of services from a brief intervention during an acute crisis, semipsychotherapeutic functions while advising critical care teams about such issues as boundary setting and stress management more generally, or as an intermediary who refers the staff member for appropriate services when needed. It has been our experience that critical care staff often suffer silently with emotional issues in part because the ICU culture encourages and, in some cases, requires the minimization of psychological reactions. In addition, the ICU culture does not allow for time-outs to regroup or process a difficult experience due to the sheer volume of need in the ICU with limited staff. Although robust psychological defenses and the ability to remain calm, focused, and clinically effective in crisis are necessary skills for the critical care provider, they can lead to denying or ignoring mounting stress and chronic issues that ultimately impact performance, relationships, team dynamics, and patient care. After developing deeper professional and even personal relationships with the psychologist, staff often are much more willing to disclose such feelings or issues and accept suggestions regarding treatment or referral options. Also, when psychologists meet with patients and families to address emotionally challenging issues (e.g., grief, anger, fear), this meeting, in some cases, may serve to offload some of the staff's overall stress load. Furthermore, the rehabilitation psychologist can provide in-services, formal or informal team meetings, and clinical insights during rounds that expose staff to the necessity for healthy stress management and the importance of recognizing early symptoms indicative of compassion fatigue or burnout.

Educational Services

Level I trauma centers and large hospitals equipped to hire a full-time psychologist are also often teaching hospitals. Psychologists can teach hospital staff, medical students, residents, and other trainees about behavioral health concepts, including the complexities of psychiatric conditions, their treatment, and the role of psychological factors in adjustment to illness or injury. For example, the first author has taught crisis prevention and intervention, and other classes for the ICU and rehabilitation staff for the past 20 years with a clear influence on select units. Moreover, the second author is part of the hospital's psychiatry clerkship in which medical students have the opportunity to shadow both the patient consults as well as ICU family groups. Thus, doctoral-level clinicians can help fulfill Accreditation Council for Graduate Medical Education training requirements while facilitating the integration of rehabilitation principles into the delivery of patient care. This parallel training, in our opinion, leads to higher quality and more comprehensive trainee preparation and patient care.

Accreditation Requirements

With regard to Level I trauma centers, it has been suggested that rehabilitation psychologists can help programs meet specific accreditation requirements by participating in research, the provision of social services, and performance improvement initiatives (Warren et al., 2013). Critical care settings also must have access to and regularly consult with mental health providers for a variety of services beyond psychiatric support, including but not limited to suicide risk assessment, need for additional mental health services, and capacity evaluations. In the future, accreditation requirements for ICUs may change; however, currently with regard to the psychologist's unique contribution, this may be more applicable to the Level I trauma center.

Research

Psychologists are uniquely qualified to collaborate with leaders in critical care to simultaneously develop new approaches to patient care and research projects to investigate their effectiveness. Publication requirements often are instituted in academic medical centers and always for American College of Surgeons Committee on Trauma Level I trauma centers. The common populations of interest for rehabilitation psychologists are similar to those treated in the ICU (e.g., the occurrence and implications of injuries that lead to disability, quality of life postinjury, psychological response to trauma, factors that can hinder or facilitate recovery, community participation following significant injury).

CONCLUSION

It seems apparent that there are wide ranging and compelling arguments to support the inclusion of rehabilitation psychologists as integrated members of the critical care team. Rehabilitation psychology training emphasizes specific competencies, such as consultation, brief bedside assessment, interprofessional collaboration, adaptation to disability, and continuity of care facilitation, that are valuable in all critical care environments. These competencies are especially valuable, though, at Level I trauma centers where survivors often transition into inpatient or outpatient rehabilitation settings after discharge. Hospital-based psychologists currently are developing or modifying assessment and intervention strategies that are effective in this fast-paced and demanding setting. In addition to clinical services, a fully integrated rehabilitation psychologist can create some consistency for the family and patient who may have difficulty keeping track of the various physicians and providers who may start but not finish the entire hospital admission with them. Indeed, the rehabilitation psychologist may be the only health care provider who continues to have contact with the patient after ICU or hospital discharge. The importance of preserving this relationship should not be underestimated; the authors have personally experienced its value in transition to the medical floor, rehabilitation unit, and outpatient rehabilitation programs. The presence of psychology in the critical care setting in turn likely increases the probability of early access to needed services on return to the community and potentially prevents unnecessary recidivism or triage decisions that may not consider the full clinical picture. However, the actual impact of early exposure to psychology services in the critical care setting remains an open area of study and no definitive statements can be made regarding cost effectiveness or how it modifies the overall quality of care received by patients and families.

Furthermore, at this time it is unclear how many psychologists in the United States are currently working in critical care settings; in addition, formal training guidelines are nonexistent. We now are in an era of increased focus on supervision, accountability, and competencies (Robiner, Dixon, Miner, & Hong, 2010). To provide competent and effective services in the critical care setting, psychologists must be familiar with more than just the biopsychosocial model and hospital-based practice. To earn the trust and respect of their medical staff colleagues, these practitioners must demonstrate a practical and sophisticated understanding of critical care and how it differs from other medical settings. In the future, we expect that leaders in the field will make efforts to answer questions such as: What qualifications or training should a psychologist have to provide or be considered competent to provide these services? Will there be a need for training standards and or formal programs in the future if the need for such psychologists increases?

We agree with others who have suggested that this is a golden opportunity to apply rehabilitation psychology principles to the critical care environment, especially considering that it is already well known that starting other rehabilitative interventions in the ICU can prevent or minimize certain complications (e.g., decubitus ulcers, contractures, debility; Musicco, Emberti, Nappi, & Caltagirone [for the Italian Multicenter Study on Outcomes of Rehabilitation of Neurological Patients], 2003). In the future, we hope that leaders in the field will conduct multisite studies that compare outcomes in critical care patients who have and have not received contact with properly trained psychologists during acute hospitalization. Specific research questions might include: Does a psychologist's acute intervention services lead to shorter length of stay, more efficient resource use, better quality of care, or reduced readmission rate? Which assessment techniques and interventions are most effective in reducing the risk for PICS, PICS-F, and other related complications? Is a psychologist uniquely qualified to provide these services or can other critical care staff be trained to provide them with equal or similar effectiveness? What incremental value do psychological services add to the program's overall effectiveness beyond value-added service and improved patient satisfaction? Future research would be helpful in clarifying these questions and whether the other points made in the body of this chapter are indeed systematically realized in hospitals throughout the country.

References

Agarwala, R., Ahmed, N., & Patil, K. (2011). An audit of adult critical care rehabilitation processes in a UK district general hospital based on NICE guidelines [Poster presentation]. *Critical Care*, *15*(Suppl. 1) P218. http://dx.doi.org/10.1186/cc9952

American College of Surgeons Committee on Trauma. (2014). *Resources for optimal care of the injured patient*. Chicago, IL: Author.

Andreoli, P. B. A., Novaes, M. A. F. P., Karam, C. H., & Knobel, E. (2001). The ICU humanization program: Contributions from the psychologist team [Meeting abstract]. *Critical Care*, *5*(Suppl. 3), P80. http://dx.doi.org/10.1186/cc1413

Archer, K. R., Castillo, R. C., Wegener, S. T., Abraham, C. M., & Obremskey, W. T. (2012). Pain and satisfaction in hospitalized trauma patients: The importance of self-efficacy and psychological distress. *Journal of Trauma and Acute Care Surgery*, *72*, 1068–1077. http://dx.doi.org/10.1097/TA.0b013e3182452df5

Azoulay, E., Pochard, F., Kentish-Barnes, N., Chevret, S., Aboab, J., Adrie, C., . . . Schlemmer, B. (2005). Risk of post-traumatic stress symptoms in family members of intensive care unit patients. *American Journal of Respiratory and Critical Care Medicine*, *171*, 987–994. http://dx.doi.org/10.1164/rccm.200409-1295OC

Bienvenu, O. J., Colantuoni, E., Mendez-Tellez, P. A., Dinglas, V. D., Shanholtz, C., Husain, N., . . . Needham, D. M. (2012). Depressive symptoms and impaired physical function after acute lung injury: A 2-year longitudinal study. *American Journal of Respiratory and Critical Care Medicine*, *185*, 517–524. http://dx.doi.org/10.1164/rccm.201103-0503OC

Cox, D. R., Cox, R. H., & Caplan, B. (2013). *Specialty competencies in rehabilitation psychology*. New York, NY: Oxford University Press. http://dx.doi.org/10.1093/med:psych/9780195389241.001.0001

Davidson, J. E., Jones, C., & Bienvenu, O. J. (2012). Family response to critical illness: Postintensive care syndrome—Family. *Critical Care Medicine*, *40*, 618–624. http://dx.doi.org/10.1097/CCM.0b013e318236ebf9

Davydow, D. S., Desai, S. V., Needham, D. M., & Bienvenu, O. J. (2008). Psychiatric morbidity in survivors of the acute respiratory distress syndrome: A systematic review. *Psychosomatic Medicine*, *70*, 512–519. http://dx.doi.org/10.1097/PSY.0b013e31816aa0dd

Davydow, D. S., Gifford, J. M., Desai, S. V., Bienvenu, O. J., & Needham, D. M. (2009). Depression in general intensive care unit survivors: A systematic review. *Intensive Care Medicine*, *35*, 796–809. http://dx.doi.org/10.1007/s00134-009-1396-5

Davydow, D. S., Gifford, J. M., Desai, S. V., Needham, D. M., & Bienvenu, O. J. (2008). Posttraumatic stress disorder in general intensive care unit survivors: A systematic review. *General Hospital Psychiatry*, *30*, 421–434. http://dx.doi.org/10.1016/j.genhosppsych.2008.05.006

Desai, S. V., Law, T. J., & Needham, D. M. (2011). Long-term complications of critical care. *Critical Care Medicine*, *39*, 371–379. http://dx.doi.org/10.1097/CCM.0b013e3181fd66e5

Deutschman, C. S., Ahrens, T., Cairns, C. B., Sessler, C. N., & Parsons, P. E. (2012). Multisociety Task Force for critical care research. *Chest*, *141*, 201–209. http://dx.doi.org/10.1378/chest.11-2629

Dowdy, D. W., Bienvenu, O. J., Dinglas, V. D., Mendez-Tellez, P. A., Sevransky, J., Shanholtz, C., & Needham, D. M. (2009). Are intensive care factors associated with depressive symptoms 6 months after acute lung injury? *Critical Care Medicine*, *37*, 1702–1707. http://dx.doi.org/10.1097/CCM.0b013e31819fea55

Dowdy, D. W., Dinglas, V., Mendez-Tellez, P. A., Bienvenu, O. J., Sevransky, J., Dennison, C. R., . . . Needham, D. M. (2008). Intensive care unit hypoglycemia predicts depression during early recovery from acute lung injury. *Critical Care Medicine*, *36*, 2726–2733. http://dx.doi.org/10.1097/CCM.0b013e31818781f5

Dowdy, D. W., Eid, M. P., Dennison, C. R., Mendez-Tellez, P. A., Herridge, M. S., Guallar, E., . . . Needham, D. M. (2006). Quality of life after acute respiratory distress syndrome: A meta-analysis. *Intensive Care Medicine*, *32*, 1115–1124. http://dx.doi.org/10.1007/s00134-006-0217-3

Dowdy, D. W., Eid, M. P., Sedrakyan, A., Mendez-Tellez, P. A., Pronovost, P. J., Herridge, M. S., & Needham, D. M. (2005). Quality of life in adult survivors of critical illness: A systematic review of the literature. *Intensive Care Medicine*, *31*, 611–620. http://dx.doi.org/10.1007/s00134-005-2592-6

Ely, E. W., Inouye, S. K., Bernard, G. R., Gordon, S., Francis, J., May, L., . . . Dittus, R. (2001). Delirium in mechanically ventilated patients: Validity and reliability of the confusion assessment method for the intensive care unit (CAM-ICU). *JAMA*, *286*, 2703–2710. http://dx.doi.org/10.1001/jama.286.21.2703

Figley, C. R. (1995). Compassion fatigue: Toward a new understanding of the costs of caring. In B. H. Stamm (Ed.), *Secondary traumatic stress: Self-care issues for clinicians, researchers, and educators* (pp. 3–28). Lutherville, MD: Sidran Press.

Finkelstein, E. A., Corso, P. S., & Miller, T. R. (2006). *Incidence and economic burden of injuries in the United States*. New York, NY: Oxford University Press. http://dx.doi.org/10.1093/acprof:oso/9780195179484.001.0001

Florida Department of Health. (2013). *Brain & spinal cord injury program: Facility designation standards*. Retrieved from http://www.floridahealth.gov/provider-and-partner-resources/brain-and-spinal-cord-injury-program/index.html

Garrouste-Orgeas, M., Coquet, I., Périer, A., Timsit, J.-F., Pochard, F., Lancrin, F., . . . Misset, B. (2012). Impact of an intensive care unit diary on psychological distress in patients and relatives. *Critical Care*

Medicine, *40*, 2033–2040. http://dx.doi.org/10.1097/CCM.0b013e31824e1b43

Girard, T. D., Jackson, J. C., Pandharipande, P. P., Pun, B. T., Thompson, J. L., Shintani, A. K., . . . Ely, E. W. (2010). Delirium as a predictor of long-term cognitive impairment in survivors of critical illness. *Critical Care Medicine*, *38*, 1513–1520. http://dx.doi.org/10.1097/CCM.0b013e3181e47be1

Gonzalez, J. S., Tanenbaum, M. L., & Commissariat, P. V. (2016). Psychosocial factors in medication adherence and diabetes self-management: Implications for research and practice. *American Psychologist*, *71*, 539–551. http://dx.doi.org/10.1037/a0040388

Granja, C., Gomes, E., Amaro, A., Ribeiro, O., Jones, C., Carneiro, A., & Costa-Pereira, A. (2008). Understanding posttraumatic stress disorder-related symptoms after critical care: The early illness amnesia hypothesis. *Critical Care Medicine*, *36*, 2801–2809. Retrieved from http://dx.doi.org/10.1097/CCM.0b013e318186a3e7

Granja, C., Lopes, A., Moreira, S., Dias, C., Costa-Pereira, A., & Carneiro, A. (2005). Patients' recollections of experiences in the intensive care unit may affect their quality of life. *Critical Care*, *9*, R96–R109. http://dx.doi.org/10.1186/cc3026

Griffiths, J. A., Barber, V. S., Cuthbertson, B. H., & Young, J. D. (2006). A national survey of intensive care follow-up clinics. *Anaesthesia*, *61*, 950–955. http://dx.doi.org/10.1111/j.1365-2044.2006.04792.x

Hall, M. J., DeFrances, C. J., Williams, S. N., Golosinskiy, A., & Schwartzman, A. (2010, October 26). *National hospital discharge survey: 2007 summary* (DHHS Pub. No. 2011-1250). Hyattsville, MD: U.S. Department of Health and Human Services, Centers for Disease Control & Prevention, National Center for Health Statistics.

Hopkins, R. O., & Jackson, J. C. (2006). Long-term neurocognitive function after critical illness. *Chest*, *130*, 869–878. http://dx.doi.org/10.1378/chest.130.3.869

Hopkins, R. O., Key, C. W., Suchyta, M. R., Weaver, L. K., & Orme, J. F., Jr. (2010). Risk factors for depression and anxiety in survivors of acute respiratory distress syndrome. *General Hospital Psychiatry*, *32*, 147–155. http://dx.doi.org/10.1016/j.genhosppsych.2009.11.003

Hopkins, R. O., Weaver, L. K., Pope, D., Orme, J. F., Jr., Bigler, E. D., & Larson-Lohr, V. (1999). Neuropsychological sequelae and impaired health status in survivors of severe acute respiratory distress syndrome. *American Journal of Respiratory and Critical Care Medicine*, *160*, 50–56. http://dx.doi.org/10.1164/ajrccm.160.1.9708059

Iwashyna, T. J., Ely, E. W., Smith, D. M., & Langa, K. M. (2010). Long-term cognitive impairment and functional disability among survivors of severe sepsis. *JAMA*, *304*, 1787–1794. http://dx.doi.org/10.1001/jama.2010.1553

Iwashyna, T. J., & Netzer, G. (2012). The burdens of survivorship: An approach to thinking about long-term outcomes after critical illness. *Seminars in Respiratory and Critical Care Medicine*, *33*, 327–338. http://dx.doi.org/10.1055/s-0032-1321982

Jackson, J. C., & Jutte, J. E. (2016). Rehabilitating a missed opportunity: Integration of rehabilitation psychology into the care of critically ill patients, survivors, and caregivers. *Rehabilitation Psychology*, *61*, 115–119. http://dx.doi.org/10.1037/rep0000091

Jackson, J. C., Jutte, J. E., Hunter, C. H., Ciccolella, N., Warrington, H., Sevin, C., & Bienvenu, O. J. (2016). Posttraumatic stress disorder (PTSD) after critical illness: A conceptual review of distinct clinical issues and their implications. *Rehabilitation Psychology*, *61*, 132–140. http://dx.doi.org/10.1037/rep0000085

Jones, C., Bäckman, C., Capuzzo, M., Egerod, I., Flaatten, H., Granja, C., . . . the RACHEL Group. (2010). Intensive care diaries reduce new onset post traumatic stress disorder following critical illness: A randomised, controlled trial. *Critical Care*, *14*, R168. http://dx.doi.org/10.1186/cc9260

Jones, C., Bäckman, C., & Griffiths, R. D. (2012). Intensive care diaries and relatives' symptoms of posttraumatic stress disorder after critical illness: A pilot study. *American Journal of Critical Care*, *21*, 172–176. http://dx.doi.org/10.4037/ajcc2012569

Kapfhammer, H. P., Rothenhäusler, H. B., Krauseneck, T., Stoll, C., & Schelling, G. (2004). Posttraumatic stress disorder and health-related quality of life in long-term survivors of acute respiratory distress syndrome. *American Journal of Psychiatry*, *161*, 45–52. http://dx.doi.org/10.1176/appi.ajp.161.1.45

Kessler, R. C., Chiu, W. T., Demler, O., Merikangas, K. R., & Walters, E. E. (2005). Prevalence, severity, and comorbidity of 12-month *DSM–IV* disorders in the National Comorbidity Survey Replication. *Archives of General Psychiatry*, *62*, 617–627. http://dx.doi.org/10.1001/archpsyc.62.6.617

Klainin-Yobas, P., Ng, S. H., Stephen, P. D. M., & Lau, Y. (2016). Efficacy of psychosocial interventions on psychological outcomes among people with cardiovascular diseases: A systematic review and meta-analysis. *Patient Education and Counseling*, *99*, 512–521. http://dx.doi.org/10.1016/j.pec.2015.10.020

Kress, J. P., Gehlbach, B., Lacy, M., Pliskin, N., Pohlman, A. S., & Hall, J. B. (2003). The long-term psychological effects of daily sedative interruption on critically ill patients. *American Journal of Respiratory and Critical Care Medicine*, *168*, 1457–1461. http://dx.doi.org/10.1164/rccm.200303-455OC

Kross, E. K., Engelberg, R. A., Gries, C. J., Nielsen, E. L., Zatzick, D., & Curtis, J. R. (2011). ICU care associated with symptoms of depression and posttraumatic stress disorder among family members of patients who die in the ICU. *Chest, 139*, 795–801. http://dx.doi.org/10.1378/chest.10-0652

MacKenzie, E. J., Rivara, F. P., Jurkovich, G. J., Nathens, A. B., Frey, K. P., Egleston, B. L., . . . Scharfstein, D. O. (2006). A national evaluation of the effect of trauma-center care on mortality. *The New England Journal of Medicine, 354*, 366–378. http://dx.doi.org/10.1056/NEJMsa052049

McAdam, J. L., Dracup, K. A., White, D. B., Fontaine, D. K., & Puntillo, K. A. (2010). Symptom experiences of family members of intensive care unit patients at high risk for dying. *Critical Care Medicine, 38*, 1078–1085. http://dx.doi.org/10.1097/CCM.0b013e3181cf6d94

McGiffin, J. N., Galatzer-Levy, I. R., & Bonanno, G. A. (2016). Is the intensive care unit traumatic? What we know and don't know about the intensive care unit and posttraumatic stress responses. *Rehabilitation Psychology, 61*, 120–131. http://dx.doi.org/10.1037/rep0000073

Merbitz, N. H., Merbitz, C. T., & Ripsch, J. P. (2012). Rehabilitation outcomes and assessment: Toward a model of complex adaptive rehabilitation. In P. Kennedy (Ed.), *The Oxford handbook of rehabilitation psychology* (pp. 96–127). New York, NY: Oxford University Press.

Merbitz, N. H., Westie, K., Dammeyer, J. A., Butt, L., & Schneider, J. (2016). After critical care: Challenges in the transition to inpatient rehabilitation. *Rehabilitation Psychology, 61*, 186–200. http://dx.doi.org/10.1037/rep0000072

Musicco, M., Emberti, L., Nappi, G., & Caltagirone, C., for the Italian Multicenter Study on Outcomes of Rehabilitation of Neurological Patients. (2003). Early and long-term outcome of rehabilitation in stroke patients: The role of patient characteristics, time of initiation, and duration of interventions. *Archives of Physical Medicine and Rehabilitation, 84*, 551–558. http://dx.doi.org/10.1053/apmr.2003.50084

National Center for Injury Prevention and Control. (n.d.). Welcome to WISQUARS™. Retrieved from http://www.cdc.gov/injury/wisqars

Needham, D. M., Davidson, J., Cohen, H., Hopkins, R. O., Weinert, C., Wunsch, H., . . . Harvey, M. A. (2012). Improving long-term outcomes after discharge from intensive care unit: Report from a stakeholders' conference. *Critical Care Medicine, 40*, 502–509. http://dx.doi.org/10.1097/CCM.0b013e318232da75

Needham, D. M., Dinglas, V. D., Bienvenu, O. J., Colantuoni, E., Wozniak, A. W., Rice, T. W., & Hopkins, R. O., & the NIH NHLBI ARDS Network. (2013). One year outcomes in patients with acute lung injury randomised to initial trophic or full enteral feeding: Prospective follow-up of EDEN randomised trial. *British Medical Journal, 346*, f1532. http://dx.doi.org/10.1136/bmj.f1532

O'Donnell, M. L., Creamer, M., Holmes, A. C. N., Ellen, S., McFarlane, A. C., Judson, R., . . . Bryant, R. A. (2010). Posttraumatic stress disorder after injury: Does admission to intensive care unit increase risk? *Journal of Trauma, 69*, 627–632. http://dx.doi.org/10.1097/TA.0b013e3181bc0923

Ottenbacher, K. J., Smith, P. M., Illig, S. B., Linn, R. T., Ostir, G. V., & Granger, C. V. (2004). Trends in length of stay, living setting, functional outcome, and mortality following medical rehabilitation. *JAMA, 292*, 1687–1695. http://dx.doi.org/10.1001/jama.292.14.1687

Ouimet, S., Kavanagh, B. P., Gottfried, S. B., & Skrobik, Y. (2007). Incidence, risk factors and consequences of ICU delirium. *Intensive Care Medicine, 33*, 66–73. http://dx.doi.org/10.1007/s00134-006-0399-8

Paul, F., & Rattray, J. (2008). Short- and long-term impact of critical illness on relatives: Literature review. *Journal of Advanced Nursing, 62*, 276–292. http://dx.doi.org/10.1111/j.1365-2648.2007.04568.x

Pochard, F., Azoulay, E., Chevret, S., Lemaire, F., Hubert, P., Canoui, P., . . . Schlemmer, B., & the French FAMIREA Group. (2001). Symptoms of anxiety and depression in family members of intensive care unit patients: Ethical hypothesis regarding decision-making capacity. *Critical Care Medicine, 29*, 1893–1897. http://dx.doi.org/10.1097/00003246-200110000-00007

Prin, M., & Li, G. (2016). Complications and in-hospital mortality in trauma patients treated in intensive care units in the United States, 2013. *Injury Epidemiology*, 3, 18. http://dx.doi.org/10.1186/s40621-016-0084-5

Robiner, W. N., Dixon, K. E., Miner, J. L., & Hong, B. A. (2010). Hospital privileges for psychologists in the era of competencies and increased accountability. *Journal of Clinical Psychology in Medical Settings, 17*, 301–314. http://dx.doi.org/10.1007/s10880-010-9203-6

Roebuck-Spencer, T., & Sherer, M. (2018). Moderate and severe traumatic brain injury. In J. E. Morgan & J. H. Ricker (Eds.), *Textbook of clinical neuropsychology* (2nd ed., pp. 411–429). New York, NY: Taylor & Francis.

Rothbaum, B. O., Kearns, M. C., Price, M., Malcoun, E., Davis, M., Ressler, K. J., . . . Houry, D. (2012). Early intervention may prevent the development of posttraumatic stress disorder: A randomized pilot civilian study with modified prolonged exposure. *Biological Psychiatry, 72*, 957–963. http://dx.doi.org/10.1016/j.biopsych.2012.06.002

Rubin, E. H., & Zorumski, C. F. (2012). Perspective: Upcoming paradigm shifts for psychiatry in clinical care, research, and education. *Academic Medicine*, *87*, 261–265. http://dx.doi.org/10.1097/ACM.0b013e3182441697

Schelling, G., Stoll, C., Haller, M., Briegel, J., Manert, W., Hummel, T., . . . Peter, K. (1998). Health-related quality of life and posttraumatic stress disorder in survivors of the acute respiratory distress syndrome. *Critical Care Medicine*, *26*, 651–659. http://dx.doi.org/10.1097/00003246-199804000-00011

Schmidt, M., & Azoulay, E. (2012). Having a loved one in the ICU: The forgotten family. *Current Opinion in Critical Care*, *18*, 540–547. http://dx.doi.org/10.1097/MCC.0b013e328357f141

Society of Critical Care Medicine. (2011). *Critical care units: A descriptive analysis* (2nd ed.). Des Plaines, IL: Author.

Stevenson, J. E., Colantuoni, E., Bienvenu, O. J., Sricharoenchai, T., Wozniak, A., Shanholtz, C., . . . Needham, D. M. (2013). General anxiety symptoms after acute lung injury: Predictors and correlates. *Journal of Psychosomatic Research*, *75*, 287–293. http://dx.doi.org/10.1016/j.jpsychores.2013.06.002

Stiers, W., Barisa, M., Stucky, K., Pawlowski, C., Van Tubbergen, M., Turner, A. P., . . . Caplan, B. (2015). Guidelines for competency development and measurement in rehabilitation psychology postdoctoral training. *Rehabilitation Psychology*, *60*, 111–122.

Stucky, K., Jutte, J. E., Warren, A. M., Jackson, J. C., & Merbitz, N. (2016). A survey of psychology practice in critical-care settings. *Rehabilitation Psychology*, *61*, 201–209. http://dx.doi.org/10.1037/rep0000071

Stucky, K. J., Kirkwood, M. W., & Donders, J. (2014). Traumatic brain injury. In K. J. Stucky, M. W. Kirkwood, & J. Donders (Eds.), *Clinical neuropsychology study guide & board review* (pp. 432–447). New York, NY: Oxford University Press.

Stucky, K. J., & Liff, C. D. (2014). Delirium. In K. J. Stucky, M. W. Kirkwood, & J. Donders (Eds.), *Clinical neuropsychology study guide & board review* (pp. 381–398). New York, NY: Oxford University Press.

Sukantarat, K., Greer, S., Brett, S., & Williamson, R. (2007). Physical and psychological sequelae of critical illness. *British Journal of Health Psychology*, *12*, 65–74. http://dx.doi.org/10.1348/135910706X94096

Tan, T., Brett, S. J., Stokes, T., & the Guideline Development Group. (2009). Rehabilitation after critical illness: Summary of NICE guidance. *British Medical Journal*, *338*, b822. http://dx.doi.org/10.1136/bmj.b822

Thornton, M., & Travis, S. S. (2003). Analysis of the reliability of the Modified Caregiver Strain Index. *Journals of Gerontology. Series B*, *58*, S127–S132. http://dx.doi.org/10.1093/geronb/58.2.S127

Ursano, R. J., Work Group on ASD and PTSD, Steering Committee on Practice Guidelines, Bell, C., Eth, S., Friedman, M., . . . Yager, J. (2004). Practice guideline for the treatment of patients with acute stress disorder and posttraumatic stress disorder. *American Journal of Psychiatry*, *161*, 3–31.

van den Born-van Zanten, S. A., Dongelmans, D. A., Dettling-Ihnenfeldt, D., Vink, R., & van der Schaaf, M. (2016). Caregiver strain and posttraumatic stress symptoms of informal caregivers of intensive care unit survivors. *Rehabilitation Psychology*, *61*, 173–178. http://dx.doi.org/10.1037/rep0000081

van der Schaaf, M., Bakhshi-Raiez, F., van der Steen, M., Dongelmans, D. A., & de Keizer, N. (2015). Recommendations for intensive care follow-up clinics: Report from a survey and conference of Dutch intensive cares. *Minerva Anestesiologica*, *81*, 135–144.

van der Schaaf, M., Beelen, A., Dongelmans, D. A., Vroom, M. B., & Nollet, F. (2009a). Functional status after intensive care: A challenge for rehabilitation professionals to improve outcome. *Journal of Rehabilitation Medicine*, *41*, 360–366. http://dx.doi.org/10.2340/16501977-0333

van der Schaaf, M., Beelen, A., Dongelmans, D. A., Vroom, M. B., & Nollet, F. (2009b). Poor functional recovery after a critical illness: A longitudinal study. *Journal of Rehabilitation Medicine*, *41*, 1041–1048. http://dx.doi.org/10.2340/16501977-0443

Warren, A. M., Rainey, E. E., Weddle, R. J., Bennett, M., Roden-Foreman, K., & Foreman, M. L. (2016). The intensive care unit experience: Psychological impact on family members of patients with and without traumatic brain injury. *Rehabilitation Psychology*, *61*, 179–185. http://dx.doi.org/10.1037/rep0000080

Warren, A. M., Stucky, K., & Sherman, J. J. (2013). Rehabilitation psychology's role in the Level I trauma center. *Journal of Trauma and Acute Care Surgery*, *74*, 1357–1362.

Weinert, C. R., Gross, C. R., Kangas, J. R., Bury, C. L., & Marinelli, W. A. (1997). Health-related quality of life after acute lung injury. *American Journal of Respiratory and Critical Care Medicine*, *156*, 1120–1128. http://dx.doi.org/10.1164/ajrccm.156.4.9611047

Weinert, C. R., & Sprenkle, M. (2008). Post-ICU consequences of patient wakefulness and sedative exposure during mechanical ventilation. *Intensive Care Medicine*, *34*, 82–90. http://dx.doi.org/10.1007/s00134-007-0829-2

Wiseman, T., Foster, K., & Curtis, K. (2013). Mental health following traumatic physical injury: An integrative literature review. *Injury*, *44*, 1383–1390. http://dx.doi.org/10.1016/j.injury.2012.02.015

Zainal, N. Z., Booth, S., & Huppert, F. A. (2013). The efficacy of mindfulness-based stress reduction on mental health of breast cancer patients: A meta-analysis. *Psycho-Oncology*, *22*, 1457–1465. http://dx.doi.org/10.1002/pon.3171

CHAPTER 29

COMMUNITY-BASED REHABILITATION

Pim Kuipers, Michele Foster, Letitia Burridge, and Elizabeth Kendall

Around the world, rehabilitation systems are responding to demands that create shifts in clinical practice, treatment models, and strategic planning. Global population changes, the prevalence of chronic illness and disability, increases in medical and care costs, shifts in public/private financing and service delivery, as well as pressure for decreased length of hospitalization are all factors that are fueling the growing trend toward community-based rehabilitation (CBR; Rivera, 2012).

Community-based rehabilitation is an approach that draws from primary health care and typically includes the provision of rehabilitation assistance in the community through the adaptation and "upskilling" of local, often informal resources; family members; and intermediate-level workers (Hartley, Finkenflugel, Kuipers, & Thomas, 2009). Within this model, it is acknowledged that the base from which a client's participation can best be maximized is the client's home and community, where he or she engages in local daily activities (Steihaug, 2015). Indeed, most rehabilitation clients prefer services to be provided in their homes and communities (Darzi, Officer, Abualghaib, & Akl, 2016). The period of inpatient or clinic-based rehabilitation is usually a small part of the person's life. It is during the return to the community that much "re-habilitation" takes place, specifically, where the client's longer term goals are achieved and functional and participation-related challenges are resolved. Most important, in terms of outcomes, community-based approaches compare favorably with hospital-based services (Barnes & Radermacher, 2001; Doig, Fleming, Kuipers, & Cornwell, 2010). As such, CBR is a vital dimension of rehabilitation and one that has significant implications for rehabilitation psychology. It also has considerable implications in terms of the competencies required of rehabilitation psychologists who practice in community settings (see Chapter 1, this volume).

HISTORY AND CONTEXT

Informal, basic rehabilitation has been practiced in the home and community for as a long as rehabilitation has existed. Not until the mid-1970s, however, was the formal model of CBR first promoted by the World Health Organization (WHO) to address the limited nature of the rehabilitation workforce in developing countries. In those settings, CBR typically is conducted through the provision of basic services at a community level and incorporates the principles of primary health care, the adoption of relevant rehabilitation practices, the use of local resources, and an emphasis on building local skills (Hartley et al., 2009).

Although the approach in developing countries has been guided by major international manuals (WHO; United Nations Educational, Scientific and Cultural Organization; International Labour

http://dx.doi.org/10.1037/0000129-030
Handbook of Rehabilitation Psychology, Third Edition, L. A. Brenner, S. A. Reid-Arndt, T. R. Elliott, R. G. Frank, and B. Caplan (Editors-in-Chief)

Organization; & International Disability Development Consortium [WHO, UNESCO, ILO, & IDDC], 2010), CBR is not uniform and is conducted in an array of styles and approaches across the world. In their definition of CBR, some Western services include outpatient rehabilitation in hospital clinics and centers (Hillier & Inglis-Jassiem, 2010) or single-discipline outpatient units (Graham, 2013). In general, however, community-based services seek to incorporate and, to some extent, engage with the unique attributes of the client's community and social context, especially the client's home and family context (Rivera, 2012). The shift toward CBR in Western countries has occurred concurrently with a number of contextual influences, including political and economic imperatives to reduce the cost of care, the changing social and structural profile of disability, and the rise of choice and control that influence practice and service design. All of these drivers have significant implications for rehabilitation psychology.

A driver that is common to health and rehabilitation systems globally is the high and increasing economic cost of delivering services during times of unprecedented demand for access. Population trends, including a growing disease burden and aging populations, ever-increasing costs associated with more complex treatments and technologies, and better informed consumers, are potent demand-side drivers that influence costs (Deloitte, 2015). As a result, traditional service delivery and professional practice models are undergoing rapid transformation on issues of location and preference toward more community-based ways of operating (Elrod & DeJong, 2008; United Nations, 2006). In the field of rehabilitation, there is now greater emphasis on early intervention to maintain quality of life and expand the opportunities for social and economic participation (Organisation for Economic Co-operation and Development, 2009). Yet there is continuing pressure to contain costs without diminishing quality or adding to inequities.

These political and economic pressures on the rehabilitation field are not new. Rather, they are compounding old problems and also creating new dilemmas and imperatives for rehabilitation practice. Indeed, 2 decades ago, Hagglund and Frank (1996) described the multiple tensions for rehabilitation psychologists due to rising costs and rationing in rehabilitation. They argued that to maintain optimal and ethical practice, it would be important to document the value of services (including community rehabilitation services) and be active in the development of guidelines (Hagglund & Frank, 1996).

In terms of a second driver, the social structural nature of disability is a key contextual factor shaping the evolution of CBR. Increasing understanding of the importance of the person–environment dimension of disability together with the effect of social and structural impediments and inequalities (WHO & World Bank, 2011) signpost the need for more localized and multidimensional solutions. The International Classification of Functioning, Disability and Health (WHO, 2001) brought attention to the importance of social and structural factors. such as services/systems and physical environments (Scheer, Kroll, Neri, & Beatty, 2003), as well as attitudes that often exclude and disenfranchise people with disability (Van Brakel, 2006). Such a focus requires rehabilitation psychologists to understand that the needs of individuals arise from complex interactions and relationships with multiple systems, including family, social, economic, legal, and political dimensions (see Chapter 1). What is called for is a more ecological approach (Germain, 1973) toward assessing how problems and needs are experienced and constructed, and intervening to influence systems for the benefit of individuals and their support networks. Such competencies are reflected across assessment, intervention, consultation, and advocacy tasks (see Chapter 1). The CBR model aligns closely with rights-based approaches and provides a useful model to guide necessary steps to address social structural issues associated with disability. For rehabilitation psychologists, it suggests the need to identify and collaborate with multiple stakeholders, across multiple systems, to build linkages that can support clients in reaching their goals. Inevitably, there will be a need to work between clinical and systemic roles, and to demonstrate capacity to work across disciplinary and organizational boundaries, thus engaging in different forms of advocacy, intervention, and activism (see Chapter 1), to derive systemic solutions to complex problems.

A third contemporary driver in CBR is the notion of user choice and control. This driver has emerged from a strong consumer and disability rights movement in which individuals no longer see themselves as merely passive recipients of services but as active consumers with status and rights who desire more responsive personalized services (J. Clarke & Newman, 2007; Yeatman, Dowsett, Fine, & Gursansky, 2008). This shift has led to a push for more localized and user-centered approaches to optimize service delivery and improve consumer experiences (MacEachen et al., 2013). Such user-centered approaches require rehabilitation psychologists to be mindful of and to take steps to manage disciplinary power and information asymmetries that can impede choice and control. This shift also is reflected in the advocacy-related dimensions of the professional competencies (see Chapter 1) and means that rehabilitation psychologists must be prepared to act as resources for individuals living with disability and their support networks. For example, rehabilitation psychologists must be ready to enable and empower those living with disability and chronic conditions through information, education, and knowledge so that those individuals may actively participate in their rehabilitation (Kendall, Muenchberger, & Catalano, 2009).

CONTEMPORARY COMMUNITY-BASED REHABILITATION

In contemporary Western settings, the scope of CBR is broad and is delivered in a variety of ways (Kendall et al., 2009). Usually initiated after hospital- or center-based care, professionalized services often are provided informally and by nontraditional service providers. Rather than relying on expert-driven, professionalized models in which the client is relatively passive, CBR generally tends occur in a partnership-oriented manner in which the consumer has an active role. Professionals and other workers operating on a transdisciplinary team provide support and develop capacity (Kendall et al., 2009), usually aiming to optimize participation, function, and quality of life. Community-based rehabilitation is not formally prescribed and coordinated (Steihaug, Lippestad, & Werner, 2016). Instead, it often relies on multiple stakeholders (Juvva & Newhill, 2011) and, unfortunately, is particularly vulnerable to fiscal constraints and organizational influence (Steihaug et al., 2016). Given this variable context, it is unsurprising that in practice, the frequency and intensity of CBR services also are highly variable over time, condition, and location.

A meaningful way of coming to terms with the variety and ambiguity of CBR in Western settings is through a classification system. Using the International Classification of Functioning, Disability and Health terminology (WHO, 2001), CBR interventions may be used to seek gains in the client's function, activities, and participation within that client's personal and environmental circumstances (see Chapter 8, this volume). As such, CBR may encompass not only health interventions and therapy services but also relationships, family, and vocational matters, including education and housing. It even may seek to influence social policy and physical infrastructure. Indeed, the consumer-directed peer support, advocacy, information, and referral services of the centers for independent living in the United States sometimes are described as CBR (Ravesloot & Seekins, 2012).

In many cases, CBR is provided in natural community settings and conducted or overseen by rehabilitation professionals (Fortune, Walsh, & Richards, 2016). Another defining characteristic of CBR is the reliance on, or involvement of, family members, community members, or intermediate-level workers to deliver interventions (WHO, UNESCO, ILO, & IDDC, 2010). Because highly specialized services typically are not available in the community, CBR approaches focus more on the needs generated by daily life, such as adapting one's way of functioning to accommodate disability, practicing rehabilitation techniques in the home, finding local resources, and accessing opportunities. A priority in CBR practice is to link with local services so that the transition to functioning within the person's natural context will be more coherent (Steihaug et al., 2016).

EVIDENCE FOR AND ADOPTION OF COMMUNITY-BASED REHABILITATION

Although CBR is evolving in a changing political, economic, and social environment, as indicated by the professional competencies (see Chapter 1), the widespread adoption and practice of CBR should arise out of a strong evidence base. Unfortunately, as Kendall and colleagues have noted, the growth of CBR has outstripped the quality of the evidence (Kendall et al., 2009). To some extent, the paucity of evidence is related to the complexity of the CBR approach. Because CBR is not a discrete intervention, outcomes are not standardized, and effectiveness is difficult to establish; therefore, the CBR "model" as a whole lacks clear evidence (Hartley et al., 2009; Roels, Aertgeerts, Ramaekers, & Peers, 2016).

Despite the limited evidence, there are a number of preliminary indications of the appropriateness of CBR for some groups. For example, home-based rehabilitation for older people with a range of conditions, including Parkinson's disease, stroke, falls, or fractured neck of femur, seems to be as effective as hospital- or center-based rehabilitation (Parker et al., 2011; Ward, Drahota, Gal, Severs, & Dean, 2008), especially if delivered intensively (Ryan, Enderby, & Rigby, 2006). For this population, community-based approaches are suited particularly to addressing the psychosocial aspects of rehabilitation, including changing beliefs and behaviors (Hurley & Carter, 2016). Likewise, for people with stroke, community rehabilitation teams have achieved at least equivalent outcomes (i.e., decreased impairment and reduced activity limitations) compared with traditional hospital-based rehabilitation (Barnes & Radermacher, 2001; Doig et al., 2010). For people with brain injuries, CBR has been associated with immediate and significant gains across physical and social domains (Curran, Dorstyn, Polychronis, & Denson, 2015).

Indeed, the growing adoption of the community-based model would seem to be related to factors beyond research evidence alone. Its continued expansion also is partly attributable to organizational, financial, and general perception factors. For instance, the CBR approach now is widely understood to facilitate early discharge from hospital and therefore is assumed to result in reduced hospitalization costs (Mayo et al., 2000; Rudd, Wolfe, Tilling, & Beech, 1997; Widén Holmqvist et al., 1998) without compromising clinical outcomes (Anderson, Ni Mhurchu, Brown, & Carter, 2002). This expansion closely aligns with many contemporary organizational priorities.

Furthermore, the popularity of the CBR model, especially postdischarge, may be the result of clinically informed reasoning. For example, in the community setting, rehabilitation focuses on daily activities, in home surroundings, and using local services (Steihaug, 2015). Therapy in CBR is more contextualized; it responds to the environments of greatest relevance to the individual: the person's home, community, and workplace (Curran et al., 2015). Acknowledging the importance of context to the transfer of skills and to the sustainability of outcomes (Booth & Kendall, 2007), it is logical for CBR to be widely adopted postdischarge, at least from a clinical perspective if not persuasively from an evidence perspective. Similarly, because clinical practice has recognized that the client's sense of community and community integration are critical to life satisfaction and well-being, clinicians have tended toward models that foster such priorities (Ditchman, Keegan, Batchos, Haak, & Johnson, 2017).

CHALLENGES TO IMPLEMENTING COMMUNITY-BASED REHABILITATION

Although to some extent these foundations have ensured continuing support for CBR, the literature also indicates a number of challenges to embedding and sustaining the community-based approach in rehabilitation. First, as governments seek greater control over health care expenditure and costs, there is an emphasis on investing in services that provide value for money while avoiding those that are of low value. This pressure results in a tendency to link financial investment to specific time-limited targets and cost-efficiency benchmarks (Turner-Stokes, 2007). The problem for CBR services is that such benchmarks often are simplistic, universal, functionally based, and unable to capture the longer term benefits that are realized in the community when dealing with quality of life outcomes (Turner-Stokes, 2007). Although some countries, such as Australia, have attempted to isolate costs and investments more clearly in a traditionally strong biomedical health care system, the less tangible CBR model does not compare favorably with clearly measurable acute care services (New & Poulos, 2008).

Second, although it is advocated that CBR should be more widely adopted and focused on a broader range of conditions (Prvu Bettger & Stineman, 2007), it is not necessarily suited to all conditions nor to all "communities." For example, CBR generally is not suited to address early impairment or the acute stages of injury or illness, but it is well suited to assisting people whose injuries and disabilities require long-term rehabilitation and care, such as neurological, congenital, and aging-related conditions (Kuipers & Doig, 2010). In addition, not all families or communities will have the resources or resilience required to be able to benefit from the CBR approach. Some rehabilitation clients may not have families. In some cases, informal care within a family places unrealistic and undue strain on women who already may bear the majority of the burden of such care (Bartolo et al., 2010). For others, a reliance on volunteers within or outside of the family will put extreme pressure on already stressed relationships (S. Clarke, Barudin, & Hunt, 2016).

A key challenge in community-based approaches, which may be particularly pronounced for rehabilitation psychologists, is the lack of standard procedures and tools for clinical measurement in CBR. This lack has profound impacts on establishing evidence and documenting the uniformity of outcomes across activities or clients, as well as constraining genuine comparison and benchmarking across services (Lukersmith et al., 2013; Mannan et al., 2012). To some extent, this shortcoming can be met by individualized goal planning, which guides a rehabilitation program in accordance with a client's needs and desires. Goals may be seen as a way of measuring outcomes aimed at achieving community reintegration and participation, which are key aims of CBR programs. Competencies in goal setting complement those of assessment and evaluation (see Chapter 1) in that the rehabilitation psychologist and intervention are focused on the individual's needs and priorities. Goal orientation also enhances the responsiveness of community rehabilitation because goals evolve over time or alter in response to client and environmental changes (Scobbie, Duncan, Brady, & Wyke, 2015). Unfortunately, although goal setting has been embedded within some CBR services and is a way of measuring client progress, actual goal setting practice has been found to vary greatly and still is considered suboptimal in CBR (Scobbie et al., 2015).

Recognizing that these limitations particularly constrain the refinement and quality of CBR, a new framework for outcome measurement and goal setting may be required that encompasses more of the breadth of community-based practice. In this regard, ethicist John Banja noted that rehabilitation should strive for outcomes that are functionally effective, personally fulfilling, and socially meaningful (Banja, 1990). *Functionally effective outcomes* are the traditional clinical outcomes that usually are the primary focus in rehabilitation; they pertain to functional performance, physical abilities, vocational pursuits, and independent living. Beyond these, and aligning strongly with the personal, social, and contextual strength of the CBR paradigm, the potential importance of personally fulfilling and socially meaningful outcomes is evident. *Personally fulfilling outcomes* reflect the extent to which an individual feels satisfied with the rehabilitation process and with his or her personal gains made during rehabilitation. *Socially meaningful outcomes* involve the extent to which individuals can engage in social relationships and perform appropriate roles in their families or other social contexts at a level and in a way that is meaningful in their specific environment (Banja, 1990). Such a framework for implementing outcome measures or indeed for setting rehabilitation goals would be highly consistent with the nature and aspiration of CBR, and would reflect the extent to which the person has been empowered to manage his or her life productively and positively.

WORKFORCE IN THE COMMUNITY-BASED REHABILITATION MODEL

The distinctiveness of the CBR model and the dynamic sociopolitical contexts within which it has evolved have significant implications for rehabilitation psychologists and other professionals and workers. From a service delivery perspective, CBR professionals rarely work in discipline-specific roles (Kendall et al., 2009). For rehabilitation psychologists, this breadth of focus aligns with competencies required to work in interdisciplinary settings (see Chapter 1) and implies the need to acquire generic rehabilitation skills, work across professional and discipline boundaries, and focus on capacity building (Kendall et al., 2009; Steihaug et al., 2016). In community rehabilitation, consultation and the sharing of professional skills across a team are vital (Steihaug et al., 2016; see also Chapter 1). However, in community settings, the team also may be geographically dispersed, so particular attention must be paid to maintaining consistent impact on the client (Steihaug et al., 2016), as well sufficiently supporting others involved in the process. A well-functioning community rehabilitation team with professionals fulfilling complementary roles also ensures support of the staff and broadens the potential range of interventions and expertise available to the client (McColl et al., 2009).

A characteristic of CBR is the emphasis on the role of family members and intermediate-level workers to deliver aspects of rehabilitation interventions. The relevant competencies required of rehabilitation psychologists emphasize the importance of working closely with family members and support networks. This emphasis places a priority on skill-sharing in which the rehabilitation psychologist provides formal and informal training to family members or support workers in the client's immediate social network. For example, family members may be involved in rehabilitation sessions for the purposes of therapy follow-up and consolidation of gains, as well as education about disability, empowerment, goal setting, support services, and the gaining of independence (WHO, UNESCO, ILO, & IDDC, 2010). The role of the professional in CBR often is as facilitator or organizer of a person's rehabilitation by promoting communication and coordination among the client, his or her family, health and community services, and all stakeholders involved in the client's journey. In some cases, this facilitation may extend to building networks of formal and informal services to create a complete response to client need.

It often is stated that CBR is implemented through the combined efforts of the client, client's family, and rehabilitation professionals, as well as appropriate health, education, vocational, and social services, and the broader community. However, this summary belies the reality that communities and families vary considerably in their capacity, their resources, and opportunities to engage. Indeed, there often are very limited services at the community level, and those that do exist tend to be piecemeal, decentralized, inconsistent, and under-resourced or privately funded, and driven by the need for profit or reimbursement. Recent studies have shown that there is generally a lack of competence and capacity in community-based practice (Steihaug et al., 2016) that will perpetuate these challenges for many years to come.

To meaningfully engage with this approach, rehabilitation psychologists will have to considerably broaden their skill base, drawing from the full complement of competencies across foundational, clinical/health, intervention/consultation, and social/community frameworks. The skills required for CBR include generic rehabilitation and trans-disciplinary skills. Community-based rehabilitation requires the capacity to share skills, facilitate, coordinate, collaborate, and advocate (Markle-Reid et al., 2011), skills that traditionally have not been core in the psychologist's toolkit but are recognized in contemporary competencies, and for which rehabilitation psychologists are well prepared, given their psychosocial orientation.

In light of the sociopolitical drivers described earlier in this chapter, rehabilitation psychologists and the CBR workforce in general also will need to be equipped to operate effectively at organizational, systems, and policy levels. Indeed, the ability of rehabilitation psychologists to develop and deliver services that address the broad spectrum of clients' personal and social needs will depend on decisions about funding and resource distribution made at the policy level (Kewman, 2001).

It is therefore imperative that rehabilitation psychologists are equipped with the capacity to work collaboratively with key stakeholders to generate and apply empirical findings to realize equitable, effective, and affordable service and system improvements. In essence, rehabilitation psychologists need to accumulate and document their frontline knowledge of service provision and work with key organizational and policy stakeholders to ensure continued service improvement (Lopez-Baez & Paylo, 2009).

The future sustainability of the CBR approach largely will depend on establishing a robust evidence base regarding outcomes and cost effectiveness (Tomlinson et al., 2009) and using that evidence to advocate and influence policy (Turner-Stokes, 2007; see also Chapter 1 or 24, this volume). As scientist–practitioners, rehabilitation psychologists will be well positioned to contribute to research on community-based programs and interventions that recognize the complexity of impairments and disabling environments, and that acknowledge the challenges of relationships, communities, access, and participation that are common globally (MacLachlan & Mannan, 2014; see also Chapter 24).

CONCLUSION

This chapter has outlined the historical origins and current evolving context of CBR. Rehabilitation psychologists need to be well informed about the scope of CBR to work alongside their multidisciplinary colleagues, clients and family, and other stakeholders in addressing the challenges generated by the complexity and disparities they will encounter. They also need to be innovative and astute frontline researchers to build rigorous evidence that will influence policy and the future directions of rehabilitation psychology.

References

Anderson, C., Ni Mhurchu, C., Brown, P. M., & Carter, K. (2002). Stroke rehabilitation services to accelerate hospital discharge and provide home-based care: An overview and cost analysis. *PharmacoEconomics*, *20*, 537–552. http://dx.doi.org/10.2165/00019053-200220080-00004

Banja, J. D. (1990). Rehabilitation and empowerment. *Archives of Physical Medicine and Rehabilitation*, *71*, 614–615.

Barnes, M. P., & Radermacher, H. (2001). Neurological rehabilitation in the community. *Journal of Rehabilitation Medicine*, *33*, 244–248. http://dx.doi.org/10.1080/165019701753236419

Bartolo, M., De Luca, D., Serrao, M., Sinforiani, E., Zucchella, C., & Sandrini, G. (2010). Caregivers burden and needs in community neurorehabilitation. *Journal of Rehabilitation Medicine*, *42*, 818–822. http://dx.doi.org/10.2340/16501977-0612

Booth, S., & Kendall, M. (2007). Benefits and challenges of providing transitional rehabilitation services to people with spinal cord injury from regional, rural and remote locations. *Australian Journal of Rural Health*, *15*, 172–178. http://dx.doi.org/10.1111/j.1440-1584.2007.00880.x

Clarke, J., & Newman, J. (2007). *Creating citizen–consumers*. London, England: Sage.

Clarke, S., Barudin, J., & Hunt, M. (2016). Ethics and community-based rehabilitation: Eight ethical questions from a review of the literature. *Physiotherapy Canada*, *68*, 197–205. http://dx.doi.org/10.3138/ptc.2015-35GH

Curran, C., Dorstyn, D., Polychronis, C., & Denson, L. (2015). Functional outcomes of community-based brain injury rehabilitation clients. *Brain Injury*, *29*, 25–32. http://dx.doi.org/10.3109/02699052.2014.948067

Darzi, A. J., Officer, A., Abualghaib, O., & Akl, E. A. (2016). Stakeholders' perceptions of rehabilitation services for individuals living with disability: A survey study. *Health and Quality of Life Outcomes*, *14*, 2. http://dx.doi.org/10.1186/s12955-016-0406-x

Deloitte. (2015). *2015 global health care outlook: Common goals, competing priorities* [Report]. Retrieved from http://www2.deloitte.com/content/dam/Deloitte/global/Documents/Life-Sciences-Health-Care/gx-lshc-2015-health-care-outlook-global.pdf

Ditchman, N. M., Keegan, J. P., Batchos, E. J., Haak, C. L., & Johnson, K. S. (2017). Sense of community and its impact on the life satisfaction of adults with brain injury. *Rehabilitation Counseling Bulletin*, *60*, 239–252. http://dx.doi.org/10.1177%2F0034355216661850

Doig, E., Fleming, J., Kuipers, P., & Cornwell, P. L. (2010). Comparison of rehabilitation outcomes in day hospital and home settings for people with acquired brain injury—A systematic review. *Disability and Rehabilitation*, *32*, 2061–2077. http://dx.doi.org/10.3109/09638281003797356

Elrod, C. S., & DeJong, G. (2008). Determinants of utilization of physical rehabilitation services for persons with chronic and disabling conditions: An exploratory study. *Archives of Physical Medicine and Rehabilitation*, *89*, 114–120. http://dx.doi.org/10.1016/j.apmr.2007.08.122

Fortune, D. G., Walsh, R. S., & Richards, H. L. (2016). Cognitive reserve and preinjury educational attainment: Effects on outcome of community-based rehabilitation for longer-term individuals with acquired brain injury. *International Journal of Rehabilitation Research*, *39*, 234–239. http://dx.doi.org/10.1097/MRR.0000000000000175

Germain, C. B. (1973). An ecological perspective in casework. *Social Casework*, *54*, 323–330. http://dx.doi.org/10.1177/104438947305400601

Graham, L. A. (2013). Organization of rehabilitation services. In M. P. Barnes & D. C. Good (Eds.), *Handbook of clinical neurology* (Vol. 110, pp. 113–120). New York, NY: Elsevier.

Hagglund, K., & Frank, R. G. (1996). Rehabilitation psychology practice, ethics and a changing healthcare environment. *Rehabilitation Psychology*, *41*, 19–32. http://dx.doi.org/10.1037/0090-5550.41.1.19

Hartley, S., Finkenflugel, H., Kuipers, P., & Thomas, M. (2009). Community-based rehabilitation: Opportunity and challenge. *The Lancet*, *374*, 1803–1804. http://dx.doi.org/10.1016/S0140-6736(09)62036-5

Hillier, S., & Inglis-Jassiem, G. (2010). Rehabilitation for community-dwelling people with stroke: Home or centre based? A systematic review. *International Journal of Stroke*, *5*, 178–186. http://dx.doi.org/10.1111/j.1747-4949.2010.00427.x

Hurley, M. V., & Carter, A. (2016). ESCAPE-into the community—A community-based rehabilitation programme for elderly people with chronic joint pain. *Perspectives in Public Health*, *136*, 67–69. http://dx.doi.org/10.1177/1757913915626351

Juvva, S., & Newhill, C. E. (2011). Rehabilitation contexts: A holistic approach. *Journal of Human Behavior in the Social Environment*, *2*, 179–195. http://dx.doi.org/10.1080/10911359.2010.525081

Kendall, E., Muenchberger, H., & Catalano, T. (2009). The move towards community-based rehabilitation in industrialised countries: Are we equipped for the challenge? *Disability and Rehabilitation*, *31*, 2164–2173. http://dx.doi.org/10.3109/09638280902939734

Kewman, D. G. (2001). Advancing disability policy: Opportunities and obstacles. *Rehabilitation Psychology*, *46*, 115–124. http://dx.doi.org/10.1037/0090-5550.46.2.115

Kuipers, P., & Doig, E. (2010). Community-based rehabilitation. In J. H. Stone & M. Blouin (Eds.), *International encyclopedia of rehabilitation*. New York, NY: Center for International Rehabilitation Research Information and Exchange. Retrieved from https://sphhp.buffalo.edu/content/sphhp/rehabilitation-science/research-and-facilities/funded-research-archive/center-for-international-rehab-research-info-exchange/_jcr_content/par/download/file.res/pdf.zip

Lopez-Baez, S. I., & Paylo, M. J. (2009). Social justice advocacy: Community collaboration and systems advocacy. *Journal of Counseling & Development*, *87*, 276–283. http://dx.doi.org/10.1002/j.1556-6678.2009.tb00107.x

Lukersmith, S., Hartley, S., Kuipers, P., Madden, R., Llewellyn, G., & Dune, T. (2013). Community-based rehabilitation (CBR) monitoring and evaluation methods and tools: A literature review. *Disability and Rehabilitation*, *35*, 1941–1953. http://dx.doi.org/10.3109/09638288.2013.770078

MacEachen, E., Kosny, A., Ferrier, S., Lippel, K., Neilson, C., Franche, R. L., & Pugliese, D. (2013). The ideal of consumer choice in social services: Challenges with implementation in an Ontario injured worker vocational retraining programme. *Disability and Rehabilitation*, *35*, 2171–2179. http://dx.doi.org/10.3109/09638288.2013.771704

MacLachlan, M., & Mannan, H. (2014). The *World Report on Disability* and its implications for rehabilitation psychology. *Rehabilitation Psychology*, *59*, 117–124. http://dx.doi.org/10.1037/a0036715

Mannan, H., Boostrom, C., Maclachlan, M., McAuliffe, E., Khasnabis, C., & Gupta, N. (2012). A systematic review of the effectiveness of alternative cadres in community based rehabilitation. *Human Resources for Health*, *10*, 20. http://dx.doi.org/10.1186/1478-4491-10-20

Markle-Reid, M., Orridge, C., Weir, R., Browne, G., Gafni, A., Lewis, M., . . . Thabane, L. (2011). Interprofessional stroke rehabilitation for stroke survivors using home care. *Canadian Journal of Neurological Sciences*, *38*, 317–334. http://dx.doi.org/10.1017/S0317167100011537

Mayo, N. E., Wood-Dauphinee, S., Côté, R., Gayton, D., Carlton, J., Buttery, J., & Tamblyn, R. (2000). There's no place like home: An evaluation of early supported discharge for stroke. *Stroke*, *31*, 1016–1023. http://dx.doi.org/10.1161/01.STR.31.5.1016

McColl, M. A., Shortt, S., Godwin, M., Smith, K., Rowe, K., O'Brien, P., & Donnelly, C. (2009). Models for integrating rehabilitation and primary care: A scoping study. *Archives of Physical Medicine and Rehabilitation*, *9*, 1523–1531. http://dx.doi.org/10.1016/j.apmr.2009.03.017

New, P. W., & Poulos, C. J. (2008). Functional improvement of the Australian health care system—Can rehabilitation assist? *Medical Journal of Australia*, *189*, 340–343. https://www.mja.com.au/journal/2008/189/6/functional-improvement-australian-health-care-system-can-rehabilitation-assist

Organisation for Economic Co-operation and Development. (2009, May). *Sickness, disability and work: Keeping on track in the economic downturn*. Paper presented at the High-Level Forum, Stockholm, Sweden.

Retrieved from http://www.oecd.org/employment/emp/42699911.pdf

Parker, S. G., Oliver, P., Pennington, M., Bond, J., Jagger, C., Enderby, P., . . . Dyer, C. (2011). Rehabilitation of older patients: Day hospital compared with rehabilitation at home. Clinical outcomes. *Age and Ageing, 40*, 557–562. http://dx.doi.org/10.1093/ageing/afr046

Prvu Bettger, J. A., & Stineman, M. G. (2007). Effectiveness of multidisciplinary rehabilitation services in post-acute care: State-of-the-science. A review. *Archives of Physical Medicine and Rehabilitation, 88*, 1526–1534. http://dx.doi.org/10.1016/j.apmr.2007.06.768

Ravesloot, C., & Seekins, T. (2012). An emerging role for the rehabilitation psychologist in community rehabilitation service delivery. In P. Kennedy (Ed.), *The Oxford handbook of rehabilitation psychology* (pp. 143–159). New York, NY: Oxford University Press.

Rivera, P. A. (2012). Families in rehabilitation. In P. Kennedy (Ed.), *The Oxford handbook of rehabilitation psychology* (pp. 160–170). New York, NY: Oxford University Press.

Roels, E. H., Aertgeerts, B., Ramaekers, D., & Peers, K. (2016). Hospital- and community-based interventions enhancing (re)employment for people with spinal cord injury: A systematic review. *Spinal Cord, 54*, 2–7. http://dx.doi.org/10.1038/sc.2015.133

Rudd, A. G., Wolfe, C. D., Tilling, K., & Beech, R. (1997). Randomised controlled trial to evaluate early discharge scheme for patients with stroke. *BMJ, 315*, 1039–1044. http://dx.doi.org/10.1136/bmj.315.7115.1039

Ryan, T., Enderby, P., & Rigby, A. S. (2006). A randomized controlled trial to evaluate intensity of community-based rehabilitation provision following stroke or hip fracture in old age. *Clinical Rehabilitation, 20*, 123–131. http://dx.doi.org/10.1191/0269215506cr933oa

Scheer, J., Kroll, T., Neri, M. T., & Beatty, P. (2003). Access barriers for persons with disabilities: The consumers perspective. *Journal of Disability Policy Studies, 13*, 221–230. http://dx.doi.org/10.1177/104420730301300404

Scobbie, L., Duncan, E. A., Brady, M. C., & Wyke, S. (2015). Goal setting practice in services delivering community-based stroke rehabilitation: A United Kingdom (UK) wide survey. *Disability and Rehabilitation, 37*, 1291–1298. http://dx.doi.org/10.3109/09638288.2014.961652

Steihaug, S. (2015). Addressing the organisation of home-based rehabilitation. *International Journal of Physical Medicine & Rehabilitation, 3*, 293. http://dx.doi.org/10.4172/2329-9096.1000293

Steihaug, S., Lippestad, J.-W., & Werner, A. (2016). Between ideals and reality in home-based rehabilitation. *Scandinavian Journal of Primary Health Care, 34*, 46–54. http://dx.doi.org/10.3109/02813432.2015.1132888

Tomlinson, M., Swartz, L., Officer, A., Chan, K. Y., Rudan, I., & Saxena, S. (2009). Research priorities for health of people with disabilities: An expert opinion exercise. *The Lancet, 374*, 1857–1862. http://dx.doi.org/10.1016/S0140-6736(09)61910-3

Turner-Stokes, L. (2007). Politics, policy and payment—Facilitators or barriers to person-centred rehabilitation? *Disability and Rehabilitation, 29*, 1575–1582. http://dx.doi.org/10.1080/09638280701618851

United Nations. (2006). Convention on the Rights of Persons with Disabilities. Retrieved from https://www.un.org/development/desa/disabilities/convention-on-the-rights-of-persons-with-disabilities.html

Van Brakel, W. H. (2006). Measuring health-related stigma—A literature review. *Psychology Health & Medicine, 11*, 307–334. http://dx.doi.org/10.1080/13548500600595160

Ward, D., Drahota, A., Gal, D., Severs, M., & Dean, T. P. (2008). Care home versus hospital and own home environments for rehabilitation of older people. *Cochrane Database of Systematic Reviews, 2008*, CD003164. http://dx.doi.org/10.1002/14651858.CD003164.pub2

Widén Holmqvist, L., von Koch, L., Kostulas, V., Holm, M., Widsell, G., Tegler, H., . . . de Pedro-Cuesta, J. (1998). A randomized controlled trial of rehabilitation at home after stroke in southwest Stockholm. *Stroke, 29*, 591–597. http://dx.doi.org/10.1161/01.STR.29.3.591

World Health Organization. (2001). *International classification of functioning, disability and health*. Retrieved from http://www.who.int/classifications/icf/en/

World Health Organization; United Nations Educational, Scientific and Cultural Organization; International Labour Organization; & International Disability Development Consortium. (2010). *Community-based rehabilitation: CBR guidelines*. Geneva, Switzerland: World Health Organization. Retrieved from http://www.who.int/iris/handle/10665/44405

World Health Organization & World Bank. (2011). *World report on disability.* Retrieved from http://www.who.int/disabilities/world_report/2011/report.pdf

Yeatman, A., Dowsett, G. W., Fine, M. D., & Gursansky, D. (2008). *Individualization and the delivery of welfare services: Contestation and complexity*. New York, NY: Palgrave Macmillan.

Chapter 30

ARTIFICIAL INTELLIGENCE AND ROBOTICS IN REHABILITATION

David D. Luxton and Laurel D. Riek

This chapter provides an overview of applications of intelligent technologies in contemporary rehabilitation practice and research. Within the context of the chapter, we focus primarily on current trends and future capabilities in ubiquitous computing, especially smart environments, intelligent mobile and wearable devices, and other assistive technologies. We also explore the application and study of robotics in rehabilitation practice and research. This is followed by a discussion of the broader implications for rehabilitation practice and research.

INTRODUCTION

Technological advances, particularly in artificial intelligence (AI) and robotics, are revolutionizing the methods and capabilities of rehabilitation research and practice. Smart homes, for example, can assist inhabitants with everyday functioning and alert care providers if assistance is required. Intelligent mobile and wearable devices are available to collect data, and provide users with information to assess health and monitor progress toward individualized rehabilitation goals. Moreover, socially and physically assistive robots can be used to help people recuperate after illness or injury, or to help bridge gaps caused by sensory, motor, or cognitive impairments. These technologies are playing an important role in helping people to improve their functional abilities, independence, and overall well-being.

Our goal with this chapter is to provide an overview of intelligent technologies in contemporary rehabilitation practice and research. We begin by summarizing current trends and future capabilities in ubiquitous computing, especially smart environments, intelligent mobile and wearable devices, and the application and study of robotics in rehabilitation practice and research. Although a comprehensive review of all intelligent technologies and evidence of their effectiveness in rehabilitation is outside the scope of this chapter, we do provide several examples of their application to demonstrate their capabilities. We also discuss *assistive technologies* (AT; equipment or systems designed to maintain or improve the functional capabilities of people), and the *human activity assistive technology model* as a basic conceptual framework for conducting research and practice. We conclude with a discussion of the broader implications for rehabilitation practice and research, including ethical considerations.

UBIQUITOUS COMPUTING AND AMBIENT INTELLIGENCE

Ubiquitous computing (also referred to as *pervasive computing*) entails embedding computational capability into everyday objects so they can communicate information (Abowd et al., 1999; Fogg, 2002; Weiser, 1993). The continual reduction in size of electronic devices (e.g., microprocessors and sensor technology),

http://dx.doi.org/10.1037/0000129-031
Handbook of Rehabilitation Psychology, Third Edition, L. A. Brenner, S. A. Reid-Arndt, T. R. Elliott, R. G. Frank, and B. Caplan (Editors-in-Chief)

as well as the use of wireless technology, make it possible to do this in such a way that systems are transparent (unobtrusive) and fully integrated (Luxton, June, Sano, & Bickmore, 2015). Ubiquitous computing systems can be designed so that data is captured *implicitly*, through passive sensing, or *explicitly*, by periodically surveying people, such as via a kiosk, smart mobile device, or through speech (voice processing).

Ambient intelligence (AmI) is a type of ubiquitous computing that refers to intelligent electronic environments that are sensitive and responsive to the presence of people within them (Aarts & de Ruyter, 2009; Aarts & Wichert, 2009; D. J. Cook, Augusto, & Jakkula, 2009; Vasilakos & Pedrycz, 2006). For example, ubiquitous computing systems embedded within a person's home or other rehabilitation setting can be aware of the needs, preferences, and functioning of inhabitants by analyzing situational data in real time, such as a person's physical location within the environment and other relevant information, such as the time of day. *Context awareness* refers to how technologies infer the current activity state of the user (e.g., smart home inhabitant) and the characteristics of the environment in order to manage information content and information distribution (D. J. Cook et al., 2009; O'Connor & Riek, 2015).

Recent gains in speech recognition, natural language processing (NLP), eye and face tracking, and gesture recognition provide users with multiple ways for interacting with intelligent technologies in a naturalistic manner. For example, it may be difficult or impossible for some people to effectively use keyboards or touch screens as an input device. Verbal interaction can allow people with physical or visual impairments to communicate with and control devices and eye trackers can enable respirator users to do the same.

AI can also assist with other basic but important "behind the scenes" functions such as preserving battery life by being aware of the situation (e.g., shutting down equipment when it is not in use). Basic functions such as battery life may be especially important when considering the use of technologies in critical health contexts, such as patient monitoring (Luxton et al., 2015), fall detection (Casilari & Oviedo-Jiménez, 2015), or when performing resuscitation (Gonzales, Henry, Calhoun, & Riek, 2016).

INTELLIGENT MOBILE AND WEARABLE DEVICES

Intelligent mobile and wearable devices make excellent data collection platforms for health-related data, as well as contextual data relevant during rehabilitation. Consumer wearable devices from companies such as Apple, Fitbit, Jawbone, or Nike can be used to collect physiologic, behavioral, environmental (e.g., from ambient sensors), biological, and self-reported assessments (Luxton et al., 2015; Patel, Park, Bonato, Chan, & Rodgers, 2012; Piwek, Ellis, Andrews, & Joinson, 2016). A principal advantage of wearable technologies, such as smart watches, is that they are in physical contact with users for extended periods of time and they do not require the user to interact with a keyboard or touch screen while wearing them (Luxton et al., 2015).

Fall detection systems (FDS; Acampora, Cook, Rashidi, & Vasilakos, 2013; Gasparrini, Cippitelli, Spinsante, & Gambi, 2014) are an example of a technology germane to rehabilitation that uses intelligent sensors placed within an environment and/or as a wearable device. The goal of these systems is to detect falls and automatically alert medical staff, emergency services, or family members if assistance is required (Casilari & Oviedo-Jiménez, 2015). Casilari and Oviedo-Jiménez (2015) pilot tested such a system that uses fall detection algorithms implemented in a smartphone app and a smartwatch (both provided with an embedded accelerometer and a gyroscope) to track and analyze movements of simulated patients. The system was designed to discriminate falls from the conventional activities of daily living by simultaneously and independently analyzing the data from the two devices (they can interact via Bluetooth connection). Machine learning algorithms allow these types of systems to learn the behavioral patterns and characteristics of individuals over time and therefore help to reduce false positives. Moreover, systems can be designed to assess environmental risks, such as household lights that are off or proximity to fall hazards (e.g., stairwells) and preemptively alert inhabitants or care providers.

A growing number of mobile apps for use in rehabilitation are now available to health care professionals, clients, and family members. These include point-of-use tools for accessing health-related information, clinical decision support tools, medical imaging, mood and behavior trackers (e.g., pain diaries), physiological monitors, and assistive tools. (For general reviews regarding available mobile health apps, see Boulos, Brewer, Karimkhani, Buller, & Dellavalle, 2014; Luxton, McCann, Bush, Mishkind, & Reger, 2011; Martínez-Pérez et al., 2014; Ventola, 2014). Mobile devices also offer a way to facilitate live chatting with health care or other support professionals, text messaging interventions (e.g., behavioral reminders), scheduling and appointment reminders, and synchronous video-based tele-rehabilitation services (Kuemmel & Luxton, 2015; Luxton et al., 2011).

Integrated systems, such as our example in Figure 30.1, may collect data seamlessly from several types of sensors and data inputs. Data can be collected from sensor networks embedded within the environment (e.g., motion sensors) or worn on the user (e.g., physiological sensors) and sent via wireless connections to other mobile devices, a desktop computer, or other central processing system for analysis. Fully automated systems can be built to analyze and monitor data 24/7 and alert health care professionals and/or family members if needed. Synchronous video-based telehealth services could also be provided. Moreover, robots that provide physical assistance functions (e.g., lifting items, opening doors), monitoring, and therapeutic social functions may also be placed in these environments (Chan, Estève, Escriba, & Campo, 2008). The Care-O-bot 4, from Fraunhofer IPA (depicted in Figure 30.1), for example, is a commercially available configurable robot designed to provide assistive functions in the home.

INTELLIGENT VIRTUAL AGENTS

An *intelligent virtual agent* (IVA) is a computer-generated, animated, artificial intelligent virtual character that can be designed to take on the visual appearance of humans, animals, or any other form imaginable (Hudlicka, 2015; Prendinger & Ishizuka, 2004). Their design can range from cartoonlike agents to highly detailed and lifelike three-dimensional agents. IVAs can been deployed on personal computers and on mobile phones and tablet computers, or even on robots (Luxton et al., 2015). Speech recognition and natural language processing (NLP) can allow the virtual agent to converse with the user through basic text interface or through verbal conversation. IVAs typically have a knowledge-engine with information that it uses

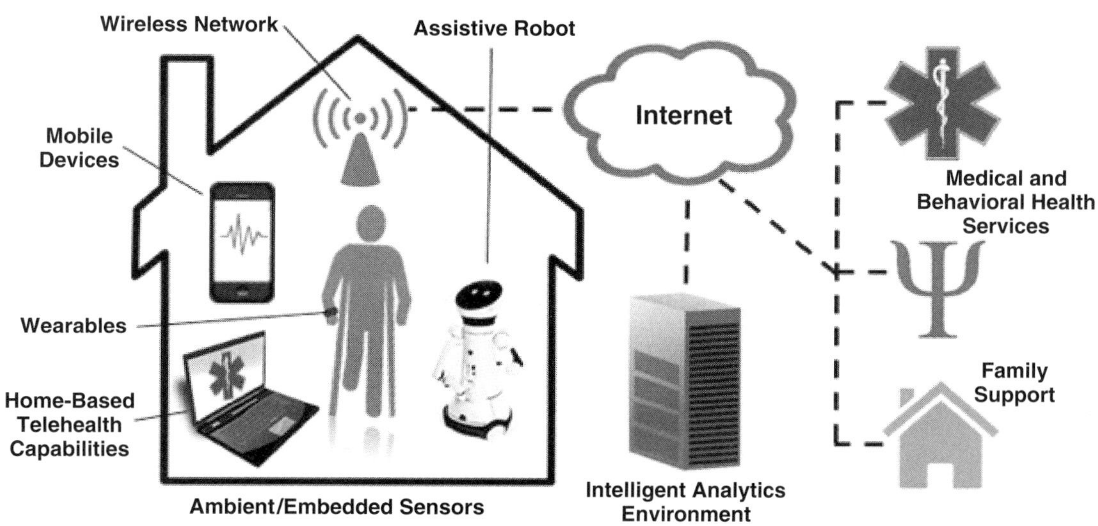

FIGURE 30.1. Integrated smart environment system.

in conversation to enable it to understand, reason, and sometimes exhibit emotions.

Virtual affective agents are IVAs that are capable of affective interaction through recognition of human emotions and expression of emotions by the agent (Hudlicka, 2015; Hudlicka et al., 2008). Systems can be designed to detect mood states through analysis of language as well as through sensors that detect nonverbal information such as facial expressions and eye gaze (Luxton, 2014a). Affective agents may also be designed with the capability to explicitly model emotions, thereby enabling the agents to display nuances of emotional and social intelligence (e.g., awareness of social cues and user goals; Hudlicka, 2015). This capability gives these systems some ability to form and maintain relationships with human users, as well as to adapt in real time to the changing states and needs of the user. IVAs with this ability are sometimes called *relational agents*. As noted by Hudlicka (2015), it is important for agent developers to balance the need for agent expressiveness, the complexity of the associated processing required for them to function, and the needs of the users within the given interaction context.

IVAs, such as virtual humans, provide many potential benefits for rehabilitation and health care in general. For example, IVAs that simulate patients can be used for training purposes (Talbot, Sagae, John, & Rizzo, 2012). They can be designed to simulate various disorders or conditions in order to allow trainees to practice their interviewing skills and gain experience. The U.S. military, for example, has tested the use of lifelike virtual military veterans with depression and suicidal thoughts to teach military clinicians and other personnel how to recognize the risk for suicide (Kenny, Parsons, & Rizzo, 2009). Virtual patient simulations used in instruction have shown to be associated with better learning outcomes compared to conventional educational methods without simulations (Hirumi et al., 2016).

IVAs have also been developed for providing clinical care and coaching tasks (Luxton, 2015). For example, Bickmore and colleagues (2010) developed and tested a virtual nurse for use in hospital discharge planning and found that patients preferred to receive the discharge planning from the virtual human because they spent more time with the patient and never seemed rushed. Other studies suggest that IVAs can make users feel better understood while also reducing social anxiety (Bailenson & Yee, 2005; Gratch, Wang, Gerten, Fast, & Duffy, 2007; Kandalaft, Didehbani, Krawczyk, Allen, & Chapman, 2013; Kang, Gratch, Wang, & Watt, 2008; Lucas, Gratch, King, & Morency, 2014).

Other advantages of IVAs who stand in for human coaches and care providers are that they will not experience burnout or fatigue, and they may potentially be more reliable than humans (Luxton, 2014b). That is, they could be programmed with and learn skills that are applied consistently while also adapting to the client/patient's needs and preferences (Luxton, 2014b). They may also be capable of sensitivity and adaptation to specific aspects of a patient's culture, such as race/ethnicity or socioeconomic status. For example, a virtual human rehabilitation psychologist could modify its physical appearance and mannerisms (e.g., eye contact), speech dialect, use of colloquialisms, and other characteristics to match a given cultural group. This capability could help the system to develop and enhance rapport with a client, contributing to improved rehabilitation outcomes.

The application of IVAs that "stand in" for human rehabilitation professionals suggests that they may become a competitive threat to the rehabilitation workforce. There is indeed growing concern and evidence in many industries, including health care, that AI will replace human professionals (Brynjolfsson & McAfee, 2012; Luxton, 2014a). It is most likely, however, that IVAs will be used to assist rehabilitation professionals and enhance what they do, rather than replace them. There are also opportunities for rehabilitation psychologists to contribute to the design and testing of IVAs and to assure that they are put to use in ways that are ethical and effective at improving outcomes for clients.

VIRTUAL REALITY, AUGMENTED REALITY, AND SERIOUS GAMES FOR REHABILITATION

Virtual reality allows people to become immersed within and interact with three-dimensional computer-generated simulated environments (Rizzo, Buckwalter,

& Neumann, 1997; see also Chapter 31, this volume). Virtual reality can be used to create virtual humans or other simulated life forms (e.g., virtual pets) that humans can interact with inside of virtual environments (e.g., in computer games). In therapeutic applications, virtual reality affords the capability to create and control environmental stimuli such that behavioral reactions to them can be practiced and recorded for clinical assessment, intervention, and rehabilitation goals (Schultheis & Rizzo, 2001). *Augmented reality* allows computer-generated virtual reality to be superimposed over live "real world" video imagery (Caudell & Mizell, 1992; Craig, 2013; Hugues, Fuchs, & Nannipieri, 2011). This allows information about the surrounding environment of the user to be available for interaction and digital manipulation in order to augment the user's perception of the world.

Virtual and augmented reality systems have been used for motor function training and recovery after stroke (Merians et al., 2002) and in pain management (Sato et al., 2010). Mirror therapy, for example, entails the use of a glass mirror to provide visual feedback to the brain. Augmented reality mirror systems use a high-resolution video screen and video cameras to simulate a mirror reflection. Thus, the technology allows a person to look into the simulated mirror to see a computer-generated image (e.g., a limb) or other images created by augmented reality. Sato and colleagues (2010) developed and tested a virtual mirror visual feedback system and applied it to the treatment of complex regional pain syndrome and found that it may be an effective alternative treatment for complex regional pain syndrome.

Serious games are computer games developed for training and learning purposes (as opposed to games designed solely for entertainment purposes; Hudlicka, 2015). In health care, serious games are used for training and education purposes for health care professionals (e.g., emergency room triage, nursing care, surgery) as well as for therapeutic and educational purposes for patients and clients (e.g., education about diet and exercise, coaching to increase physical activity, pain management, social skills training; Horne-Moyer, Moyer, Messer, & Messer, 2014). The skills to be learned or practiced are embedded within the game tasks and can be customized to the user's specific learning needs or therapeutic goals. The game aspect provides the benefit of motivating users (i.e., behavioral reinforcement) while also making the training or tasks more engaging.

One example of serious gaming for rehabilitation are exergames. These are video game—like simulations that allow a user to, for example, relearn basic motor skills by practicing them in a virtual environment. By combining a virtual mirror therapy component, these simulations can allow users to observe their own movements "in the game."

Desai and colleagues (2016) developed and tested an exergame for rehabilitation that uses low-cost, commercially available cameras such as Microsoft Kinect V2, to create a 3D model of the person and immersing the model in interactive virtual environments. These researchers designed games, such as a bowling simulation and a shotput game as well as a virtual trivia game requiring elbow rotation movement. Results of their initial test on ten participants (with no known disabilities) showed the games to be fun and realistic, and at the same time engaging and motivating for performing exercises. This example, while a preliminary test of this technology for rehabilitation, shows promise as a cost-effective tool for both in-office and in-home rehabilitation. Desai and colleagues (2016) also noted that this particular system does not require sensors to be worn by the user, thus it is less cumbersome and restrictive of physical movements.

ROBOTICS TECHNOLOGY IN REHABILITATION

Robots are "physically embodied systems capable of enacting physical change in the world" (Riek, 2015, p. 185). They enact this change with effectors which can move the robot (locomotion), or objects in the environment (manipulation). Robots typically use sensor data to make decisions. They can vary in their degree of autonomy, from fully autonomous (the robot makes all decisions itself) to fully teleoperated (an operator makes all decisions for the robot), though most modern systems have mixed initiative, or shared autonomy. More broadly, *robotics technology* includes affiliated systems, such as related sensors, algorithms for processing data, and so on (Riek, 2015).

Robotics is a field of study that began in the industrial domain, studying the "intelligent connections between perception and actions" (Siciliano & Khatib, 2008, p. 2), though in the past few decades it has shifted to supporting people across nearly every human environment and exploring problems relating to teaming with real people in the real world (Iqbal & Riek, 2017; Riek, 2015).

This shift has been referred to in the literature as *human-centered robotics*, and an emerging area in the past decade focusing on problems in this space is known as *human-robot interaction* (HRI; Riek, 2015).

In health care, robots have tremendous potential to help people receiving rehabilitative care and their caregivers, as well as the clinical workforce itself. Robots can provide both physical and cognitive support to these individuals, across multiple types of care settings, and across the lifespan (Riek, 2017). These applications are discussed within the context of rehabilitation below.

Physically Assistive Robotics

Robots have been used extensively in physical rehabilitation applications across multiple clinical areas, including helping patients recover motion after a stroke (Johnson, Rai, Barathi, Mendonca, & Bustamante-Valles, 2017; Matarić, Eriksson, Feil-Seifer, & Winstein, 2007), recovering or supplementing lost function (Maciejasz, Eschweiler, Gerlach-Hahn, Jansen-Troy, & Leonhardt, 2014), and supporting mobility (van den Heuvel, Lexis, Gelderblom, Jansens, & de Witte, 2016). For example, Lancioni, Sigafoos, O'Reilly, and Singh (2012) described several robot-based intervention studies that aimed to increase activity engagement and ambulation among a small number of participants (*n* 8 56) with severe physical and cognitive disabilities. The mobile robots used in the studies helped to improve participants' engagement with the physical world while also increasing their independence. Other recent advancements have included providing care receivers with additional physical reach, such as with wheelchair-mounted robot arms or smart, on-body prostheses, and multisetting mobility capabilities, such as via exoskeletons or accessible personal transportation devices (Riek, 2017).

Another key area for physically assistive robots is as an aid to the clinical workforce itself. This is a population often overlooked in the technology literature, yet who are under constant physical and cognitive overload, and are at great risk for burnout and suicide (Card, 2018). They could greatly benefit from additional assistance in their work. For example, physically assistive robots can be used to help health care providers accomplish nonvalue-added tasks that detract from care delivery, such as removing waste, fetching supplies, cleaning rooms, or helping lift patients (Riek, 2017). Robots can also help treat patients with highly infectious diseases, which can further protect the clinical workforce (Kraft, Chu, Hansen, & Smart, 2016). Recent work in robotics has explored ways that robots can physically adapt to people in real time, by modeling their motion and altering their movement accordingly, as well as by predicting future behavior (Iqbal, Rack, & Riek, 2016; Nikolaidis, Forlizzi, Hsu, Shah, & Srinivasa, 2017). These concepts may prove particularly useful in future robots that provide physical rehabilitative support to people with disabilities, as well as to clinicians, by providing affordances for intuitive human-robot/human-agent teaming.

Socially Assistive Robotics

Socially assistive robotics represent a juncture between assistive robotics and socially intelligent robotics (Riek, 2015). As can be seen in Figure 30.2, socially assistive robots can be designed to be anthropomorphic, animal-like (zoomorphic), or machinelike (Riek, Rabinowitch, Chakrabarti, & Robinson, 2009). Roles that these robots can take in health care, and specifically in rehabilitation, include companion, coach or instructor, or play partner (e.g., in play therapy). Paro, for example, is a robotic baby seal used to provide therapy for patients with dementia (Shibata & Wada, 2011) and RoboKind's Milo is a small anthropomorphic robot that teaches social behaviors for young persons with autism.

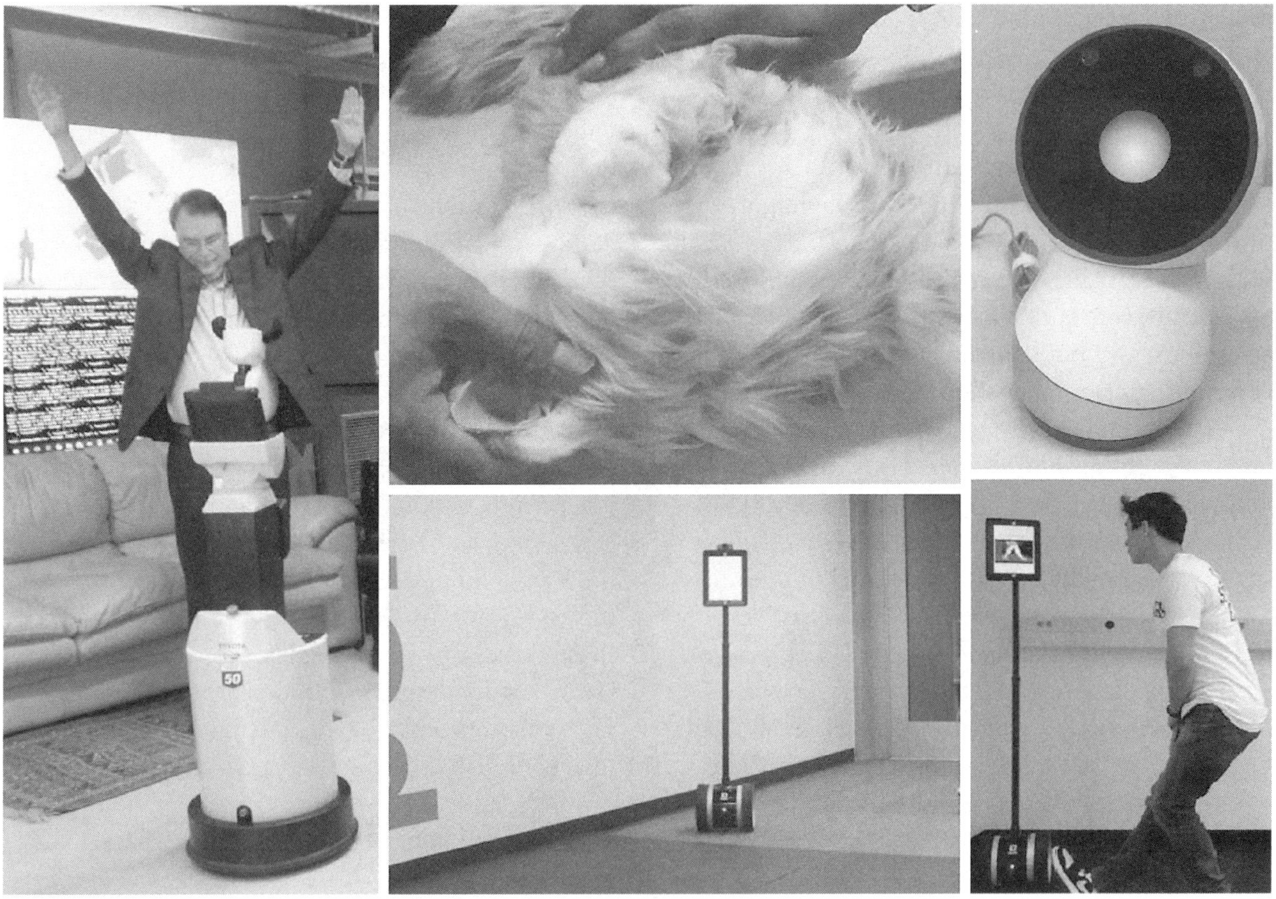

FIGURE 30.2. Example robots used for rehabilitation from Dr. Riek's lab. Clockwise from left: (a) the Toyota Human Service Robot is a mobile robot used to encourage activity in older adults and to assist with activities around the house; (b) stuffed animal robots, like the Hasbro companion pet robot, are often used to alleviate symptoms of loneliness and depression; (c) table top social robots, like Jibo, are being used to provide cognitive support to people with autism and dementia; and (d) mobile telepresence robots, like the Double (shown at the bottom center and right), provide prehabilitation support to workers. For more information, see Lee and Riek (2018) and Woodworth, Ferrari, Zosa, and Riek (2018). Parts a–c copyright 2018 by L. D. Riek. Reprinted with permission. Part d from "Preference Learning in Assistive Robotics: Observational Repeated Inverse Reinforcement Learning," by B. Woodworth, F. Ferrari, T. E. Zosa, and L. D. Riek, 2018, *Proceedings of Machine Learning Research*, *85*, p. 11. Copyright 2018 by B. Woodworth, F. Ferrari, T. E. Zosa, and L. D. Riek. Reprinted with permission.

Application domains of socially assistive robotics include support for older adults, individuals with physical recovery/rehabilitation and training needs, and individuals with cognitive, developmental, and social disorders (Tapus, Mataric, & Scassellati, 2007). Socially assistive robotics are highly useful for facilitating active rehabilitation exercises (Tapus et al., 2007). For example, Eriksson, Mataric, and Winstein (2005) tested a "hands-off" therapist robot that assists, encourages, and socially interacts with patients who have suffered a stroke. These authors note that the shared physical context and physical movement of the robot, encouragement, and continuous monitoring supported patient compliance with rehabilitation exercises.

IMPLICATIONS FOR REHABILITATION PRACTICE AND RESEARCH

The development, evaluation, and practical use of technologies in rehabilitation require the identification and measurement of relevant outcomes. As noted by Smith (2016), there is great complexity around outcomes in the field of rehabilitation in general, so target outcomes must be simplified and well organized. The multitude of emerging technologies used in diverse rehabilitation contexts and populations adds to this complexity.

The Need for Conceptual Models

Conceptual models are useful for rehabilitation professionals because they can provide a theoretical basis for advancing research and improving practice. Specifically, conceptual models can help to classify areas of inquiry (and outcomes), evaluate design and alternatives, and analyze data across different populations and contextual circumstances (Lenker & Paquet, 2003). The *human activity assistive technology model* (HAAT; A. M. Cook & Hussey, 1995) is one longstanding conceptual model involving assistive technologies (for review of additional models, see Lenker & Paquet, 2003). Assistive technologies (AT) can range from low-tech devices, such as a walker, to high-tech devices, such as sophisticated smart room environments (A. M. Cook & Polgar, 2015; Mihailidis, Boger, Craig, & Hoey, 2008). Formal definitions of AT, such as from the United States, The Assistive Technology Act of 1998 (amended in 2004) and from the World Health Organization (WHO) focus on individuals with disabilities—a fact that some have argued is based too strictly on the medical model (Hersh & Johnson, 2008). ATs are also described in the context of rehabilitation and in educational settings, which are not limited to "disabled persons" or older persons. The primary difference is the applicability to broader populations and the goals concerning the use of the technology. For education, the principal goal is enabling participation and learning. For rehabilitation, it is the restoration of functioning.

As shown in Figure 30.3, the HAAT model has four components: the human, the activity, the assistive technology, and the context in which these three components exist. Essentially, the HAAT model describes an AT system in terms of a person (human) who is using an AT device to accomplish a desired task (activity) within a

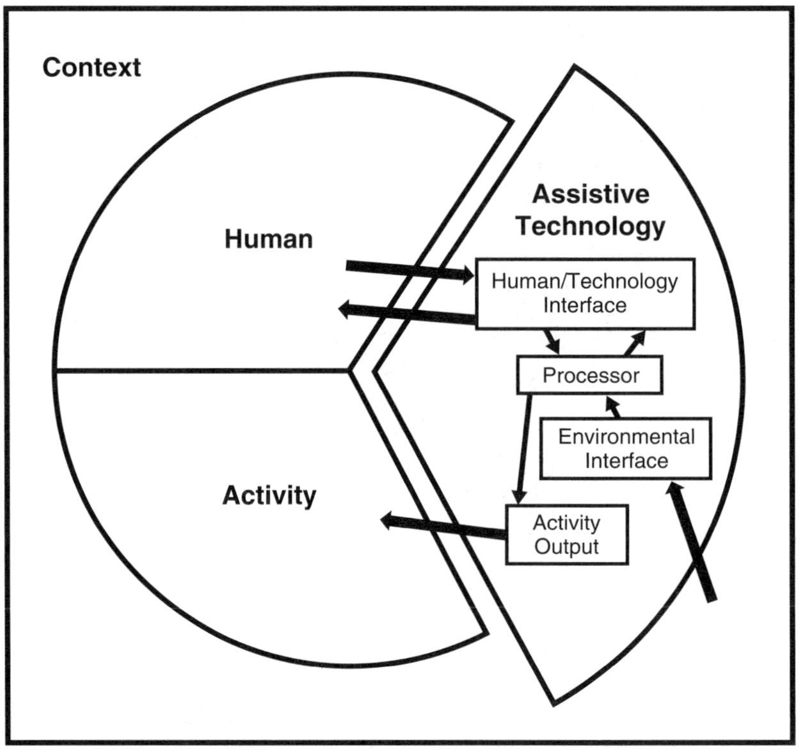

FIGURE 30.3. The human activity assistive technology model showing the assistive technology component. From *Assistive Technologies: Principles and Practice* (4th ed., p. 26), by A. M. Cook and J. M. Polgar, 2015, St. Louis, MO: Elsevier Mosby. Copyright 2015 by Elsevier Inc. Adapted with permission.

particular context (environment). Each component should be considered both independently and in combination with the others when designing, selecting, applying, and evaluating AT devices (Lenker & Paquet, 2003).

According to A. M. Cook and Hussey (1995), the *human* element refers to physical, cognitive, and affective aspects of the participant. The *physical* element has to do with the physical attributes and functioning of a person, such as their coordination, strength, balance, and physical structure (i.e., anatomy). The *cognitive* element refers to measurable constructs such as attention, alertness, and problem-solving abilities, as well as other varying deficits of attention, judgment, insight, and so on. The *affective* element may include attitudes associated with the experience (e.g., frustration) as well affective symptoms associated with psychiatric conditions such as depression. The *activity* component refers to the process of doing something, such as daily living activities (e.g., dressing, hygiene, mobility), work activities (e.g., home management, educational, vocational activities), or play and leisure activities (e.g., activities related to enjoyment, relaxation, and self-expression). The *context* refers to social and cultural contexts, as well as environments and physical conditions. Lastly, the *AT technology* component (i.e., the device or devices) is described as having a human-technology interface, a processor (typically, an electronic computer or a mechanical device), and an activity output (Lenker & Paquet, 2003).

As noted by Lenker and Paquet (2003), the HAAT model aims to characterize system performance, rather than confining focus to human or device performance. The approach also considers aspects of human factors engineering and occupational therapy: the former entails analysis of how task characteristics of and environments influence human performance and the later aims to improve human performance in purposeful activities.

Quality of Care and Economic Considerations

The development of intelligent technologies in rehabilitation and health care in general has the potential to improve the quality of care while also providing economic benefits. One way that these technologies can improve overall quality of care is by the amount of health-related data that can be collected to assess patient outcomes. As noted earlier, mobile devices such as smartphones and ambient home technologies can collect data in real time, with more frequent data collection, and in the environments that people live in, thus providing richer data to measure improvements in functioning and outcomes of treatments. These technologies also have the potential to improve adherence to treatment and rehabilitation plans by providing users with behavioral reminders (e.g., to conduct a daily exercise regimen) and feedback regarding use and progress toward goals (Luxton et al., 2015). Moreover, assistive technologies can also improve safety outcomes by providing real-time monitoring and alerts when increased assistance is needed.

Intelligent technologies in rehabilitation and health care can also provide significant economic benefits for health care providers and consumers of services. The increased accessibility and lower costs of intelligent technologies that provide services may make available opportunities for longer term treatments that might otherwise be restricted by managed-care costs (Luxton, 2014b). Thus, patients will have the opportunity to participate in longer term therapies and also receive periodic checkups that improve outcomes while also greatly reducing costs.

While initial development costs of fully interactive, intelligent rehabilitative systems may presently be high, depending of the complexity of the system, they can provide economic benefits. For example, they can potentially address treatment access gaps and be part of stepped care—the process whereby the least resource intensive care is provided to the most people first, with more intensive care provided to patients who need it the most (Bower & Gilbody, 2005). Clients could seek initial consultation and be assessed or screened by a virtual human and referred to more intensive care if needed.

Privacy and Data Security Considerations

The technologies presented in this chapter entail specific privacy and electronic data security requirements that may need to be met, such as those enforced by the Health Insurance Portability and

Accountability Act (HIPAA) in the United States. With HIPAA, the health care service provider must assure compliance whenever a user is to transmit protected health information to a health care provider (if they are considered a covered entity). Although business associate agreements (BAAs) are required, they do not remit clinicians or their employers of all responsibility if consumers are harmed (Luxton, Nelson, & Maheu, 2016). HIPAA requires that several standards be met, including the availability of "audit trails" that make records of interactions accessible to authorities when needed, as well as "breach notification tools" that inform clinicians of breaches, such as when a transmission is illegally hacked.

It is important to note that physiological data that are collected, stored, and transmitted by ubiquitous computing technologies could also be used to identify a person (Luxton, Kayl, & Mishkind, 2012). This extends far beyond video and audio data—even basic actigraphy can reveal identifiable health information, and even "anonymized" data can be easily de-anonymized (Piwek, Ellis, Andrews, & Joinson, 2016). Thus, systems that collect such data, whether mobile apps, ambient intelligence systems or robots, might fall under the same regulatory requirements when used in the context of health care. Moreover, the technologies that we have discussed in this chapter also pose privacy issues associated with third parties (e.g., bystanders, family members). For example, cameras or microphones in smart environments may also collect images and sounds from residents and guests who are not aware of the data collection (Luxton, June, Sano, & Bickmore, 2015).

To help address these ethical quandaries, researchers and practitioners are encouraged to consult resources such as the Connected and Open Research Ethics (CORE) tool, a dynamic online resource which provides ethical practices and guidelines (Torous & Nebeker, 2017). Other professional organizations have also recently released codes of ethics guiding research practice in these technologies, including the IEEE, which may also provide a valuable resource to researchers (Chatila, Firth-Butterflied, Havens, & Karachalios, 2017; Riek & Howard, 2014).

CONCLUSION

The technologies and methods presented in this chapter provide many exciting opportunities to enhance rehabilitation services and research. Improvements in existing technologies and future ones not yet developed will further advance rehabilitation capabilities and methods. These systems can provide numerous benefits to rehabilitation professionals, care providers, and clients.

While all of the specific technologies presented in this chapter can be expected to advance the field of rehabilitation psychology, it is likely that the integration of these technologies will provide the most significant opportunities for the field in the years ahead. For example, assistive robots with onboard IVAs can facilitate interactive communication and therapeutic bonds with the client. The system could also receive information (e.g., physical activity) from an ambient sensor network at home and, through the use of machine learning techniques, predict and adapt interventions that optimize rehabilitation outcomes, safety, and user satisfaction. The integration of these technologies also poses some challenges, including the need to design for interoperability and additional privacy risks (e.g., data security). Researchers and clinicians will need to consider the additional complexities and requirements of these systems.

Several limitations warrant mention. More research, especially clinical trials, are needed to evaluate the effectiveness of these technologies in the rehabilitation context. Unfortunately, the clinical trials that are needed to make informed decisions about the efficacy and benefits of various technologies can take many years to go through funding, implementation, and results and simply cannot keep up with the rapid evolution in many types of technology. Disruption technologies (or disruptive innovations) present a particular problem. New technologies and methods are constantly being brought to the marketplace, and while this progress is a good thing, it also requires new research and sometimes entire paradigm shifts in how care or services are provided. Technology access limitations is a related issue. Some people will simply not have access to technologies due to lack of economic resources and infrastructure (e.g., Internet access). This presents an ethical issue that needs to be considered by policy makers, researchers, and practitioners.

References

Aarts, E., & de Ruyter, B. (2009). New research perspectives on ambient intelligence. *Journal of Ambient Intelligence and Smart Environments*, *1*, 5–14.

Aarts, E., & Wichert, R. (2009). Ambient intelligence. In H. J. Bullinger (Ed.), *Technology guide* (pp. 244–249). Berlin/Heidelberg, Germany: Springer. http://dx.doi.org/10.1007/978-3-540-88546-7_47

Abowd, G., Dey, A., Brown, P., Davies, N., Smith, M., & Steggles, P. (1999). Towards a better understanding of context and context-awareness. In H. Gellerson (Ed.), *Handheld and ubiquitous computing* (pp. 304–307). Berlin/Heidelberg, Germany: Springer.

Acampora, G., Cook, D. J., Rashidi, P., & Vasilakos, A. V. (2013). A survey on ambient intelligence in health-care. *Proceedings of the IEEE*, *101*, 2470–2494. http://dx.doi.org/10.1109/JPROC.2013.2262913

Bailenson, J. N., & Yee, N. (2005). Digital chameleons: Automatic assimilation of nonverbal gestures in immersive virtual environments. *Psychological Science*, *16*, 814–819. http://dx.doi.org/10.1111/j.1467-9280.2005.01619.x

Bickmore, T. W., Mitchell, S. E., Jack, B. W., Paasche-Orlow, M. K., Pfeifer, L. M., & Odonnell, J. (2010). Response to a relational agent by hospital patients with depressive symptoms. *Interacting with Computers*, *22*, 289–298. http://dx.doi.org/10.1016/j.intcom.2009.12.001

Boulos, M. N. K., Brewer, A. C., Karimkhani, C., Buller, D. B., & Dellavalle, R. P. (2014). Mobile medical and health apps: State of the art, concerns, regulatory control and certification. *Online Journal of Public Health Informatics*, *5*, 229.

Bower, P., & Gilbody, S. (2005). Stepped care in psychological therapies: Access, effectiveness and efficiency: Narrative literature review. *The British Journal of Psychiatry*, *186*, 11–17. http://dx.doi.org/10.1192/bjp.186.1.11

Brynjolfsson, E., & McAfee, A. (2012). *Race against the machine: How the digital revolution is accelerating innovation, driving productivity, and irreversibly transforming employment and the economy*. Retrieved from http://ebusiness.mit.edu/research/Briefs/Brynjolfsson_McAfee_Race_Against_the_Machine.pdf

Card, A. J. (2018). Physician burnout: Resilience training is only part of the solution. *Annals of Family Medicine*, *16*, 267–270. http://dx.doi.org/10.1370/afm.2223

Casilari, E., & Oviedo-Jiménez, M. A. (2015). Automatic fall detection system based on the combined use of a smartphone and a smartwatch. *PLoS One*, *10*(11), e0140929. http://dx.doi.org/10.1371/journal.pone.0140929

Caudell, T. P., & Mizell, D. W. (1992). Augmented reality: An application of heads-up display technology to manual manufacturing processes. *Proceedings of the 25th Hawaii International Conference on System Sciences*, 2, 659–669. http://dx.doi.org/10.1109/HICSS.1992.183317

Chan, M., Estève, D., Escriba, C., & Campo, E. (2008). A review of smart homes—Present state and future challenges. *Computer Methods and Programs in Biomedicine*, *91*, 55–81. http://dx.doi.org/10.1016/j.cmpb.2008.02.001

Chatila, R., Firth-Butterflied, K., Havens, J. C., & Karachalios, K. (2017). The IEEE global initiative for ethical considerations in artificial intelligence and autonomous systems [standards]. *IEEE Robotics & Automation Magazine*, *24*, 110. http://dx.doi.org/10.1109/MRA.2017.2670225

Cook, A. M., & Hussey, S. M. (1995). *Assistive technologies: Principles and practice*. Baltimore, MD: Mosby.

Cook, A. M., & Polgar, J. M. (2015). *Assistive technologies: Principles and practice* (4th ed.). St. Louis, MO: Elsevier Mosby.

Cook, D. J., Augusto, J. C., & Jakkula, V. R. (2009). Ambient intelligence: Technologies, applications, and opportunities. *Pervasive and Mobile Computing*, *5*, 277–298. http://dx.doi.org/10.1016/j.pmcj.2009.04.001

Craig, A. B. (2013). *Understanding augmented reality: Concepts and applications*. San Francisco, CA: Elsevier.

Desai, K., Bahirat, K., Ramalingam, S., Prabhakaran, B., Annaswamy, T., & Makris, U. E. (2016). Augmented reality-based exergames for rehabilitation. *Proceedings of the 7th International Conference on Multimedia Systems*, 232–241. http://dx.doi.org/10.1145/2910017.2910612

Eriksson, J., Mataric, M. J., & Winstein, C. J. (2005). Hands-off assistive robotics for post-stroke arm rehabilitation. *Proceedings of the IEEE 9th International Conference on Rehabilitation Robotics*. Retrieved from http://robotics.usc.edu/publications/media/uploads/pubs/452.pdf

Fogg, B. J. (2002). *Persuasive technology: Using computers to change what we think and do*. San Francisco, CA: Morgan Kaufmann.

Gasparrini, S., Cippitelli, E., Spinsante, S., & Gambi, E. (2014). A depth-based fall detection system using a Kinect® sensor. *Sensors*, *14*, 2756–2775. http://dx.doi.org/10.3390/s140202756

Gonzales, M. J., Henry, J. M., Calhoun, A. W., & Riek, L. D. (2016). Visual task: A collaborative cognitive aid for acute care resuscitation. *Proceedings of the 10th EAI International Conference on Pervasive Computing Technologies for Healthcare*, 45–52.

Gratch, J., Wang, N., Gerten, J., Fast, E., & Duffy, R. (2007). Creating rapport with virtual agents. In C. Pelachaud, J. C. Martin, E. André, G. Chollett, K. Karpouzis, & D. Pelé (Eds.), *Intelligent virtual agents* (pp. 125–138). Berlin/Heidelberg, Germany: Springer. http://dx.doi.org/10.1007/978-3-540-74997-4_12

Hersh, M., & Johnson, M. A. (Eds.) (2008). *Assistive technology for visually impaired and blind people*. Berlin/Heidelberg, Germany: Springer.

Hirumi, A., Kleinsmith, A., Johnsen, K., Kubovec, S., Eakins, M., Bogert, K., . . . Cendan, J. (2016). Advancing virtual patient simulations through design research and interPLAY: Part I: Design and development. *Educational Technology Research and Development*, *64*, 763–785. http://dx.doi.org/10.1007/s11423-016-9429-6

Horne-Moyer, H. L., Moyer, B. H., Messer, D. C., & Messer, E. S. (2014). The use of electronic games in therapy: A review with clinical implications. *Current Psychiatry Reports*, *16*(520). http://dx.doi.org/10.1007/s11920-014-0520-6

Hudlicka, E. (2015). Virtual affective agents and therapeutic games. In D. D. Luxton (Ed.), *Artificial intelligence in mental and behavioral healthcare* (pp. 81–116). San Diego, CA: Elsevier.

Hudlicka, E., Lisetti, C., Hodge, D., Paiva, A., Rizzo, A., & Wagner, E. (2008). Artificial agents for psychotherapy. *Proceedings of the AAAI spring symposium on emotion, personality and social behavior* (pp. 60–64). Menlo Park, CA: AAAI.

Hugues, O., Fuchs, P., & Nannipieri, O. (2011). New augmented reality taxonomy: Technologies and features of augmented environment. In B. Furht (Ed.), *Handbook of augmented reality* (pp. 47–63). New York, NY: Springer. http://dx.doi.org/10.1007/978-1-4614-0064-6_2

Iqbal, T., Rack, S., & Riek, L. D. (2016). Movement coordination in human–robot teams: A dynamical systems approach. *IEEE Transactions on Robotics*, *32*, 909–919. http://dx.doi.org/10.1109/TRO.2016.2570240

Iqbal, T., & Riek, L. D. (2017). Human-robot teaming: Approaches from joint action and dynamical systems. In A. Goswami & P. Vadakkepat (Eds.), *Humanoid robotics: A reference* (pp. 2293–2312). Dordrecht, The Netherlands: Springer.

Johnson, M. J., Rai, R., Barathi, S., Mendonca, R., & Bustamante-Valles, K. (2017). Affordable stroke therapy in high-, low- and middle-income countries: From Theradrive to Rehab CARES, a compact robot gym. *Journal of Rehabilitation and Assistive Technologies Engineering*, *4*. http://dx.doi.org/10.1177/2055668317708732

Kandalaft, M. R., Didehbani, N., Krawczyk, D. C., Allen, T. T., & Chapman, S. B. (2013). Virtual reality social cognition training for young adults with high-functioning autism. *Journal of Autism and Developmental Disorders*, *43*, 34–44. http://dx.doi.org/10.1007/s10803-012-1544-6

Kang, S. H., Gratch, J., Wang, N., & Watt, J. H. (2008, May). Does the contingency of agents' nonverbal feedback affect users' social anxiety? *Proceedings of the 7th International Joint Conference on Autonomous Agents and Multiagent Systems* (Vol. 1, pp. 120–127). Liverpool, England: International Foundation for Autonomous Agents and Multiagent Systems.

Kenny, P. G., Parsons, T. D., & Rizzo, A. A. (2009). Human computer interaction in virtual standardized patient systems. In J. A. Jacko (Ed.), *Human-computer interaction: Interacting in various application domains* (Part IV, pp. 514–523). Berlin/Heidelberg, Germany: Springer.

Kraft, K., Chu, T., Hansen, P., & Smart, W. D. (2016). Real-time contamination modeling for robotic health care support. *Proceedings of the IEEE/RSJ International Conference on Intelligent Robots and Systems*, 2249–2254. http://dx.doi.org/10.1109/IROS.2016.7759352

Kuemmel, A., & Luxton, D. D. (2015, February). *Best telehealth practices with rehabilitation populations: Ethical, legal, privacy, and safety considerations*. Paper presented at the meeting of Rehabilitation Psychology, San Diego, CA.

Lancioni, G. E., Sigafoos, J., O'Reilly, M. F., & Singh, N. N. (2012). *Assistive technology: Interventions for individuals with severe/profound and multiple disabilities*. New York, NY: Springer.

Lee, H. R., & Riek, L. D. (2018). Reframing assistive robots to promote successful aging. *ACM Transactions on Human-Robot Interaction*, *7*, Article 11.

Lenker, J. A., & Paquet, V. L. (2003). A review of conceptual models for assistive technology outcomes research and practice. *Assistive Technology*, *15*, 1–15. http://dx.doi.org/10.1080/10400435.2003.10131885

Lucas, G. M., Gratch, J., King, A., & Morency, L. P. (2014). It's only a computer: Virtual humans increase willingness to disclose. *Computers in Human Behavior*, *37*, 94–100. http://dx.doi.org/10.1016/j.chb.2014.04.043

Luxton, D. D. (2014a). Artificial intelligence in psychological practice: Current and future applications and implications. *Professional Psychology: Research and Practice*, *45*, 332–339. http://dx.doi.org/10.1037/a0034559

Luxton, D. D. (2014b). Recommendations for the ethical use and design of artificial intelligent care providers. *Artificial Intelligence in Medicine*, *62*, 1–10. http://dx.doi.org/10.1016/j.artmed.2014.06.004

Luxton, D. D. (Ed.). (2015). *Artificial intelligence in behavioral and mental health care*. San Diego, CA: Elsevier/Academic Press.

Luxton, D. D., June, J. D., Sano, A., & Bickmore, T. (2015). Mobile, wearable, and ambient intelligence in behavioral health care. In D. D. Luxton (Ed.), *Artificial intelligence in behavioral and mental health care* (pp. 137–162). San Diego, CA: Elsevier Academic Press.

Luxton, D. D., Kayl, R. A., & Mishkind, M. C. (2012). mHealth data security: The need for HIPAA-compliant standardization. *Telemedicine and e-Health, 18*, 284–288. http://dx.doi.org/10.1089/tmj.2011.0180

Luxton, D. D., McCann, R. A., Bush, N. E., Mishkind, M. C., & Reger, G. M. (2011). mHealth for mental health: Integrating smartphone technology in behavioral healthcare. *Professional Psychology: Research and Practice, 42*, 505–512. http://dx.doi.org/10.1037/a0024485

Luxton, D. D., Nelson, E., & Maheu, M. (2016). *A practitioner's guide to telemental health*. Washington, DC: American Psychological Association.

Maciejasz, P., Eschweiler, J., Gerlach-Hahn, K., Jansen-Troy, A., & Leonhardt, S. (2014). A survey on robotic devices for upper limb rehabilitation. *Journal of Neuroengineering and Rehabilitation, 11*(3). http://dx.doi.org/10.1186/1743-0003-11-3

Martínez-Pérez, B., de la Torre-Díez, I., López-Coronado, M., Sainz-de-Abajo, B., Robles, M., & García-Gómez, J. M. (2014). Mobile clinical decision support systems and applications: A literature and commercial review. *Journal of Medical Systems, 38*(4). http://dx.doi.org/10.1007/s10916-013-0004-y

Matarić, M. J., Eriksson, J., Feil-Seifer, D. J., & Winstein, C. J. (2007). Socially assistive robotics for post-stroke rehabilitation. *Journal of Neuroengineering and Rehabilitation, 4*(5). http://dx.doi.org/10.1186/1743-0003-4-5

Merians, A. S., Jack, D., Boian, R., Tremaine, M., Burdea, G. C., Adamovich, S. V., . . . Poizner, H. (2002). Virtual reality-augmented rehabilitation for patients following stroke. *Physical Therapy, 82*, 898–915.

Mihailidis, A., Boger, J. N., Craig, T., & Hoey, J. (2008). The COACH prompting system to assist older adults with dementia through handwashing: An efficacy study. *BMC Geriatrics, 8*(28). http://dx.doi.org/10.1186/1471-2318-8-28

Nikolaidis, S., Forlizzi, J., Hsu, D., Shah, J., & Srinivasa, S. (2017). *Mathematical models of adaptation in human-robot collaboration*. Retrieved from https://arxiv.org/pdf/1707.02586.pdf

O'Connor, M. F., & Riek, L. D. (2015). *Detecting social context: A method for social event classification using naturalistic multimodal data*. Retrieved from https://cseweb.ucsd.edu/ψlriek/papers/fg2015-oconnor-riek.pdf

Patel, S., Park, H., Bonato, P., Chan, L., & Rodgers, M. (2012). A review of wearable sensors and systems with application in rehabilitation. *Journal of Neuroengineering and Rehabilitation, 9*(21). http://dx.doi.org/10.1186/1743-0003-9-21

Piwek, L., Ellis, D. A., Andrews, S., & Joinson, A. (2016). The rise of consumer health wearables: Promises and barriers. *PLoS Medicine, 13*(2), e1001953. http://dx.doi.org/10.1371/journal.pmed.1001953

Prendinger, H., & Ishizuka, M. (Eds.). (2004). *Life-like characters: tools, affective functions, and applications*. Berlin/Heidelberg, Germany: Springer.

Riek, L., & Howard, D. (2014). A code of ethics for the human-robot interaction profession. *We Robot, 2014*. Retrieved from https://www.researchgate.net/publication/286220724_A_Code_of_Ethics_for_the_Human-Robot_Interaction_Profession

Riek, L. D. (2015). Robotics technology in mental healthcare. In D. Luxton (Ed.), *Artificial intelligence in behavioral health and mental health care* (pp. 185–203). San Diego, CA: Elsevier. http://dx.doi.org/10.1016/B978-0-12-420248-1.00008-8

Riek, L. D. (2017). Healthcare robotics. *Communications of the ACM, 60*(11), 68–78. http://dx.doi.org/10.1145/3127874

Riek, L. D., Rabinowitch, T. C., Chakrabarti, B., & Robinson, P. (2009). Empathizing with robots: Fellow feeling along the anthropomorphic spectrum. *Proceedings of the 3rd International Conference on Affective Computing and Intelligent Interaction and Workshops*, 1–6. http://dx.doi.org/10.1109/ACII.2009.5349423

Rizzo, A. A., Buckwalter, J. G., & Neumann, U. (1997). Virtual reality and cognitive rehabilitation: A brief review of the future. *The Journal of Head Trauma Rehabilitation, 12*(6), 1–15. http://dx.doi.org/10.1097/00001199-199712000-00002

Sato, K., Fukumori, S., Matsusaki, T., Maruo, T., Ishikawa, S., Nishie, H., . . . Morita, K. (2010). Nonimmersive virtual reality mirror visual feedback therapy and its application for the treatment of complex regional pain syndrome: An open-label pilot study. *Pain Medicine, 11*, 622–629. http://dx.doi.org/10.1111/j.1526-4637.2010.00819.x

Schultheis, M. T., & Rizzo, A. A. (2001). The application of virtual reality technology in rehabilitation. *Rehabilitation Psychology, 46*, 296–311. http://dx.doi.org/10.1037/0090-5550.46.3.296

Shibata, T., & Wada, K. (2011). Robot therapy: A new approach for mental healthcare of the elderly—A mini-review. *Gerontology, 57*, 378–386. http://dx.doi.org/10.1159/000319015

Siciliano, B., & Khatib, O. (Eds.). (2008). *Springer handbook of robotics*. Berlin/Heidelberg, Germany: Springer. http://dx.doi.org/10.1007/978-3-540-30301-5

Smith, R. O. (2016). The emergence and emergency of assistive technology outcomes research methodology. *Assistive Technology Outcomes and Benefits, 10*(1), 19–37.

Talbot, T. B., Sagae, K., John, B., & Rizzo, A. A. (2012). Sorting out the virtual patient: How to exploit artificial intelligence, game technology and sound educational practices to create engaging role-playing simulations. *International Journal of Gaming and Computer-Mediated Simulations, 4*(3), 1–19. http://dx.doi.org/10.4018/jgcms.2012070101

Tapus, A., Mataric, M. J., & Scassellati, B. (2007). Socially assistive robots [Grand Challenges of Robotics]. *IEEE Robotics & Automation Magazine, 14*, 35–42. http://dx.doi.org/10.1109/MRA.2007.339605

Torous, J., & Nebeker, C. (2017). Navigating ethics in the digital age: Introducing Connected and Open Research Ethics (CORE), a tool for researchers and institutional review boards. *Journal of Medical Internet Research, 19*(2), e38. http://dx.doi.org/10.2196/jmir.6793

van den Heuvel, R. J., Lexis, M. A., Gelderblom, G. J., Jansens, R. M., & de Witte, L. P. (2016). Robots and ICT to support play in children with severe physical disabilities: A systematic review. *Disability and Rehabilitation: Assistive Technology, 11*, 103–116. http://dx.doi.org/10.3109/17483107.2015.1079268

Vasilakos, A., & Pedrycz, W. (2006). *Ambient intelligence, wireless networking, and ubiquitous computing.* Norwood, MA: Artech House.

Ventola, C. L. (2014). Mobile devices and apps for health care professionals: Uses and benefits. *Pharmacy and Therapeutics, 39*, 356–364.

Weiser, M. (1993). Some computer science issues in ubiquitous computing. *Communications of the ACM, 36*(7), 75–84. http://dx.doi.org/10.1145/159544.159617

Woodworth, B., Ferrari, F., Zosa, T. E., & Riek, L. D. (2018). Preference learning in assistive robotics: Observational repeated inverse reinforcement learning. *Proceedings of Machine Learning Research, 85*, 1–19.

Chapter 31

VIRTUAL REALITY AND REHABILITATION

Sebastian T. Koenig, Denise Krch, Belinda S. Lange, and Albert "Skip" Rizzo

Virtual reality (VR) technology has seen a recent surge in market adoption for video games, movies, broadcasting of live events, and industries such as real estate and health care. A report from Goldman Sachs (2016) placed health care as the second largest projected market for VR and augmented reality (AR) in 2025 with an estimated 3.4 million users. The underlying technological advances and financial backing of large corporations such as Google, Apple, Samsung, Microsoft, and Facebook have transformed VR hardware from bulky, expensive systems to affordable, accessible consumer devices. While the entertainment industry is rapidly adopting new VR systems, clinical use of VR technology is still in its infancy. With such a fast-paced market, this chapter will focus on evidence and technology released within the past 5 years to avoid discussing outdated or discontinued VR systems.

Recent reports and systematic reviews have provided detailed accounts of VR's potential for motor rehabilitation (Howard, 2017; Laver, George, Thomas, Deutsch, & Crotty, 2012; Levin, Weiss, & Keshner, 2015), neuropsychological assessment (Parsons & Phillips, 2016), treatment of phobias and posttraumatic stress disorder (Botella, Serrano, Baños, & Garcia-Palacios, 2015; Rizzo & Shilling, 2017), chronic pain (Trost et al., 2015) or acute pain (Hoffman et al., 2011). Meanwhile, little attention has been paid to the state of VR in rehabilitation psychology, including questions of when and how VR will see widespread adoption in this clinical field.

This chapter provides a pragmatic overview of VR technology, including its strengths and limitations, recent research and system development, and future perspectives. The strengths of VR for clinical application have seen extensive debate and documentation. Opportunities that were identified over the past 2 decades (Rizzo & Buckwalter, 1997; Rizzo & Kim, 2005), have finally become a reality in the design of modern VR systems. The widespread appeal of VR in society, untethered hardware, and integration of VR accessories, tracking devices, and psychophysiological monitoring are among the topics that have pushed VR into the spotlight, even in nontraditional VR markets such as rehabilitation psychology.

While rehabilitation psychologists work with a wide range of patient populations with various disabilities and health conditions, they serve as part of a multidisciplinary team to help patients achieve optimal physical, psychological, and cognitive outcomes. We have chosen to focus on the aspect of rehabilitation psychology associated with cognitive outcomes. VR can serve as a valuable tool for assessing and treating cognitive impairments, thereby maximizing the health, welfare, independence, functional abilities, and social and vocational engagement of the patient.

http://dx.doi.org/10.1037/0000129-032
Handbook of Rehabilitation Psychology, Third Edition, L. A. Brenner, S. A. Reid-Arndt, T. R. Elliott, R. G. Frank, and B. Caplan (Editors-in-Chief)

WHAT IS VIRTUAL REALITY?

Virtual reality can generally be defined as "the use of advanced technologies, including computers and various multimedia peripherals, to produce a simulated (i.e., virtual) environment that users perceive as comparable to real world objects and events" (Weiss & Jessel, 1998, p. 277). This definition includes commercially available gaming systems and active-assisted robotic devices. It further includes nonimmersive, flat screen—based systems, fully immersive systems, and anything in between. VR systems are not defined by any specific hardware configuration and can be composed of a wide range of display and interaction devices.

Nonimmersive VR can best be compared to the experience of playing a video game. VR content is displayed on a computer monitor or TV without any occlusion of the outside world. Users interact with a simulated environment through gamepads, joysticks, mouse and keyboard, or other specialized interface devices such as treadmills and tracked hand controllers.

Immersive VR is characterized by a user experience that attempts to shut out the outside world and engage the user in a compelling virtual world through head-mounted displays (HMDs) or surrounding wall-projection systems (i.e., cave automatic virtual environments, or CAVEs). Sensory content can also be delivered via headphones, surround audio systems, motion platforms, or even scent machines. The user can interact with such systems through a myriad of tracking and input devices as outlined later.

Mobile VR has become widely accessible through smartphone-enabled HMD systems such as Google Daydream and Samsung Gear VR. Despite their simplicity, mobile VR systems occlude the outside world and can be considered immersive. However, compared to desktop VR systems, mobile VR devices have less graphical fidelity and lower field of view due to their smaller form factor and reduced processing power. These devices provide low-cost, accessible options for clinicians to administer VR-based assessments and treatments to their patients or for patients to independently access clinician-supervised treatment options from the comfort of their home.

The terms *multisensory* and *interactive* have often been included in definitions of VR. Only over the past few years, as the hardware to support such experiences has become widely available and more affordable for VR consumers, have naturalistic user interfaces through hand and eye tracking, and even natural locomotion, become part of the VR landscape. Five years ago, such features would have been exclusive to custom VR systems, designed for industrial or laboratory use, costing tens, if not hundreds of thousands of dollars. This has changed dramatically with high-quality HMDs appearing on the market for \$300 to \$600, that would have cost over \$20,000 just 5 years ago. Moreover, while new HMDs and display solutions have received the primary focus in the popular media, the development and market for novel and intuitive VR interface devices and body-tracking systems is now also emerging.

This chapter focuses on interactive simulations that are customized for the rehabilitation setting and do not provide active assistance (i.e., robotic devices are excluded). We further exclude off-the-shelf commercial VR games from our discussion, even though we recognize the future potential of the commercial market for VR games using the Oculus Rift, PlayStation VR, HTC Vive, Samsung Gear VR, and Google Daydream. Although initial reports are appearing on the adaptation of these new VR hardware systems for delivering custom-built rehabilitation software (Holmes, Charles, Morrow, McClean, & McDonough, 2016; Just, Sterling, Ros, Naghdy, & Stapley, 2016; Kim, Darakjian, & Finley, 2017), the bulk of the published VR rehabilitation research has been conducted using older gaming systems such as Microsoft Kinect, the Nintendo Wii (including Balance Board), and the PlayStation EyeToy.

WHAT MAKES VR IDEAL FOR REHABILITATION PSYCHOLOGY?

The advantages of VR technology for rehabilitation have been discussed extensively over the years (Rizzo & Kim, 2005; Rizzo & Koenig, 2017; Rose, Brooks, & Rizzo, 2005). This section provides an updated view of VR as a natural fit for clinical use, highlighting key features that can positively impact rehabilitation outcomes and address social and vocational aspects of cognitive rehabilitation.

Ecological Validity

Ecological validity is one of the most frequently reported strengths of VR. It is commonly referred to as the degree of similarity that a test or training has compared to the real world (Neisser, 1978). The underlying assumption in favor of ecological validity is its association with high predictive validity for real-world function (i.e., veridicality) and transfer of learned skills to patients' everyday lives. However, ecological validity is referred to as a *multidimensional construct* (Schmuckler, 2001), and thus, virtual environments, virtual stimuli, and user interaction can independently vary in their degree of ecological validity. For example, virtual environments and virtual stimuli can be gamelike and of low graphical realism while user interactions, tracked movement, and cognitive task requirements can closely resemble interactions in the user's daily life (e.g., reaching for objects, looking around for orientation). Moreover, the graphical fidelity of VR content does not always seem to be of primary importance relative to believable user interaction and relevant task content. This ability of VR treatments to evoke "suspension of disbelief" has been reported frequently in exposure-based therapies for addiction, posttraumatic stress disorder, and anxiety disorders (Bordnick, Yoon, Kaganoff, & Carter, 2013). That is, users report high subjective levels of discomfort and distress when exposed to evocative stimuli, despite many early VR interventions being of low graphical quality (Costanzo et al., 2014; Norrholm et al., 2016).

One crucial element for cognitive tasks is their complexity and how closely they mimic the multimodal demands that people encounter in their daily lives. Most situations of daily living require the concurrent processing of many different stimuli as well as inhibition, flexibility, and complex motor responses. The controlled simulation of such complexity is one of the least understood and most critical elements of VR applications that requires further investigation. It has already been demonstrated that the complexity of virtual environments can have a significant effect on test performance (Parsons, Carlew, & Sullivan, 2015) by providing distractions and influencing psychophysiological state. Traditional neuropsychological tests frequently target cognitive constructs as opposed to functional behavior (Burgess et al., 2006), thus focusing on the complexity and intensity of stimuli within a single cognitive domain instead of exploring more complex, varied, and integrated stimulus compositions. VR applications can dramatically increase the complexity of stimulus presentation while still maintaining precise control over stimulus exposure, intensity, timings, and distractions. However, such complexity does not easily compare to the basic conceptualization of cognitive domains that is represented by traditional paper-and-pencil tests. An intuitive example of a complex functional task is that of making breakfast in a virtual kitchen. The patient must correctly sequence the individual steps to prepare food, search for utensils, cook eggs and bacon, make coffee and toast, feed the cat, listen to the weather forecast, prepare sandwiches for lunch, and get interrupted by several phone calls as well as the sound of the neighbor mowing the lawn. All of this can be precisely simulated in a VR scenario and implemented with full motor interaction to complete each subtask. The amount of data collected in such a scenario is orders of magnitude more complex than a full battery of neuropsychological and motor tests. Kinematic data from any sensor that tracks the user's movement, combined with psychophysiological measures, behavioral data, and log files of the stimuli triggered in the VR scenario create rich data sets that require more sophisticated data processing and analyses compared to the scoring of neuropsychological tests and behavioral ratings of motor tasks. This complexity can be successfully applied to cognitive rehabilitation by carefully varying the co-occurrence and timing of cognitive subtasks and supplementing them with distractions that increase in intrusiveness as the patient progresses through the training.

Simulating social interactions is another way to enrich virtual scenarios and increase their relevance for the daily lives of patients undergoing rehabilitation. The successful implementation of virtual humans (VHs) in clinical assessments, treatments, and trainings has been demonstrated for the following use cases: simulating virtual patients to train novice clinicians; clinical interviewing to reduce stigma and encourage seeking treatment (Rizzo & Talbot, 2016); job interview training for young adults on the autism spectrum (Bresnahan et al., 2016); and as health care guides and clinical support agents (Rizzo, Shilling, et al., 2015). We further believe this social element of VR tools to be of particular value in enhancing VR's ecological validity for rehabilitation psychology. Imagine an impatient friend who distracts or stresses the patient without any regard for the patient's cognitive deficits. Patients will need to be prepared for such situations in their everyday lives, and there is a lot of potential in simulating such socially challenging scenarios during rehabilitation. We therefore encourage researchers and developers to add more social interactions to VR assessments and trainings in the future.

These complex design elements complicate the validation of VR tests and trainings and demand a stronger focus on predictive validity and functional outcomes in the context of patients' everyday lives. A trend toward functional VR scenarios opens up opportunities for transdisciplinary design and development of VR tools, including experts in clinical research and rehabilitation, computational neuroscience, computer science, biomedical engineering, human computer interaction, and statistics. Imagine exposing patients to adaptive, dynamic training scenarios based on machine learning that challenge each user at just the right level of difficulty to maximize rehabilitation outcomes and transfer to real-world functional or vocational tasks.

Motivation

Despite the critical importance of compliance with rehabilitation exercises for recovery, adherence is frequently low (Jack, McLean, Moffett, & Gardiner, 2010). Patients often struggle with adherence to lengthy training protocols, especially during unsupervised training outside of the clinic. Motivation is a critical determinant of initiation and maintenance of treatment, with greater motivation leading to increased practice and improved outcomes (Maclean, Pound, Wolfe, & Rudd, 2002; Winkels, Kottink, Temmink, Nijlant, & Buurke, 2013).

The motivating nature of VR applications is one of the driving factors for their implementation in clinical practice. Compelling environments, story-driven content, virtual characters, relevant feedback, and engaging user interactions are common elements of modern game development, which, when combined with evidence-based task design promote user motivation and engagement (Lange, Flynn, Proffitt, Chang, & Rizzo, 2010; Lange, Flynn, & Rizzo, 2009). Virtual environments are thus experienced more like a game and less like a testing or training scenario, leading patients to naturally be more engaged, less self-conscious and anxious in testing scenarios, and more motivated to adhere to long training protocols (Gamito, Oliveira, Santos, et al., 2014). The feasibility of translating traditional evidence-based interventions into computer gaming formats is increasingly being recognized by clinicians and scientists as a methodology for exploiting the features of games for therapeutic change (Fleming et al., 2017). Thus, VR's potential in health care and the field of "Games for Health" is evidenced by an evolving scientific literature and conferences focused on this topic.

Ideally, VR applications promote an effective motivation style, characterized by persistence and continuous effortful engagement (Granic, Lobel, & Engels, 2014). This spurs patients to work toward a meaningful goal and persevere in the face of challenges and failures. Optimal motivation and patient performance is attained by striking a balance between the level of challenge and frustration, with sufficient experiences of success and accomplishment (Engeser & Rheinberg, 2008; Granic et al., 2014). Concrete immediate feedback regarding effort informs the patient of where they are along this continuum. VR applications that adjust dynamically to the patient's abilities can potentially achieve this balance seamlessly, providing a more naturalistic training scenario. The proper motivation is even more critical for cognitively impaired patients whose deficient initiation and goal-setting decrease the likelihood of treatment adherence.

User motivation does not always need to be achieved through gamification or gamelike content. For patients undergoing rehabilitation, simulation of a meaningful environment such as a home, classroom, or workplace can be highly motivating and engaging. Learning methods that focus on motivational enhancement are well established in improving attention and the outcome of skills training. That is, motivation engenders effective acquisition of new information and new skillsets, which is critical to the transfer of skills targeted during rehabilitation to other contexts. VR interventions designed with consideration of learning and motivation principles will foster improved adherence, user satisfaction, and enjoyment (Kizony, 2011).

Bending the Rules of Reality

VR training scenarios can purposely ignore realism and introduce training mechanisms that are not easily accessible in the real world. For example, tracking a patient's impaired limb can be manipulated to show more pronounced or even mirrored virtual movement compared to the patient's real movement (Regenbrecht, Hoermann, Ott, Müller, & Franz, 2014). Similarly, physical properties of virtual objects or even time can be manipulated in virtual scenarios. Tasks can be paused or slowed down to provide performance feedback, discuss treatment strategy, and encourage errorless learning. Visual and audio cues can be provided that are not available during real-world training. Self-cueing is an innovative feature that asks patients to record feedback or encouraging phrases prior to engaging in a VR scenario. At specific points during the scenario, such as when committing an error or surpassing a threshold of the patient's monitored heart rate, the prerecorded feedback is played as guidance or a source of calmness. The design possibilities for VR are literally endless and still mostly unexplored. Although exciting, this makes the design, implementation, and evaluation of VR rehabilitation content an extremely challenging task, as there are few existing best practices or past success stories on which to build.

Cost and Accessibility of VR Systems

VR has demonstrated promising results for assessing and treating a wide range of psychiatric and neurological disorders. However, even the most promising VR applications need to be accessible and affordable for consumers in order to have a positive impact.

The games industry and technology companies such as Facebook, Google, Samsung, HTC, and Microsoft have been the drivers for substantial investments in advancing VR technology for the consumer market and thus, dramatically reducing the cost for VR hardware, smartphones, and PCs. A complete VR system with PC, HMD, and hand-tracking devices can be purchased for approximately $2,000. Mobile VR systems merely require a recent smartphone and a mobile VR viewer (e.g., Google Daydream, Samsung Gear VR), together available for around $500 to $750. This rapid growth of consumer VR technology has set the stage for a VR accessories market, aimed at VR gaming, but also immensely important for rehabilitation applications. VR eye-tracking systems, hand trackers, EMG and EEG sensors, treadmills, fitness trackers, and various other tracking devices have been developed to engage consumers in unique VR gaming experiences. The availability of many hardware devices not only benefits the end users (i.e., patients, clinicians, researchers), it also gives developers of VR systems a much wider choice of affordable hardware and development tools. For VR treatments that can be used at the patient's home, affordable hardware opens up additional possibilities for including family members and friends in the rehabilitation process. This transition of VR treatments from clinic to community-based rehabilitation will become easier as VR hardware becomes standard in households around the world. "It is probable that VR devices will become like toasters in the next few years—although they won't necessarily be used every day, every household will have one" (Rizzo, 2016). Goldman Sachs (2016) estimated that the number of VR/AR users for video games and entertainment will combine to exceed 300 million by 2025.

WHAT SYSTEMS ARE AVAILABLE FOR USE IN REHABILITATION PSYCHOLOGY?

A wide range of VR applications for neurorehabilitation have been reported in the literature. One might incorrectly assume that publications with "rehabilitation" in the title refer to treatments. Upon closer inspection, the vast majority of VR tools that have been reported in the literature are in fact VR assessments that target motor and/or cognitive domains. We can only speculate as to the reasons for this, but the effort to design a series of VR assessment tasks does pale in comparison to the substantial amount of virtual training content required to build a complete intervention. It seems logical that researchers and companies would start by validating tasks within the limited scope of an assessment, and if successful, extend the virtual scenario to an intervention by adding content, progression, and potentially a storyline. We have experienced such progression of a VR tool ourselves by building an assessment for executive functions (Krch et al., 2013) and extending it to a comprehensive, yet focused, higher-level attention training over the past 4 years with pilot results and development methodology to be published soon. Given this trend in existing research and commercial VR tools, we summarize current VR systems and highlight their attributes and applicability, differentiating assessments from treatments. Distinctions are made between construct-driven systems and function-driven systems.

OVERVIEW OF RESEARCH ON COGNITIVE ASSESSMENTS

Early efforts to apply VR to rehabilitation assessments concentrated on translating existing evaluations of discrete cognitive constructs to simulated environments. These VR tools were meant to extend the ecological validity of existing assessments. One of the most successful examples of one such tool is the virtual classroom paradigm, a virtual version of the computerized Continuous Performance Test (CPT), designed to assess and diagnose attention disorders. The basic VR classroom scenario consists of a child seated at a desk in a virtual classroom, facing the blackboard. The child is asked to sustain attention and respond to stimuli presented on the blackboard, while ignoring distractors. The Virtual Classroom, created in 1999 by Rizzo and colleagues, used an HMD-based VR system that allowed for the occlusion of distractions from the outside world, an important detail that is required to prevent unrelated stimuli from interfering with the attention evaluation (Rizzo et al., 2006). Indeed, research demonstrated that children with attention-deficit/hyperactivity disorder (ADHD) were found to miss targets due to looking away from the virtual blackboard during 25% of the trials relative to normal subjects who only looked away less than 1% of the time. Trackers afford the ability to capture head and body movement, providing data on motor hyperactivity, which is simply not possible using traditional assessment methods. Findings from motion tracking indicated higher activity levels on all metrics in children with ADHD relative to controls, and higher activity levels in children with ADHD in a distraction condition relative to nondistraction (Rizzo et al., 2006).

In recent years, multiple research groups have produced varying classroom paradigms. AULA Nesplora (Climent, Banterla, & Iriarte, 2010) is one such successful example (Díaz-Orueta et al., 2014). The AULA differs from previous versions in that the target stimuli are presented both visually and aurally. It also deliberately presents a no-go paradigm (i.e., press a button when the target stimulus is not perceived) prior to a go paradigm (i.e., press a button when the target stimulus is perceived), reasoning that this sequence more accurately reproduces the problem faced by children with low self-regulation in adaptation to new environments after performing an overstimulating activity. The AULA is notable for its methodological rigor and the vast scale of normative data that has been collected on it, which is more commensurate with the validation seen in commercially available neuropsychological tests.

Construct-driven VR assessments adapted from traditional neuropsychological tests, such as two Stroop paradigms (the Virtual Classroom Bimodal Stroop and the Virtual Reality Stroop Task) and the Virtual Reality Paced Auditory Serial Addition Test have been developed with the goal of providing unique information untapped by traditional attention and executive functioning tasks (Parsons & Carlew, 2016; Parsons & Courtney, 2014; Rizzo et al., 2006). The Virtual Classroom Bimodal Stroop can be deployed using an HMD or monitor with a tracker to track head movements. The assessment takes place in a virtual classroom and is comprised of a color block task and a word-based task, each of which have nondistraction and distraction conditions. In the block-based tasks, a series of colored rectangles (red, blue, green) appear on the virtual blackboard while a female voice states the names of the colors. Participants are instructed to click the mouse as quickly as possible when the color spoken matches the color of the rectangle on the virtual blackboard and to refrain from responding when the color spoken and the color shown do not match. In the word-based condition, color words are presented on the virtual blackboard in different ink colors. Stimuli are congruent and incongruent, comparable to the colored rectangles. The colors are again stated in a female voice and participants are to click on the mouse when the spoken word matches the color of the word. If the spoken and written words do not match, participants refrain from responding. The Virtual Classroom Bimodal Stroop and an apartment Stroop paradigm developed by Henry, Joyal, and Nolin (2012) were recently evaluated for feasibility and efficacy as a treatment (Salisbury, Dahdah, Driver, Parsons, & Richter, 2016).

The Virtual Reality Stroop Task can also be administered in a Humvee within a military-relevant assessment. Stroop stimuli appear on the windshield, while the user navigates the Humvee through alternating zones of low threat (e.g., driving down a desert road) to high threat (e.g., stressors such as gunfire and explosions). The varying degrees of threat allow for the evaluation of attention processing at different levels of arousal (Parsons et al., 2011). The Virtual Reality Paced Auditory Serial Addition Test (VR-PASAT) evaluates calculation ability, auditory information processing speed, and flexibility. The VR-PASAT is presented on an HMD in conjunction with a tactile transducer. While varying degrees of background chatter are presented, the participant must add each new digit to the one immediately prior. This work is an important step toward evaluating the effect of contextual factors such as environmental complexity, emotional valence of virtual content, and distractors on patient performance. The systematic evaluation of this combination of functional context- and construct-driven tasks paves the way for more function-led VR assessments and treatments in the future (Parsons et al., 2015).

A much more recent development in the field has been the appearance of strictly function-driven assessments. These are of potentially greater interest to rehabilitation psychologists given that rehabilitation models focus on return to functional activities. Copland and colleagues, in collaboration with Katana Simulations, developed a unique evaluation tool, the Cognitive Assessment for Aphasia App (C3A; Wall, Cumming, Koenig, Pelecanos, & Copland, 2018), to evaluate cognitive function in individuals with aphasia secondary to stroke. Aphasic patients are often excluded from validation trials and from the VR design process due to their decreased ability to communicate and provide feedback (see Wall et al., 2015). The C3A decreases emphasis on language by providing short, simple verbal instructions, a computerized visual demonstration, practice prior to testing, and a variety of auditory and visual feedback techniques to facilitate learning. The test includes a simple reaction time task to assess psychomotor speed, a visual search task to assess neglect and attention, a sequence copy task to assess visual memory, and a functional kitchen task to assess executive functioning. The C3A is deployed on an Android tablet with touch screen interface for easy navigation (Wall et al., 2018). In a feasibility study conducted with 64 individuals poststroke (35 with aphasia and 29 without) and 32 controls, the authors found that out of all participants with stroke, only one with aphasia was unable to complete all aspects of the C3A, suggesting that the C3A may offer a significant advantage over paper-and-pencil cognitive tests in the evaluation of planning, sequencing, and problem-solving (Wall et al., 2018). Inclusion of aphasic patients and a multidisciplinary team of stakeholders in the development, design, and validation of VR systems is important to adequately treat the wide range of symptom profiles and deficits in neurological disorders.

One of the most methodologically rigorous VR-based assessments found in the literature is the Virtual Reality Functional Capacity Assessment Tool (VRFCAT), a VR-based assessment of functional abilities (Ruse et al., 2014) developed and sold by NeuroCog Trials (NeuroCog, 2015). Specifically, the VRFCAT evaluates activities of daily living, including navigating to and from the grocery store via bus, shopping for and purchasing items at the store, and completing a recipe. Thus, the mini scenarios target transportation, finances, household management, and planning functional measures. Six different versions of these scenarios are available, and the software is deployed within a nonimmersive environment. The assessment measures the amount of time subjects spend completing 12 different objectives, and how many errors are committed in the process. Research in individuals with schizophrenia has demonstrated that the assessment possesses good test-retest reliability (ICC 8 .81), good convergent validity, minimal practice effects, strong sensitivity in differentiating healthy controls from schizophrenia and high, positive correlations with cognitive performance (Keefe et al., 2016). Strong psychometric properties of the alternate test versions have supported repeat assessments in clinical trials. Although the software was designed and marketed as an evaluation tool in schizophrenia clinical trials, the authors suggest that it may prove widely applicable to assessing functional capacity in a range of central nervous system disorders, including mood disorders, mild cognitive impairment, and Alzheimer's disease. Additionally, the assessment has been culturally adapted for use in the United Kingdom and Canada.

Within the realm of functional assessments, the Virtual Library Task (VLT; Renison, Ponsford, Testa, Richardson, & Brownfield, 2012) expands assessment of executive function, a construct traditionally complex and challenging to evaluate using traditional measures, into a novel library environment. The VLT is a nonimmersive VR role-play task that is deployed using Xbox and a PlayStation-compatible handset. Participants are required to perform several specific tasks associated with day-to-day running of a library while adhering to a set of rules. Functional tasks are designed to reflect seven components of executive function, including task analysis, strategy generation and regulation, prospective working memory, interference and dual task management, response inhibition, and time- and event-based prospective memory. Thirty participants with moderate to severe traumatic brain injury (TBI) and executive difficulties were evaluated using the VLT. Additional measures collected included a behavioral rating scale of everyday executive functioning, performance on a real-world library task, a functional executive function task, and other traditional neuropsychological measures. Whereas only one of the five traditional neuropsychological measures distinguished performance between individuals with TBI and healthy controls, performance on four of the five VLT subtests and the functional task of executive functioning distinguished these groups. Further, scores on the VLT were highly positively correlated with those on the real-world library task (Renison et al., 2012). The findings from this study established feasibility in administering VR-based assessments to individuals with moderate to severe TBI and provided evidence for good construct and ecological validity of the VLT, suggesting improved sensitivity of the VR measure relative to traditional measures.

The Complex Shopping Mall (CSM), a large urban virtual shopping mall based on a real mall, was created by Weiss and colleagues to assess functional performance. The CSM was created as part of a larger multidisciplinary effort to establish a "Rehabilitation Living Lab" to optimize social inclusion of persons with disabilities in enabling physical and social environments (Sangani et al., 2012). A four-item shopping task was adapted and modified from previous studies investigating the use of a virtual supermarket (Rand, Katz, & Weiss, 2007). Users navigated to a store and purchased items on a list and were evaluated for task completion time and navigation path (Sangani, Fung, Kizony, Koenig, & Weiss, 2013). The CSM was implemented on an advanced locomotor system that combined the virtual environment with a self-paced treadmill mounted on a motion platform in order to determine the feasibility of evaluating motor performance. Data collected from healthy younger and older adults in Canada and Israel showed that younger adults took less time to complete the task and their path took a smoother trajectory relative to older adults. The locomotor task increased engagement, but changing direction in the mall proved difficult as it required the participant to stop in order to rotate their view before continuing (Sangani et al., 2013). A follow-up study evaluating the Virtual Multiple Errands Test in the CSM simulation showed that, again, performance of younger adults was more efficient and faster than that of older adults. Gait parameters were not significantly different between the age groups (Kizony et al., 2017). This paradigm allows for the simultaneous assessment of cognitive and motor functioning while performing a functional task. Furthermore, the ability to carry out a Virtual Multiple Errands Test in the CSM allows for comparison with the traditional real-world Multiple Errands Task (Shallice & Burgess, 1991), providing a strong use case.

OVERVIEW OF RESEARCH ON COGNITIVE TREATMENTS

Although assessments tend to fall into either construct- or function-driven approaches, treatments are predisposed to be function-driven, perhaps because rehabilitation tends to focus on functional outcomes and virtual environments lend themselves to a storyline.

Based on the concept of the original classroom paradigm, Gawrilow and colleagues, in collaboration with Katana Simulations, created an immersive virtual classroom training to treat attention-deficit/hyperactivity disorder (ADHD; Blume et al., 2017). Lighting in the virtual classroom provides the participant with feedback that they have increased or decreased activation in a target neuroanatomical area. An upward arrow on the blackboard indicates that the child should increase activation and a downward arrow indicates that the child should decrease activation. The authors are currently evaluating the efficacy of a near infrared spectroscopy (NIRS) feedback training in conjunction with the virtual classroom in children with ADHD (Blume et al., 2017). It is hypothesized that the virtual classroom scenario will facilitate self-regulation skills obtained in the NIRS feedback training. Ninety children with ADHD will be randomized to an NIRS-based training in the VR classroom, an NIRS-based training in a 2D classroom, or an electromyogram-based training in VR. This clinical trial is ongoing.

Gamito (2013) and colleagues established a VR toolkit, the Systemic Lisbon Battery (SLB), a portfolio of 17 serious games (in Portuguese). The games can be played online or deployed on tablets. The SLB is a small virtual town in which participants are free to walk around and engage in instrumental activities of daily living and digital games. The virtual town contains a house, where users can engage in home-based activities (e.g., personal hygiene, dressing, preparing meals), a supermarket, an art gallery, a pharmacy, and a casino. Tasks address all domains of cognitive function, including memory, attention, and executive function. The SLB tasks can be used both as assessments and treatments. Normative data have been collected for the Virtual Kitchen Test (Gamito et al., 2015), which is part of the SLB, in a sample of individuals with alcohol dependence. Additionally, normative data for three subtests (i.e., fruit matching, supermarket, art gallery) from the SLB has been collected in a sample of 243 healthy college students (Gamito et al., 2016). However, this portfolio of games can also be used as treatments and the authors have established clinical efficacy in stroke and alcohol and substance use disorders (Gamito, Oliveira, Coelho, et al., 2017; Gamito, Oliveira, Lopes, et al., 2014, 2017). In each of these intervention trials, treatment consisted of two to three 60-minute sessions occurring over a 4- to 6-week period of inpatient stay for each patient population. The cognitive training protocol consisted of exposing participants to several SLB tasks with increased level of difficulty across sessions. The control groups received treatment as usual. In all three studies, the patient group receiving the SLB improved performance in the target cognitive domain relative to the control groups. The consistent improvement that patients have shown when training with the SLB is very promising. Important next steps for future research with the SLB should be the inclusion of more functional-based outcome measures in order to establish ecological relevance for patients' everyday lives.

Man and colleagues developed a 12-session VR-based cognitive rehabilitation program using everyday prospective memory activities as training content for application in Chinese patient populations (Yip & Man, 2013). Participants carried out event- and time-based prospective memory training tasks in a virtual convenience store. The treatment was evaluated in 37 subjects with acquired brain injury. Outcome measures included a VR-based assessment of prospective memory, a real-world behavioral measure of prospective memory, a standardized paper-and-pencil assessment of prospective memory, and several traditional neuropsychological tests. Results demonstrated improvements from pre- to posttreatment in the VR-based test of prospective memory in the treatment group. As the VR-based test was not administered to the control group, no between-group comparisons could be made. Individuals in the treatment group showed significantly better performance on event-based, but not time-based, real-life behavioral prospective memory tasks relative to the control group. A similar pattern was seen on the standardized prospective memory assessment; however, this difference between groups was not significant. The accuracy of real-life event-based prospective memory tasks moderately correlated with most of the items in the VR-based prospective memory tasks. A commendable feature of the research design of this study is the assemblage of a battery that not only includes traditional measures, but behavioral measures and VR-based functional measures as well. Results were likely limited by the small sample size and the fact that the training content was fixed, making it inappropriate for individuals with varying skill levels. Additionally, the psychometric properties of the VR- and behavioral-based prospective memory tasks created for the purpose of evaluating the treatment are unknown (Yip & Man, 2013).

Klinger and colleagues (2013) created a configurable and upgradable tool for the creation of individualized therapeutic applications in cognitive rehabilitation. AGATHE allows therapists to assess specific cognitive constructs (e.g., executive function, memory) through a functional approach, and offers the potential to train a wide range of instrumental activities of daily living. The core of the program consists of a virtual neighborhood comprising a studio, a post office, and a supermarket, with the possibility to be scalable to add new places and new tasks. AGATHE is another example of a training tool that was created with input from various stakeholders, including patients, researchers, and therapists from different disciplines (e.g., physicians, neuropsychologists, occupational therapists). The interface allows the clinician to set tasks, and to manage instructions and cues delivered to the patient during the session. A second interface allows the clinician to supervise the patient's activity in real time and to replay the patient's activity. Preliminary pilot trials established feasibility and usability (Klinger et al., 2013). The authors intend to conduct further efficacy trials and later commercialize the software.

Krch, Spero, and Koenig (2018), in collaboration with Katana Simulations, created Wonderkin Wonderworks, a nonimmersive VR treatment system that targets divided attention and set shifting impairments. Development was informed by patients, clinicians, and research rehabilitation experts using an iterative design approach. Wonderworks takes place in a virtual office environment, wherein the user carries out various tasks following the storyline of an internship across eight 30-minute modules. The length of each session was chosen to fit the treatment duration that is most common in clinical practice. Some of the treatment's tasks might be encountered in a real office (e.g., managing faxes and photocopies), but some are imaginary (e.g., monitoring animated toy animals) in keeping with the fictional storyline of the internship. Each module is comprised of the primary tasks that take place in the virtual world, complemented by content at the beginning and end of the module that engages the patient in psychoeducation, exposure to practical real-world examples, and review of prior modules and assigned homework. The software is designed to be appropriate for individuals with a wide range of attention skills, which is accomplished through the use of adaptive difficulty that adjusts to performance level by changing the pace, timing of stimuli, and number of distractions. Adaptive difficulty automatically adjusts the difficulty level according to the patient's skill, ensuring that the difficulty level is challenging, but not frustrating. Wonderworks is deployed on a Windows PC and controlled through mouse or touch screen. This software has shown preliminary efficacy in a small double-blind randomized controlled pilot trial in individuals with TBI and attention impairments. Importantly, outcome measures selected for the pilot trial included not only traditional neuropsychological tests, but also self-report assessments of psychosocial functioning, functional abilities and limitations, and more real-world functional assessments. Future steps are to conduct a large-scale randomized controlled trial and to commercialize the treatment.

WHAT ARE THE CURRENT LIMITATIONS OF VR IN REHABILITATION PSYCHOLOGY?

Recent meta-analyses have extensively reviewed studies pertaining to VR rehabilitation. Without exception, each of these reviews concludes with similar remarks.

There is a lack of sufficiently powered, randomized, well-controlled clinical trials (Bogdanova, Yee, Ho, & Cicerone, 2016; Larson, Feigon, Gagliardo, & Dvorkin, 2014; Ogourtsova, Silva, Archambault, & Lamontagne, 2017; Parsons & Phillips, 2016; Pietrzak, Pullman, & McGuire, 2014; Valladares-Rodriguez et al., 2016). Some trials exist, but these are the exception rather than the rule. Instead, the bulk of the research consists of small single-case studies, pilot trials, and underpowered clinical trials of varying methodological quality, preventing researchers from drawing meaningful conclusions about the efficacy and psychometric properties of VR rehabilitation treatments and assessments.

Standardization is severely lacking in every aspect of VR rehabilitation. This lack of standards negatively impacts VR software development (Valladares-Rodriguez et al., 2016), choice of assessment and treatment characteristics, and evaluation methodology, as well as selection of outcome measures.

With such unanimous conclusions of these recent reviews, the importance of the identified issues can only be stressed repeatedly, with recommendations made to address these problems. There is no consensus on the critical components of VR treatments and assessment and to what degree they contribute to successful rehabilitation outcomes. VR intervention characteristics such as treatment intensity, user interaction, feedback delivery, stimulus selection, and task and environmental complexity have seen only isolated investigations with very few conclusive reviews emerging in the literature. It also remains unclear how different patient populations of varying deficit profiles are benefiting from different choices of treatment characteristics (De Luca, Calabrò, & Bramanti, 2018). As the field moves forward, rigorous methodological design will allow investigators to critically evaluate the variables important to successful evaluation and treatment tools.

The vast heterogeneity of study designs, applied methodology, and reported outcome measures is limiting the progress of VR for rehabilitation considerably. Several systematic reviews recommend a stronger focus on functional outcomes and evaluation of real-world skills instead of relying on traditional tasks that have low relevance for patients' ability to function in their daily lives (Coyle, Traynor, & Solowij, 2015; Negut, Matu, Sava, & David, 2016; Ogourtsova, Silva, Archambault, & Lamontagne, 2017). One of the biggest cases for using VR technology as a treatment tool in the first place is to improve on the limitations of our current treatments. How can we promote ecologically relevant treatments if we measure change on outcome measures not designed to capture function? Our traditional measures do a stellar job in many aspects of evaluation, but fall short when it comes to appraising complex skills required in activities of daily living or occupational settings. Underscoring this point, Krch and colleagues (2013) demonstrated in both multiple sclerosis and TBI populations statistically equivocal performance on standard cognitive tests relative to healthy controls, while both patient groups performed significantly worse on VR-based measures of cognition. With this in mind, researchers evaluating VR-based treatments are encouraged to include VR-based assessments (when available), as well as functional and real-world tests along with the traditional measures.

Considering that psychology as an independent science has been around for about 125 years with a focus on studying human behavior and interaction in the physical world, it makes sense that it may take a few more years to evolve the science for how humans behave and interact in the virtual world. Thus, there is plenty of good science that will need to be done to specify the areas in which VR adds value over existing traditional methodologies.

Need for Hardware-Agnostic Design

Hardware manufacturers are releasing new VR hardware, controllers, and tracking devices at a much higher pace than researchers and clinicians can design, develop, and validate VR rehabilitation tools. Clinical validation, user-centered design, and medical device approvals are time-intensive processes that can take several years from first design to commercial use. By the time a first clinical trial of a research prototype commences, the hardware that was proposed at the project start may already be outdated. Consequently, researchers and software developers should focus on hardware-agnostic design of treatments and assessments to avoid using hardware that might not be available to consumers anymore (e.g., Microsoft Kinect for Windows).

There are two encouraging trends that can potentially alleviate this concern. First, VR hardware and software manufacturers are putting more emphasis on integrating their products. Thus, VR developers can more easily integrate new hardware into their products and potentially improve existing applications or keep them relevant for the consumer market for longer periods of time. Second, initiatives like WebVR and OpenVR provide platforms that can operate with a wide range of VR hardware, and thus make VR rehabilitation more accessible and less hardware-dependent. We encourage all stakeholders to avoid fixating on specific hardware, and instead design VR applications with hardware flexibility in mind and focus on the therapeutic characteristics that can maximize each application's impact on rehabilitation outcomes.

Need for Cost–Benefit Analyses

Reimbursement by payers is a large facilitator for widespread clinical adoption of new treatments and assessments. Each health care system has different requirements and regulations, but generally, treatment efficacy, assessment validity/reliability, feasibility, safety, and cost–benefit analyses are important factors considered by payers in determining reimbursement. Cost–benefit analyses have rarely been mentioned in VR publications over the past two decades (Lloréns, Noé, Colomer, & Alcañiz, 2015; Schultheis & Rizzo, 2001). It remains an underrepresented topic in the VR rehabilitation literature, considering that the final and most important step for most clinical VR tools should be widespread adoption in international health care markets. We therefore encourage researchers, clinicians, and developers to more openly share the expected and actual costs of delivering VR therapy and assessments and how these costs compare with more traditional neurorehabilitation approaches.

Ethical Considerations

There are several concerns regarding the ethical use of VR technology for rehabilitation psychology and more broadly for clinical use. First, there are general issues such as simulator sickness, provocative content, and addiction to VR content that are not specific to clinical VR tools and require a more in-depth discussion that is beyond the scope of this chapter. The reader is referred to publications by Madary and Metzinger (2016); Rizzo, Schultheis, and Rothbaum (2003); and Yellowlees, Holloway, and Parish (2012) for details on ethical VR use. We believe the following topics of ethical VR use in rehabilitation psychology to be of relevance.

VR assessments and treatments are novel tools that require specialized training for clinicians to safely administer to patients. Therapists need to be aware of all the software and hardware features that are relevant for clinical use, in particular, how these will impact patient comfort and safety, and what unique VR features contribute to treatment success. Certification of proficiency to administer VR rehabilitation tools seems to be an obvious solution.

There is a need for more research and documented evidence of the efficacy of VR interventions. Future VR tools will require a sound theoretical foundation and scientific evidence of clinical benefits before being marketed. In an emerging area like VR where unique and specific guidelines have yet to be established, the practitioner must be fully transparent about the evidence base for the approach and take precautions to preserve the patient's safety and integrity. This may require regulatory oversight to avoid false advertisement by VR companies, as well as an effort by clinicians to keep informed about existing evidence of their VR tools of choice.

Self-treatment and self-diagnosis can be problematic when VR rehabilitation tools become freely available to patients without proper regulation to restrict access to well-trained clinical providers. We already see a similar trend with so-called brain training apps or apps that promise self-help for phobias and anxiety disorders. Such self-treatment could discourage patients from seeking proper help with qualified clinicians and may lead to worsening of a patient's condition by using improper treatment approaches. Again, regulatory oversight over apps and VR tools promising clinical treatment should alleviate this problem.

Safety and confidentiality of patient data is of central importance to any health-related discipline. Many software applications save user data in the Cloud, from Spotify playlists to Amazon purchase histories, Facebook and Twitter feeds, credit card information, and even GPS tracking using smartphones. VR applications are no different and can potentially save rehabilitation results or other sensitive, identifiable data to the Cloud. To our knowledge, many VR research prototype applications simply avoid saving data to online databases, due to both the cost and the complexity of integrating data output with hospital IT policies or even electronic medical records. Data can be saved on a local computer and printed out or sent via email (after de-identification) if needed. When data are saved online, security standards should be adhered to and data should ideally be saved with a hosting service that uses security standards that comply with patient protection guidelines. Unfortunately, most eHealth-related applications do not seem to employ data safety measures, even basic encryption of data, thus exposing critical client data (ePrivacy, 2015). Guidelines for data safety and patient confidentiality and medical device laws should be adhered to. However, enforcement of these guidelines and laws and effective oversight over rapidly growing markets such as mobile (VR) apps is a challenge. A method for educating and informing VR development companies on the regulatory landscape, and for providing cost-effective solutions that meet all regulations while not stifling innovation is needed.

HOW CAN THE POTENTIAL OF VR IN REHABILITATION PSYCHOLOGY BE REALIZED?

Virtual rehabilitation is a young and promising field with many individual projects that suggest the potential for a positive impact on the lives of those undergoing rehabilitation. It is the lack of a coherent collaborative strategy, as well as missing standards in design and evaluation methodology, that are slowing down progress in developing innovative VR assessments and treatments for rehabilitation. Clinical trials that assess feasibility and efficacy of VR tools are sparse, often underpowered, and of varying methodological quality and scientific rigor. Reviews of the virtual rehabilitation field have consistently concluded that VR rehabilitation tools possess a lot of potential but require additional adequately powered, well-controlled trials to provide evidence for their efficacy and cost-effectiveness (e.g., De Luca, Calabrò, & Bramanti, 2018; Hill et al., 2017; Pietrzak, Pullman, & McGuire, 2014). We can only underscore these recommendations as we strongly believe that a more coordinated effort to develop standards, best practices, and validated, robust rehabilitation tools is needed for general clinical use and specifically for rehabilitation psychology.

The following trends and recommendations are critical for VR research and development in order to push VR toward widespread adoption in rehabilitation.

VR hardware will advance at a continued rapid pace, making VR even more affordable, untethered, and accessible for low-end computers and smartphones, thus reaching a broad audience. Instead of attempting to keep up with the pace of new VR hardware, researchers and developers should instead focus on the general components of functional tasks and treatments, promoting hardware-agnostic design and best practices, and prototypes.

While construct-driven approaches have their place in a comprehensive rehabilitation plan, virtual rehabilitation needs to unchain itself from strictly construct-specific task content and mere translations of traditional rehabilitation content to the new VR medium. Innovations should consider function-driven and construct-function hybrid approaches as well. Further, innovation should not just occur in creating VR environments, but also in task and interaction design, and data collection, integration, and analysis. The prospect of highly adaptable rehabilitation scenarios that consider patient history, current patient performance, rehabilitation goals, and social and vocational context are on the horizon, but need substantial research and design efforts from transdisciplinary teams to become a reality.

The assessment and training of spatial abilities is still a somewhat underrepresented topic in the VR literature. Spatial orientation in virtual environments has been addressed regularly, either in large, open virtual spaces (Cogné et al., 2017), buildings (Koenig, Crucian, Dalrymple-Alford, & Dünser, 2011), or in artificial scenarios such as the Virtual Morris Water Maze (Astur, Taylor, Mamelak, Philpott, & Sutherland, 2002). However, the perception of speed and distance in virtual space is still not well understood, and VR users seem to consistently underestimate distance and sometimes speed when exposed to virtual environments (Kemeny & Panerai, 2003; Koenig et al., 2011; Plumert, Kearney, Cremer, & Recker, 2005; Renner, Velichkovsky, & Helmert, 2013). This should motivate researchers to further explore human perception in virtual environments, especially with modern VR hardware that can produce photorealistic scenarios on consumer-grade VR systems. The prospect of leveraging cues, feedback, and dynamic, complex virtual scenarios with task-related stimuli and distractors can profoundly change the way spatial abilities are assessed and rehabilitated. Clinical use cases for such VR tools include assessment and training of driving performance, hemispatial neglect, and spatial disorientation.

There are few VR-related technologies that we expect to go beyond incremental change and instead fundamentally impact the way we use VR tools for rehabilitation.

There is large potential for personalized VR rehabilitation by using 360-degree panoramic images and videos. Customized content creation is expected to get much easier over the next few years to the point where our environments are fully digitized and available as 3D models (e.g., Google Earth), eventually with sufficient quality for photorealistic VR content. Even today, consumer-grade 360-degree cameras can easily capture patients' familiar environments and expose them to scenarios that are crucial for living independently after inpatient rehabilitation ends (cf. Koenig, 2012). Filmmaker Bruce Branit (2009) provided a vision for how VR content can provide meaningful, personalized context to rehabilitation.

Eye-tracking systems are becoming the latest trend to enhance existing VR tools (Lutz et al., 2017). Eye tracking is expected to fulfill a dual role of lowering hardware requirements through a technique called foveated rendering (Patney, Kim, Salvi, Kaplanyan, & Wymona, 2016), and acting as an innovative data collection and feedback tool for rehabilitation. The benefit of eye-tracking technology will be especially evident in applications addressing the rehabilitation of visual deficits, spatial attention, and specifically, hemispatial neglect.

Improvements in markerless tracking of hands and their integration in existing VR hardware will enable more natural interactions and increase ecological validity for VR rehabilitation scenarios, specifically for dual tasks that target cognitive *and* motor demands. While such tracking sensors are already available, their integration in consumer-grade HMDs will set a new standard for human interaction with virtual environments and strengthen the case for holistic rehabilitation that targets cognitive and motor deficits simultaneously.

CONCLUSION

Researchers, clinicians, and companies have spent the past 25 years fighting technological barriers, distorted public perception, and a lack of experience in designing VR rehabilitation tools. Developed VR tools were predominantly replications of traditional assessments and trainings that originated in real-world assessments (e.g., Multiple Errands Test) or paper-and-pencil tests (e.g., Stroop Task, Wisconsin Card Sorting Test, Continuous Performance Test; Parsons et al., 2015). However, the past 5 years have brought a massive shift in VR technology from expensive research-grade systems to affordable consumer-grade products. Therefore, the field of virtual rehabilitation is at a tipping point where the technology has finally caught up to the high expectations of the media and potential users in the rehabilitation setting. With a concerted research effort to identify the active ingredients of VR tools and how they affect rehabilitation outcomes in a wide range of clinical populations, we anticipate that VR technology will become an indispensable tool for rehabilitation psychology. This will become evident through new VR scenarios that simulate activities of daily living while also including social elements, either in multiplayer environments that include family and friends or through interactions with virtual human characters. Such scenarios could play out in schools, home environments, or workplaces such as offices, warehouses, supermarkets, and restaurants. The potential and possibilities for innovative VR rehabilitation tools are endless and only limited by our imagination and our capacity to scientifically evaluate their added value.

References

Astur, R. S., Taylor, L. B., Mamelak, A. N., Philpott, L., & Sutherland, R. J. (2002). Humans with hippocampus damage display severe spatial memory impairments in a virtual Morris water task. *Behavioural Brain Research*, *132*, 77–84. http://dx.doi.org/10.1016/S0166-4328(01)00399-0

Blume, F., Hudak, J., Dresler, T., Ehlis, A. C., Kühnhausen, J., Renner, T. J., & Gawrilow, C. (2017). NIRS-based neurofeedback training in a virtual reality classroom for children with attention-deficit/hyperactivity disorder: Study protocol for a randomized controlled trial. *Trials*, *18*, 41. http://dx.doi.org/10.1186/s13063-016-1769-3

Bogdanova, Y., Yee, M. K., Ho, V. T., & Cicerone, K. D. (2016). Computerized cognitive rehabilitation of attention and executive function in acquired brain injury: A systematic review. *Journal of Head Trauma Rehabilitation*, *31*, 419–433.

Bordnick, P. S., Yoon, J. H., Kaganoff, E., & Carter, B. (2013). Virtual reality cue reactivity assessment: A comparison of treatment- vs. nontreatment-seeking smokers. *Research on Social Work Practice*, *23*, 419–425. http://dx.doi.org/10.1177/1049731513482377

Botella, C., Serrano, B., Baños, R. M., & Garcia-Palacios, A. (2015). Virtual reality exposure-based therapy for the treatment of post-traumatic stress disorder: A review of its efficacy, the adequacy of the treatment protocol, and its acceptability. *Neuropsychiatric Disease and Treatment*, *11*, 2533–2545. http://dx.doi.org/10.2147/NDT.S89542

Branit, B. (2009, February 24). *World builder* (high quality). Retrieved from https://www.youtube.com/watch?v=VzFpg271sm8

Bresnahan, T., Rizzo, A. A., Burke, S. L., Partin, M., Ahlness, R. M., & Trimmer, M. (2016, September). *Using virtual interactive training agents (VITA) with adults with autism and other developmental disabilities.* Paper presented at the International Conference on Disability, Virtual Reality and Associated Technologies, Los Angeles, CA.

Burgess, P. W., Alderman, N., Forbes, C., Costello, A., Coates, L. M-A., Dawson, D. R., . . . Channon, S. (2006). The case for the development and use of "ecologically valid" measures of executive function in experimental and clinical neuropsychology. *Journal of the International Neuropsychological Society*, *12*, 194–209. http://dx.doi.org/10.1017/S1355617706060310

Climent, G., Banterla, F., & Iriarte, Y. (2010). Virtual reality, technologies and behavioural assessment. In G. Climent & F. Banterla (Eds.), *AULA, ecological evaluation of attentional processes* (pp. 19–28). San Sebastian, Spain: Nesplora.

Cogné, M., Taillade, M., N'Kaoua, B., Tarruella, A., Klinger, E., Larrue, F., . . . Sorita, E. (2017). The contribution of virtual reality to the diagnosis of spatial navigation disorders and to the study of the role of navigational aids: A systematic literature review. *Annals of Physical and Rehabilitation Medicine*, *60*, 164–176. http://dx.doi.org/10.1016/j.rehab.2015.12.004

Costanzo, M. E., Leaman, S., Jovanovic, T., Norrholm, S. D., Rizzo, A. A., Taylor, P., & Roy, M. J. (2014). Psychophysiological response to virtual reality and subthreshold posttraumatic stress disorder symptoms in recently deployed military. *Psychosomatic Medicine*, *76*, 670–677. http://dx.doi.org/10.1097/PSY.0000000000000109

Coyle, H., Traynor, V., & Solowij, N. (2015). Computerized and virtual reality cognitive training for individuals at high risk of cognitive decline: Systematic review of the literature. *American Journal of Geriatric Psychiatry*, *23*, 335–359. http://dx.doi.org/10.1016/j.jagp.2014.04.009

De Luca, R., Calabrò, R. S., & Bramanti, P. (2018). Cognitive rehabilitation after severe acquired brain injury: Current evidence and future directions. *Neuropsychological Rehabilitation*, 1–20.

Díaz-Orueta, U., Garcia-López, C., Crespo-Eguílaz, N., Sánchez-Carpintero, R., Climent, G., & Narbona, J. (2014). AULA virtual reality test as an attention measure: Convergent validity with Conners' Continuous Performance Test. *Child Neuropsychology*, *20*, 328–342. http://dx.doi.org/10.1080/09297049.2013.792332

Engeser, S., & Rheinberg, F. (2008). Flow, performance and moderators of challenge-skill balance. *Motivation and Emotion*, *32*, 158–172. http://dx.doi.org/10.1007/s11031-008-9102-4

ePrivacy. (2015). *Whitepaper: Datensicherheit und Datenschutz von Apps* [Whitepaper: Data security and privacy for apps]. Retrieved from https://www.eprivacy.eu/datensicherheit-und-datenschutz-von-apps/

Fleming, T. M., Bavin, L., Stasiak, K., Hermansson-Webb, E., Merry, S. N., Cheek, C., . . . Hetrick, S. (2017). Serious games and gamification for mental health: Current status and promising directions. *Frontiers in Psychiatry*, *7*, 215. http://dx.doi.org/10.3389/fpsyt.2016.00215

Gamito, P. (2013). *LabPsiCom: Laboratório de Psicologia Computacional*. Retrieved from http://labpsicom.ulusofona.pt

Gamito, P., Morais, D., Oliveira, J., Ferreira Lopes, P., Picareli, L. F., Matias, M., . . . Brito, R. (2016). Systemic Lisbon Battery: Normative data for memory and attention assessments. *JMIR Rehabilitation and Assistive Technologies*, *3*, e5. http://dx.doi.org/10.2196/rehab.4155

Gamito, P., Oliveira, J., Caires, C., Morais, D., Brito, R., Lopes, P., . . . Santos, C. (2015). Virtual Kitchen Test: Assessing frontal lobe functions in patients with alcohol dependence syndrome. *Methods of Information in Medicine*, *54*, 122–126. http://dx.doi.org/10.3414/ME14-01-0003

Gamito, P., Oliveira, J., Coelho, C., Morais, D., Lopes, P., Pacheco, J., . . . Barata, A. F. (2017). Cognitive training on stroke patients via virtual reality-based serious games. *Disability and Rehabilitation*, *39*, 385–388. http://dx.doi.org/10.3109/09638288.2014.934925

Gamito, P., Oliveira, J., Lopes, P., Brito, R., Morais, D., Caçoete, C., . . . Oliveira, H. (2017). Cognitive training through mHealth for individuals with substance use disorder. *Methods of Information in Medicine*, *56*, 156–161. http://dx.doi.org/10.3414/ME16-02-0012

Gamito, P., Oliveira, J., Lopes, P., Brito, R., Morais, D., Silva, D., . . . Deus, A. (2014). Executive functioning in alcoholics following an mHealth cognitive stimulation program: Randomized controlled trial. *Journal of Medical Internet Research*, *16*(4), e102. http://dx.doi.org/10.2196/jmir.2923

Gamito, P., Oliveira, J., Santos, N., Pacheco, J., Morais, D., Saraiva, T., . . . Barata, A. F. (2014). Virtual exercises to promote cognitive recovery in stroke patients: The comparison between head mounted displays versus screen exposure methods. *International Journal on Disability and Human Development*, *13*, 337–342. http://dx.doi.org/10.1515/ijdhd-2014-0325

Goldman Sachs. (2016). *Virtual & augmented reality: The next big computing platform?* Retrieved from http://www.goldmansachs.com/our-thinking/pages/virtual-and-augmented-reality-report.html

Granic, I., Lobel, A., & Engels, R. C. (2014). The benefits of playing video games. *American Psychologist*, *69*, 66–78. http://dx.doi.org/10.1037/a0034857

Henry, M., Joyal, C. C., & Nolin, P. (2012). Development and initial assessment of a new paradigm for assessing cognitive and motor inhibition: The bimodal virtual-reality Stroop. *Journal of Neuroscience Methods*, *210*, 125–131. http://dx.doi.org/10.1016/j.jneumeth.2012.07.025

Hill, N. T., Mowszowski, L., Naismith, S. L., Chadwick, V. L., Valenzuela, M., & Lampit, A. (2017). Computerized cognitive training in older adults with mild cognitive impairment or dementia: A systematic review and meta-analysis. *The American Journal of Psychiatry*, *174*, 329–340. http://dx.doi.org/10.1176/appi.ajp.2016.16030360

Hoffman, H. G., Chambers, G. T., Meyer, W. J., III, Arceneaux, L. L., Russell, W. J., Seibel, E. J., . . . Patterson, D. R. (2011). Virtual reality as an adjunctive non-pharmacologic analgesic for acute burn pain during medical procedures. *Annals of Behavioral Medicine*, *41*, 183–191. http://dx.doi.org/10.1007/s12160-010-9248-7

Holmes, D. E., Charles, D. K., Morrow, P. J., McClean, S., & McDonough, S. M. (2016, September). *Usability and performance of leap motion and Oculus Rift for upper arm virtual reality stroke rehabilitation*. Paper presented at the International Conference on Disability, Virtual Reality and Associated Technologies, Los Angeles, CA.

Howard, M. C. (2017). A meta-analysis and systematic literature review of virtual reality rehabilitation programs. *Computers in Human Behavior*, *70*, 317–327. http://dx.doi.org/10.1016/j.chb.2017.01.013

Jack, K., McLean, S. M., Moffett, J. K., & Gardiner, E. (2010). Barriers to treatment adherence in physiotherapy outpatient clinics: A systematic review. *Manual Therapy*, *15*, 220–228. http://dx.doi.org/10.1016/j.math.2009.12.004

Just, M. A., Sterling, D., Ros, M., Naghdy, F., & Stapley, P. J. (2016). A comparison of upper limb movement profiles when reaching to virtual and real targets using the Oculus Rift: Implications for virtual reality enhanced stroke rehabilitation. *Journal of Pain Management*, *9*, 277–281.

Keefe, R. S. E., Davis, V. G., Atkins, A. S., Vaughan, A., Patterson, T., Narasimhan, M., & Harvey, P. D. (2016). Validation of a computerized test of functional capacity. *Schizophrenia Research*, *175*(1–3), 90–96. http://dx.doi.org/10.1016/j.schres.2016.03.038

Kemeny, A., & Panerai, F. (2003). Evaluating perception in driving simulation experiments. *Trends in Cognitive Sciences*, *7*, 31–37. http://dx.doi.org/10.1016/S1364-6613(02)00011-6

Kim, A., Darakjian, N., & Finley, J. M. (2017). Walking in fully immersive virtual environments: An evaluation of potential adverse effects in older adults and individuals with Parkinson's disease. *Journal of Neuroengineering and Rehabilitation*, *14*, 16. http://dx.doi.org/10.1186/s12984-017-0225-2

Kizony, R. (2011). Virtual reality for cognitive rehabilitation. In N. Katz (Ed.), *Cognition, occupation and participation along the life span: Neuroscience, neurorehabilitation and models for intervention in occupational therapy* (3rd ed., pp. 143–158). Bethesda, MD: AOTA Press.

Kizony, R., Zeilig, G., Krasovsky, T., Bondi, M., Weiss, P. L., Kodesh, E., & Kafri, M. (2017). Using virtual reality simulation to study navigation in a complex environment as a functional-cognitive task; A pilot study. *Journal of Vestibular Research*, *27*, 39–47. http://dx.doi.org/10.3233/VES-170605

Klinger, E., Kadri, A., Sorita, E., Le Guiet, J. L., Coignard, P., Fuchs, P., . . . Joseph, P. A. (2013). AGATHE: A tool for personalized rehabilitation of cognitive functions based on simulated activities of daily living. *IRBM*, *34*, 113–118. http://dx.doi.org/10.1016/j.irbm.2013.01.005

Koenig, S., Crucian, G., Dalrymple-Alford, J., & Dünser, A. (2011). Assessing navigation in real and virtual environments: A validation study. *International Journal on Disability and Human Development*, *10*, 325–330. http://dx.doi.org/10.1515/IJDHD.2011.050

Koenig, S. T. (2012). *Individualized virtual reality rehabilitation after brain injuries*. Christchurch, New Zealand: College of Engineering, University of Canterbury.

Krch, D., Nikelshpur, O., Lavrador, S., Chiaravalloti, N. D., Koenig, S., & Rizzo, A. (2013, August). Pilot results from a virtual reality executive function task. In *Virtual Rehabilitation, 2013 International Conference on Virtual Rehabilitation* (pp. 15–21). IEEE.

Krch, D., Spero, R., & Koenig, S. T. (2018). *Preliminary efficacy of Wonderworks: A VR-based attention training for individuals with TBI*. Unpublished manuscript.

Lange, B., Flynn, S., Proffitt, R., Chang, C. Y., & Rizzo, A. S. (2010). Development of an interactive game-based rehabilitation tool for dynamic balance training. *Topics in Stroke Rehabilitation*, *17*, 345–352. http://dx.doi.org/10.1310/tsr1705-345

Lange, B., Flynn, S., & Rizzo, A. A. (2009). Initial usability assessment of off-the-shelf video game consoles for clinical game-based motor rehabilitation. *The Physical Therapy Review*, *14*, 355–363. http://dx.doi.org/10.1179/108331909X12488667117258

Larson, E. B., Feigon, M., Gagliardo, P., & Dvorkin, A. Y. (2014). Virtual reality and cognitive rehabilitation: A review of current outcome research. *NeuroRehabilitation*, *34*, 759–772.

Laver, K., George, S., Thomas, S., Deutsch, J. E., & Crotty, M. (2012). Cochrane review: Virtual reality for stroke rehabilitation. *Stroke*, *48*, 523–530.

Levin, M. F., Weiss, P. L., & Keshner, E. A. (2015). Emergence of virtual reality as a tool for upper limb rehabilitation: Incorporation of motor control and motor learning principles. *Physical Therapy*, *95*, 415–425. http://dx.doi.org/10.2522/ptj.20130579

Lloréns, R., Noé, E., Colomer, C., & Alcañiz, M. (2015). Effectiveness, usability, and cost-benefit of a virtual reality-based telerehabilitation program for balance recovery after stroke: A randomized controlled trial. *Archives of Physical Medicine and Rehabilitation*, *96*, 418–425.e2. http://dx.doi.org/10.1016/j.apmr.2014.10.019

Lutz, O. H.-M., Burmeister, C., Ferreira dos Santos, L., Markisch, N., Dohle, C., & Krüger, J. (2017). Application of head-mounted devices with eye-tracking in virtual reality therapy. *Current Directions in Biomedical Engineering*, *3*(1), 53–56.

Maclean, N., Pound, P., Wolfe, C., & Rudd, A. (2002). The concept of patient motivation: A qualitative analysis of stroke professionals' attitudes. *Stroke*, *33*, 444–448. http://dx.doi.org/10.1161/hs0202.102367

Madary, M., & Metzinger, T. K. (2016). Real virtuality: A code of ethical conduct. Recommendations for good scientific practice and the consumers of VR-technology. *Frontiers in Robotics and AI*, *3*, 3. http://dx.doi.org/10.3389/frobt.2016.00003

Negut, A., Matu, S. A., Sava, F. A., & David, D. (2016). Virtual reality measures in neuropsychological assessment: A meta-analytic review. *Clinical Neuropsychology*, *39*, 165–184. http://dx.doi.org/10.1080/13854046.2016.1144793

Neisser, U. (1978). Memory: What are the important questions? In M. M. Gruneberg, P. E. Morris, & R. N. Sykes (Eds.), *Practical aspects of memory* (pp. 3–24). London, England: Academic Press.

NeuroCog. (2015). *Virtual reality functional capacity assessment tool—VRFCAT*. Retrieved from http://www.neurocogtrials.com/products/virtual-reality-functional-capacity-assessment-tool-vrfcat/

Norrholm, S. D., Jovanovic, T., Gerardi, M., Breazeale, K. G., Price, M., Davis, M., . . . Rothbaum, B. O. (2016). Baseline psychophysiological and cortisol reactivity as a predictor of PTSD treatment outcome in virtual reality exposure therapy. *Behaviour Research and Therapy*, *82*, 28–37. http://dx.doi.org/10.1016/j.brat.2016.05.002

Ogourtsova, T., Silva, W. S., Archambault, P. S., & Lamontagne, A. (2017). Virtual reality treatment and assessments for post-stroke unilateral spatial neglect: A systematic literature review. *Neuropsychological Rehabilitation*, *27*, 409–454. http://dx.doi.org/10.1080/09602011.2015.1113187

Parsons, T. D., Carlew, A., & Sullivan, E. (2015). A case for the development and use of virtual reality measures for assessment of executive function. In P. Cipresso & S. Serino (Eds.), *Virtual reality: Technologies, medical applications, and challenges* (pp. 177–193). Hauppauge, NY: Nova Science.

Parsons, T. D., & Carlew, A. R. (2016). Bimodal Virtual Reality Stroop for assessing distractor inhibition in autism spectrum disorders. *Journal of Autism and Developmental Disorders*, *46*, 1255–1267. http://dx.doi.org/10.1007/s10803-015-2663-7

Parsons, T. D., & Courtney, C. G. (2014). An initial validation of the Virtual Reality Paced Auditory Serial Addition Test in a college sample. *Journal of Neuroscience Methods*, *222*, 15–23. http://dx.doi.org/10.1016/j.jneumeth.2013.10.006

Parsons, T. D., Courtney, C. G., Arizmedi, B., & Dawson, M. (2011). Virtual Reality Stroop Test for Neurocognitive Assessment. In J. D. Westwood et al. (Eds.), *Medicine meets virtual reality*, 18. http://dx.doi.org/10.3233/978-1-60750-706-2-433

Parsons, T. D., & Phillips, A. S. (2016). Virtual reality for psychological assessment in clinical practice. *Practice Innovations*, *1*, 197–217. http://dx.doi.org/10.1037/pri0000028

Patney, A., Kim, J., Salvi, M., Kaplanyan, A., & Wymona, C. (2016, July). *Perceptually-based foveated virtual reality*. Paper presented at the SIGGRAPH 2016 Emerging Technologies, Anaheim, CA.

Pietrzak, E., Pullman, S., & McGuire, A. (2014). Using virtual reality and videogames for traumatic brain injury rehabilitation: A structured literature review. *Games for Health Journal*, *3*, 202–214. http://dx.doi.org/10.1089/g4h.2014.0013

Plumert, J., Kearney, J., Cremer, J., & Recker, K. (2005). Distance perception in real and virtual environments. *ACM Transactions on Applied Perception*, *2*, 216–233. http://dx.doi.org/10.1145/1077399.1077402

Rand, D., Katz, N., & Weiss, P. L. (2007). Evaluation of virtual shopping in the VMall: Comparison of post-stroke participants to healthy control groups. *Disability and Rehabilitation*, *29*, 1710–1719. http://dx.doi.org/10.1080/09638280601107450

Regenbrecht, H., Hoermann, S., Ott, C., Müller, L., & Franz, E. (2014). Manipulating the experience of reality for rehabilitation applications. *Proceedings of the IEEE*, *102*, 170–184. http://dx.doi.org/10.1109/JPROC.2013.2294178

Renison, B., Ponsford, J., Testa, R., Richardson, B., & Brownfield, K. (2012). The ecological and construct validity of a newly developed measure of executive function: The Virtual Library Task. *Journal of the International Neuropsychological Society*, *18*, 440–450. http://dx.doi.org/10.1017/S1355617711001883

Renner, R. S., Velichkovsky, B. M., & Helmert, J. R. (2013). The perception of egocentric distances in virtual environments—A review. *ACM Computing Surveys*, *46*, 1–40. http://dx.doi.org/10.1145/2543581.2543590

Rizzo, A. A. (2016). *With the release of Oculus Rift, what's next for virtual reality*? Retrieved from https://news.usc.edu/97921/

Rizzo, A. A., Bowerly, T., Buckwalter, J. G., Klimchuk, D., Mitura, R., & Parsons, T. D. (2006). A virtual reality scenario for all seasons: The virtual classroom. *CNS Spectrums*, *11*, 35–44. http://dx.doi.org/10.1017/S1092852900024196

Rizzo, A. A., & Buckwalter, J. G. (1997). Virtual reality and cognitive assessment and rehabilitation: The state of the art. *Studies in Health Technology and Informatics*, *44*, 123–145.

Rizzo, A. A., & Kim, G. J. (2005). A SWOT analysis of the field of virtual reality rehabilitation and therapy. *Presence*, *14*, 119–146. http://dx.doi.org/10.1162/1054746053967094

Rizzo, A. A., & Koenig, S. T. (2017). Is clinical virtual reality ready for primetime? *Neuropsychology: Special Issue on Assessment and Intervention*. http://dx.doi.org/10.1037/neu0000405

Rizzo, A. A., Schultheis, M. T., & Rothbaum, B. O. (2003). Ethical issues for the use of virtual reality in the psychological sciences. In S. C. Bush & M. L. Drexler (Eds.), *Ethical issues in clinical neuropsychology* (pp. 243–280). Lisse, Netherlands: Swets & Zeitlinger.

Rizzo, A. A., & Shilling, R. (2017). Clinical virtual reality tools to advance the prevention, assessment, and treatment of PTSD. *European Journal of Psychotraumatology*, *8*, http://dx.doi.org/10.1080/20008198.2017.1414560

Rizzo, A. A., Shilling, R., Forbell, E. D., Scherer, S., Gratch, J., & Morency, L.-P. (2015). Autonomous virtual human agents for health care information support and clinical interviewing. In D. D. Luxton (Ed.), *Artificial intelligence in mental health care practice* (pp. 53–80). Oxford, England: Academic Press.

Rizzo, A. A., & Talbot, T. (2016). Virtual reality standardized patients for clinical training. In C. D. Combs, J. A. Sokolowski, & C. M. Banks (Eds.), *The digital patient: Advancing medical research, education, and practice* (pp. 255–272). New York, NY: Wiley. http://dx.doi.org/10.1002/9781118952788.ch18

Rose, F. D., Brooks, B. M., & Rizzo, A. A. (2005). Virtual reality in brain damage rehabilitation: Review. *CyberPsychology & Behavior*, *8*, 241–262. http://dx.doi.org/10.1089/cpb.2005.8.241

Ruse, S. A., Davis, V. G., Atkins, A. S., Krishnan, K. R., Fox, K. H., Harvey, P. D., & Keefe, R. S. (2014). Development of a virtual reality assessment of everyday living skills. *Journal of Visualized Experiments*, *86*, e51405. http://dx.doi.org/10.3791/51405

Salisbury, D. B., Dahdah, M., Driver, S., Parsons, T. D., & Richter, K. M. (2016). Virtual reality and brain computer interface in neurorehabilitation. *Baylor University Medical Center Proceedings*, *29*, 124–127. http://dx.doi.org/10.1080/08998280.2016.11929386

Sangani, S., Fung, J., Kizony, R., Koenig, S. T., & Weiss, P. L. (2013, August). *Navigating and shopping in a complex virtual urban mall to evaluate cognitive functions*. Paper presented at the International Conference on Virtual Rehabilitation, Philadelphia, PA.

Sangani, S., Weiss, P. L., Kizony, R., Koenig, S. T., Levin, M. F., & Fung, J. (2012, September). *Development of a complex ecological virtual environment*. Paper presented at the International Conference on Disability, Virtual Reality and Associated Technologies, Laval, France.

Schmuckler, M. A. (2001). What is ecological validity? A dimensional analysis. *Infancy*, *2*, 419–436. http://dx.doi.org/10.1207/S15327078IN0204_02

Schultheis, M. T., & Rizzo, A. A. (2001). The application of virtual reality technology in rehabilitation. *Rehabilitation Psychology*, *46*, 296–311. http://dx.doi.org/10.1037/0090-5550.46.3.296

Shallice, T., & Burgess, P. W. (1991). Deficits in strategy application following frontal lobe damage in man. *Brain: A Journal of Neurology*, *114*, 727–741. http://dx.doi.org/10.1093/brain/114.2.727

Trost, Z., Zielke, M., Guck, A., Nowlin, L., Zakhidov, D., France, C. R., & Keefe, F. (2015). The promise and challenge of virtual gaming technologies for chronic pain: The case of graded exposure for low back pain. *Pain Management*, *5*, 197–206. http://dx.doi.org/10.2217/pmt.15.6

Valladares-Rodriguez, S., Peréz-Rodgriguez, R., Anido-Rifón, L., & Fernández-Iglesias, M. (2016, December). Trends on the application of serious games to neuropsychological evaluation: A scoping review. *Journal of Biomedical Informatics*, *54*, 296–319. http://dx.doi.org/10.1016/j.jbi.2016.10.019

Wall, K. J., Cumming, T. B., Koenig, S. T., Pelecanos, A. M., & Copland, D. A. (2018). Using technology to overcome the language barrier: The Cognitive Assessment for Aphasia app. *Disability and Rehabilitation*, *40*, 1333–1344. http://dx.doi.org/10.1080/09638288.2017.1294210

Wall, K. J., Issacs, M. L., Copland, D. A., & Cumming, T. B. (2015). Assessing cognition after stroke. Who misses out? A systematic review. *International Journal of Stroke*, *10*, 665–671. http://dx.doi.org/10.1111/ijs.12506

Weiss, P. L., & Jessel, A. S. (1998). Virtual reality applications to work. *Work*, *11*, 277–293. http://dx.doi.org/10.1016/S1051-9815(98)00044-8

Winkels, D. G., Kottink, A. I., Temmink, R. A., Nijlant, J. M., & Buurke, J. H. (2013). Wii-habilitation of upper extremity function in children with cerebral palsy: An explorative study. *Developmental Neurorehabilitation*, *16*, 44–51. http://dx.doi.org/10.3109/17518423.2012.713401

Yellowlees, P. M., Holloway, K. M., & Parish, M. B. (2012). Therapy in virtual environments—Clinical and ethical issues. *Telemedicine and e-Health*, *18*, 558–564. http://dx.doi.org/10.1089/tmj.2011.0195

Yip, B. C., & Man, D. W. (2013). Virtual reality-based prospective memory training program for people with acquired brain injury. *NeuroRehabilitation*, *32*(1), 103–115.

AFTERWORD

Robert G. Frank and Timothy R. Elliott

As John Corrigan (2010) predicted in the final chapter of the second edition of this handbook, rehabilitation psychology—and all of health care—has experienced a fundamental paradigm change. In the United States, health care spending per capita has increased from $9,163 in 2013 to $11,504 (estimated) in 2018 (Kaiser Family Foundation, 2014), leading to concerns about the ever-escalating cost of health care. In addition, the Patient Protection and Affordable Care Act (2010) has increased pressure on health care providers and organizations to be accountable for their patients' health care outcomes. At the same time, the American predilection toward early adoption of and reliance upon expensive technology has increased, and new horizons in precision medicine promise personal, though likely more expensive, solutions to individual illnesses. Precision medicine is "an emerging approach for disease treatment and prevention that takes into account individual variability in genes, environment, and lifestyle for each person" (National Institutes of Health, National Library of Medicine, 2018).

At the intersection of technology and health care, the next decade is likely to see a coalescing of key trends related to high-technology care that have been apparent over recent years. The field of rehabilitation has historically prioritized the consumer or patient; this has not been the case in other areas of health care. The ascendency of the consumer will be made possible by the optimization of technology, which will increase patients' knowledge and their ability to participate in decision-making regarding their health care. Empowering consumers with more information will not only improve efficiency of the system but also provide more impetus for patients to manage their own health. More care will occur at home with improved self-monitoring.

Second, technology will influence approaches to the provision of health care. The growth in the use of data analytics will lead to better decisions, to innovations in health care, and to more effective population health management. Data analytics will help clinicians identify precursors to disabling conditions. With this knowledge, and more understanding of the environment–genome interaction, novel interventions and more directed self-management approaches will be possible. As connectivity increases, electronic medical records will likely become truly portable, breaking the silos that discourage collaboration between providers, and reducing the number of often-redundant tests. Artificial intelligence and augmented-reality devices will change the management and diagnosis of many health conditions (Askay, Patterson, & Sharar, 2009). Genomics may change health care through personalized medicine, genetic manipulation, and predictive diagnosis. Smart applications will use evidence-based practice to change clinical workflow and enhance consumer self-management.

Finally, the configuration of health care systems is also evolving. Payment for health care will continue

http://dx.doi.org/10.1037/0000129-033
Handbook of Rehabilitation Psychology, Third Edition, L. A. Brenner, S. A. Reid-Arndt, T. R. Elliott, R. G. Frank, and B. Caplan (Editors-in-Chief)

the transition from a volume-based, fee-for-service model to a quality-focused episode-of-care approach. Innovations in payment methods will encourage the bundling of services, risk sharing, and capitation of health payments, requiring providers to work in novel ways. Fiscal pressures will create mergers among health systems and move the locus of care out of expensive hospitals to clinics and health malls. More care will be managed via smartphones that will be able to measure many health outcomes. Care will move to lower cost providers such as physician assistants, nurse practitioners, master's level counselors, and pharmacists, who are less costly than doctoral providers. Family members of individuals with chronic or disabling health conditions will likely experience an increase in expectations and responsibilities for assistance and participation as informal extensions of the health care team. Optimally, health communities, such as chat groups dedicated to diagnoses or advocacy groups, will come together to provide support, knowledge, and enhanced healthy lifestyles.

For rehabilitation psychologists, these changes are likely to emphasize increases in activities that resemble data review and coaching instead of diagnosis and treatment. As physicians have moved to practices bolstered by midlevel practitioners (physician assistants and nurse practitioners), psychologists must identify a similar model or risk becoming the midlevel practitioner.

We also anticipate that the move toward precision medicine will lead to substantial progress and to opportunities for health care practitioners prepared to embrace the changes. Precision medicine, with its consideration of the person–environment interaction, is compatible with models used by rehabilitation psychologists. In addition, the primary hope of precision medicine is that it will allow broad diagnostic categories such as coronary artery disease (CAD) to be subdivided according to "driving pathways" that can be addressed by a distinct intervention. Yet, an alternative model of precision medicine, and one that may also have great promise, is that a disease is manifested by a qualitative mix of causal risk factors that blend together in each individual (Khera & Kathiresan, 2017).

CAD provides an opportunity to determine whether either of these approaches is a better model, and efforts are underway to examine these possibilities. Khera and Kathiresan (2017) proposed that both approaches apply—though for most people, the qualitative approach describing a broad blend of causal factors will be most applicable. Thus, precision medicine will likely identify small groups of individuals that constitute a "subgroup" for which genetic therapies may provide radical improvement, while for most individuals "a quantitative blend of causal genetic and environmental factors underlies the majority of CAD cases" (Khera & Kathiresan, 2017, p. 1006). Shaywitz (2017) proposed that if Khera and Kathiresan are correct, precision medicine may not lead to customized individual cures, but will better illustrate the complex genetic architecture of disease. Undoubtedly, subtypes of disabling conditions will emerge that will fundamentally alter the understanding of and responses to clinical conditions. In this scenario, the skills of rehabilitation psychologists will be relevant for many years to come, but the surrounding context of providing services will change notably.

For rehabilitation psychologists, the future requires dedicated sensitivity to pursuing, and understanding, the evolution of the delivery of health services. Too often, psychologists have chased the expiring model of health care, only to be marginally prepared for the evolved replacement to the previous model (see Frank, 2017, for more detail). In 2015, Kassler, Tomoyasu, and Conway (2015) noted that improving health requires adoption of population health models that focus on the health of all people in a given geographic area. They also emphasized that population health goes beyond the biomedical paradigm to include the community and social determents of health. It is critical to act on the "causes of the causes of ill health" (Jong-wook, 2005, p. 1006).

Notably, population health differs from public health, which has also been identified as an important perspective and point of intervention for rehabilitation psychologists (Elliott & Frank, 2000). *Population health* is

> the health outcomes of a group of individuals, including the distribution of such outcomes within the group. These populations are often geographic regions, such as nations or communities, but

> they can also be other groups, such as employees, ethnic groups, disabled persons, or prisoners. Such populations are of relevance to policymakers. In addition, many determinants of health, such as medical care systems, the social environment, and the physical environment, have their biological impact on individuals in part at a population level. (Kindig & Stoddart, 2003, p. 382)

In contrast, *public health* refers to the collective actions taken to promote health for the public. Population health mirrors the changes in the health care system created by the move toward value purchasing. Population health also considers determents of health, which is congruent with the tenets of rehabilitation psychology.

The predicted transition to a population health perspective will finally herald the long-promised integration of health services with behavioral health. Indeed, the emerging population health paradigm will likely go further than the mere integration of medical services and behavioral health. As population health interventions and a better understanding of, and ability to predict, the social determinants of health evolve, the health delivery system will dynamically fuse behavioral health and the biomedical model. With this fusion, many environmental barriers for people with disabilities, from transportation to neighborhood access, will gain more attention. The promise of the World Health Organization's International Classification of Functioning, Disability and Health (2001; known commonly as ICF) model of integrating environmental, individual, and health factors for understanding health and behavior outcomes will be advanced. Individuals—patients in the biomedical treatment paradigm—will become consumers who engineer their health with extensive data and input from health professionals.

So how does a discipline prepare for a wave of diffuse social and intellectual changes? For rehabilitation psychologists, and psychologists of all types, to prosper in the years ahead it will be necessary to recognize that in times of change, boundaries blur. Economic and social mobility opportunities will occur that require rethinking historic divisions. The person–machine interface will undoubtedly expand, as more machines are used to assist both simple and complex human functions. The notion of "disability" will be reconsidered as the person–machine boundary becomes less clear and machines (or genetic modification) are used to address disabling factors. This person–machine boundary issue will be an exemplar of advances in the changed health care delivery world, with information being the driving force.

These challenges and opportunities require a thoughtful evaluation of the boundaries, allegiances, and traditional activities and roles associated with rehabilitation psychology. As we have seen throughout the chapters in this third edition, rehabilitation psychologists are well equipped to propose, develop, and evaluate home- and community-based programs (see Chapter 29, this volume) that may facilitate the health and well-being of individuals with disabling conditions (including their family members). Application of new or evolved technologies will likely alleviate disparities individuals with disability face in gaining access to quality services. Rehabilitation psychologists can take the lead in adapting new transdiagnostic approaches for use in community, home-based, and primary care settings to efficiently treat the mechanisms common across emotional disorders (e.g., emotional dysregulation, cognitive biases, inflexibility, ineffective and avoidant coping; Barlow & Farchione, 2017) experienced by individuals living with disability.

For home- and community-based services to be cost-effective, however, low-cost nondoctoral-level service providers will likely be on the front lines, ideally in programs administered and supervised by psychologists (Callahan, 2010). Rehabilitation psychologists have a stake, then, in the deliberations now occurring within the American Psychological Association in defining and accrediting health service psychology master's programs. The lack of a viable presence of rehabilitation psychologists in accredited doctoral programs may require strategic efforts to influence these discussions. Moreover, influential policy and program initiatives that capitalize on the changes in the health care system (value purchasing, machine–human interface, precision medicine) may benefit rehabilitation psychology. Huge changes are coming in the health care delivery and financing system. For rehabilitation psychology as a discipline to benefit from understanding the complex changes ahead, individual rehabilitation psychologists must be willing to take the risk of assuming leadership positions in health care entities. This may be difficult for colleagues who are committed to organizational structures and institutional settings that limit their practice and scholarship and relegate their roles to the traditional rehabilitation enterprise (Elliott & Andrews, 2016). New alliances and collaborations with other professions may be necessary.

We ended the first edition of the *Handbook of Rehabilitation Psychology* by saying,

> Psychologists have a bright future as catalysts of change in health care. Maintenance of the current paradigm inevitably weakens the profession. Recognizing the importance of chronic health issues, developing theory-driven models of psychological health, and harnessing innovation all provide the keys to the success of the discipline. (Elliott & Frank, 2000, p. 651)

With the health care evolution that has since occurred and the opportunities that remain on the horizon, these ideas have retained their veracity and continue to show the way for rehabilitation psychology. Rehabilitation psychologists are positioned to participate in proposing, developing, and implementing policies that initiate and support the kinds of services and programs that effectively and efficiently promote quality of life for individuals with disabilities.

References

Askay, S. W., Patterson, D. R., & Sharar, S. R. (2009). Virtual reality hypnosis. *Contemporary Hypnosis, 26*, 40–47. http://dx.doi.org/10.1002/ch.371

Barlow, D. H., & Farchione, T. J. (2017). *Applications of the unified protocol for transdiagnostic treatment of emotional disorders*. New York, NY: Oxford University Press.

Callahan, C. (2010). Rehabilitating the health care organization: Administering psychology's opportunity. In R. G. Frank, M. Rosenthal, & B. Caplan (Eds.), *Handbook of rehabilitation psychology* (2nd ed., pp. 459–466). Washington, DC: American Psychological Association. http://dx.doi.org/10.1037/15972-033

Corrigan, J. D. (2010). Afterword: Of bins and arrows. In R. G. Frank, M. Rosenthal, & B. Caplan (Eds.), *Handbook of rehabilitation psychology* (2nd ed., pp. 477–482). Washington, DC: American Psychological Association.

Elliott, T. R., & Andrews, E. E. (2016). Physical rehabilitation facilities. In J. C. Norcross, G. R. VandenBos, D. K. Freedheim, & M. M. Domenech Rodriguez (Eds.), *APA handbook of clinical psychology: Vol. 1. Roots and branches* (pp. 509–524). Washington, DC: American Psychological Association. http://dx.doi.org/10.1037/14772-029

Elliott, T. R., & Frank, R. G. (2000). Afterword: Drawing new horizons. In R. G. Frank & T. R. Elliott (Eds.), *Handbook of rehabilitation psychology* (pp. 645–653). Washington, DC: American Psychological Association. http://dx.doi.org/10.1037/10361-032

Frank, R. G. (2017). Hither and thither: How do we innovate? *Rehabilitation Psychology, 62*, 1–6. http://dx.doi.org/10.1037/rep0000114

Jong-wook, L. (2005). Public health is a social issue. *The Lancet, 365*, 1005–1006.

Kaiser Family Foundation. (2014). *National health care expenditures per capita, 1960–2023*. Retrieved from https://www.kff.org/health-costs/slide/national-health-expenditures-per-capita-1960-2023/

Kassler, W. J., Tomoyasu, N., & Conway, P. H. (2015). Beyond a traditional player—CMS's role in improving population health. *The New England Journal of Medicine, 372*, 109–111. http://dx.doi.org/10.1056/NEJMp1406838

Khera, A. V., & Kathiresan, S. (2017). Is coronary atherosclerosis one disease or many? Setting realistic expectations for precision medicine. *Circulation, 135*, 1005–1007. http://dx.doi.org/10.1161/CIRCULATIONAHA.116.026479

Kindig, D., & Stoddart, G. (2003). What is population health? *American Journal of Public Health, 93*, 380–383. http://dx.doi.org/10.2105/AJPH.93.3.380

National Institutes of Health, National Library of Medicine. (2018). *What is precision medicine?* https://ghr.nlm.nih.gov/primer/precisionmedicine/definition

Patient Protection and Affordable Care Act, 42 U.S.C. § 18001 et seq. (2010).

Shaywitz, D. (2017, October 24). *Why precision research may lead to blockbuster, not customized, medicines*. Retrieved from https://www.forbes.com/sites/davidshaywitz/2017/10/24/why-precision-research-may-lead-to-blockbuster-not-customized-medicines/#5eb21b4d6e85

World Health Organization. (2001). *International classification of functioning, disability, and health*. Geneva, Switzerland: Author.

Index

About the Editors

Lisa A. Brenner, PhD, ABPP, is a board-certified rehabilitation psychologist; a professor of physical medicine and rehabilitation (PM&R), psychiatry, and neurology, the University of Colorado, Anschutz School of Medicine; and the director of the Veterans Administration Rocky Mountain Mental Illness Research, Education, and Clinical Center. She is also the research director for the Department of PM&R, as well as a past president and fellow of APA Division 22 (Rehabilitation Psychology). Dr. Brenner is an associate editor for the *Journal of Head Trauma Rehabilitation*. Her primary areas of research interest are traumatic brain injury, comorbid psychiatric disorders, and negative psychiatric outcomes including suicide. Visit her website (https://www.mirecc.va.gov/visn19/staff/brenner.asp) and follow on twitter @LisaABrenner.

Stephanie A. Reid-Arndt, PhD, ABPP, is associate dean for academic affairs in the School of Health Professions at the University of Missouri, Columbia. She is a fellow of the American Psychological Association and is board-certified in rehabilitation psychology. She is widely published, and she currently serves on the editorial boards of the *Journal of Head Trauma Rehabilitation* and *Rehabilitation Psychology*. Dr. Reid-Arndt's research focuses on understanding how psychosocial factors and neuropsychological functioning influence health outcomes and quality of life for individuals with chronic medical conditions, particularly traumatic brain injury and breast cancer. She lives in Columbia, Missouri. For more information, visit her website (https://healthprofessions.missouri.edu/personnel/stephanie-reid-arndt/).

Timothy R. Elliott, PhD, ABPP, is a university distinguished professor in the Department of Educational Psychology and executive director of the Telehealth Counseling Clinic at Texas A&M University. He is a past president of APA Division 22 (Rehabilitation Psychology), current editor of the *Journal of Clinical Psychology*, and a past editor of *Rehabilitation Psychology*. His research examining adjustment processes among people living with chronic health conditions contributed to innovations in telepsychology services for underserved communities. He is a recipient of several awards and honors, including from APA Division 22. Dr. Elliott lives in Fischer, Texas. For more information, visit his website (http://telliott.education.tamu.edu/).

Robert G. Frank, PhD, is director of the Center for Innovation in Health and Education at the University of New Mexico. He formerly served as president at the University of New Mexico, as provost at Kent State University, and as dean of the College of Public Health and Health Professions at the University of Florida. Throughout his career, Dr. Frank has been highly involved with health policy at both federal and state levels, working with numerous initiatives and policymakers. Dr. Frank is a past president of APA Division 22 (Rehabilitation Psychology). He lives in Albuquerque, New Mexico. Visit his website (http://nmcup.us/council-members/robert-frank.html) and follow @RG_Frank25.

Bruce Caplan, PhD, ABPP (CN, RP), has received two Distinguished Service Awards and the Lifetime Practice Excellence Award from APA Division 22 (Rehabilitation Psychology). He previously served as president of Division 22 and as editor of *Rehabilitation Psychology*, the Division's journal. Dr. Caplan is senior editor of the *Journal of Head Trauma Rehabilitation*, a member of the editorial board of *Topics in Stroke Rehabilitation*, and a founding member of the American Board of Rehabilitation Psychology. He coedited two editions of the *Encyclopedia of Clinical Neuropsychology* and was sole editor of the *Rehabilitation Psychology Desk Reference*. Currently in independent practice in Wynnewood, Pennsylvania, he was formerly chief psychologist in the Department of Rehabilitation Medicine at Jefferson Medical College.